A Professional Legacy

The Eleanor Clarke Slagle Lectures in Occupational Therapy, 1955–2010

3rd Edition

Edited by
René Padilla, PhD, OTR/L, FAOTA, LMHP
Yolanda Griffiths, OTD, OTR/L, FAOTA

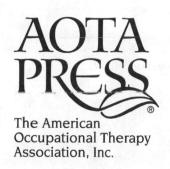

AOTA PRESS®

The American
Occupational Therapy
Association, Inc.

AOTA Centennial Vision
We envision that occupational therapy is a powerful, widely recognized, science-driven, and evidence-based profession with a globally connected and diverse workforce meeting society's occupational needs.

Vision Statement
AOTA advances occupational therapy as the pre-eminent profession in promoting the health, productivity, and quality of life of individuals and society through the therapeutic application of occupation.

Mission Statement
The American Occupational Therapy Association advances the quality, availability, use, and support of occupational therapy through standard-setting, advocacy, education, and research on behalf of its members and the public.

AOTA Staff
Frederick P. Somers, *Executive Director*
Christopher M. Bluhm, *Chief Operating Officer*

Chris Davis, *Director, AOTA Press*
Ashley Hofmann, *Developmental/Production Editor*
Victoria Davis, *Production Editor/Editorial Assistant*

Beth Ledford, *Director of Marketing*
Emily Zhang, *Technology Marketing Specialist*
Jennifer Folden, *Marketing Specialist*

The American Occupational Therapy Association, Inc.
4720 Montgomery Lane
Bethesda, MD 20814
Phone: 301-652-AOTA (2682)
TDD: 800-377-8555
Fax: 301-652-7711
www.aota.org
To order: http://store.aota.org

Disclaimers
This publication is designed to provide accurate and authoritative information in regard to the subject matter covered. It is sold or distributed with the understanding that the publisher is not engaged in rendering legal, accounting, or other professional service. If legal advice or other expert assistance is required, the services of a competent professional person should be sought.
—*From the Declaration of Principles jointly adopted by the American Bar Association and a Committee of Publishers and Associations*

It is the objective of the American Occupational Therapy Association to be a forum for free expression and interchange of ideas. The opinions expressed by the contributors to this work are their own and not necessarily those of either the editors or the American Occupational Therapy Association.

ISBN: 978-1-56900-297-1

Library of Congress Control Number: 2011924614

Design by Debra Naylor, Naylor Design, Inc., *Washington, DC*
Composition by Maryland Composition, *Laurel, MD*
Printed by Automated Graphics Systems, Inc., *White Plains, MD*

Contents

Introduction to the Third Edition

On the Way to the *Centennial Vision*

A couple of summers ago, my oldest son left home to attend law school in the nearby city of Lincoln, Nebraska. We loaded my car full of furniture for his new apartment, and when we were ready to leave I realized the view in my mirror was obstructed—I could not look backward in order to pull out from my driveway. My son had to get out of the car and verbally guide me. During the whole drive through the Omaha streets and later on the freeway, I was constantly shocked into attention when I looked through the rearview mirror and all I could distinguish was the back of a dresser. While I could see where I was headed, I felt very uneasy with no real sense of what was coming from behind or my place in the flow of traffic. On a couple of occasions I tried to move around slow traffic, but the sound of a horn caused me to pull back in line and pray that the dawdling truck ahead of me would soon leave the main road and clear my way. Many drivers sped by me. However, I felt it safest to stay in my lane and not to take risks to pass other drivers. The trip took almost twice as long as it should have, and by the time we arrived at our destination, I was nearly too tired from the tension to unload the car.

In 2006 the Representative Assembly of the American Occupational Therapy Association (AOTA) adopted a *Centennial Vision* to guide the work of the association and its members for the year 2017 and beyond. This vision, intended to help set strategic directions and deepen our personal resolve to shape our common future, states that "We envision that occupational therapy is a powerful, widely recognized, science-driven, and evidence-based profession with a globally connected and diverse workforce meeting society's occupational needs" (AOTA, 2007, p. 613).

Looking ahead at occupational therapy's 2017 Centennial year can be much like driving without a rearview mirror if we do not continually look back, get a sense of where we have been, glimpse what is coming, and discern where we are in the flow of history. While without such a reflection we can no doubt move forward, it is likely that we will do so without knowing when it is best to change course or speed up and move ahead of others. Without such grounding from our past we are prone to retreat to the safety of following others. The likely result of such a journey is that when we arrive at our destination, if we do so at all, we will be exhausted and, most certainly, very late.

Using the Slagle Lectures to Imagine the *Centennial Vision*

Kathleen Barker Schwartz (2009) noted in a recent lecture that "the *Centennial Vision* does not represent a new set of values but rather builds on values that the profession has held since its inception in 1917." A review of the Eleanor Clarke Slagle Lectures in occupational therapy contained in this volume can provide a rearview mirror to inform our future travels as a profession. We will soon discover that the *Centennial Vision* itself was also being articulated in these lectures. Each honoree, in his or her unique way, has challenged us to continue shaping our future and to fulfilling this vision. Each dimension of the vision is identifiable as a theme in the lectures. In the pages that follow, the *Centennial Vision* is illustrated with statements from the lecturers. Each lecturer is identified by name and the year of his or her lecture. The illustrations are by no means exhaustive, and readers are encouraged to review the lectures in depth to further mine them for connections to the *Centennial Vision*.

Powerful

The philosophy of action that underlies the core concept of occupation is the most salient feature of our expression of power as a profession as articulated by the Slagle lecturers. Florence Stattel (1955) reminded us that such power comes from the knowledge that "our specialty field is related to helping the human being." Ruth Brunyate (1957) added that our power comes from "the ability to appreciate the commonplace, to note a touch of beauty in the midst of squalor, or be aware of tenderness even in frugal living . . . this is the trait that refreshes and strengthens." She added that our familiarity with occupation is "a knowledge of how to support as well as how to lead." Mary Reilly (1961) noted that the commonplaceness of occupation "is and always will be the pride . . . of our profession." She articulated one of the most inspiring descriptions of the power of occupation, that "man, through the use of his hands as they are energized by mind and will, can influence the state of his own health. . . . It falls in the class of one of those great beliefs which has advanced civilization."

In turbulent times in society, Slagle lecturers have reminded us that we have the power to "make a decision as to our future course" (Naida Ackley, 1962) and to remain viable by continually assessing "the place of the profession in society and its service to the individual in relation to that society" (Gail Fidler, 1965). Irene Hollis (1979) affirmed our identity by reminding us that "occupational therapy is commonplace and unsophisticated often, and therapists are frequently apologetic about this aspect. Instead, we should take pride in our use of the ordinary and commonplace to bring about desired results when more sophisticated modalities have failed."

Elizabeth Yerxa (1966) emphasized that "professionalism is much more than appearance and intellectual accomplishments. It means being able to meet real needs. It means being unique. It means having and acting upon a philosophy. It also means being 'authentic.'" The gaining of power as a profession has a specific purpose. Wilma West (1967) asserted as much when she said that "the primary orientation of the profession is to the community interest, there must be concern for all people on the basis of equal opportunity and with a standard of the highest possible quality that it is within our ability to provide."

Mary Fiorentino (1974) brought our attention to a potential loss of effectiveness by asking, "Are we ready to be challenged by the ongoing advances being made in medicine and research and changes in health care brought about by federal and state regulations?" Carolyn Baum (1980) declared that "occupational therapists' tremendous commitment to Man and to his ability to shape his destiny through activity and accomplishment puts us in a very favorable position because we provide a service that the health care system is recognizing to assure it is delivered." She then urged us to take a leadership position by asking, "When are we going to stop following the grazing trail and develop the technology to plant our own fields?"

Elnora Gilfoyle (1984) affirmed that occupational therapy, like other "allied health fields dominated by women, will be recognized not as allied but as independent health profession. Transformation to an integrative power of technology and touch within medicine will further shake the foundations of occupational therapy," and therefore, she encouraged us to remain constant in the development of our unique identity rather than be swayed by a hierarchical view of health care. Ann Grady (1994) saw that our unique contribution was "leading the development of inclusive community is right for occupational therapy, and we all have it in us to do it." David Nelson (1996) continued to encourage our unique strengths and urge our growth by saying that "persons from other professions are coming late to the table and claiming credit for dome of the great ideas of occupational therapy. These ideas deserve the most careful . . . scrutiny. As occupational therapists, we need to own these ideas while enlightening other disciplines as to their usefulness." Janice Posatery Burke (2010) urged us to look deeply at the basic social interaction that defines our profession. She described the source of the unique therapeutic power of the profession by noting that "Occupational therapists conduct the business of therapy within a distinct frame of improving performance. Occupational therapists use physical space, therapeutic objects, their bodies, their voices, and their reasoning skills to create an interaction that produces therapeutic outcomes."

Widely Recognized

For the lecturers, power as a profession comes from being recognized for what we do. As Brunyate (1957) noted, "the patient is the reason we exist." Reilly (1961) argued that "the value of occupational therapy exists in a controversial state" because of changes in society and our shyness in announcing our contribution. She wondered rhetorically if "occupational therapy [is] a sufficiently vital and unique service for medicine to support and society to reward" and affirmed that indeed, occupational therapy could be one of the 20th century's great ideas.

Professionalization has been a constant theme in the Slagle lecturer's exhortations. Ackley (1962) plainly stated, "if we want the recognition and status of professional personnel we must function on that level." Fidler (1965) extended this theme by stating that the occupational therapy professional must be "able to share with others a concern for and a dedication to the welfare of all peoples and thus to share freely and work collaboratively with others in the service of human welfare." Yerxa (1966) also noted that "a profession obtains wide recognition of the need for the services which it can perform" and asked, "How widely is the need for occupational therapy recognized?"

Geraldine Finn (1971) lecture expounded on the theme of recognition through professionalism. She argued that "in order for a profession to maintain its relevancy it must be aware of the times, interpreting its contribution to mankind in accordance with the needs of the time." She articulated a vision for the future, stating that occupational therapy is a profession possessing the knowledge necessary to maintain the health of people. She added that "to move from therapists to health agent demands us to change but to change in a forward, positive way. We do not have to give up what we know; rather, we must instead be willing to know more." Jerry Johnson (1972) continued the theme, stating that we "need to expand our concept of professionalism to meet criteria we establish and to develop an organizational strategy which enables us to relate to and interact with other professions and disciplines in positive and constructive ways, without sacrificing the concepts in which we believe."

Lorna Jean King (1978) remarked that "as we look toward an era of increasing specialization, we are soberly aware that without a unifying theory to insure cohesiveness, specialization could easily become fragmentation." Baum (1980) made the call, "As a profession and as professionals, let us put our resources, intelligence, and emotional commitment together and work diligently toward the ascent of our profession. The health care system, the clients we serve, and each of us individually will benefit from our commitment."

Robert Bing (1981) warned that we would not move forward until we took the "time to assiduously locate our profession's diggings, to excavate what is relevant, and, then, to learn from what has been unearthed." At a time when it seemed the profession was questioning its identity and value, Gilfoyle (1984) noted that "Occupational therapy has not left the past behind, but has not quite embrace the future either. Thus, our profession is in a time of parenthesis that brings us many uncertainties." She further encouraged us by arguing that "Uncertainties, however, can be our opportunity. We need only make use of the challenge and possibilities that are part of our dynamic present. Transformation is a time to direct our own future."

Anne Mosey (1985) urged us to continue looking to the future with determination. She argued that while "the understanding and appreciation of our history is important . . . to use it to substantiate a number of different ideas of what we are or ought to be is a questionable practice." She urged us to strive to be updated, relevant in the present, and posed for the future. Lest the profession completely loose its grounding in the past, Kathryn Reed (1986) asked, "Is occupational therapy losing its heritage or keeping up with the times?" Claudia Allen (1987) noted, echoing the thoughts of the Slagle lecturers that preceded her, that "Difficulties in explaining the value of using activity as a treatment method have been with us from the beginning," and affirmed that we should continue to rest on our application of occupation as a therapeutic activity because of its power to "compensate for disability by utilizing remaining capabilities to accomplish desirable activities with satisfactory results."

Susan Fine (1990) urged us to advance toward clearer client and occupation-centered practice. She claimed that "as a group we are far more effective at defining reality and assessing and promoting performance than we are at assessing and making use of patients' views of themselves and their situation. Although our clinical power has grown greatly, we are too often committed only to present manifest performance." She also noted that "our responsiveness to the inner lives of others can add perspective to our professional assumptions and enhance our understanding of human performance capacity."

Nelson (1996) later commented that occupational therapy as a profession "will flourish over the next century for the same reason that it has flourished over the past century. Real human beings needed therapeutic occupation in the days of Eleanor Clarke Slagle; they need therapeutic occupation in our times; and they will continue to need it beyond our days." Recognition would be granted, he noted, because "We are the profession uniquely devoted to helping persons help themselves through their own active efforts." He further added that his vision for the 21st century "is that occupational therapy will take its rightful place among the major professions in our society. The powers and complexities of occupation justify the sanctioning of a major profession." He concluded that "the ultimate statement of pride and confidence in the profession will be the full adoption of the term *occupation* in the language of the profession, with each occupational therapist taking personal responsibility for explaining to the world why we are called occupational therapists."

Anne Fisher (1998) carried the theme and added, "We need to recognize the need to set goals and document efficacy in terms of occupational performance and not impairments of performance components." Charles Christiansen (1999) further emphasized that "occupational therapy is positioned uniquely to meet the challenges confronting people whose identity is threatened by impairment, limitations to activity, and restrictions to their participation as social beings." Betty Hasselkus (2006) noted that occupational therapists have the potential to "be an exception to the generalized invisibility of everyday occupation in people's lives." She emphasized that this could accomplish this by "awakening to its already existing presence in our philosophy, in our education, in our research, and in our therapeutic practices." She explained that this awareness in the public "an awareness such as this will contribute toward broader and deeper insights into the importance and meaning of everyday occupation in the social fabric of our lives, thereby helping people find value in their everyday practices."

Jim Hinojosa (2007) discussed how occupational therapy practitioners must respond to rapid and unpredictable change in order to remain relevant and recognized as valuable. He exhorted that "we must become innovators to meet our responsibilities as therapists and as individuals. Our profession's future depends not on what AOTA develops but on how each of us creates lives as modern professionals. The future of occupational therapy is in our control."

Science-Driven and Evidence-Based

According to the lecturers, recognition of our worth is related to our ability to demonstrate the effectiveness of our services. The importance of being a science-driven profession has been a long-lasting theme in the lectures. Stattel (1955) inaugurated the lectures by noting that "Study of the vast amount of material that is available in the medical field will result in research that will bring answers and improved treatment techniques in occupational therapy. Our educational backgrounds provide us with a basic philosophy along with knowledge and skill to carry it out." She also alluded early to the need for our practice to be based on sound evidence. She stated that "knowledge . . . can be secured by correlating and strengthening our beliefs with facts. Empirical methods should be tested when possible, and reasonable doubt should be eliminated." Margaret Rood (1958) addressed some challenges to carrying out that research. She pointed out that "in the majority of occupational therapy schools, the scientific preparation in physical disabilities is less than in physical therapy schools when functional activities would seem to require as great a knowledge of structure and function if not more." Ackley (1962) added that "the ability to recognize and understand factors which contribute to or precipitate disability, and the acquisition of knowledge and security in using remedial techniques is the justification for the long and expensive education of the occupational therapist."

Jean Ayers (1963) dedicated her lecture to advancements in research and noted that "there is a long gap between these basic research data and the assurance that a treatment procedure is effective. We need many studies to test, scientifically, the hypotheses suggested by the theories." Fidler (1965) commented that criteria for professional identity included "an infinite commitment to the advancement of learning, to research as an attitude, and to the maintenance of critical, evaluative, and creative thinking, is still another criteria of professional identity." She emphasized the importance of research because "a profession must base its technique of operation upon principles rather than rule of thumb procedures or routine skills." Yerxa (1966) also addressed the importance of research by stating that "a body of knowledge is essential. This body of knowledge must be based upon research. Occupational therapists are becoming increasingly involved in planning, conducting, and publishing the results of their own research studies." Answering practitioners' possible trepidations, she added that "the scientific attitude is not incompatible with concern for the client as a human being but may be one of the best foundations for acting upon that concern."

West (1967) directly challenged practitioners by asking if "can we rely on the work of a small but increasing number of researchers among us to confirm the scientific basis of our practice? . . . Decidedly not." Lela Llorens (1969) exemplified the professional committed to advancing knowledge through research. Her lecture addressed "premises which express the developmental theory of occupational therapy . . . outgrowth of my own experience and research."

Finn (1971) provided encouragement by noting that "after years of intuitive service to the sick and disabled we have now begun to define our practice and validate our clinical impressions through research studies." Alice Jantzen (1973) particularly encouraged educators, suggesting that "occupational therapy faculty should take leadership in the research activities for our profession. Further, I suggest that we who are university faculty members should begin to demand that university administration support us in these endeavors."

King (1978) proposed a theoretical framework that could give direction to research. She suggested that the adaptive process could provide such a framework because it "can be applied to all the specialty areas as a unifying concept; that it will differentiate occupational therapy from other professions; that it is readily explainable to other professionals and consumers; and that it is adequate in depth to allow for scientific elaboration and refinement."

Joan Rogers (1983) noted that "the clinician functions as a scientist, ethicist, and artist," and Gilfoyle (1984) added that "to maintain our upward spiral, our profession must re-examine the scientific view and value system that has been the basis of present concepts regarding activity and focus on future concepts based on a science of occupation and an art of purposefulness." Reed (1986) admonished educators in particular to teach why a medium or method is used as well as how. She noted that "researchers need to provide more information as to why certain media and methods became part of our tool kit." She further advised that "practitioners would be wise to follow the statement, 'If you know how, be sure you know why and be sure the why is consistent with the philosophy of occupational therapy.'"

Anne Henderson (1988) noted that clinicians had an essential role in the advancement of research because "from the knowledge of the treatment strategies that clinicians have found to work, as well as from the findings of intervention research, the theorists can begin the process of developing, classifying, and abstracting general principles from the practice knowledge." Florence Clark (1993) continued to call the profession to a commitment to research. She stated that "innovative and unique methods . . . need to be developed to tackle the research questions posed by occupational science" and encouraged the use of life histories as unique ways in which research could approximate the collaboration that exists between clients and occupational therapy practitioners. She noted that "interpretive occupational science research speaks to practice, not by discovery of general laws of principles, but by providing thick descriptions of actual cases that practitioners can refer to as they submerge themselves in practice."

Catherine Trombly (1995) introduced her lecture by saying, "My goal is to spark and explosion of research concerning therapeutic occupation." She went on to describe the complex ways in which occupation motivates action and concluded by saying, "research is needed to verify each of these hypothesis, I hope each occupational therapist will be joining me in taking responsibility to contribute to that effort." Nelson (1996) reminded the profession that "the founders thought of occupation as a method, not just a goal. They believed that occupation could have thera-peutic effects on the human being, and they wanted to document these effects through scientific research." He added that such a vision was not yet fulfilled and recommended a continued impetus toward "research for occupational therapists conducted by occupational therapists and those who understand occupational therapy. Our primary focus should be to examine the power of occupation as therapy."

Margo Holm (2000) reminded occupational therapy practitioners about their commitment to competency: "What is necessary for continued competence in research and for our professional survival is for all of us to increase the number and level of our research competence—not just to 'maintain competence' as the wording in our *Code of Ethics*, but, rather, to improve our competence." She concluded with a pointed question for the profession to con-sider in the new millennium, "Can we meet this challenge today?" Holm also explicitly introduced evidence-based practice to the lectures, noting it should be part of the basic competence of professionals: "Although the evidence for what we do and how we do it may be difficult to find, we have an obligation to become competent in, and make a habit of, searching for the evidence, appraising its value, and presenting it to those we serve in an understandable manner." She re-emphasized her point be adding that it is our obligation "to develop the habit of using those com-petencies in everyday practice, and to advance the evidence based of occupational therapy in the new millennium."

Winnie Dunn (2001) echoed the notion that occupational therapy practitioners must understand research inti-mately. She stated that "we might characterize our role as translator: We stand in the space between abstract con-structs (i.e., research) and application to practice, looking back and forth, translating for each group what the other has to say." Charlotte Royeen (2003) added that in addition to "translation," the challenge to the profession was to "discern the pattern of occupations giving rise to varying conditions or states such as health, disease, injury, or hap-piness" and proposed the use of chaos theory as a way to liberate our thinking "from a linear view of reality, which does not match practice."

Finally, Wendy Coster (2008) explored the "tensions inherent in the assessment process in a profession that is holistic and humanistic in its orientation." She proposed that "in order for assessment to serve our goal of support-ing health and participation through engagement in occupation we must accept the uncertainty and be vigilant about the biases in thinking that are inherent in our measures." Thus, she called for renewed efforts for the profes-sion to develop its own measures rather than continue borrowing them from medicine, education, psychology, and education. She related these efforts to evidence-based practice by noting that "we need to challenge interpretations of research evidence that draw inappropriate conclusions from the measures that were used, particularly when those interpretations are used to restrict occupational therapy practice or to establish overly narrow service guidelines." Finally, Schwartz (2009) noted that a concern for "engagement in and dissemination of scientific research that sup-ports the effectiveness of occupational therapy" was an explicit part of the *Founding Vision* articulated at the begin-ning of the profession in 1917.

Globally Connected Workforce

This theme perhaps appears explicitly with less frequency in the lectures because the basic purpose of the Eleanor Clarke Slagle Lecture award is to recognize the contributions of the awardees toward the advancement of the pro-fession as a whole. Essentially, all lectures were directed to all occupational therapy practitioners. Stattel (1955) spoke about our inherent unity as a profession: "We are all occupational therapists first, reduced from our specialties by the common denominator, the human being who needs our help." June Sokolov (1956) reinforced this sentiment by adding, "Our common aim of helping people help themselves."

Rood (1958) spoke about the importance of diversity in the profession: "All occupational therapists should add to our store of knowledge and general growth. . . . Each must contribute at his own level so that the whole may be more complete, since each with different backgrounds and interests will see different facets of the same problem." Ackley (1962) expressed concern for integrating new perspectives into the profession brought by students and new professionals, noting that "continuance of a profession depends upon the generation to come."

Johnson (1972) acknowledged that "our lives are becoming more complex, more interrelated, and more inter-dependent" and affirmed such interdependence was needed for us to "develop a strategy and organize ourselves, as a profession, so that we can conduct negotiations and transactions with the larger social system in which we exist, thereby ensuring the provision of our services to those who have need of them." King (1978) also reinforced the need for unity by stating that "splintering into small professions (specialization) results in watering-down of job devel-opment effectiveness, the scattering of progressively scarcer financial resources for education, and the loss of politi-cal 'clout.'"

Mosey (1985) believed that unity is not synonymous with single-mindedness or adherence to a narrow set of beliefs and theories. She argued that "a pluralistic identity gives us freedom to grow and progress. It gives us the opportunity to engage in practice and scholarly pursuits unencumbered by tradition, authority, or ideology . . . and would prepare us to meet the needs of those we seek to help." Henderson (1988) later also noted that "We need to be unified in our fundamental assumptions, but diverse in our technical knowledge."

Dunn (2001) pointed to the productive outcome of a diverse profession, noting that "The discipline of occupa-tional therapy has had a collective interest in sensory processing across the entire evolution of the profession. We have generated and continue to generate a wealth of information about how persons process sensory information and how those methods guide choices."

Suzanne Peloquin (2005) illuminated our *ethos*—the beliefs that guide us as a single, identifiable profession—as the intention "to advance into the future embracing the ethos that has characterized occupational therapy since its inception is to reclaim the profession's heart." Our interconnectedness comes from, she argued, the common beliefs that ground us as occupational therapy professionals:

> The ethos of occupational therapy restores our clear-sightedness so that we see what is essential: We are pathfind-ers. We enable occupations that heal. We co-create daily lives. We reach for hearts as well as hands. We are artists and scientists at once. If we discern this in ourselves, if we act on this understanding every day, we will advance into the future embracing our ethos of engagement. And we will have reclaimed a magnificent heart.

Burke (2010) also affirmed that a unique source of our professional identity id related to our ability to interact uniquely with clients. She noted that "The conduct of an interaction is endlessly fascinating. It's a riddle. It is always different, yet it includes the same parts and structure each time."

Schwartz (2009) noted that the *Centennial Vision* was essentially an extension of the values articulated in the *Founding Vision* almost 100 years ago. She stated that the *Centennial Vision* can thus "can give practitioners of today a sense of continuity and community with earlier generations of occupational therapists."

Meeting Society's Occupational Needs

This, perhaps, has been the universal theme of all Slagle lecturers. While each addressed the profession internally, the context was the advancement of our service to society. Stattel (1955) inaugurated the Slagle lectures by stating that "We have been given a wonderful professional heritage of courage and wisdom and as we continue to extend our hand to benefit mankind, may we continue to believe and search for further knowledge."

Sokolov (1956) expounded on the role of the administrator as one through whom "the service to those who need the care that only occupational therapy can provide is extended." Brunyate (1957) recounted the birth of occu-pational therapy and the commitment of its founders to serve the needs of society and recalled Jane Adams's address to the third annual occupational therapy convention in 1919 as stating, "you are really the vanguard on the line of philanthropic effort and you are beginning at the bottom as all great social experiments have always done."

Rood (1958) titled her lecture *Every One Counts*, referring not only to members of the profession but also to peo-ple with disabilities seeking to make their way in society. Lilian Wegg (1959) highlighted the development of occu-pational therapy's contribution to meeting vocational (i.e., productive) needs of members of society, and Muriel Zimmerman (1960) encouraged us to "remain eager to participate in any way where the vision of others or our own vision can create a better world for the disabled." Reilly (1961) further noted that "American society in general, and medicine in particular, has need of a profession which has as its unique concern the nurturing of the spirit of man for action" and warned that "If we fail to serve society's need for action, we will most assuredly die out as a health profession."

As quoted earlier, Ackley (1962) argued that the cost of educating occupational therapy professionals was justified by the knowledge we poses about factors that contribute to or precipitate disability. Ayers (1963) summarized her work in developing effective treatment approaches for the growing population of members of society with perceptual–motor dysfunction, and Fidler (1965) reminded us that "professional roles are set forth by the needs of the society to be served, circumscribed by the profession's delineation of the extent to which it may be expected to fulfill such needs."

Noting the basic needs of all human beings to find their place in society, Yerxa (1966) stated that "Our broad purpose is to produce a reality orienting influence upon the client's perception of his physical environment and his social and psychological self, to the end that he can function in his environment with self-actualization." Later, West (1967) pointed out that "one fact is virtually undeniable today: comprehensive health care, among others of man's needs, is beyond individual attainment for far too many people." She then added that "if we accept this fact, we can accept the organization of increasingly costly and complex programs designed tor reduce disease and disability among victims of economic disparity and to raise the health standards of our country as a whole."

Llorens (1969) described occupational therapy as "a facilitation process which assists the individual in achieving mastery of life tasks and the ability to cope as efficiently as possible with the life expectations made of him." She noted that the profession needed to be keenly aware of society's demands because "the occupational therapist serves as the enculturation agent for the conditions of . . . health in which the developmental level being experienced . . . is unequal to the age-related demands made on this organism as a result of natural or traumatic incident."

Finn (1971) acknowledged that "The needs of our times are now asking us to contribute to the preservation of each person's right to achieve his highest level of human functioning," and Johnson (1972) exhorted us to "utilize knowledge . . . to help us predict social change and anticipate the consequences of such change." Jantzen (1973) noted that occupational therapy existed for the delivery of our particular kind of health care services to patients or clients and that our education "should be aimed at meeting the needs of society in our own particular way."

Fiorentino (1974) likened the development of the occupational therapy professional to the scheme through which children develop into adults and noted the culmination was a professional who can "meet the changing world of medicine, the controls of government, the demands of professionalism, and the obligations of competence." Josephine Moore (1975) also noted our professional responsibility to maintain high competence and a positive public image, stating that we would "fail unless the individual being treated is motivated and has faith in those who are helping him."

Joy Huss (1976) described the basic human need of a caring touch and noted that if we "begin to use touch in a caring manner, in time we could make a difference in our culture." King (1978) noted that occupational therapy professionals are uniquely qualified to address needs that others in society are not. One example is "hospital-induced sensory deprivation that is of critical importance in rehabilitation or therapy." Another example is the adaptive response to change or stress, which she noted was "a growing concern in society."

Hollis (1979) encouraged the profession to view clients' problems as opportunities that stimulate or spark better performance. In her view, occupational therapy was uniquely disposed to serve the human need to "interest the whole mind, the aggregate nature of man more continuously and more deeply." Baum (1980) argued that "our responsibility as a profession is to implement a broader perspective of health care delivery—one that places its values on individuals as they accept the responsibility for their own health status," and Bing (1981) celebrated the long tradition of the profession expressed in "the ideal that those who are sick and handicapped can regain, retain, and attain some semblance of function within the fundamental limitations of the human organism and the expectations of the society in which all must exist." Rogers (1983) stated throughout her lecture that occupational therapy was concerned with discerning "the intentions and potentials of chronically disabled patients." She noted that the profession's ultimate social responsibility was to elicit such intentions and potentials "and use them to help patients discover health within themselves."

Gilfoyle (1984) dedicated her lecture to explaining why and how the profession should take advantage of opportunities to be transformed in order to meet the needs of society, and Mosey (1985) proposed that a pluralistic approach to our professional identity would best support our ability to meet those needs. Reed (1986) provided an overview of the evolution of the media occupational therapy has used since its inception and argued that during each period, such media revealed a rationale that ultimately helped the profession meet the social needs of the particular time in history. Allen (1987) likewise argued that the most unique contribution the profession could make to society was the elucidation of activity as treatment method, adding that "because occupational therapists use activity as a treatment method, they are in a position to see the social meaning of a disability and witness the formation of a personal sense of the disability." She noted that occupational therapy professionals could help fill the gap between the patient's desirable activities and society's expectations, acceptance, and operational barriers by helping the person compensate for disability by using remaining capabilities.

Henderson (1988) emphasized in her lecture that the profession needed to maintain an ongoing commitment to theory building that would continually guide practice so that the profession could fulfill its mission to serve specific social needs. Likewise, Shereen Farber (1989) encouraged the ongoing incorporation of advances in neuroscience into the practice of occupational therapy as they offered fresh new insight into ways in which occupational needs are normally satisfied and, thus, how we might support patients who have impairments satisfy them by alternative means.

Fine (1990) argued that the very nature of human beings was to search for meaning and purpose and that in our use of occupation as a medium "we will find ourselves far better able to help our patients refine their adventures, find meaning and purpose in their ordeals, discover there is more to themselves than current circumstance suggests, and transform the dross of their adversity into the gold of their accomplishment." Likewise, Clark (1993) argued the relevance of the profession lies on its acknowledgment of the "centrality of occupation in the lives of people." Grady (1994) noted that, as the result of the civil rights movements in the previous decades, "a new sociopolitical environment is developing in which persons with disabilities are taking or creating social and political actions on their own behalf." This new environment promoted changes in society regarding opportunities for inclusion of all persons in all aspects of living, and in her view, were the focal points for exploring occupational therapy's role in building inclusive community.

Trombly (1995) asserted that occupational therapy was founded on the belief that engaging in occupation brought about mental and physical health, and thus, the social need we served was helping people regain health through the use of occupation as means and as end. Nelson (1996) noted that a future role for occupational therapy "is in the solution of some of our society's chronic social and public health problems, such as drugs, violence, unprepared motherhood, unemployment, and homelessness." Fisher (1998) described occupational therapy's contribution to societal needs as "enable[ing] . . . clients to seize, take possession of, or occupy the spaces, time, and roles of their lives."

Christiansen (1999) noted that "one of the most compelling needs that every human being has is to be able to express his or her unique identity in a manner that gives meaning to life." Asserting that "occupations are key not just to being a person, but to being a particular person, and thus creating and maintaining identity," he concluded that "the ultimate goal of occupational therapy services is well-being, not health. Health enables people to pursue the tasks of everyday living that provide them with the life meaning necessary for their well-being."

Holm (2000) argued that the interventions we used to meet societal needs needed to be supported by empirical evidence and called professionals to increase their competence in research knowledge and skills. Dunn (2001) stated that "occupational therapists can advance thinking about the contribution of sensory processing to our understanding of the human experience both in the typical course of the day and as it might interfere with living a satisfying life," and Royeen (2003) stated that "occupational therapists see the surreal in order to help people get real. We can see what is not possible, and through occupation can create and adapt the world to make things doable with meaning."

Zemke (2004) said that "The occupational health of individuals and of societies is linked together—the problems of an economic recession resulting in widespread unemployment is a societal health problem and to the individuals affected a personal occupational one as well, resulting in occupational insufficiency or deprivation." She noted, therefore, that "A society that enables occupation for all will require not only health care change, but political, economic, and other social change."

Peloquin (2005) noted that our charge was to help vulnerable people open paths to occupation in ways that foster dignity, competence, health, and engagement, and that we did so through a blend of artistry and science that expressed care. Hasselkus (2006) sought to raise awareness of "the complexity and 'delicate layerings' of everyday occupation, its theoretical and conceptual underpinnings" as well as the "consequences of severe occupational constraints to health and well-being," because such understanding clarified the relevance of occupational therapy and occupational science to the world. Hinojosa (2007) challenged us to "become innovative, reflective practitioners who embrace life in an era of hyperchange" in order to serve society's occupational needs. Coster (2008) argued our goal is to support health and participation through engagement in occupation, and to do that "we must accept the uncertainty and be vigilant about the biases in thinking that are inherent in our measures." Schwartz (2009) pointed out that both the *Founding Vision* and the *Centennial Vision* "share a focus on . . . successful promotion of occupation as a vital force to meet society's needs," thus demonstrating that this concern has been at the core of the profession since its inception.

Burke (2010) summarized the unique contribution of occupational therapy toward serving societal needs by casting our work as future-oriented, as optimistic and hope-filled:

> Occupational therapy is interpersonal interaction. Although the space that each of us creates as an occupational therapist reflects unique experiences and training, our profession's unifying commitment to the interactional relationship drives all of us to focus on the same priorities: providing our patients and their families with glimpses of what is possible, what can be done, and what it will take to get there.

Conclusion

British politician Henry St. John Lord Bolingbroke wrote that "History is philosophy teaching by example and also by warning" (as cited in Kramnick, 1992). The Slagle lectures aptly fit that description. Collectively they capture past, present, and future of the profession and as such offer us the long view needed for strategic planning (Schwartz, 1996). These lectures encourage, exhort, remind, and lead. They offer multiple perspectives of the source of our power, our potential to be widely recognized, our responsibility to develop our science and support our practice with evidence, our need to be a globally connected workforce, and our commitment to serve the occupational needs of society. They are, therefore, shining examples of the values that inspired the *Centennial Vision* and will propel us to our next 100 years of existence.

Organization and Use of the Third Edition

This volume maintains similar organization as the second edition with some changes. To set the stage of the lectures, the volume begins with recognition of the person for whom the honor was named. We reprint here an address presented by Adolf Meyer in honor of the retirement of his colleague, Eleanor Clarke Slagle, in 1937.[1] Then, to aid in reflection and discussion, the text is organized according to decades, each decade preceded by a brief historical account of the events taking place in the world and in the United States at the time. After this his-

---

[1]Originally published in 1985 in *Occupational Therapy in Mental Health, 5*(3), 109–113.

torical account, the Slagle lectures for the decade are reprinted.[2] Again, each decade is closed by a series of suggested learning activities and discussion questions. We have expanded this section with questions related to the *Centennial Vision*. The historical account of happenings in the world and in the United States since the beginning of the new millennium has been updated, and six new lectures have been included in this latest edition. Likewise, biographies and bibliographies of the lecturers have been updated whenever possible (see Appendix A). Updates were provided either by the lecturers themselves or resulted from extensive searches of databases and publication listings.[3] Those lecturers who were able to contributed special comments about the *Centennial Vision*. Bibliographies of world and U.S. history (see Appendix B), history of occupational therapy in the United States (see Appendix C) and around the world (see Appendix D), and a list of every AOTA president (see Appendix E) also have been updated.

References

American Occupational Therapy Association (2007). AOTA's *Centennial Vision* and executive summary. *American Journal of Occupational Therapy, 61,* 613–614.

Kramnick, I. (1992). *Bolingbroke and his circle: The politics of nostalgia in the age of Walpole.* Ithaca, NY: Cornell University Press.

Schwartz, P. (1996). *The art of the long view: Planning for the future in an uncertain world.* New York: Doubleday.

---

[2]The majority of Eleanor Clarke Slagle Lectures were first published in the *American Journal of Occupational Therapy.* The original publication reference is included with each lecture.

[3]Databases searched included Medline, CINAHL, PsychINFO, Ageline, Web of Science, ERIC, Academic Search Premiere, Humanities International Index, PubMed, and OT Search. Other sources included Books in Print, Google Scholar and Google Books. In addition, special searches were conducted through the index listings of journals including *The American Journal of Occupational Therapy, Occupational Therapy Journal of Research, Occupational Therapy International Physical and Occupational Therapy in Pediatrics, Occupational Therapy in Mental Health, Occupational Therapy in Healthcare,* and the *Journal of Occupational Science.*

Introduction to the Second Edition

Historical Context of Scholarship and Leadership in Occupational Therapy

This book contains, as its title suggests, a true legacy in the tradition of one of the greatest occupational therapy pioneers, Eleanor Clarke Slagle (1876–1942). The American Occupational Therapy Association (AOTA) recognized this pioneer's influence by establishing its highest award in her honor in 1953. Slagle "continually reaffirm[ed] her strong convictions in research and study as *the* fundamental mortar for building our practice and our continuing contributions to the health of those we serve" (Cromwell, 1977, p. 645, italics in original). Slagle was "legendary for the political and administrative expertise she demonstrated as executive secretary of the AOTA" (Schwartz, 2003, p. 6). She was described as someone who "shaped the philosophy and practice of occupation for generations to come" (Bing, 1997, p. 220) through "unusual modesty and gentleness . . . the embodiment of example and principle" (Meyer, 1985, pp. 111–112) and, ultimately, "the consummate [occupational therapy] professional" (Metaxas, 2000, p. 57).

The Eleanor Clarke Slagle Lecture was first awarded in 1955 and, since its inception, candidates are nominated by the general AOTA membership and chosen by the Recognitions Committee. The purpose of the lectureship is

1. To honor a member of the Association who has creatively contributed to the development of the body of knowledge of the profession;
2. To acknowledge the development of improved methods and techniques in the practice of occupational therapy that improve service to clients or the public and that foster public awareness of the profession;
3. To recognize contributions to the profession made by or through research, education, and practice in occupational therapy;
4. To enable members to benefit from new or revised knowledge and developments in the profession; and
5. To give Occupational Therapists, Registered, and Certified Occupational Therapy Assistants the opportunity to express and publish the results of their studies and to share their knowledge and experience with the membership. (AOTA, 1985, p. v)

2005 marks the 50th anniversary of the first Eleanor Clarke Slagle Lecture in Occupational Therapy. All of these lectures, most of which were first presented at the AOTA Annual Conference and then published in the *American Journal of Occupational Therapy,* represent individual and collective achievement that indeed honor occupational therapy as a profession. They contain history, leadership, mentoring, encouragement, admonishment, philosophy, and practical guidance. Above all, however, they reflect Slagle's vision of integration of theory, philosophy, and spirit (Meyer, 1985) from which all of us—practitioners, educators, and students—can draw inspiration.

This volume presents 41 Eleanor Clarke Slagle Lectures, from the first one in 1955, through the 2004 lecture (no awards were made in 1964, 1968, 1970, 1977, 1982, 1991, 1992, 1997, and 2002). While the lectures individually stand firm on their own as solid examples of scholarship, when read sequentially they demonstrate that "leadership and learning are indispensable to each other" (Kennedy, 2000, p. 103) and form a unique record of the steady progress and increasing sophistication of occupational therapy.

—*René Padilla, PhD, OTR/L, FAOTA, LMHP*
Associate Professor, Department of Occupational Therapy
Creighton University
Omaha, NE

References

American Occupational Therapy Association. (1953). [Minutes of the AOTA House of Delegates and Board of Management, November 16 and 19, 1953]. New York: Author.

American Occupational Therapy Association. (1985). *A professional legacy: The Eleanor Clarke Slagle Lectures in Occupational Therapy, 1955–1984*. Rockville, MD: Author.

Bing, R. (1997). "And teach agony to sing": An afternoon with Eleanor Clarke Slagle. *American Journal of Occupational Therapy, 51*, 220–227.

Cromwell, F. (1977). Eleanor Clarke Slagle, the leader, the woman. *American Journal of Occupation-al Therapy, 31*, 645–648.

Kennedy, J. F. (2000). *The greatest speeches of President John F. Kennedy*. Bellingham, WA: Titan.

Metaxas, V. (2000). Eleanor Clarke Slagle and Susan E. Tracy: Personal and professional identity and the development of occupational therapy in Progressive Era America. *Nursing History Review, 8*, 39–70.

Meyer, A. (1985). Address in honor of Eleanor Clarke Slagle (delivered September 14, 1937). *Occupational Therapy in Mental Health, 5*, 109–113.

Schwartz, K. B. (2003). The history of occupational therapy. In E. Crepeau, E. Cohn, & B. Shell (Eds.), *Willard and Spackman's occupational therapy* (10th ed.). Baltimore, MD: Lippincott Williams & Wilkins.

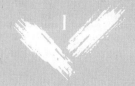

THE 1950s

Launching a New Tradition

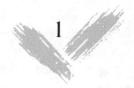

Setting the Stage—Address in Honor of Eleanor Clarke Slagle

Adolph Meyer

It is a great privilege to have an opportunity to speak on this occasion, which honors a friend and long-time co-worker, our Mrs. Eleanor Clarke Slagle, as a person and as the personification of occupational therapy. Presidents and officers have come and gone, but for 20 years Mrs. Slagle has brought into the field just that kind of personality which proved highly fruitful and auspicious: she has been, not a dictator, not a boss, but a leader by example, a human being and human factor among human beings, a cultivator of human relationships, in gathering around herself co-workers and in making co-workers of the patients. Such is the human being Mrs. Slagle and what she means to us and to the thousands of patients who have been and are still reached by her and her pupils. And inseparable from this personal human side, there stands before us the nature and character of the product of her work and the spirit and philosophy her life and life-work exemplify, that which brings us together in this assembly and in this large and impressive organization.

This gathering and the work achieved by this body with Mrs. Slagle as the head worker are enough of a testimonial for a cause and its leading and stabilizing captain. Obviously Mrs. Slagle has had her ideal not only in perpetuating herself in a special role but in training a rank and file ever able to furnish timber for leadership from the ranks and in the ranks, and growth from the ranks.

For 20 years, from the beginning of our organization, Mrs. Slagle has, as treasurer and secretary, done that work of continuity which with changing presidents and changing topics represents the very constitution of this growing force in the ranks of dealing with those who, for a time and sometimes for good, are forced into that army that needs shelter and protection and among whom the work of restoring health and better ways of prevention and achievement of the handicapped brings care and cure.

In these days in which we are perhaps too much inclined to look upon leadership as a profession, and upon professional agitators as the reapers of honor and power, it is a tremendous satisfaction to see one of the chief workers completing 20 years in that office which personifies the very constitution of this body. Mrs. Slagle and Dr. Dunton have been the spirits in the ranks and from the ranks and for the ranks, not imposed managers, but the souls of the essence of the work, giving freely of their time and experience while carrying on the work itself.

In the great division of labor we need continuity and examples that survive the changes and are embodiments of the very essentials which only the best workers can perpetuate in steady growth, in stability of motion and promotion, those who see that ever new deals are fair deals, deals embodying the wisdom of those who do and actually work and never cease to grow and to create.

Growth and work and achievement and attainment are all a function of that one virtual commodity—time, that steady rhythm of day and night, of seasons and years, not a mere eternal return but eternal progression. No 2 days can be quite the same, and no 2 years; but there has to be an element of continuity and cohesion; and for this it takes

Originally published 1985 in *Occupational Therapy in Mental Health, 5*(3), 109–113.

those starting with enough personality, capable of maintaining themselves and of remaining forces and centers of growth. And as in the nature of humanity, generation follows generation, the young work beside the old and the old work beside the young, those capable of being the bearers of continuity are few and rare and, we are glad to see, honored and sought as the very essence of progress.

Mrs. Slagle comes from the same source and soil that gave me my first opportunities and encouragement: the opportunity to realize the need for more, the need for growth, the opportunity to find similarly minded forces and the spirit of action that has to go with knowledge and vision to make it both fertile and practical: Illinois, large needs and large enterprises, a whole group of aspiring forces and engaging problems, needs in practice and needs in hospitals, close to Missouri, wanting to be shown and shown by actual work and performances. The educator, the social worker, and the physician were bound to get together. Miss Lathrop was one of the great links. As the great gardener Froebel in education and his pupil Grossman in the therapeutic training of psychopaths by work recognized the need of a setting for work and for therapy in sound use of time, so there was the shaping of an atmosphere of work and action at Kankakee, encouraged by the social spirit about Hull House, all working for the training by action and not only by word. The old ideal of the Middle Ages, pray and work, took real form in the union of one's best thought and work, and when we opened the Phipps Clinic for action, Miss Lathrop was able to lend us Mrs. Slagle as the model and instigator of workmanship in the service of therapy. That the greatest benefit for the sufferer was to come from the philosophy of time and its use and from the right person to exemplify it was natural in the pragmatic atmosphere of the middle west and Mrs. Slagle brought the fruit of experience to our new center. She started us and, like all good workers, inspired others, so that, when she was needed for more and more training of new forces, she left with us the workers who carried on while she was drawn into that field of training and teaching and organizing, that did so much in the emergencies of that international madness called war and again for the needs arising from the madness and the immaturity and blunderings even in peace. As a contributor to the philosophy of time and life, as a cultivator of life and health in activity, Mrs. Slagle has become a guide, philosopher, and friend of hundreds and hundreds, and as I said, the embodiment of example and principle. What she has added in the nearly 25 years since she came to help us is a proud record, a rare fulfillment of a life still growing and still progressing.

The demands of actual life and work where it is most needed have wrought a wonderful change in turning psychology from esoteric contemplation into the service of actual life. Real needs and real opportunities have led us into modern psychobiology and a science of human nature and behavior. And the basis of this modern psychobiology is not mere analysis and preaching of license, but a study and cultivation of the person and action. This is how the old principle of engaging patients in activity has become the basic setting of all modern therapy. Pathology is no longer a kind of gloating over what can be found at autopsy. It is the study of the mistakes and maladjustments, the failures of man to use his best sense and opportunities. Mistakes become damage and damage becomes disease and disease in turn has to be brought back to where it is treated as "poor work" to be replaced by good and helpful work. This is the role of occupational therapy, not merely making a lot of stereotyped articles but releasing or implanting and fostering action with the reward and joy of achievement. I heard Mrs. Slagle quote from a passage in the first paper I ever wrote on the treatment of nervous and mental disorders, addressed to the Chicago Pathological Society in February, 1893, nearly 45 years ago, in which I asked my colleagues for the discussion of the kind of work which could be expected from and recommended to American ladies. I do not know why I picked on the ladies; I suppose because the doctors present were all men and I felt I knew them. I said: 'Experience alone can give suggestions in this line.' I called it mental hygiene, foreshadowing what I now mean by "mind," the person in action, good or bad, helpful and effective or mere restlessness, often overactive only as the result of fatigue and mismanagement.

I should like to be able to voice adequately what so many of my patients have gained through Mrs. Slagle and her pupils and what it all means not only for the sufferer but also for the healthy of our time. When the development of machinery supersedes the driving power of necessity in the development of habits and possibilities of work, we turn to the ingenuity of those who know the creative possibilities available not only for the sick but for the rank and file of those with "time on their hands."

From reveling in thoughts of eternity, we now have the great task to inject again the joys of activity of the day so that we may make a return of the pleasure of the day's work an efficient competitor with the mere pleasure and glamour of night life. We are grateful to Mrs. Slagle and her pupils and co-workers for their devotion and skill and creative zeal and achievements in the furtherance of the joy and rewards of work and creation.

It must be a great satisfaction to Mrs. Slagle to see the onward march of what had but slender beginnings. There is a need of leisure for the spreading of the wisdom that has come from the wide experience under difficult conditions. As wisdom grows there comes the demand for a spreading into wider usefulness. Today we have come into a period of prostitution of the capacity and love for work to the service of the something and the somebody else of mere wages. We have more and more cause to search for the natural inducements to work and the opportunities for new creative principles. We have to study work for its own rewards and to honor and cherish it and to cultivate it so as to make it deserve the honor and joy. Working under the difficulties met by the psychiatric occupational worker should and will give us much material for a usable knowledge of the relation of person and work, worker and work, and worker and leadership.

What is the work one can love and live with and live on? What are the conditions of work that are needed if the worker is to love the work and to live on and through it?

I shall never forget the deplorable words of a Secretary of Labor in a discussion of immigration. He told us we needed some immigration to get labor to do the dirty work which no American parent would want his children to do.

We occupational workers know that there is no work that cannot be shaped so as to find its worker able to get satisfaction from the doing and the result.

In these days in which continuity of purpose seems overshadowed by doctrines of change and where leadership in a democratic sense threatens to be belittled and to degenerate in other lands into high-power dictatorships, it is a matter of great joy and cheer to see respect and honor brought to a leader of unusual modesty and gentleness.

In the midst of talk and reality of change we see careers of continuity of progress, of action and creativeness in the ranks, and as part of the ranks.

We see those natural and inspiring instances in which a rare individual becomes a live and effective example of ideas and ideals as the living and active person, and persons expressive of ideals.

And we are glad to see those persons who become living symbols of great movements and realizations, in the midst of the younger and the budding generations, sharing with them the experience of a lifetime and the spirit of everbudding youth.

It is the pride of democracy to cherish its leaders as parts of the ranks, as influence by example, and as recipients of recognition and of fellowship in the rank and file.

We like to see it brought home that a lifetime of work and service and devotion and leadership in a cause also finds its recognition, and recognition and esteem its expression.

2

Historical Context

Around the World

During World War II (1939–1945), the Soviet Union, the United States, and Great Britain allied against their common enemies—Germany, Italy, and Japan, known as the Axis Powers. However, by 1947 the animosity between these allies had re-emerged, and the Cold War had begun. Drawn along the sharp ideological line between capitalism and communism, the United States and the Soviet Union accused each other of expansionist schemes. Great Britain's Prime Minister, Winston Churchill, called this ideological line the "Iron Curtain," spanning Eastern Europe from the Baltic Sea to the Adriatic Sea along the western borders of Poland, East Germany, Czechoslovakia, and Hungary, leaving countries east of this curtain increasingly under the control of the Soviet Union. In a speech to Congress on March 12, 1947, U.S. President Harry S Truman set the stage for what would become the American ethos of the 1950s and most of the 1960s:

> The seeds of totalitarian regimes are nurtured by misery and want. They spread and grow in the evil soil of poverty and strife. They reach their full growth when the hope of a people for a better life has died. We must keep that hope alive. The free peoples of the world look to us for support in maintaining their freedoms. If we falter in our leadership, we may endanger the peace of the world—and we shall surely endanger the welfare of our own nation. (*Congressional Record, 93*, p. 1981)

While Europe had lost its position of dominance in the world, and most of its colonies successfully nurtured independence movements, the two new superpowers began a form of neo-colonialism in a race to reduce each other's influence over less powerful nations. The nations avoided open war by building up armed forces and, in particular, nuclear weaponry. Each side aimed to have the upper hand with greater military force to keep the other's power in check in a cold war that would last 4 decades.

In 1950, China and the Soviet Union signed a treaty of friendship, alliance, and mutual assistance and named Japan and the United States as common enemies. Soon after, Communist forces from North Korea, backed by Soviet and Chinese resources, invaded South Korea. The United Nations, formed in 1945 at the end of World War II, urged its members to support South Korea and put American General Douglas MacArthur in command of the U.N. forces charged with containing the Korean conflict. This ignited the Korean War, which involved 16 nations fighting the "Communist threat." After high casualties on both sides, an armistice agreement was signed in 1953, but tensions in the area remained. Indochina became the next ideological hot spot, with the initiation of a civil war in South Vietnam that lasted for the rest of the decade and beyond.

The Cold War included fronts around the world, although the United States and Soviet involvement generally was more disguised. For example, in 1954, Guatemala stopped participating in the Inter-American Conference, called to draft human rights laws across nations, over a resolution to bar communism from the Western

Hemisphere, which led to a U.S. boycott that lasted 3 months. Suspecting that its neighbor Nicaragua was planning an invasion with tacit consent from the United States, Guatemala turned to Communist sources for the purchase of arms, touching off decades of covert operations by both the United States and Soviet Union in the region.

Similarly, after Egypt seized the Suez Canal from the British and Israel invaded the Gaza Strip in 1956, the United Nations sent an international force heavily backed by the United States to the region and brokered a cease-fire between Jordan and Israel. The Soviet Union and China declared that the presence of U.S. troops in the area was a violation of the U.N. charter and announced their support of the Middle East "against Western aggression." This added significantly to the tension that was already brewing and that remains unresolved today.

Another example of Cold War antagonism in the 1950s was the Cuban revolution of 1959. Guarding its economic interests, the United States had supported the dictatorship of Fulgencio Batista for 7 years while the Soviet Union supported rebel forces lead by Fidel Castro. Castro's success brought the "Communist threat" very close to U.S. soil and would become the focus of a major crisis in the 1960s.

As previously noted, an important trend in the 1950s was the gaining of independence for many countries once colonized by European nations, especially Great Britain and France. International politics was heavily loaded with the rhetoric of human rights and self-determination. Not all countries were fully successful, however. A prime example of this struggle was South Africa, whose Department of Interior color-classified its residents in 1951 and issued them with cards to prove whether they were White, Black, or Colored in a move to enforce its apartheid policies. In 1953, the South African Parliament gave Prime Minister Daniel F. Malan dictatorial powers to oppose Black and Indian movements, which led to a deeply repressive string of governments that ruled until the 1980s. A similar struggle for civil rights took place in the United States with markedly different results.

In the United States

The "Communist threat" that fueled the Cold War also fueled many trends within the United States during the 1950s. Although both World War II and the Korean War exacted heavy tolls, an economic boom was unfolding, motivated greatly by a national cause to "beat the Communist foe." Nuclear weapons were touted as the ultimate force to protect the nation, and people accepted nuclear tests being conducted on American soil. After the Soviet Union launched the first humanmade satellite, Sputnik I, technological development in the United States increased with a fury. Computers were developed to handle sensitive information at incredible speeds. Technology developed for the military began being applied to civilian industry, and soon most homes had television sets, dishwashers, vacuum cleaners, and myriad other appliances. "National defense" was pursued in education as well, and the government poured millions of dollars into the educational system to strengthen science, mathematics, and foreign language instruction. Roads were built to enhance communication across the country, and the automobile industry boomed. An important goal was to stay ahead of the Soviet Union at all levels.

The fear of the "Communist threat" created a form of collective paranoia in the country. In 1950, Senator Joseph McCarthy of Wisconsin started a Communist "witch hunt" that would last 4 years. His campaign gained momentum in 1951, when Julius and Ethel Rosenberg were executed for transmitting U.S. atomic secrets to the Soviet Union. Anyone with Communist sympathies was suspect, and many people, particularly those in the entertainment industry, were blacklisted and barred from working or entering the country. Finally, in 1954 the Senate censured McCarthy for misconduct after he leveled a vicious charge against an assistant of the lawyer representing the Secretary of the Army, whom McCarthy had accused of concealing evidence.

Although technological advances represented a rise in the American standard of living, Black Americans in the country remained far behind, segregated in education, marginalized from economic advancement, and often barred from voting and other rights. The Ku Klux Klan violently retaliated against any protesters throughout the

South. However, the decade was marked by several victories for the civil rights movement in U.S. courts. For example, in 1954 the U.S. Supreme Court ruled in *Brown v. Board of Education* that racial segregation in public schools was unconstitutional. In 1955, Rosa Parks was arrested for refusing to yield her seat to a White man on a Montgomery, Alabama, bus, triggering a 10-year campaign by Black Americans to end segregation laws. The following year, the Supreme Court outlawed segregation on interstate public transportation. Despite these landmark gains, segregation continued, and across the country the civil rights movement began taking shape. A Black clergyman, the Reverend Martin Luther King, Jr., organized peaceful protests against discrimination, whereas a Muslim leader, Malcolm X, advocated more forceful resistance.

Finally, there were many noteworthy advancements in the area of health care during this decade, particularly in the development and use of medications and in the understanding of diseases. Penicillin began to be widely used, and the polio vaccine was perfected. Dramatic evidence emerged that smoking was hazardous to health, and Prednisone was introduced for the treatment of arthritis and other conditions. Oral contraceptives were developed, although not widely distributed. Researchers began describing the minute components of human genetic makeup. Tranquilizer drugs that eliminated anxiety and excitement without causing drowsiness were developed. The use of Thorazine in the treatment of psychosis was pioneered, and a shift toward community mental health services soon was under way while people left mental institutions.

Although the 1950s were characterized by much growth, the decade was also a time when the gap between rich and poor grew rapidly. By the end of the decade, more than 5 million people were unemployed, and a clear migration toward the suburbs was leaving inner cities in ruins. Use of LSD and other illegal drugs began to be noted as a growing public health concern, particularly in the inner cities.

Even into the 1950s, laws in some states prohibited people "diseased, maimed, mutilated, or in any way deformed so as to be an unsightly or disgusting object" from appearing in public (Flecher & Zames, 2001). However, efforts were made on several fronts to change the lives of people with disabilities. Legislatively, the Social Security Amendments of 1950, precursors of the Social Security Disability Insurance program, established a federal–state program to aid people with permanent and total disabilities. In 1952, President Truman established the President's Committee on Employment of the Physically Handicapped, a permanent organization reporting to the President and Congress. In 1954, Congress passed the Vocational Rehabilitation Amendments to the Social Security Act, which authorized federal grants to expand programs, including university programs, available to people with physical disabilities. Finally, the Social Security Amendments of 1956 (P. L. 84–880) created a Social Security Disability Insurance program for workers with disabilities ages 50 to 64 years. The benefits of this program were later extended in 1958 to dependents of workers with permanent disabilities.

Important service programs for people with disabilities were founded in the 1950s. Howard Rusk, a physician, opened the Institute of Rehabilitation Medicine at New York University Medical Center in 1951. This center, the first of its kind, included people with disabilities on its payroll and was dedicated to the development of technological innovations such as electric typewriters, mouth sticks, improved prosthetics, and other adaptive aids for people with severe disabilities. In 1952, Henry Viscardi, a man with disabilities, took out a personal loan to found Abilities, Inc., in New York, a jobs training and placement program for people with disabilities. At a time when people with disabilities were all but excluded from the workforce, Abilities, Inc., was a revolutionary concept that demonstrated that people with disabilities could—and should—be productive contributors to society. Within a few years, Abilities, Inc., was winning contracts from such defense industry giants as Northrop Grumman, General Electric, and IBM, as well as the U.S. Department of Defense.

The 1950s saw a resurgence of activism on behalf of people with disabilities. For example, in 1950 representatives of various state associations of parents of children with mental retardation established the Association for Retarded Children of the United States (later renamed the Association for Retarded Citizens, and then The Arc) in Minneapolis. In 1957, the first National Wheelchair Games in the United States were held at Adelphi

College, Garden City, New York. That same year, Little People of America was founded in Reno, Nevada, to advocate on behalf of dwarfs or little people. And in 1958, the National Association of the Physically Handicapped, Inc., was formed in Grand Rapids, Michigan. This organization, which remains active, proposes and supports legislation to provide educational and rehabilitation opportunities, tax relief, employment, and other benefits for people with physical disabilities.

Reference

Flecher, D., & Zames, F. (2001). *The disability rights movement: From charity to confrontation.* Philadelphia: Temple University Press.

3

1955 Eleanor Clarke Slagle Lecture

Equipment Designed for Occupational Therapy

Florence M. Stattel, MA, OTR

It is difficult to find words that would adequately express my feelings and appreciation for the honor which you have extended to me in electing me to present the first Eleanor Clarke Slagle lecture. With deep humility and profound professional pride, I thank you for this privilege.

Occupational therapy had its conception in the faith and convictions of our early founders. It developed as a profession because of strong beliefs. Eleanor Clarke Slagle, along with the men and women who shared her convictions, is responsible for our presence here today as the American Occupational Therapy Association. We have been given a wonderful professional heritage of courage and wisdom and as we continue to extend our hand to benefit mankind, may we continue to believe and search for further knowledge.

This knowledge, in our present age, can be secured by correlating and strengthening our beliefs with facts. Empirical methods should be tested when possible, and reasonable doubt should be eliminated. When we consider beliefs we find that they are formations of ideas. Most ideas are really very old. They are rediscovered and formulated and incorporated into one's philosophy and thinking. New ideas are rare, and in a lifetime few individuals are fortunate to accumulate them in even single numbers. In preparing this paper on equipment designed for occupational therapy, it is important to note that the ideas may be old. The newness lies in the formulation of the idea into equipment that has a purposeful use in occupational therapy. The keynote to good design of any type is simplicity that will afford real and effectual usefulness. The refinement of design, structure and engineering aspects of the equipment to be discussed were achieved by close cooperation and consultation with the Franklin Hospital Equipment Company and their staff of technical experts. Three pieces of equipment will be discussed in this paper:

1. Tilt table
2. Standing table
3. Bilateral tilt tables.

The first two pieces of equipment you are no doubt familiar with. The tilt table and the standing table will be discussed briefly in relation to the design which has afforded broader usefulness in occupational therapy. The major portion of the lecture will be devoted to the thinking behind the design and use of the bilateral tilt tables, which are a new treatment concept.

Tilt Table

In recent years we have been increasingly aware of the emphasis which the medical profession has placed on early weight bearing and ambulation. Man's physiological functions improve when he is in an upright position, and

Originally published 1956 in *American Journal of Occupational Therapy, 10,* 194–198.

his mental attitude is often reflected in improved behavior. The physiological and psychological importance of the vertical position is equally important to all patients, ranging from the temporarily disabled to the permanently disabled.

The tilt table is familiar to you. It is a piece of equipment that permits the patient to be gradually elevated to the supported upright position with full weight bearing. Orthopedists have long reported the importance of weight bearing on the long bones of the body to prevent osteoporosis. Neurologists indicate the reinforcement of complex series of reflexes called postural reflexes which control muscle groups so that the upright position can be maintained. Hellebrandt and associates,[1] in 1949, reported on the effects on the cardio-vascular respiratory systems and the action of the heart in preventing gravity shock when subjects were gradually brought from a horizontal to a semi-vertical position. As we go through the list of medical specialists, to name a few, the urologist, plastic surgeon, cardiologist, internist, we find further agreement as to the physiological improvement associated with the upright position.

Prescribed degrees of angulation and time are indicated by the physician in the use of the tilt table. The physical therapist reports

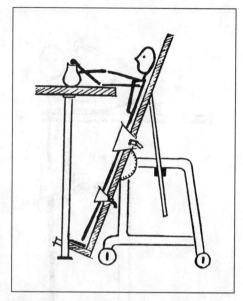

Figure 3.1. Tilt table—secures correct body positioning, frees upper extremities for treatment activities.

increased time and angulation tolerance in the severely involved cases. When the patient has been stabilized at a particular angle and can work in that position using his upper extremities, he can be wheeled on the tilt table into occupational therapy. In cases that are routine, without precautionary factors, the patient can be started on the tilt table for the time prescribed by the physician. The *availability of a tilt table with wheels which incorporates a secure lock device,* and the *attachment of suspension slings,* broadens the uses of this piece of equipment and makes it valuable in occupational therapy.

Many patients who normally would not be referred for early treatment in occupational therapy can be started on programs of early specific exercise and self care. The effect upon the patient when he is employed in an activity instead of being a spectator is instantaneous. To name a few diagnoses which can benefit by the use of the tilt table in occupational therapy: quadriplegics, rheumatoid arthritics, muscular dystrophics, multiple sclerotics and cardiacs.

The tilt table permits the exercise of the upper extremities and the skeletal muscle from the waist up. This increases muscular activity, forces the blood through vertical channels, increases heart rate and metabolic processes. For the severely disabled patient, permanent or progressive, it provides psychological as well as physiological benefits in being changed from the supine to the supported upright position. Occupational therapists have long related the use of the full body support in treatment of children in the vertical position. The idea is not new; however, the design and mobility of the tilt table with its added accessories make it invaluable in broad usefulness in occupational therapy.

Standing Table

The standing table is a natural piece of equipment which follows progressively the use of the tilt table in treatment. This particular standing table was designed to consider the following:

1. Adjustable frontboard which extends from the mid portion of the rib cage to approximately two-thirds of the femur beyond the hip joint. This board acts as a support to the abdominal muscles and diaphragm when the pelvic support is adjusted. In the lower extremities it prevents and corrects flexion contractures due to muscle tightness or spasm;

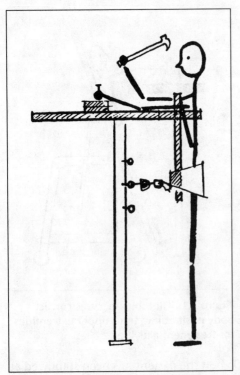

Figure 3.2. Standing table—frontboard, elbow supports and pelvic band aid in body positioning and stability when standing.

2. Adjustable elbow supports are provided for quadriplegic, ataxic and other patients who need support for anterior, posterior and lateral balance. These elbow supports are not for body weight bearing but for shoulder and shoulder girdle support;

3. The table is firmly bolted to the floor or a planked platform and affords structural security for the patient. A height of 46" from the floor is suggested;

4. The pelvic support is a heavy canvas binder with a leather strap end which snaps, with a double and nautical sail buckle, to one of three eyelets on the metal upright of the table. This support tilts and stabilizes the pelvis against the front board. When the feet are spread to provide a broad base, this stabilization provides correct positioning and enables the patient to use his upper extremities freely.

The table has been used successfully with and without pelvic support. When the support is not used, anterior/posterior balance may be the prime objective. When there is a loss of one or more extremities or where a neuromuscular dysfunction exists, balance must be considered in body compensations. Brunnstrom's[2] article on "The Center of Gravity Line in Relation to the Ankle Joint in Erect Standing" is recommended reading on the subject of posture. Occupational therapists should be aware of the body mechanics involved in maintaining the upright position, as the stability or instability influences the usefulness of the upper extremities in purposeful activities in self care and vocational objectives.

Bilateral Tilt Tables

This piece of equipment is new in design and incorporates the use in exercise of unilateral, bilateral, reciprocal and alternate motions and considers the total body concept in treatment.

For centuries man has postulated on the relationship of mind and body, and sought answers in the study of the physical and psychic development of man. An awareness of the natural process of physical and mental growth has resulted in consideration of treatment of the total man rather than in single entities. This is further reflected in the term neuromuscular, which denotes the close integration of neurology and kinesiology. The exercise treatment of the isolated muscle has been challenged repeatedly as a physiological impossibility. More and more attention is being devoted to movements and patterns of movements.

In a new born baby, movements and patterns of movements are exhibited entirely by reflex. Ford[3] states that a number of these motor reactions are present in the first few months when they are not inhibited by cerebral function. When volitional activity develops the reflex reactions are obscured. These reactions may be elicited thereafter only in pathological conditions. The neurologists know that at birth the anatomical development of the nervous system is not complete. In 1950, Gesell[4] reported on "Tonic Neck Reflex and Symmetro-Tonic Behavior." In his comment he states "In spite of his bilateral construction, man does not face the world on a frontal plane of symmetry. He generally confronts it on an angle." He also felt that the tonic neck reflex behavior reflected three important principles of development: principle of developmental direction, principle of functional asymmetry and the principle of reciprocal interweaving. Ontogenous organization does not move along evenly. Periodic fluctuation of dominance takes place.

In the period 1947–1950 and 1951, Hellebrandt and her associates reported on cross education as related to contralateral, homolateral, ipsilateral effects of exercise.[5, 6, 7] Bilateral, unilateral, alternate and reciprocal exercises were studied to observe the functional capacity. The vast amount of work covered in these three papers cannot be condensed and they are references for further thought. For the purposes of this lecture, selected comments are brought in to illustrate the influence this work had on the design of the bilateral tilt tables. The therapeutic use of cross education was indicated and the validity of the single muscle test was questioned when considered as a criterion of functional capacity. In the study of bilateral, unilateral, alternate and reciprocal exercise, the effect of the exercise on the functional capacity of the weakened limb was noted. Contractile power and endurance was reportedly increased. The report of 1951 indicated the lack of justification of limiting treatment to the affected side. Hellebrandt referred to postural reflexes as reported by Magnus and Walshe. Reciprocal and alternate exercise and the influence of facilitating mechanisms were considered. In the subjects used for the study it was noted that some gave up because of psychological and not physiological reasons and the reverse was also true. The body will follow

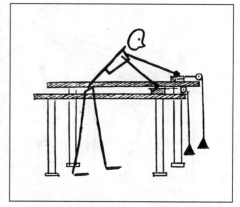

Figure 3.3. Bilateral tilt tables—alternate bilateral exercise, broad base.

the dictates of the mind and the mind will follow the dictates of the body when it is fatigued, but the subject controls both and close observation was made to detect differences. In 1952, Levine and Kabat[8] reported on the "Dynamics of Normal Voluntary Motion in Man." The concept that we must think of movement rather than isolated muscle activity was presented. Interdependence of distantly located muscles was stressed. Significant to the bilateral tilt tables was the report that inherent in all movements is the inclusion of the rotation of the trunk and pelvis. Levine and Kabat discussed the purpose of maximum achievement with importance of proprioception, patterns of movement and cocontractions in voluntary movement in man. Eberhard, Inman and Bresler, 1954,[9] in the study on locomotion, report that muscles do not act in the traditional anatomical sense, they fit into the whole pattern of motion. In walking there is rotation of the trunk and pelvis and independent of this, rotation of the femur and tibia.

The premise for the functional design and use of the bilateral tilt tables evolved from the above readings and clinical observation of patients in occupational therapy and are listed as follows:

1. Reflex patterns of movement that are present at birth and are lost when voluntary activity takes over can be elicited in pathological conditions;
2. Functional asymmetric development is found in man and reciprocal correspondence or interweaving of opposite sides takes place;
3. Contractile power and endurance of muscles could be increased by use of bilateral and unilateral alternate and reciprocal exercise, in prescribed rhythmic beat and maximum resistance;
4. Rotation of the trunk and pelvis are inherent in all movements;
5. In locomotion, muscles tend to fit into the whole pattern of motion rather than function in the traditional anatomical sense.

The tables were constructed to permit adequate space for standing or sitting. The tilt is provided by the telescoping mechanism on the forward portion of the tables which permits an angulation of 45°. A series of 21 adjustments permit the desired range of motion of the extremities from 0° to over 90° starting from the horizontal position. Surface of the table is a plastic non-friction finish. Full width clamps slide together to wedge and hold project or work of the patient. Small end clamps with pulleys permit the occupational therapist to add resistance or assistance in particular movements. Attachments for a belt support are provided on the stable, upright posts. An audiovisual metronome can be used to establish the rate of speed at which the patient can work and to have a check on the amount of exercise accomplished.

The positions of the feet when standing are:

1. Standing, feet close together—small base;
2. Standing, feet spread—broad base;
3. Standing, one foot ahead of other in pace position.

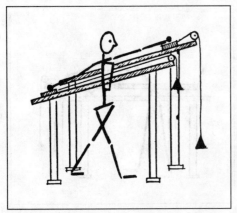

Figure 3.4. Bilateral tilt tables—reciprocal bilateral exercise, pace position.

Exercise patterns of the upper extremities:

1. Unilateral—pertaining to one side;
2. Bilateral—pertaining to both sides;
3. Alternate—complete pattern of movement on one side one or more times; complete pattern of movement on the opposite side, one or more times. Complete pattern of movement on both sides;
4. Reciprocal flow of exercise from one side to another in a continuous pattern of movement. Flow of continuous pattern of movement on one side.

Position of head:

1. Directed toward the involved extremity to reinforce extension pattern;
2. Directed away from the involved extremity to reinforce flexion pattern;
3. Head in mid position.

In occupational therapy many activities are bilateral and unilateral. In the use of these tables, woodworking, weaving and ceramics have been set up in the exercise patterns described above. Finger painting has also worked out successfully. The element of interest which is stimulated by the craft acts as a motivation for the patient to work and achieve and the sometimes inhibiting psychological factor is less apparent.

The audiovisual metronome was mentioned earlier. This instrument provides a sound beat and a simultaneous flash of light. To the patient who has extensive cerebral damage it is advisable to present as many stimuli as possible and this instrument can be used to present this stimulation. The eyes and ears are in this instance reached and the pattern of movement is established along with the stimulus. In all instances it can be used to establish the speed and endurance of a patient to a particular exercise; for example, the patient is set up at the bilateral tilt tables in a selected position, the metronome is set for 40 strokes a minute. If the exercise is unilateral, the 40 strokes would indicate the amount of exercise; if the exercise was bilateral, it would indicate that 20 strokes for each extremity had been accomplished. By setting a timer the occupational therapist could be certain how much the patient had accomplished in exercise at the end of 1, 5 or 10 minutes or more. The metronome can often be used to set the exercise pace and through its use it is possible for the patient to maintain the established rhythm.

In preparing this paper, an attempt has been made to cover a vast amount of material which represents condensed thinking. The bilateral tilt tables and the premise on which they were designed are presented. The piece of equipment now needs testing in clinical application to remove reasonable doubt and provide facts in terms of its usefulness. It also needs further exploration as to its functional value in other than the physical disability field.

Some of the thoughts that were postulated when the bilateral tilt tables were completed, were as follows:

1. *Mentally Ill.* Would the physical approach in calling into action the primitive pattern of movement be beneficial to the mentally ill patient?

   Would the audiovisual metronome assist in establishing early rhythmic patterns of movement in craft activities with varied tempo and duration?

2. *Cardiac, Tuberculosis.* Can improved work classifications result in timed, specific work output under supervision of the occupational therapist?

   Could vital capacity be improved through prescribed, closely observed, selected activities which would be closely timed and amount of exercise recorded?

3. *Prevocational Exploration.* Should testing be done in patterns of movements?

   Would it be possible to test motor fatigue and gauge sensory fatigue?

   Would minimum effort and maximum achievement result in analyzing patterns of movements in job demands?

As each selected field of occupational therapy seeks to improve its clinical application, it is earnestly hoped that more questions will be the result. Study of the vast amount of material that is available in the medical field will result in research that will bring answers and improved treatment techniques in occupational therapy. Our educational backgrounds provide us with a basic philosophy along with knowledge and skill to carry it out. Some occupational therapists have selected the psychiatric field, others the tuberculosis field and so on down the list of specialties. Their efforts in selected fields have increased their knowledge and skill in that field. However, it must be remembered that any knowledge or information in any specialty field is related to helping the human being. Our basic philosophy in occupational therapy embraces in treatment the physical and emotional makeup of the total person. With this thought in mind we are all occupational therapists first, reduced from our specialties by the common denominator, the human being who needs our help.

Early in this paper the beliefs of the pioneers in our profession were mentioned. Our profession is a stimulating and deeply satisfying one, which has grown because of our individual and united beliefs. It is sincerely hoped that this lecture will stimulate broad thinking and that indications of individual and group studies of professional importance will develop; that the growth of a national research laboratory in occupational therapy will result as in individual instances and as an organization, we continue to extend our hand to benefit mankind as we search for knowledge.

References

1. Hellebrandt, F. A. and associates. "The Relative Importance of the Muscle Pump in the Prevention of Gravity Shock," *The Physical Therapy Review,* 29:1 (Jan.), 1949.
2. Brunnstrom, Signe. "The Center of Gravity Line in Relation to the Ankle Joint in Erect Standing," *The Physical Therapy Review,* 34:3 (March), 1954.
3. Ford, Frank R., M.D. *Diseases of the Nervous System in Infancy, Childhood and Adolescence,* Springfield, Ill.: Charles Thomas, 1952.
4. Gesell, Arnold, M.D., Ames, Louise, Ph.D. "Tonic Neck Reflex and Symmetro-Tonic Behavior," *The Journal of Pediatrics,* 36:2 (Feb.), 1950.
5. Hellebrandt, F. A., M.D., Parrish, Annie M., Houtz, Sara Jane. "The Influence of Unilateral Exercise on the Contralateral Limb," *Archives of Physical Medicine,* 28 (Feb.), 1947.
6. Hellebrandt, F. A., M.D., Houtz, Sara Jane. "Influence of Bimanual Exercise on Unilateral Work Capacity," *Journal of Applied Physiology,* 2:8 (Feb.), 1950.
7. Hellebrandt, F. A., M.D. "Ipsilateral and Contralateral Effects of Unimanual Training," *Journal of Applied Physiology,* 4:2 (Aug.), 1951.
8. Levine, Milton G., Ph.D., Kabat, Herman, M.D. "Dynamics of Normal Voluntary Motion in Man," *Permante Foundation Medical Bulletin,* 10 (Aug.), pp. 1–4, 1952.
9. Klopsteg, Paul E., Ph.D., Wilson, Philip D., M.D., *Human Limbs and Their Substitutes,* New York: McGraw-Hill Company, Inc., 1954, Chapt. 15, p. 437.

Bibliography

Floyd, W. F., Welford, A. T. *Human Factors in Equipment Design.* London: H. K. Lewis and Co., Ltd., 1953.

Floyd, W. F., Welford, A. T. *Fatigue.* London: H. K. Lewis and Co., Ltd., 1953.

Levens, A. S., Inman, V. T., and Blosser, J. A. "Transverse Rotation of the Segments of the Lower Extremity in Locomotion," *Journal of Bone and Joint Surgery,* 30A:859, 1948.

Magnus, R. *Korperstellung.* Berlin: Julius Springer, 1924 (Sectional translation by Signe Brunnstrom).

4

1956 Eleanor Clarke Slagle Lecture

Therapist Into Administrator:
Ten Inspiring Years

June Sokolov, OTR

Foreword

To my peers and colleagues: You have seen fit to confer upon me a high award, the symbol of your respect and affection. I have been awed by this honor. I spent many hours deliberating a fitting subject for my discourse with you today and settled finally, not without some misgiving, upon the core of those philosophical beliefs which have been tempered during the past ten rewarding years of practice as a therapist and administrator. I am not an innovator; what I say here is far from new. I would only have you know that what I humbly share with you is representative of the deepest convictions I hold as a therapist, as an administrator, as a human being.

Therapist Into Administrator:
Ten Tempering Years

Some ten years ago the writer sat in a classroom attempting to assimilate and commit to indelible memory an impossible array of facts about the practice of occupational therapy. We were being prepared, in time-honored fashion, for the registration examination. From today's vantage point it is difficult to refrain from comparing that process with those rituals which accompany tribal customs. Certainly we resembled the uninitiated in all respects too closely for the comfort of either teachers or pupils.

Today, undeniably older if questionably better informed as a result of exposure to practical considerations, it is possible to recognize with some degree of equanimity that the makers of that first registration examination undoubtedly faced its trial run with something of the same apprehension that dogged the students who were soon to provide the test of its validity. However, ten years ago, such reasoning was at least temporarily denied to me. I could sense only considerable foreboding, reproach myself for my lack of faith in teachers and God and return to the fine print of the almighty text books there to search unremittingly for the meanings to puzzles which persisted in eluding me. What accounted for the sudden and bewildering synergistic action of a muscle which, up to a point, had behaved in calculable fashion as a prime mover? What nature of chemical compound was known to remove printer's ink from some spot where it had no official business? (And, wouldn't it be more efficacious in this instance to remove one's offending self from the premises as rapidly as possible?) What precautions did one observe with a sixty-five year old hemiplegic complicated by total aphasia, cardiac insufficiency and diabetes mellitus? Or, more to the point, what kind of occupational therapy program did one offer because, of course, there had to be one. This major faith, at least, in the unlimited scope and authority of one's chosen profession was unshakable.

Originally published 1957 in *American Journal of Occupational Therapy, 11*, 13–19.

So we pondered the technicalities of our profession, secure only in the one, irrefutable fact that all this was worthwhile and even possible because it would eventually permit us to realize our common aim of helping people to help themselves. What a rude surprise then, as we sat in that relatively peaceful classroom, to be singled out for the prediction that within three years' time I should have left the practice of occupational therapy for the province of administration. Impossible! Cold, forbidding word and world of topside decision and responsibility, devoid of all patient—nay, all human contact. How could one help but react with immediate rejection of such a fate? This could not happen to me. I wanted nothing to do with boards and committees, community action, finances, services and all the rigamarole of executive responsibility. I wanted to work with people. (Heaven forgive me and ascribe to the naivete of youth my repudiation of communities and their citizenry as something other than people. For among these were later to be found the generous affirmation of a personal faith.)

I have wondered since how many young people draw the same faulty inference. And, if they do, may our incorrect assumptions be traced to certain common administrative practices we meet as we move toward maturity and responsibility, as well as to our human way of prejudicing a situation by seeing it in the narrow framework of imperfect knowledge rather than against the unlimited horizon we can flush with a little vision.

The predictions of our teacher were painfully accurate. Were I not so well acquainted with her discerning and judicious approach to life, I might well have suspected her of consulting a crystal ball or dabbling in extra-sensory perception. Almost three years to the day after taking up my duties as an occupational therapist, I found myself involved in administrative functions and by the time five additional years had elapsed, this had become the provocative and rewarding substance of my working existence.

I have no inclination here to propound the role of the administrator in scholarly or detailed fashion. The accepted texts devoted to this subject are adequate if not overwhelming. It shall be my pleasure (and yours, I hope) to dwell for a while on the art of administration which is essentially an art of working with people to encourage and assure those personal and group satisfactions which tend to result in affirmative, effective performance.

The great American myth of the push-button executive to the contrary, executives in social agencies, at any rate, must work chiefly with and through people. Some measure of their success may be noted in the degree to which this capacity for working through the medium of people bears fruit in the improved and even inspired performance of staff and the consequent greater good that accrues to those served. Obviously, we subscribe to a definition of success which pivots upon the quality of our human relationships. We are not primarily concerned with the size and scope of endeavors, the number and variety of personnel, the roster of services, the soaring annual budget, indicative as these may be of growth and development. Such attributes seem to be all too easily come by in an era of prosperity when rehabilitation of the ill and injured receives almost as much daily attention from the press as the political scene receives in an election year. The trick becomes how to avoid a mushrooming growth and hold to a realistic operation, a qualitative service, to moderate change that suits the circumstances and is not dictated by the artificial stimulus of a current trend.

What, then, are some of the values one perceives, infers and confirms in the process of working with and through people to achieve group goals?

If one tends to be inherently a "doer," a prime but difficult lesson to master and practice is the restraint and rechanneling of energies. The goal changes from personal performance to eliciting increased assumption of responsibility from others. For many people (therapists not excepted) doing comes easier than talking about it. In consequence, we may resort to showing or performing rather than sketching in a backdrop or opening a door, as it were. As has been said, a good teacher is one who leads the pupil to the threshold of his own mind and bids him enter. While more difficult to achieve, this is the procedure of choice and tends to ensure more lasting satisfactions and greater gains in personal stature.

In any case, the pangs of relinquishing proof of personal competence are lessened at the earliest observation of staff satisfactions. And these staff satisfactions are the natural corollary of expanded horizons and the chance to come to grips with new and more challenging responsibilities. The first time one is suffused in a glow of pure pleasure because a staff member has ventured into new and untried territory to emerge either bruised and questioning or victorious and wiser, becomes the memorable date of a new romance with the art of administration. This is the moment when one feels the bite of conviction and knows where the greatest rewards will henceforth lie.

We hear frequently that young people of today do not crave responsibility—that they seek freedom from the burden of responsible choice and decision. As always, one does well to be chary of such generalizations. In those rare cases where the glove fits, we should perhaps be quicker to recognize true personality disturbances instead of chalking the response up as yet another "sign of the times." In our admittedly limited experience, an atmosphere in which the premium is placed on achieving personal satisfaction through exploring, investigating, making mistakes, finding out why, pooling group thinking and reaching out constantly to new accomplishment in the name of commonly cherished ideals, exerts the irresistible tug of a strong current and carries the worker with it magnetically. There is no substitute for the exercise of reason and self-trust and the reward thereof is constant. Given the basic aim of wanting to help people help themselves, human beings tend to gravitate toward those ways of life which promise to transform their intangible aims into realities. The administrator is on the scene to provide this opportunity, to set the stage for personal growth and to allow the accomplishment of group and agency objectives. How does he go about his role of catalyst?

One significant contribution he can make is to free the work atmosphere of irritating fears and tensions. We readily acknowledge that no one works successfully or happily in an atmosphere charged with constant anxiety or apprehension. Yet the evidences of such circumstances are legion. The writer has frequently been called on to define and analyze the reasons for ineffectual performance and poor standards of work, only to find that something akin to staff demoralization exists which freezes into immobility every healthy human and professional impulse. A change of leadership is contemplated, staff cutbacks are being considered, financial problems loom, a new order is in the making but no one has thought it necessary or fitting to discuss these crucial problems with the people intimately concerned. An undertow of panic results.

Let us illustrate the administrative function in such a situation. A new worker has been added to a well-integrated and functioning staff. This worker has left a secure position in the highly organized and orthodox field of education to seek new opportunities and horizons in the field of rehabilitation. He represents an unexplored aspect of service in the agency and brings with him a host of techniques, talents, beliefs, practices and prejudices which are new to the staff. He brings with him, also, a natural concern about the merits of his decision which was perhaps arrived at somewhat rapidly. It seemed like a good idea at the time. After a few days in a totally new environment and some encounters with unfamiliar practices, he's not so sure. During the orientation to the agency's services and the people behind them, it becomes fairly obvious that he is unable to listen, absorb, assimilate. He appears preoccupied, concerned with other things. He catches at details and misses concepts—sees the grain of sand but not the world mirrored therein. These symptoms readily communicate themselves to other staff members. Mental images are stored, calculations and reservations are made. It is time for administration to intervene in an attempt to rectify the situation before the staff begins to reflect an established group attitude which is apt to anchor these early responses. Informal conferences with the worker are aimed at clearing the air. These are not effective. The administrator takes another avenue. He consults with supervisory staff (department heads) about the problem. The possible and probable causes of the worker's reactions are weighed and considered and a potentially influential group attitude is forged. The staff concludes that the new worker deserves all the help they can muster to convert his energies and will to the job at hand. They agree that his unease is, undoubtedly, temporary. To a man, they go forth determined to offer extra assistance, encouragement and support to help channel responses and criticisms to appropriate sources for consideration. Within a very brief period results may be measured in the new staff member's relaxed manner, receptiveness to suggestion and participation in group thinking and planning. After a month or two, he is working with obvious satisfaction and making a substantial contribution to the agency's objectives in terms of his personal endowment. A group of people who have worked toward and achieved a common set of goals have succeeded in communicating their good-will, enthusiasm and positive experience to another human being.

The link is forged into the chain. Administration has helped to refocus group energies on meeting client needs. Similar examples abound. Every department, every agency is the scene of innumerable tensions, group and personal. They are a part of the fabric of existence and no more to be frowned upon than the rind we discard with the eating of an orange. But they must be recognized and evaluated for potential damage. Sensitivity to impressions, recognition of a disturbed environment, proper timing, analysis of the problem and bringing to bear upon it the powerful antidote of group acceptance are implicit in the administrative function.

The cultivation of impressions or intuitions is worth a moment's digression. While we may not rely indiscriminately upon a single impression, many such perceptions constitute the genesis of all ideas, the basis for achievement. Henry James has summed this up exquisitely in *The Art of Fiction and Other Essays*.[1] He discusses the business of writing from experience and says, "Experience is never complete; it is an immense sensibility, a kind of huge spiderweb of the finest silken threads suspended in the chamber of consciousness and catching every airborne particle in its tissue. It is the very atmosphere of the mind; and when the mind is imaginative—much more when it happens to be that of a man of genius—it takes to itself the faintest hints of life, it converts the very pulses of the air into revelations. The power to guess the unseen from the seen, to trace the implications of things, to judge the whole piece by the pattern, the condition of feeling life in general so completely that you are well on your way to knowing any particular corner of it—this cluster of gifts may almost be said to constitute experience . . . . If experience consists of impressions, it may be said that impressions are experience, just as they are the very air we breathe . . . ." And he goes on to admonish "Try to be one of the people on whom nothing is lost."[1]

One of the major fears which confront occupational therapists as administrators is an expressed or implied fear about the value of occupational therapy itself. Like most fears, this one if suspected must be taken out and viewed in that strong daylight which does so much to dispel shadows and reduce problems to size. Conversely, when it has been examined and analyzed for the benefit of all concerned, doubt and distrust should be dispersed by the active, intensive and changing practice of our profession. The Overstreets speak convincingly of learning to call an episode finished when it is over with, and label this "the art of rescuing the present and the future from the tyranny of the past."[2] If occupational therapists persist in some of the breast-beating and loud self-recrimination which have attended us too regularly in the past eight to ten years, we cannot expect the world to look upon us with either respect or trust. No one denies that we must examine the reasons which invest our practices. We might, however, do well to remember that T. V. Smith, the eminent philosopher, upon his retirement thanked God publicly for the right of old age to "withstand all easy commitment." "All my life," says Mr. Smith, "I have been abashed at having to decide things in the name of reason for which there were no adequate reasons. I know there were not, because equally reasonable men are always deciding such things differently. And the more important the issues, the more differently they get decided. . . . Indeed, I myself incline to the view . . . that there are never adequate reasons for doing anything."[3]

All of us have heard and perhaps uttered the cry of frailty: occupational therapy will not live to see another decade if it is not perfected as a science; if we do not recruit more therapists; if we do not settle the problem of unregistered personnel. All these qualifications are dependent on which crisis looms largest in the group addressing itself to the problem of our future. These are problems we must deal with, yes, but they do not constitute a final threat to the life and vitality of occupational therapy any more than the rising cancer rate threatens the life or continuous practice of medicine or the hazards of the road threaten the use of the automobile. The seriously debilitating factor is our own lack of faith and conviction about what occupational therapy has to offer the patient. Nothing will erase this basic fault except the cultivation and practice of a genuine belief and its substantiation in the daily revelation of efficacy.

A good deal of our discomfort and uneasiness may stem from the fact that we, along with other disciplines, are living through an attempt at conversion to a more exact science. This is a painful process at best and can be devastating to a profession burdened with amorphous beginnings which lend themselves all too easily, in the hands of the unselective, to branding occupational therapists with currently unacceptable labels, such as "do-gooders."

Daily we are impressed with the revival of interest in religion, the revanescence of handcrafts, the renewed emphasis on a liberal arts education. All about us are signs of the swing of the pendulum from crass materialism to a renewed acknowledgment of man's continuing need for human kindness and compassion, for individual creative effort. What could be more reassuring to people engaged in the practice of healing through doing?

With an apology to our psychiatric colleagues who, I suspect, have always known and held to this conviction, it behooves us to emphasize and underscore the significance of effective human relationships implicit in the practice of occupational therapy whether we are talking to a physiatrist or a psychiatrist. Regardless of our tools, it is primarily by virtue of our interest, enthusiasm and concern that we shall bridge the chasm of illness to draw the patient back into the mainstream of active participation which signifies the return to life and hope.

This is in no sense a repudiation of the effort to improve our practices, sharpen our professional tools, better our methods of work. It is dictated by a deep-seated belief that the medium we use is always secondary to the motives and drives which direct our actions.

The administrator becomes an important avenue for the unequivocal voicing of such sentiments since his attitudes and beliefs will unfailingly be sensed and transmitted to the staff. His is the job, then, of conditioning the atmosphere so that unspoken fears may be voiced, group attitudes reshaped and fused, healing action taken to correct the profound debilitation caused by irritating doubt.

Patient evaluation sessions, used as a teaching device, may provide a useful vehicle for crystallizing group attitudes about occupational therapy. It is more than a passing impression that, given the opportunity to comment on the function of occupational therapy, the therapist too often remains passive and silent only to fester later under an impossible assignment doled out by the attending physician. Administration has a responsibility for overcoming such deadlocks. A leading question directed to the physician, the therapist or both, may instigate the conversational give and take that is essential to the forging of individual ideas, the art of selling them to others, the grace of retreating with good countenance and heart when fairly defeated and the satisfaction of having actively contributed to decisions about the purpose and function of one's own métier. The old, if somewhat impertinent, remark about "put up or shut up" has its merits applied to this situation. Staff members must learn to charge, parry, thrust, defend or retreat in the intellectual arena much as they have previously learned the rules of the game in the sports arena.

Clearing the air of basic fears about the value of occupational therapy is an on-going process. Self-recrimination should give way to the more purposeful activity of meeting problems as they arise for these are the stuff of life and ours the incomparable privilege of rising to their eternal challenge.

The art of administration supposes, also, acknowledgement and cultivation of an atmosphere in which a premium is placed on the making of courageous errors. We do well to recall often the sense of peace and freedom to be found in reviewing our identification with the family of man, that curious groper after knowledge, that colossal maker of mistakes. How comforting to know that one is entitled to try and fail, that it is upon this shifting foundation that all human advances are achieved. From *The Mind Goes Forth*, we take heart in the following quotation: "The deeply civil person knows life as imperfect, flawed, limited, self-contradictory; as unfinished; often immature, raw on the edges, unfulfilled; but as remarkable in fact and possibility and as structured for growth. With all these aspects the truly civil person feels at home."[2]

Administration generally has responsibility for inaugurating teaching programs. The example set by first-class hospitals leaves little doubt that clinical teaching enriches and improves services rendered to the client. The new knowledge, the fresh perspective, the spirit of inquiry the student brings with him illuminate the scene and stimulate the staff to their best creative effort. To the degree that all experience is grist to the human mill, we may assume the student also profits. In attempting to qualify the returns to the student over a period of years, certain basic ingredients of a teaching program parade before us for review.

Young people often come to us hemmed in by the safe margins of the knowledge they have assimilated well. They will not readily push these margins out unless we commend the pioneering spirit and, indeed, breast the frontiers ourselves. This should not be promptly equated in the listener's mind with study and research, applicable though they be. It is much more an attitude, a state of mind which invests our every action, from shifting a schedule to tossing out a traditional method for some new system. It is, we believe, a refreshing jolt for the new student who arrives on the scene primed for performance (with the mental image of the rating scale never far away) to be assured that he will be rewarded for imagination and invention, that his supervisor will cherish trial and error rather than past performance according to text book specifications.

Gradually, we have had the temerity to question the fine line drawn between the status and responsibility accorded the student and the therapist. It seems to us that this is a chimera which cannot be perpetuated if we hope to give to student and patient that sense of security and authority which are prerequisite to a positive relationship. In seeking to create for the student a level somewhat below that of staff prestige, yet to demand from him those things expected of a staff member (with the possible exception of ultimate responsibility to administration), we seem to be pursuing an unrealistic, if not unattainable objective. In good government we underwrite responsibility with authority. The student in training is anywhere from one to nine months short of his first job. Overnight, he will be expected to drop the pose of subservience and assume the mantle of adulthood. Since few of us are quick-change artists when it comes to personal development, the outcome of such a system will generally be an additional year of growing into responsible performance. Yet the current situation demands prompt assumption of leadership and mature judgment from the new therapist. This is often deplored but I suspect it is something we might cease to deprecate. In many of the established giant businesses of today this golden option for personal responsibility has been severely curtailed. Thousands of young clerks and typists seem never to move beyond the immediate assigned task, be it filing the card meticulously under "C" or typing the letter neatly and accurately. The card may bear information of keen significance to the boss and the letter may read like gibberish but there will too seldom be an attempt to check on the information or to read the letter for sense. This is not necessarily the sign of a dull mind but rather of a dependent one which has been denied the God-given opportunity of thinking for itself, of questioning, of investigating even at the risk of appearing foolish.

To a degree our schools perpetuate this state of dependency. We still persist in spoon-feeding substance to students, examining them regularly and all but lifting them through the business of learning with methods and devices as adroit as they are stultifying. We forget or overlook the fact that education in its deepest sense is "lifelong discipline of the individual by himself."[4] We assume self-discipline will set in, like grey hair, after the student is on the job.

If the therapist–administrator seeks to engender a dynamic and rewarding teaching program he will do well to examine this dichotomy and establish the student as a full-grown person of whom is expected the creative effort, natural error, renewed curiosity and growing capacity for responsibility which we associate, whether rightly or wrongly, with the finished therapist. In place of the smothering pat of authoritative approval, we may substitute the listening ear—the sounding board against which the student may try the "ping" of his ideas. While this may play some havoc with established efficiency, it will assuredly contribute to personal and professional growth.

We are reminded of an episode which may illumine these abstractions. A student was treating an emotionally labile hemiplegic woman of middle age. The physician in charge was carried away with the importance of self-care for this patient and somewhat arbitrarily emphasized this in his prescription to the exclusion of other activities. In the manner of many busy doctors, he had found little time to examine the background of the case which indicated a long career of drudgery interrupted for the first time in many years by the respite of illness. The student was vaguely aware of this implicit contradiction but failed (in traditional fashion) to verbalize it to the doctor. Instead, she proceeded to carry out the orders to the letter. The patient broke down and sobbed uncontrollably on the day she was first able to master her shoelaces alone. The student, shocked, discussed the situation with a therapist who, neither condemning nor approving, helped the student to voice her desire to try a less orthodox approach. Utilizing a spark of interest the patient had revealed for drawing and painting as a stimulus to other activities, the student encountered some success. She was asked to present the results to the physician, who, in the face of the evidence and the student's new-found assurance, was moved to adjust his recommendations. Much was learned; a small world was conquered. Had the therapist, at the outset, issued warnings about deviating from the prescription, we might have succeeded solely in perpetuating a blind and mulish adherence to rule.

Physicians who enjoy the practice of medicine as art and science, rather than the artificial prerogatives bestowed by overawed humanity, tell us that they are neither qualified nor interested in planning discrete occupational therapy programs. They alone can and will set the guidelines for us, indicating the pitfalls and dangers inherent in treatment. We must heed this advice and also the ring of inner conviction which tells us that we alone can create, devise and adjust the program of therapeutic work which is our contribution to the healing process.

The cult of objectivity in human relationships has occasioned a good deal of fanfare in our teaching and clinical training settings. Random observations in our own field and allied situations moved us to examine this precept and to cast our vote with those who believe it is neither possible nor desirable to establish antiseptic relationships with people, to divest our relationships of some degree of emotionality. Undoubtedly some of the existing confusion we experience here rests upon problems of semantics. The word "emotional" is often viewed in the narrow sense of uncontained feeling. It appears to the writer that what we bring to patient or staff relationships rests largely upon our ability to manifest a warm interest in individuals as people. An axiom of our profession is the importance of our approach to people. Just what do we mean by this? Is it a kind of come-on that we hold out as bait until the fish is hooked, then to withdraw rapidly into our shell of cool aloofness? Or does it mean that we are able to convey to people at all moments of our relationship that they are important and valuable to us, that we have an investment in their future, that we care considerably what happens to them. If we accept the evidence that what we do and say often influences even momentary or fleeting relationships, how much more obvious is this potential in daily association? As members of the genus *homo sapiens* we all move in a constant search for understanding. As human beings we are not constituted to live together without involvement. We have learned that events across the span of oceans and continents affect us, that we are in more than an abstract sense our brothers' keepers. This is no less true of our more intimate associations with patients and colleagues. To the degree that these feelings are neither unrecognized nor unmanageable, they are, we submit, the most powerful tool we have for evoking response and encouraging movement forward. And, if we should err, let us remember that we were not meant to be omnipotent. People will forgive us the errors made in the name of earnest belief more readily than the achievements which result from calculated planning. We should differentiate this kind of response to others from the casual benevolence that rests upon familiarity with the size and fortunes of Joe Doake's family as the base of association. The kind of interest we propose as a part of the administrative armamentarium is an enlightened concern with personal growth and achievement.

In this role of helping people to achieve commonly held objectives, nothing is more rewarding than our deepening awareness of human strength and frailty. One learns to hold aloft the ideal, to expect from people the most and the best of which they are capable yet to respect human frailty and hence to treasure the least of the offerings. As the staff family grows from a few people who have learned to harmonize "exceeding sweet" to a whole chorus which is more apt to give out with a sour note from time to time, there is, for the administrator, the endless fascination of reading an increasingly complex score. The bass are the conservative element, holding the line, providing the foundation; the tenors are the mercurial element, given to temperamental sallies and sudden bursts of melody; the contraltos are the mediators creating a blending of voices; the sopranos carry the design ever onward. All have their inalienable place and the whole is the less for any loss or absence.

The importance of expecting the best from people is illustrated by the remarks of a famous dancer who, as she exhorted young and very green converts to attempt greater feats, pointed out that few of us know even the inside limits of our endurance, nor do we take the time or trouble to find this out except when life itself calls the turn. I remember that we students had been complaining that we could not run any longer. The artist dared us to test this statement. She suggested that we run until we dropped of breathlessness or a stitch-in-the-side. Some of us took the dare and learned, in the process, an illuminating lesson about the depth of our endurance and physical powers.

This can be translated into mental efforts. People may gripe and complain about being stimulated and provoked to new and greater efforts but, in our humble opinion, they respond to challenge as the hound to the hare. This is no more nor less than a reflection of man's eternal striving after perfection. Attainment may, indeed must, in many instances fall far short of the goal. This is secondary. It is the reaching that counts; not the thing we grasp. The sense of joy and accomplishment, of participation, are to be found on the march. The goal, achieved, has already altered and is elusively beyond us again.

Another lesson to be mastered in this complex and provocative business of working with people is the sharpening and refinement of the sense of timing. How easily one loses the golden opportunity to communicate an idea or advance a plan when the time is either too soon or too late. We might speculate lengthily that timing is the essence of success in all things great and small. Certainly it has a place in successful administration. The atmosphere of a staff or board meeting, the readiness of people for a concept or plan, the degree of skepticism, the point at which this turns to argument, the introduction of personal motives and consequent loss of focus on the objective, all these are as significant to the development of the administrative sense as the scent of smoke on the air is to a present danger for animals of the forest. Reactions like these are not to be overlooked in the ardor of one's own beliefs. Personal conviction and zeal spice an offering but they must be preserved within the framework of group readiness much as a treble phrase plays a counterpoint against a holding base.

While the sense of timing can be enhanced with experience, it has in common with all true things an intuitive basis. We say of the gifted politician that he can sense the mood or will of the people, and uses this to introduce advanced ideas and doctrines. This is equally applicable to the administrator who, seeking to inaugurate a new policy with staff or board, must consider group structure, mood and will. Long ago Shakespeare immortalized this idea when he said, "There is a tide in the affairs of men which, taken at flood, leads on to fortune . . . ."

By way of example, a staff may resist the introduction of a timesaving procedure for the exchange of routine information. They are unmoved by the suggestion that such measures will reduce the burden of frustration upon individuals. The matter is discussed and, wisely, tabled for the present. Soon the moment for which our administrator has been waiting arrives. Several staff members register complaints about the lag in communication. While this irritation is prominent the staff is convened to hear an expression of the problem by its own members. Together the group seeks an answer and happens, magically, upon the plan originally proposed by administration. The time is right; the goal is realized. Astute members of the group recognize some semblance of coincidence, to others this is not yet revealed. This is unimportant. With faithful practice, everyone is eventually in on the secret and common obstacles may be hurdled with the speed and co-ordination that endow the polished athlete.

The tempering years have sustained our conviction that the goal of harmonious group performance, per se, is a false idol. One insurgent and gifted human being is worth twenty robots who have been chastened into the uncomplaining performance of assigned tasks. New ideas, new people, new projects may threaten to disrupt equilibrium, upset patterns, create temporary dissensions. Do we decide for or against their injection into our midst?

Some of our social scientists have been preaching that "the whole is greater than its parts, that the system has a wisdom beyond the reach of ordinary mortals." William H. Whyte, Jr., writes tellingly of this quandary in *Is Anybody Listening.*[5] Says Mr. Whyte, "The individual can be greater than the group and his lone imagination worth a thousand graphs and studies. He is not often a creator, but even as spectator, as the common man, he can rise in ways his past performance would not predict. To aim at his common denominators in the name of ultimate democracy is to despise him, to perpetuate his mediocrities and to conceive him incapable of responding to anything better than the echo of his prejudices. . . . It is not in the nature of social engineering to be creative; it must necessarily be based on what is already existent. It can measure what is or what was . . . . It cannot dream or conjure; it cannot find out from people whether they would like something new, something untried, because people cannot judge what they do not know. And they will not know until someone is damn fool enough to stick his neck out and have faith in his intuition, his perception and his hunches."

There is room for rugged individualism within the staff framework; room for these insurgents, these uncommon men and women to make their contribution to the patient and the agency and to claim in return the honest respect of other personnel. To the administrator falls the challenging job of placing such people in optimum positions to insure their productiveness, of providing the environment which will foster their creative effort.

The incomparable privilege of working with people, lay and professional, leads inevitably to a reaffirmation of principles expounded by great men in every era. Man hungers after beauty, goodness and truth. He seeks to experience life first-hand and in so doing develops a personal independence and esteem which sustain him through trial and tribulation. He seeks also to identify with mankind, to give and receive warmth, affection and love. He is a problem-solver and so dispels, inch by painstaking inch, the fears which beset his way. He responds to the challenge of perfection yet craves acceptance of his frailty. Although actually he may present a less than admirable figure, he is potentially superb. The practice of administration, like the practice of occupational therapy, is another way of recognizing these truths.

References

1. James, Henry. *The Art of Fiction and Other Essays.* New York: Oxford University Press, 1948.
2. Overstreet, Harry and Bonaro. *The Mind Goes Forth.* New York: W. W. Norton and Company, Inc., 1956.
3. Smith, T. V. "The Leisure of the Theory Class," *The Saturday Review,* August 25, 1956.
4. Barzun, Jacques. *Teacher in America.* Garden City, New York: Doubleday Publishers, 1954.
5. Whyte, William H., Jr. *Is Anybody Listening.* New York: Simon and Schuster, Inc., 1952.

Powerful Levers
In Little Common Things

Ruth W. Brunyate, OTR

Preface

Madam president, occupational therapists and guests. It is with great pride, an overwhelming sense of inadequacy and profound humility that I accept the award you have conferred upon me. It is strange how small one feels in perhaps his biggest hour.

Worthiness for such an honor is never singly earned. An occupational therapist is, after all, merely a tool through which the doctor treats his patient. The value of the therapist can be judged only on the soundness of his contribution to treatment—for this is the culmination of his professional training. The therapist who participates in the administrative phases of a treatment program is again a tool through which the patient receives his treatment. The value of an administrative therapist can be judged only by the extent to which he is able to mold professional knowledge with sound business practice in such a way as to hold the patient in true perspective—for this is the culmination of his nonprofessional training.

These values are learned through formal education and experience but above all through the inspiration of others. I would, therefore, acknowledge the three people beyond my own family who have most affected the development of my abilities: Miss Helen S. Willard, Doctor Winthrop M. Phelps and Mr. Christopher H. Wiemer. Under Miss Willard's guidance I developed my philosophy of occupational therapy and my faith in my profession. Under Dr. Phelps' leadership I have developed my philosophy and techniques of treatment of the cerebral palsied and a concept of education as a continuing process based on simplicity, honesty, patience and diligence in the approach to complex problems. Under Mr. Wiemer's counsel I am beginning to learn the value of the individual in the ordered structure of the treatment unit, and a faith in oneself to see that value, to nurture it and direct it.

You have given me a very beautiful gift which I shall always treasure. I thank you each individually and pray that the hours of deliberation and the final thoughts presented here may be worthy of your trust.

Foreword

Forty years ago, on September 3, 1917, the first annual meeting of the National Society for the Promotion of Occupational Therapy was held in New York City. The meeting was called to order by the vice-president, Mrs. Eleanor Clarke Slagle. Who was this woman leading a pioneer group dedicated to a new profession? Occupational therapists who were active prior to 1942 had the privilege of knowing her. Some had met her, others knew her intimately. But for those who knew her not at all we would like to review her life, that each may understand why an award has been established to perpetuate her memory and why we value our Slagle heritage.

Originally published 1958 in *American Journal of Occupational Therapy, 12,* 193–202.

Eleanor Clarke Slagle was born just eighty-one years ago this October 13th in Hobart, New York.[1] Her brother was one day to become a prominent United States Senator from their native state. Mrs. Slagle was educated by tutors, then attended Claverack College, summer school of Columbia University and graduated from the Chicago School of Civics and Philanthropy. Here, as early as 1908, and largely through the inspiration of Julia Lathrop and Rabbi Harris, a course in invalid occupation was offered to attendants and nurses from hospitals for the insane. Dr. Adolf Meyer, professor of psychiatry at Johns Hopkins Hospital, gave continued advice and encouragement to the course.

In 1913, when the Henry Phipps Psychiatric Clinic of the Johns Hopkins Hospital was opened, Mrs. Slagle became the director of occupational therapy. This position she continued to hold until 1917 when she became director of the Henry B. Favill Memorial School in Chicago. She returned to New York in 1922 to become director of occupational therapy of the New York State Hospital Service to which she devoted her energies until her death.

In March of 1917 at Consolation House, Clifton Springs, New York, the National Society for the Promotion of Occupational Therapy, forerunner of the American Occupational Therapy Association, was founded. Incorporation papers were drawn and later signed by five people, two of whom, Dr. Dunton and Mrs. Slagle, are familiar to even the youngest of our present members. Mrs. Slagle became vice-president in 1919, president in 1920 and was secretary-treasurer from 1922 to 1937.

When she resigned in 1937 she retired to Tarrytown, New York, but continued her work in the state program where she established the practice of holding annual institutes for chief therapists to discuss problems and review new methods. She, in a sense, pioneered the very type of conference that we have only this year perfected. The last ten years of her life were complicated by a heart problem which was greatly taxed by a fall and back injury in 1940. Her insistence on continuing to practice her profession undoubtedly contributed to her death on September 18, 1942.

Reports of the early meetings of our Association tell us much of Mrs. Slagle and of the spirit which fostered our early development.[2] Forty years ago at our first annual conference the treasurer noted receipts of $109, expenses of $72.36 and an indebtedness of $150 to the lawyer for the cost of incorporation. The Society numbered 39 members of whom 26 attended this first meeting to enjoy a program including papers entitled, "Comparative Methods of Hospital Teaching," "Arts and Crafts in Medicine," and "The Teacher in Occupational Therapy." A review of patients followed and is notable, for it presented a depressed patient and an apparent case of paralysis, thus contradicting the now popular belief that early interests were devoted only to psychiatry. Finally a banquet was announced with great enthusiasm and later reported with equal interest, though Dr. Dunton tells us that it was a very sad occasion, for only three people appeared at Keen's Chop House to bolster their spirits and show their faith in a future profession. One of the three, of course, was Mrs. Slagle.

At the second annual meeting of the National Society for the Promotion of Occupational Therapy, September 2–4, 1918, in New York, Mrs. Slagle again played a prominent role and, again as vice-president, she presided. The treasurer reported a balance of $38.73 and noted that with the aid of a loan of $30 the costs of incorporation had been paid, for the lawyer was growing impatient. He also noted there was owing this Society $64 in unpaid dues.[3] (Perhaps we have inherited some early weaknesses?) Twenty-five members attended this meeting and heard papers on "The Problems of the Invalid Occupations in War Hospitals," "The Principles of Occupational Therapy," and "The Remuneration of the Teacher." The word "teacher" in the early literature refers to the one who teaches the patient, thus the therapist. The speaker here suggested that his topic was untimely "since more than half the world is giving its all in sacrifice,"[4] but continues that we are assured a "laborer is worthy of his hire." The topic initiated much discussion and the consensus was that the average salary for the occupation teacher seemed to be from forty to fifty dollars a month with maintenance. The salaries offered for re-construction aides averaged $1350 for home service, $1500 for head aide with ten assistants, and $1800 for supervisors. Post-Depression graduates will note how this compared with their initial salaries of $1300 with maintenance.

Another note of interest is Mrs. Slagle's comment on training for occupational therapy. She stated that after considerable experience the speaker felt that two months of crafts training and three months of practice teaching in hospitals made an ideal arrangement for a short course. The candidate should have college education or its equivalent in other experience.[5]

The third annual meeting was held September 8–11, 1919, in Chicago at the Favill School, probably the first of all occupational therapy schools. The Favill School had for three years been housed by Hull House and the renowned Jane Addams greeted the convention and congratulated the Society "because you are really the vanguard on the line of philanthropic effort and you are beginning at the bottom as all great social experiments have always done."[6]

At this meeting Mrs. Slagle was elected president and so formally began her many years of leadership in our profession. As time goes by fewer therapists will be able to recall her personality, for fewer will have known her. Future therapists will instead have to do as we have done, turn to her letters, the minutes of meetings in which she participated and the memories of her friends to learn of the heritage she left to them. They must read of her dominant personality, her sense of humor, her abiding interest in children, her ability to be outstanding in any situation, her dignity and handsome manner of dress and carriage, her astute mind, and her ability to rise above adversity. These traits of character were forceful factors in her influence on the growth of our profession as she moved from office to office and helped determine the framework of our present American Occupational Therapy Association.

But Mrs. Slagle's greatest contribution was to the practice of occupational therapy, not to its organization. This phase of her work is less known perhaps because it is a more personal thing or because it is less tangible and more difficult to study. She was tremendously interested in students, in their education and growth and in the direction of their work that they might share her enthusiasm in patient treatment. To perpetuate her memory we will now turn to this her greatest heritage and, using her own writings as a point of departure, will incorporate some of our own thoughts on student training and its meaning to the individual student, to the director of his course and to the members of this Association.

As we begin this third Slagle lecture we would use her own words from the presidential address of 1920, "this happens to be my turn and, like the measles and mumps or various and numerous other labelled states of mind or body, you wish me well, and hope it will be over soon."[7]

"Powerful Levers—In Little Common Things"

Clinical training is an outmoded phrase. We now speak of student affiliation and indeed date ourselves when we fail to do so, yet the original phrase has meaning for us as a review of definitions will show. The dictionary defines "clinic" as "medical instruction at the bedside of the patient," and defines the word "train" as "to bring to a required standard of knowledge or skill to give education by instruction and discipline." Since education is "the systematic development or cultivation of natural powers by inculcation or example," the concept of clinical training immediately implies apprenticeship. In clinical training one is assigned to a clinic to apprentice or "serve in order to learn." Initially then our choice of the phrase "clinical training" was to describe that period of the professional education devoted to serving another that through instruction and discipline one would cultivate his own natural abilities.

More recently we have adopted the phrase student affiliation. A student is "a person engaged in a course of study especially an advanced scholar—one who closely examines or investigates." To affiliate is "to receive on friendly terms, associate with—to adopt as a child." And here we would better cease to quote for the dictionary goes on to say "to associate with, usually reflexively or passively,"[8] and we know of few training experiences which could be called passive. Our new phrase "affiliate" has, we believe, a meaning too often overlooked, namely, to receive on friendly terms—to adopt. Our traditional concept of clinical practice is usually in terms of an assigned period spent in each of four or five clinics in which the student bridges the gap from the classroom to the job, a period of trial under supervision, a period in which to practice all that has previously been theory, thus the climax of academic experience.

We would think of student affiliation in a far broader sense for we believe that it is a period of transition to a whole new way of life. In an early paper Mrs. Slagle said, "A study of the greatest teaching personalities is a revelation of the powerful levers they found in little common things to lift their pupils up and out into a fuller life, and it is to the study of such methods that the most successful teacher will look for help."[9] Mrs. Slagle was using this thought to describe a therapist's work with a patient for she again used the word "teacher" as we now use the word "therapist." We feel, however, that this same key to success in treatment is the real key to success in teaching and indeed even the key to success in the performance of all of our daily tasks.

The nine month period of clinical affiliation must be a period of time in which the student gains far more than the opportunity to put his new knowledge into practice. It must be above all else a period of time in which those who teach "lift the student up and out and into a fuller life." Those who direct the student do not perform their roles successfully until they place the development of the individual in true perspective—above the importance of interpreting the theory and practice of occupational therapy in a particular disability area. The student who enters the affiliation period just to become proficient in applying his professional skills fails miserably if he does not first develop the personality and character through which the professional skills receive their most potent meaning.

Too often we forget that the majority of occupational therapy students are gaining their college education and professional training at one and the same time. We try to graduate a professional tool for the doctor and lose sight of the basic need of all college students to find time to grow as they learn.

The period of affiliation is, we feel, the most important of all educational experiences for it is true education lifted beyond the framework of what is purely academic. It is a practical experience and a period of transition in which the student must gain the ability to live as an independent person—which is to say he must begin to jell his own philosophy of life, of work and of his profession.

Sometimes those who teach are so preoccupied in following the essentials set down by the American Medical Association that they fail to see that a student is also trying to live with himself and others. Each affiliation must have a "well-defined program to interpret the function of occupational therapy in its own area or type of service,"[10] but of more permanent value is the atmosphere and personalities through which this program is introduced. People are more important than things. Personalities are remembered long after course content is forgotten. In the clinical field even more than in the formal setting of the professional school, the character of the teacher makes a lasting impression, for here there is daily contact under all sorts of conditions, here there is a sharing of responsibilities, here there is an apprenticeship. The importance of the individual therapist in training a student in any one affiliation will be notable to you if you will but for a moment recall your own affiliations. Is it not true that even those of you who have been out of school for "generations" can recall to this day the individual personalities of those who counselled you in each affiliation while you may have forgotten some once favored classroom professor. We remember the things we do rather than the things we hear about. We remember the things we see rather than the things about which we are told. We remember the things we feel rather than those we experience only through others.

For these reasons therapists involved in student affiliation programs must evaluate themselves as well as their staffs and programs with utmost care. We should have a very sound philosophy of student training if we are to accept the challenge and privilege of student education. This philosophy must enable us to give to the student through our own example an opportunity to develop a wisdom, an acceptable law by which he will live his adult life. It must give him, too, an appreciation for and thus the desire to share our own way of living, of working, of practicing our profession. If we teach these things we are successful in student training. As a guide to teaching them we would now suggest some factors so common and so little that they have a tremendous effect upon us all. Let us enumerate a few as an index for individual thinking.

The ability to make one's way alone. College is the time when a young person makes the transition to independence—independence of action and of thought. It is the time when personality is developed and character molded, the time when he must realize that he becomes an adult and must make his way alone. This transition is a difficult one and yet must occur while the student is under the stress of study. All such experiences are learned under stress, for this is when one uses the ultimate of his own discipline, and discipline is innate to the process of education. If a student learns to habituate himself to his environment he will have matured tremendously, for his environment is only temporary and will always change as long as he shall live. If he learns to adjust himself to living with his own kind and with those who differ in every way he will achieve some measure of both success and happiness.

The acceptance of things you do not condone or choose. Along with growth in independence must come the realization that things cannot always go according to one's own choosing. This is perhaps the most difficult of all experiences which occur when youth accepts adulthood, and many individuals of senior years bring unhappiness to themselves or others through never having understood the lesson. Students have so recently acquired freedom from the dictums of others that they have a false security in the justifiability of their own ideas and wishes, and so resent having to accept again a control even in this new form—self discipline and tolerance. Sir William Osler, the famous physician, once said, "Things cannot always go your own way. Learn to accept in silence the minor aggravations, cultivate the gift of taciturnity and consume your own smoke with an extra draught of hard work, so that those about you may not be annoyed with the dust and soot of your complaints."[11] This attitude once acquired becomes ingrained and is the fountain from which we gain our ability to understand others and so to be comfortable in our work with them. It must become part of an individual before he is able to follow direction and share departmental responsibility and it must be so inherent in his personality that it is no longer a conscious thing if he is to be successful in the direction of others.

A willingness to listen. This is another trait which must develop in college years and crystallize at the time of student affiliation. Too often freedom from the classroom, assigned reading and prearranged group participation gives an exaggerated feeling of importance and fosters an eagerness to express oneself and a restlessness which leaves no time for reflection. New found information is assumed to be seasoned knowledge which the owner is impatient to share—or at least reiterate. Quietness or meditation and attentiveness are scorned as the shy attributes of the inexperienced and are accepted only with embarrassment unless the student is given the opportunity to practice them and encouraged to realize their value. Today's students are being groomed for a world geared to the pace of group dynamics and the workshop exchange of ideas. They will lose half the value of participating if they have not first learned to listen. Sometimes it would appear we are all afraid of a moment of silence.

A willingness to seek advice. Perhaps this is felt to be a feminine trait yet some of the biggest men in history personify it. It begins again in little things, the recognition that we cannot know everything, that we are human and therefore even forget part of what knowledge we have acquired. One must learn to turn to others when the need arises but to turn cautiously and select our source wisely, then meld the counsel with our own experience and thus accept it as advice, not as a directive or decision. Mrs. Slagle once wrote to a friend, "I seek advice—I also seek to please."[12] Some would say this is a contradiction and that she was in a sense just trying to see-saw by herself and was thus running from the seat at one end to that at the other. Others would feel she was straddling an issue, thus standing over the fulcrum and so successful in see-sawing alone. We feel that the two thoughts frequently go hand in hand, for seeking the thoughts of others often results in giving pleasure to both of the individuals involved. At any rate there seldom, if ever, comes the time when we arrive at the point of never needing the help of others.

An ability to appreciate the commonplace. An occupational therapist will always work with people from all walks of life. Frequently he is pulled far from his own native environment and thrown into the problems of varied standards of living. Sometimes the sordid, the filthy, the crude come hand-in-hand with illness and disability and overwhelm the inexperienced. The ability to appreciate the commonplace, to note a touch of beauty in the midst of squalor or be aware of tenderness even in frugal living, this is the trait that refreshes and strengthens the individual as he is introduced to the ways of others. Osler once said, "Nothing will sustain you more potently than the power to recognize in your own humdrum routine as perhaps it may be thought, the true poetry of life—the poetry of the commonplace, of the ordinary man, of the plain, toilworn woman, with their loves and their joys, their sorrows and their griefs."[13]

The ability to retain the buoyance of youth. The young have a wonderful zest for living which carries them through many a difficult hour. Unfortunately, as we take our place in the working world we gradually lose that enthusiasm, that eagerness and spontaneity. The student who learns to modify it yet retain it will be well repaid. True, the exuberance and clumsiness of the puppy, particularly the big puppy, is humorous but not continuously desirable nor is it compatible with the dignity of maturity. However, who will deny the strength derived from the ability to rebound after rebuff, or the desire to adventure after mishap—and are these qualities not rooted in buoyance and vivacity?

An understanding of the value of time. Our modern world is time conscious and we are keyed to schedules and to a rapid pace, that we may accomplish the utmost immediately. We know a doctor who mourns that people no longer have time to be sick, nor to get well. He says that we used to crawl into bed and suffer our colds for four or five days but now must have a shot of this or a dose of that to stay on our feet. This trend is infectious and our students soon catch the disease. We must, through our own example, give them a truer concept of the value of time. Each day is a very real and integral part of one's life, for each individual is but the sum total of each day's experience. The student, busy with each affiliation, is keenly aware of blocks of time—four weeks here, eight weeks there—and prone to work through those blocks. If he will pause to realize that that which he adds to each day becomes the sum total of all his days, he will build a far better life. This is particularly true if he thinks he does not like the area to which he is currently assigned and is anxious to get on to another disability area. Someone has said, "Time is not always something to beat, it is also something to linger through and enjoy."[14] If we check off the days, we lose time, if instead we take each in turn and add to the day, we profit.

A realization that privilege is bound in duty. Traditionally as one moves up in status to more responsible positions he is granted more privileges. Those who are just learning the structure of an institution and the relative rank of services and positions frequently see the privileges that go with increased rank and perhaps even envy those who have found them. It is again at the student level that we must begin to realize that privilege and duty are closely interrelated. The apparent freedom of hours, of expression, of entrance and exit, carry a duty which should outweigh the privilege. One of the early members of the Dupont dynasty taught his sons that "no privilege exists that is not inseparably bound to a duty."[15] Privilege must be recognized by the one who receives it, must be guarded, never flaunted, must be doubly repaid through the sense of obligation that others in turn may respect it.

An equanimity of mental and moral outlook. Each student has lived through years of counsel from his elders, his family, his minister, his professors, but there comes a time when he must realize that the problems of the great moral issues of his time are now his own to solve. Many of our occupational therapy students attended college in areas close to their own homes, even perhaps commuting from their family residences. For them the affiliation period is the first real break, particularly if they are not receiving maintenance, for now they find themselves in a strange city completely independent. Those of us who are busy with such a student in duty hours frequently forget that he may be experiencing for the first time the pressure of living the moral code that he has inherited. We must somehow help him to see that while mores change, fundamentals do not. This is the time in which an innate sense of the fitness of things becomes his own possession rather than a hand-me-down. If he gains an appreciation of the good which is inherent in every fellow being whatever his station in life, and a commiseration for the evil again in every human being whatever his claim to godliness,[16] then he will be able to secure his own personal code of behavior upon which he will operate for the rest of his days. This phase of a student's adjustment to life is a very personal one and does not routinely come under the scrutiny of his director, for a student lives this in his own privacy as he justly should. Let us then just be aware that it is going on and that the atmosphere which we create in our own living can aid and abet it.

A desire to represent the best in manhood and womanhood. This is perhaps the summation of all the factors we have named. In this period of transition a student may easily struggle against that which his seniors expect of him. Now he is preoccupied with trying to become a good therapist, he is bombarded with tangible things, patients, techniques of treatment, records, supplies, and we must not so emphasize them that he fails to realize that becoming a good therapist is dependent upon first becoming a good person.

These are but a few of the common little things which the director of student affiliation and his junior staff members must hold in their consciousness if they are to give the student the best of any training experience. These are the little things which should be part of our own lives given through example that a student may develop his own philosophy of living—an acceptable law by which he will live each day of his life.

The student affiliation must also create an atmosphere in which the student may evolve his own philosophy of work and of his profession. This again is not a tangible thing taught in lecture or through supervised patient treatment but it is a very real factor in graduating successful therapists. There are many elements in our working lives which go to make up our philosophy of work and of our profession. Most of these are common to all paramedical or ancillary services. Some are peculiar to occupational therapy alone and are so taught in our theory classes on ethics and etiquette. We feel, however, that there are certain basic concepts which the affiliation centers exemplify and would again enumerate a few in random order, for they too are the common little things which collectively make the big person if he will encompass them in his philosophy of work.

A dedication to the patient. The patient is the reason we exist. This maxim is so true and common that frequently it is forgotten. In our big clinics, particularly in our teaching clinics, the patient is frequently outnumbered twenty to one. He is surrounded by doctors, nurses, technicians, social workers and therapists and though he is always the focus of the group, he is not always given his rightful place. In our eagerness to teach we frequently categorize patients, lump them into groups and label with symptoms to tag for specific modalities. Here the student comes to prominence and the patient recedes. In our anxiety to give full treatment we surround the patient with a mass of records, tests, reports and schedules even to the point of eclipsing the human element. We tell ourselves too frequently that patient welfare has priority over all else and then we busy ourselves with the myriad of mechanical details related to his care. Mrs. Slagle was acutely aware of this and always directed her attention to the patient first. Even as she became more and more involved with the administrative phases of her department she kept her patient in proper perspective. This is a trait seen in all great physicians even as their work calls them into teaching and research fields. The ability to understand the patient and his human problems as well as his physical or mental handicap is always the clue to successful treatment.

An appreciation of where the textbook ends. In many fields we have accumulated a vast amount of knowledge and so have devised given treatment routines. In arts and crafts we have inherited through the ages acceptable techniques and methods. These have been formalized and expounded in textbooks. Usually it is true that a subject is not taught until texts are available and we are accustomed to this type of learning; it is comfortable and gives us security as we practice the knowledge so gained. Yet there comes the time when textbooks do not validate what is practiced, where techniques cannot be defined in print, and it is here that experience has the advantage over mere education. It has been said that the successful person is not always the one who envisions an idea, but rather the one who is able to sell that idea to others. Freedom from established fact or directive is gained through the years but respect for it should start in college. In helping her students understand the approach to patients Mrs. Slagle said, "There can be no set of rules or theories applied; simple tact, patience and common sense assist more than anything else."[17]

Here again is one of the reasons we support the apprentice type of learning experience. Let us encourage students to examine and observe the staff in its performance of duty, and foster a respect for things that are successful through experience, not alone through the textbook. A staff member should not be embarrassed if he cannot always produce a fact to support his premise or his act, if execution of that idea is successful in its end effect on the patient.

An avoidance of overconfidence in our methods. In her report as president in 1920, Mrs. Slagle said, "Much valuable time, no doubt, was lost in the beginning by an over-agitation of standards—nothing is more stultifying to progress than standardization in a comparatively new field of service—keep your program flexible—let us have ideals always, fine, strong and true to the proper development of the individual patient but let us not be overconfident of our methods yet. A great many of us have opinions concerning the proper way of administering occupational therapy, all, no doubt, perfectly good opinions, but the chief point for us to remember is that we are still representing only a small part of the treatment given . . . ."[18] Continuous re-evaluation is a must.

A willingness to get in step with each institution. Preconceived ideas seldom helped anyone or any situation. Each clinic has its own problems, its own idiosyncrasies, its own weakness and strength. As we move from one to another we must be slow to criticize and quick to analyze. We must be willing to learn and to understand before we venture to change. Again Mrs. Slagle said that "we must carefully get in step and in line with the individual problems presented by each situation in which we serve, that the emotion toward our particular branch of work does not determine its force."[19]

A knowledge of how to support as well as to lead. Some say that leaders are born, others that they are developed, yet whatever you hold to be true you must grant that leaders follow before they lead. A supporting role is inglorious yet can be the most satisfying of experiences. We cannot graduate a profession of leaders for immediately we have nothing to lead. We must instead give proper respect and recognition to those who follow. In a treatment situation the individual who contributes the most is the one who quietly goes his way treating his patients with sincerity and compassion without an overlay of wishing to do otherwise. The being of the clinic lies with the patient, the greatest contribution to its functioning lies immediately with those who work closest to the patient, for as they are successful the clinic justifies its very reason for existence. The routine treating therapist is the backbone of the whole program as is the duty nurse. Such a therapist contributes in other ways too—through his enthusiasm for his job, his optimism in difficult times, his flexibility in accepting assignments, his willingness to do the menial if needed, his "acknowledgment of the dignity of the cure of disease,"[20] his assumption that he must give beyond what he receives.

A recognition of the average, not just the superior. We cannot create a profession peopled only with the outstanding, the superior, the talented, but instead must remember that the majority of us will have average ability. We must respect this average and recognize it as our balance wheel for frequently it will prevent us from wandering at a tangent. We must develop a respect for the average and not give it a stigma by apparent oversight in our eagerness to acknowledge those who have unusual capabilities. We must appreciate it and encourage those who have this status, that they too may have the security of knowing that they contribute to our profession.

An acceptance of learning on the job. We cannot graduate experienced therapists. A new staff member cannot be proficient in all disability areas nor is he qualified to meet every situation presented in daily treatment. We are vocative in complaining that our young therapists do not know this or that fact or technique so vital to our own job or disability area. We fret because schools and training centers do not supply this needed skill. We should instead expect a new graduate to continue to learn—always, if he is wise. We must provide that opportunity and consider his first few years of employment as a continuation of professional training. We are each morally obligated to give this training whether or not our department has an active teaching program.

An awareness that facts need no embellishing. Again we quote Mrs. Slagle whose comments on record writing are pertinent. "From the beginning of hospital practice students are taught the value of accurate notes, that a fact needs no embellishing in the way of narrative."[21] This art is almost impossible to teach without benefit of practical experience and is one that we continue to learn for many years. We would interpret Mrs. Slagle's words another way, too, and apply them to the problem of argument versus the expression of opinion. A student must learn that a staff member must always supply facts to support his position or ideas but must never embellish them by narration which then turns the situation into an argument. This is true when any staff member is asked to inform his seniors of a given problem. If that staff member does not like the situation he is justified in reporting the fact of his dislike and may support that fact with comments to prove its logic. He may, however, never go beyond that point to argue or harangue for in so doing he only weakens his own position. Facts accurately presented stand alone and are well interpreted whether they apply to treatment progress or to a working situation.

An enthusiasm for small job benefits. As jobs become more plentiful in our profession and therapists continue to be short in supply, we frequently find ourselves trying to sell our vacancies. This is done through formal job analysis, or an advertisement or a letter. Let us never forget the value of the unsolicited selling which is done in the daily performance of the job. Our own enthusiasm for fringe benefits, our loyalty to the institution, or interest in our chosen field, these frequently form a more impressive bit of information than does the listing of hours, pay scale, increments and the like.

A recognition of the value of extra-professional interests. Not every therapist is a so-called career therapist. Some practice their profession with less enthusiasm than others. Those who devote added hours to their profession and exhibit an extensive interest in its organization become mechanical participants unless they have learned to add other outside interests. There are only so many hours per day and the therapist who works and then participates in extracurricular professional activities must be particularly alert to other interests. Again we turn to Osler who said, "No man is really happy or safe without a hobby, and it makes precious little difference what the outside interest may be—botany, beetles or butterflies, roses, tulips or irises, mountaineering or antiquities—anything will do so long as he straddles a hobby and rides it hard."[22]

These are but a few of the common little things that we must cherish in our philosophy of our profession. There are many more but these will serve to indicate why we feel that the concept of student affiliation must be in the broadest sense an apprenticeship. These things are learned by example, by experience, they become part of an individual as he sees what they have meant to others and so accepts them himself. This then is why we must today adopt a student for we must inculcate by example that through us a student will increase his own self-discipline and thus multiply his chances of enjoying his profession.

Many occupational therapists are concerned directly with the problems of student training and develop an amazing enthusiasm for this phase of our work which tends to overwhelm those therapists not so involved. This is understandable for it is a dynamic problem and a tremendous responsibility. Most of us are so absorbed with the vastness of it all that we tend to get it out of all proportion to the total practice of our profession. We would do well to think on the implications of this for a moment. There has developed, we fear, an aura which surrounds that occupational therapy department which trains students as compared to one enjoying a similar program but without students. As we educate more and more students and particularly as we see them go through the same clinical centers, we build up a whole wedge of our profession intimately familiar with a limited number of departments and their staffs. If a student has enjoyed his affiliation he carries with him a deep and genuine respect for those who taught him. As he attends his initial conferences he feels strange and young and unrecognized. It is natural then for him to welcome the familiarity of those with whom he trained.

We feel that the total membership of the American Occupational Therapy Association should carefully evaluate several current trends which we believe are directly related to this perhaps inordinate attention on the training departments. We have the greatest respect for our schools and their personnel and for the student affiliation directors and their staffs. We would, however, sound a word of caution that we of AOTA must not put undue emphasis on them in conducting our national affairs. The 1957 Yearbook lists 1,257 agencies which have occupational therapy departments. Of these, 250 are recognized student affiliation centers used by the accredited schools. These departments employ 973 OTR's and the school staffs number approximately 86 OTR's, hence a total of 1,059 OTR's associated with students. The Yearbook lists 4,762 registered therapists of whom 3,138 are known to be working. Only one fifth of our departments and one third of the OTR's are participating in student education. A review of our Association shows that twelve out of thirteen standing committee chairmen, twenty-three of thirty-seven members of the House of Delegates, fourteen of the seventeen Board members and all of the officers are now, or were at the time of election or rise to national prominence, involved in student training.

We apparently choose our leaders from the schools and student affiliation groups and probably do so because they are familiar as well as capable people. Whether or not this is healthy is not for discussion here, but we would suggest that it should prompt those who are in training units to direct the attention of our students to the non-training departments. You of these departments can help. You can do so by your very active participation in local associations so that your names and abilities may become familiar to the students we bring to these meetings. Your expression of opinion on local and national matters is a vital factor in maintaining the proper balance. It is your key to gearing the policies of the Association to the particular needs of your departments. Your willingness to express yourselves clearly at local meetings will enable the student to understand the problems of the non-training departments in which they will more than likely find their initial employment.

A quick review of a recent issue of *AJOT* shows that seven out of ten of the papers written by OTR's were written by training personnel. So, too, were seven out of ten of the letters to the editor. Does this reflect the day-to-day practice of our profession? Where is the lone therapist who works without other registered occupational therapy staff members and without students? The common thought is that student affiliation staff members have more time, more freedom to write, more secretaries at their disposal. We suggest that they are simply prompted by their habit of teaching and by the very students who take up their time. A well-directed affiliation is never a labor-saving device for it takes hours of staff time and energy if it is properly guided. The non-training therapist has just as much time if he will but seek it. We urge that every practicing therapist consider it his duty to evaluate his work and to contribute some portion of it to professional literature. The expression of an idea or an opinion will do if there is neither time nor material for a full paper.

The non-training therapist can help offset the prominence of the affiliation center in many ways just as can the center itself. The combined efforts of both, and of the schools, must arouse a greater respect for the lone therapist and a greater opportunity for him to participate, perhaps through attendance at student affiliation council meetings or at institutes. Whatever the method may be it must develop in an atmosphere which encourages the value of non-academic learning and this atmosphere can be created by all training and school personnel. Let us not formalize everything to the point of overlooking the value of the individual. What we need most of all is a contributing membership to the American Occupational Therapy Association, not in the financial sense of a paid membership, but rather as an inherent part of each registered therapist's practice of his profession.

We have endeavored to present here our thoughts on student affiliation and its meaning to the individual student, to his director and to the members of this Association. In summary we would say that education belongs to the individual who receives it and, as we were once told, it is not to bank, to hoard, nor to squander, but is to ease the rigors of one's existence. If we would share our education we would do well to look to the little common things to lift one up and out and into a fuller life. As we earn our own education or guide others as they attain it, let us, however, always hold it secondary to a far greater thing—service—for service is the real meaning of our lives and of our careers. To it we must be dedicated or we do not live our profession. And with this thought we would give you one closing quotation from Mrs. Slagle, for we feel it is the true theme of all our lives, both personal and professional. "If we look to service, not to reward, we shall see in our own day, OUR work ministering to the highest needs of man."[23]

References

1. Slagle, Eleanor Clarke. Editorial, *Occupational Therapy and Rehabilitation,* 21:6 (December), 373, 1942.
2. Proceedings of the first annual meeting of the Nat. Soc. for the Promotion of OT. Spring Grove State Hospital. Sheppard Pratt Hospital Press, 1918.
3. Proceedings of the second annual meeting of the Nat. Soc. for the Promotion of OT. Sheppard and Enoch Pratt Hospital Press, 1918.
4. *Ibid.*
5. *Ibid.*
6. Addams, Jane. Proceedings of the third annual meeting of the Nat. Soc. for the Promotion of OT. Sheppard and Enoch Pratt Hospital Press, p. 41, 1919.
7. Slagle, Eleanor Clarke. Proceedings of the fourth annual meeting of the Nat. Soc. for the Promotion of OT. Spring Grove State Hospital and Sheppard Pratt Hospital, p. 1, 1920.
8. *Funk and Wagnall's Desk Standard Dictionary.* New York: Funk & Wagnalls, 1946.
9. Slagle, Eleanor Clarke. "Development of Occupations for the Insane." *Maryland Psychiatric Quarterly,* IV:1 (July), p. 19, 1914.
10. "Essentials of an Acceptable School of Occupational Therapy." *The Yearbook.* New York: American Occupational Therapy Assoc., 1957.
11. Cushing, Harvey. *Life of Sir William Osler,* Vol. I, Ch. 22. New York: Oxford University Press, 1940.
12. Slagle, Eleanor Clarke. Letter to William Rush Dunton, Jr., M.D.

13. Cushing, *op. cit.,* Vol. II, Ch. 26.

14. Etting, Gloria Braggiotti. "Go by Sea." *Town and Country,* August, p. 96, 1957.

15. Dupont (Irene Dupont's father, 1784). "The Duponts of Wilmington." *Life,* 42:8, p. 101.

16. Brunyate, William L. Letter to daughter, 1935.

17. Slagle, Eleanor Clarke. "Development of Occupations for the Insane." *Maryland Psychiatric Quarterly,* IV:1 (July), p. 19, 1914.

18. Slagle, Eleanor Clarke. Proceedings of the fourth annual meeting of the Nat. Soc. for the Promotion of OT. Spring Grove State Hospital and Sheppard Pratt Hospital, p. 1, 1920.

19. *Ibid.*

20. Pledge and creed for occupational therapists.

21. Slagle, Eleanor Clarke. "Training Aids for Mental Patients." *Archives of Occupational Therapy,* 1:1 (February), p. 17, 1922.

22. Cushing, *op. cit.,* Ch. 29.

23. Slagle, Eleanor Clarke. Report of president, proceedings of the fourth annual meeting of the Nat. Soc. for the Promotion of OT. Spring Grove State Hospital and Sheppard Pratt Hospital, p. 1, 1920.

6

1958 Eleanor Clarke Slagle Lecture

Every One Counts

Margaret S. Rood, MA, OTR, RPT

Introduction

As the activation of every reflex is necessary in the proper sequence toward coordinated effortless muscular control, so the activation and learned control of basic reflexes in developmental order are necessary for the highest level of emotional maturity. Intellectual maturity, independent thinking, can never be achieved by stuffing the mind with rote learning or facts without progressing onward to individual comprehension and application to original contributions based on the work of others.

If emotional and intellectual maturity are developing dynamically, then professional maturity can be attached happily and wisely for the warmest interaction of all, to secure the best treatment for the patient. And if we are truly maturing, then the needs of others will be our guide in the considerate give and take of professional life.

And as we come to the full realization of the need for stress for growth, so we must realize that the attitude toward stress will make it a challenge toward increased development or a block to our progress. Unlike the school situation where a grade remains static on the record, in living one has a chance to try again. Having achieved, that record counts as does the strength gained from trying.

The course was charted for us a long time ago. Each individual is a product of his heritage, his experiences. We benefit by the drive and vision of those who have gone before, and we in turn have a responsibility to add our particular share whatever it may be. And as Eleanor Clarke Slagle had the vision and selfless devotion in the initiation and development of our professional organization, we must build on that foundation to pass on an improved heritage to those to come.

In turn may I discuss briefly the physical, emotional, intellectual and professional aspects in relation to selected principles of muscle reaction.

Physical Development

Activation of muscles proceeds from reflex or involuntary stimulation to voluntary control. In the loss of voluntary control of muscles from many causes it may be possible to reactivate muscles if the cause is physiological discontinuity and not anatomical destruction. But it is necessary to stimulate the first reflex pattern. Therefore, the sequence is important and the total pattern within the sequence. If balanced development does not occur early the problem of treatment will always be more difficult because there will be parts of many reflexes acting in an imbalanced pattern.

For efficiency of a part, interaction with an antagonist is necessary for (primary) shortening and (secondary) lengthening before cocontraction of both at the same time is possible. If one of a pair of muscles does not function

Originally published 1958 in *American Journal of Occupational Therapy, 12,* 326–329.

in reciprocal innervation, eventually the normal one will be seriously affected. Gravity or stress is essential for the stimulation of the heavier work muscles and for bone growth. Cocontraction or static support positions are essential before heavy work movement is effective. As in cocontraction for support—whether on elbows, all fours or standing—the distal segment is stable, so too the heaviest work a muscle does in movement in its biological purpose is with the distal segment stable. One of the most difficult muscle problems is the lengthening reaction of heavy work one-joint muscles such as the soleus, vasti and anconeus. Slow knee bends with heels flat will get both lengthening and shortening reaction of the vasti and soleus. This is different work from the lighter guiding (lengthening) reaction of the longer muscle passing more joints. Lengthening reactions are important to flexibility as well.

As an example of this approach to muscle action, we might contrast the Delorme heavy resistance at ankle for knee extension versus squatting, which is the normal functional use of the muscle.

The quadriceps loom or kick wheel which embodies this same principle is excellent for the rectus femoris but not for the vasti which is our major problem usually.

In squatting the feet are on the floor or, in other words, the distal segment is stable and the muscles must pull the rest of the body into alignment, a heavier job than just moving the distal end of the extremity.

In life, the rectus femoris comes into play in walking which is a lighter work demand. Therefore in actuality, occupational therapy procedure involving squatting is more effective than kicking if it is the vasti which needs strengthening.

In learning patterns or movement to reproduce at will, the individual must do his own learning. As therapists we must give sufficient stimulus but prevent ourselves from helping too much. Passive action is not the answer. Light work patterns of skill require cortical or voluntary attention. The shoulder rotator cuff muscles of a patient with subluxation of the humerus may be activated by heavy work grip of the hand but not by light work.

Postural cocontraction for erect position can be gained by dental dam rubber resistance to top of head or over each shoulder following appropriate stimulation. Therefore, rather than asking for voluntary correction of posture or traction, resistance is used to cause postural cocontraction without conscious thought. During passive activity such as TV viewing, no attention need be paid because there are more reflex feedbacks below the level of consciousness for heavy work. Stimulus from the muscle spindles found in heavy work muscles pass only as high as the cerebellum for integration. Also repetitive, rhythmical patterns will release top level control after patterns have once been learned. Therefore rhythmical music is the most effective tool; not the metronome with its interrupted tone which requires a more cortical response.

The last two examples would give some indication that fatigue is involved not in the muscle but the cortical control of the pattern. These same points might well serve to illustrate developmental reactions in emotional, intellectual and professional growth.

Emotional Development

As the give and take of shortening and lengthening reactions of muscles is necessary for the health of both, so the giving and receiving of love and of stress is necessary for healthy emotional reactions, and these must be in the sequence of normal development. The baby receives care, love and protection. From this early selfish taking he should progress to wise receiving and giving. That which an individual desires and that which is most ego satisfying to the giver may create or prolong dependence. There will be many, many steps in human relations with definite sequences and experiences necessary for full maturity. Accepting one's parents as interesting individuals on their own merit is one of the higher steps.

The facing of stress is essential to full emotional maturity. Sympathetic nervous system arousal needs repetition so that it can be assessed as non-critical, and therefore may result in a controlled learning experience rather than an uncontrolled emotional reaction. Some withdraw from hurt, others become aggressive. The former is more serious since the damage is to self while the exterior signs do not bring forth the social disapproval attendant to aggression.

Aggression, or any pressure of ideas, begets resistance, so care should be used in pushing ideas. Attitude on the part of the recipient toward stress will determine whether it be a healthy challenge to growth or a stimulus for withdrawal in an unhealthy pattern. Comprehension of the fact that insecurity breeds resistance will allow for more intelligent handling of such problems. Holding firm under stress is important also for the individual to learn.

Muscles need light and heavy work patterns in movement and holding to keep in the best equilibrium. Making a point of having friends of all ages is one of the surest ways to prevent atrophy or contractures of the spirit.

Careful selection of most important things will prevent the hyperkinesia of too great superficial stimulation. Heavy work stimuli lead to relaxation and renewal of the body. The physical and emotional are interdependent. It is important that there be a balance of gross physical activity when the mind creates tensions. Likewise the joys of simple as well as the more complex, pleasures should be kept and fostered.

Dependence on outward approval may be too strong. There is a need for developing one's own goals and these may be higher than those set by others. Insecurity requires constant repetition of approval. A secure person realizes that if a decision is thoughtful and right insofar as one knows, one must try to face without bitterness the criticisms which will inevitably come. There is adaptation of the sensory receptors only if the situation is too static or repetitive, however there is some slight adaptation of the sensory receptors to the criticism; nevertheless the criticism should be listened to carefully and the soundness of it judged in the light of what one knows. The interference of emotional reflex reaction will not allow sound judgment, as reflex emotion and intellect are at variance.

Intellectual or Educational

Thinking too must have the reciprocal innervation of give and take to be of the greatest value. Light and heavy work will give an appropriate balance.

Rote learning or easy receiving is supposed to be at its peak up to fourteen years of age. Are we continuing it beyond this age unnecessarily? One knows how hard it is to set students free to think. It is easier in the beginning of professional life, but if set patterns have been established, insecurity and emotional reactions will delay the establishment of new habit patterns. The new student can more easily relate principles to the basic sciences since he does not have old techniques to uproot.

In professional life, are we properly stimulating our therapists in give and take at small unit meetings as part of our association activities? Individual study assignments to key free-for-all discussions would stimulate greater effort than the more standard passive reception of lectures, worthwhile though they be. Efforts on this line have been more notable on the national than the state level.

Although study and reading with a specific goal is difficult initially, repeated exposure provides its own self-ignition because of the interest created, and if done in relation to a patient's problems, solutions are easier. Answers to the theoretical questions which might take months to secure can be found far more quickly if they relate to a specific patient's problem. Not as much cortical driving is necessary since many of the clues are there at hand and certainly the motivation. Comprehension gained this way is more rounded and better remembered since it need not be translated learning.

In the majority of occupational therapy schools, the scientific preparation in physical disabilities is less than in physical therapy schools when functional activities would seem to require as great a knowledge of structure and function if not more.

Professional

As supervisors are we preventing growth by too much supervision? Are we allowing others to help set their own goals? Dependence does not develop strength in staff, students or patients. By setting sights, we risk setting lower goals than they might set for themselves. The safety and security of well-defined boundaries such as specific assignments, authority over ideas as well as work, prevents individual development. Once exposed to the headiness of individual projects rather than merely satisfying someone else, the exposure usually takes.

All occupational therapists should add to our store of knowledge and general growth, not suffer technique and equipment contractures. We have a tendency to be dependent when there is need to exercise our muscles of initiative. Each must contribute at his own level so that the whole may be more complete, since each with different background and interest will see different facets of the same problem. The richness of research material and its application to treatment techniques has been slow to seep to the therapy level. Our responsibility is to read widely and observe, to think and bring to the doctor's attention those things which might affect the patient. Therapy will be only as good as the therapist.

The establishment of an advanced study treatment center should be contemplated, not in conjunction with any school of therapy but of and for the Association and its members. This would provide for dynamic interaction of minds under medical guidance. Some of the points to be considered in relation to such a center would be:

1. Inclusion of small groups of occupational therapists and allied professional groups. In the physical disabilities area, the physical and occupational therapist would be the basic interacting unit.
2. A nucleus of top therapists each with special abilities that all might learn from one another.
3. Therapists selected should have five or more years' experience.
4. Theory and its application and practice must be integrated with enough time for studying, thinking and thoughtful application.
5. Individual courses for special weaknesses (such as written and oral communication) could be secured in other facilities.
6. This might be a central bureau for the proper consideration of new developments in the field, including testing of new treatment procedures and equipment ideas as well as evaluating existing procedures.
7. Preparation of abstracts and papers for professional publications should be a requirement.

Support could come from grants from numerous foundations, and quarters are secondary to personnel and ideas.

Summary

It is important in development and growth that there be stimulation from without and from within so that autogenetic or self-igniting facilitation and inhibition be developed. There are many steps along the road but heavy work patterns of effort and stress must be faced and overcome before the finer, higher level patterns are possible. Both movement and holding are necessary. In the past we have performed reciprocal innervation patterns for movement only, without the cocontraction patterns against stress. We have been assisting weak muscles and giving them the lightest work when a heavier work pattern given first would make the skilled pattern possible or easier. To change to the thought of heavy work patterns will be difficult, but by knowing all of the sensory stimuli for the appropriate sensory receptors it is possible to aid the desired pattern through the nervous system. Thought is necessary in order to put patterns of muscle work through the proper sequential order of normal development. Any omission or transposition of order will prolong the process or make the results imperfect.

The most important points in all of our developmental patterns are sequential order, activation for primary and secondary action in movement, and the resistance to stress. These apply to emotional, intellectual and professional development as well as physical growth. With mastery of these points will come the auto-inhibition and facilitation so necessary for functioning alone as a human being within the total group. We will then add our share to the heritage which has been given to us by others and which will be carried on in the future by many more. May our journey as explorers in life be fruitful and satisfying, and increasingly stimulating mentally. Our physical age of maturity has definite limits but our mental and spiritual age need not.

7

1959 Eleanor Clarke Slagle Lecture

The Essentials of Work Evaluation

Lilian S. Wegg, OTR

Preface

The principles of occupational therapy established by our pioneer occupational therapists, and most particularly Eleanor Clarke Slagle, have given us the foundation upon which to build advanced techniques and approaches.

Although pre-vocational occupational therapy is a recognized part of our work, it seems apparent that there is still a need for a discussion of the basic principles and practices essential to such a program.

The essentials which will be considered today are the expression not only of myself, but also of the members of the work evaluation team of the May T. Morrison Center for Rehabilitation. The recognition you have given to me must, in truth, go to this team as a whole.

Introduction

In the consideration of vocationally oriented occupational therapy, it is essential to provide an effective means of determining needs, measuring abilities and predicting capacities of an individual. One of the most effective means is through the use of tests. Experience in helping to develop a work evaluation service has taught me that tests are basic to such a service and that the work tests developed in occupational therapy are the very essence of such a program.

It is, therefore, this subject of tests which will be our primary consideration today; what a test is, what a test should do and the role of the occupational therapist as a tester.

In the field of physical disabilities, certain tests have become standard to good treatment. Some of these are range of motion tests, muscle examinations and functional activity tests. Initially, we use these various evaluations as a way of establishing tentative goals. Throughout the course of treatment, we use them as a means of measuring progress or abilities.

The work evaluation team, in an examination of the vocational needs of the patient, realized that these tests did not reveal, to any practical extent, the person's ability and capacity for work. The need for a more thorough appraisal and accurate prediction of vocational capacities was evident. It was appropriate that an approach be developed which would attempt to deal with this need and which would be suitable for all diagnostic areas.

In work evaluation, tests using the reality situation or work sample method have proven to be such an approach.

Statement

If we recognize that tests play a part in determining needs and act as a guide to the attainment of goals, then we can assume that the purposes of a work evaluation program are the testing and evaluation of work abilities, including

Originally published 1960 in *American Journal of Occupational Therapy, 14*, 65–69, 79.

skills; the testing and predicting of work capacities, including the level of employment expected; and the testing and exploration of interest and work aptitudes.

More specifically, the objectives of the tests are:

(1) To evaluate ability as related directly to recommended and specific job tasks. The evaluation of the person's learning ability, retention of skill through tests and recall of skills on re-tests should be considered.

(2) To determine capacity to perform job tasks. Such factors as production and proficiency in terms of the specific samples should be carefully evaluated.

(3) To evaluate such physical and psychological factors as work tolerance and work habits.

    (a) To evaluate work tolerance, such factors as ability to work in the required physical position for the required length of time; tolerance to job demands, such as noise, dust, people and tools; tolerance to routine, repetitive work or skilled work should be considered.

    (b) To evaluate work habits, such factors as responsibility, cooperation, attention span, response to authority and criticism, method and manner of performance, mood and relationship to others, should be examined.

(4) To devise and evaluate work simplification methods as indicated.

(5) To provide the patient with an opportunity to participate in a realistic work program.

In order to meet these testing objectives based on vocational needs, it is necessary to have media closely related to job demands. Work sampling and evaluation is job-oriented, not disability-oriented. We are evaluating the ability of a person to work. Because the individual is vocationally in need, our media and our roles must have a vocational orientation. The fact that a medical diagnosis rendered the person in need of vocational rehabilitation means that we must be aware of the diagnosis in the work program. We are dealing, then, with a medical and a vocational program, with consideration of the former but emphasis on the latter. This change of emphasis influences the role of the occupational therapist.

To understand this clearly, we first need to know what a test is and what a test should do. A test is defined as "a means of measuring the skill, knowledge, intelligence, capacities or aptitudes of an individual." In preceding remarks, it was mentioned that a work testing program should provide a reality situation, an accurate measurement of abilities, and an accurate prediction of capacities.

Let us keep the definition of a test and these essentials of testing in mind and determine how work tests should be organized to accomplish the objectives.

Many of you will be familiar with the *Dictionary of Occupational Titles*. This publication has been prepared by the Division of Occupational Analysis, of the United States Employment Service. It has provided a suitable framework upon which to organize the structure of work tests. This structure allows for division and selection of appropriate work samples according to the major job families, such as: technical work, clerical and sales work, service work, mechanical work and manual work.

The test should measure as nearly as possible the movements required on the job. In addition, such intensity factors as the distance walked, directions reached, and weights lifted and carried should be evaluated. It should be of sufficient length to evaluate both ability and endurance. This means that the test should involve normal units of work rather than single units which would evaluate only the momentary capacity. If, under normal working conditions, the individual would be required to work with 500 or 1,000 parts for a given period of time, then the work sample should be set up accordingly.

The tests should be provided in a special atmosphere which is tailored to fit the demands of the various job families and which is in keeping with the demands of a testing situation. Unless group testing has been specifically recommended, the tests should be administered in a room separate from the occupational therapy department or workshop area.

The test should provide both an objective and a subjective analysis and standardization in all tests is a recognized goal. Standardization does not relieve the occupational therapist of interest, ingenuity or initiative. On the contrary, as each client varies so greatly from the next, the tester's entire thought and time will be directed to the evaluation of that particular person's performance in terms of the test objectives established for him. Without standardization of the testing procedures, there would be no reference point or base line for the tester, there would be no opportunity to accumulate reliable data and, indeed, the entire process would lose the scientific concept.

The test should be easily administered. Each test should have a test kit indexed according to the occupational classification and titled with the test name itself. For example: handwriting is classified under the major heading of "Clerical Work, General Recording," with the numerical classification of 1-X2-0. Assembly, packaging and sorting of miscellaneous items is classified under the major heading of "Manual Bench Work" with the numerical classification of 6-X4-3.

Each test kit should contain a test outline composed of a description of the test in industrial terminology, the purpose of the test, the physical demands of the task, the psychological factors to be considered, a list of the equipment and supplies required, a detailed explanation of how to prepare the work place, an explanation of the exact information to be given the client, and full instructions as to what should be included in the timings and what items should be recorded as errors. The equipment, tools and supplies should be assembled in a portable kit if possible.

The test results should be readily evaluated. This requires a standard and quick method of scoring and checking for accuracy. Several systems for the latter can be used, such as: special marks, numerical codes, or answer sheets. When evaluating craftsmanship, models for comparison should be used. When evaluating work samples classified as repair work, the tester should be sure that the finished project works. Discussion of scoring will come later in the paper.

The test should be acceptable to the individual taking it. This is not a problem if there is rigid adherence to the reality situation. There is some danger when devising a work sample to make something do for the sake of economy in time and money. This is false economy. It results in the test appearing silly to the client and thus losing its predictive value.

The test should be available to facilities and occupational therapists at a moderate initial outlay. Replacement or maintenance should not be costly.

The use of work evaluation tests means that the occupational therapist must be a work tester and, as such: is assuming a function of more vocational emphasis than medical. This change in emphasis, however, does not change our functions radically. The following outline of the essential functions of the tester will indicate that these are basically the same as the defined and accepted functions of the occupational therapist. The items with which we work, the factors which we consider, the terminology which we use, the goals which we set, may be adapted to fit the need. The basic or fundamental things that we do, however, have not changed.

Essential Functions of the Tester

Referral. Included in the referral for work evaluation should be as many known factors as possible, such as: the work history, the medical, social and educational histories and the results of psychological evaluations. There should be a recent physical examination or medical approval of the program. In our facility, it has been the occupational therapist and the rehabilitation counselor who have procured and assembled this data.

Acceptance. Once this information is obtained, the referral should be followed by a staff review for determination of acceptance and choice of work samples. At the May T. Morrison Center, we have termed this review the work sample prescription conference. The occupational therapist, the physiatrist and the rehabilitation counselor select the appropriate tests. If the referral comes from the Vocational Rehabilitation Services, the counselor active in the case attends the conference. The selection of tests is based on the client's physical capacities, personality appraisal, social history, vocational interests and aptitudes and the tentative vocational objective.

The occupational therapist should assist in recommending the actual tests to be used. He should suggest whether or not re-tests or equivalent tests seem indicated and at what stage these should occur in the program. Re-tests refer to the same tests done more than once and can be administered within the first tryout period or scheduled for a later date. Re-tests given within the initial period will evaluate the individual's ability to recall skills. If given at a later date, re-tests will not only evaluate re-call but also will serve as a measurement of progress in abilities. Equivalent tests refer to tests which are similar to others in that they can evaluate similar factors but will differ in such things as the test outline, the instructions or the tools. These are generally done within the initial tryout period. Such tests are useful when evaluating the client's tolerance to working with a variety of materials, such as wood as opposed to metal or vice versa.

Preparation. In the planning stage, preparation refers to the scheduling of the client. Various social, psychological or physical factors enter into the choice of time and days. The time of the day, the day of the week, the time of the month, the attitude of the family can, and will, influence the client's participation in the testing program.

Pre-Testing

Preparation. The equipment should be kept in working order, the supplies should be adequate for each testing period and the work room should be properly arranged for the client and the job.

Presentation. In the explanation of the testing program, it is important to orient the client to the purpose of the testing and of the tests. Terminology should be used which is in keeping with the job and suited to the client's needs, such as in the case of the deaf, blind or the brain injured. Initial contact will structure the total testing atmosphere.

Instructions will be oral, written or schematic depending on the nature of the job. Instructions should be kept to the test outline as they have been carefully worked out according to normal job conditions.

Demonstrations of the movements required and the various methods needed to complete the work sample will be necessary. This is particularly true in jobs requiring a high rate of production. Our test outlines are written for the non-handicapped person and adapted as necessary for each client. This adaptation would be required in the case of a functionally one-handed individual performing a task normally requiring the use of two hands.

Tryout phase. The client should be allowed to try out part of the test to learn the procedures and to allow the tester to observe his capacities. The learning time should be recorded for comparison with the average learning time. The need for accuracy should be stressed during this phase and all errors should be corrected and discussed with the client as they occur.

Test

Administration. An accurate administration is essential otherwise the scores cannot be validated. Strict adherence to the work samples as prescribed, however, should be up to the discretion of the tester—a judgment which is used constantly in the treatment of patients.

Instructions and comments should be confined to the testing situation. The performance must be by the client's own efforts in this phase. Unnecessary words or actions will disturb the worker.

Observation. Both direct and indirect methods of observation should be used. An example of the direct method would be the close observation essential to note the number and types of errors which the client makes. Very often an individual will make consistent errors. These could be due to an oversight during the instruction period, or something that the client has failed to comprehend or something that he is prone to do. Without close attention to this detail, the wrong conclusion could be made. An example of the indirect method would be the subtle observation of manifestations of behavior.

Recording and evaluation. When making observations, it is easy to overlook certain factors, forget certain details or emphasize unimportant events. Therefore, for recording and evaluating, it is recommended that the tester use a work test sheet, check list (work sample prescription) and stop watch. A slide rule is optional.

The work test sheet is an ideal place for recording the client's name, diagnosis, date, numerical classification and title of test. It also allows space for a description of the client's performance and his production, proficiency and final ratings. If this sheet is carefully written, it can serve as a part of the final report. Only the most significant material should be recorded. This places additional importance on the work sample prescription as the testing objectives will then serve as a guide.

To evaluate performance, it is necessary that some method of scoring be established. The Morrison Center has a norm for each work sample test. This norm was established by methods used by our industrial engineer, Mr. Paton B. Crouse. The norm is set up so that 100% represents the normal good performance of non-handicapped workers familiar with the job and working at a tempo that would be required in competitive employment.

These norms, written in decimal figures, are recorded in each test kit. If the test involves several parts, each part will have a norm. A decimal stop watch is used to record the client's time. At the conclusion of the test, the norm is divided by the time achieved by the work. This establishes a percentage and is known as the production rating. To obtain a proficiency rating, a certain percentage is then deducted for errors. This percentage is based on the degree of skill needed and the quality required by the job. All final ratings are based not only on the production and proficiency ratings, but also on the subjective analysis of the client's coordination, attention and interest for that particular job. These ratings are expressed in terms of "good," "fair," or "poor" depending on where they fall in the numerical scale of 100–0. For example 0–30 represents poor or questionable performance and means that the client is capable of selective work in the sheltered shop area or noncompetitive employment. A score of 30–50 represents a fair performance and means that the client is capable of sheltered shop work at that time with the potentiality for competitive employment with training or adjustment. A 50–75 score represents good and means that the client is an adequate worker for competitive employment. A 75–100 score represents superior and means that the client is a good to exceptional worker and capable of competitive employment.

The final evaluation must also be based on the atmosphere and deviations which have been allowed by the tester. These deviations may or may not be acceptable from the vocational viewpoint. It is imperative that this be determined before the tester ventures too far from the standard procedure. This again is one reason why a discreet choice or prescription of samples is so essential. If the elements of a test have to be varied to such a degree that the test loses its identity, then an appropriate work sample was not selected.

Reporting

Quite detailed and structured reports should be prepared. Adoption of standard terminology by the team is essential. To avoid unnecessary repetition when preparing the report, our evaluation service has adopted a standard organization of the report and standard phrases for certain parts. For example, the opening paragraph always states:

> The following work samples were selected on the basis of the client's education and employment history, psychological test results and physical (or psychiatric) information in order to evaluate his physical ability and capacity, his emotional tolerance and capacity, his interest and aptitude to engage in the following work.

The prescribed or selected work samples are then listed, after which is a description and evaluation of the client's performance on each test. A summary of the overall performance relating directly to the testing objectives with recommendations for future course of action or possible areas of placement concludes the report. Whatever the organization of the report, however, the tester must strive to be objective in his remarks. The tester must not be influenced by previous evaluations. His opinions must be based solely on the observations during the testing period.

The preceding essentials form the scientific basis of a work evaluation program. The success of such a program depends on the most important essential of all—that is, the tester. It is obvious that there are certain traits that a tester should possess. First, the tester should be one who can perform concise analyses, both of a qualitative and quantitative nature. As he will be confronted with varying abilities, diagnoses and degrees of intelligence, he must be one who can react consistently and objectively. He must be sensitive to the needs of the client during the testing—needs which could result in a shift in the task or the atmosphere. The tester should be one who can adopt and maintain a scientific concept. He should be one who is willing to work in harmony with a team. He must be one who is interested in learning new concepts, in developing new programs and in the broadening of his education.

The opinion of the work evaluation team at the Morrison Center is that the occupational therapist is the natural choice for the work tester. An occupational therapist's training and work experience is geared to dealing directly with human beings—not just for a few brief moments, or in an hour's interview, but hour after hour throughout a day. An occupational therapist's thoughts and techniques provide him with a unique approach. This approach is ideal for, and essential to, a testing situation.

Before concluding, there are certain other practical considerations which should be noted at this time. First of all, one should not assume that a vast number of tests are required for a work evaluation service. There are four major job classifications which are most commonly requested. These are: clerical and sales work, service work, skilled mechanical work, semi-skilled to unskilled manual work. Of these four classifications, the first and the last are the most used and the most practical from the standpoint of placement areas for handicapped individuals.

Although our tests number 83, only 26 of these are most commonly used. These 26 are:

Clerical and Sales Work

1. Computing work using the calculator machine
2. Handwriting
3. Simple book-keeping
4. Typing
5. Checking of equipment, invoices
6. Routine recording work, using adding machines
7. Classifying work
8. Filing
9. Clerical machine operation
10. Collating
11. Telephone and switchboard work
12. Cashiering and vending machine

Service Work

1. Kitchen helper
2. Domestic worker

Skilled Mechanical Work

1. Electrical equipment repairing
2. Radio repairing

Semi-skilled to Unskilled Manual Work

1. Inspection
2. Electrical unit assembling
3. Wood unit assembling and woodworking machine operation
4. Miscellaneous bench work
5. Metal bench work
6. Miscellaneous metal working
7. Miscellaneous paper work: assembling, cutting, sorting
8. Light elemental work: simple routine, repetitive jobs
9. Elemental service work: janitorial or dishwashing jobs
10. Miscellaneous physical work. This is work requiring simple, routine tasks such as might be found on construction projects or in maintenance areas and which would range from light to medium to heavy in degree.

A second major consideration is the number of days suitable for testing. We have found that a period of three days is quite adequate. This is a concentrated period, lasting all day, with one occupational therapist handling one client at a time. Such an arrangement is ideal, but this period must be solely confined to testing and not include training or adjustment. It is my feeling that there is a time and a place for testing, and a time and a place for adjustment or training. An attempt, on the part of one occupational therapist, to do both of these simultaneously loses the scientific approach. This is not to say that adjustment and training cannot be scientific, but in the combination of the two, the true purposes become obscured. The purpose of the testing is to diagnose and evaluate the client's ability and capacity for work but not to condition him for employment. Testing is required to determine the area of training, the level of training and, indeed, if training should be considered. The purpose of a work adjustment program, on the other hand, is to adjust and condition the client to the demands of work by providing opportunities for him to develop work habits or improve such work assets as were noted in the testing situation. The opportunity to participate in a testing program, with close relation to an adjustment program, has made me realize that similar but not identical evaluations can be gained. It would seem apparent, therefore, that both a work testing and a work adjustment program is needed to provide a thorough vocational appraisal. These programs must be coordinated in a team approach. As the work training or adjustment program should occur in a variety of places depending on the results of the work tests, a coordinated team approach implies the integration of an in-center and an out-center team.

There is one last consideration. This is the implication of a testing and evaluation program to our patients, our media and our selves. It means that we are able to offer a more thorough program to our patients by determining their vocational needs and assisting in their fulfillment. It means that occupational therapy can offer a scientific approach. It means that the occupational therapist has a new and stimulating concept. All of these factors have a far-reaching implication as they extend to the potential occupational therapist, our students, a challenge to enter our profession.

In conclusion, certain basic essentials must be considered and adopted in order to provide an effective work evaluation program. It is apparent that such a program must be composed of several phases. The phase which has been discussed today, namely work sample testing, is just one step towards the determination of the patient's ultimate vocational objective. This paper has been an attempt to outline work evaluation essentials and to show the effectiveness of occupational therapy when planned with a group of experts and executed with a goal in mind.

8

The 1950s: Discussion Questions and Learning Activities

The Lectures

Stattel, F. M. (1956). Equipment designed for occupational therapy (1955 Eleanor Clarke Slagle Lecture). *American Journal of Occupational Therapy, 10,* 194–198.

Sokolov, J. (1957). Therapist into administrator: Ten inspiring years (1956 Eleanor Clarke Slagle Lecture). *American Journal of Occupational Therapy, 11,* 13–19.

Brunyate, R. W. (1958). Powerful levers in little common things (1957 Eleanor Clarke Slagle Lecture). *American Journal of Occupational Therapy, 12,* 193–202.

Rood, M. S. (1958). Every one counts (1958 Eleanor Clarke Slagle Lecture). *American Journal of Occupational Therapy, 12,* 326–329.

Wegg, L. S. (1960). The essentials of work evaluation (1959 Eleanor Clarke Slagle Lecture). *American Journal of Occupational Therapy, 14,* 65–69, 79.

Learning Activities

1. Investigate the occupational profile of most Americans in the 1950s. Some useful bibliographical references to explore appear in Appendix B.
   - What was the average family size?
   - What was the average salary? What were some typical jobs?
   - What did homes cost?
   - What were the clothing styles of the decade?
   - What was significant about the popular culture of the decade (e.g., music, film, books)?
2. If you have access to a complete collection of the *American Journal of Occupational Therapy,* scan the table of contents for each issue. What were some common topics? Can you identify any patterns in these topics? How do these relate to the messages of each Eleanor Clarke Slagle Lecture?
3. Try to summarize each Eleanor Clarke Slagle Lecture in a sentence that captures the main theme. Complete the sentence "This lecture was about. . . ."
4. Consider each lecture. Are there common threads among them that you identify? Are there common themes that emerge when you consider these lectures together?
5. Review the biography of each lecturer of this decade (see Appendix A). Read some of the other work by the lecturer to gain an insight to the reasons why each one received this honor.
6. Consider what was happening in the history of the occupational therapy profession at the time of each Eleanor Clarke Slagle Lecture. Appendix C provides some useful bibliographical references for the history of the profession in the United States, and Appendix D has references for the global history of the profession.

7. Review what each president of the American Occupational Therapy Association presented as his or her vision for the profession at the time of each Eleanor Clarke Slagle Lecture. (A list of these presidents appears in Appendix E.) How do the lectures relate to these visions? The presidents addressed the profession through several forums, including columns in the *American Journal of Occupational Therapy,* such as "President's Address," "Nationally Speaking," and "The Issue Is."

8. Review each lecture in light of the *AOTA Centennial Vision.* What themes of the *Vision* stand out the most? What additional insights into the *Vision* do the lecturers offer?

Discussion Questions

1. Toward the beginning of her lecture, Stattel stated that "knowledge . . . can be secured by correlating and strengthening our beliefs with facts. Empirical methods should be tested when possible, and reasonable doubts should be eliminated." Evaluate how Stattel illustrated this in her lecture. What empirical support did she give for the equipment about which she spoke?

2. Consider the equipment you use in your practice. What empirical support is there for its use? How might knowing this empirical evidence affect what you do in practice?

3. While discussing bilateral tilt tables, Stattel stated, "The body will follow the dictates of the mind and the mind will follow the dictates of the body when it is fatigued, but the subject controls both." Explain what she meant by this statement, and describe 2 examples from your practice that illustrate or contradict this statement.

4. A main philosophical value of occupational therapy is the belief that meaningful activity connects a person's efforts with the product of his or her hands. Explain how Stattel built upon this philosophical value in her lecture. Then explain why you agree or disagree with her perspective.

5. Another fundamental value of occupational therapy is the concept of "holism" (or "wholism"). How did Stattel's lecture represent this value? Did she refer to it directly, or was the value implied? How do you think the use of equipment in the profession has (or has not) contributed to the survival of this value in contemporary occupational therapy practice?

6. Sokolov called for action from fellow occupational therapists in several areas throughout her lecture. Select 1 area and discuss its relevance then and today. What has changed since then? What is the same?

7. Sokolov spoke about the medium used in occupational therapy being secondary to the motives and drives directing the actions of occupational therapists. Do you think this way of thinking has changed? Where do you see those changes, or in what ways do you think this view remains?

8. Compare the role of the administrator that Sokolov described with how you have experienced administration in occupational therapy in the present. How can you explain any differences or similarities?

9. In the second paragraph of her lecture, Brunyate stated, "An occupational therapist is, after all, merely a tool through which the doctor treats his patient. The value of the therapist can be judged only in the soundness of his contribution to treatment—for this is the culmination of his professional training." What do you think about this statement, and why do you think Brunyate stated this?

10. Brunyate listed 20 different factors "so common and so little that they have a tremendous effect upon us all." Choose the 3 you think are the most important to consider today and explain why you believe so.

11. How did Rood use the concepts of reciprocal innervation, following developmental sequences, and resistance to stress to explore aspects of physical, emotional/spiritual, intellectual, and professional development?

12. What were Rood's views on theory versus technique? How would these views impact occupational therapy student education today if they were implemented?

13. In the first paragraph of her lecture, Wegg stated, "The principles of occupational therapy established by our pioneer occupational therapists, and most particularly Eleanor Clarke Slagle, have given us the foundation upon which to build advanced techniques and approaches." Do you think work evaluation truly

depicts what the founders intended occupational therapy to be? In what ways do you think work evaluation supports the foundation, or is in conflict with the foundation? Provide examples from the literature to support your argument.

14. Wegg spoke of many changes to the role of occupational therapists, specifically of a shift from medical to vocational programs. How did the role she described compare to the role established by the founders of the profession, and how does it compare to the current role of occupational therapists? How do you think this "shift" influenced the relationship of occupational therapy with other professions?

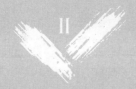

II

THE 1960s
Theoretical Flourishing

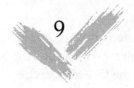

9

Historical Context of the 1960s

Around the World

The Cold War continued to dominate the international scene during the 1960s, marked with escalating standoffs around the globe that brought the United States and Soviet Union to the brink of direct warfare. Although Cuba, East Germany, and Vietnam were the most serious hot spots, smaller confrontations took place elsewhere as well.

In 1960, Prime Minister Fidel Castro of Cuba signed an agreement with the Soviet Union for $100 million for sugar and credit against future purchases. The United States dramatically cut its import of Cuban sugar, and U.S. President Dwight Eisenhower vowed never to permit a regime "dominated by international Communism" to exist in the Western Hemisphere. To counter this "American economic aggression," Castro nationalized American banks and large businesses in Cuba (Ambrose & Brinkley, 1997, p. 371). The United States responded with an embargo on all Cuban exports, and Soviet Prime Minister Nikita Khrushchev threatened to use his country's rockets to protect Cuba from potential U.S. intervention. Despite this threat, newly elected U.S. President John F. Kennedy supported a Cuban invasion at the Bay of Pigs in 1961 undertaken by 1,600 Cuban exiles trained by the CIA to overthrow Castro. The invasion was a dismal failure, and the invaders suffered heavy losses.

Tensions between the United States and Soviet Union peaked the following year when aerial surveillance showed Soviet offensive nuclear missile and bomber bases in Cuba. Kennedy ordered that Cuba be surrounded and quarantined to prevent further Soviet shipments from reaching the island. The Soviet Union promised to remove its missiles from Cuba if the United States removed its nuclear missiles from Turkey. Although President Kennedy publicly rejected the proposal, the missiles in Turkey were quietly removed. The Cuban blockade ended, and the Soviets dismantled their missile sites. The American embargo of Cuba continues to this day.

By the late 1960s, numbers of missiles and warheads were so high in both the United States and the Soviet Union that each country was quite capable of destroying the other's infrastructure. Thus, a balance of power system known as "mutually assured destruction" came into being. It was thought that the possible consequences of a general thermonuclear war were so deadly that neither power would risk initiating one. The two countries kept each other in check by maintaining this balance.

By 1960, West Germany's recovery from World War II was touted as an economic miracle when its industrial production reached 176% of prewar levels. However, U.S., British, French, and Soviet forces continued to occupy Berlin. After Kennedy asked Congress for a dramatic boost in number of troops and financial resources to "meet the worldwide Soviet threat" (Kennedy, 2000, p. 21), East German authorities, under pressure from the Soviet Union, closed the border between East and West Berlin in 1961. To stop the mass exodus of East Berliners to the West, the East German government built the Berlin War in August of that year. In a visit to Germany later that year, President Kennedy pledged support for efforts to defend West Berlin from Communist encroachment and to some day reunify. The Berlin Wall stood for more than 30 years.

Vietnam's civil war increasingly caused international concern. Late in 1960, after losing the presidency to a military coup, the Vietcong (Vietnamese Communists) organized the National Front for the Liberation of South Vietnam. The following year money provided by the United States helped South Vietnamese government forces launch operations to eliminate Vietcong guerillas. At the same time, reports emerged suggesting that Communist North Vietnam was supporting the Vietcong. When American forces in the region came under attack in 1963, U.S. President Lyndon B. Johnson ordered covert U.S. naval actions in North Vietnam and in 1964 ordered the bombing of North Vietnamese bases in retaliation for continued attacks on U.S. forces, under the Gulf of Tonkin Resolution.

The United States continued to pour military resources into South Vietnam to restrain the mounting infiltration of the Vietcong. In 1965, building on the Tonkin Resolution, Johnson announced that the United States would stand next to the South Vietnamese people in resisting the Communist North Vietnamese aggression and adopted a policy of massive bombing on Vietcong targets. By July of that year, 125,000 U.S. troops were in Southeast Asia, and Johnson had announced a doubling of draft calls. Although U.S. popular sentiment was increasingly turning against involvement in Vietnam, the war continued with heavy casualties for several more years until a partial ceasefire in 1968 after the Tet Offensive in January of that year, which had been intended to speed peace talks in Paris. However, the following year the more than 600,000 U.S. and allied troops in the region escalated the war in Vietnam when peace talks failed to progress.

Although the Cold War was a dominant concern of this decade, it was not the only important current of the 1960s. The movement for independence and formation of self-directed governments of colonized Africa continued amid much localized turmoil. Critics argue that these events garnered little international attention because they did not represent major threats to the economic interests of either superpower. However, these events evolved into crises of international proportion in later decades. Civil war was already imminent in many countries, including Congo, Ethiopia, Burundi, Rhodesia, Ghana, Sudan, and Somalia.

In addition, tensions between Arabs and Israelis escalated and several violent military confrontations took place, including the Six-Day War in 1967, which resulted in the closing of the Suez Canal for eight years. Most of these crises brewed slowly out of sight of most of the world and eventually became humanitarian catastrophes in later decades. Further, a cultural revolution was begun by the government in China to assure the growth of "actual socialism" in the nation. By 1966 the Chinese education system had ground to a halt. University entrance exams were canceled during this period, and a very reduced number of people, mostly men, were allowed to advance to tertiary education. Many dissident intellectuals were purged or "sent down" to rural labor camps to be "re-educated."

The political situation around the globe caused the Roman Catholic Church to question its relevance in the world. The Second Vatican Council was probably the most profound event in the modern era of the Roman Catholic Church. Opened by Pope John XXIII in October 1962 and closed by Pope Paul VI in December 1965, the council produced 16 written documents, including four major constitutions. These documents, touching virtually every aspect of the Church's life, were a wellspring of renewal for the church in the modern world. Significantly, mass was no longer conducted in Latin, greater participation of the laity in matters of the Church was encouraged, and clerics became actively involved in social and political struggles around the globe.

In the United States

The 1960s was a crucial decade in the life of the United States. Fear of the "Communist threat" spurred by the Cold War paradoxically grew at the same time that popular sentiment increasingly turned against military action on foreign soil. Lee Harvey Oswald, a Communist sympathizer, shot President John F. Kennedy in November of 1963, spurring rumors of a broader plot that persist to the present. Five years later, Kennedy's brother, Robert F. Kennedy, was assassinated during his presidential bid by Jordanian sympathizer Sirhan Sirhan. Violence on American soil seemed to be an everyday occurrence. However, the civil rights movement was probably the most significant legacy of this decade.

The civil rights movement became increasingly organized throughout the 1960s. A major victory was won in Congress with the passing of the Civil Rights Act in 1960 (P.L. 86–449). However, much work remained to make enactment of this legislation a reality. Black Americans began a series of sit-ins to desegregate lunch counters, and Freedom Rides were staged to press for desegregation on interstate buses. These rides, like most other Black demonstrations, brought violent reprisals from Southern White people. Support for the movement was growing in the North, and the brutal assault by Birmingham police on nonviolent marchers in early 1963 increased the outcry for government action. Kennedy pushed for a more comprehensive Civil Rights Act (P.L. 86–449), which was eventually passed in 1964 and outlawed discrimination in any public facility. In 1965, Congress enacted a tough Voting Rights Act (P.L. 89–110), enabling full participation by Black Americans in federal and local elections.

Discrimination remained after the passing of this legislation but was more economic and informal than legal. The civil rights movement became splintered with disagreements between proponents of nonviolent and more militant tactics. The murder of two important Black leaders, Malcom X and Martin Luther King, Jr., as well as localized race riots in many cities across the country toward the end of the decade, combined to undermine wide support for the movement, and by the end of the 1960s, it had lost some of its impetus. However, the decade saw the appointment of the first Black Supreme Court justice, Thurgood Marshall, by President Johnson.

Suppression in 1964 of a free speech movement at the University of California at Berkeley began a long period of U.S. campus unrest that developed into an antiwar movement that lasted well into the next decade. As military action in Vietnam increased, so did the number of antiwar rallies across the country. University enrollments swelled as young men took advantage of draft deferrals to escape the escalation of war, and campuses were tense with unrest. In 1967, the U.S. government announced that students who participated in antiwar demonstrations would lose their draft deferments. By the end of the decade, radicals had broken off from the peaceful student movement and began planting bombs to protest the continuing war in Vietnam.

Other national movements were boosted or originated in the 1960s. By the beginning of the decade, more than 34% of U.S. women older than age 14 and 31% of all married women were in the labor force. In 1963, Congress voted to guarantee women equal pay for equal work, but little was done to enforce the law. Activists founded the National Organization of Women in 1966 to help gain equal rights.

A national Indian movement increasingly gathered energy for resistance and came to the forefront in 1969 when Indian militants seized Alcatraz Island in the San Francisco Bay and demanded it be given to the Indian community as an initial reparation to all the treaties with Indian Nations the U.S. government had violated over the past century.

A gay rights movement was violently launched in 1969 at New York's Stonewall Inn as homosexuals, bolstered by the free speech movement sweeping the country, protested a police raid on a gay dance club and bar.

As African Americans, women, and other social minorities gained political influence in the 1960s, so, too, did people with disabilities. A pivotal event took place in 1962 when Ed Roberts, paralyzed from the neck down because of a childhood bout with polio, overcame opposition and gained admission to the University of California at Berkeley. Soon several other men and women with disabilities joined him on campus and, with a grant from the U.S. Office of Education, they created the Physically Disabled Students Program, the first of its kind on a college campus. It was, in effect, the beginning of the independent living movement.

As in the previous decade, the Cold War continued to be an incentive for technological development in the country. Privately financed nuclear power plants began to operate, and computers began to be distributed more widely to business offices, universities, laboratories, and other buyers. The laser (*l*ight *a*mplification by *s*timulated *e*mission of *r*adiation) was perfected and used in industry. Reportedly 90% of American households had a television, and the American Broadcasting Corporation began broadcasting in color. The Xerox™ copier began a revolution in paperwork reproduction. In a race to outdo the Soviets, who had already sent a manned flight into space on April 12, 1961, the National Aeronautics and Space Administration launched the first U.S. manned space expedition commanded by Alan B. Shepherd on May 5 of the same year. Three months later the Soviets launched a manned expedition that orbited the earth 17 times. John Glenn made the first U.S. flight to orbit Earth three times the following

February, but it was not until July 21, 1969, that U.S. astronauts Neil Armstrong and Edwin "Buzz" Aldrin became the first humans to walk on the moon.

The 1960s saw continued development of psychotropic medications. Librium sales outdid those of other meprobamates in 1960, but in 1963 Valium was introduced and was more widely prescribed than Librium because of the lack of known side effects. Methadone began being used to help rehabilitate heroin addicts. In spite of this, heroin addiction grew consistently and remained a serious source of crime in many cities.

In 1962, the first successful measles vaccine was produced, although it was not released until 1966. In addition, this decade saw the initial successful attempts to use artificial hearts during surgery (1963) and to transplant human hearts (1967). The Medicare Act (P.L. 89–97) was signed by President Johnson on July 30, 1965, setting up the first government-operated health insurance program for more than 25 million senior citizens. Overall, the cost for health care in the United States escalated because billing went unchecked and physicians ordered countless tests to protect themselves from lawsuits.

With expanded use of psychotropic medications, there was a major reform in public mental health services, and the medical community continued its movement toward community mental health. Deinstitutionalization was an effort to dismantle and close state mental hospitals and to supplant them by a network of community-based mental health services. Not all communities were ready to receive these people, however, and in many instances, deinstitutionalized patients were forced to live in rooming houses, inner-city hotels, nursing homes, and chronic-care facilities. The few remaining state hospitals saw severe budget cuts, with funds redirected to community-based programs or out of the mental health system altogether. Substandard conditions at institutions for people with mental retardation were exposed in the media, and in 1961 President Kennedy appointed a special President's Panel on Mental Retardation to investigate the status of these people and make reforms in the services they received. In 1963, Congress passed the Mental Retardation Facilities and Community Health Centers Construction Act (P.L. 88–164), authorizing federal grants for the construction of public and private nonprofit community mental health centers.

Although there were some advances in mental health services, conditions remained particularly dismal for people with developmental disabilities. In 1966, Burton Blatt and Fred Kaplan published a landmark book, *Christmas in Purgatory*, documenting the appalling conditions at state institutions for people with developmental disabilities. During this decade 25 states still had sterilization laws for people labeled mentally retarded, and in the majority, sterilization was compulsory. Although in some states such laws were repealed, such sterilization continued well into the 1970s.

Although changes in attitudes and services for people with mental illness were slow to change, the 1960s saw several significant advances in the way in which people with physical disabilities participated in society. Social Security Amendments in 1960 (P.L. 86–778) eliminated the restriction that disabled workers receiving Social Security Disability Insurance benefits had to be younger than age 50, and the Social Security Amendments of 1965 (P.L. 89–97) established Medicare and Medicaid to provide federally subsidized health care to disabled and elderly Americans covered by Social Security.

In 1961, the American National Standard Institute, Inc., published the *American Standard Specifications for Making Buildings Accessible to, and Usable by, the Physically Handicapped*. This landmark document became the basis for all subsequent architectural access codes, and in 1963 South Carolina passed the first statewide architectural access code. The Urban Mass Transportation Act of 1964 (P.L. 88–365) required that systems accepting federal monies authorized under the act must make those systems accessible to elderly people and people with physical disabilities. Finally, in 1968 the Architectural Barriers Act (P.L. 90–480) required that all buildings built with federal funds must be accessible to people with physical disabilities.

When Ed Roberts became the first student with severe disabilities at the University of California at Berkeley in 1962, more attention was directed toward issues in education of people with disabilities in general. Soon other students across the country joined Roberts, and the University of Illinois initiated its Disabled Students' Program that same year, becoming the first program to facilitate community living for people with severe disabilities. These changes in higher education brought questions about the desirability of separate special education programs in grade schools and high schools. In 1965, parents of children with autism founded the Autism Society of America in response to discrimination, lack of educational services, and the prevailing view of medical "experts" that autism was a result of poor parenting rather than a neurological disability.

References

Ambrose, S., & Brinkley, D. (1997). *Rise to globalism: American foreign policy since 1938.* New York: Penguin.

American National Standard Institute. (1961). *American standard specifications for making buildings accessible to, and usable by, the physically handicapped.* New York: Author.

Kennedy, J. F. (2000). We seek peace but we shall not surrender: Radio and television report to the nation on the Berlin crisis, 1961. In J. F. Kennedy, *The greatest speeches of President John F. Kennedy* (pp. 21–30). Severna Park, MD: Titan.

10

1960 Eleanor Clarke Slagle Lecture

Devices:
Development and Direction

Muriel E. Zimmerman, OTR

Preface

As the sixth occupational therapist to receive the Eleanor Clarke Slagle award, I find myself not without a feeling of great humility as well as one of pride. I am respectful of the achievements and high standards of my predecessors and also of the many other occupational therapists who have made and are making a fine contribution to our profession. Thus I am most honored by this confidence you bestow upon me and hope I shall be worthy of it.

I should be remiss if I did not say that whatever I have learned has not been due solely to my own efforts nor to my own inspiration nor to what I am. For I have been fortunate in knowing and working with so many very wonderful people, each of whom has played a significant role in my growth and understanding. To all of them I am deeply indebted for their faith, encouragement, counseling and guidance which have directed my path. My only regret is that it is not possible to name them here; the list is long and I could not be happy with any omitted. To both professional and personal friends, and to my own understanding family who have suffered growing pains with me, I wish to express my deepest gratitude.

Foreword

We need no temple gong, village bell, television commercial or other fanfare to quicken the pulse and the pace or to get attention for a discussion of the use of mechanical devices or aids which have become by now an integral part of the rehabilitation procedure. We are no longer skeptical as to whether this ought to be the concern of the occupational therapist. We know only too well what has been and can be accomplished for the physically disabled patient by the application of mechanical inventions. And we are fortified in our enthusiasm by rapid technical advances.

Just why we should have waited so long to consider the fact that man has always made use of such skills to help himself is perplexing. It might in part have come when it was recognized that we did not necessarily do the patient a service by doing things for him and that we aided only when we helped him to help himself. Perhaps it could simply have been the result of man's inventiveness coming to his rescue out of necessity, in this area of his life as well as in others. By whatever circumstances it evolved, we can only be delighted that it happened and comforted that from mankind's tragedy came also his means of escape.

Yet not every therapist may have as much time at his disposal as he would like for participation in such helpful procedures. He may also still be meeting some frustration in the form of lack of cooperation from staff in other services and lack of referral. And there may be others who seek more and better ways for advancing the knowledge and skill already available.

Originally published 1960 in *Proceedings of the 1960 Annual Conference,* 17–24, New York: American Occupational Therapy Association.

It is then at this time my pleasure to present a discussion of this exciting aspect of treatment.

During these past ten years of investigation and search into practical and satisfactory devices to help achieve independence for the physically disabled, a basic philosophy and a technical approach to selection of the proper devices have been a natural development. Trial and error methods, if carefully observed and studied, must lend direction to further pursuits. In 1956 I presented to this same body, at the annual conference in Minneapolis, some of my first organized findings. The analysis discussed at that time consisted of the following approach: (1) evaluation of the patient's physical needs; (2) evaluation of the psychological factors involved in use of special devices; and (3) selection and design of suitable materials and methods of fabrication in relation to the first two factors.

It is not my intent to repeat what I have said before, but to present any additional findings that have refined and improved former methods and which still leave a challenge for future growth.

The study of physical needs by analysis of motions used in the performance of various activities has pinpointed for us the specific losses to be compensated for, either wholly or in part. Through observation, the process of eating has been described and charted. This has shown us which motions are used and for what purpose. We have had some indications also as to relative importance of each of the motions, the extent used and whether it is an "active" motion or a "holding" or "stabilizing" motion.

Such studies are naturally based first on motions as observed in a "normally" functioning arm. As such, our analysis seems relatively simple—especially as we all have very similar habits and patterns, due to our common anatomical structure and the fact that we have all been taught a similar way of accomplishing various activities.

We must realize, however, that even normal functioning varies, and since the upper extremity is fitted to perform many activities, the motions that we use for one activity do not necessarily require ALL the movements available. Thus, if we are minus some of the usual motions in eating, for example, we may still easily be able to manage quite satisfactorily. This we can observe frequently in many of our patients. Often the substitutions or variations are hardly discernible or are performed with such efficiency and ease that we are not quick enough to detect them immediately. This is apt to be true when the loss is minimal or when it is confined to only one location or joint. Here, substitution of either another body motion or use of a device is relatively easy to achieve.

But let us take the patient who may have multiple weaknesses or losses, the one who may be classified as having so much and yet so little. Here the dynamics of motion become much more complex. Let me illustrate with the problem as presented by a rather typical disability limitation such as is often found in the patient with quadriplegia as the result of a spinal cord injury. Upon examination it is found that elbow flexion tests good, extension is zero, shoulder flexion is poor or trace, but abduction is fair plus to good minus, supination and pronation are fair, wrist extension is poor plus to fair minus and grasp is zero. There are no range of motion limitations. This patient, if left to his own resources, might be able but for lack of grasp to feed himself, if he were so motivated. But you would probably observe a rather bizarre pattern of motion. The arm would be raised outward by shoulder abduction to shoulder height, then the hand brought in toward the mouth. (One must also remember that in such patients trunk balance is apt to be very poor, so that they cannot bend forward to meet the hand; and wearing a neck collar will further lessen their ability to compensate in this direction.) Another reason why you will find such patients using more shoulder motion than elbow flexion, even though the shoulder is weaker, is that by so doing they eliminate the problem of hitting themselves in the face. This situation is due to lack of triceps muscle, which comes into play after the forearm is raised to a vertical position and then drops toward the face.

According to this report, it would seem that only a substitute for grasp and some assist for shoulder flexion would provide the needed aid and the preferred eating motions. A simple device such as a leather utensil holder or a built-up handle will provide a substitute for grasp. Either an overhead sling with one support under the elbow or a ball-bearing arm support with "flying saucer" used as elbow rest (both standard devices) may be used for providing shoulder flexion positioning.

Such devices, however, have been found to enable only partially satisfactory performance. Too often I have found that the shoulder assist as described above did not accomplish what was expected of it: rather, the patient was frustrated and hampered. Instead of using the support, he is apt to revert to his own substitution; and this bizarre pattern may put undue strain on the shoulder, often bringing on early fatigue and sometimes pain. Why is not the flexion assist as described helpful? We have observed two principles of dynamics which seem to contribute to this happening. One is the result of the type of device used to substitute for grasp. In equipping a patient with a holding device, we must remember that the most frequently used devices position the utensil as though held with a hook grasp rather than pinch grasp. This is not the usual grasp of adults. Also, hook grasp positions the forearm in pronation rather than the mid-supination used in pinch grasp. As a result, when picking up the food, because further rotation of the forearm is impossible, some rotation and abduction of the shoulder is usually necessary. This automatically lifts the elbow from any support provided. Once lifted, the natural tendency is not to lower the elbow to the support and use elbow flexion to bring the hand to the mouth, but to continue shoulder abduction and, as described before, bring the hand to shoulder height and then toward the mouth.

What then should be done? A holding device utilizing pinch grasp may be provided, although thus far any device made for this purpose is far more complicated than those designed for the hook type of grasp. If a fork is used, the tines can be turned down rather than up. Or the fork end can be bent downward. This works very well unless the food is too soft or slippery in which case it may be lost before the fork is partially raised. Some wrist flexion and ulnar deviation may be used as a substitute, and the normal individual would employ these other motions. But when some weakness of the wrist is present, wrist strength is apt to be utilized mainly for a stabilizing force, which is also one of its purposes. The presence of a wrist splint may impose further limitations.

Of the two shoulder flexion positioning assists, I have found the overhead sling with elbow supports the most helpful. The sling ought to be equipped either with a spring of the correct length and tension or with a device to provide similar action. Then, as the elbow is raised up and away from the body, the sling shortens, thus keeping the elbow-piece under the elbow, ready to support it and encourage its use by lowering the elbow before raising the hand to the mouth. This sling support is simple, but it is also conspicuous. Moreover, there must be some conscious effort and cooperation on the part of the patient to make use of the support as intended.

It is rather obvious from the above-presented description of dynamic functioning that we are still in need of better assisting devices. It should remind us that we are dealing with a part of the body in which more than fifty muscles, wonderfully constructed, are working together for an integrated performance. When the loss of function is minimal and confined to one joint or motion only, the problems arising are relatively uncomplicated. Also, when total function is lost, a fairly satisfactory substitute performance can be achieved through a contrived mechanism. Yet, to aid satisfactorily when there is a multiple combination of varying degrees of loss of function, and to keep pace with adjustments needed as function improves, meanwhile making certain that undesirable motion patterns or substitutions are avoided, requires careful evaluation and proper selection of equipment.

Let us further examine this human tool, the upper extremity. To assist mechanically the functioning of all the components of hand and arm requires as varied an approach as mathematical law dictates for possible combinations of the many units involved and the varying degree of participation of each.

An early study made by the engineering department of the University of California was entitled "Studies to Determine the Functional Requirements for Hand and Arm Prostheses." Because of the need to sort out of all of these movements those that would be most useful, the kinematic analysis of the motions of the activities of daily living was one of the main aspects of the study. Those conducting the study scientifically determined, through many engineering processes, the most useful types of hand grasp. Of the two needs, (1) to pick up an object and (2) to hold objects, it was found that the pick-up motion most frequently used a lateral grasp (58 to 34) with the thumb against the lateral aspect of the index finger. The hold-for-use motion most frequently employed a palmar prehension grasp (64.5 to 34) with the pads of the thumb tip and first two finger tips together. It was found that both grasps were about equally employed. However, it was also found that palmar grasp could be used to substitute for picking up many objects normally using lateral grasp. It was not so with substituting lateral grasp for palmar. Therefore the hand prosthesis was designed to provide a palmar prehension as the most useful motion for the hand.[1]

These hand activity requirements would be the same whether a prosthesis or a splint is desired. Hand splints are also designed to provide a palmar prehension type of grasp. This is true of both the Warm Springs type of opponens hand splint and the flexor hinge tenodesis hand splint.

So far, this last analysis has considered only the hand or terminal device. While it can be studied separately, it is also dependent upon arm function for placing it in a position of use. Let us consider each of the arm parts and its contribution to the total hand-arm functioning.

The wrist as a positioning device is well known. Most persons agree that either a neutral or a slight cock-up position, if there need be any limits set, is the most useful. This is perhaps true. However, depending upon the type of object grasped and at what height it is in relation to the body, other factors must be considered in any analysis, such as whether other accommodations are possible, as supination and pronation, internal and external rotation of the shoulder or trunk, or body bending. Again, citing the study by Boetler, Keller, Taylor and Zahn as an example, it takes 42 degrees of supination of forearm for picking up a plate. The action can be accomplished if only 30 degrees of supination are present; however, there must be additional compensations, such as depressing the arm or bending the body to the right.[1] Nevertheless, while this compensation may be anticipated as a possible and satisfactory accommodation in the average amputee, it generally is not possible to expect many persons with frail upper extremities resulting from poliomyelitis or a spinal cord injury to do this.

Elbow flexion and extension are obviously important in most activities and are provided for fairly easily. The motions or various positionings of the shoulder are complex and again, as in the hand, realistic replacement of all of them is almost impossible, at least today. Stabilization against the force of gravity, some flexion and abduction and some internal and external rotation are probably the most useful.

Let us go back for a moment to the selection of a suitable design for a functional splint for the hand. The pinch type of grasp has seemed to prove the most useful, yet the design as now used does not seem to be totally adequate. In various patients we have tested with this device we have found that many objects are still difficult to pick up. The difficulty seems due, largely, to lack of ability to position the hand. And if we observe an amputee using a hook we will find that even with his many arm and body accommodations he may have to pre-position the article. If these accommodations or the ability to position the hand are impossible, then we must often accept limited performance. Just recently a patient whom we were fitting with a splint was experiencing some of these difficulties, and he offered us a suggestion for possible improvement in the present flexor-hinge hand splint, which was designed to position and stabilize the thumb in abduction and hold the interphalangeal joints of the first two fingers in slight flexion. Motion (of a hinge type) is provided at the metacarpal–phalangeal joints. When the wrist is in a cock-up position, picking up objects is difficult. If, however, pinch grasp were provided by stabilization of just the interphalangeal joints of fingers and thumb, while motion (opening and closing of grasp) occurred in both fingers and thumb, then pick up might be easier. This means another moving part and usually that complicates any device. However, the suggestion as mentioned to us is being tried experimentally and a sample splint has been constructed with very good mechanical results at the time of this writing.

We have not had time to use this splint on a patient. Therefore, it is only a first-test model and cannot be classified as good, poor or bad. Rather, it is being shown as an illustration of how, when a specific problem is defined, an attempt may be made to solve it (Figures 10.1, 10.2, 10.3, 10.4). The only results we can state at this moment are that less wrist motion is used and more opening of grasp is obtained. Wrist motion required in the original model was approximately 70 degrees. In the new design, it is 25–30 degrees, or less than half. Opening of grasp was increased from 2 ½ to 2 ⅜ inches. It is possible, however, that the new design may call for greater strength for operation, which could negate the advantages.

Again, we have presented another functional problem to illustrate the extent to which our present knowledge and efforts are still limited, in terms of our needs. A helpful procedure to follow would be (1) to evaluate for loss of necessary motions for a specific activity; (2) to select devices to compensate or substitute for lost motion; (3) to note whether devices provide for a normal functioning of the specific part or whether they

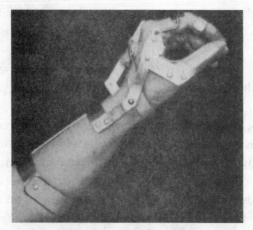

Figure 10.1. Hand splint (old design) with wrist extended and fingers closed.

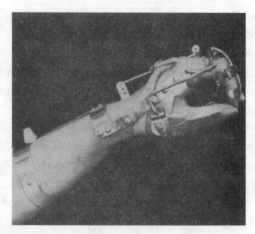

Figure 10.2. Hand splint (new design) with wrist extended and fingers closed.

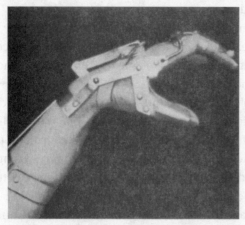

Figure 10.3. Hand splint (old design) with wrist flexed and fingers open.

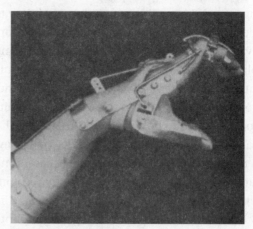

Figure 10.4. Hand splint (new design) with wrist flexed and fingers open.

impose abnormal patterns; and, (4) to note substitute motions imposed because of abnormal patterns and adjust the equipment accordingly.

Such studies as are currently being undertaken by the University of Michigan in their research program on orthotics should be most helpful to all of us concerned with this field of rehabilitation. One in particular[2] is the study of total arm function for specific activities in relation to space, a study being made on a much broader scale than ever before attempted. A parallel might be drawn here with motion studies made in the field of homemaking in which it was shown that the most frequent trips made in the kitchen are between the sink and the stove. The resulting energy-saving principle arising from this situation is that these two pieces of equipment should be placed in close proximity. When this is not done, ways and means of compensating must be provided.

Thus far I have discussed only additional problems of one factor, namely, that of the study of motion in relation to physical needs. The second factor is that of the psychological implication of devices to the patient.

Many of the responses of the patient are the same as those he exhibits toward the disability itself and are, of course, the psychologist's concern to evaluate, not ours. But we can recognize also some attitudes directly related to the devices and we ought to be aware of why they make an additional emotional impact. I believe the sociological attitudes of our society are greatly at fault for much of what occurs. The term independence to most of us, for example, is apt to mean sheer physical strength. And in today's world this is not so strange, as often the non-disabled are hard put to keep pace with work and leisure activities of a busy and highly competitive culture. Here, however, is a paradox. Although man thinks of himself as physically capable of taking care of himself, he at the same time strives to help himself more and more with mechanical inventions.

Let us look for a moment at the busy executive. He gathers information, communicates it, and directs much of his business via the telephone, intercommunications system, dictaphone and possibly TV or radar viewing screens. Most of the time while doing this he sits behind a desk in a chair. Physical energy used is at a minimum. This same person, as a good many other citizens of today, probably whisked himself out of bed in the morning, got ready for the day and traveled to work using many other mechanical devices such as modern plumbing, which provides instant hot water at the turn of a tap; an electric razor, electric stove, automatic coffee maker; packaged or frozen foods; a bus, taxi, automobile or subway; and an elevator to lift him from the ground floor to wherever his office is located. Whenever I am in our workshop and glance out for a moment to the towering structure of the Empire State Building, I am reminded of the fact that without elevators this building would be only an empty structure, except for a few rugged individuals; and they would undoubtedly be found on the first ten floors, with just possibly an isolationist above, rejoicing in his ivory tower.

Man has continually striven to extend his power beyond his own physical ability. Could we learn of the heavens beyond our reach without our great telescopes? And now we are designing rockets to take us to these great outer spaces. From the beginning of the discovery of flint and the invention of the wheel, man has steadily reached forth for new and better ways to help himself.

This being so, why should any person resist using devices just at the very time they can mean so much to him? Let us look at the other side of the picture. The ideal of the anatomically perfect person is shouted at us from the pictures and slogans of advertising, from road signs, magazines, radio and television. So the need for outside assistance is like adding insult to injury. If any of us has any doubt of the real importance of this trauma to the ego of the individual, I can ask you to reflect on how so many of us react to the more or less accepted use of eyeglasses, hearing aids and even certain easily recognized styles of clothing. Spectacles are given all sorts of added glamor in the form of color, shape and decoration; or contact lenses deny the presence of glasses altogether. Hearing aids are mounted behind the ear, some on the ends of spectacle bows to make them less conspicuous. I have come across an advertisement by a hairdresser in which he showed hair styles designed to hide a hearing aid. And certainly the manufacturers of our nationally advertised commodities make use of a real or fictitious person who represents the American ideal to enhance selling appeal. Have you ever noticed how often this person is a handsome Adonis or a rugged outdoor sportsman or both? Why do we cling to such ideals? Probably because physical perfection represents strength and beauty. We still need reminding that there are other types of strength and beauty besides that which we see—goodness, truth, achievement and thoughtfulness.

It is all too infrequently that we see an advertisement representing these other qualities. But we do have them occasionally. One that I clipped showed the "egghead" modeling a new style boy's shirt. A well-known magazine, which is famous for typifying the American public, showed on its cover the college campus with the girls clustering around the top science student while the football hero passed by unattended. And some of my colleagues may have heard me comment on one of the cigarette ads which purports to appeal to the "thinking man." (Even so, the "thinking man" shown usually has a spectacular hobby.)

We must remember that ages ago, when many of these concepts had their origin, brute strength was important. Survival often depended upon it. And we must admit that in those days it was man's greatest attribute. The person who survived by his wits was rare. Because of these occasions brains were given a high regard even then. But there was little opportunity to use them and physical labor was paramount. Today, we live in a different age, a highly mechanized one. We employ all our ingenuity and skill to improve our lot. Is there really much difference between the robot arm which aids the man in the atomic laboratory to handle radio-active material and the artificial muscle and CO_2 which enable a powerless hand to pick up and hold the objects necessary to his daily activities? There is nothing really unique in the dependence of the physically disabled upon equipment except in the degree and type of design for operation. And it would be helpful to all of us if we could remember the philosophy of Antoine de Saint Exupery that just as man has created these many tools that he uses, he is also master of them and slave only when ignorance and prejudice keep him from trying to help himself.[3]

It may seem that I have been talking rather at length concerning man's use of mechanical aids. However, if we are going to be working with patients who need such equipment, then we cannot lightly ignore such influences but must deal with them. We do our patient no service by stating merely, "He is uncooperative" or "He does not wish to help himself," and by feeling that he must automatically consider us the angel of deliverance from his problems.

What can we do then to make these devices acceptable to the disabled? I believe there are several definite courses of action to take. One method of making equipment more palatable is to introduce it into the treatment program as early as possible. This takes away from that stigma of being "the last resort," which is inevitable if devices are sought only after all other measures have failed. It is easier to accept help in the beginning with the hope that it may be discarded later—as well it may be, for recovery comes for some—and it has been found that devices can have some part in enhancing the possibility of recovery of skills. Also, familiarity with equipment can lessen the threat of its continued use, if such is the need. Let me give one example to illustrate the early use of devices.

Sometime last spring I was confronted with a challenging situation which called for definite action. A patient in his early twenties, a first-year medical student and a victim of Guillain-Barre syndrome, was referred to the service for evaluation in terms of supports and other self-help equipment for the upper extremities, both of which had very little muscle power in shoulders or elbows. The wrists and hands were fairly good, although not completely normal.

I first introduced myself and explained the function of our service. Whereupon the patient turned to me and stated very positively, "Of course, you realize I shall have no need of your services because by September I shall be completely well and back in medical school!"

Before I could make any comment he continued, "And I may as well tell you that in the other hospital, where I was before coming here, the occupational therapist tried to rig me up in all sorts of contraptions, treating me like a hopeless cripple."

I gulped inwardly, thought fast, and then replied, "Well, you are quite right in that devices are designed to help the person who is or may be permanently disabled to become independent; but they are used in other ways as well. They can be set up as therapeutic agents to provide independence while one is working on a treatment program. Can you, for instance, feed yourself now?"

The reply was, "No." So I explained that I could provide him with a device with which he could do this. The device, if properly set up, would do nothing for him that he could do for himself. It would only substitute for those motions that he could not make now. And as soon as any progress was made, adjustment would be made in the device accordingly, to gradually lessen the assistance as he became able to take over. He was then asked whether he would like to see the equipment. He agreed and was willing to give it a test. He was fortunately so impressed that we were able to set up the equipment for his use. For several days he was visited regularly to check whether everything was satisfactory. He was then left to continue its use. Later, at an opportune time, I visited him again to see whether any changes were needed. When I remarked that possibly we might consider some lessening of the assistance, the reply was, "Oh, let's not do it yet!" The patient continued to use the equipment and gradually less and less assistance was needed. Today, fortunately, the patient does not need any aid for the upper extremities. It is not to be inferred that the apparatus provided was solely responsible for return of strength and function. Many other treatment measures were being provided simultaneously. But the patient was able to start performing many activities very early, and it can be assumed that the devices were contributory and did enhance other programs by providing early coordinate use of the arms and build-up of tolerance and skill.

In addition to the early use of devices, there are other measures that can be taken to insure their success and value. We can and should make the best devices possible. We must first be certain they will really serve the purpose for which they are intended; the study of motion, as described, helps to determine this. Then we must ask ourselves whether the device is performing as efficiently as possible. Is its operation simple? Free from breakdown or need of frequent adjustment? Within the understanding and grasp of the operator after a minimal amount of practice and supervision? Or is it inconspicuous, so as not to attract undue attention? Is it as near to the accepted mode as possible without being freakish? Is it cosmetic and attractive? In regard to the improvement made in eyeglasses, for instance, it should be recognized that not all the recent advances are a result of our need for ego-building or just to keep up with the Joneses, although we cannot deny this aspect of the picture. The use of color is pleasing and satisfying, and that, as well as the shape, can either add to or detract from one's appearance. And perhaps most important is design for function. Contact lenses certainly were originated with that purpose in mind. They are much more simplified than glasses and reduce the breakage hazard. They eliminate possible discomfort from pressure irritation on the nose or ear as well as interference of vision from the frames.

Modern designers are more and more alert to function and efficiency. While they do not yet advertise many of their products as designed for the person with a physical limitation, they do promote the fact that they require only one hand to operate and thus will take less effort to do the job. The development of improvements in kitchen and household equipment has been a real boon to any homemaker whether physically impaired or not. The major reason we have been so happy about our new Functional Home for Easier Living is that its selection and adjustment of features do provide easier living for anyone.

If you wish to remind yourself some time of these various requirements of equipment, let me suggest a simple method. Just ask yourself what you would demand. Let us look at clothes. Function and versatility: as few pieces as possible to serve as many needs as possible; easy and quick to put on and take off; design or style in keeping with today's fashion trends; becoming to you; wearability and ease of care; "travel-a-bility"; and, of course, a price within your budget.

These are high goals and to provide all of these answers is not yet totally within our scope. But if we try to do our best, so may the patients be more willing to try also.

There are two other brief thoughts that I cannot exclude. One is that although we must do everything possible to provide equipment to aid our patients, if this is the answer to their problems, we should never try to impose anything upon anyone just because it is one way of giving assistance. All equipment has its limitations and must be judged according to its usefulness and the need for it as against the disadvantages. Socio-economic factors also must be considered. A favorite story of ours at the Institute is that of the patient referred to ADL for dressing activities who finally said, "But do I have to learn to dress myself now when I've always had and will have a valet to do it for me?" Electric wheel chairs, as helpful as they are, are not the answer for persons going home to remote areas or underdeveloped countries where as yet no facilities for repairs or adjustments are available.

The last factor is that of patient participation. Full explanation from us of what is to be accomplished, leading to understanding by the patients, is the easier road to acceptance. In these busy days we often let lack of time rob us of this responsibility. Also needed is the willingness to listen to the patient, to his ideas or complaints. The patient not only feels that you are interested in him, but you may discover many interesting facts and learn better ways of doing things. For after all, it is the patient who is experiencing the satisfactions or difficulties of devices made for his help.

The third and last factor in selection and provision of equipment is the fabrication or construction of the device itself. Again, this is an area that I have already covered previously and therefore I shall not make more than a brief resume.

It is important to know something about materials and principles of construction design and to evaluate this information in terms of the tools, the time, and the personnel and skill at our disposal. While devices are becoming more and more available as more people enter the field professionally, the occupational therapist, I believe, still has a role to play, if not in construction, then in understanding so as to improve his ability to work with the team in evaluating, testing and training.

The engineer does not select or choose at random the various materials he uses, nor create a design out of idle fancy. He uses fundamental principles regarding properties of materials and laws of mathematics and physics. Even the clothing designer relies on more than just the need for a new fashion. As it was expressed to me by a well-known dress designer, a sure sense of such things as the very "feel" of a material, which suggests the "hang" and "hinge" of the weave—the pull and tension of the threads themselves—is basic to good design.

And we can make another contribution. This is to seek and find the different types of devices that will meet the needs of many different disabilities and many activities and will satisfy the various other demands of a majority of the disabled, their therapists, doctors and families. Upon such a basis, and by means of the production line, manu-facturers will eliminate some of the higher costs of today's individual construction. At present, because some pro-duction is limited and prices therefore high, we have a tendency to complain that this goal is not being achieved. But we must remember that their inability to provide us with lower costs is in large part directly related to our own inability to accomplish the above and thereby come into some accord on what we want.

To appreciate fully the manufacturer's problem, let me give you a simple illustration. I asked our staff to tell me how long it would take them to make an ordinary spring-clip clothespin. Estimated time was from one-and-a-quarter to six hours. Obviously, various levels of skill are represented here and must affect the cost of labor which, if figured accordingly, would run from $1.75 to $6.00 for this one simple, dime-a-dozen clothespin. Man-ufacturing costs also are high for a single clothespin, for making the necessary jigs may take longer than to make a whole clothespin. The only answer to this lies in quantity production.

This can only be desirable, for it is also an answer to helping more patients. We must recognize and accept with standardization, however, the fact that there will always be the extreme deviations from the average or norm, which will leave us with some unanswered problems requiring special solutions. And, as with all standardization, we must never fall into the trap of believing we have found our final goal. There must remain the challenge of further improvement.

It is within this last framework of thought that I would like to call attention, before I close, to the contribu-tions of research and special studies and the place of the occupational therapist in these endeavors. When I, as an occupational therapist, entered the field of self-help devices, there were no specific boundaries or limitations as to who should be doing this work or how it was to be done. With time, we are lending direction to how it should be done and, to a certain extent, by whom. The role of the occupational therapist is being defined. It seems necessary, as we shift from the unique to the standard, to fit into the pattern and scheme of organization and teamwork.

Nevertheless, when one problem or set of problems has been solved, automatically new goals are set, new needs discovered. I like to recall the words of Robert Browning.[4]

"Ah, but a man's reach should exceed his grasp,
Or what's a heaven for?"

For occupational therapists looking for new worlds to conquer, there is always one waiting at our finger tips. And while we may not recognize at first where the path lies, if we seek we shall find it.

At a time when there came a deeper recognition of the need for stepped-up development and use of self-help or assistive devices, occupational therapists along with others made available their talents and skill to help find the answers. And out of all these efforts there has been achieved a beginning science of this new field. We recog-nize that we have certain techniques at our disposal: (1) the study of motion requirements for specific activities and how these relate to the possibilities of the total functioning of an individual and to limited function; (2) the understanding of the patient's psychological needs and ways of meeting them and (3) the understanding of mechanical requirements through study of materials and fabrication processes. And, finally, we can come to deter-mine how and where our contributions as occupational therapists will serve most potently in the total process.

Most probably it will be in testing for selection of devices, check out for use, and training. Sometimes, depending upon need and suitability, occupational therapists' skill may be used in fabrication.

In conclusion, we have met our responsibility to the patient who needs devices by lending our resources to this field. We must continue to meet these responsibilities so long as there remains a need for our skills. And finally, we must remain eager to participate in any way where the vision of others or our own vision can create a better world for the disabled.

References

1. Boetler, Keller, Taylor, & Zahn. *Studies to Determine the Functional Requirements for Hand and Arm Prostheses.* Los Angeles, Calif.: Department of Engineering, University of California, July 25, 1947.
2. University of Michigan, Ann Arbor. Orthetics Research Project.
3. Saint Exupery, Antoine de, *Wind, Sand and Stars.*
4. Browning, Robert, *Andrea del Sarto.*

11

1961 Eleanor Clarke Slagle Lecture

Occupational Therapy Can Be One of the Great Ideas of 20th-Century Medicine

Mary Reilly, EdD, OTR

Specifying the Theme

As an occupational therapist honored by her peers, I join my Eleanor Clarke Slagle predecessors in feeling the awesome responsibility of the award. The occasion, it seems to me, makes it obligatory for an awardee to objectify a lifetime experience and then speak of an issue of concern to all. With this in mind, I have elected to present an issue which impinges upon the very root meaning of our existence. In developing the idea I have sought to reflect it against the changing background of the world in which we live. My hope is that its exploration will add to an understanding of the profession which we practice.

The question I would like to speak to is one which each one of us has asked at some time or other in our professional lives. Some of us have asked it many times. It has been raised in different ways and expressed in different words, both within and outside our field. In all probability, it will continue to be asked by those who follow us. I am referring to an anxiety about our value as a service to sick people. This theme I have identified by the question: *Is occupational therapy a sufficiently vital and unique service for medicine to support and society to reward?*

The anxiety begins in a primitive form when we stand before our first patient and sense the enormous demands that a treatment problem makes upon the occupational therapy brush, hammer or needle. The wide and gaping chasm which exists between the complexity of illness and the commonplaceness of our treatment tools is, and always will be, both the pride and the anguish of our profession. Anxiety accumulates as we become increasingly involved in treatment, teaching and research, and even more sophisticated questions tend to arise from that same source to plague us.

The theme of today's presentation is focused, therefore, on the critical appraisal of the essential worth of occupational therapy. I say critical because the technique of criticism will be the method by which the issue will be explored. The subject was selected because I found from my experience that the value of occupational therapy exists in a controversial state. Among any group of my colleagues who have practiced long and well, I found that this question of value constituted a continuous and almost lifelong dialogue.

The Theme Converted to an Hypothesis Test

Where and how does one begin to make dependable and hence usable judgments about value? Taking full advantage of the freedom inherent in the Slagle lectureship, I reasoned that the idea most basic to our practice ought to be searched out and then converted into a kind of a question which might be answerable to some degree. This search,

Originally published 1962 in *American Journal of Occupational Therapy, 16*, 1–9.

I further reasoned, should begin in the time of our earliest days. I began there and found that there was a single root idea embedded deep in our foundation and this deeply embedded belief is what we call occupational therapy. In the stormy years between then and now, I found that there were few opportunities given to examine the roots of our foundation and to consider the growth which sprang from it.

My re-examination of our early history revealed that our profession emerged from a common belief held by a small group of people. This common belief is the hypothesis upon which our profession was founded. It was, and indeed still is, one of the truly great and even magnificent hypotheses of medicine today. I have dared to state this hypothesis as: *That man, through the use of his hands as they are energized by mind and will, can influence the state of his own health.* This is the inherited occupational therapy hypothesis passed on for proof by the early founders.

The splendor of its vision goes far beyond rating it as an idea conceived once in a lifetime or even once in a century. Rather, it falls in the class of one of those great beliefs which has advanced civilization. Its magnificence lies in the optimistic vote of confidence it gives to human nature. It implies that there is a reservoir of sensitivity and skill in the hands of man which can be tapped for his health. It implies the rich adaptability and durability of the central nervous system which can be influenced by experiences. And more than all this, it implies that man, through the use of his hands, can creatively deploy his thinking, feelings and purposes to make himself at home in the world and to make the world his home.

For a profession organized around this hypothesis it sets few limits to its growth. It merely endows a group with the obligation to acquire reliable knowledge leading to a competency to serve the belief. Because this is an hypothesis about health, it requires that this knowledge be made available for the guidance of physicians and that it be made applicable to a wide range of medical problems.

The Role of Criticism

Before preparing a brief for its validation I would like to make a detour into a description of the method whereby the issue will be explored. The method is in harmony with my temperament because, by choice, I am neither a conservative nor am I a conformist. I am a devout and practicing, card-carrying critic. Since criticism as a technique of public discussion has yet to emerge in our association affairs, I feel a need to define and describe it. Its philosophy, techniques and tactics will constitute the point of view from which I will speak.

The public use of criticism by a profession has been spelled out best by Merton[1] who sees it as a prevailing spirit within a group necessary to maintain a group's progress. Its greatest usefulness is that it acts to repudiate a smugness which assumes that everything possible has already been attained. Its presence commits an association to keeping its members from resting easily on their oars when they are so inclined. In general, Merton finds that criticism stings a profession into a new and more demanding formulation of purpose and maintains a policy position of divine discontent with the state of affairs as they are.

A disciplined person in either the sciences or the professions uses critical thinking as a personal tool of reality testing and problem solving. When a professional organization as a whole accepts criticism as the dominating mode of thought, then indeed, theorizing flourishes and the intellectual atmosphere of their gatherings is characterized by sweeping controversies. In this atmosphere of controversy, progress becomes somewhat assured.

But a card-carrying critic must do more than merely engage in critical thinking. Judgments made by a critic must emerge from a discreet use of techniques which are difficult to master and dangerous to apply. Basically, the skill is dependent upon an ability to analyze, interpret and synthesize. A critic must have a sharply developed capacity to see deficiencies in data and fallacies in interpretation. The best stock in trade that any critic has is a discerning eye for trends and an ability to pattern and verbalize them. Whether a critic is worth listening to is usually decided by an ability to use language well, by a creativeness in synthesizing new relations and by courage to propose provocative hypotheses. Ultimately, however, a good critic rests his case upon how well he has been able to restructure the issue so that the necessary powers for its resolution can be freed. These idealistic but difficult standards are the ones I hope to follow in restructuring the issue of how valuable is occupational therapy.

Design of the Presentation

Having discussed the point of view from which I will speak, it is now necessary to describe the plan of attack which will be made on this global theme. For the sake of this presentation let us suppose that the hypothesis I have proposed is the wellspring of our profession and that it is worth proving. It would not follow necessarily from this that it is provable. A large part of the power to act on the hypothesis, of course, resides with us, the members of the American Occupational Therapy Association. But the society in which our profession lives holds power too and can rule on its growth. Even before we begin the validation, we must look at the probability that this idea may not be capable of proof in this century. I plan to ask first whether the American culture can tolerate such an hypothesis. Next I shall question whether the 20th Century is the right time for the test. The most crucial aspect of the presentation will be an attempt to identify the point at which the process of proof ought to begin. This will be followed by an attempt to identify the basic pattern of our service by which the hypothesis will be proven. Finally, I shall comment on some ongoing crises which the hypothesis is undergoing and then leave for history its continuing proof.

Is America the Place to Test the Hypothesis?

Let us first consider the tolerance in America for the occupational therapy idea. In his social history, Max Lerner[2] identified certain dynamic forces which impelled the greatness of this country. He cited in the American mind two crucial images present since the beginning. One was the self-reliant craftsman, whether pioneer, farmer or mechanic. He was the man who could make something of the American resources, apply his strength and skill to nature's abundance, fashion new tools and machines, imagine and carry through new constructions. Without taking himself overseriously, Max Lerner's American has generally regarded the great engineering, business, government and medical tasks as jobs to be done. Progress in technology was seen simply as agenda for the craftsman.

The second image Lerner drew was from the American environment. It was that of a vast continent on earth, as in space, waiting to be discovered, explored, cleared, built-up, populated and energized. Lerner contends that our culture is dominated by an American spirit which hates to be confined. A drive toward action, he postulated, is a part of the American character.

This drive towards action seems to me to make reasonable the American idea of a patient. Our cultural concept of the man of action suffers little change when an American moves into a hospital community. It has been supported by a series of principles which merged and fused into what we now call rehabilitation. Early in this century, there emerged the principle in medical management that patients were easier to handle when they were occupied with mild tasks. Later when it was found that an active patient tended to recover faster, early ambulation became an acceptable principle of physiology and blended well with the principle of patient occupation. Concern for the psychological nature of patients brought forth the widespread acceptance of craft, recreation and work programs in hospitals. The need to train patients in self-care became almost a crusade to insure the rights of patients to be independent. Within the community, laymen cooperated in ventures to assure the handicapped's right to return to work. Now we are implementing in full swing the socio-economic principle that it is good business for society to support such programs with public monies.

There are some obvious things which can be concluded about America's tolerance for the occupational therapy hypothesis. It would seem almost axiomatic that the American society in general, and medicine in particular, has need of a profession which has as its unique concern the nurturing of the spirit in man for action. In every way it knows how, America has said that this spirit must be served and served in a special kind of way when it has been blocked by physical or emotional ills. That this need will be persistent in American culture seems fairly certain. That occupational therapy will persist is not quite so certain. It is true, however, that if we fail to serve society's need for action, we will most assuredly die out as a health profession. It is also most assuredly true that if we did dissolve from the scene, in a decade or so, another group similarly purposed and similarly organized and prepared would have to be invented. I believe, therefore, that the occupational therapy hypothesis is a natural one to be advanced in America.

Is the 20th Century the Time?

The timeliness of the hypothesis is the next question I should like to raise. Are we the people and these the times for the test? We are all deeply entangled in the forces and events of the century in which we live. But if this entanglement commits our energies to the endless treadmill of survival, then the hypothesis cannot get off the ground. The social scientists tell us that the world we live in is in a state of indigestion from too much change. We have yet to absorb the disorganizations brought on by a depression, two wars and an ongoing massive technological revolution. This change is being reflected by society into all its component institutions. It follows naturally that we feel its reflection in our professional lives.

But our state of turmoil was not always so, because occupational therapy was born in the quieter times of this century. In the first several decades of our existence, medicine offered us a tranquil and supportive setting. Our literature reveals that physicians tended to nurture the development of our schools and clinics. In these earlier times we were helped to meet the challenges of contributing to the ongoing medical scene. The last several decades, however, have put excessive stress for expansion upon a profession whose role had been barely defined. We have seen our practice organized into specialty fields by the demands of World War II. Our clinicians have only recently been systematized into team behavior by the pressures of rehabilitation. Now in the sixties we are confessing to a mounting sense of confusion and voicing a need for direction. We are keenly aware of the conflicting demands being made upon our practice. The problems that our schools face in digesting the accumulating technical knowledge which practice demands is a matter of growing distress. Caught up in these forces, how free can we be to control our growth?

If we are anxious today, the social scientist offers the explanation that it is because we are now aware that the hopes we had cultivated in gentler times of the past are being threatened by the pace of the world around us. Historians, however, are quick to counter that when times of great change appear, they are forecasting a death to the old and a birth to a new way of life. It is inconceivable that we or any other group with organized intelligence would stand idly by and permit the random destruction of the old and encourage blind birth to the new. Fortunately, most institutions have centralized their action for controlling change through planning groups variously called the Task Force, Master Plan Committee or the Role Definition Study. Our national association has not remained aloof from such efforts and is currently involved in three change controlling studies. As many of us know well, the studies involve professional curriculum and clinical practice, the functions of the organization and the future development of the profession.

We may conclude that we have shown by our action that we have felt the buffeting of great change and are attempting to control it. But how can we know whether the efforts we are making are sufficient and are of the right kind? This difficult question has some partial answers. One common sense answer is that we must recognize the fact that we have grown and have changed as we grew. In our forty years of existence our sense of purpose, our anchorage points have shifted. It is only logical to reason that we will not rediscover a sense of purpose by merely reflecting within our professions the problems of the larger society in which we exist. Few rewards are granted to those who are content to reflect problems. Society demands that its problems be answered. Therefore, to any group which aspires to be a profession, there is placed before it a clear-cut mandate. This mandate says that if we wish to exist as a profession we must identify the vital need of man which we serve and the manner in which we serve it.

I contend that this is the point at which the proof of the occupational therapy hypothesis begins. The reality of our profession depends upon an identification of the vital need of mankind that we serve. How free we are in these troubled times to reconstruct our thinking at this basic level I do not know. But I do know that the crucial nature of our service cannot be spelled out in the loosely constructed way that it is today. I personally have little trust that we can continue to exist as an arts and crafts group which serves muscle dysfunction or as an activity group which serves the emotionally disabled. Society requires of us a much sharper focus on its needs. As the next step in the development of the theme it becomes necessary to make a critical examination of what, if any, vital need we serve.

What Vital Need Is Served?

As the first order of the business at hand we ought to have it clearly in mind what constitutes a vital need. Of all the descriptions of the need states of man which I have heard I like Eric Fromm's[3] the best. He says that needs are an indispensable part of human nature and imperatively demand satisfaction. The need we serve must fall within this category. He says further that they are rooted in the physiological organization of man and consist of hunger, thirst and sleep and that in general they all belong to self-preservation. He proposes a simple, forthright formula of self-preservation which is directly applicable to occupational therapy. According to Fromm, when man is born the stage is set for him. He has to eat, drink, sleep and protect himself from his enemies. Therefore, for his self-preservation he must work and produce. Work, in the Eric Fromm sense, is a physiologically conditioned need and therefore a need to work is postulated as an imperative part of man's nature.

In our forty years of practice we have accumulated some fascinating odds and ends of understanding about the need to work. For example, early in my training I was taught that work was good for people. All people needed to work and sick people even more so. This kind of justification of service reminds me of the old story about the man who died and woke up surrounded by all kinds of delights which were his for the mere bend of the finger. After he had satiated himself well, he called for the headman, expressed his appreciation for the manner in which he was treated and then said, "Now that I have pleasured myself well, it is my wish to do something. My good man, what is there for me to do in this paradise?" The answer given to him was, "You are doing it now." "But," replied our man, "I must do something or else my stay in heaven will be intolerable." "Who" replied the headman firmly, "said that you were in heaven?" In the past I have been guilty of believing and having my patients persuaded that work was good and heaven would prove me right. The rationale that man works because it is good for him, regardless of its comfort to us, makes little contribution to our understanding of work as a basic need.

During the thirties, the economic depression gave us an unparalleled opportunity to learn that when able people could not find work, certain psychological disorganization occurred. These changes were deemed to be over and above the changes which could reasonably result from economic loss. We are able to generalize from the depression that human nature does not thrive in idleness. In the last several decades we have accumulated a few more broad generalizations. One is that the stress of work produces psychosomatic conditions in modern businessmen. Another generalization which is now being formulated is that when people retire from their work, they retire from life itself.

A vital need to be occupied however, is not to be inferred from such global generalizations. It is being left to the more rigorously controlled experimentations to do this. Now under laboratory conditions man's need-state for action is being rigorously investigated. In the United States and Canada basic research is going on in an area called sensory deprivation. The work began in reaction to the Russian brainwashing attempts. The research was designed on the principle of restricting man's interaction with the ongoing world of reality. Under controlled conditions of isolation man was found to suffer profound disturbances of his thought processes. In isolation men regressed to unrealistic and prelogical modes of behavior. The sensory deprivation findings suggest strongly that the concepts of man's response to his environment must be sharply revised. The behavioral aberrations which were observed in the idleness of depression and retirement, and the stress of overwork, appear to have been confirmed by the laboratory induced sensory deprivations. The data were checked out by neurologists, psychiatrists, biochemists, pharmacologists, mathematicians and engineers.

The final sensory deprivation report sums up to a concept that the mind cannot continue to function efficiently without constant stimuli from the external world. The central nervous system is now seen as a complex guessing machine oriented outward for the testing of ideas. The experimenters postulate that each individual constructs a different development pattern with respect to strategies for dealing with reality. Jerome Brauner,[4] as one of the researchers, concluded that early sensory deprivation prevents the formation of adequate models and strategies for dealing with the environment. Later sensory deprivation in normal adults, he suggests, disrupts the vital evaluation process by which one constantly monitors and corrects the strategies one has learned to employ in dealing with the environment.

To summarize at this point, it seems to me that the American drive toward action as identified by Max Lerner and the human drive toward work as identified by Fromm have been verified in the laboratories. I believe that we are on safe ground right now to say that man has a vital need for occupation and that his central nervous system demands the rich and varied stimuli that solving life problems provides him and that this is the basic need that occupational therapy ought to be serving.

What Is the Unique Service?

A profession, however, must do more than identify the need it serves. There is a twin obligation to spell out its unique pattern of service. The next gigantic task which this presentation faces and with some trepidation, because of the limitation of time, is an attempt to identify the basic pattern of our service by which the hypothesis may be proven. The charge is gigantic because it makes it obligatory to define the occupational therapy body of knowledge, its treatment process and techniques.

A search for valid content, process and methods has been my preoccupation in the past ten years of reading, study and practice. If I had the ability to do all this with any degree of clarity, I would not be here talking about it. I would be in a clinic doing it. However, I am now admitting to a rising sense of satisfaction in the project and a receding sense of frustration. At no time in technological history have the behavioral scientists been producing so much knowledge directly applicable to our field as they are now. The material is emerging from sources as divergent as neurological theory, animal psychology, developmental and personality theory and from psychologists as diverse as Allport, Murphy, Harlow, Hebb, Goldstein, Piaget and Schlachtel.

In order to plunge directly into this material I am going to have to make use of a device in logic known as a First Principle. For if we were to have a First Principle in occupational therapy it would provide us with a way to specify our knowledge. To those who may not be familiar with the meaning of First Principle, it is a device in reasoning to account for all that follows. For instance, the idea of God is a First Principle which accounts for the Universe. There has been a First Principle postulated to explain the nature of man. We are told that the first duty of an organism is to be alive. Medical science derives its premise from this first law of life. If it were not desirable to cure disease and prolong life, the rules of science and the skills and practice of medicine would be irrelevant. The second duty of an organism is to grow and be productive. Occupational therapy ought to derive its premise from the second law of life. If it were not desirable to be productive, the skills and practices of occupational therapy would be irrelevant.

These two laws merge into a concept of function which asserts that both the existence and the unfolding of the specific powers of an organism are one and the same thing. This concept of function is expressed as: the power to act creates a need to use the power, and the failure to use power results in dysfunction and unhappiness. The validity of the First Principle is easily recognizable in the physiological functions of man. Man has the power to talk and move, therefore, if he were prevented from using the power, severe physical discomfort would result. Freud utilized this First Principle to build a powerful theoretical position from which emotional illness was so successfully attacked. He accepted man's biological necessity to produce and generalized that when sexual energy was blocked, neurotic disturbances resulted. He endowed sexual satisfaction with all-encompassing significance. He developed his theory of sexual satisfaction into a profound symbolic expression of the fact that man's failure to use and spend what he has is the cause of sickness and unhappiness. The Freudian theory that human action is primarily sexually based has thrown a strong but restrictive shadow over other behavioral fields. It has been only lately that attention has been given to human productivity in non-sexual areas. Occupational therapy's focus, it is asserted here, lies in the non-sexual area of human productivity and creativity.

In Gardner Murphy's[5] brilliant defense of human productivity he makes us aware that there is a distinct path which leads to becoming human. This path is not seen as being sexually directed. The direction lies largely in the enrichment and elaboration of the sensory and motor experience and the life of symbolism which depends upon them. He maintains that the sheer fact that we have a nervous system, the sheer fact that we can learn, means that we can prolong and complicate sensory and motor satisfactions, can make them richer, can give them more connections, can avoid boredom, can recombine them, can feed upon them, can become immersed in them and make them a part of ourselves. In all these respects, Murphy says man is most completely human. His primary thesis is that man achieves satisfaction in using what he has, in using the equipment that makes him human; and this entails not only the sensory and motor equipment but that central nervous system upon which the learning and thinking processes depend.

Murphy's spirited description of the conditions necessary for being human can provide the basis for an occupational therapy First Principle. This logic constitutes our mandate to discover and organize our body of knowledge; to develop a treatment process; and to devise techniques for its application to the health of man. The logic of occupational therapy rests upon the principle that man has a need to master his environment, to alter and improve it. When this need is blocked by disease or injury, severe dysfunction and unhappiness result. Man must develop and exercise the powers of his central nervous system through open encounter with life around him. Failure to spend and to use what he has in the performance of the tasks that belong to his role in life makes him less human than he could be. With this principle in mind I would like to summarize my thoughts of the last several years of work on our body of knowledge, our treatment process and techniques.

Regarding the Body of Knowledge

Because our profession is focused on influencing the health of people there will always be a need to include in our body of knowledge the fundamental material of anatomy, neurophysiology, personality theory, social processes and the pathological states to which these functional areas are subject. However, I do not feel this is our unique content. We should have as a special contribution a profound understanding of the nature of work.

Knowledge of work capacity lies scattered over many behavioral fields. We do know, for instance, that man's ability to work has been developed in the long evolutionary process. It began when man hunted and fished for his food and continued as he grew his food and fabricated objects for his comfort. The lot of man was considerably improved when he freed himself from arduous labor through tools and machinery. His comfort was immeasurably assured by the social institutions he built and operated with increasing skill over the centuries. It is my contention that this evolutionary process, plus a bit more, is present, symbolically expressed in today's culture. The concept of work capacity as being an outgrowth of an evolutionary process I call the phylogenesis of work. I believe that cultural history of work ought to be deeply embedded in the occupational therapy body of knowledge and its phylogenetic nature considered particularly in program building.

We know that as a child grows, he recapitulates the history of his race in the stages through which he himself must pass enroute to maturity. The need to pass through phylogenetic experiences in work is necessary for mature work capacity to be developed. There is historical evidence that a child's ability to play, to explore his environment, to exercise his motor skills are the foundation for his later school experiences. The problem-solving processes and the creativity exercised in school work, craft and hobby experiences are the necessary preparations for the later demands of the work world. Because we know that the random movements of the infant progress in developmental sequence toward the job competencies of the mature adult, I postulate an ontogenesis of work. I believe that the ontogenetic nature of work ought to be considered in the case study approach to each treatment problem.

The occupational therapy body of knowledge should include therefore, an understanding of the developmental nature of the sensory-motor systems, the patterning of aptitudes, abilities and interests, the nature of the learning process involved in the acquisition of skills. It should include also an understanding of the developmental nature of the problem-solving process and process of creativity. My epistemological conclusion is that the biological, psychological or social knowledge we select as part of our thinking content must be intermeshed deliberately with the knowledge of work-phylogenesis and work-ontogenesis.

Regarding the Treatment Process

The capacity to work develops in the long socialization process through which a child becomes an adult. It proceeds along the path of growth as man learns to intermesh his motor with his intellectual functions and adapt this integration to the tasks of his life which satisfy his need to control his environment. Work capacity, in this sense, can be said to develop out of the struggle with gravity for motor control, the struggle with learning for manual and mental skills and the struggle with people and people purpose for economic and social control. When the struggle is great, the personal involvement is high; although conflict and frustration are high, so, too, is work satisfaction high. It follows, too, that when involvement is low, work satisfaction is low. The occupational therapy process becomes primarily concerned with that special aspect of the socialization process called work satisfaction. Its approach in treatment is biographical because work satisfaction is, by its nature, the result of past experiences expressed in the present ability to cope with the environment. Its focus is on the meaningful involvement in problem solving tasks or creative performances. The parameters of its concern are the ability to experience pleasure in achievement, to tolerate the frustrations of struggle, to sustain the burden of routine tasks and to maintain the level of aspiration within the reality level of work skills. The goal of the process is to encourage active, open encounter with the tasks which would reasonably belong to his role in life. The process is paced and guided by the supervision of the prescribing physician.

Regarding Treatment Techniques

Techniques which would emerge from the body of knowledge and the professional process as just described would be concerned with program and treatment execution. Methods would include all those administrative techniques of program building which would provide a laboratory setting for human productivity. The treatment technique would be all those procedures associated with modifying sensory-motor dysfunctions, perceptual difficulties and the difficulties inherent in coping with the world of play, work and school. It is suggested in terms of today's thesis that in the merging of our content, process and methods, the unique pattern of our function will be spelled out. If this pattern is focused strongly on man's need to be occupied productively and creatively, the hypothesis will grow stronger.

Major Tests of the Hypothesis

Of all the ongoing tests of the occupational therapy hypothesis, I have selected a few major ones upon which to comment. The first and obvious one is whether a need to accumulate substantial knowledge about human productivity and creativity will be recognized and acted upon in our schools and clinics. The problem of balancing our knowledge has been with us for some time. Until now our attention has been preoccupied with the medical science which supports the application of our craft knowledge to medical conditions. But medical science knowledge is a means for the application of our service and not an end in itself. A profound knowledge of human dynamics of productivity and creativity is the end to which our knowledge ought to be designed. As far as our practice today is concerned, we have more medical science knowledge than we know how to apply and we are applying more knowledge about human productivity than we actually have on hand.

The second, and not so obvious test, is the delimiting effect that psychoanalytical practice has on the promotion of a non-sexual concept of human productivity. The fundamental doctrine of the Freudian pleasure principle is that the essential movement of a living organism is to return to a state of quiescence and that primary pleasure is sought in sensual gratification. A fundamental principle of work is that primary pleasure can be sought through efficient use of the central nervous system for the performance of those ego integrating tasks which enable man to alter and control his environment. In this sense psychoanalytical theory is seen to focus on subjective reality while work theory becomes largely concerned with objective problem-solving reality. It is not that these points of view run counter to each other. They simply do not meet or interact except under very special conditions of intimate supervision by a psychoanalyst.

In 1943 Hendrick[6] raised this issue in the *Psychoanalytic Quarterly*. He argued that the psychosocial activities of the total organism are not adequately accounted for by the pleasure and reality principles when these are defined, in accordance with Freudian tradition, as immediate or delayed response, respectively, to the need for sensual gratification. He suggests that work is not primarily motivated by sexual need or associated aggressions, but by the need for efficient use of the muscular and intellectual tools, regardless of what secondary needs (self-preservation, aggressive or sexual) a work performance may also satisfy. Hendrick postulated a need for a work principle which asserts that primary pleasure is sought by efficient use of the central nervous system for the performance of well integrated ego functions which enable the individual to control or alter his environment.

In psychoanalytic practice today sexual satisfaction is seen as being influenced by ontogenetic, phylogenetic and biographical considerations while no such considerations are seen needed for work satisfaction. Although many analysts have agreed that sexual capacity correlates highly with work capacity, the idea has not been developed much beyond the statement. Work is seen as a kind of experience a patient ought to have and whatever satisfaction he derives from it will be dependent upon his subjective state. As a result, extensive activity programs have grown up around psychiatric treatment which have been designed for participation, but not specifically for ego involvement. These programs are now being called activity programs and those implementing them are called activity therapists.

Such activity programs encourage the participation of large groups and usually appeal to the automatic, learned patterns of behavior. However, activity programs so designed deny the dignity of a human being to struggle, to control his environment as witness the fact that they tend to make man quiescent within the hospital community. They tend to depersonalize, institutionalize and, in general, debase human nature. The occupational therapy hypothesis makes the assumption that the mind and will of man are occupied through central nervous system action and that man can and should be involved consciously in problem solving and creative activity. It is believed that psychoanalytical theory and the occupational therapy hypothesis can profitably co-exist if a work principle is postulated and executed. This will be even more true if occupational therapy deepens its understanding of the phylogenetic and ontogenetic nature of work and make a case study approach to ego involvement of patients. It is not so possible, however, that activity therapy and occupational therapy can co-exist. It is believed that the major crisis in the proof of our hypothesis will not be how to co-exist with psychoanalytical theory but to know the difference between activity and occupation and to act on the knowledge of this difference.

The last major test which I will discuss has to do with the physical disability field. In this specialty we have been placing heavy emphasis upon muscle efficiency and enabling devices. There is a long, perilous and complex ladder to be scaled between neuro-muscular efficiency and work satisfaction. The ontogenetic reconstitution of motor behavior is a tedious process and must be done step by step. It begins at the reflex muscle action stage and proceeds to the development of complex patterns of motor skills which are utilized in a rich variety of work skills. These, in turn, must be disciplined to a sustaining level of tolerance for routine labors. It is upon this broad pattern that human tolerance for working with people in people affairs is built. If any of these steps are missing, they must be re-fashioned and the whole pattern re-shaped accordingly. The proof of the occupational therapy hypothesis in the physical disability field will depend upon how much we know about the process of restoring work capacity. It cannot be done from prescriptions based upon a narrow understanding of human productivity. It cannot be done in cramped clinics dependent upon scrap material. Nor can it be done from our present ignorance of the world of industry for which we believe we are preparing patients. The challenge to the hypothesis in this area is severe, yet provocative. The technical literature of our profession is indicating that this challenge is not being ignored.

Summary and Conclusion

In summarizing the many ideas I have touched or expanded upon in this thesis, I once again return to my original question: *Is occupational therapy a service vital and unique enough for medicine to support and society to reward?* In answering it, I have said that we have had a magnificent hypothesis to prove and if it could be proven, even to some degree, the answer would be that we are valuable to medicine and to society. The hypothesis that I presented for evidence of proof was that *man, through the use of his hands as they are energized by mind and will, can influence the state of his own health.* I asked if this were a kind of idea that America could subscribe to and to that I replied with a resounding yes. I wondered about the stress that the terrible 20th Century was putting on this idea and worried some about the energy left to us to advance it. I suggested the hypothesis would begin its proof when we identified the drive in man for occupation and would continue as we shaped our services to fill that need. I speculated on some of the crises the hypothesis was now undergoing and left the decision not in the lap of the gods but in our own laps for us to think and act upon in our daily practice.

I have said that our profession has a magnificent medical purpose. Whether we shall fulfill it or whether it shall ever be fulfilled I have not said because I do not know. But this I can say from personal experience, that we belong to a profession that requires the mind to look at the history of man's achievements throughout civilization. It requires the spirit to respond to the wonders of what man has accomplished with his hands. It gives us a mandate to apply this knowledge and more to help man influence the state of his own health.

References

1. Merton, Robert K. "The Search for Professional Status." *American Journal of Nursing,* March, 1959.
2. Lerner, Max. *America as a Civilization.* New York: Simon and Schuster, 1957.
3. Fromm, Eric. *The Fear of Freedom.* London, England: Routledge and Kegan Paul Ltd., 1960.
4. Solomon, Philip, & etc. *Sensory Deprivation.* Cambridge, Massachusetts: Harvard University Press, 1961.
5. Murphy, Gardner. *Human Potentialities.* New York: Basic Books, 1958.
6. Hendrick, Ives. "Work and the Pleasure Principle." *Psychoanalytic Quarterly,* Vol. VII:3, 1943.

Bibliographical Notes

Work has been studied from the viewpoint of economics, philosophy, sociology and psychology, and although the literature is considerable, and is being added to constantly, it is a comparatively recent focus for scholars. So far no general study of work has been written, but to some extent a student in this field need not be left entirely without guidance. He needs to remember, however, that the literature is too extensive for one individual to investigate thoroughly. This bibliography noting is designed to serve as an introductory guide. Many of the recommended writings also include full bibliographies of the topic with which they are concerned.

Anyone who seeks to be a student of human occupation should attempt first to build a historical perspective of the field. *A History of Technology,* edited by Charles Singer, E. J. Holmyard and A. R. Hall, is a massive five-volume series published by Clarendon Press in Oxford from 1954 to 1958 and provides a general historical background as far as science, economics and technology is concerned. An account of the effect of labor and technology on the culture of the west is set forth in another series titled *The History of Civilization,* edited by C. K. Ogden and published in New York by Alfred A. Knopf, 1926 to 1929.

The sociological nature of work may be approached through a study of the socialization process and the field of industrial social psychology. This aspect of study is excellently covered in *The Handbook of Social Psychology,* edited by Gardner Murphy and published in two volumes by Addison-Wesley Company in 1952. A recent perceptive and illuminating view of the social and economic nature of work and the worker is presented by *Theories of Society,* Vol. I and II, edited by Parsons, Stills, Naegele and Pitts published by the Free Press of Glencoe, Inc., in 1961.

The specific classics regarding human occupations are exemplified by: Theodore Caplow's *The Sociology of Work* (Minneapolis: The University of Minnesota Press, 1954); Eli Ginzberg's *Occupational Choice: An Approach to a General Theory* (New York: Columbia University Press, 1951); Anne Roe's *The Psychology of Occupations* (New York: John Wiley and Sons, 1956); Donald Super's *The Psychology of Careers: An Introduction to Vocational Development* (New York: Harper and Brothers, 1957) and John Darley and Theda Hagenah's *Vocational Interest and Measurement: Theory and Practice* (Minneapolis: The University of Minnesota Press, 1955).

The classics concerned with human creativity are: Viktor Lowenfeld's *Creative and Mental Growth,* revised edition (New York: The Macmillan Company, 1952); Edwin Ziegfeld's *Education and Art: A Symposium* (Paris: 19 Avenue Kleber, United Nations Educational, Scientific and Cultural Organization, 1953) and Harold Anderson's *Creativity and its Cultivation* (New York: Harper and Brothers, 1958).

The author further recommends: Robert Gagne and Edwin Fleishman's *Psychology and Human Performance* (New York: Henry Holt and Company, 1959); Ernest Schachtel's *Metamorphosis* (New York: Basic Books, 1959); Gordon Allport's *Personality and Social Encounter* (Boston: Beacon Press, 1960); Hannah Arendt's *The Human Condition* (New York: Doubleday Anchor Books, 1959); Erich Fromm's *Man for Himself* (New York: Rinehart and Company, 1945); Gerald Gurin, Joseph Veroff and Sheila Feld's *Americans View Their Mental Health: Number Four* (New York: Basic Books, 1960); and Frederick Herzberg, Bernard Mausner and Barbara Snyderman's *The Motivation to Work* (New York: John Wiley and Sons, 1959).

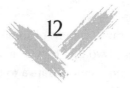

12

1962 Eleanor Clarke Slagle Lecture

The Challenge of the Sixties

Naida Ackley, OTR

It is with feelings of trepidation and humility as well as pride that I take my place in the lengthening procession of Eleanor Clarke Slagle lecturers. Although deeply honored to be the recipient of this award, I feel you have not so much honored me as an individual as that you have chosen me as a symbol, a representative, for all the occupational therapists who have devoted their interest and professional competence to the treatment of the mentally ill.

Changing Roles

I would like to use this time to examine with you some of the current developments in psychiatry in the United States of America which have implications for us and for our future practice. Many changes are taking place in the whole field of psychiatry. Long established and accepted concepts of care and treatment are being critically evaluated; different types of in and out patient treatment facilities are being established; traditional roles are changing as professional and nonprofessional groups review their qualifications and patterns of operation in order to improve their current function or assume new roles. Social scientists and anthropologists are contributing new insights, and the role of the community in all aspects of the mental health problem is increasingly recognized.

These changes have vital implications for occupational therapists in psychiatric practice which we must recognize and act upon. The decisions we reach and the action we take during the next few years will determine the future of occupational therapy. We must finally answer the question "What is the function of occupational therapy in psychiatry?" There is no consensus today; opinion and practice range from dynamically oriented treatment programs to ones which are very broad in scope and general in application. My personal and professional conviction has always been that occupational therapy is treatment. In psychiatry it is a form of treatment which utilizes activities and the relationship developed around and through these activities to assist the patient in finding more acceptable patterns of relating to others, and more mature ways of dealing with and solving his problems.

Utilizing Occupational Therapy

The education of the occupational therapist is designed to prepare personnel equipped to carry out this treatment function under medical direction, but many institutions do not use their occupational therapists in this capacity. This may be due to the orientation of the hospital itself. *Action for Mental Health* documents an impressive number of institutions which are not treatment oriented.[1] It may be due to the quality and immaturity of the occupational

Originally published 1962 in *American Journal of Occupational Therapy, 16,* 273–281.

therapists it employs. Or it may be due to the unwillingness of some physicians to accept allied medically trained personnel as co-therapists. Whatever the reason, I wonder how much longer we can persuade young occupational therapists to enter the psychiatric area if we do not demonstrate a role and function for them which is commensurate with their professional preparation. The ability to recognize and understand factors which contribute to or precipitate disability, and the acquisition of knowledge and security in using remedial techniques is the justification for the long and expensive education of the occupational therapist. Today the need for personnel with medical or medically related professional training is so acute, that it is difficult to justify the use of such personnel in any capacity which does not utilize their professional preparation to the fullest possible extent.

Future Responsibilities

There are many situations where the occupational therapist is a respected member of the treatment team and where occupational therapy makes an important contribution to treatment. These include private hospitals, psychiatric services in general hospitals, state hospitals, Service and Veterans hospitals. Since my experience has been primarily in state hospitals I shall discuss treatment focused occupational therapy in that setting. Many influential people in psychiatry feel the state hospital will be superceded by other kinds of treatment facilities for all types of mental illness. Others, equally authoritative, feel the state hospital provides the best facilities for the treatment of major mental illness and will continue to do so for many years. There is general agreement that many changes will be made, but again there is a difference of opinion about the degree of these changes and the form they will take. I am no crystal gazer and can certainly make no predictions about the future size or specific function of the state hospital, but I feel safe in saying that the future of occupational therapy in psychiatry is in our hands as it has never been before.

We, in common with other professional groups, are being asked to review and evaluate our practice, to determine objectively which of our current functions could be delegated to less highly trained workers so that professionally trained personnel can devote more of their time to specific patient treatment. This request is predicated on the well-documented assumption that professional staff shortages will exist for a long time to come, and it is thus imperative that current professional staff be relieved of every duty, administrative or treatment-focused, which could be performed by less highly trained workers. This is in no way an effort to reduce services to patients. It is rather an effort to relieve physicians and allied medical personnel of routine or administrative duties and minor responsibilities and functions which have become associated with their positions over the years, so that they will have time and energy to use their specialized skills in more meaningful patient treatment. The request to re-evaluate professional functions also takes cognizance of the development and use of volunteer groups and the services which they render, the availability of personnel with specialized activity skills, the increasing emphasis on vocational rehabilitation and after care services, and the use of ward personnel in ward activity programs.

Occupational therapists should recognize the implications in this request and should act to formulate a statement of role and function which will justify the continued inclusion of occupational therapy as one of the allied medical services of the hospital. If we want the recognition and status of professional personnel we must function on that level. We must be prepared to participate actively in patient evaluation, treatment planning and disposition conferences. We must understand the concepts and terminology of the psychiatrist, psychologist and social worker, and we must be able to discuss the contribution of occupational therapy in terms that are meaningful to them. Our treatment objectives must be carefully formulated and psychiatrically meaningful if we wish to have them incorporated in the overall treatment plan for the patient. If individual occupational therapists do not feel adequately prepared to function at this level or if their institutions want to use the program for diversional activity or as a management device, the program should not be called occupational therapy but should be given another designation which does not carry treatment implications.

The continuing shortage of qualified occupational therapists makes it almost mandatory that we relinquish all activity functions which can be performed by other personnel who are more readily available. To do so will permit us to fulfill treatment responsibilities which have been too often curtailed or neglected in the effort to supply activity programs for large numbers of patients. At one time occupational therapists were almost the only group able to meet activity needs, but today this is not true. There are trained personnel in the areas of recreation, music and library; volunteers conduct many activities and make available community contacts and cultural and diversional opportunities which institutional personnel could not duplicate. The increasing recognition of the importance of an attractive stimulating ward atmosphere has emphasized the need for activity programs conducted by ward personnel. These developments should be welcomed and supported by occupational therapists as each allows us to assume more of the treatment functions for which we are prepared.

This is important as the number of qualified personnel in mental health professions is not increasing. An extensive study of man power trends, made by Dr. George W. Albee for the Joint Commission, presents a discouraging picture. He is not optimistic about solving personnel problems through increased recruitment efforts, as he relates the shortage of candidates for all mental health careers to the shortages in other categories of professional man power. He documents the fact that there are not enough candidates to begin to meet the needs of the various professions.[2] One might say we are all fishing in an inadequately stocked pool. Those of us who hoped the population bulge would solve our staffing problems have apparently been entertaining an illusion. There may be more personnel but there will be more patients who are also part of the bulge. Since we cannot realistically expect to expand professional staff to any marked degree we must utilize those we have to the greatest advantage.

Changing Treatment Goals

Today occupational therapy has to be geared to the concepts and tempo of contemporary psychiatry. Modern treatments have radically changed the character of the mental hospital which now has a quieter, more purposeful atmosphere. More patients are receiving active treatment and many more are now accessible to and can profit from psychotherapy. The goal of a short period of hospitalization is stressed and patients are encouraged to maintain their interest in and contact with the community. Techniques and procedures which alleviate acute symptoms and promote control and the ability to function are given priority while ones based on long periods of hospitalization are being used less frequently. Generally speaking there is less emphasis on individual analytical psychotherapy but much more emphasis on group techniques of treatment. These procedures utilize the attributes of group identification and interaction to develop a degree of insight which will permit the patient once again to adjust in the community. Similarly where individual psychotherapy is used, it is often short term in nature and directed toward assisting the patient in reintegration of ego functions and the development of a sufficient degree of insight to facilitate social and work adjustment in the community.

The insidious factors in hospitalization are being identified and the more noxious are being removed or ameliorated as rapidly as possible. It is interesting to note that many of these factors are ones which occupational therapists have long recognized as being undesirable and have tried to counteract in their work with patients. They have seen the development of apathy and loss of self-respect as the patient succumbed to ward and hospital procedures which stifled him in routine and protected him from all decision-making. They have observed disturbed behavior subside in the permissive atmosphere of the occupational therapy clinic and they have fostered and nurtured any sparks of initiative and creativity which could be awakened. They have encouraged patients to accept responsibility for their own work and they have trusted them with dangerous tools and expensive equipment. These few examples among many possible ones are not recent developments in occupational therapy. They are based on insights which the occupational therapist has utilized for many years. The occupational therapist has had little difficulty in accepting the idea of a therapeutic community—in many aspects it is only an extension to the hospital as a whole of attitudes and concepts which are traditional in our clinics.

Correlating Treatment

Contemporary occupational therapy cannot exist in a vacuum or on the outskirts of medical awareness. To make an effective contribution in today's intensive treatment schedules it must correlate its treatment skills with other treatment effort, and it must contribute its observations and insight for the use of all team members. The organization of professional staff to achieve this focusing of treatment resources and knowledge will vary with the type of service but the importance of good communication in good treatment is universally recognized. Today the psychologist, social worker, psychiatric nurse and occupational therapist under the leadership of the psychiatrist, pool their collective knowledge to work out and implement effective treatment for patients assigned to their care.

The functions of occupational therapy in a dynamically oriented center are determined by the needs of the patient and the other treatments he is receiving. It may be used as a form of psychotherapy to augment psychotherapy or it may be used to facilitate the process of repression and restitution of ego functions. It may be evaluation, either initial or ongoing, used by itself or in conjunction with other diagnostic procedures, or it may be used to determine a patient's response to special treatment procedures or over-all therapy. The patient may be referred for occupational therapy upon admission, at any stage of treatment or for evaluation for readiness and suitability for vocation rehabilitation, community placement or intra-hospital transfer.

If occupational therapy is to discharge these functions, adjustments must be made by other services and divisions of the hospital. Large numbers of patients needing supportive activity cannot be included in occupational therapy groups where therapists are trying to establish meaningful interpersonal relationships and provide corrective emotional experiences for the active treatment of patients. The size of the occupational therapy groups has to be determined in accordance with the severity of the patients' symptoms and the goals of the treatment, and usually comprises from 6 to 15 patients per therapist. The occupational therapy department has to have an adequate budget. It cannot rely on a revolving fund supported by the sale of projects, and the department should not be expected to function as an interior decorating service or the source for small items of equipment or furniture for the hospital. These functions are generally not compatible with the needs of the patients, and might be considered as a continuation into the present of the era when patient labor was basically for the benefit of the institution.

Intensive Treatment Program

Many hospitals consider the primary function of occupational therapy as work with the nonverbal, regressed patient who cannot be reached by treatments which are based on group participation or words. It is true that occupational therapists are often very effective with these patients, but I cannot agree that this is our primary function. Such patients are only one of a number of types of patients who are included in an intensive treatment program. When these regressed, withdrawn patients are referred to occupational therapy they are assigned to clinics where a small number of patients (usually 6 to 8 at one time) are treated in an atmosphere that is warm, friendly and undemanding. A limited number of activities are available but these include both those that are structured and can be used to give support and security, and those which are unstructured and projective in nature and may be used by the patient to express his problems and anxieties. Interpersonal demands are kept at a minimum, but at all times the therapist provides support, reassurance and acceptance. The patient is encouraged to participate in an activity which may provide the staff with insight into his problem, but often the complete freedom of projective techniques is too threatening. In that event structured activity is substituted. This permits guidance from the therapist and may be the first step in a meaningful relationship which the patient could not tolerate without the activity to provide the justification for instruction and guidance. If the therapist has been sufficiently accepting and undemanding, and has tried to understand the non-verbal communication, the patient will generally become more relaxed and less frightened. As this occurs he can relinquish some of his more extreme defenses and may begin slowly to establish verbal contact with the therapist. This should be quietly accepted and unobtrusively utilized to deepen the relationship. When the patient can tolerate awareness of the others in the group, or when he begins to show any interest in them, the therapist will then try to encourage a relationship with another patient or patients.

Observation and Evaluation

As the process of re-integration continues, the team may decide on other forms of therapy which may either take the place of or supplement occupational therapy. This illustrates another point in the team concept of treatment. Although all disciplines are represented, under the supervision and direction of the psychiatrist, any member of the treatment team may become the dominant therapist. This role will pass from one discipline to another as the patient is able to utilize the special skills of each. This approach provides a continuous, coordinated but flexible program under medical direction which can be adjusted to meet the changing needs of the patient during his period of treatment.

Newly admitted patients are often referred to occupational therapy for observation and evaluation. The rationale for this procedure is based on the concept that all of a patient's behavior and reactions are significant and are directly related to the problems which cause his illness. Occupational therapy is one of the most normal situations which the hospital provides in which to observe characteristic behavior and patterns of defense, and the observation which the occupational therapist can supply for the use of the psychiatrist or the team in evaluating the patient's condition and determining procedures of treatment will become an increasingly important function of occupational therapy. Current emphasis on the desirability of psychotherapy for increasing numbers of patients has meant that psychologists, as one of the groups best able to meet this need, are devoting more and more time to this function, with a corresponding decrease in the number of psychological evaluations which they can provide. I do not mean to imply that information which the occupational therapist can supply is a substitute for the psychologist's evaluations which are based on standardized test procedures and protocols. Rather it is a means of evaluating the functioning level of the patient in a reality oriented situation where he can be as active or passive in participation in activities and relationships as he chooses.

The occupational therapy clinic looks like a well-equipped home workshop, a familiar kitchen, a hobby shop or a pleasant club room such as one finds in various community centers. The atmosphere is relaxed and there is little to remind one of a hospital. In this environment the patient is invited to select and participate in an activity. The type of activity he chooses, the way he goes about the task, the nature and degree of help he seeks and his movement towards completion all indicate his habitual approach to problems and their solution.[3] Since observation and reporting of characteristic patterns of behavior is the objective of the referral, the occupational therapist cannot interfere in the situation in any way except to protect the patient or other patients in the groups from serious physical injury. He cannot offer guidance (unless the patient requests it,) he cannot protect the patient from the results of faulty judgment or patterns of behavior, for to do so would influence the patient's choice and/or normal pattern of behavior and thus invalidate the information obtained. In this type of situation the patient is exposed to the personnel, patients and available activities and allowed to proceed on his own initiative. The way he reacts in the situation usually reflects his patterns before hospitalization. If these patterns have been such as to court or insure failure, this will be demonstrated. If his behavior has been such as to invite rejection or retaliation, this will probably be forthcoming from other patients, or the occupational therapist may recognize the wish to reject or retaliate in his own feelings. Through such observations the occupational therapist will gain concrete, "on the spot" examples of the patient's usual behavior and reactions which will clarify his problems. The occupational therapist has an advantage when evaluating not generally shared by the psychiatrist, social worker or psychologist, who more frequently evaluate through interview or other techniques in a one-to-one situation. The occupational therapist, on the other hand, generally evaluates the patient in a situation where other patients are present. This permits observation of the patient's responses in situations which can generate sibling rivalry, dependence or other characteristic behavior in relating to people.

Evaluating Purpose

It is desirable to distinguish between evaluation, which is a preliminary to planning treatment, readability and the ongoing evaluative process, which is an integral part of treatment. It is advisable to differentiate when occupational therapy is to be used as an instrument of evaluation and when it is to be used as treatment. When occupational therapy is used as an evaluation procedure, the therapist is as passive and non-intervening as possible. No effort is made to inhibit self-defeating behavior. The faulty patterns of relationship or performance which have created difficulties for the patient prior to hospitalization tend to be repeated within the occupational therapy setting. This repetition of destructive or inappropriate behavior may be a detriment to later treatment, but this is not the case if the patient is placed on a type of psychotherapy designed to uncover unconscious motivations and to foster the development of insight. Patients who are receiving other forms of therapy usually appear to derive more benefit in occupational therapy from activities and techniques which permit the therapist to give them a great deal of personal attention with enough firmness and control to provide support and security in the situation.

The period of observation and evaluation is followed by the initiation of an individual program of treatment. Should this program include any of the somatic therapies it is very helpful if the occupational therapist has had an opportunity to observe the patient's pre-treatment reactions, since somatic therapies tend to have a repressive effect which masks psychotic symptoms. In addition there may be organic reactions directly related to these therapies which affect the patient's response in occupational therapy. Immediate treatment objectives are limited, being directed primarily to the relief of confusion, strengthening contact with reality and assisting the patient to regain self-confidence and security. Treatment procedures and activities are simple, structured and of a nature which permits and encourages frequent contact with the occupational therapist to supply the support and reassurance which the patient needs. Later the goal should be to facilitate restitution of ego function and the satisfaction of emotional needs, with no specific attempt to provide insight, since somatic therapies are not primarily designed to uncover underlying or unconscious material. This approach requires just as much psychiatric knowledge on the part of the occupational therapist as one involving the development of insight, since he must be able to recognize the dynamics which underlie symptoms, the importance of different patterns of relationship, and the way in which activities may be used to satisfy unconscious emotional needs.

If the patient is assigned to a treatment program emphasizing the development of insight, the function of occupational therapy will be quite different. I should like briefly to describe two such programs, one designed for residents of a hospital and the other for day hospital patients.

The residential program is focused around an open ward in the men's division of the hospital which is made as attractive and home-like as possible. Treatment includes group psychotherapy and occupational therapy and is supplemented by industrial assignments. Adequate library and recreational facilities are available. The psychotherapist and the social worker, who have their offices on the ward, and the ward personnel offer support and encouragement, but responsibility for planning diversional activities, meeting individual assignments and ward housekeeping are delegated to the patients. In order to maintain or develop normal social interaction, the men go for lunch each day to the comparable women's ward. At least once a week these women spend the evening on the men's ward where they play cards or converse and there are frequent dances. Activities away from the hospital are sponsored by volunteers.

Coordinating Program

Occupational therapy and group psychotherapy are closely coordinated. The psychotherapist meets once a week with the occupational therapy personnel in the occupational therapy clinic, to examine the patient's work and discuss all significant developments which have occurred in either locale. In addition a weekly meeting is held with the social worker, ward personnel and occupational therapist to share information, review and revise treatment goals and evaluate new developments. Occupational therapy is directed toward providing both individual and group experiences for the patient and facilitating his ability to appraise more accurately the demands of, and react appropriately in, both types of situations. Since the majority of these patients are psychotics with considerable variation in age and background, it is sometimes difficult to find group activities which are generally acceptable, but wherever possible they are selected by the group and worked out with the guidance of the occupational therapist.

The day hospital group is composed of patients who are primarily neurotic or borderline psychotics. The majority come from the community each day, although some in-patients are assigned for a transitional experience before complete separation from the hospital. All patients have group psychotherapy daily and most are seen in individual therapy sessions. These patients attend occupational therapy as a group and often use part or all of the session as an extension of their psychotherapy hour. In order to facilitate appropriate identification and to provide as nearly a normal situation as possible there are both a woman occupational therapist and a man who is a certified industrial arts instructor in the clinic. The personnel have to play many roles and assume many responsibilities, perhaps the most difficult being to keep the group active and therapeutically effective. The personnel must have confidence in the value of dynamic group interaction and they must not impede the group process with their opinions, advice or interpretations. There must be meaningful communication and correlation of effort between the occupational therapists and the day hospital nurse and psychotherapist. Personnel in both situations must be informed about all developments and reactions as they occur in order to maintain consistency in attitude and to frustrate the patients' efforts to manipulate the situation and embroil the personnel in dissension. Where good correlation exists, each group experience (psychotherapy or occupational therapy) enhances and strengthens the effectiveness of the other. Occupational therapy provides an opportunity for reinforcement and testing of insight, release of tension created but not expressed in the psychotherapy session, and stimulation of enough tension and anxiety to keep the patients working and talking in group therapy. The occupational therapist must frustrate the group's dependency, which is expressed by trying to force her into a position of leadership, consistently handing all responsibility for insight, opinions, judgments and solution of problems back to them as individuals or as a group.

However the occupational therapist cannot therapeutically ignore all dependency needs. Activities provide one area where the patient is justified in seeking assistance and instruction and where the occupational therapist can accept and fulfill the dependency needs, symbolically, through concern and attention expressed in her instruction and supervision. A good variety of activity should be available but there should be no overt pressure to participate. The atmosphere of the clinic and the example of other patients is usually enough to motivate the patient to start a project. Once started, the patients soon utilize the activities in the clinic to externalize and express unconscious material. The atmosphere is one of controlled permissiveness with sufficiently defined limits to protect the patients from unrestrained acting-out. For example, patients may be verbally aggressive but they are not permitted to indulge in assaultive acting-out. They can destroy their own projects but they may not destroy other patients' work or clinic property.

Developing Insights

The occupational therapist must be constantly aware of transference reactions, interpersonal relationships and the way the patient uses, or does not use, the group and activity. The response by occupational therapy personnel to the misconceptions and distortions expressed in behavior and verbalization are determined by the patient's needs and his treatment plan. For one this might be an interpretive statement, "This is the way you would like to treat your father." Another may need to be confronted with reality, as, "But I am not your sister," while in many instances the group itself will confront the patient with an interpretation. The patient uses the clinic, the activities, the personnel and the group to work through and test developing insights, to practice new patterns of relating to people and reacting to frustration and pleasure, and to demonstrate to himself the greater satisfaction derived from more mature and objective ways of facing and solving his problems.

Evaluation Service

Following completion of formal treatment and during the state of consolidation and convalescence, occupational therapy is called upon to supply another type of service. This relates to preparing the patient for his return to work and the community. Since the "work" of most women patients is still home-making, a unit is provided utilizing skills such as food shopping, cooking, cleaning, laundry and sewing for the home as modalities. The patients receive instruction and practical experience in such activities as budgeting and efficient home management, menu planning and food service, home decorating and personal grooming. This program has demonstrated its value in helping the patient make the transition from hospital to home duties without undue anxiety and often with increased security and competence.

This period of the patient's hospitalization is also used to evaluate suitability for vocational rehabilitation if this is needed. Occupational therapy does not provide vocational rehabilitation services but it does provide a preliminary evaluation and screening service for the vocational rehabilitation counselor which is not available from other hospital services.

Supportive Activity

I have talked about the functions of a treatment focused occupational therapy program in a dynamically oriented state hospital, but I have not mentioned two groups of patients who must receive attention, the chronic and the geriatric. I have purposely left these groups until now as I believe they need a program of supportive activity rather than specific treatment. The chronic patients have generally received all appropriate treatment which the hospital provides without evidencing sufficient improvement to permit their return to the community. Occupational therapy for these patients should be directed toward maintaining the level of improvement which has been achieved, providing the support and reassurance which encourages further progress, and preparing them to function at their maximum level of adjustment within the hospital community. The same goals apply to the geriatric patient, except that ability to function in the hospital community is often more limited.

Many occupational therapists consider that this type of program is also treatment. I cannot agree. I believe that a program can be valuable and perform an essential function within the hospital structure without having to bear the label "treatment." In fact I feel that the indiscriminate labeling of everything which occurs within the hospital as "therapy" or "treatment" has devalued the term, and has made the thoughtful physician sceptical about most non-medical so-called "therapies." It is commonly said that we treat the whole man and that we want to return him to his community as a functioning individual with the insights gained through treatment enriching his capacity to live. Do we want to send him back to the community with the concept that his work is a treatment, his recreation a treatment, if he reads a book or attends a concert he is engaged in a form of treatment? I am of the opinion that the provision of components of normal life situations within a hospital is no more a part of specific treatment than is the provision of an adequate diet or heat in the winter time. The fact that recreation, library and music enrich our lives, and that work is an essential activity in our culture, does not make participation in them treatment per se. I am in favor of providing as many types of activity as we can for patients; all I ask is that we do not slip into the fallacy of labeling activity "treatment" just because it is carried on within the hospital boundaries.

Re-evaluation

I called this paper "The Challenge of the Sixties" and I should like to restate the challenge as I see it. We, along with other mental health professions, need to re-evaluate our role and function in the care and treatment of patients suffering from mental illness. We need to undertake this re-evaluation in the interests of providing better treatment for more patients. Can we as a professional group meet these needs? In order to re-evaluate the role and function of occupational therapy in psychiatry, we should reach a broad agreement on what our role and function is. Certainly re-evaluation can be carried out on a departmental basis, but this is not resolving the confusion which exists concerning the role of occupational therapy as a professional entity. Vacillation in coming to grips with this problem and in working out a solution has in turn inhibited our ability to work towards the solution of related problems which call for action. We have all expressed the feeling that physicians should receive more orientation to occupational therapy in medical schools. Even if time were made for it in their crowded curriculum, whose concepts should be presented? We look forward to the day when we can have accreditation of clinical centers, but what will form the basis of accreditation? We wish students were better prepared for practice in the clinical area, but for which type of program should they be prepared?

Professional roles are changing. Social workers, nurses and psychologists have been engaged in studies of their role and function for some time and already changes are in evidence. Some of these came about rapidly; others have occurred almost imperceptibly. Think for a moment of nursing and what seems to have happened in the last five years. Practical nurses now perform most of the bedside functions which registered nurses used to carry out, registered nurses now perform some procedures previously restricted to physicians, and a whole new category of workers has come onto the scene as ward secretaries, cleaners, porters, food servers, and so forth.

Changes are also occurring in the physician's role. In order to meet the needs of patients who could benefit from psychotherapy there has been a rapid increase in the use of group therapy techniques and the utilization by the physician of allied personnel as co-therapists, group leaders or as primary therapists. In the capacity of team leader the physician functions as a consultant and adviser who supports his team in their work with patients. While medical responsibility for diagnosis and treatment is vested in the physician, he uses the specialized training and competence of his team to assist him in both functions, and through the team's effort more patients are treated than could be reached through the physician's efforts alone.

The greatest challenge for occupational therapy is to define our own role in terms of present day psychiatry, and to determine which of our current functions actually require professional preparation and which could be adequately performed by less expensively prepared personnel. If the function does not require professional preparation it should be relinquished. This is not going to be easy, but if we do not accept this responsibility we shall not long retain our identity as members of the institution's professional staff. Today the graduate occupational therapist is considered part of the professional medical staff in many treatment oriented centers and service at this level should be the goal of all occupational therapists in psychiatric practice. We should utilize our training in the medical aspects of treatment and remember that at this time we are one of the few groups which have such qualification. Many psychiatrists recognize and value the contribution which occupational therapy currently makes to patient treatment and are willing to provide guidance and support if we demonstrate our readiness to accept increased responsibility. When the psychiatrist is willing and prepared to use the occupational therapist to the extent of his education and ability to assist in treating patients, there remains the problem of supplying therapists to use in this manner. If occupational therapy is to be a significant part of psychiatric treatment, we must attract with some degree of consistency competent and enthusiastic recent graduates to our centers. This can be accomplished only if we provide challenging opportunities for them to work in treatment situations which demand all of their professional knowledge. Recent graduates are not interested in nor attracted to positions which require primarily activity or even administrative skills.

Student Training

It is more than possible that disinterest or lack of attraction has its roots in the clinical affiliation in psychiatry, and what has just been said of the recent graduate is equally applicable to the student in affiliation. Indeed it is my belief, that if a student's clinical experience in psychiatry takes place in a department where occupational therapy is an activity program and where the graduate occupational therapists function only as administrators, the future graduate is already lost to psychiatric practice. The student in affiliation who has had an unfavorable experience in one clinical area generally avoids undergoing a corrective experience as a staff member in the same area.

Fortunately it should be easier to provide the affiliating student with an effective experience of occupational therapy used as treatment in a psychiatric program than it is to provide this same experience for a young staff member. The students, performing directly under close supervision by a qualified occupational therapist who serves as preceptor, desirably will observe, comprehend and practice occupational therapy as treatment through the example, discussion and constructive criticism of the occupational therapist. The staff member, on the other hand, does not often enjoy such immediate guidance and may be said to have to light his own way.

All students in psychiatric affiliation are entitled to the following positive experiences. (1) They should be shown the different ways that patients use activity to satisfy their emotional needs. (2) They should be shown how the occupational therapist not only facilitates this use of activity by the patient but can also help the patient gain insight into his feelings and behavior through his reaction to activity. (3) Students should be shown the various patterns of relationship which the occupational therapist uses to achieve treatment goals for individual patients or for the functioning group. (4) Finally students should be shown how to observe, analyze, evaluate and formulate appropriately the factors pertinent to planning or reporting treatment for a psychiatric patient.

These experiences should not be left to chance and the native awareness and skill of the student. The supervising occupational therapist should make certain that the student observes accurately the actual patients in the clinic, understands the significance of what he sees and his own reactions to it, can set realistic goals in occupational therapy for the patient and arrive at a feasible program to achieve them. The student should progress from the role of observer (by way of discussion and practice) to active participant in the therapeutic situation and finally to that of therapist, with all the responsibility that this implies. A student who has had this type of experience during the psychiatric affiliation becomes a young staff member who is prepared to administer treatment and who will continue to grow in professional skill through constant self-evaluation of his practice.

Specific mention must also be made of one other experience which is of great value to the young staff occupational therapist, which should also be shared by the affiliating student wherever possible. This is participation in conferences of the psychiatric treatment team. In this situation the occupational therapist has an opportunity to judge for himself the significance of occupational therapy's contribution as it is seen by other disciplines. Moreover, there is no better preservative or restorative of the sense of proportion than genuinely working with members of other professions in treating the same patient or group of patients.

Conclusion

My summary is not lengthy but it is as sincere and heartfelt as anything I have ever said in my lifetime as an occupational therapist in psychiatric practice. We occupational therapists in psychiatry must now make a decision as to our future course. On one hand we can strive to turn out many occupational therapists to be the personnel responsible for carrying out or supervising programs of activity for large numbers of patients as an instrument of patient management. Unfortunately it does not seem realistic to anticipate the necessary numbers of these personnel resulting from the current educational pattern of the registered occupational therapist. On the other hand we may work to produce a more limited number of occupational therapists who will perform a strictly treatment role for selected patients, having relinquished non-treatment or routine treatment aspects of previous occupational therapy functions to other personnel (even including supervision of non–occupational therapists). These specialists will find that their practice utilizes all their professional preparation and indeed demands continually increasing competence. Young persons who are considering a career of service in a health-related profession respond to challenge, and it is with confidence that I predict an adequate, although always limited, supply of good students and recent graduates to meet the demands of the psychiatrist who uses occupational therapy as treatment. In the last analysis, continuance of a profession depends upon the generation to come. So long as occupational therapy in psychiatric practice continues to attract vital recruits, so long will it maintain the worthy tradition of service to patients laid down by pioneers like Eleanor Clarke Slagle.

References

1. Joint Commission on Mental Illness and Health. *Action for Mental Health,* 19–23.
2. Albee, George W. "Mental Health Manpower Trends—1959." *Action for Mental Health,* 154–158.
3. Ellis, Madelaine and Arthur Bachrack. "Psychiatric Occupational Therapy: Some Aspects of Role and Functions." *American Journal of Psychiatry,* 115:319–322, 1958.

13

1963 Eleanor Clarke Slagle Lecture

The Development of Perceptual–Motor Abilities:
A *Theoretical Basis for Treatment of Dysfunction*

A. Jean Ayres, OTR, PhD

Central to the concept of occupational therapy are the evaluation, enhancement and use of skilled motor actions. While many central nervous system processes are involved in skilled movement, one aspect of sensorimotor function has come under particular attention lately as a large determinant of fine motor facility. That aspect is perceptual–motor functions, formerly called "eye–hand" coordination. Deficits in this domain are most easily and frequently observed in the patient who can accomplish simple grasp and release with apparent ease yet who cannot accomplish with comparable dexterity such tasks as tying shoes, handling tools or manipulating objects. The possible nature of that dysfunction is described in this paper and hypotheses presented regarding related developmental processes.

One of the more generally accepted postulates on which treatment of motor dysfunction is based is the recapitulation of the sequence of development. Accordingly, theories regarding the ontogeny of perceptual–motor abilities provide a basis for treatment of dysfunction in this area of human behavior. The data to which the theoretical system is anchored come largely from a research project conducted at the University of Southern California. (This investigation was supported in part by PHS research grant MH06878-01 from the National Institute of Mental Health, Public Health Service.) Results of published research by neurophysiologists have served as additional sources of knowledge. Although well supported with scientific facts, the highly provisional nature of the theoretical framework must be kept in mind. It has been necessary to force considerable structure onto the data (largely by omission of detail) in order to make them manageable. As our conceptual formulations become more familiar and secure, we will undoubtedly find that they have oversimplified the true nature of perceptual–motor function and it will be necessary for us to restructure them on a more complex basis.

Method of Obtaining Information

A brief review of the method by which the major research data were gathered is needed for their interpretation. One hundred children of approximately six and seven years of age who were suspected of having perceptual deficiencies were administered a battery of tests covering visual, tactile, and proprioceptive perception and some motor skills. Auditory and language functions were not included. None of the children carried a medical diagnosis of cerebral palsy; all of them had or had had learning or behavioral problems. The battery of tests was selected on the basis of descriptions in the literature of areas of perceptual–motor dysfunction. The scores made by the children on the tests were correlated and then subjected to R-technique factor analysis in order to determine the possible existence of associations among symptoms that would justify hypothesizing the presence of

Originally published 1963 in *American Journal of Occupational Therapy, 17,* 221–225.

taxonomic categories or syndromes of dysfunction. Establishment of factors is a means of summarizing and simplifying masses of confusedly interrelated observations, a function not possible by the human brain alone. A factor is a process which accounts for differences in a domain of behavior under observation—the domain in this case being perceptual–motor function. For example, among cerebral palsied children, certain neurophysiological processes account for the behavioral manifestation called spasticity, different processes determining athetosis, and another type of dysfunction causing ataxic behavior. These different neurophysiological processes are used to identify the neuromuscular problem of the patient. Understanding the process has served as a basis for establishment of treatment procedures.

In essence, this study has attempted a comparable categorization of a domain of neurological dysfunction, with reliance not upon subjective human judgment, but the objective accuracy of statistical computations. Nevertheless, a major limitation to this type of study lies in the fact that the emergence of a syndrome and its nature is dependent upon the type of data gathered. A serious omission in data collection will result in a gap in the results. Consumers of the information must be alert to this limitation.

Since the data were gathered from children with learning or behavioral disorders, we can expect to find similar syndromes of dysfunction among other children with comparable difficulty. Although cerebral palsied and definitely mentally retarded children were not included in the sample population, it is not unreasonable to expect these data to apply to children with those disorders. Caution must be used, however, in assuming that comparable clinical syndromes might be manifested in the individual sustaining brain injury as an adult.

Areas of Perceptual–Motor Function

Some of the types of perceptual–motor functions covered in the test battery are shown in Figure 13.1. In some instances, an area of function represents several tests. In these cases the mean factor loading of a group of tests was

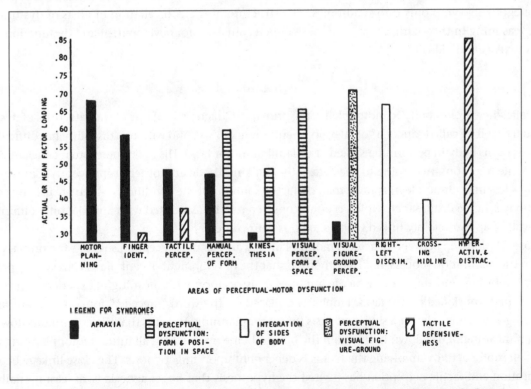

Figure 13.1. Factorial content of five major clinical syndromes of perceptual–motor dysfunction.

obtained by taking the square root of the mean of the squares of the factor loadings of several tests, all of which had significant loadings on that factor.

Motor planning was evaluated by (1) how well a child could draw a line with a pencil on top of another line, (2) the degree of quickness and accuracy with which the child could assume a posture demonstrated by the examiner, and (3) the ability to manipulate an object. Finger identification was evaluated by the identification by the child of which of his fingers the examiner touched. Tactile perception was based on (1) the accuracy with which the subject could localize a tactile stimulus on hand or forearm, (2) his ability to discriminate between one and two tactile stimuli in the finger tips, (3) the degree to which he could perceive two simultaneously administered tactile stimuli to cheek and/or hand, and (4) his accuracy in identifying simple figures drawn on the back of the hand. Manual perception of form was tested by visual recognition of a geometric form held in the hand. The accuracy with which the child could return his hand to a position previously assumed with the help of the examiner was the basis for the score on kinesthesia. Visual perception of form and space included Frostig's tests of form constancy, position in space, and space relations. Ability to identify superimposed and imbedded pictures of objects made up the test of figure-ground perception. Right–left discrimination refers to the child's identifying his right and left sides as well as those of the examiner. Reluctance to cross the mid-line of the body was evaluated by whether or not the child would spontaneously put his hand on a part of the body on the opposite side and, in addition, pick up objects placed on the other side of the body's mid-line. Hyperactive, distractible behavior is self-explanatory.

The Major Syndromes and Their Hypothesized Development

The statistical analysis of the data gathered by the method described above (and to be described in statistical detail elsewhere) leads to postulating the existence of five major syndromes of perceptual–motor dysfunction. These syndromes, which emerged from the analysis as factors, and the mean or actual factual loadings of the tests of perceptual–motor function on each factor are shown in the diagram. The most important general observation to make is that different syndromes are represented by different constellations of deficits of function. This fact provides the basis for categorizing symptoms into syndromes. The structure of the constellation of areas of dysfunction also directs our reasoning in theorizing about the nature of perceptual–motor development and dysfunction. Each factor will be discussed individually.

Apraxia

Because a deficiency in the ability to motor plan is the primary characteristic of one of the categories of dysfunction, it is suggested that it be called "apraxia" or "developmental apraxia." A child with this disability has difficulty directing his hands or his body in performing skilled or unfamiliar motor tasks. His major perceptual deficiency lies quite clearly in tactile functions. According to the data gathered, kinesthetic and other proprioceptive sources of information play a less important role in apraxia than do tactile sources. Of the conditions which are usually considered aspects of body scheme disturbance (which is often considered to be associated with apraxia) only diminished finger identification appears closely linked with apraxia, as defined here.

The close relationship between deficits in motor planning and tactile perception suggests the primacy of tactile functions in the maturation process. It is hypothesized that the development of central nervous system processes of organizing, inhibiting, and augmenting tactile impulses in association with meaningful experiences must precede the ability to perform skilled motor tasks. Emphasis is placed on the word "precede," for concomitant tactile perception during a motor task is not a sufficient basis for motor planning. It seems that the continuous flow of tactile sensations, if meaningful, lay down in the brain the body scheme upon which all future motor planning is based.

Skill in all motor activity involving the hands is dependent upon finger gnosis. The close linkage between finger identification and tactile perception has invited the hypothesis that finger agnosia is, at least partially, a function of a disordered tactile system.

Our approach to treatment of the child with apraxia must focus on normalizing the tactile functions as well as training in motor skill.

Perceptual Dysfunction: Form and Position in Space

Another important syndrome reflects a deficit in perception of form and position in two-dimensional space. As shown in the diagram, perception refers, here, not only to visual perception, but also to tactile perception of form and kinesthetic perception of the position of the hand in space. It is the grouping of these three sensory modalities that provides us with a major clue regarding the development of visual perception. It is hypothesized that the visual perception of form and position in space is preceded developmentally by the purposeful response to tactile and kinesthetic sensations carrying information about form and space. If a child feels with assurance where his hand is, how his fingers are positioned, and what they are holding, he will be better able to visually cope with form and space, such as is required in tasks as simple as setting a table or as complex as drawing designs, reading, or assembling an object on the production line. The relationship may not be an inevitable one, however, for relationships among perception of form and space in the three sensory modalities may be a function of a common neurological process.

The implication for treatment, again, is to first normalize, as much as possible, tactile and kinesthetic sensation, followed by the enhancement of perception in these modalities and of visual stimuli.

Deficit of Integration of Function of the Two Sides of the Body

From the research data emerged a syndrome with characteristics to which reference has been made in the literature for many years. However, the grouping of symptoms into a single dimension of central nervous system development and organization appears not to have been suggested prior to this time. The two most distinguishing aspects of behavior of this syndrome are a tendency of the hands to avoid crossing the mid-line of the body when engaged in motor tasks and difficulty in learning to discriminate and identify the right and left sides of the body, the latter type of behavior being the best representative of the syndrome. It is possible that there are other, more effective means of identifying this type of dysfunction. Studying those aspects of perceptual–motor dysfunction which showed close association with crossing the mid-line and right–left discrimination suggests a basic clinical syndrome of inadequate integration of the two sides of the body. Whenever the motor function of one side of the body is related to activity of the other side, the function of the two sides requires coordinating by a central nervous system mechanism of unknown type which is clearly vulnerable to disorder. Thus, successful participation in rhythmic activities requiring a temporal interrelationship of the two hands or two feet is partially dependent upon this central nervous system mechanism even though the mid-line is not crossed. Similarly, jumping with both feet simultaneously and performing reciprocal motions with the extremities are affected. It even seems likely that having to draw on one side of a page a duplicate of a design appearing on the other side of the page involves integration of the two sides of the body. The ability of the eyes to cross the mid-line of their respective ranges of motion is part of this behavioral dimension.

The sensory component of the syndrome is obscure, but, again the significant correlations between scores on tests of tactile perception and crossing the mid-line or right–left discrimination suggest the importance of tactile stimuli in the developmental process. It is hypothesized that crawling or creeping has found favor among therapists and psychologists as a therapeutic process partly because it is one of the most basic and ontogenetically early sensorimotor patterns requiring and enhancing integration of function of the two sides of the body. It is interesting to note that at the age of six or seven years, the degree to which the right and left sides could be correctly identified was apparently a function of the maturation of a specific area of sensorimotor development, as contrasted with verbal skill. This syndrome is deserving of much attention from the occupational therapist. As in the case of most of the other syndromes, it requires treatment with controlled sensation and bilateral motor activity. The effect of some of our bilateral activities begins to take on new significance.

The fact that diminished body balance is associated with poor integration of sides of the body leads to wondering whether there is a neurophysiological deficit basic to both balance and body side integration or whether balancing on one foot involves the kind of neuromuscular integration diminished in children with inadequate functional interrelationship of the two symmetrical halves of the body.

Identification of the pattern of dysfunction in the cerebral palsied child may be very difficult. It is not likely that it would have been detected statistically in a cerebral palsy population. Our inability to detect it does not preclude its presence, and we must be alert to its manifestation and response to treatment.

Perceptual Dysfunction: Visual Figure-Ground

Deficiency in visual figure-ground perception has been identified as a clinical condition for many years. The disability emerged from the research data as a specific and independent syndrome, although some of the children with apraxia also demonstrated disturbance in figure-ground perception. Inspection of correlations between scores on tests of visual figure-ground perception and other perceptual–motor tests suggests that the neurological process basic to figure-ground perception is also basic to all other types of perceptual–motor ability. Somatic perception is closely associated with visual figure-ground perception, the latter even appearing within the apraxia syndrome. The relationship may lie in mutual dependence upon the discriminatory functions of the non-specific processes of the reticular formation and thalamus. The developmental process underlying visual figure-ground perception is far from clear.

A neurophysiological approach to treatment of this syndrome remains to be investigated. The most fruitful approach will likely be through influencing the function of the non-specific reticular system by control of sensory input. If we can enhance the discriminatory function of the general system, figure-ground perception will likely improve. The area is a fertile field for investigation by therapists.

Tactile Defensiveness

The last major syndrome to be described is one brought to our attention for the first time by our research at the University of Southern California. It is characterized by deficit in tactile perception, by hyperactive, distractible behavior, and by a defensive response to certain types of tactile stimuli. It is interesting to note that hyperactive and distractible behavior carried a significant loading on only one syndrome, suggesting that this troublesome behavior problem may, in these children, be linked to a specific neurophysiological mechanism. The syndrome is closely and directly associated with emotions. These data, when taken into consideration with other neurophysiological information, have led to a fruitful theory described in detail elsewhere. In essence, the developmental process suggested by the syndrome reflects the phylogenetic primacy of tactile stimuli as messages warning the organism of danger and to prepare to flee or fight. This type of interpretation of tactile stimuli leads to the over-alertness of distractibility, the flight-like behavior of hyperactivity, and a tendency toward negative affect (fight). The presence of the syndrome interferes with the development of perceptual–motor ability. It was found primarily in association with the other syndromes and not as an isolated condition.

Identification, at least hypothetically, of a neurophysiological basis for certain types of hyperactivity gives us a cue for another approach to treatment of the dysfunction—the approach being a normalizing of tactile functions.

General Discussion

Attention must be drawn to the fact that the five syndromes may not be expected to appear in pure states in any child. Correlation among scores on perceptual–motor tests warrants the expectation that a child who is perceptually deficient in any one area is likely to be deficient in all other areas but he is not necessarily so. From the statistical analyses emerged many other syndromes of lesser clarity and accounting for less of the source of variance among the children. Additional research may indicate their significance.

Although tactile functions emerged as highly significant, the apparent comparative lesser role of the proprioceptors may be purely a matter of inadequate evaluation of their function or an inability to interpret the results.

While emphasis has been placed on a neurophysiological understanding and approach to treatment, the cognitive approach is certainly not excluded as an important aspect of treatment. The two approaches are really ends of the same continuum. It is strongly suggested, however, that treatment based primarily on influencing basic neurophysiological integration, through control of sensorimotor behavior, and secondarily on intellectual processes will be the most effective approach. There is a long gap between these basic research data and the assurance that a treatment procedure is effective. We need many studies to test, scientifically, the hypotheses suggested by the theories.

14

1965 Eleanor Clarke Slagle Lecture

Learning as a Growth Process:
A *Conceptual Framework for Professional Education*

Gail S. Fidler, OTR

An honor such as that which is mine today seldom represents the single achievement of one individual but rather a synthesis of the knowledge, ideas and experiences of many. I am deeply indebted to associates and others in related fields but particularly to those colleagues and students with whom I have been privileged to work and whose creative thinking and imaginative experimentation has contributed so much to my knowledge and to the development of occupational therapy. What I shall say regarding the nature and scope of professional education is neither new nor unique but is an attempt to relate these theories to the education of the occupational therapist in such a way as to hopefully increase our skill and knowledge as therapists and educators and enhance our growth into a profession.

The rapidly changing, complex world of today creates new and increasing demands upon and expectations for the professions. The development and maintenance of a vitality essential to the existence of a profession and to the fulfillment of its obligations to society is inextricably bound to its philosophy of education and those processes directed toward attaining professional competency.

In a changing society, roles need to be constantly assessed and a profession must continually ask itself how it may impart to the learner a given body of knowledge and nourish the development of skills in such a way as to motivate the developing professional to creatively elucidate and expand concepts; develop and test new hypotheses; continually enhance and refine skills and thus contribute to the growth and maturation of that profession.

It is axiomatic that the scope and function of a profession, its role and definition determine its educational objectives. Since educational objectives are delineated in relation to the scope and function of a profession, they can be defined and pursued only insofar as the nature and role of that profession is clearly conceptualized.

Professional roles are set forth by the needs of the society to be served, circumscribed by the profession's delineation of the extent to which it may be expected to fulfill such needs. It therefore follows that the responsibilities assumed by a profession define the nature and quality of the particular knowledge and skills required of its members.

Assumption of professional responsibility involves both privileges and obligations, and it is these which constitute a professional identity and provide a basic frame of reference for those learning experiences which may be expected to prepare the student to fulfill such obligations. A profession is characterized by the nature and quality of its body of knowledge and skills, the capacity to discern when the application of such knowledge and skill is indicated and the ability to make reasonable predictions regarding the outcome of such application.

A second identifying characteristic of a profession is the existence of a definable set of principles, concepts and attitudes basic to its functions but which also transcend the confines of that profession to the extent that the professional is able to share with others a concern for and dedication to the welfare of all peoples and thus to share freely and work collaboratively with others in the service of human welfare.

Originally published 1966 in *American Journal of Occupational Therapy, 20,* 1–8.
Please note that there was no Eleanor Clarke Slagle Lecture in 1964.

An infinite commitment to the advancement of learning, to research as an attitude and to the maintenance of critical, evaluative and creative thinking, is still another criterion of professional identity. Furthermore, a service profession is characterized by its inherent belief in the integrity of man, in the capacity of the human being for growth and change and in those attitudes and feelings which make possible appropriate and satisfying interpersonal relationships. A fifth criterion may be stated as a deep and objective commitment to the growth of the profession as a human welfare service and to the maintenance of the unique identity of that profession.

Finally, a profession is identified by a practice wherein authority and privilege are derived from the requirements which the profession sets regarding knowledge and practitioner skills. Thus power and privilege stem from the profession itself and exist in relation to the standards of that profession rather than emanating from sources outside itself.

Such criteria suggest that more is at stake in educating for the professions than the accumulation of facts and data or the teaching of skills per se. Professional preparation requires that the educational process be concerned with teaching a body of principles and concepts rather than routine skills or "slide rule approaches." Ralph W. Tyler[1] warns against cluttering professional curriculum with activity courses that can be learned on the job. He emphasizes that a profession must base its technique of operation upon principles rather than rule of thumb procedures or routine skills. Charlotte Towle[2] in discussing the general objectives of professional education states that, "it is characteristic of professional education that it teach a body of principles and concepts for differential use. In short, it endeavors to set in operation a learning process that will endure and wax strong throughout the years of professional activity. Such a focus makes possible the achievement of self-dependent, professional thinking and functioning rather than the more limited technical 'how or what-to-do' approach."

A second aim of professional education is to develop in the student the capacity and drive to learn; the ability to think critically, creatively and analytically; to teach the process of logic and thus to enable the learner to develop and refine problem-solving and decision-making skills. An attitude of scientific inquiry, the ability to analyze, synthesize and generalize require an open mindedness, a freedom to explore and accept new ideas and different ways of thinking. The educator and thus the educational process must then be committed to change as the outcome of learning providing the incentive and opportunity for such change. Furthermore, such perspectives place high value on the ability and right of the individual logically to arrive at his own conclusions. Thus sound professional education needs to provide the opportunity to develop capacities for independent thought and action. Walter Lifton[3] speaking to this point warns against teaching a repertoire of typical responses and suggests that, "it is only when we are not sure that our answer is best that we fear having a person seek his own best solution."

A third objective in the advancement of learning is to nurture a set of attitudes and feelings which will enhance the student's capacity to think and function appropriately. Such an objective points up the importance of understanding self and others and emphasizes the need for learning experiences which provide opportunity for the student to become aware of his attitudes and feelings, how these influence his own behavior and the response of others and finally to work toward necessary attitudinal changes.

Students bring to the learning experience a variety of attitudes, values and previously learned responses. Some of these will need to undergo change, others be enhanced and broadened if the learner is to achieve the personal growth and the critical human perception essential for meeting the requirements of a profession. The capacity to effectively alter or change attitudes is dependent upon being able to look at one's set of values and beliefs critically and objectively, to come to have some understanding of self, developing an identity and integrity sufficient to enable learning and growth to occur. Thus learning needs to occur within a setting and in such a manner as to support and foster these perspectives and concomitant growth. Self awareness for the sake of self awareness is never an aim of professional education but is the means whereby a student may develop those capacities and that breadth of knowledge essential for professional fulfillment.

Another goal in training for the professions is the development of a capacity to engage in appropriate, mutually satisfying interpersonal relationships. The ability to work collaboratively with others, to establish and sustain relationships is in proportion to one's understanding of and respect for self and others. Achievement of such understanding and respect emanates from a receptivity to self awareness and understanding and thus the educational process aims to increase such receptivity and to provide interpersonal learning experiences which will enable the student to use this appropriately and productively.

In addition, a sense of security and integrity generated by an increasing capacity to think logically and independently and comprehension of the basic set of principles indigenous to the profession contributes immeasurably to collaborative and interpersonal skills. In essence, the capacity to establish and maintain interpersonal relationships represents the ability to think and feel appropriately and evaluatively with minimal biases regarding self and others. Charlotte Towle[4] succinctly describes what is involved in such relationships when she states: "Decisive also in establishing and maintaining purposeful working relationships will be the readiness to assume and sustain responsibility, the capacity to meet the dependency of others without taking the management of affairs out of their hands, the willingness to play a minor or subordinate role as well as a major one and the ability to separate one's self from another so that one's own feelings, attitudes and needs are not blindly projected onto others."

Finally, professional education must teach a perspective regarding the place of the profession in society and its service to the individual in relation to that society. This perspective should make possible firm commitment to the maintenance of the professional identity but also generate an ongoing constructively critical evaluative attitude regarding that profession. While a profession is recognized by a given body of knowledge which makes possible a distinguishable service, objective appreciation of its unique contributions, as well as its limitations, can be achieved only through an understanding of the significance of other professions and the needs which they serve.

Attainment of these educational goals can become a reality only insofar as the learning experience is conceptualized as a growth process directed toward the development of a professional person. Within this context, the educative process stresses integrated learning in preference to cognitive as the means whereby new functions are integrated and growth and change consolidated. This frame of reference brings the teaching-learning experience into focus as a dynamic human relationship and underlines the need to evolve an effective teaching-learning theory.

Development of a dynamic teaching–learning theory requires understanding the nature of the integrative learning process, perceptual organization and the way in which a function becomes an integral part of the self.

Pearce and Newton[5] define growth as the integration of a new function or the expansion of a function. They emphasize that in order for new learning to become an integral part of the self system such learning, including a synthesis of prior and current experiences, must come clearly into awareness at the time of integration and be consensually validated with a person or persons of significance. This concept of growth points up the importance of bringing all aspects of new learning experiences into clear awareness and building a student-teacher relationship which will maximize the necessary synthesis and consensual validation. The implications of these theories for the teaching-learning relationship have been outlined in an earlier paper which explores concepts relating to professional learning and defines a frame of reference for such learning and growth.[6]

Identifying growth and change as the ultimate aim of education, Leland P. Bradford[7] points out that a deeper and broader goal than cognitive learning must exist if growth and change is to occur. He comments that learning which remains merely cognitive and does not become part of one's internal systems and external behavior, becomes compartmentalized and of little value. He stresses the importance of consensual validation in the learning process, emphasizing that one learns under conditions in which relevant, accurate and acceptable feedback is provided.

An effective teaching-learning process requires understanding of the role of the learner and of the teacher, what each brings to the transaction and how each influences that transaction. The needs, attitudes, biases and expectations of both student and teacher regarding learning, knowledge and growth play a significant role in defining the nature and quality of the learning experience. What are the learner's concepts regarding himself, how does he conceptualize his potential for learning, for growth? What does learning mean to him and on the basis of his past experiences what expectations does he bring to the transaction?

The teacher needs to be aware of his own particular needs and attitudes. Arthur Jersild[8] suggests that the teacher needs to deal with his anxieties relative to his role of authority and/or benefactor. Bradford[9] articulately defines the importance of the teacher's awareness and understanding of his own needs and motivations when he asks, "to what extent does the teacher's need to control people, to maintain dependency upon himself or to seek love and affection distort and disturb his function and thus the learning transaction? To what extent does his fear of hostility develop repression in the learner so that healthy conflict as a basis of learning is lacking? To what extent does his fear of relationships with people keep the learner at arm's length and thus reduce the possibility of an effective teaching-learning transaction?"

Recognition of the significance of human needs, respect for the integrity of man, belief in his capacity for growth, change and self-dependent functioning are essential ingredients for an effective teaching-learning relationship. Productive learning will in good measure be determined by the extent to which these attitudes are an integral part of the teacher's self system and become evident in his transactions with students.

Theories concerning the nature of the learning process need also to relate to resistance to learning. The importance of anxiety both as a change inducing agent and as a response to the threat of change must be recognized. The new and unknown, the expectation that old safe patterns and attitudes will need to undergo change and alteration is understandably anxiety provoking. Anxiety associated with change, however, is at the same time in conflict with man's innate drive toward growth. The teacher needs to understand the nature of this dilemma and through such understanding provide the appropriate measure of support to diminish blocks to learning, nurture receptivity to changes and guard against intellectualization or cognitive rote learning as a defense.

Finally, an effective teaching-learning theory recognizes the dynamics of the group and the dyadic relationship as forces for learning, as interactional, growth-inducing processes.

Generative engagement in the teaching-learning transaction requires more than knowing about human behavior and learning theories. It demands a sensitivity to ongoing relationships and skill in using this perception in creating a culture conducive to integrated learning and more concretely in directly facilitating the integration of a function. The teaching-learning relationship must provide sufficient freedom and help to enable the student to learn to reason and function independently and collaboratively; to increase his capacity for creative original thinking; to translate such thinking into productive action; to assume responsibility for making decisions as well as the results of such decisions and finally to make mistakes and find support in learning from these.

Teaching then is conceptualized as the process of making opportunities available for the development of a body of knowledge, skills and attitudes in such a way as to enhance the learner's capacity to function creatively, with skill, understanding and discernment; the nature of such a process constituting an interpersonal transaction conducive to growth and concomitant change.

Such a definition of teaching also rightfully describes the nature and goal of the therapist-patient interaction, for if we are to teach students to become skillfully engaged with patients or clients in a helping-growth process, the students' learning experience must itself then be a helping growth process.

Appreciation of learning as a growth process inevitably points up the need to re-examine and carefully scrutinize our methods of education, both in the didactic and clinical spheres. First, however, we must define our expectations regarding educational experiences. What are we to teach in occupational therapy? What growth do we hope for; what knowledge, skills and attitudes do we expect the learner to integrate? Are we willing and able at this time to commit ourselves to the development of occupational therapy into a profession? Or, is such a commitment incongruous to our definition of its role and function? Professional responsibilities cannot be compromised. As Charlotte Towle so aptly states,[2] "there cannot be an admixture of limited goals and high goals. Professional education cannot be designed to train a few to lead, many to follow and others to permanently serve under the guidance of more competent members. It is to be remembered that a profession's leaders cannot advance it beyond the level of its common practice."

Answers to these questions will define the nature and quality of the learning experiences we structure for our students. If we can consensually define our goal as the growth of occupational therapy into a profession and if we are willing to accept the responsibilities inherent in such a decision, we must then clearly define our professional role and scope and reassess those procedures and experiences which we provide as the developmental process for the occupational therapist.

Expectancies for undergraduate and graduate learning will need to be redefined within the context of the level at which one can train for professional competency. It is perhaps understandable that as a young, developing discipline, education in occupational therapy has had to be primarily concerned with the needs for a multiplicity of subjects at the sacrifice of depth of content and dynamic teaching-learning theories. It has, however, been evident for some time that adequate preparation of the occupational therapist for today's practice requires graduate level education. One must seriously question the concept that education to fulfill professional expectations can be achieved at an undergraduate level, regardless of the nature of that profession. As disciplines or quasi-professions have moved toward professional roles each has found this to be evident. The depth and breadth of specialized knowledge and skill required of today's professional cannot be achieved at the undergraduate level and development of occupational therapy into a profession is contingent upon recognition of this fact. Undergraduate experiences may be structured to provide a broad base upon which professional education may build but they can no longer be perceived as professional preparation.

Learning occurs at several different levels and should progress from the perceptual to the most complex one of conceptual integration. Education for professional responsibility requires that learning proceed through each stage and be integrated at each organizational level. It is this process which differentiates cognitive from integrated learning and makes self-dependent, continued learning possible. By and large, the average educational experience does not train for perceptiveness and there are few disciplined opportunities for developing sensitivity awareness. The ability to conceptualize and to make theoretical constructs operant has its foundation in learning at the primary level of perceptual organization. Thus we might perceive our undergraduate education as learning experiences preparatory to professional education, with a focus on teaching the young student to become more acutely aware of sensations and building skill in perceptual organization processes. Professional education could then rightfully place greater emphasis on learning at higher levels of integration.

These frames of reference relating to professional identity and education suggest that the classroom needs to be viewed as a potential for dynamic human interaction and thus for learning in an experiential way the perceptiveness, the human interactional skills and the principles and concepts generic to theories of occupational therapy. The practicum is conceptualized as a continuing growth process, as a laboratory for integrating, consensually validating and consolidating those functions inherent in professional competency. Within this context, it would seem useful to briefly explore learning experiences both in the classroom and practicum which may complement such definitions.

Traditional lecture methods have generally been the procedure of choice when didactic material needs to be mastered, while group discussion has been reserved for dealing with content relating to feelings and attitudes. It would seem that such is the case since too frequently the seminar or group discussion is perceived as a permissive, unstructured experience concerned primarily with opinion sharing and attitudinal change. Such criticism should in no way be perceived as generally applicable to the small group experience wherein group process is used to facilitate personal growth and attitudinal change. Such groups have been used and studied extensively and there is little doubt that with skillful leadership they are effective, growth-inducing experiences. However, mastery of didactic material presents a somewhat different problem.

Learning complex didactic material is not maximized by permissive unstructured approaches. However, when skillfully planned, the classroom discussion group can become an effective, dynamic way of learning even the most difficult material. It is essential to recognize that in using the classroom discussion group approach the teacher is involved with group process skills as well as subject matter teaching. Thus the teacher needs to acquire facility in group work skills if the classroom is to provide experiential learning concomitant with mastery of didactic material.

William Faucett Hill has developed a creative and functional method for structuring the classroom discussion group to achieve this goal. His monograph, "Learning thru Discussion"[10] including his cognitive group map presents well organized and lucid guidelines for dynamic learning experiences within the classroom. The cognitive group map provides a procedural outline for didactic content analysis and group interactional processes. This method enables mastery of subject matter using group process as the milieu, wherein integrated learning of didactic material becomes possible and group development is used simultaneously as a learning and growth experience. Presenting the rationale for such an approach, Dr. Hill emphasizes a well known fact of learning theories that isolated, unassociated facts are the first to be forgotten and that knowledge must not only be accumulative and integrated but also have personal value and significance to the student. He states, "Subject matter mastery should enhance feelings of ego mastery. Acquired knowledge that is not internalized and remains ego-alien is either readily forgotten or if it is retained results in the creation of arid scholasticism or mere pedantry." The lecture method approach frequently encourages little more than cognitive learning.

In addition to the use of Hill's cognitive group map procedure, other methods have been found to be effective in maximizing the potential of the classroom group as a setting for learning and growth. Role playing and use of the critical incident provides opportunities for students to test the efficacy of newly acquired knowledge and concepts, practice problem-solving and diagnostic skills and synthesize that which is being learned. When other students function as observers or alter egos to the role playing or critical incident analysis, additional experience is provided for synthesizing as well as developing insight into the influence of feelings on perception, thinking and behavior. These techniques have been especially useful in helping the student develop a perceptive understanding of the dynamisms of interpersonal and group transactions, evaluative and observational procedures and many other facets of the occupational therapy experience. However, carefully structured, well organized planning is essential if mastery of subject matter is to be achieved. Too frequently role playing, like the group discussion or seminar, is too loosely structured and permissive to teach complex material or depth of content.

The spontaneous panel offers additional opportunity for integrating complex theoretical material, dealing with content analysis in a personally significant way and developing vital skills in verbal communication. These experiences are most effective when panels are formed spontaneously and the students expected to discuss and think through a given problem or issue without pre-planning their presentations. Such methods facilitate conceptualization of occupational therapy theories and provide essential experience in the use of logic and analysis.

If we are to teach a set of principles from which critical discernment and professional skill may emerge then our methods of teaching must be analogous to content so as to firmly consolidate an appreciation of the reciprocal relationships among theories and functions. There are inherent correlations between interpersonal theories and skill, group process, self awareness, psychiatric theory and the meaning and use of objects. Our teaching needs to conclusively demonstrate the dynamic interrelatedness among these and others and thus guard against simply learning isolated facts or skills per se.

Adaptations of a technique used by Blake and Mouton[12] have been effective in combining the learning of didactic subject matter and group process skills. This method requires that each student prepare a solution to a given problem or critical incident, presenting this to his small discussion group. The group is then expected to arrive at one solution after which each student's answer is given a numerical scoring by the group. Ratings are based on content mastery and process of logic. Finally each group is asked to critique how it functioned as a group in arriving at a consensus regarding both a solution and individual scoring. Total classroom discussion then centers around the accuracy of solutions and group interactional processes.

Use of the task-oriented group pattern is still another procedure for maximizing the potential of the classroom as a dynamic setting for experiential learning of didactic material as well as interpersonal and group process skills. This procedure calls for the formation of small working groups whose membership remains constant throughout the course. Each group is responsible for completing several content related assignments and presenting these to the class group for critique. Each group is also expected to present at the end of term a process analysis of their group. It has been found that in addition to actively engaging the student in learning content, these leaderless groups provide an excellent experience in group development and constructively increase awareness of the impact of one's feelings and behavior on others.

An awareness of oneself as an interacting, dynamic force in all human transactions and the capacity to develop and use this potential are fundamental to professional competency. Thus throughout our educational program, appropriately related opportunities need to be provided in order to enhance self-awareness and give impetus to growth and change.

Personal diaries or logs in which feelings and responses to learning experiences are recorded provide a means for self-evaluation and an opportunity to increase one's understanding of self and others, perceive changing attitudes as well as blocks to learning and growth. Personal diaries have been used by many persons, in a number of settings to enhance self-awareness and sharpen perceptiveness of cause and effect relationships. Two well formulated discussions of this method may be found in the works of Lifton[11] and Wechler and Reisel.[12] The use of such diaries in conjunction with the occupational therapy classroom seminar and the task-oriented group experience has demonstrated their value in helping the student to consolidate new insights, attitudes and concepts.

The use of students as process observers during classroom sessions creates opportunity for learning techniques of observation, for increasing awareness of interaction and enhancing the student's ability to identify pertinent and related occurrences. Consensual validation and practice of communication skills is possible when the student-observer reports his observations to the class for discussion.

The activity laboratory is an experience which helps to develop an appreciation for and understanding of the meaning of objects and activities and the impact of these on feelings and behavior by engaging the participant in a sequence of activities and object creations. As the activity is pursued, students are encouraged to identify feelings which occur, explore the specific characteristics of both the action and objects which seem to elicit such feelings and discern how feelings are manifested in behavior and in the content of productions. Involvement such as this teaches in a personally significant way the very basic concepts of occupational therapy, initiates a receptivity to self awareness, sharpens sensitivity and understanding and thus creates the basis for an ultimately more accurate and sensitive appreciation of patient response.

Teaching methods need always be related and appropriate to the material being taught. They also reflect basic attitudes regarding ourselves, our students and growth. If we are to approach the aims of professional education, our teaching theories must indeed mirror such objectives and our methods facilitate rather than obstruct or dull the innate drive of the student to learn and grow.

One student commented in her diary, "I wonder sometimes if this course is not to teach us so much as it is to make us able to learn—it would seem that what I am learning is how to learn and teach myself—this conviction grows stronger each week."

A second student wrote, "I'm beginning to get the impression that Mrs.———doesn't really care half as much about what we think as that we think." Another commented, "It's infuriating! Think and reason, think and reason—I'm sick of these words! Seven weeks and no hard cold facts! The assumption that students can answer their own questions is ridiculous. Why do we come to college in the first place?" Near the end of the semester this same student wrote, "It's taken a long time but I finally seem to be getting the message—things are beginning to fall into place and what's so exciting is that *I* have put them there—not some teacher who *'told me!'*"

The practicum or clinical experience is an additional opportunity for growth, for learning to apply knowledge, develop and test clinical skills, consensually validate and thus consolidate those functions which comprise professional competency. Within this frame of reference self-dependent thinking becomes a primary objective. A sense of professional responsibility needs to be created and decision-making skills developed by allowing the student to assume realistic responsibilities with sufficient freedom to make decisions rather than limiting these on the basis of unrealistic expectations. Collaboration with others is best taught by expecting and supporting collaborative roles rather than passive–dependent ones. Latitude to think and function in this manner, however, will be consistent with theories and goals of the professional educative process only if supervision is an integral part of the learning-growth process. Time and a multiplicity of experiences are not the primary agents for growth but rather skillful teaching which nurtures the development of the professional person.

Generally the concept of supervision seems to be in the literal sense of Webster's definition, "to oversee, to direct or inspect with authority." However, as a growth process in professional education, supervision is conceptualized as a dynamic teaching-helping relationship committed to the learning and growth of the student or supervisee. This learning experience has as its focus the exploration, analysis and synthesis of the ongoing functions of the learner to the extent that theoretical knowledge may emerge as professional skill. It exists on the basis that learning must be a conscious process in order for integration to be maximized and that self-awareness and understanding is the substructure of professional maturation and competency. Supervision in this sense then becomes the primary modus operandi in fulfilling the educational aims of the clinical experience and such is the contract which binds supervisor and learner together.

Frequently individual supervisory sessions are perceived as occurring only when specific problems or questions arise. However, this helping-teaching process needs to be an ongoing occurrence, regularly scheduled and proceeding in a logical sequence related to the learner's individual capacities and what is to be learned. Although what the student brings to the learning experience has an influence on the transaction, fulfillment of the supervisory contract will depend in great measure upon the attitudes and skill of the supervisor. The teaching-helping relationship, in the context of preparation for meeting professional expectations, has as one of its major goals increased self awareness and understanding—perception and understanding of self not as a goal in itself but for the purpose of developing a coherent, definable set of constructs concerning the dynamics of interpersonal relationships and the assimilation of these into basic attitudes and modes of functioning. The supervisor therefore must be sufficiently secure and free from biases to be able to approach situations realistically. He must possess an openness and receptivity to looking at feelings and their impact on behavior and have enough self awareness and understanding to provide the assurance and objectivity so necessary to exploring and understanding ongoing function and catalyzing appropriate change.

In conceptualizing supervision as a learning-growth process, it is important to understand the difference between this experience and therapy. Therapy is that process which has as its primary focus the alteration or diminution of psychopathology and thus is frequently concerned with the unconscious and genetic forces motivating pathological thinking and behavior. Supervision is directed toward learning and explores feelings and behavioral responses only in relation to the facilitation of learning and the development of professional skills. Extensive or depth exploration of personal feelings and their causative factors has no place in supervision. Personal problems which seriously interfere with learning and growth may well need to be worked through in therapy before the goals of supervision can be realized but the supervisory session is not therapy and the resolution of these problems belongs in another setting. For example, a student who has difficulty in helping a patient deal with his angry, hostile impulses needs to explore with the supervisor the nature and quality of the problem and come to have some understanding of how his own attitudes regarding such feelings have an impact on what transpires between himself and the patient. However, the personal, historical basis for such attitudes on the part of the student and working these through in depth does not belong in the supervisory session.

Charlotte Towle[13] presents some excellent formulations on the nature and scope of the supervisory relationship and Margaret Williamson[14] in her description of supervision makes useful comparisons between such processes, psychotherapy and counselling.

The terms *administration* and *supervision* are frequently used interchangeably. However, the concept of supervision as presented here emphasizes that the two, although related, are essentially different processes. Supervision is a dyadic relationship committed to the learning and growth of the individual. Administration is perceived as those procedures which are directed toward creating a milieu or culture, an organizational pattern, which may be expected to maximize attainment of the goals of a given institution or organization. Supervision is concerned with the professional development of the individual, administration with maximizing goal achievement of organization. Such a differentiation points up the relatedness of these two processes and at the same time brings into focus an appreciation for the different modes of operation within each. While the needs of the learner are served by each it is important to understand their particular differences in order to keep in focus the set of values and frames of reference unique for each setting in which learning occurs.

Development of the learner as a professional person requires that the teaching-learning process be perceived and understood as a dynamic human interactional growth process. In order for a profession to fulfill its obligations to the society it serves, learning must be a continuing, ongoing process. Education for the profession does not stop at the time of graduation. We must teach in such a way that learning will result in a research attitude; a way of thinking so that questioning, investigation and constructively critical evaluation become a way of life and thus learning and growth a continuing process. In addition, professional education should assure the maintenance of change, the learning transactions being of such a nature as to provide the developing professional with a sense of ego mastery so that his new set of values and concepts are not dangerously compromised once the teaching-helping relationship has been terminated.

Perhaps at no other time have there existed for us the opportunities we face today. Modern medicine with its developing sociologic focus creates new and exciting expectations for all professions. The concept of the whole man as a social interacting being brings more sharply into focus the significance of those concepts and practices indigenous to occupational therapy. Man's innate drive to fulfill his needs for self identity and self realization through productive transactions with his object and interpersonal world is and has been the corner stone of occupational therapy.

It is the privilege and responsibility of a profession to define the kinds of learning which will develop its students' potential for the fulfillment of its educational aims. May we have the courage, the knowledge and the sensitive discernment to measure up to the greatness of this challenge and to prepare professional leaders for tomorrow's practice.

References

1. Tyler, Ralph W. "Educational Problems in Other Professions," in Bernard R. Berelson (ed.), *Education for Librarianship.* Am. Library Assn., 1949.
2. Towle, Charlotte. *The Learner in Education for the Professions.* Univ. of Chicago Press, 1954, pp. 5, 10.
3. Lifton, Walter. *Working with Groups.* John Wiley and Sons, 1961, p. 5.
4. Towle, Charlotte, op. cit. p. 10.
5. Pearce, Jane, and Newton, Saul. *Conditions of Human Growth.* The Citadel Press, 1963.
6. Fidler, Gail S. "A Guide to Planning and Measuring Growth Experiences in the Clinical Affiliation." *AJOT,* XVIII:6, 1964.
7. Bradford, Leland P. "The Teaching–Learning Transaction," in *Forces in Learning,* Selected Reading Series Three, Nat'l Training Laboratories. Nat'l Ed. Assn., Wash., D.C., 1961, p. 8.
8. Jersild, Arthur. *"When Teachers Face Themselves."* N.Y. Bureau of Publications, Teachers College, Col. Univ., 1955.
9. Bradford, Leland, Op. cit.
10. Hill, William Faucett. *Learning thru Discussion.* Youth Studies Center, Univ. of Southern California, 1962.
11. Lifton, Walter, Op. cit.
12. Wechsler, Irving R., and Reisel, Jerome. *Inside a Sensitivity Training Group.* Institute of Industrial Relations, Univ. of California, 1960.
13. Towle, Charlotte, op. cit.
14. Williamson, Margaret. *Supervision—New Patterns and Processes.* Association Press, 1961.

15

1966 Eleanor Clarke Slagle Lecture

Authentic Occupational Therapy

Elizabeth June Yerxa, OTR

In the spring of 1963 I attended the "Workshop on Graduate Education in Occupational Therapy" held in the Ozark Mountains of Missouri. The air was heavy with the fragrance of a million dogwood blossoms. I was just settling into a mood of peacefulness when my tranquility was abruptly shattered by Earnest Brandenburg, dean of the University College of Washington University. Dean Brandenburg said, "It is my candid judgment that the field of occupational therapy in 1963 is *not* regarded and probably should not be identified as one of the professions."[1]

What image do you see when you think of a professional? A person who always wears clean white shoes or someone who can spout off the origins and insertions of every muscle in the body or one who can discuss Freudian theory with a psychiatrist? No, professionalism is much more than appearance and intellectual accomplishments. It means being able to meet real needs. It means being unique. It means having and acting upon a philosophy. It also means being "authentic."

Steps Toward Professionalism

In 1966, occupational therapy is moving with speed and accelerating self-confidence toward true professionalism. In the past we often dwelled upon our insecurity about who or what we were to the point that we were paralyzed into inaction. Remember how much time we used to spend in masochistic soul-searching? One of my favorite cartoons from the *Saturday Review* shows two bearded meditators sitting side by side on a mountain top. One says to the other, "There must be more to life than pursuing the meaning of life." Our growth toward appropriate confidence as professionals indicates that we have discovered there is much more to occupational therapy than contemplating its meaning.

What are some of the significant steps we have taken toward professionalism? In discussing the characteristics of a profession, Dean Brandenburg emphasized that a body of knowledge is essential. This body of knowledge must be based upon accepted research. Occupational therapists are becoming increasingly involved in planning, conducting and publishing the results of their own research studies. Clinicians are developing unique tools of evaluation and specialized methods for recording data. Treatment programs have thus not only become based upon sounder thought but have been sufficiently organized and objectified to be studied.

A few years ago our conferences relied primarily on physicians and other professionals from outside our field to identify what was important to our practice. Now our annual conferences plus workshops, seminars and study courses are loaded with excellent papers conceived and presented by occupational therapists. We have learned to look within our field for provocative thought and inspiration. We have found it in abundance.

Originally published 1967 in *American Journal of Occupational Therapy, 21*, 1–9.

Perhaps most significant for the future development of our body of knowledge is the increased awareness that the scientific attitude is not incompatible with concern for the client as a human being but may be one of the best foundations for acting upon that concern. This awareness is demonstrated by our students of today who are much more critical of the thinking of their elders, much more objective in assessing their own performance and much more likely to be able to frame a question which can lead to research than the students of ten years ago. Yet, if anything, today's students have gained in their capacities to care about the client.

The development of a body of knowledge in a professional carries with it considerable personal responsibility for making both rational (scientific) judgments and intuitive (artistic) decisions according to Dean Brandenburg. Occupational therapists are accepting greater responsibility to contribute to the pool of knowledge about the client, to exercise judgment as to how our skills can best be used to fulfill his needs, to assess the client's responses and communicate our unique findings to other professionals who need them in order to fulfill their responsibilities. The written prescription is no longer seen by many of us as necessary, holy or healthy. Instead our relationship to the referring physician is becoming much more communicative and collaborative. The pseudo-security of the prescription required that we pay a high price. That price was the reduction of our potential to help clients because we often stagnated at the level of applying technical skills.

Dean Brandenburg suggested that in order for occupational therapy to merit recognition as a "true" profession we needed to carry out a continuous evaluation and revision of our educational curricula. Do you realize that the past three years have constituted an educational revolution in occupational therapy? Since 1962, when we published the findings of our own curriculum study, we have engaged in an overwhelming amount of educational revisions of our curricula. For example, we held a workshop on graduate education in occupational therapy, revised the Essentials of an Acceptable Curriculum in Occupational Therapy, completed a study on the implications of the curriculum study including the formulation, for the first time in history, of a thought-provoking set of proposed educational objectives for occupational therapy. Two of our curricula have started pilot programs by which students can become registered occupational therapists and earn their master's degrees simultaneously. For a profession which frequently perceives itself as moving slower than a snail going uphill against the wind, this is astounding educational progress made in three years. If I were a faculty member I think I would be tempted to say to my students, as I stood before the class, "Don't worry about today's lesson, what you will learn in tomorrow's will make all of this obsolete."

The real significance of our educational progress lies on a deeper level than studies completed and changes initiated. Clinicians and educators have worked more closely together on this process of educational self-assessment than at any time in our past history. As a result, each has learned to respect the contribution of the other. It is as if theory and practice have finally touched hands and found that they respect and need each other. This unity will lead to basic education for our students which is a unified and continuous process.

Many of these changes have been hammered out through vigorous argument and the obstinate patience of occupational therapists who defended their educational philosophies in meetings lasting far into the night. I am certain at such times many of them longed, in their secret hearts, to rely upon some outside "authority." But they did not choose the easy way. As a result we can point with pride to the fact that *we* have taken the initiative and responsibility to evaluate and upgrade our total educational system using our unique resources. As Dr. Mary Reilly put it, "Like Rumpelstiltskin, we have taken the straw and woven it into gold."

A profession obtains wide recognition of the need for the services which it can perform. How widely is the need for occupational therapy recognized? Remember how we used to laugh, rather painfully, about the persons who would smile politely and say "oh isn't that nice" when we told them we were occupational therapists? For we knew they had no idea of what we did. To make matters worse we were not at all sure that we could tell them. We still experience similar responses but they occur less and less.

More significantly, the people and agencies who can recognize the need for our services and *do* something about it are well aware of how much they need us. The Medicare bill and corresponding state legislation recognize the need for occupational therapy in hospitals, home health services and extended care programs. These bills and regulations write our profession into the law as one criterion for an acceptable program. For the first time in history, these bills recognize our own registration process and graduation from an acceptable curriculum as the criteria for professional qualification.

Convalescent homes, out-patient facilities, rehabilitation centers and schools are clamoring for our services. One of our greatest problems of the future is not going to be how to bring about a greater awareness of the need for our services but rather to provide for the need which already exists with a level of service of which we can be proud.

An organization for a profession is also widely recognized, Dean Brandenburg stated. How widely recognized is the American Occupational Therapy Association? Our leaders have been sought for advice and counsel in writing the regulations for "Medicare." Many professions are most cognizant of the educational and organizational changes we have instituted, including our pilot programs on a master's level. A physician said to me recently, "You are far ahead of many other health professions educationally. Your organization is progressive. It looks toward the future." At a recent workshop for faculty members from schools of social work I was astounded at the reaction of intense interest and admiration for our foresight in both developing and having in operation certified occupational therapy assistants training programs.

Since 1963, occupational therapy has made important progress toward true professionalism by further identifying and substantiating our body of knowledge, developing the research attitude and tools for research among practitioners and students, accepting the responsibility for using judgment and making scientific and intuitive decisions, obtaining increasing recognition of the need for our services, maintaining standards for admission to the profession and obtaining legislative recognition of our own registration process as the criterion of professional qualification and undertaking a continuing evaluation and revision of our educational curricula.

This substantial progress does not mean that we have made it. For professionalism, by its very nature, requires our continual efforts to progress in all of these areas, particularly in identifying our own body of knowledge. Through our faith in the efficacy of our practice we have resisted pressures that would regress us to the level of technicians, pressures to drop our dual educational emphasis upon the behavioral and biological sciences, pressures to disavow in practice what we were unable to prove at the moment. In resisting these pressures we have acted in the present while maintaining a vision of the future.

Purpose of Occupational Therapy

It is all fine and good to talk about our steps toward true professionalism but what is the purpose of occupational therapy? I believe that our broad purpose is to produce a reality-orienting influence upon the client's perception of his physical environment and his social and psychological self, to the end that he can function in his environment with self-actualization. This purpose is certainly not unique to occupational therapy. It is shared by many professional groups who are motivated to provide altruistic service to the client.

If this broad purpose is a shared one, then how are we unique? When it comes to identifying even a part of the uniqueness of occupational therapy we frequently behave as though we belonged to the school of Chinese philosophers called Taoists. Substitute the words occupational therapy for the word Tao in the following poem and you will see the parallel. "The thing that is called Tao, is elusive, evasive. Elusive, evasive, yet latent in it are forms. Elusive, evasive yet latent in it are objects. Dark and dim yet latent in it is the life force."[2] We are often afraid that by defining our own elusive, evasive qualities we shall make our profession too small in concept.

For the purpose of provoking your thought and in full awareness of the dangers of limiting us, may I propose a concept? Occupational therapy is unique because we use the choice of self-initiated purposeful activities to produce a reality-orienting influence upon the client's perception of himself and his environment so that he can function. Let us examine four key phrases which help identify our uniqueness: choice; self-initiated, purposeful activity; reality-orienting; and perception.

Choice

First, the factor of *"choice."* Occupational therapy has been unique, historically, because of the client's participation in his own treatment. Choice has been so fundamental to our thinking that we have questioned whether procedures which are done *to* the person, over which he has no control, should be called occupational therapy. Choice has been encouraged in the client's selection of media, his unique interaction with our media and, most importantly, in setting the objectives for his treatment program.

Since self-initiated activity is our "stock in trade" and since it is impossible to force any human being to initiate without his choosing to do so, choice is one of the keys to our unique therapeutic process. It is also a necessity if we are to achieve the ultimate goal of occupational therapy, that is, the ability of the person to function in his environment with self-actualization. For no matter how well-conceived the therapeutic program, the resulting achievement of the client's function depends both upon his capacities and his *choice* to use them.

Our everyday vocabulary reveals our attitudes. We ask, "What would you like to accomplish with your arm brace?" or, "Would you prefer to plan your kitchen today or concentrate on bathing the baby?" We say we "work with the client." We do not "do" the client or "care for" the client or "manage" him.

Does the emphasis on choice mean that occupational therapists abdicate responsibility for the client's welfare, that our milieu is one of anarchy or that we are less knowledgeable than other professionals who "know" what is best for the client and treat him accordingly? Not on your life! Our client's choice is based upon exposure to our therapeutic process which encourages him to make a series of decisions leading to progressing degrees of independence.

Occupational therapists use their knowledge, skills and personalities to enable the client to experience his possibilities. He must be given the chance to choose on the basis of reality, not fantasy. He is not adequately informed to make choices until he can anticipate the results of his choices.

The occupational therapist identifies the small steps necessary to attain the client's larger goal, the purposes of the media and what the client might expect to accomplish or fail to accomplish, depending upon his choices. The occupational therapist's personal conviction may be an important means of eliciting the client's participation in an activity which he initially rejects because the experience of success, which the therapist knows he can attain, is not initially a fact to him. Many "motivation" problems occur because the client is afraid to fail and cannot anticipate the gratification of success.

This active role of the occupational therapist in helping the client delineate his choices takes more knowledge, skill and sensitivity plus more faith in the individual than an authoritarian role of "you must do this because it is good for you."

Rose Meyer, medical social worker, in her article "Dependency as an Asset in the Rehabilitation Process" said, "the rehabilitation process may be a long and dynamic struggle that influences and is influenced by the dependency–independency conflict."[3] She felt that the patient's ability to *use* his initial physical and psychological dependency could move him increasingly toward independence, similar to the evolution of his earlier life. Miss Meyer gave the following case history of a forty-year-old engineer who had recently become paraplegic: At first the patient rejected the dependency created by his injury. He tried to master his situation by learning all about his condition, his prognosis and how he could immediately participate in his own care. His aggressive, though reasonable attitude was overbearing to the nursing staff, for the progress he desired was always a bit ahead of reality. His behavior deteriorated to stubbornness and disinterested compliance. By the time he started his occupational therapy program he was threatening to leave the hospital in order to carry out many of his own ideas for developing independence. He was frustrated by the lack of opportunity to participate actively in his own program. When given the opportunity by the occupational therapist to make a choice for his treatment from several modalities for an explained purpose, he found structure for his move toward independence, not only in his own treatment but in his investment in the program of other patients for whom he designed appliances and work projects.

As Miss Meyer stated, "He could depend upon the occupational therapist's knowledge and skill to act as a catalyst for his own creative investment."

The occupational therapist thus serves as a catalyst by which the client moves toward increasing self-direction. The process begins with the client's acceptance of a reasonable degree of dependence upon the therapist's skill and knowledge, moves toward his understanding of the reality of his condition, his formulation of goals based upon that reality and his selection of media within a category of choices appropriate to the goals.

But what about the patient who is too incapacitated, physically and/or emotionally, to make *any* choice. Sister Madeline Clemence, in her moving essay, "Existentialism: A Philosophy of Commitment," dealt with this question in relation to nursing. "Whenever the nurse takes an initiative which should have been the patient's, she should understand that it is only a temporary measure and that it should be ratified by the patient."[4] The same principle applies to the occupational therapist.

Self-Initiated, Purposeful Activity

The second key phrase in investigating our uniqueness is *"self-initiated, purposeful activity."* Self-initiated refers not only to psychological choice but to sensory-motor participation. Dr. Karl Smith, professor of psychology at the University of Wisconsin has criticized behavior theory for its past emphasis on physiological drive states as the basis for human motivation. He states, "Yet much of ordinary human behavior—verbal and graphic skills, patterns of work, artistic and recreational pursuits—which we observe in ourselves and others seem to bear little relation to hunger, thirst, sexual drives and the like."[5] Dr. Smith feels that perceptual motivation or activity motivation should be considered of primary importance in behavior organization. "The nature of this motivating force can be described specifically in terms of the intrinsic make-up of the regulatory mechanisms of motion, for the neurogeometrically organized motion systems drive the individual to action as relentlessly and more consistently than hunger or thirst."

Self-initiated activity, specifically verbal and graphic skills, patterns of work, artistic and recreational pursuits—activity of concern to occupational therapists—is of primary importance in human motivation, if we accept Dr. Smith's theory.

Motion is patterned according to the spatial and temporal demands of the environment as the individual reacts to differences in stimuli. In resolving these differences, the individual continually and by his own movements produces new differences to which he must react. Thus self-initiated activity is both a response to sensory stimulation and a source of additional stimulation by which the individual develops patterns of adaptive behavior. Passive movements apparently do not result in the same degree of adaptation.[5] The individual must respond dynamically to changed stimulus relationships in order to adapt.

Dr. Jean Ayres called occupational therapy's emphasis on purposeful activity the factor which unites our profession in its practice for patients with emotional as well as physical conditions. She said, "If purposeful activity is one of the distinguishing functions of occupational therapy, it might well be asked if it is necessary for the treatment of motor disability." Then she answered, "In the life of the neurologically normal individual, activity is not random but purposeful, i.e. directed toward the accomplishment of a goal. It is generally this *goal* that is the basis for activity in the central nervous system and therein lies its value."[6]

A year ago I helped evaluate a brain damaged client's function. She was asked to open her hand. No response occurred, except that she was obviously trying. Next she was moved passively into finger extension while the occupational therapist demonstrated the desired movement. This time the client responded with increased finger flexion. In frustration she cried, "I know, I know." Finally she was offered a cup of water. As the cup was perceived, her fingers opened almost miraculously to grasp it. Only the factor of purpose could produce the desired response.

Purposeful activity is activity which has meaning to the client, not just to the occupational therapist. Our clients are individuals who have differing ideas of purpose. Some individuals are deeply imbued with our cultural admonition that "work is virtue." Such persons may respond with greater motivation to resistive exercise than to an elaborately adapted craft activity given for the same reason. For persons with lower motor neuron disease for whom the objective is increased muscle strength which will be translated into function, such exercise, providing that it constitutes purposefulness for the client, may be the most effective physiological and psychological method for producing the desired result.

Conversely and most particularly for patients with central nervous system impairment, straight exercise might not only be purposeless to the client but through its demand for attention upon the movement and not upon the goal, might produce an undesirable response. Craft activities or other creative, goal-directed pursuits may, in such instances, elicit a neuromuscular response which cannot be attained through other means. These activities also have the advantage of distracting the patient's attention from pain thus reducing the muscular splinting or neuromuscular alienation that often accompanies pain.

Reality Orientation

Third, the factor of *"reality orientation."* In occupational therapy the patient experiences the reality of his physical environment and his capacity to function within it. Our clinics may be chambers of horror for some individuals as they confront their physical disability for the first time by trying to do something, perhaps as simple as self-feeding. Yet, if the individual is to function with self-actualization he must discover both his limitations and his possibilities. We meet our responsibilities to the client when we provide him with opportunities to readjust his value system through the development of both new capacities and the ability to substitute for some lost capacities. We are like mirrors which can reflect, without the distortion of wish-fulfillment or self-deprecation, a true image of the client's potential.

Perception

Fourth, *"perception."* Occupational therapy produces a reality-orienting influence upon the client's perception of his physical environment as well as his psychological and social self. In the area of physical perception our media produce sensory stimuli which are perceived and reacted to by the client. Our professional literature is presently concerned with identifying syndromes of perceptual-motor dysfunction, the development of evaluation tools for identifying specific problems of perceptual-motor function and the development of theories upon which to base treatment programs to improve these functions. Because our media require the use of postural movements, transport and fine manipulation and because they allow us to stimulate many sensory modalities, we are appropriately and deeply concerned with perceptual-motor function. Dr. Ayres and others from our profession have contributed significantly to the available literature in this area.

It has been found in experiments of displaced or delayed sensory feedback that many normal individuals react to their resulting perceptual-motor discoordination with considerable emotional disturbance.[5] Similarly, persons with perceptual-motor dysfunction may exhibit severe behavior problems. Psychotic episodes have been associated with the use of such perception distorting drugs as LSD. These findings indicate the existence of a link between perceptual-motor function and emotional responses. This link, with further study, might serve to bridge another apparent gap between our practice with the physically disabled and that with the emotionally disabled person. We are one of the few professions whose education prepares us to visualize the perceptual-motor function of man as a psychobiological unity.

In addition to perception of a neurophysiological nature, the individual also perceives himself as a psychological entity and a social being. Occupational therapy provides an everyday environment in which the individual can determine, through choice, his own particular identity.

The following is an example of the kind of self-perception we sometimes deal with:

Look at me, look at me
What do you see?
A thing made of plaster, metal and skin.
Look at me, look at me
How can this be?
They make me exist in the place that I'm in.
Look at me, look at me
Help me to flee
From this world of blindness to that of the seeing.
Look at me.

This young lady, who is severely paralyzed, is pleading for help to escape from her own self-concept into the world of the "seeing," that is, a world in which she would perceive herself as being recognized, not as a "thing" but as a feeling, thinking, valuable human being.

Exposure to our media means a confrontation with objects and an opportunity for the individual to discover what he can and cannot do with them. Exposure to our professional spirit means that the individual confronts both our knowledge of his capacities and our faith that he has the right to control what happens to him.

Being a "thing" leads to social relationships based upon dependency, hostility or pity. As James Colbert, a paraplegic, said in his essay *A Study Establishing the Disabled as a Minority Group,* "pity can be referred to as a sort of sequence mechanism: disease or accident—hospitalization—disability—I am very sorry." Jim observed, "This attitude may, in fact, be responsible for motivating the disabled to stay apart from their [previous] social group and to act and interact mainly with their own [disabled] group."[7] Pity implies the socially-sanctioned classification of the disabled into a minority group and with that classification comes dismissal from the stream of "normal" society. Occupational therapy which leads to the client's ability to function in his environment can help alter other people's perception of him as the object of pity and reduce their need to classify him apart from themselves.

Occupational therapists, in my experience, are remarkably free of the sort of cynicism and expediency which might result in the client perceiving himself as a "thing." Our positive attitude has been characterized as "regulated optimism" by one occupational therapist. Another fine occupational therapist said, "Occupational therapy begins when everyone else has given up." She meant it humorously. But like most humor it had a strong core of truth. Both of these statements reflect our faith in the client.

Being able to help the client confront himself is perhaps the most sensitive, personally and professionally demanding task of the occupational therapist. For it requires courage on the part of the client, emotional support on the part of the occupational therapist and a continual mutual testing and communication of what reality is.

Just as our emphasis on "purposeful activity" unites our practice for patients with emotional as well as physical conditions, so does our emphasis upon helping the patient grasp the reality of his life situation in order to move toward increasing degrees of self-direction. For even in such a seemingly physically oriented activity as teaching a patient to dress himself, our ultimate goal is a psycho-social one. That is, by increasing the client's capacity to be independent we help him perceive himself as possessing worth. He is not a "thing" to be manipulated helplessly by others but is a human being who can exercise some control over his environment, even in being able to put on whatever shirt he wants to put on when he wants to do it.

Occupational Therapy's View of Man

The psalmist phrased the question: "What is man that thou art mindful of him?"[8] That question has been repeated over the centuries. Although fragment by fragment has been added to our knowledge of man's nature, through the sciences and historical experience, our understanding remains incomplete. For man is mysterious. He defies definition.

Yet, in spite of this mystery, our profession has chosen unique methods to help the client function with self-actualization. Both our methods and our goals imply that we have a point of view regarding man's nature. For if we are to be helpful to him, we must conceive of what is valuable to him. This takes us into philosophy.

Our particular view of man agrees considerably with that of some existential thinkers. Unfortunately, existentialism has been associated with anti-intellectualism, egocentricity, irresponsibility and anarchy. It therefore frequently conveys mental pictures of bearded beatniks who wallow in pools of self-pity, bewailing the meaninglessness of the universe, while regularly collecting their unemployment insurance checks. These associations are superficial.

According to David E. Roberts,[9] existentialism is not an organized philosophical system but rather it represents a protest against all views which tend to regard man as though he were a *thing,* that is, only an assortment of functions and reactions. It stands against philosophies or social theories in which the mass mentality stifles the spontaneity and uniqueness of the individual person. In occupational therapy's recognition of the client as one who ought to participate in his treatment and be given the opportunity to make choices, we are as Martin Buber would say, "taking a stand" in relation to him. We are viewing the client, not as an object or thing to be manipulated, controlled or made to conform but as a unique individual whose very humanness entitles him to choices in determining his own destiny. For if the client interprets himself as a thing (one thing among others in the world) he might sacrifice his selfhood and neither recognize nor realize his potentials.

Existentialists see man as involved in the process of becoming. What he becomes is shaped by himself, in response to his life experiences and relationships to others. Heidegger, the philosopher who contributed significantly to existential thinking, made a distinction between "authentic" and "inauthentic" existence. He felt that in the world of everyday experience man comes to terms with what he is only by coming to terms with his possibilities or potentialities. If he lives mainly in terms of "what one does" or what one "does not do" and is therefore merged in conventional mass reactions, he is emerged in inauthentic existence. Authenticity is achieved to the degree that the individual reaches true selfhood by rising out of mass reactions, taking the initiative in discovering the meaning of his own existence and disposing of his own potentialities accordingly. In order to achieve authentic existence man must have resolve to become his true self.

For the client who is hospitalized the institution may inadvertently represent the "mass mentality" with its pressures of what "one does" or what "one doesn't do." Louis Worth, the sociologist, once remarked that the only good institution is a dead institution.[10] His comment was provoked by the common tendency of institutions, implicitly or explicitly, to regard their own survival as a major goal thus losing sight of the client's individuality in the process.

Bill was the "ideal" patient. He kept all of his appointments religiously and worked diligently on every aspect of his treatment. He accepted the wisdom of the physicians who directed his rehabilitation program. He carried out his therapeutic activities without question. He used every piece of self-care equipment which was ordered for him. He attained an amazing degree of physical independence prior to discharge to the point that he became an example to inspire other patients. Six months after his discharge he came back to hospital for a clinic visit. His facial expression was passive and lifeless. He had gained thirty pounds, had developed a pressure sore and had become dependent in all activities except for minimal self-feeding. Obviously Bill had conformed to the hospital's value system temporarily but once out of the institutional environment had become primarily a dependent and passive being. In that sense he had lived an "inauthentic" existence while hospitalized. Instead of encouraging his adherence to the value system of the institution, how much better it would have been if his behavior had been recognized as conformity. The occupational therapist might then have provided him with opportunities to question, complain and become emotionally involved in his rehabilitation program. Often the clients who distress the hospital staff the most by not behaving as "patients" become the most self-directed after discharge.

Earlier I mentioned the client's confrontation with the reality of his disability in occupational therapy. This confrontation with pain, suffering, loss of function and the high anxiety associated with it are realities about which he can begin to determine the meaning of his life's experiences. In other words, the pain and deep stresses of such an experience may lead to resolve. For such traumatic experiences, which cannot be ignored, can transform the individual's existence from that of a day to day contact with superficial, meaningless events to a "mind and heart" involvement in being. Instead of regarding himself as surrounded by circumstances and chance events, he can begin to see himself in a situation which is something to be mastered. Action on his part can become, instead of mainly a series of external, practical activities, a development of inner resources which can be stronger than mere happenings.

The particular reality of the occupational therapy clinic involves not only the client's disability but his opportunity to make the kinds of choices by which he can discover, for himself, the meaning of his own existence and realize his potentials in accordance with that meaning. Our clinics are one of the few environments within institutions in which the client can make such choices.

Existentialism also makes a firm distinction between subjective and objective truth. It does not deny that through common sense, science and logic men are able to arrive at genuinely objective truth. But, it insists that in connection with ultimate matters it is impossible to lay aside the impassioned concerns of the *individual*. In the search for ultimate truth, the whole man, not just his reason and intellect, are involved. His emotions and his will must be aroused and engaged so that he can live the truth he sees. As Heidegger put it, "The scientist pursues one legitimate way of studying what is, but he makes an extra-scientific assertion when he adds, 'That's all there is. There isn't anymore.'"

In occupational therapy we are providing a milieu in which the total man, not just his reason, is involved. Our purposeful media, our emphasis upon the discovery of the client's potential, the necessity for him to act in occupational therapy and his relationship to us deeply involve his will and emotions, providing that we can be authentic in relation to him.

Authentic Occupational Therapy

What then, is authentic occupational therapy? Authentic occupational therapy is based upon a *commitment* to the client's realization of his own particular meaning. The authentic occupational therapist recognizes that although initial dependency might require a temporary suspension of the patient's right to choice, the therapeutic experience is primarily an opportunity for self-actualization. Therefore, the occupational therapist does not force his value system upon the client. But rather, through using his skills and knowledge, exposes the client to a range of possibilities which constitute his external reality. The client is the one who makes the choice.

Authentic occupational therapy means *involvement* of both the client and the occupational therapist. Through the use of media the client is involved intellectually and emotionally in discovering what is purposeful to him. He is also involved in relation to objects, actions and persons. Through these relationships he is helped to come to grips with his particular reality including his disability, his emotional reactions, his will and his potential.

Professional authenticity in occupational therapy means that the occupational therapist in every professional *act* defines the profession. For example, he may believe that it is important to perform clinical research but that belief has no meaning until he *acts* upon it by initiating research activity.

As a professional, the authentic occupational therapist recognizes his responsibility to be a lifelong student and to contribute to the body of knowledge. He also recognizes that an important part of what he will learn and contribute will be subjective, that is, concerned with feelings and human motivation. He will not expect science to provide him with all the answers but he will respect what science has to contribute.

Personal authenticity as an occupational therapist means that the therapist allows himself to feel real emotion as he enters into *mutual* relation with the client. In a mutual relationship as Martin Buber said, "My thou affects me as I affect it. We are molded by our pupils and built up by our works."[11] The authentic occupational therapist is involved in the process of caring and to care means to be affected just as surely as it means to affect.

William Barrett in his superb book *Irrational Man* cites the example of the successful businessman who flies to the country for the weekend, is whisked off to golf, tennis, sailing; who entertains his guests successfully, all on a split-second schedule and at the end of the weekend flies back to the city without ever having the desire to lose himself by walking down a country lane. Such a man, we say, is marvelously organized and really knows how to manage things; but the point is that he has mastery over beings but not Being. "He never has contact with Being. He goes to the country and returns without ever *really* being there."[12] We cannot really help clients unless *we are there*; that is we feel, we encounter, we take time, we listen and we *are* ourselves.

The authentic occupational therapist is open to the client's ideas and feelings and real in responding to them. He does not give in to the temptation to insulate himself against feeling because if he does so he will lose his capacity to be there. "Being there" also means being able to separate his feelings for the client as a human being from projections of how *he* would feel if he had experienced the client's disability. For the authentic occupational therapist knows that the client is the only one who can discover his own particular meaning. Stephen Becker in his essay *On Being a Patient* put it this way. "One man's hangnail is another man's broken neck."[13] He went on to say that once the disabled person has decided to live he must stop asking "why me?" He must reject pity and singularity with equal and absolute indifference. Mr. Becker, as a result of his experience of being a patient, reaffirmed his philosophy that nature never rejoices and never mourns.

In the new dimension of 1966, occupational therapy is becoming a true profession. This is a time to be proud of what we have accomplished. Our service to the client is unique in its application of choice, self-initiated, purposeful activity and its emphasis upon the goal of function with self-actualization. Our media have been identified as those activities which are at the very source of human motivation. Philosophically we do not see man as a "thing" but as a being whose choices allow him to discover and determine his own Being. Our media, our emphasis upon the client's potentials, the necessity for him to act and the mutuality of our relationship with him provide a milieu in which his suffering can be translated into the resolve to become his true self.

This is also a time for each of us to determine our own authenticity as professionals. The degree to which we can maintain faith in our profession and still strive to improve it by our own acts, the degree to which we can maintain faith in our clients while becoming involved in the process of helping them will determine the future authenticity of our practice. We are ever becoming.

Rainer Maria Rilke wrote:

> "Out of infinite yearnings rise
> finite deeds like feeble fountains,
> that early and trembling droop.
> But those, else silent within us,
> Our happy strengths—reveal themselves
> in these dancing tears."[14]

Acknowledgment

The author wishes to express her appreciation for the thoughts and support contributed by the following persons: Lois Barber, OTR; Jerry Johnson, OTR; Janet Stone, OTR; Doris Kroulek, OTR; and the staff and students of the Occupational Therapy Department at Rancho Los Amigos Hospital.

References

1. Brandenburg, Earnest. "Building Toward Professionalism." *Proceedings of Workshop on Graduate Education in Occupational Therapy*, April, 1963.
2. Yutang, Lin (ed.). "The Manifestations of Tao." *The Wisdom of China and India*, Random House, 1942.
3. Meyer, Rose. "Dependency as an Asset in the Rehabilitation Process." *Rehab Lit*, XXV:10 (Oct.), 1964.
4. Clemence, Sister Madeline. "Existentialism: A Philosophy of Commitment." *Amer J Nurs*, March, 1966.
5. Smith, Karl U. *Perception and Motion.* W. B. Saunders, 1962.

6. Ayres, A. Jean. "Occupational Therapy for Motor Disorders Resulting from Impairment of the Central Nervous System." *Rehab Lit,* October, 1960.

7. Colbert, James. "A Study Establishing the Disabled as a Minority Group." Unpublished paper, UCLA.

8. Psalm VIII, verse 4, *The Bible.*

9. Roberts, David E. *Existentialism and Religious Belief.* Oxford University Press, 1960.

10. Richardson, Stephen A. "Some Unintended Consequences of Current Rehabilitation Practices." *Staff Reprint,* Association for the Aid of Crippled Children, 1959.

11. Buber, Martin. *I and Thou.* Charles Scribner's Sons, New York, 1958.

12. Barrett, William. *Irrational Man.* Doubleday Anchor Books, 1962.

13. Becker, Stephen. "On Being a Patient." *The Atlantic,* July, 1966.

14. Norton, M. D. Herter. *Translations from the Poetry of Rainer Maria Rilke.* The Norton Library, 1938.

16

1967 Eleanor Clarke Slagle Lecture

Professional Responsibility in Times of Change

Wilma L. West, MA, OTR

We are now convened for the final day of a conference in celebration of the 50th anniversary of our professional life. Behind us lie five decades of individual and group endeavor—endeavor to develop a profession, to define and refine a service, to improve an image and extend its acceptance, to recruit others to our ranks and train them for perpetuation of our ideals, to research new and better ways of accomplishing our goals.

At this milestone in our history, one could be tempted to look back through the years and analyze the functional relationship between endeavors and accomplishments. Such stock-taking would surely yield an inventory of assets in many areas of effort in which we might feel mutual pride. It would also, however, show liabilities for which we remain collectively responsible. Still other accounts might appear as outstanding or receivable, thus implying the necessity for continued effort in the commitment to further progress. Depending on the perspective and purpose of the individual doing the analysis, this measure of our first fifty years might be impressive, discouraging or inconclusive with respect to net accomplishment.

Santayana has warned that "He who neglects history will be condemned to repeat it." However, awareness and understanding of effort input with reference to success or failure of outcome are most functional when new approaches are being brought to the solution of old problems. If, on the other hand, changing or new conditions prevail and hence a different set of problems is presented, there is diminishing value in more than brief review of the methods of other people and times. The example of the inadequacy of conventional defenses in a nuclear age is the obvious one, but professional personnel in medical and educational fields today face a dilemma equal to that of the military in recognizing that old ways of solving problems are no longer adequate.

Let us turn, then, from any comfortable reflection on our past to the infinitely more exciting exercise of projecting our future. Wisely approached, this can be as scientific as a retrospective analysis and surely it is a more dynamic course if we wish to have a part in determining our future rather than merely accepting one on assignment or default of others.

One cannot be in the practice of any of the health professions today without being keenly aware of the many forces shaping his future roles and responsibilities. Nor can he neglect his duty to examine the implications of these forces in three dimensions: for himself as a professional person, for the profession of which he is a member, and for the professional organization which represents and promotes his individual and group interests. In brief, the questions currently confronting us are: What is happening in both our immediate and larger worlds? and, What does this mean to us?

The general stage for this discussion may be set by an analogy from another field that is strikingly similar to that of medicine. Francis Keppel, former commissioner of the Office of Education, Department of Health,

Originally published 1968 in *American Journal of Occupational Therapy, 22*, 9–15.

Education, and Welfare, says that America is entering a third revolution in education. In the first revolution, education of the masses was achieved by the establishment of the public school system. Later, equality of education for all people became the rallying cry for school reform. Now the astounding advances in technology demand specialized and high-quality education for all regardless of race, creed, or social class.[1]

Today this country is well into a similar multistaged reorganization of health and medical care in which equal availability and high quality of health services are sought for all people. The bipartisan endorsement of providing services to meet two of man's most fundamental needs—for education and health care—has removed the question from the arena of welfare and politics and placed it in the larger domain of basic human development.

Whether one agrees with these trends wholly, partially, reluctantly, or not at all, one fact is virtually undeniable today: comprehensive health care, among others of man's needs, is beyond individual attainment for far too many people. If we accept this fact, we can accept the organization of increasingly costly and complex programs designed to reduce disease and disability among victims of economic disparity and to raise the health standards of our country as a whole.

"Governmental involvement (then) in the financing and organization of health services is here to stay and there is every indication that it will increase."[2] I submit, however, that governmental participation and individual responsibility are neither incompatible nor mutually exclusive. In fact, we must go even further in pursuit of a rationale that is in tune with both our changing times and a high standard of personal and professional integrity. I therefore tend to agree with another commentator on this subject who has said that "placing health in the category of the rights of man involves the transformation of a social desire into a moral imperative."[3] This imperative has been stated as follows by the New York Academy of Medicine: "That *all people* should have . . . *equal opportunity* to obtain a *high quality* of *comprehensive health care.*"

It is difficult to see how anyone could mount an argument against the humanitarian elements of this high goal. In the sense that the primary orientation of the professions is to the community interest, there *must* be concern for all people on the basis of equal opportunity and with a standard of the highest possible quality that it is within our ability to provide. Implications of most of the key phrases in this all-encompassing objective are clear. However, the last dimension—comprehensive health care—bears elaboration because it is with reference to this focus that we will examine how our profession can best adapt its philosophy and practice to future requirements.

At our annual conference in Minneapolis last year, the theme was "Dimensions of Change." Many of us, I am sure, recall the message of several thoughtful speakers who helped us read signs among today's maze of medical plans and programs that are as complex and confusing as the newest multistory interchange of highways around our large cities. I hope we also recall the repeated emphasis on *health,* as well as illness, on *prevention* of disease and disability, in addition to seeking the cures not yet discovered, on *maintenance and promotion of well-being,* not just being satisfied that there is an "absence of infirmity,"[4] on *continuity of care,* in lieu of only episodic attention to emergency conditions, and on *comprehensive health services* that must replace the diagnostic or categorical approach of conventional medicine.

The trends in these directions are unmistakable. They are also irreversible. To recognize them, however, is only the first step. We must also interpret their meaning for each of our specialty areas and aggressively adapt or redesign our roles to provide a more viable future service.

No one person can or should do this for all facets of his profession. Each must, however, do it for his own focus of interest and with all the professional outlook and insight he can muster. I can best relate these changing trends and their implications to the field of pediatrics, with which I have been most closely involved in recent years. I shall attempt to do so in the general framework of comprehensive health care for children and, more specifically, with reference to selected groups which present us with some very challenging opportunities to develop a preventive role for our profession. I shall conclude with some thoughts on the implications of these and other changes for the profession as a whole.

Comprehensive Health Care for Children

What is meant by comprehensive health care for children? This is a term that is variously defined, but on the conceptual level, I prefer the following statement to all others that I have read: "By comprehensive, we mean a constellation of health services that focuses on the patient as an individual human being rather than as a collection of assorted organ systems, some of which are diseased."[5] On the practical level, we believe this ideal must be translated into programs which include health supervision in the various parameters of growth and development and the regular use of specific devices for screening deficits and dysfunctions. Comprehensive health care for children, we feel, is committed to enhancing normal development as insurance against disease or, failing that objective, to the earliest possible casefinding of those conditions which have their origin in prenatal causes or in the disabling illnesses of infancy and the preschool years.

Both the number and scope of programs designed to provide health care for children are greater today than ever before. The idea behind them, however, is hardly a new one. For it was in 1890 in France that the first nursing conferences and milk stations were established to provide preventive health services for lower socioeconomic segments of the child population. At that time the motive was to reduce the enormously high infant and preschool child mortality, but from these early beginnings, clinic services of similar types have developed throughout the world. In the United States, the milk stations of the World War I era subsequently became known as well-baby clinics and today, in many areas, are called child health conferences.

It is interesting to trace the broadening philosophy of these forerunners of modern comprehensive health care for children. Since such enterprises were designed to provide health supervision of well children, one of their primary functions was to screen children for evidence of abnormality or illness that might warrant referral for care.

A classic text on preventive medicine and public health[6] tells us that the child health conference was originally necessary because a large segment of the population was unable to pay for health supervision. However, it also goes on to point out that even today such services cannot be transferred to the private practitioner. The reason, the authors state, is that education and training of medical students is still largely oriented to the patient with cellular pathology, with the result that many practitioners today have limited interest in and knowledge of the principles and techniques of health supervision of growing children. Furthermore, child health personnel even in recent years have been largely preoccupied with the development of treatment and training programs for handicapped children.

And so, it seems, have occupational therapists in pediatrics. Thus we, too, have been slow to develop a role in prevention that might greatly enhance our total professional contribution to health care. Although our traditional commitment to medicine and our orientation to illness and treatment are understandable, our greater development of a preventive role, which is "an integral part of all medical practice, wherever it may be and under whatever auspices"[7] is long overdue.

There is even a sense of urgency to the situation that cannot be escaped. Consider for example the number and diversity of settings in which new health care programs for children are constantly being developed. The well-child clinics or child health conferences that have already been mentioned are standard services of state and local health departments, but they are only one of several locales where continuing health supervision of children is assuming ever greater importance.

Probably the best known among others that I will discuss here are the Head Start programs that have received extensive publicity in the brief two years since their inception. Although the initial focus of these efforts was on enrichment of experience in preparation for school, a spin-off benefit of major importance has been identification and treatment of health deficits. It is of significance to us that the range of these deficits goes far beyond the dental and nutritional problems inevitable in the target populations and includes a high incidence of retarded or deviant physical and psychosocial development. As we well know, the chances for remediation of many such problems are infinitely better at age three or four than at beginning school age which, until now, has provided our earliest largescale screening opportunity.

Another very new program of the Office of Economic Opportunity which was launched late this past summer could provide an even richer locus for occupational therapy in a preventive role. This is the development of Parent and Child Centers that is currently taking place in thirty-six American communities to provide services for disadvantaged families who have preschool children. A prime objective of these centers will be the use of techniques and processes both to prevent deviations and deficits and to stimulate development to the maximum potential. Among the skills and experience sought for staff are the ability to recognize and understand the developmental stages of young children and prescribe a plan for progress to meet each child's individual needs.[8]

To pediatric occupational therapists who have been concerned with the larger objective of optimal child growth and development as well as with restoration of impaired function, the possibilities inherent in these new centers must indeed be exciting. Think, for example, of the broad range of activities that could be used to provide multisensory input directed to the development of intellectual, emotional, social and physical skills. The graded and guided use of activities for such purposes is so integral a part of occupational therapy that this would seem to be a most fitting application of our skills to plan, elicit, interpret and modify both performance and behavior.

There are other groups of children for whom health surveillance could provide either prevention or earlier treatment. Sparked by the increasing prevalence of daytime employment of both parents or the absence of one parent and employment of the other, day care facilities have become a way of life for thousands of young American children. The larger of these, the day care centers, are units with seven to seventy-five or more children, a staff of one or more persons, and an organized program. In these settings today, ages of children usually range upwards from two and a half years, this being the minimum age for most children to participate in group play or other organized activities. What an opportunity there is here to prevent, restrict or retard development of problems we now see only when they are entrenched and disabling, often to a severe degree.

A final example is a group of children which has received special attention during the past year and is already providing the occupational therapist with a role in screening, evaluation and programming as well as in treatment. This is the group served by the Children and Youth projects sponsored by the Children's Bureau.

Organized in areas of economic and social disruption, these projects are designed to provide comprehensive health care for large numbers of children who, under existing circumstances, have only marginal opportunity to develop a healthy mind and body. Now, however, a broad range of health professionals is being assembled to provide services which should greatly improve their future outlook.

Included in the authorized core staff for children and youth projects is an occupational therapist whose job description reads quite differently from the specifications for other pediatric roles. If a few of these promising new positions can be filled by therapists with vision as well as skill, there are few limits on the extent to which they will be permitted to develop a broader role. For example: in New York City, two pediatric neurologists on a children and youth project added an occupational therapist to assist them in screening for neurological deficits; in Dallas and in Denver, pediatricians directing diagnostic clinics use their therapists to evaluate motor performance and behavior adjustment and to participate in programming based on team findings and recommendations; and in several other areas of the country, therapists are involving children in activities which permit assessment in numerous areas of function and providing selected experiences to promote development of neuromuscular, emotional and intellectual competencies of children.

These, then, are some of the programs made possible by the federal-state alliance to extend and improve health services for increasing numbers of people. They require of all professions a careful appraisal of changes that may be necessary as we jointly seek creative and workable solutions to both old and new problems. Although we have centered attention on one specialty of our profession, it is intriguing to think about how the number and kinds of changes in pediatrics today will inevitably, in time, affect every other age group and specialty field of occupational therapy.

Furthermore, there are equally radical changes occurring simultaneously in patterns of delivering health and medical services to all people. Witness, for example, the burgeoning community mental health programs and consider the implications of trends in that specialty of our profession. Are there not elements here, paralleling the new kinds of community-based services in pediatrics, which are dictating programs concerned with the maintenance and promotion of health as well as the treatment of illness? And hence, are there not here, too, strong indications for increased emphasis on the preventive role of occupational therapy?

Of course there are, and many progressive occupational therapists in both these and other specialties of our profession have already taken steps to keep pace with trends that require new or expanded roles. Furthermore, they have done so with such effectiveness that they have created roles and functions that greatly improve the image of our profession. In a sense, therefore, my commentary only reflects what I consider to be the best abroad in practice today, with a few thoughts on where, how and why it seems particularly urgent that we intensify our efforts in these directions and at this time.

I fear, however, that there are yet too many among us who do not sufficiently appreciate current trends and who therefore are not lending their efforts to hasten and make credible more functional roles throughout the profession. The platform at a general session of our Annual Conference and assured publication in our professional journal lend temptation to speak frankly to one's colleagues. And, the occasion of a golden anniversary provides a good point at which to cross the treacherous terrain of prophecy and hazard a glimpse of where our best future directions may lie. He who does so will always run the chance of suggesting some wrong turns, but he who does not has missed both an opportunity and a responsibility to share with others his views on areas of mutual concern.

We Are Committed to Our Profession as a Whole

I would like, now, to discuss some ramifications of these thoughts in terms of the profession as a whole rather than in the framework of any one or more specialty areas of practice. For, regardless of our individual concerns with separate fields, it is to the whole profession that we are jointly committed and for which we must cooperatively work. My remaining remarks will explore some of the reasons why it seems important that this be so.

What is the relevance to us as a professional group of the changes I have discussed, of other changes that are taking place in patterns of providing health services, and of the implications these have for traditional and transitional roles in our profession? Is it enough that there is a growing number of clinicians in each of our specialty fields who are continually sharpening conventional skills and also developing new ones? Can we rely on the work of a small but increasing number of researchers among us to confirm the scientific basis of our practice? Does the greater sophistication of today's authors sufficiently raise the level of our professional literature? Will the growing number of our members who are obtaining graduate degrees insure a higher quality of performance in the future? Are changes that are being effected by the more progressive among our educators adequate to the preparation of tomorrow's therapists? In short, will the leadership of these and other significantly contributing individuals suffice? Indeed, should it have to?

Decidedly not. What is absent from this kind of thinking is the concept of group responsibility—responsibility for awareness and interpretation of those changes which affect any part of our profession, and responsibility for whatever group action is appropriate to facilitate or hasten adjustment to change. Thus, although we clearly recognize that "All occupations are dependent on the individual contributions" of those who practice them, we must also realize that "the effectiveness of an occupation is not gauged by individual efforts alone; the total efforts of occupational members working together with some degree of cooperation must also be considered. The public image of an occupation, then, is in part individual and in part collective. . . . Moreover, the goals of an occupation are only in a limited sense individual, for the individual responsibility of practitioners and a consciousness of the aims of the occupation are very much a function of collective action."[9]

There are, of course, many terms for the kind of collective action here referred to. Among them is what I shall call professional consciousness and responsibility. This is an attribute that we in occupational therapy have to a quite considerable degree. It has served us well in the fifty years of our professional development to date, primarily, I believe, because we have used it more in the sense of professional responsiveness to public interest and need than for purposes of protecting or promoting our constituent individuals and groups. These two major purposes of a profession—meeting external obligations to society on the one hand, and internal loyalties to members on the other—may often be in conflict. That they have not created serious problems or dichotomies for us up to this time may be viewed as a mixed blessing, for readings in the sociology of development of the professions make it clear that it is only a matter of time until they do. Factors which may have delayed this apparently inevitable process include our extremely small size and the relative homogeneity of a profession with only incompletely developed specialties.

Trend Toward Decreased Professional Unity

With the passage of time, however, we are experiencing both an increase in size and a proliferation of special skills among our members. As these two dimensions grow, we become increasingly subject to the influence of factors which will tend to decrease professional unity and promote segmentation in accordance with divergent interests and strengths as they develop among us. Although it will undoubtedly create some problems, this trend is by no means undesirable. On the contrary, it usually brings with it both an improved service, which results from increased knowledge and skill of specialists, and a growing professional influence which can be used to improve the status of those who provide that service.

There are signs that the era of segmentation is already upon us; witness for example, the increasing number of special interest meetings and concurrent sessions scheduled at this year's Annual Conference. While neither deploring the problems nor lauding the advantages an increase in this trend will bring, I hope that we will retain an attitude of general professional consciousness and concern for as long as we exist. Conviction of the need for this lies in the belief that "the chief factor . . . in the accomplishments of any profession is the unified, aggressive efforts of its members."[10]

Numerous theories have been put forth to explain why persons pursuing an occupation come together and associate in a formal manner. These include everything from the likely initial motivation for exchange with those doing the same work, to such presently accepted objectives as raising standards of competence, formulating codes of ethics, improving education, undertaking protective and promotional activities, and many others. The activities of associations as major interest groups which participate in planning and policy decisions on matters of concern to them are generally thought of as a development of recent years undertaken to counter the influence of governmental regulations on professional activities; in fact, however, these date back at least three centuries when, as one writer says, "it was characteristic of the times that powers and duties of so extensive a nature were granted to vocational associations that they may be regarded as organs of the state."[11] Thus they are illustrative of the influence a well-organized profession can have on public decisions and policies.

I make no case for our professional association to aspire to this degree of power. I do, however, believe that both as individuals and as a professional group we should be assuming a far more frequent and contributing part in the planning of health services. It will, in fact, be mandatory that we do so if, as I said earlier, we are to have a part in shaping our own development.

Izutsu believes that "it is not too late to achieve positions of leadership that will determine the future" of our profession.[12] However, he also lists several steps that we must take if we are to remain equal to changing patterns in the organization and delivery of health services. Among these are the development of leaders not only to plan for therapy but to think in the broad spectrum of social planning; training of therapists in public health principles and procedures; and exposure, in our training, to community-oriented settings and other health team members in lieu of training primarily in hospital settings.

Professionally, We Often Resist Change

I do not suppose any of us knows, with any degree of certainty, the ideal future course for our profession. We do, however, see many signs that it must keep changing if it is to stay abreast of the larger world of which it is a part. Change is seldom easy or comfortable. Yet there is little about the world in which we live today that is more characteristic of it than the continual and fast-moving changes which transcend every aspect of our lives.

Although each of us makes the necessary adaptation to these changes as they affect our personal concerns and activities, we are slower as a group to adjust our professional directions and developments to that which is new. We are often, in fact, resistant to the suggested need for change and all that it implies in the necessity for new learning and the establishment of new roles and functions. We are also reluctant to explore new potentials, to experiment, to take an occasional risk.

From Therapist to Health Agent

Increasingly, today, I believe we should identify with the field of health services, thus broadening our traditional, more limited identification with medicine. We should enlarge our concept from that of being a therapist to one of functioning as a health agent with responsibility to help insure normal growth and development. We should think more about roles in prevention as well as in treatment and rehabilitation, about socioeconomic and cultural as well as biological causes of disease and dysfunction, and about serving health needs of people in many other settings than the hospital.

One occasion on which this was expressed in a very effective way by a number of our colleagues was the conference on research in occupational and physical therapy held last February in Puerto Rico. In one of the discussion groups there was studied avoidance of the term "patient," which many felt limited their concern to illness, and a plea for consideration of health as only one aspect of the developmental process of man which should not be isolated from other factors impinging on life. This kind of thinking and discussion culminated in the group's consideration of its topic in the framework of what they called "the continuum of health services which reflect the needs of man in his environment."[13]

A broad frame of reference? Admittedly, but it is also entirely in keeping with our traditional philosophy of concern for the person rather than just his disability. For us, therefore, the idea possesses what might be called "instant validity." It now needs rapid if not instant implementation.

We are living today in a world that is vastly different from that when occupational therapy began. It matters not so much that it has taken fifty years to reach this day, as that the next fifty see more, and more rapid, progress than the last. It matters less that we are still struggling to define our profession than that we build a broader base for the better definition that will one day be written. It matters most of all that we recognize the responsibility of the profession to change with changing demands for its services, to adapt via new approaches, to assume different roles, to develop the preparation for them and to recruit in a new mold rather than by recasting the prototype of an earlier time.

On the eve of her retirement from active work in our national organization, Eleanor Clarke Slagle was paid the following tribute:

> Those of us who have been privileged to follow the winding trail of those years know of struggles, of courage in facing criticism, of disappointments and rewards, of patient waiting, persistent faith and devoted work. The questing youth of our profession accepts both with commendation and condemnation what has been so painstakingly accomplished through this quarter century. But when they too can look back over an equal span of service in this field, they, and occupational therapy, will still be moving to the measure of the thought of Eleanor Clarke Slagle.[14]

That "equal span of service" has now passed so we, too, are looking back over the second quarter of a century which immediately precedes the present day. It seemed fitting that we do so in the context of both our practice to which she gave so much, and our professional association which she helped to organize, served as an officer in four capacities, and directed as its executive for many years. I, for one, hold to much that she obviously held high among her goals for the profession. Among those goals, I feel sure, was one related to the need for professional responsibility at all times. In times of change such as these, that need and our response to it will be of great importance in determining the next fifty years of our professional life. At the turn of the 21st century, when yet another generation looks back on these times, may they see that ours was a dynamic posture of professional consciousness and responsibility.

References

1. Keppel, Francis. *The Necessary Revolution in American Education.* New York: Harper and Row, 1966.
2. Burns, Evalina. "Policy Decisions Facing the United States in Financing and Organizing Health Care." *Public Health Reports, 81:*8 (Aug.) 1966.
3. Dearing, W. P. "Prepaid Group Practice Medical Care Plans." *Public Health Reports, 77:*10 (Oct.) 1962.
4. Preamble to the Constitution of the World Health Organization.
5. Kissick, William L. "Trends in the Utilization of Rehabilitation Manpower." *Manpower Utilization in Rehabilitation in New York City.* New York: New York City Regional Interdepartmental Rehabilitation Committee, Sept., 1966.
6. Sartwell, P. E., ed. *Maxcy–Rosenau Preventive Medicine and Public Health,* 9th ed. New York: Meredith Publishing Co., 1965.
7. Freeman, Ruth B. "Impact of Public Health on Society." *Public Health Reports, 76:*4 (April) 1961.
8. *Criteria for Parent and Child Centers.* Washington, D.C.: Office of Economic Opportunity, July 19, 1967.
9. Vollmer, Howard M., and Mills, Donald L. *Professionalization.* Englewood Cliffs, New Jersey: Prentice-Hall, Inc., 1966.
10. Stinnett, T. M. "Accomplishments of the Organized Teaching Profession." *The Teacher and Professional Organizations.* Washington, D.C.: The National Education Association, 1956.
11. Carr-Saunders, A. M., and Wilson, P. A. "The Rise and Aims of Professional Associations." *The Professions.* Oxford: The Clarendon Press, 1933.
12. Izutsu, Satoru. "The Changing Patterns of Patient Care." (A Position Paper). *Research Conference in Occupational Therapy and Physical Therapy.* New York: American Physical Therapy Association, 1967.
13. Group Report. "Research in Patient Care." *Proceedings of the Research Conference in Occupational Therapy and Physical Therapy.* New York: American Physical Therapy Association (to be published).
14. "In the Past, Pride—In the Future, Faith." A Documentary of the Heritage, Growth and Outlook of the American Occupational Therapy Association. Produced by the Association for its Forty-First Annual Conference, New York, New York, October 21, 1958.

1969 Eleanor Clarke Slagle Lecture

Facilitating Growth and Development:
The Promise of Occupational Therapy

Lela A. Llorens, MA, OTR

Preamble

To be the recipient of the Eleanor Clarke Slagle Lectureship is indeed an awesome honor. Preparing for this moment has been an arduous task. Many of my colleagues and friends have checked periodically on my progress during the year and the answer most often given was, "We're living with it." We, including my family, have literally lived with the "Lecture" this year and the breakthrough that I was struggling for did not come until late summer during our trip to West Africa. When it did, it came in the form of ten premises which express a developmental theory of occupational therapy.

The theory which I am presenting has been an outgrowth of my experience and research in the field of psychiatry, both pediatrics and adult, and more recently in pediatric general medicine and community health. In order to do justice to the formulation, however, I have spent considerable time in consultation with my colleagues in physical medicine and rehabilitation and with their patients. These experiences as well as the fortunate opportunities I have had to participate in a number of seminars and workshops over the past several years have stimulated my desire to think through the function and purpose of occupational therapy as I have experienced it.

Introduction

In this paper, a conceptual model for understanding the knowledge that presently supports the practice of occupational therapy is presented with a discussion of how and where occupational therapy fits into the scheme of human development.

My thesis is simply this: that occupational therapy is a facilitation process which assists the individual in achieving mastery of life tasks and the ability to cope as efficiently as possible with the life expectations made of him through the mechanisms of selected input stimuli, and availability of practice in a suitable environment. The occupational therapist serves as the enculturation agent for the conditions of physical, social and psychological health in which the developmental level being experienced by the individual in any one of a number of parameters of development is unequal to the age-related demands made of that organism as a result of natural or traumatic incident.

Originally published 1970 in *American Journal of Occupational Therapy, 24,* 93–101.
Please note that there was no Eleanor Clarke Slagle Lecture in 1968.

Developmental Theory of Occupational Therapy

The theory is based on these premises:

1. That the human organism develops horizontally in the areas of neurophysiological, physical, psychosocial and psychodynamic growth and in the development of social language, daily living and sociocultural skills at specific periods of time;

2. That the human organism develops longitudinally in each of these areas in a continuous process as he ages;

3. That mastery of particular skills, abilities and relationships in each of the areas of neurophysiological, physical, psychosocial and psychodynamic development, social language, daily living and sociocultural skills, both horizontally and longitudinally, is necessary to the successful achievement of satisfactory coping behavior and adaptive relationships;

4. That such mastery is usually achieved naturally in the course of development;

5. That the fundamental endowment of the individual and the stimulation of experiences received within the environment of the family come together to interact in such a way as to promote positive early growth and development in both the horizontal and longitudinal planes;

6. That later the influences of extended family, community, social and civic groups assist in the growth process;

7. That physical or psychological trauma related to disease, injury, environmental insufficiencies or intrapersonal vulnerability can interrupt the growth and development process;

8. That such growth interruption will cause a gap in the developmental cycle resulting in a disparity between expected *coping behavior and adaptive facility* and the necessary skills and abilities to achieve same;

9. That occupational therapy through the skilled application of activities and relationships can provide growth and development links to assist in closing the gap between expectation and ability by increasing skills, abilities and relationships in the neurophysiological, physical, psychosocial, psychodynamic, social language, daily living and sociocultural spheres of development as indicated both horizontally and longitudinally.

10. *That occupational therapy through the skilled application of activities and relationships can provide growth experiences* to prevent the development of potential maladaptation related to insufficient nurturance in neurophysiological, physical, psychosocial, psychodynamic, social language, daily living and sociocultural spheres of development both horizontally and longitudinally.

This in my opinion is the promise of occupational therapy. In order to pursue this theory further, let us look at the various areas of knowledge which support the continuum of human development including behavior and ability expectation.

Current Knowledge of Human Development

The life span of the individual encompasses several phases of physical growth, neurophysiological, psychological, social and emotional development as well as a gradual decline in many of these life processes, particularly physical development, as the individual ages requiring continued growth in the adaptive abilities of the organism. Ayres has contributed greatly to our knowledge of neurophysiological development from infancy to adolescence.[1] Gesell has contributed specifically to our knowledge of the physical development of children through this same age span, as well as to our knowledge of the development of social language, sociocultural and daily living skills in this age group.[2] At the present time, however, such specific details of the physical development of adults is not easily available for either the young or the aging. Erikson has given us in his "Eight Ages of Man" some insight into the psychosocial development of the individual in terms of his behavior both at the time of initial emotional experience and at the time of reexperience of early development in adult life.[3] He spans the life cycle from infancy to old age and emphasizes the continual growth conflicts which are inherent in living. He cautions against believing that any level of developmental achievement, once achieved, becomes a permanent part of the psychological makeup of the individual as the individual is a dynamic, changing, developing organism. Freud has provided us with an understanding of child development as it relates to personality in its organization and dynamics.[4, 5]

In the process of development the human organism expects and is expected to achieve specific adaptive behaviors which equip him to cope with life. These specific behaviors assist him in the larger task of getting on in the world. In his *Developmental Tasks and Education*, Havighurst presents us with a concept of developmental tasks as being midway between an individual need and a societal demand.[6] Meeting societal demands requires adaptive skills and mastery of self and the environment. The adaptive skills correlative to this formulation have been developed from the work of Pearce and Newton and the work of Mosey. Pearce and Newton give us some insight into how residuals of early patterns of development become a part of the personality structure as an adult as well as how early patterns of development contribute to adaptation, the ability for and style of coping with life demands.[7] Mosey has defined for us specific adaptive skills required by the individual to adjust to his internal needs as well as to the external demands.[8] These are the areas that constitute horizontal and longitudinal development.

At any point in time, the human organism experiences simultaneous growth (horizontally) in the areas of physical, neurophysiological, psychosocial, psychodynamic, sociocultural development, and in the skills of daily life and social language. As he matures, he experiences longitudinal growth in each of these areas. In order for the individual to achieve in the adaptive areas of functioning it is necessary for him to experience satisfaction and mastery both horizontally and longitudinally in the developmental spectrum.

For emotional growth to proceed in a natural and spontaneous way, it must be nurtured with affection, understanding, security and discipline, and be stimulated by achievement and social acceptance. It is necessary, too, that children gain satisfaction in their relationships with others so that they may develop the feeling that they are lovable, that their individuality is respected and that they can have confidence in their own strength and capability as a person. As the child develops he explores his environment, establishes relationships and acquires knowledge and skills which enable him to successfully adapt to his world.[9]

In adolescence the activities of the period expand into social, intellectual, literary and artistic interests. Intense relationships as with a chum are particularly important to this period. Physical changes occur which must be incorporated into the self-image. It is necessary for the adolescent to have the support and understanding of his family as he reaches for adulthood.

"The primary conditions for growth for the adult are crucially different from the conditions of growth of the developmental eras of pre-adulthood. These differences relate to the adults' responsibility to initiate and consolidate experience, and also to the new significance of sharing."[10]

Middle age requires reorganization of several factors of one's life. Emotional responsibilities of parents become less demanding as children leave home and ongoing financial responsibility becomes finite and predictable. Physical and physiological changes occur which must figure in the adaptation of the individual.

Not enough information has been documented concerning physical growth and development in old age. Cultural cliches hold that growth does not take place in the aging years, that the quality of life in those years tends to be strongly determined by the nature of the outcome of the middle-aged crises.

Each stage of development in this longitudinal process is dependent upon the successful resolution of the developmental "crises" related to each growth stage. Physical or psychological trauma experienced in any one of the horizontal parameters at any particular time in the longitudinal process can interrupt the developmental cycle.

Facilitating growth and development during and following traumatic experiences is the task of occupational therapy. Understanding the needs of the individual as they relate to the determination of function and dysfunction and the choice of activities and relationships to ameliorate or modify dysfunction, to enhance remaining function and to facilitate continued growth consistent with the individual's developmental stage are the tasks of the occupational therapist.

There are sensorimotor activities, developmental play activities, symbolic activities and interpersonal relationships which are specifically significant to particular age ranges in the longitudinal process. There may be specific reason to emphasize one or another of this range of activities as well as relationships at any one given point in time depending on the horizontal area of development most affected by trauma. I wish to stress that although emphasis may be placed on the facilitation of growth in one particular parameter, simultaneous though perhaps less attention must be given to all of the other areas of growth as well in order for an integrating growth experience to take place.

Developmental Theory Illustrated

In an effort to illustrate this concept in graphic form Sections I and III of Figure 17.1 have been developed to show the areas of developmental growth as described by Ayres, Gesell, Erikson and Freud and the areas of expectation and adaptation as described by Havighurst, Mosey, Pearce and Newton. In order to demonstrate relevance to age, age ranges have been imposed. Caution must be observed in interpreting the age ranges as they are suggestive rather than absolute. The imposition of age ranges is particularly useful in correlating development horizontally as well as longitudinally but has its limitations in application which must be considered.

Section II of Figure 17.1 illustrates the tools of occupational therapy which are utilized in the process of facilitating growth and development. The age ranges are suggested by position also in a correlative fashion.

Let us look at the implications of Section I. During the first two years of life the human organism is developing sensory perception of the tactile, vestibular, visual, auditory, olfactory and gustatory functions; physical-motor behavior and body integration; is developing a balanced sense between "trust and mistrust" through these same functional areas which manifests itself in ease of feeding, depth of sleep and relaxation in elimination and is nurtured by consistency, continuity and sameness. At the same time that these areas are developing, the oral "stage" related to dynamic development as seen in dependency, initial aggression and oral erotic activity is evident. Sociocultural development at this age is centered first around the individual mothering relationship and later extends to the immediate family group. Social language is beginning first with small sounds, then coos, vocalization, listening, speaking words and responding to simple verbal directions. Activities of daily living, including early recognition of the source of food, beginning to hold feeding objects and, later, controlling elimination, are developing.

We see that there is overlap in these stages, that development does not occur in neat segments. As the infant learns to motor plan, which encompasses the first four years of life beginning with the discovery of the hands and feet, he progresses to all fours then to walking, climbing, balancing, developing hand preference and coordination of eyes and hands and eyes and feet. The development of the body scheme, knowledge of body parts, development of a sense of two integrated sides with a front and back can be seen. During this period a balance between "autonomy and shame and doubt" are being developed and manifested in conflictual behavior between emotionally "holding on" and "letting go." The anal "stage" is evident in independent, resistive, self-assertive, narcissistic and ambivalent behavior. Magical thinking and anal preoccupation are also characteristic of this stage. Sociocultural development during this period centers around parallel relationships in play, isolated play and the importance of extended family. Social language is expanding into the verbal identification of objects, asking "why" and putting words together in short sentences. Feeding himself, helping to undress, recognizing simple tunes and controlling night time wetting become important activities of everyday life.

Between the ages of three and seven the sensory functions are refined, coordination becomes more graceful, muscles become stronger, skills are developed. At the same time a balance is being developed between "initiative and guilt" manifest in aggressiveness, manipulation and coercion.

The genito-oedipal stage is evident in the interest the child shows in his own genitals and those of the opposite sex, his possessiveness of the opposite sex parent, antagonism to the same sex parent and in castration fears or disappointment. Sociocultural development during this period centers around the companionship of others, learning to make decisions, learning to play successfully with other children, learning to play alone, taking turns and

Figure 17.1. Schematic representation of facilitating growth and development.

SECTION I				
DEVELOPMENTAL EXPECTATIONS, BEHAVIORS & NEEDS				
(Selected for illustrative purposes)				
NEUROPHYSIOLOGICAL-SENSORIMOTOR Ayres	PHYSICAL-MOTOR Gesell	PSYCHOSOCIAL Erikson	PSYCHODYNAMIC Grant/Freud	SOCIO-CULTURAL Gesell
0-2 Sensorimotor Tactile functions Vestib. functions Visual, Auditory, Olfactory, Gustatory	0-2 Head sags Fisting Gross motion Walking Climbing	Basic Trust vs. Mistrust/Oral Sensory Ease of feeding Depth of sleep Relax. of bowels	1-4 Oral Dependency Init. aggres. Oral erotic activity	Individual mothering person most important Immediate family group important
1-4 Integration of Body Sides Gross motor plan. Form & space perc. Equil. resp. Post. flex. Body sch. dev.	2-3 Runs Balances Hand pref. established Coordination	Autonomy vs. Shame & Doubt/ Muscular-Anal Conflict between holding on & letting go	1-4 Anal Independence Resistiveness Self-assertive- ness Narcissism Ambivalence	Parallel play Often alone Recognizes extended family
3-7 Discrimination Refined tactile Kinesth., Visual, Auditory, Olfact., Gustatory funct.	3-6 Coordination more graceful Muscles devel. Skills develop	Initiative vs. Guilt/Locomotor- Genital Aggressiveness Manipulation Coercion	3-6 Genital-Oedipal Genital interest Poss. of opp. parent Antag. to same parent Castration fears	Seeks compan- ionship Makes decisions Plays with other children Takes turns
3- Abstract Thinking Conceptualization Complex relat. Read, write, numbers	6-11 Energy develop- ment Skill practice to attain proficiency	Industry vs. In- feriority/Latency Wins recognition thru productivity Learns skills & tools	6-11 Latency Prim. struggles quiescent Init. in mastery of skills Strong defenses	Group play & team activities Independence of adults Gang interests
	11-13 Rapid growth Poor posture Awkwardness	Identity vs. Role Confusion/Puberty & Adolescence Identification Social roles	11- Adolescence Emancip. from parents Occup. decisions Role experiment Re-exam. values	Team games Org. important Interest in opposite sex
		Intimacy vs. Isolation/Young Adulthood Commitments Body & Ego mastery		
		Generativity vs. Stagnation/ Adulthood Guiding next generation Creat., pro- ductive		
		Ego Integrity vs. Despair/Maturity Acceptance of own life cycle		

(continued)

Figure 17.1. Schematic representation of facilitating growth and development *(cont.)*.

		SECTION II FACILITATING ACTIVITIES & RELATIONSHIPS (Selected)				SECTION III BEHAVIOR EXPECTATIONS & ADAPTIVE SKILLS	
SOCIAL-LANGUAGE Gesell	ACTIVITY OF DAILY LIVING Gesell	SENSORI-MOTOR ACT.	DEV. PLAY ACT.	SYMBOLIC ACT.	INTER-PERS. RELAT.	DEVELOPMENTAL TASKS Havighurst	EGO-ADAPTIVE SKILLS Mosey, Pearce & Newton
Small sounds Coos Vocalizes Listens Speaks	Recognizes bottle Holds spoon Holds glass Controls bowel	Tact. stim. Ident. body parts Sounds Objects	Dolls Animals Sand Water Excursions	Biting Chewing Eating Blowing Cuddling	Individual Interaction	Learning to Walk Talk Take solids	Ability to respond to mothering Mastering of gross motor responses
Identifies objects verb. Asks "why?" Short sentences	Feeds self Helps undress Recog. simple tunes No longer wets at night	Phys. exer. Balancing Motor planning	Pull toys Play grnd. Clay Crayons Chalk	Throwing Dropping Messing Collecting Destroying	Individual Interaction Parallel play	Elimination Sex difference To form concepts of soc. & phys. reality To relate emotionally to others	Ability to respond to routines of daily living Mastery of 3 dimen. space Sense of body image
Comb. talking and eating Complete sent. Imaginative Dramatic	Laces shoes Cuts with scissors Toilets indep. Helps set table	Listening Learning Skilled tasks & games	Being read to Coloring Drawing Painting	Destroying Exhibiting	Individual Interaction Play small groups	Right Wrong To devel. a conscience	Ability to Follow directions Tol. frustrations Sit still Del. gratification
	Enjoys dressing up Learns value of money Responsible for grooming	Reading Writing Numbers	Scooters Wagons Collections Puppets Bldg.	Controling Mastery	Individual Interaction Groups Teams Clubs	Learn phys. skills Getting along Reading, writing Values Soc. attitudes	Ability to perceive, sort, org. & utilize stimuli Work in groups Mas. of inanimate obj.
	Interest in earning money		Weaving Machinery tasks Carving Modeling		Individual Interaction Groups Teams	More mature rel. Social roles Sel. occupation Achieving emot. independence	Ability to accept & discharge resp. Capacity for love
						Selecting a mate Starting family Marriage, home Congenial social group	Ability to function indep. Control drives Plan & execute Purposeful motion Obtain, org. & use knowledge Part. in primary group Part. in variety of relationships Exp. self as accept. Part. in mutually satis. heterosex. relations
			Arts Crafts Sports Club & interest groups Work		Individual Interaction Groups	Civic & social responsibility Econ. standard of living Dev. adult leisure act. Adj. to aging parents	
						Adj. to decr. phys. health, retire., death Age group affil. Meeting social obligations	

(Vertical label between first two columns and the next section: E V A L U A T I O N)

sharing. Social language development sees the child combining talking and eating, using complete sentences, expressing his imagination and creativity. His activities of daily living include shoe lacing, cutting with scissors, toileting independently and helping with chores such as setting the table and making his bed.

Beginning at about three years of age, becoming more refined around five and six and continuing on throughout life, the functions of abstract thinking, conceptualization, reasoning, the development of complex relationships and the ability to read, write, count and figure numbers develop. Physically around six the child becomes more energetic and proficient in the mastery of skills through practice. The balance between "industry and inferiority" is developing and is manifest in attempts to win recognition through productivity and learning skills and tools. The "latency" stage is evident as the primitive struggles quiet, the interest in mastery of skills becomes predominant, toleration of competitiveness, identification and acceptance of reality become important and strong defenses develop. Sociocultural development during this period centers on group play and team activities, developing independence of adults and interest in "gang" activities. Activities of daily living include joy in dressing up, learning the value of money and developing responsibility for personal grooming.

Physically, rapid growth takes place between eleven and thirteen accompanied by poor posture and awkwardness. During the adult years some physical growth, though less rapid, continues. Around eleven the balance between "identity and role confusion" is developing, manifest in identification with social roles. The "stage" of adolescence in dynamic terms is evident in the emancipation from parental control, the making of occupational decisions, role experimentation, difficulty with compromise, intensification of feelings and the re-examination of societal values. The sociocultural development of this period is centered around organized team activities and interest in the opposite sex. Activities of daily living include interest in earning money.

Adult development as described by Erikson places the struggle for balance between "intimacy and isolation" in young adulthood. This period is characterized by the capacity to commit oneself to concrete affiliations and partnerships and to abide by such commitments. Ego and body mastery must predominate. Adulthood is characterized by the struggle to maintain balance between "generativity and stagnation" which is manifest in behavior directed toward guiding the next generation, one's own creativity and productivity. Maturity is characterized by the balance between "ego integrity and despair" and manifest by the acceptance of one's own life cycle as "something that had to be."

These developmental expectations, behaviors and needs characterize the cycle of human development. Successful growth and mastery in all of these areas is the basis on which the developmental tasks of life are achieved as found in Section III of Figure 17.1. The developmental tasks as described by Havighurst and ascribed to the first six years of life include learning to walk, talk, take solids, control elimination, understand sex differences, form adequate concepts of social and physical reality, relate to others at an emotional level, distinguish right from wrong and develop a conscience.

The ego-adaptive skills developing simultaneously during this period are the abilities to respond to mothering, to respond to routines of daily living, to follow directions, tolerate reasonable amounts of frustration, sit still, delay gratification, share and take turns. As with longitudinal development, there are also overlaps in the horizontal plane. In this discussion the developmental tasks and adaptive behavior delineations serve to summarize the human growth continuum.

Beginning at about six years of age, learning physical skills, building wholesome attitudes towards oneself, getting along with others, learning appropriate masculine and feminine social roles, achieving personal independence, reading, writing, developing values and acceptable social attitudes are important developmental tasks. The correlative adaptive skills include the ability to accurately perceive, sort, organize and utilize stimuli and the ability to work cooperatively in groups and individually.

Adolescent developmental tasks include achieving more mature relationships with others, developing appropriate social roles, selecting an occupation, achieving emotional independence of adults while the adaptive skill most predominant is the ability to accept and discharge a certain amount of responsibility.

Young adulthood developmental tasks may include selection of a mate, starting a family, learning to manage a home and developing a congenial social group. The tasks of adulthood include the expansion into accepting responsibility for civic and social conditions, developing and maintaining an economic standard of living, developing adult leisure activities and adjusting to the reality of aging parents. The developmental tasks of maturity require adjustment to decreasing physical health, retirement and death; developing appropriate age group affiliations and meeting appropriate social obligations.

The adaptive skills correlative with this period from young adulthood through maturity are the abilities to function independently; control drives and select appropriate objects; plan and execute purposeful motion; obtain, organize and use knowledge; participate in a primary group; participate in a variety of relationships; experience self as acceptable; and participate in mutually satisfying heterosexual relationships.

In the course of human development, should the individual experience physical or psychological trauma related to disease, injury, environmental insufficiencies or manifest intrapersonal vulnerability which interrupts the natural process, a gap thereby develops resulting in a disparity between expected coping behavior and adaptive facility as illustrated in Section III of Figure 17.1 and the necessary basic skills in growth and development as illustrated in Section I. Occupational therapy through the skilled application of activities and relationships can provide the necessary links to assist in closing the gap by facilitating basic growth and development, increasing skills, abilities and relationships in the neurophysiological, physical, psychosocial, psychodynamic, social language, daily living and sociocultural areas of development both horizontally and longitudinally.

Let us now look at Section II of Figure 17.1 which illustrates selected activities and relationships which are the tools of occupational therapy utilized in facilitating the growth process. Evaluation is the first step in the process of intervention, the process by which a determination is made relative to the need for as well as the primary objectives for occupational therapy intervention. Evaluation including testing, interviewing, record review, and systematic clinical observation should take into account the areas of basic growth and development represented in Section I and the expected behaviors and adaptive skills represented in Section III.

The activities and relationships available to the occupational therapist have been categorized as sensorimotor activities; developmental "play" activities, symbolic activities and interpersonal relationships and have been assigned an age relationship correlative to the basic developmental functions and adaptive behaviors by position. These positions, however, as with development, cannot be considered absolute.

During the first two years of life, activities which facilitate development of sensorimotor functions include touching; being touched, cuddled, hugged; moving, exploring, looking, hearing, tasting, smelling, identifying, sounds and objects. Developmental play media which incorporate these stimuli include blankets, dolls, animals, sand, water, books, blocks, food, and trips of various kinds. Symbolic activities of this age require biting, chewing, eating, blowing and cuddling. All of these "activities" must be practiced in an individual "mothering" relationship, the relationship of choice, to be maximally useful to the individual.

Beginning in the first year and extending through the third, the sensorimotor activities include physical exercise, balancing and motor planning; the developmental play materials include gross movement toys, pull toys, "play ground" type equipment, clay, crayons and chalk; symbolic activities of the period include throwing, dropping, messing, collecting, and destroying; and the interpersonal relationships of choice are individual interaction and parallel "play."

Between the three- and six-year span, the sensorimotor activities include listening, learning, practicing skilled tasks and games; the developmental play activities include being read to, coloring, drawing and painting; symbolic activities include destroying and exhibiting, and the interpersonal relationships of choice are individual interaction and parallel "play" in small groups. During the six to eleven year span; sensorimotor activities include the high level cognitive tasks of reading, writing and numbers; developmental play activities include scooters, wagons, collections, puppets, and building tasks; symbolic activities of the age are characterized by control and mastery and the interpersonal relationships of choice include individual interaction, groups, teams and clubs.

Adolescent developmental "play" activities include weaving and other home crafts, machinery tasks, carving and modeling and the interpersonal relationships of choice are individual interaction, group and team relationships.

Practice and continued development of competence in sensorimotor functions are assumed to take place until the organism begins to decline in neurophysiological function, the exact time of which will vary from individual to individual. The activities engaged in in leisure as well as in work from adulthood through maturity facilitate this continued development. Affective growth continues with the availability and responsiveness of the individual to interpersonal relationships as well as his ability to receive gratification through symbolic processes which continue to reactivate as the organism grows and develops.

Implications for Practice

This theory states that physical or psychological trauma related to disease, injury, environmental insufficiencies or intrapersonal vulnerability can interrupt the natural process of growth and development and that such growth interruption will cause a gap in the developmental cycle resulting in a disparity between the development of expected coping behavior and adaptive skills and the necessary basic skills and abilities to achieve such growth. It implies that the incongruence in developmental functioning evident in illness and disability is similar to conditions experienced by the individual at an earlier level of developmental functioning which requires relearning of skills, working through of emotional conflicts and re-development of many functions which may have been previously mastered. Further that it is the task of the occupational therapist to determine at what level the individual is functioning in the various aspects along the developmental continuum and to program for facilitating growth and development in each of these areas in accordance with the needs of the individual and the demands of his age. The use of selected relevant activities and relationships appropriate to his level of functioning would be indicated.

In order to assist the individual in his movement toward the development of a comfortable adaptive relationship to life it is necessary to meet his needs at his developmental level as a beginning. Through careful monitoring of the treatment process and careful attention to clues that signify movement to a higher level and therefore readiness for change in programming needs of the patient, we can move toward providing an integrating treatment experience. My experience suggests that to provide activity and relationship processes for a level higher than the individual's ability to cope is to heap stress on an already overwhelmed system and to do relatively more harm than service. The permissive school of treatment within occupational therapy practice has had on its side the natural instincts of the individual to seek his level of need and therefore lead the therapist into appropriate interaction at a point of toleration for the patient provided this level could also be tolerated by the therapist. The symptom-oriented school of thought has also had some success in that symptomatology often points to needs which may indicate a level of development at which the individual is functioning provided the leads are accurate and the therapist is "listening." The disability-oriented school of treatment has had some measure of success in restoring function, however, may fail in having the restored function integrated for use if careful attention is not paid to other related levels of development.

The implications of this theory for the preservation of health and the prevention of potential maladaptation related to insufficient nurturance in the various aspects of growth and development are related to the belief that intervention at a stage that can be identified before trauma becomes overwhelming will allow the individual to continue his growth process with a minimum of interruption and continue toward the achievement of ego-adaptive skills. In cases of permanent residual or chronic physical or psychological disability, achievement of developmental tasks and ego-adaptive skills must be guided within the individual's limitations and geared to a realistically attainable level.

This formulation does not provide a recipe for practicing occupational therapy. It simply orders some of the factors relevant to a developmental theory for practice that must be validated. It provides a framework in which to understand the contribution of the various testing, systematic observation and other evaluation tools that are available to us in relationship to occupational therapy intervention, a framework in which to understand our selective use of activities and relationships and a system which speaks both to horizontal and longitudinal growth.

Within the practice of our profession, there are predictable aspects relative to cause and effect in the use of activities and the application of relationships which must be identified, applied repeatedly in a systematic manner, analyzed and documented in order to establish their validity. There are also measurable phenomena related to change relative to occupational therapy intervention which must be studied and documented as well.

Looking at our profession from a developmental point of view, one might say that we have mastered the sensorimotor levels of development and have achieved body integration, learned to walk and talk, have worked through our needs for dependency, although there may be remaining conflicts between holding on and letting go. We recognize the need for reading and writing and are developing our skills accordingly. We appear to be on the threshold of abstraction and conceptualization and working toward mastery of the understanding of the essence of our profession. This is my impression by observation; more careful evaluation would be necessary to determine the truth of these observations as well as to elicit others. In order to move us toward mastery, selected relevant activities and relationships will be needed to nurture our continued growth and development.

In closing, I would like to share with you a rather startling discovery that I made some time ago. It was, that "they," whoever "they" were, that I felt should be doing something to objectify our knowledge and raise the level of our practice included "me." I, herewith, challenge each of you to join me in that task so that "we" can move toward facilitating growth and development and fulfilling the promise of occupational therapy.

This study was made possible under Children and Youth Health Service Grant #640, Children's Bureau, Department of Health, Education and Welfare.

References

1. Ayres, A. Jean. "Perceptual–Motor Training for Children." Lecture given during 1962 WFOT Study Course VI—*Approaches to Treatment of Patients with Neuromuscular Dysfunction.*
2. Gesell, Arnold, and Armatruda, Catherine. *Developmental Diagnosis.* New York: Harper and Row, Inc., 1967.
3. Erikson, Eric. *Childhood and Society.* New York: W. W. Norton and Co., 1963.
4. Hall, Calvin S. *A Primer of Freudian Psychology.* New York: The New American Library, 1964.
5. Grant, Quentin R. Unpublished lecture notes.
6. Havighurst, Robert J. *Developmental Tasks and Education.* New York: David McKay Co., Inc., 1967.
7. Pearce, J., and Newton, S. *Conditions of Human Growth.* New York: Citadel Press, 1963.
8. Mosey, Anne C. *Occupational Therapy: Theory and Practice.* Medford, Mass.: Pothier Brothers, 1968.
9. Llorens, Lela A., and Rubin, Eli Z. *Developing Ego Functions in Disturbed Children.* Wayne State University Press, 1967.
10. Pearce, J., and Newton, S., op. cit., p. 119.

The 1960s: Discussion Questions and Learning Activities

The Lectures

Zimmerman, M. E. (1960). Devices: Development and direction (1960 Eleanor Clarke Slagle Lecture). In *Proceedings of the 1960 Annual Conference* (pp. 17–24). New York: American Occupational Therapy Association.

Reilly, M. (1962). Occupational therapy can be one of the great ideas of 20th-century medicine (1961 Eleanor Clarke Slagle Lecture). *American Journal of Occupational Therapy, 16,* 1–9.

Ackley, N. (1962). The challenge of the sixties (1962 Eleanor Clarke Slagle Lecture). *American Journal of Occupational Therapy, 16,* 273–281.

Ayres, A. J. (1963). The development of perceptual–motor abilities: A theoretical basis for treatment of dysfunction (1963 Eleanor Clarke Slagle Lecture). *American Journal of Occupational Therapy, 17,* 221–225.

Fidler, G. S. (1966). Learning as a growth process: A conceptual framework for professional education (1965 Eleanor Clarke Slagle Lecture). *American Journal of Occupational Therapy, 20,* 1–8.

Yerxa, E. J. (1967). Authentic occupational therapy (1966 Eleanor Clarke Slagle Lecture). *American Journal of Occupational Therapy, 21,* 1–9.

West, W. L. (1968). Professional responsibility in times of change (1967 Eleanor Clarke Slagle Lecture). *American Journal of Occupational Therapy, 22,* 9–15.

Llorens, L. A. (1970). Facilitating growth and development: The promise of occupational therapy (1969 Eleanor Clarke Slagle Lecture). *American Journal of Occupational Therapy, 24,* 93–101.

Learning Activities

1. Investigate the occupational profile of most Americans in the 1960s. Some useful bibliographical references to explore appear in Appendix B.
   - What was the average family size?
   - What was the average salary? What were some typical jobs?
   - What did homes cost?
   - What were the clothing styles of the decade?
   - What was significant about the popular culture of the decade (e.g., music, film, books)?
2. If you have access to a complete collection of the *American Journal of Occupational Therapy,* scan the table of contents for each issue. What were some common topics? Can you identify any patterns in these topics? How do these relate to the messages of each Eleanor Clarke Slagle Lecture?
3. Try to summarize each Eleanor Clarke Slagle Lecture in a sentence that captures the main theme. Complete the sentence "This lecture was about. . . ."

4. Consider each lecture. Are there common threads among them that you identify? Are there any common themes that emerge when you consider these lectures together?

5. Review the biography of each lecturer of this decade (see Appendix A). Read some of the other work by the lecturer to gain an insight to the reasons why each one received this honor.

6. Consider what was happening in the history of the occupational therapy profession at the time of each Eleanor Clarke Slagle Lecture. Appendix C provides some useful bibliographical references for the history of the profession in the United States, and Appendix D has references for the global history of the profession.

7. Review what each president of the American Occupational Therapy Association presented as his or her vision for the profession at the time of each Eleanor Clarke Slagle Lecture. (A list of these presidents appears in Appendix E.) How do the lectures relate to these visions? The presidents addressed the profession through several forums, including columns in the *American Journal of Occupational Therapy,* such as "President's Address," "Nationally Speaking," and "The Issue Is."

8. Review each lecture in light of the *Centennial Vision.* What themes of the *Vision* stand out the most? What additional insights into the *Vision* do the lecturers offer?

Discussion Questions

1. What do you think of Muriel Zimmerman's statement, "Many of the responses of the patient are the same as those he exhibits toward the disability itself and are, of course, the psychologist's concern to evaluate, not ours." Do you agree with this statement? Why or why not?

2. Zimmerman pointed to the paradox of humanity and stated that "Although man thinks of himself as physically capable of taking care of himself, he at the same time strives to help himself more and more with mechanical interventions." Why is this a paradox?

3. Discuss several ways in which, on the basis of Zimmerman's lecture, you believe occupational therapists and occupational therapy assistants can help clients accept assistive devices.

4. What are Zimmerman's opinions of the role occupational therapists should play in research and specialized studies?

5. Explain what Mary Reilly meant by the statement, "The wide gaping chasm which exists between the complexity of illness and the commonplaceness of our treatment tools is, and always will be, both the pride and anguish of our profession." Explain what Reilly meant by this statement, and discuss whether or not you believe this to be true for occupational therapy today. Explain your position.

6. Reilly stated that "the value of occupational therapy exists in a controversial state." What did she mean by that? What parallels are there between the 1960s and the early 2000s that could make this true for today?

7. Explain what Reilly meant by "the need for public criticism" for the profession. Include in your explanation a discussion about the profession's ability to (1) analyze, (2) interpret, and (3) synthesize criticism. What, in your opinion, does that mean for practice today? Does this criticism occur in our profession at present? How? Explain why or why not you believe public criticism of our profession is necessary today.

8. Summarize Reilly's description of the vital and unique service of occupational therapy. How has this vital service changed in the 40+ years since this lecture was presented? What, in your opinion, is the vital service to society we can provide now and in the future?

9. How did Nadia Ackley argue in favor of the need for occupational therapy services in the mental health field? How would her arguments reflect today's reality in that practice area?

10. Ackley used the phrase "the challenge of the sixties" in the title of her lecture. What was that challenge? What do you think the challenge for occupational therapy is in the present decade?

11. In what areas did Jean Ayres call on occupational therapists to do more research? What in her presentation might motivate therapists to do research?

12. Compare Ayres's presentation of this lecture with those you have already studied. Identify any common themes. What do you believe was the purpose of her format, if any?

13. Toward the beginning of her lecture, Gail Fidler named 6 characteristics of professions. Choose 3 of those characteristics that you find particularly important, and give an example in the current practice of the profession of that characteristic. Discuss aspects in which the profession lives up to the characteristic well and ways in which the profession does not fully exemplify the characteristic.

14. Explain what you believe Fidler meant by the phrase "integrated learning." Why should this form of learning be preferred over cognitive learning? How could this make a difference to the profession as a whole, not only to the individual doing the learning?

15. Elizabeth Yerxa implied that occupational therapy is educationally "progressive." Do you agree with this statement? How do you think Yerxa would perceive the new national requirements regarding postbaccalaureate entry–level programs and the curriculum itself?

16. How would you answer the questions "[Should] procedures which are done to the person over which he has no control . . . be called occupational therapy?" and "Should client choice be required to define intervention as occupational therapy?"

17. Yerxa gave 2 examples that support and refute the idea of using "resistive exercise" in practice. Do you think she makes a case for or against the use of adjunctive methods in occupational therapy? How so?

18. The very last sentence of Wilma West's lecture reads as follows: "At the turn of the 21st century, when yet another generation looks back on these times, may they see that ours was a dynamic posture of professional consciousness and responsibility." As a reader at this threshold, what do you think? Would she applaud occupational therapy's progress, or would she encourage occupational therapists to persist in reaching some goals?

19. Brainstorm ideas regarding the "new mold" and potential areas in the community, public health, or prevention in which occupational therapy could play a vital role in the spirit of West's lecture. Be creative. Share at least 2 fairly developed ideas (more than just "Occupational therapists could work in _____"). Give an example of what type of intervention occupational therapists would do.

20. In the introduction to her lecture, Lela Llorens stated as part of her thesis that "The occupational therapist serves as the enculturation agent for the conditions of physical, social, and psychological health in which the developmental level being experienced by the individual in any one of a number of parameters of development is unequal to the age-related demands made of that organism as a result of natural or traumatic incident." In your own words, explain what she meant by this statement. What did she mean by "enculturation agent?" How does the therapist serve as an enculturation agent for the conditions Llorens mentioned?

21. Llorens described some of the tools of occupational therapy available at the time of her lecture. How do those tools reflect the tools occupational therapists use today? Are there others in use now? Have therapists stopped using some? Use your practice experience to draw out examples of the appropriate and inappropriate use of these tools from a developmental standpoint.

22. Llorens classified schools of treatment in occupational therapy as "permissive," "symptom-oriented," and "disability-oriented." Explain each of these approaches, and analyze possible strengths and limitations of each. Also discuss which, in your opinion, is the predominant school of present practice.

III

THE 1970s
Growth and Expansion

19

Historical Context of the 1970s

Around the World

The situation in Vietnam continued to be of great concern around the world during the 1970s. In response to mounting international and national pressures regarding the rising casualties, the United States reduced its troop strength to 400,000. The crisis, however, extended across the borders of Vietnam into Cambodia and Laos when North Vietnamese forces entered both countries in 1971. U.S. President Richard M. Nixon ordered military support for the South Vietnamese army, which mounted a massive move into the neighboring countries. After heavy casualties, the South Vietnamese were driven out of Laos in early 1972. The United States continued to slowly reduce its forces in the area.

In March 1972, Nixon traveled to the People's Republic of China to end hostilities that had persisted between the United States and China since 1949. However, within a month, U.S. planes resumed bombing North Vietnamese cities, and China, the Soviet Union, and Mongolia sped aid to the North Vietnamese. After heated debate in the Senate, the United States removed its last ground troops from the Vietnam conflict March 29, 1973. U.S. bombing of Cambodia continued until all prisoners of war were repatriated. The death toll had reached 1.3 million Vietnamese and nearly 56,000 American lives. As North Vietnamese forces closed in on Saigon in April 1975, American helicopters evacuated the last Americans and some 5,000 Vietnamese, thus officially ending the war.

After the South Vietnamese and American departure from Laos, the Communist Khmer Rouge established a new regime backed by China. This government undertook the wholesale slaughter of anyone suspected of dissension or past cooperation with Vietnamese or U.S. forces. This massive genocide went unnoticed by most of the world until Vietnamese troops, armed by the Soviet Union, invaded Cambodia in late 1978 and captured the capital, Phnom Penh. Khmer Rouge forces dispersed to the mountains and attempted to organize guerilla warfare but disappeared by the 1990s. Vietnamese occupying forces, which had been hardened by the brutalities of the Vietnam War, were shocked as they discovered the legacy of the Khmer Rouge. Throughout the countryside, Cambodia was marked by sunken depressions of dirt that marked mass graves. Estimates suggest that nearly 2 million people died at the hands of the Khmer Rouge.

The years of the conflict in Southeast Asia resulted in the mass migration of refugees from the region across the world. Approximately 100,000 Vietnamese, 195,000 Cambodian, and 135,000 Laotian refugees left their homelands. Nearly half settled in the United States.

The 1970s witnessed other violent events around the world. Anti-American sentiment rose sharply in the Middle East after the United States refused to sanction Israel for illegal seizure of Palestinian land in 1967. In the 1970s, Arab nations began using profitable U.S. oil investments in their land as leverage to resolve the conflict. In spite of U.S. efforts to broker a peace agreement, Israel attacked guerilla bases in Lebanon and bombed Jordanian army posts. Civil war in Jordan ensued, and the Palestinian Liberation Organization (PLO), which had mounted the strongest resistance against Israel, was forced to move to Lebanon. The world began to realize its vulnerabilities when PLO terrorists murdered 11 Israeli athletes at the Olympic games in Munich, Germany, in the summer of 1972.

The Arab–Israeli conflict escalated into outright war along the Suez Canal and Golan Heights. After the Soviet Union announced it would assist the Arab effort to regain its territory, the United States announced it had begun supplying military equipment to Israel. With United Nations involvement, a tenuous ceasefire was reached, and a U.N. buffer zone was created between Egypt and Israel. The Camp David Accords between Egypt and Israel, brokered by the United States, were agreed upon on September 17, 1978, thus ending the state of war that had existed between those two countries for nearly 30 years.

Peace in the region was very short lived, however. The PLO had been using refugee camps in southern Lebanon as bases for guerilla incursions into Israel, and Israel retaliated, causing heavy bloodshed among Lebanese citizens. This ignited civil war in Lebanon between Christians and leftist Muslims who supported the PLO. Although the United Nations continued to push for Israeli withdrawal from Arab territories and the formation of an independent Palestinian state, civil war continued in Lebanon and threatened to involve Jordan, Egypt, Libya, Saudi Arabia, and Syria. Under an Arab League mandate, Syria's army took control of Lebanon in 1976. In April of that year, the U.S. ambassador to Lebanon was killed, and American citizens were advised to leave the region. Although the civil war had ended, unrest continued for several months.

Instability in the rest of the Middle East became increasingly apparent in the late 1970s. After a year of high civil unrest, the Shah of Iran fled the country in January of 1979 and exiled Shiite Muslim leader Ayatollah Ruholla Khomeini returned to take charge of the government. He accused the United States of fomenting disunity in the country and crushed any group seeking autonomy. On November 4, 1979, Iranian terrorists captured the American embassy, taking 53 hostages and demanding the extradition of the shah, who was in exile in Mexico. These hostages were held for 444 days, and their release would become one of the important events of the 1980s.

Although attention of the world was on Southeast Asia and the Middle East, significant occurrences in Latin America once again confirmed the global scale of the Cold War. One such occurrence was the election by democratic majority of a Marxist president, Salvador Allende, in Chile in 1970. Allende extended recognition to Cuba and proceeded to nationalize the country's large industrial firms. It was not until after a bloody military coup in 1973 that it became apparent that the United States had attempted to block his election through covert actions by the Central Intelligence Agency (CIA). Allende reportedly took his own life when the government palace was under attack, but many believe military personnel backed by the United States killed him. General Augusto Pinochet was named president and, vowing to exterminate Marxism from the country, began a repressive 16-year dictatorship.

A second occurrence was the persistent civil war in Nicaragua, which threatened to extend through Central America. In August 1978, leftist guerillas who called themselves Sandinistas seized the National Palace in the capital, Managua, in a bid to oust dictator Anastasio Somoza, who had enjoyed tacit U.S. support for many years in spite of his well-known corruption. Unable to oust Somoza, the guerillas negotiated safe passage to Panama, where they sought political asylum. Later that year, the publisher of a newspaper who had bitterly opposed Somoza was gunned down, an event that gained popular support for the Sandinistas. Guerilla skirmishes increased into a full-fledged civil war, and finally, in July 1979, Somoza fled to Miami with 45 aides. The Sandinistas set up a five-man junta government, which struggled in the next few years to overcome the economic ruin in which the country had been left. A counterrevolutionary movement backed by the United States would become a major focus of scandal in the following decade.

Not all U.S. relations with Latin America were strained. In an effort to signal a new era in U.S.–Latin American relations, in 1978 U.S. President Jimmy Carter succeeded in gaining Senate approval to sign a treaty for phasing out U.S. control of the Panama Canal. The treaty establishing neutrality of the canal, and a 20-year transition of control went into effect the following year. Control of the canal eventually was handed to Panama on December 31, 1999.

In the United States

The 1970s proved to be very eventful in American society. The backdrop continued to be the Cold War and the military actions in Southeast Asia. It was a decade of scandal and disappointment in the government marked by growing civil unrest. Some experts argue that by the late 1970s, U.S. citizens had been living with the threat of mutually assured destruction so long that it had become deeply ingrained into popular culture. Whereas for some it signaled the need to aggressively defend the country at all costs against any socialist threat, for others, especially young adults, it was a source of despondency and fatalism. The "flower movement," a phrase coined the previous decade to signify the ideals of nonviolent resistance, increasingly became a crusade of self-indulgence, experimentation, and unconstrained freedoms.

By the 1970s, stories of atrocities committed by American soldiers in Vietnam had begun to surface. Accusations of rape and murder were compounded with evidence of the army's lack of action in the matter and attempts to suppress information. Soldiers returning home from the war were antagonized, berated, or simply ignored. The mounting casualties, the inflationary consequences, and the government's lack of acknowledgment that it was fighting an undeclared war in Southeast Asia spurred strong antigovernment feeling, particularly among university students, whose protests were met with increasing force. When President Nixon announced the widening of the war in Cambodia and Laos, National Guardsmen shot and killed four students participating in an antiwar rally at Kent State University in Ohio. Many colleges and universities were closed for the remainder of the term as students coordinated strikes and demonstrations.

An antagonistic tone between Nixon and university students remained until December 1973, when Gerald Ford replaced Vice President Spiro Agnew, who resigned after pleading no contest to charges of income tax evasion. By then the government had become increasingly embroiled in scandal as evidence surfaced that the Commission to Re-elect the President (CREEP) had broken into the Democratic Party's national headquarters in the Watergate building in Washington, DC. Nixon initially denied any knowledge of the break-in. However, when a former CIA employee implicated Republican Party officials and *Washington Post* reporters Bob Woodward and Carl Bernstein reported a financial trail linking the break-in to CREEP, a special prosecutor demanded the White House turn over 64 tape recordings implicating Nixon with obstruction of justice. On July 30, 1974, the House Judiciary Committee adopted three articles of impeachment, and on August 9, 1974, Nixon resigned. Gerald Ford was sworn in as president the same day and one month later granted Nixon a "full, free, and absolute pardon." Most experts believe this cost Ford his bid for reelection, and in 1977 he was defeated by Jimmy Carter.

Several other events of the 1970s are worthy of note. The Supreme Court declared the death penalty unconstitutional in 1972 because the way in which it was administered was considered "cruel and unusual punishment." By 1976, Congress and most states drafted new death penalty laws for murderers, and the Supreme Court upheld them. Also on the legislative front, in 1972 the Equal Rights Amendment, originally submitted in 1923 and considered in every Congress since then, was passed. This constitutional amendment was designed mainly to invalidate many state and federal laws that discriminate against women; its central underlying principle was that gender should not determine the legal rights of Americans. It was submitted to state legislatures for final ratification within 7 years but, despite a deadline extension to June 1982, was not ratified by the requisite majority of 38 states. In spite of several attempts to reintroduce the amendment to Congress, it has not been ratified to date. In 1973, the Supreme Court ruled in *Roe v. Wade* that abortion should be a decision between a woman and her physician and that her right for privacy should be protected.

The 1970s were also characterized by a prolonged energy crisis exacerbated by an Arab oil embargo in 1972. By 1977, Carter proposed a national energy program, but millions of Americans believed the energy crisis had been fabricated by oil companies to obtain price increases. The drop in oil production in Iran in 1979 directly affected the United States, where motorists had to line up at filling stations for the first half of the year and often were unable to obtain more than a few gallons of gas at a time.

In spite of the apparent chaos in the world and in the country during the 1970s, health care continued to advance. In 1971, Nixon signed the National Cancer Act (P.L. 92–218) into law, appropriating $1.5 billion a year to combat the nation's second leading cause of death. The computed axial tomography (CAT) scanner gained wide usage in 1974, not only for diagnosing brain damage but also for whole-body scanning. The first laboratory-made monoclonal antibodies opened a new era in diagnostic and therapeutic medicine in 1975. That same year, Karen Ann Quinlan went into a coma after drinking alcohol mixed with Librium and Valium. She was fed through a nasal tube and kept alive for more than 8 years even after being removed from a respirator. Her case raised continuing arguments about the right to die. In 1977, the first magnetic resonance imaging (MRI) scanner was introduced to detect cancer and other abnormalities without exposing patients to radiation. Finally, physicians' fees and hospital rates hiked almost every year as U.S. insurance companies raised their rates on malpractice policies.

The 1970s was the decade in which the independent living movement began in earnest. This movement was a grassroots effort by people with disabilities to acquire new rights and entitlements and control over their own lives. The decade also saw changes in the relationship between people with disabilities and physicians and other rehabilitation professionals, particularly with the emergence of a disability rights movement that located "disability" problems not in the individual but in the environment. These environmental disabling conditions included attitudes, barriers, lack of services, and lack of opportunities in general. The independent living movement was sparked in 1972 with the opening of the first center for independent living, located in Berkeley, California. This service agency was run by and for people with disabilities. Soon other centers across the United States and the world were founded.

The movement was further strengthened with passage of the Social Security Amendments of 1972 (P.L. 92–336), which created the Supplemental Security Income program, relieving families of the financial responsibility of caring for their adult children with disabilities. With the Rehabilitation Act Amendments of 1978 (P.L. 95–602), Congress finally provided funds for every state to be able to provide independent living services.

Disability activists continued to fight for accessibility to services, buildings, and transportation. The Rehabilitation Act of 1973 (P.L. 93–112), considered to be the civil rights act for people with disabilities, prohibited discrimination against individuals with disabilities in any program or activity receiving federal assistance. It also broadened the power of people with disabilities to jointly draw up rehabilitation plans with professionals. This act became a powerful tool in generating such central disability rights concepts as reasonable modification, reasonable accommodation, and undue burden, which formed the framework for subsequent federal law, especially the Americans With Disabilities Act of 1990.

Despite advances for people with physical disabilities, including the passage in 1970 of the Developmental Disabilities Services and Facilities Construction Amendments (P.L. 95–602) and the passage in 1975 of the Developmental Disabilities Assistance and Bill of Rights Act (P.L. 94–103), few substantial changes took place for this group of people. The lack of an enforcement mechanism within these bills rendered them virtually useless to disability rights advocates. Finally, in 1979, parents of people with mental illness founded the National Alliance for the Mentally Ill, which in later decades became a significant force behind legislative changes for improved services for people with mental illness.

In 1975, the Education for All Handicapped Children Act (P.L. 94–142) was passed, establishing the right of children with disabilities to a public school education in an integrated environment. In the next two decades, millions of children with disabilities were educated under its provisions, radically changing the lives of people in the disability community.

20

1971 Eleanor Clarke Slagle Lecture

The Occupational Therapist in Prevention Programs

Geraldine L. Finn, OTR

Social Change

In order for a profession to maintain its relevancy it must be aware of the times, interpreting its contribution to mankind in accordance with the needs of the times. When social change was slower it was possible for a profession to make this transition gradually; to proceed in a process of evolution, with new ideas and methods slowly replacing formerly held concepts and practices. However, in our era in history, this process of adjustment has had to be accelerated in order to keep pace with the rapidity with which our society is changing. In today's world, the demand to act is often presented to us before we have had sufficient time to understand and assimilate the meaning and significance behind the demanded actions. This is a tenuous position in which to be placed. One is presented with the need and the pressure to respond to that need but without the time to reflect on the knowledge and skills required to respond effectively. Reality, today, is continually outdistancing our preparation to respond to it.

Until the twentieth century, the pace of change allowed the average person the opportunity to incorporate change while feeling a sense of stability. But during this century the scope, the scale, and above all, the pace of change have been accelerated: Change in our society has developed a visibility it did not possess in former times. C. P. Snow comments, "Until this century social change was so slow that it could pass unnoticed in one person's lifetime."[1] Such is no longer the case. Alvin Toffler in his book, *Future Shock,* addresses himself to the current phenomenon of accelerated change and its impact on man's ability to adapt. Toffler reflects on the exhaustion which can engulf the individual as he reaches an overload in his capacity to adjust to the new.[2]

Occupational Therapy and Social Change

This concern about modern change is particularly applicable to the profession of occupational therapy in 1971. For at this moment in our professional history we are being asked to expand our role identity from that of therapist to health agent. Because of the change in emphasis on the delivery of health services we are being asked to move beyond the treatment of patients into the arena of health planning and the development of prevention programs: "to broaden our traditional, more limited identification with medicine . . . to enlarge our concept from that of being a therapist to one of functioning as a health agent with responsibility to help insure normal growth and development"[3] within the lives of all the people in a community.

This is a demand that needs to be acted on immediately if we are to take our place with others involved in the health problems of our day. Yet it is a demand that will require extensive reorganization of our current practices; changes we have not had the time to explore fully. To expand our services beyond the clinic into health planning

Originally published 1972 in *American Journal of Occupational Therapy, 26,* 59–66.
Please note that there was no Eleanor Clarke Slagle Lecture in 1970.

for the community requires changes in the interpretation of our current knowledge, the addition of new knowledge and skills, the abdication of learned behavior patterns, and the revision of our educational process.

This expansion of role identity will require us to give up something we know for something new and unknown. Our education has trained us to work with the disabled person, usually within an institutional setting. Our knowledge, our training, our experience have all formed us to function within a clinical model—evaluating, treating, and rehabilitating the disabled person. We know the problems of today's society as they are reflected in the life of a particular patient but that is quite different from dealing with the problem at a community level. Yet we are faced with the request to change. Not to change gradually over a period of years but to change now; to be relevant to the needs of the times in which we live we must change our model of practice.

We find ourselves in the position of having to act while simultaneously trying to gain the knowledge necessary to act within our new role identity. The printed words in the books written about change in today's society have come alive for us. In our professional life we are actually *experiencing* the words. In today's world the demand to act is often presented to us before we have had sufficient time to understand and assimilate the meaning and significance behind the demanded action. We are living in a professional reality that is outdistancing our preparation to respond to it.

Faced with the drama of this situation we have a choice as individual occupational therapists. We can deny the urgency of the need to become involved in health planning and prevention programs and go on with our everyday activities; we can accept the importance of the mandate but feel that we can contribute more to the service of mankind by remaining in our present role as clinician; we can admit the concept of role identity change and ponder its significance in isolation away from the daily realities of practice; or we can accept the challenge and begin to change the emphasis of our practice, implementing new programs as increased knowledge and understanding are achieved.

As a clinician and administrator I chose the route of expanding my own identity to incorporate the role of health agent, and assumed the responsibility of reorganizing an occupational therapy department according to the new emphasis in health services. This reorganization has now been in progress for two years. In preparation for this lecture I attempted to study this process of change; not to report to you an autobiographical journey but rather to share with you some of the issues that became evident during this experience—issues we need to understand if we are to develop comprehensive prevention programs and revise our curricula to prepare the future occupational therapist in the role of health agent.

Practice of Occupational Therapy—1960 to 1970

In order to understand these issues as they relate to the process of expanding services into the community, it is necessary to relate these issues to the practice of occupational therapy and the changes within the health services.

To understand the position of occupational therapy practice at this particular moment when changes are being demanded of it, we need to consider the developments within our practice during the past decade. The mandate for expansion of our services into health planning comes at a time when we are just beginning to develop our full identity as a profession within a therapy role. We have progressed from technician receiving a prescription from the physician to our present position as principal agent in the treatment of patients who require an intervention process employing the therapeutic use of activities.

After years of intuitive service to the sick and disabled we have now begun to define our practice and validate our clinical impressions through research studies. During the decade of the 1960's we began, in earnest, to study the process of normal growth and development and to interpret this knowledge as it applied to the patient with developmental deviations or fixations. We studied the theorists in cognition and began to refine our understanding of the role which specific activities and experiences play in the development of perceptual–motor–cognitive skills.[4] We probed deeper into the psychological aspects of activities. We increased our knowledge of group process and the use of task-oriented groups in developing one's interpersonal skills.[5] We began to communicate to others the debilitating effects of disability on the satisfaction of these basic needs. We no longer had to apologize for our association with the practical activities of daily life because we had reached the level of awareness that it was through these activities that the disabled person was able to maintain his sense of human identity: to keep that sense of self-dignity and independence that can be so quickly lost in an institutional setting. We took our new understanding of human functioning and started to develop evaluation and treatment methods to correct specific deficits impeding the ability of the patient to fulfill these basic human needs. We responded to the permanently disabled person's need to maintain a normal way of life within the limitations of his disability, and helped him develop his social, vocational, and avocational interests.

The 1960's were productive years in the maturation of occupational therapy and the advent of the 1970's could be looked upon as the time for greater refinement in our clinical practice. At last we were beginning to define clearly the contribution of activities to the treatment of the sick and disabled. We had grown beyond the need to seek our identity by simulating the services or appearances of another profession. Therefore, as we entered the 1970's, there stretched out before us an array of avenues to follow in analyzing activities, in refining our evaluation procedures, and in developing more effective treatment techniques.

Change in Delivery of Health Services

But the needs of a particular period in history do not wait upon a timetable of priorities. Emphasis was being placed on developing prevention programs in the fields of mental health and pediatrics. Starting in the 1960's concern was centered on the importance of preventing disorders in children through the implementation of special programs. Well-baby clinics were established in local communities, Head Start for the preschool child was introduced, and more attention was given to the child with learning disabilities.[6] In the field of mental health the trend away from large state institutions and the establishment of community mental health centers was developing. Although these centers provided clinical services to people in a particular geographical area, specific attention was directed toward the establishment of collaborative relationships with other institutions in the community as a means of developing primary prevention and early intervention programs. In the field of public health there was growing concern for the increased numbers of people suffering from long-term chronic conditions such as arthritis, diabetes, mental retardation, and alcoholism.[7]

Fully recognizing the continuing need of many people for direct clinical and treatment services, there was the growing realization that many of the problems dealt with daily in the clinic could be prevented or modified if only earlier intervention had been available. Those within our society who had studied the health demands of today were saying that, for both human and economic reasons, we must expand our efforts to create an environment that would prevent serious illness and disability. The time had come to recognize that unless we began to refocus our attention on keeping people well, we would never be able to stem the tide of human suffering in our country.

The era of maintaining the health of a community through the control of communicable and infectious diseases was behind us. We had the knowledge to conquer these destroyers of human life and we must now move on to those chronic and disabling conditions that do not cause immediate death but, rather, years of human suffering and waste of human potential. In public health we had passed the time when all our energies had to be focused on the most basic physical health needs of the people. We were now able to devote our attention to the social disorders which not only affect the physical life of the individual but also have social, psychological, and economic ramifications for the individual, his family, and the society at large. Sudden illness and death have been replaced by disorders spanning an extended period of disability. Many chronic conditions limit the individual's ability to function for years. It is the length of time involved in these chronic disorders, the variety of services required, and the large numbers of people affected by them which have made chronic disorders such a major health problem today.[8]

Realizing, therefore, the need to counteract the amount of disability in our society, and recognizing that the most viable way to stop this amount of disability was through preventing it from occurring, emphasis was placed on prevention. In addition to this desire to prevent disability was the desire to provide an environment in which each person would be free to reach his fullest potential of human development. The achievement of this supportive environment was seen as an extremely complex task but it was felt that the effort made to reach this goal would be worthwhile. The need to improve the quality of all aspects of life was seen as part of the responsibility of health planning because health problems are interrelated with all the other aspects of life. It is not possible to consider the solution of health problems without being aware of the influence of other social factors, such as, economics, housing, and family life, on one's state of health.

The interrelationship of health issues and the other social forces in the community is illustrated graphically by the current problem of the elderly in our society. The control of communicable disease and the advance of medical science have combined to allow the individual of today a longer life span. This extension of life has presented complications when considered in relationship to other forces in our society. The technological advances have created a trend toward urban living, with smaller houses, constant mobility, and the separation of the nuclear family from its extended members. As a result of this life pattern there is usually no room for the aging parent in the home of the child. Housing, therefore, becomes a major concern for the elderly. Even if the elderly remain in their own homes, neighbors change so often that the sense of security among friends is often missing. Further, the cost of living continues to rise in our society. Financial retirement plans made twenty or thirty years ago are no longer sufficient to sustain the older person. Although many elderly people are still capable of working, the retirement policies of business and industry force inactivity on the older individual. Unable to work, concerned about finances, and often alone, the older person begins to withdraw from life experiences. Depression, poor eating habits, and inactivity often result. Then again protection from disease has not completely eliminated the degenerative conditions that often result from the aging process—conditions that require the older person to receive assistance with his daily life. Too often, however, the needed services which would allow the person to remain in his own home are not available. As a result, the older person must be placed in an institution. Here care is available but the expense is great. Institutions, no matter how comfortable, can never replace one's own home, and the elderly person begins to develop a sense of hopelessness. Often the children are concerned but are so caught up in coping with our rapidly changing environment that feelings of resentment begin to develop against the parent. Financial assistance beyond the family is usually needed and the care and expense of the older person becomes society's responsibility. The problem of aging becomes, therefore, not simply a health problem but a complex social problem.[9]

Issues to Consider in Prevention Programs

Supported by a growing body of knowledge in occupational therapy clinical practice and aware of the need and priority of health prevention service, it is now necessary to begin the examination of the kinds of issues to be considered by occupational therapists, as we accept the mandate to move beyond the role of therapist and become health agents and progress along the continuum from hospital and clinical services to the community and health programs.

Issue One

The first issue relates to the environment in which one carries out his practice. Prevention programs are carried out in the community, with the primary institutions—such units as the family, the school, the law, places of business, the health center, and the church. Each of these institutions makes a contribution to a person's life to one degree or another. They provide each person with the opportunities to gain the "increments of ego strength and personality robustness"[10] which enable him to cope with the demands and pressures of daily life. To maintain the sense of well-being of the people in the community and to allow them the opportunity to develop their human potential, these primary institutions must respond adequately to the needs of the people. If they do respond in effective ways then the environment provides the nurturing elements needed for human growth and happiness. Unfortunately, the perfection of these institutions has not been attained and one of the responsibilities of those engaged in prevention work is the development of programs and services that will contribute to the perfection of these institutions.

Included in the list of primary institutions are ones which have usually been outside the professional interests of the occupational therapist. Little concern has been given, for example, to the functioning of local industries, or the overall administration and policies of the school system. Until the present time the occupational therapist has limited himself primarily to the health center. Even here, though, the occupational therapist has related more to the internal functioning of the health center rather than concerning himself with the health center's role and responsibility in the community. The occupational therapist is familiar with what goes on within the walls of the health center, but the remaining primary institutions in the community are often perceived only at the level of vague general awareness.

When moving, therefore, into community programs it is necessary for the occupational therapist to become knowledgeable about these other institutions, to understand more fully their functions, their goals, their policies, and their methods of operation. It is only in this way that the occupational therapist can begin to develop appropriate communications with the primary institutions. In collaborative efforts with these primary institutions the occupational therapist must discern those areas in which he can make his contribution.

Issue Two

Consideration of this factor of collaboration introduces us to a second issue. Before the occupational therapist reaches out to the primary institutions he must have a clear understanding of the services he has to offer. Although the occupational therapist has been responsible for delineating the kinds of services he has to offer to the patients within a clinical setting, treatment programs have had the advantage of years of experience in relating specific treatment services to a particular disability. Prevention programs are new for occupational therapists and there are no traditions upon which to base one's actions. It is possible to try to reinterpret clinical programs so that they fit the particular needs of a community but it must be remembered that the clinical programs were developed for the person with a specific pathology. The programs in the community have to relate to the maintaining of a person's health. Therefore, in considering community programs the occupational therapist must have an understanding of health in order to develop appropriate prevention programs.

Dubos notes that, "solving problems of disease is not the same thing as creating health . . . the task of health demands a kind of wisdom and vision which transcends specialized knowledge of remedies and treatments and which apprehends in all their complexities and subtleties the relation between living things and their total environment."[11] Health is far more than just the absence of disease. The word *health* is an abstract term that has been given to a highly complex, multivariable condition of man. Those who have attempted to define health have come up with a series of characteristics. Gordon Allport suggests six principal characteristics of the healthy personality. First, he considers the capacity of the individual to extend himself to interests outside his own body and material possessions. The second characteristic Allport attributes to the healthy personality is self-objectification. This is the capacity of the individual to achieve a spatial and temporal quality in his orientation to life. The third attribute is a unifying philosophy of life. Allport states that this philosophy of life may, or may not, be religious, but in any event it has to be a frame of meaning and responsibility into which life's major activities fit. Fourth, Allport sees a healthy person as one who is capable of relating to other human beings in a warm and profound manner. Fifth, Allport attributes an importance to the possession of realistic skills, abilities, and perceptions with which to cope with the practical problems of life. And sixth, Allport considers the capacity to possess a compassionate regard and respect for all men and the willingness to participate in common activities that will improve the human lot.[12]

Using Allport's six characteristics as a foundation, let us attempt to develop a definition of a healthy person. A healthy person is one who is accepting of himself, responsive and concerned about other people, sees meaning in his existence, and is capable of productively fulfilling the daily demands of his life. Now, no definition of health, however, completely expresses the full understanding of this concept, but such a definition as the above does provide a basis upon which to develop a more comprehensive understanding of the subject.

It is significant to note in Allport's description of the healthy personality the role played by one's involvement in active participation in his environment. The healthy person does not remain preoccupied with self-interests but extends himself to others and relates to them in a productive manner within the daily events of life, accomplishing this through the use of his skills and abilities.

The healthy person is an active person. This fact has been recognized by philosophers and psychologists searching for a greater understanding of man. Aristotle stated that virtue is activity, by which he meant the exercise of the functions and capacities that are peculiar to man. Happiness to Aristotle was the result of activity and use, it was not a quiescent state of mind.[13] According to Erich Fromm, "man is not only a rational and social animal . . . he can also be defined as a producing animal, capable of transforming the materials which he finds at hand, using his reason and imagination; not only can man produce, he must produce."[14]

Issue Three

Armed with a realization of the concept of health, and particularly the aspect of human activity and man's relationship to the activities in his environment maintaining his sense of health, the occupational therapist must begin to reinterpret his body of knowledge. He must begin to relate his understanding of the ways in which man, throughout the stages of his life and in his active interactions with his environment, develops the characteristics that define health. He must begin to consider ways in which he can apply this knowledge within the primary institutions within the community. One example would be the association of play experiences in the cognitive and emotional development of the preschool child, and the application of this knowledge to the education of child-care workers in a community day care center.

Issue Four

This reinterpretation of the occupational therapist's body of knowledge and skills brings us to the next issue—the importance of thinking creatively. In order to meet the challenge of developing effective prevention programs we must begin to exercise our imaginations. The imagination is a mental process which, all too often in our technological society, has been dulled. We have been trained to take facts and put them together logically without the benefit of our own mental images. In our educational process the imagination has too often been relegated to a creative writing course, or a literature course, and omitted from our more scientifically-oriented courses. Yet how do people begin to see associations that have not been perceived before if they do not use their imaginations?

We are often amazed at the way a poet seems to see inside a situation and extract from it the richness of its essence. One reason for this skill rests on the development of his imagination; on his capacity to think in mental images. One poet I know refers to the specialization process in education as training people to put their knowledge into boxes. If one gets a thought that does not fit the criteria of the box, then it is discarded. A poet instead has transcended the box mentality and is open to all aspects of reality, manipulating them mentally into new images and associations.

It is this process of creative thinking which is required of us, as occupational therapists, in order to interpret our knowledge about human performance, growth and development, work, play, and human relations so that it becomes functional material for developing prevention programs in the service of maintaining the health of a community. It is necessary for us to begin to think creatively about our particular understanding of man's needs and to start to build new images around this knowledge.

Issue Five

Once we have begun the process of recombining our knowledge it is necessary to consider ways in which this knowledge can be translated into actual programs. This brings us to another issue—the development of a method to translate one's plan into action. Over a period of years we have broken down our units of knowledge and applied them in the treatment situation. For most of us in our professional careers, we entered practice with associations already established between a plan and the act. In our educational process we have studied man physically and psychologically, learned the various ways in which his functioning may be pathological because of a disease or disability, and have practiced the methods employed to treat the problem. Therefore, in our clinical practice the process of proceeding from a plan to an act has centered on the particular patient coming to us for service. We have adapted our general knowledge to translating a plan into an act for a particular patient. The situation in the community, however, is quite different. Instead of working with a single patient, we are working with a primary institution or several primary institutions possessing a litany of complexities far beyond the problems of a single person. The primary institution does not have a single, well-defined problem which is seeking solution. The primary institutions are coping with a wide variety of factors impinging on the health of people in the community. The task that is presented to us is the establishment of a method of processing the needs of the primary institutions and the services the occupational therapist has to offer.

A method which has proved satisfactory consists of conceptualizing ideas and plans into progressively more specific conceptual units until one is able to express his thoughts in action-oriented terms. This process requires the mental discipline to continue to breakdown a thought until it can be translated into a specific action relating directly to the initial idea. When dealing with such broad concepts as human performance, health, and social systems there is a tendency to forget that these words represent a complex association of facts that must be analyzed carefully if the particular components of these concepts are to be combined so that a definite plan can be carried out. Without breaking down these concepts, a chasm which cannot be crossed exists between the thought and the act. Everyone sometime in his life has had the experience, I am sure, of being able to speak knowledgeably and at length about a particular concept, but finds that he is totally lost when asked to express this concept in a concrete act. In this situation the person has not conceptualized his knowledge in action terms. But once he has broken down the concept into units of action he is able to act.

Issue Six

Once we have broken down our concepts it is possible to act—to begin to take our knowledge of activities and their significance to man and develop new programs. The implementation of new programs brings with it a recognition of risk-taking, which is the next issue to be discussed. We are most comfortable when we know the route and the expected outcome of our actions. In the process of developing new programs within a new environment it is not possible to know fully the route which the program will take or the specific details of the final outcome of the plan. Over the years we have become familiar with the expected behaviors of those working within a medical institution and have been able to transfer this information to new staff and students. Health planning, however, requires us to relate to people from nonmedical settings and from different organizational structures. Often one is involved with people from various settings simultaneously. Without the comfort of knowing the behavioral responses to expect, anxiety and apprehension can become overwhelming feelings. To cope with the need to become comfortable in unfamiliar situations we must begin to develop new skills in interpersonal relationships; to become more acutely sensitive to the behavioral cues of others as well as more conscious of our own patterns of relating.

Issue Seven

Of particular importance in dealing with new situations is a deeper understanding of the communication process. Through our professional education we have embraced a style of relating technical information comprehensible only to others trained in medically-oriented fields. We have developed a way of thinking about certain information and often assume that everyone else thinks in the same frame of orientation. When we speak, for example, about the stages of development we are thinking about the process of development—the particular process by which a person progresses along the developmental continuum. Many teachers, however, see stages of development from a static frame of orientation. They think about the child at age five, or age six, or age seven but not about the process by which the child grows from age to age.

In order to communicate with parents, teachers, Golden Age directors, clergymen, and the like we must be able to communicate our ideas in language that is understandable to the other person. This requirement forces us to admit those areas of our knowledge which remain vague and ill-defined under the mantle of the professional term. For example, unless one fully understands the psychosexual stage of orality it is very difficult to help a neighborhood recreation leader realize the particular needs of a boy in his sports group fixated at this stage of emotional development.

Issue Eight

Clear communication provides an important step in the introduction of new ideas or programs. The introduction of new ideas, new programs, or new ways of thinking and acting in a primary institution represents the core issue in prevention work. As clinicians we are used to having patients come to us for help. The person is in need and seeks our assistance. In prevention work the occupational therapist goes to the people in the primary institutions. The significance of this reversal of roles must be fully understood. It is necessary to demonstrate to the other person or group of people the feasibility of accepting the plan, the idea, the program, or the service offered by the occupational therapist. Unless the occupational therapist fully understands the service he has to offer, believes in the value of the service, and can explain how that service will benefit the other person, the desired collaboration will not occur. In order to present appropriate programs and communicate clearly about them, therefore, a great deal of thought and planning must go into the preparatory work for prevention programming.

Because the other people sometimes do not see the worth of the proposed plan, or are hesitant to accept the plan because of internal organizational factors, the element of frustration accompanies the implementation of prevention programming. Most clinicians have had the experience of a patient refusing to attend occupational therapy and know the feelings of frustration and futility that such an experience can arouse. In developing prevention programs these feelings are magnified because of the amount of preliminary work that has had to go into each plan and the endless variations in the problems and obstacles encountered. As Leonard Duhl says, "The input of information constantly redefines the situation, the problem, and the possible range of solutions."[15] Therefore, a well-defined, well-planned program may have to be revised a dozen different ways before there is agreement on the details of the plan.

Issue Nine

Because of the complexity of factors involved in developing prevention programs the morale of the staff becomes our final issue. Effective prevention work is carried out at the grass-roots level of the community. If change is to take place within the primary institutions in a community it is not sufficient that the person at the head of the institution, such as the school superintendent for example, be in agreement with the ideas. The people who actually carry out the daily action plans are the ones who must be enthusiastic. In order to maintain this kind of willingness to change on the part of others the occupational therapist must be able to maintain his sense of objectivity and interest in the project. To do this the occupational therapist must have the opportunity to look at his own feelings and also see the personal growth opportunities in the experience. To accomplish these things the occupational therapist must be receiving assistance in sorting out his own feelings and obtaining guidance in continuing his own personality development. It is for these reasons that staff supervision becomes a crucial part of any prevention-oriented program. The supervision must relate to the individual needs of each staff member for specific knowledge and skills, for the ability to deal with one's feelings, and for the development of a professional identity as an occupational therapist in the role of health agent. Because of the need for the development of a supportive system for staff involved in the pioneering work in health planning and prevention programming, a hierarchy of supervision can be developed where each staff member receives supervision from a more experienced therapist while in turn supervising a less experienced therapist. This method provides for the development of a network of support, and through this process the individual occupational therapist begins to learn ways in which he can find support for his efforts within himself, and is able in time to relinquish the great need for external support.

Summary of Issues

We have now concluded the discussion of the specific issues which began to crystallize as we proceeded through the process of expanding an occupational therapy department from an inpatient service to include prevention programs. Nine separate issues were extracted from the process data gathered over the past two years of developing prevention programs. To restate them again, they include (1) the function of primary institutions in maintaining the health of the people of a community and the need for occupational therapists to understand the functions, goals, and policies of these primary institutions; (2) the planning of appropriate programs and services based on man's need to engage in interaction with the objects in his environment in order to maintain his health throughout his life; (3) the need to reinterpret the body of knowledge available within the profession of occupational therapy in order to apply it in the service of keeping people healthy rather than in helping people minimize their disabilities; (4) the creation of new associations of our available knowledge in order to respond more accurately to the pressing reality needs of today; (5) the establishment of an organizational model which will allow translation of abstract plans about activities, human action, and the delivery of health services into concrete actions; (6) the presence of risk-taking and its ramifications on one's ability to function and persevere when faced with an unfamiliar environment; (7) the necessity of reexamining communication patterns to insure real communications among people; (8) the need to create a climate of acceptance for a planned program and the development of the skills needed to assist others in seeing the value of these programs; and (9) the role of supervision in maintaining the performance and professional growth of the staff members.

Community Programs

Before proceeding to the concluding section of my presentation I would like to share with you the kinds of programs that provided the process material from which these issues were extracted. These programs include early intervention programs for children, ages 4 to 12 years, who are beginning to present the first indications of behavioral and learning problems; a consultation service to teachers; an inservice education program in developmental screening and program planning for teachers in day care centers; an outreach program to community agencies assisting the elderly; a workshop for mothers and preschool children in early childhood development and parent-child relationships; an inservice education program on perceptual-motor development for mental health workers; development of new models of parent education and counseling; and the introduction of knowledge about developmental levels in human performance in a community drug program.

Curriculum Changes

Having localized some of the issues arising out of prevention programming we are now faced with their significance in the mandate to occupational therapists to move beyond the role of therapist to health agent. In discussion of each of these issues I have alluded to the change that must occur in the education of occupational therapists both at the level of academic professional education and at the level of continuing education for practicing occupational therapists.

In order to expand into the areas of health planning and prevention programs, occupational therapists must possess a comprehensive knowledge and understanding of the meaning and significance of activities in the development of man's fullest potential. It is natural for man to be active; to interact with the objects in his environment, to develop his physical, cognitive, and psychosocial abilities.

Man must exist in an environment which provides him with the opportunities to grow and develop as a total human being through his interaction with people and with the activities and objects in the environment if he is to remain healthy. The study of activities and the application of this knowledge to provide man with a better way of life are the essences of the profession of occupational therapy. Therefore, as the profession with this charge, we must move beyond the confines of focusing our attention on the value of a specific activity to achieve a specific result and include a more comprehensive understanding of activities and human action. It is only with such an understanding that we will be able to respond to the needs of the primary institutions in our communities and develop the kinds of particular services these institutions require in order to maintain the health of the people in the community. We must not give up the knowledge we now possess in activity analysis as it applies to the physically and psychologically disabled person, but rather we must expand this knowledge.

Secondly, we must develop our ability to become leaders; to move with confidence into the community and collaborate in the creation of a healthier environment, contributing our knowledge of activities and human action. We need, therefore, to be able to problem-solve, to understand the factors involved in complex social systems and define the problems where we can make a contribution.

And thirdly, we must increase our knowledge about the society in which we live. We must understand the effect of technology on man's way of life today, to realize the reasons behind the young people's push to return to a more human-oriented life style, to understand the economic, political, and social forces that predominate in today's society.

Summary

The trend, today, in health services is toward the prevention of disability. We are a profession possessing knowledge that is particularly necessary to maintain the health of people. To move from therapist to health agent demands us to change but to change in a forward, positive way. We do not have to give up what we know, rather, we must instead be willing to know more.

For years we have been concerned with the disabled person's right to maintain his dignity and self-worth by reaching his maximum level in human functioning. The needs of our times are now asking us to contribute to the preservation of each person's right to achieve his highest level of human functioning.

References

1. Toffler, A. *Future Shock*. New York: Random House, 1970.
2. Ibid.
3. West, W. L. "Professional responsibility in times of change." *Am J Occup Ther 22*:231–249, 1968.
4. Llorens, L. A. "Facilitating growth and development: The promise of occupational therapy." *Am J Occup Ther 24*:93–101, 1970.
5. Fidler, G. S. "The task-oriented group as a context for treatment." *Am J Occup Ther 23*:43–48, 1969.
6. West, W. L. "The growing importance of prevention." *Am J Occup Ther 23*:226–231, 1969.
7. Smolensky, J., and Haar, F. B. *Principles of Community Health*. Philadelphia: W. B. Saunders Company, 1967.
8. Ibid.
9. Berezin, A. B, and Stotsky, B. A. "The geriatric patient," in The *Practice of Community Mental Health*. Boston: Little Brown Company, 1970.
10. Bower, E. M. "Primary prevention of mental and emotional disorders: A conceptual framework and action possibilities." *Perspectives in Community Mental Health*. Chicago: Aldine Publishing Company, 1969.
11. Ibid.
12. Allport, G. W. *Personality and Social Encounter*. Boston: Beacon Press, 1960.
13. Fromm, E. *Man for Himself*. New York: Rinehart and Company, Inc., 1947.
14. Ibid.
15. Duhl, L. J. "Planning and predicting: Or what to do when you don't know the names of the variables." *General Systems Theory and Psychiatry*. Boston: Little Brown Company, 1969.

1972 Eleanor Clarke Slagle Lecture

Occupational Therapy:
A *Model for the* Future

Jerry A. Johnson, EdD, OTR

Introduction

Occupational therapists repeatedly throughout our history have demonstrated concern for the individual and a strong belief that through involvement in the occupational therapy process, those individuals who cannot contribute to or fully participate in society's marketplace can determine the quality and style of life they seek and can thereby influence their health. Mrs. Eleanor Clarke Slagle associated such concern and belief with occupational therapy when she refused an offer to go to France in 1918 to head a hospital for "shell-shock cases." Instead, she elected to remain in Chicago where she had started courses in occupational therapy as she felt her efforts could best be devoted to meeting the needs of wounded veterans in that fashion.[1]

While concern for the individual has been demonstrated consistently, our knowledge of individual behavior and social behavior has expanded so that our efforts to promote and support man's desire for health through the occupational therapy process have shifted from sole focus on the individual to recognition that equal focus must center on helping man learn to achieve a satisfying interaction with his social system or environment.

Defining the occupational therapy process has been difficult. Early in our development we found success when we employed the concepts of "moral treatment" with psychiatric patients.[2] Within this framework we were concerned with the whole man, and we attempted to provide wide-based, health-oriented services to individuals which were consistent with and responsive to society's needs. At the same time we were able to retain our belief in the individual and to demonstrate the value of his involvement in occupation to restore function and promote healing.

At other times we have lost sight of man as a whole and have concentrated on mechanics, media, or techniques, usually in an effort to influence pathological processes.[3] When we put aside our strong orientation toward health, we seem to be less successful and to harbor more doubts about the viability of occupational therapy.

At this point in time, we, as a profession, are faced with the challenge of making critical decisions which may well determine not only our success—but our survival—as a profession in the future.

This presentation will attempt to delineate a model to serve as a guide in our decision-making process as we develop a strategy for the future. I will discuss five elements, all interrelated as part of our decision-making process. I will also raise questions for our mutual consideration as we move toward decision-making.

The five elements in the decision-making process are: organizational behavior and societal change; the occupational therapy product; the marketplace for occupational therapy; the marketing process; personnel requirements.

The terminology and concepts utilized herein are derived primarily from business and biology, rather than from medicine, because we must examine many models before we can select those which are most appropriate for our professions.

Originally published 1973 in *American Journal of Occupational Therapy, 27,* 1–7.

Organizational Behavior and Societal Change

History reveals that our desire to provide services of professional status and quality has prompted us to accept and seek to fulfill the criteria of professionalism defined by medicine and also accepted as "the authority" by other professions, who also view the physician as the "professional par excellence."[4]

Fidler[5] and Yerxa[6] in their respective Eleanor Clarke Slagle lectures identified and examined our progress in fulfilling these professional criteria in our educational and practice systems. Among the criteria they examined were the following:

- Acceptance by the profession of a body of knowledge, supported and substantiated by research;
- Establishment and enforcement of ethical standards for membership behavior;
- Acceptance of responsibility for making independent judgments and for operating autonomously;
- Establishment of and control over educational standards for admission of members into the professional association; and
- Identification of services associated by the public with occupational therapy.

Our desire to move from competence to excellence has been equated with fulfilling the above criteria of professionalism. This has led us to direct our primary attention to internal matters over which we could exert some degree of control. This behavior was demonstrated in an era in which professions were distinct and often isolated entities. Lawrence and Lorsch, in their studies of organizational behavior, found that this was a generally accepted pattern of organizational behavior and that it represented a method whereby organizations could find "the one best way to organize."[7]

While we and other professions have spent most of our efforts and energy focusing on internal change and revision, and have erected organizational structures reflective of the past, the very foundations which govern all aspects of our lives have shifted. Drucker, among others, writes that in a very short period of time society has emerged from an era of experience into an era of knowledge. One of the most dramatic changes resulting from this societal transition is that the requirement for every job—skilled or unskilled—will be knowledge-based. Schooling, rather than apprenticeships, will provide job foundations because the worker's productivity will depend upon his ability to employ concepts, ideas, and theories.[8]

The moon shots exemplify this point for we had no previous experience upon which to build as we sent men to the moon. Rather, we had knowledge and technology which enabled us to anticipate and approximate experience and consequences of decisions.

A side effect, or consequence, of the emerging era of knowledge is the decreasing amount of isolationism and the increasing interrelatedness and interdependence which is found in all areas of life today. Individuals, as well as professions and organizations, are equally affected.

A case in point is that of the alcoholic whose life typifies complexity and interrelatedness in that his drinking affects his life, the lives of his family, and society at large. His behavior can endanger the lives of others. His children demonstrate more pathology than do children from nonalcoholic homes. His family as a whole seems to feel a greater sense of guilt than do other families. Ultimately, society may have to assume responsibility for both the alcoholic and his family.

Similar examples of increasing complexity, interrelatedness, and interdependence are found in the areas of health, ecology, conservation, and pollution, for we are learning that our behavior and actions may have consequences extending far beyond any which could have been conceivable in earlier times.

For example, the October 1, 1972 issue of the Washington, D.C., *Sunday Star and Daily News* reported that "thousands of men and women who worked in shipyards during World War II are threatened by a rare form of cancer stemming from exposure to asbestos . . . . The disease, a tumor affecting the lining of the chest or abdomen—has only recently begun to appear, 30 years after exposure . . . until the last decade mesothelioma was so rare that it did not warrant separate classification as a cause of death . . . . Now it is possible that 32,500 to 225,000 of the 3.25 million World War II shipyard workers still living could be killed by the disease . . . which is invariably fatal."

As demonstrated by the above examples, our lives are becoming more complex, more interrelated, and more interdependent. With the rapid advancement of technology and the availability of increasing amounts of knowledge, the importance of experience diminishes as we move into areas in which man has had no experience. It becomes necessary to rely upon knowledge to help us anticipate the future and predict more accurately the consequences of our decisions and behavior.

There are two direct and immediate implications for occupational therapy which emanate from the knowledge era. The first implication relates to an expansion of the populations which we can service. The second implication relates to our need to expand our concept of professionalism to meet criteria we establish and to develop an organizational strategy which enables us to relate to and interact with other professions and disciplines in positive, constructive ways, without sacrificing the concepts in which we believe.

Drucker supplies evidence upon which we can predict an expansion of the populations we serve when he says that our present manpower shortage will increase because marginal and unemployed individuals frequently lack, and perhaps cannot acquire through the educational system, the habits, tools, and skills which are prerequisites for employment today.[9]

If we believe Reilly's hypothesis as proposed in her Eleanor Clarke Slagle lecture, "that man, through the use of his hands as they are energized by mind and will, can influence the state of his own health,"[10] we have a responsibility to expand our service base. Dubos provides substantiative support for Reilly's hypothesis in that he proposes the distance of a direct relationship between meaningful occupation and health.[11] We as occupational therapists can offer valuable services to those individuals who are cut off from the main stream of society because they cannot effectively utilize our educational channels or compete in life's marketplace. These individuals need opportunities for experience, which are no longer readily available to them, to learn and to help them find an outlet for their skills and abilities.

The occupational therapist's knowledge of individual behavior, social behavior and occupational (or experiential) behavior as these components influence health leads to an understanding of the contribution of the occupational therapy process as it is relevant to present-day individual and societal needs.

The second implication emerging from the knowledge era is that it is not sufficient to attend to standards for the development of individual professional occupational therapists, as we have traditionally done. Now we must go beyond concern for the individual therapist to develop a strategy for the profession of occupational therapy as a whole. This strategy will need to be concerned with the interrelationships and interrelatedness between occupational therapy and other professions. It may also require that, as Lawrence and Lorsch suggest, we develop several different organizational characteristics and behavioral patterns, responsive to differing external conditions, if we are to be a successful organization in the context of societal change.[12] Finally, it may require us to develop our own criteria for professionalism and excellence.

In summary, we can utilize knowledge to anticipate and predict change in the larger social context and to identify the implications of those changes for occupational therapy as they affect our service functions and our organizational behavior. Examination of the social system thus enables one to take a fresh look at the product of occupational therapy.

The Product

Occupational therapists share a common goal in their desire to influence occupational performance in the knowledge that the individual's involvement in occupation bears direct relationship to the state of his health. Occupation is defined as any goal-directed activity meaningful to the individual and providing feedback to him about his worth and value as an individual and about his interrelatedness to others. Occupational performance consists of components of emotional, biological, cognitive, and social behavior. Each of these behavioral elements can be viewed separately, but to fulfill the goals of occupational therapy the components must ultimately be viewed in terms of their interrelatedness. Dubos lends his support to this approach by saying that the most pressing problems of humanity can be resolved only as we study "systems as a whole in all of the complexity of their interactions." He also challenges science to move from an atomistic, reductionist approach to one which deals with the responses of the "total organism to the total environment."[13]

Because occupational therapists have traditionally viewed man as a total organism seeking to influence his state of health through occupational pursuits, we have also been able to see the need for the occupational therapy process to be concerned with individuals, their social systems, and their occupations. The client and the therapist participate in a collaborative process or transaction whereby the therapist provides an experiential learning environment in which the client can initiate or participate in occupational performance meaningful to him. As a result of this learning experience, the individual should develop a sense of competence and mastery as he learns to cope with, adapt to, and conduct negotiations and transactions with his social system, thereby facilitating mutual change.

The crucial test comes when the individual is required to perform in his own social system. If we have fulfilled our responsibilities adequately, the individual should succeed for it will be possible for him and the social system to produce changes and adaptations necessary for compatible coexistence. In summary, through this process man learns to make decisions about the quality and style of life he seeks to achieve and to influence his health.

Viewed in this light, occupational therapy is an applied social science, eclectically drawing upon the biological, social, and behavioral disciplines for our basic understanding of man, occupation, and social–organizational systems.

- In summary, our product is basically a service, emanating from the following knowledge:
- That each individual has some capacity to be involved in meaningful occupational performance;
- That occupational performance provides feedback, conveying a sense of dignity, worth, and competence to the individual; and
- That through the use of occupations and his attitude toward them, the individual can determine his life style and influence his state of health.

The opportunity for individuals in our society to learn from experience is diminishing and may be gone. Through the services provided by occupational therapists, those individuals who require experience to acquire and utilize knowledge can continue to have opportunities which enable them to make decisions about their lives, and to cope with, adapt to, and negotiate with their social environments.

The above description of our product is broad and purposefully aimed at the commonalities in our professional activities. This was done in the belief that attitudes about roles and functions should be built upon a professional foundation rather than predicating the profession's future upon the role of the therapist in any given marketplace.

The Marketplace

Given the fact that our product is a service, where should we market it?

Traditionally, the hospital has been our marketplace. Should we continue, in light of the changing social context and the product as it may be defined, continue to be hospital-based and medically related?

Will the changing structure of hospitals permit us to remain there even if we wish to do so? Will our own professional goals permit us to retain our primary affiliation with medicine?

Two particular changes occurring within the spectrum of health care prompt me to question the retention of our primary ties with medicine. In the first instance, there is increasing discrepancy in health needs and expectations as identified by the public and in the needs identified by medicine. Until recently, the scope of medical care (with the exception of public health) was limited by the "germ theory." Theoretically, this theory suggested that the cause of illness or disease was a germ. If the germ could be identified, a cure could then be effected through medication, surgery, or some other prescribed regime.[14]

In contrast, the concept of illness now extends to include persons with social or behavioral problems. These problems, once considered to be of a legal or moral nature, were handled by judges or ministers who prescribed punishment or forgiveness. Now persons with such problems are candidates for health care.

The second change occurring within health care is the emergence of a new relationship between the "patient" and health professionals. The relationship involves (1) a difference in degree of patient involvement in the treatment process; (2) a movement away from the dependence and compliance required earlier of patients; and (3) a desire on the part of the patient to know more about the rationale for and consequences of the treatment program. Perhaps this change results from the greater incidence of chronic conditions and the different approaches required to change behavior.

In many instances, the cure, eradication, or control of health problems becomes a function of the contract and relationship negotiated between the health professional and the individual participating in the service program. Many of these individuals do not require hospitalization, nor will the regimented schedules and dependency states fostered of necessity by hospitals produce the desired behavioral changes necessary to enable the individual to live in relative harmony with himself and his social system.

If we are to successfully provide our services to patients, we need time which is a commodity not readily available in most hospitals. Thus, we either have to seek to change the hospital system or move into other environments. There are many other changes in medical care which cause me to question whether we can even realistically see ourselves as desiring to retain a primary affiliation with medicine and hospitals, but these instances highlight my concern.

With the changing social context, the product as I have defined it, the needs of our potential service population, and the time required to produce behavioral change, occupational therapy's greatest contribution may be other than hospital settings. We might be located in sheltered environments where opportunities for experiential learning are provided or in the individual's own social system, whereby he learns to cope with its demands, adapt to its requirements, and enter into a transactional arrangement with it.

Thus, the most ideal marketplace for occupational therapy may be in community health centers, school systems, day care centers, early child-care facilities, institutions for the chronically ill or for persons requiring long-term care as a result of either biological, social, cognitive, or behavioral problems, industrial settings, environments designed to reverse the cycles of poverty and welfare, vocational settings, or in specified medical settings where medicine and occupational therapy share or jointly seek common goals.

The decision or decisions related to the most appropriate marketplace have yet to be made, but we must explore, and evaluate all possible alternatives in order to determine whether our product can be effectively marketed in any of the marketplaces identified above.

Product Marketing

As we consider a change in the marketplace, one of our first orders of business will be to identify sources of financial support. Examination of the medical profession reveals that any movement toward a new service delivery system is accompanied by plans which insure a solid base of support for physicians. The interest in prepaid medical plans, as a means of insuring financial security, is so great that lawyers, dentists, and insurance companies are exploring the feasibility of utilizing this approach on a widespread basis.

Occupational therapy faces a more difficult problem than does medicine, dentistry, or law in that our name is not yet associated by the public with the services we provide. In reality many of the needs and problems identified by society are those for which we maintain that we can provide services. Yet a gap exists between our perception of our services and the public's ability to recognize those services as being provided by occupational therapy. Evidence also suggests that we are identified by our media, rather than by our goals and functions, and we seem to perpetuate this image by many of the advertisements which appear in our professional literature and at our professional conferences.

One of our greatest challenges is to clearly identify our product or services for ourselves and the public, particularly if we wish to achieve success in marketing them.

The inadequate solution to this challenge utilized by therapists moving into new environments has been to relinquish their professional identity to obtain jobs. It is only after they have succeeded in their jobs that they may admit that they were successful because their education and experience prepared them to contribute to the solution of certain problems. If we persist in this pattern, we run the risk of losing many excellent therapists. This is a loss we cannot afford.

We have made some inroads into marketing our product through our increased reliance upon public information systems, public relations, and development of educational brochures and materials, and our efforts to influence and utilize the legislative process. These have been tentative, hesitant steps, and we must find a way to more directly and more forcefully close the gap between our perception of our services and the public's perceptions of our services.

Drucker, in addressing the issue of marketing as business views it, defines it as the systematic purposeful organization of work to sell a product, deliver it to the customer, and receive pay for it. The purpose of marketing is to translate knowledge or technology into products or services which are economically productive. Questions he raises are: (1) What are the needs, satisfactions, and expectations of the customer? (2) What can the customer afford? and (3) Who is the customer?[15] The purchaser of the service and the consumer of the service may be different and the distinction is an important one. It certainly has relevance for occupational therapy because we have traditionally been paid by hospitals to provide services to patients—and the implications of this method of financing upon our professional behavior may not yet be clear to us. I tend to believe however that financial dependency does little to help therapists become either advocates or activists.

In essence, as we think of marketing our product, the questions proposed by Drucker may be important ones for us to consider.

Personnel Requirements

As we consider a reorganization of the delivery of occupational therapy services, the personnel required to market the occupational therapy product becomes a primary focus of consideration. We must decide how to provide, maintain, and retain experienced practitioners who provide service, and we must decide whether we will attempt to provide manpower to fill all of the positions or first try to identify and fill critical positions.

Our profession has been slow to recognize the true value of our practitioners, and while we establish standards to improve the level of practice, we have done little to increase the prestige, status, financial rewards, or opportunities for advancement within the clinical field of our experienced therapists. Our competent practitioners have to leave clinical practice to advance or to fulfill the goals of occupational therapy. Our most distinguished researchers have difficulty obtaining grants and financial support to conduct the studies to substantiate professional knowledge. If this trend continues, the most vital component of our profession—the practice of occupational therapy—may be left in the hands of young, inexperienced, or unknowledgeable therapists, of assistants and aides, and of therapists who may be complacent with competence but who do not aspire to excellence.

This is a critical problem for which we must find resolutions quickly. We must create opportunities within areas of clinical practice so that clinicians can move up in terms of professional responsibility, financial reward, and prestige without having to "move out to move up." Part of the solution to this problem may well relate to the identification of our marketplace and our ability to find sources of economic support and financial security for occupational therapists.

If clinical practice is to be assured of its rightful place within our profession, our educators have special responsibilities. We need to overcome "town–gown" attitudes of medicine for we do ourselves and our profession a serious disservice when we indulge in such negative attitudes. These attitudes are reflected in the form of criticism, frequently without apparent recognition of the fact that clinicians are the product of our educational institutions. If our clinicians fail to meet our expectations, we must examine the criteria against which we are judging their performance. We must ask why, in view of the knowledge we have imparted to them, they do not meet our expectations. Perhaps we fail to help students learn to identify for themselves, the external forces to which they must be responsive, the occupational therapy product, the marketplace in which services can be delivered, and ways of seeking financial support for our product or service.

We may fail as educators, just as therapists fail with their patients, when we focus on the product and forget the market. The patient must be able to survive in his social system. He must find a sense of satisfaction, a sense of achievement, a sense of mastery and competence—much of which is fed back to him through his occupational performance. The clinical therapist (as well as the administrator, the researcher, or the educator) must also find these satisfactions in his social system through occupational performance, and thus it behooves us to help them learn how to transact the necessary negotiations with the system in which they live and/or work in order to provide the full benefit of our services to patients.

The second way in which we demonstrate negative attitudes toward clinical therapists is perhaps most evident but not limited to university teaching hospitals. We utilized two sets of standards in hiring academic and clinical faculty and the salaries may reflect a considerable differential between academic and clinical faculty members. There is frequently reluctance on the part of academic faculty members to include the clinical faculty members in the decision-making process concerning the curriculum and the educational process. There are differing recognition and reward systems for academic and clinical faculty members. I appreciate the fact that funding for these two groups of faculty members frequently comes from different sources, but that does not relieve us of the responsibility for attempting to find alternatives and resolutions.

Clinical occupational therapists are the core of our profession—they provide the services which we value and in which we believe. It is to educate clinical therapists that our educational system exists. Research becomes necessary to improve the quality, content, and direction of practice and education, and administrators provide the facilities and other resources needed by our practitioner.

We must find ways to enable our most experienced clinical therapists to remain in the field and this is a challenge for the whole profession.

Other personnel-related issues to be anticipated as change occurs in our product, our marketplace, and our marketing process include change in professional behavior and increased conflict as we come to grips with the occupational therapist as generalist or the occupational therapist as specialist. Freidson, in studies of the medical profession, found that the nature of practice determines physician behavior. More specifically, he identified "client-dependent" and "colleague-dependent" practices. In the "client-dependent" relationship, the physician must be responsive to patient needs and expectations if he wishes to retain his patients and his income. In the latter instance, the "colleague-dependent" physician (the radiologist, pathologist, etc.) receives patients by referral from other physicians and so he is primarily responsive to their expectations, rather than the expectations of the patient.[16] This concept has relevance for occupational therapists in that we are just recognizing the implications for our behavior that are inherent in the constraints imposed by the marketplace in which we work and the source of financial support for our services. Certainly movement into new areas, often with loose or few affiliations to medicine, may be reflective of the fact that it is necessary to be employed by, or in, an environment in which there is a shared philosophy and a shared goal—or in which there is opportunity to create with others the goals which are to be shared. To be employed, without an opportunity to influence or negotiate with one's social system, is seldom satisfying. Thus, as we seek new marketplaces we may anticipate change in professional behavior, reflected by our determination to define for ourselves the standards of professionalism we wish to attain; change in our professional behavior will also reflect our growing ability to exert force, influence, or political power to see that our clients have access to adequate services. Increased conflict as an anticipated issue may arise in response to the argument to prepare generalists versus specialists. This issue has plagued occupational therapy for years, and the prospect of expanding our horizons into new service areas may intensify the conflict.

One alternative to a discussion of the merits of the generalist versus the specialist is suggested by Lawrence and Lorsch, and Dubos, respectively, as differentiation and integration or universality and diversity. Drawing from systems theory, we know that as organizations grow, they differentiate into parts which must be integrated if the entire system is to be viable. In biology, the human body follows a similar process through its differentiation into various organs, all of which are integrated through the nervous system and brain. Each system, whether in business or biology, is concerned with differentiation, integration, and adaptation to the outside world in order to survive. Both differentiation and integration are necessary for successful interaction with and achievement in any given environment, but the unavoidable consequence is conflict. According to organizational researchers, the organization's success ultimately depends upon how well it tolerates and resolves conflict so that integration is facilitated without sacrificing the need for differentiation.

For us, as occupational therapists, it will be necessary to think of our common goals as our point of integration, while specialization may be centered upon the behavioral components (biological, social, emotional, or cognitive) of occupational performance—or related to the areas in which to work. Again, our own future success may well depend upon our ability to tolerate and resolve conflict in order to facilitate integration without sacrificing needed differentiation within occupational therapy.

These issues—retention of experienced practitioners in the service areas, changes in professional behavior, and conflict resolution—demand attention now and will continue to occupy our time and energy, particularly as changes occur in our product, marketplace, and marketing process until we can find appropriate solutions to them.

Summary

In summary, I have raised several challenges to which I believe our profession must respond:

1. How can we utilize knowledge, rather than rely solely upon experience, to help us predict social change and anticipate the consequences of such change for occupational therapy?

2. Can we develop a strategy and organize ourselves, as a profession, so that we can conduct negotiations and transactions with the larger social system in which we exist, thereby ensuring the provision of our services to those who have need of them?

3. Can we identify clearly—for ourselves and for the public—the product or services we can provide? Can we identify the purchasers of our services, and can we, in actuality, provide those services?

4. Can we decide where our product should be marketed, and can we anticipate and plan for the changes which might occur as we move into new environments? In relation to this, can we define for ourselves the criteria for professionalism we seek to fulfill?

5. Finally, can we ensure the necessary support for clinical therapists who represent our larger corporate body?

The challenges I have identified are ones for which I have no ready answers—but recognition and awareness often precede problem-solving. I cannot help but believe that the wider our base of operations, the more responsive we will be to social needs, and the more responsible and accountable we will become. Furthermore, if we can identify our services as meeting identified public health needs, support may be forthcoming from many sources: from school systems, industry, proprietary as well as voluntary agencies providing a wide variety of human health services. Possibly even physicians and insurance companies will contract with us to deliver specific services to their patients. I feel that economic independence may not only facilitate but promote the move toward professional growth if we can identify how we wish to market our product. I also believe that the answers for a profession come not so much from individuals as from collective attempts and wisdom to identify problems, to resolve the conflict inherent in them, and to consider and select the alternatives which offer the most appropriate solutions.

In conclusion, I feel comfortable leaving these challenges unanswered because I believe in the ability of occupational therapists, based on demonstrated convictions about the worth of occupational therapy to clients, to help in the process of finding answers to these challenges.

Acknowledgment

The author wishes to express appreciation and gratitude for the contributions and assistance given by my colleagues, students and secretarial staff at Boston University; by Anne Henderson, OTR; Lela Llorens, OTR; and Elizabeth Yerxa, OTR; and by my mother.

References

1. Dunton, W. R. National society for the promotion of occupational therapy. *Maryland Psychiatr* Q 8:55–56, 1918.
2. Bockoven, J. S. Legacy of moral treatment: 1800's to 1910. *Am J Occup Ther 25*:223–225, 1971.
3. Mosey, A. C. Involvement in the rehabilitation movement—1942–1960. *Am J Occup Ther 25*:234–236, 1971.
4. Freidson, E. *Professional Dominance*. New York, Atherton Press. Inc., 1970, p. 51.
5. Fidler, G. S. Learning as a growth process: A conceptual framework for professional education. *Am J Occup Ther 20*:1–8, 1966.
6. Yerxa, E. J. Authentic occupational therapy. *Am J Occup Ther 21*:1–9, 1967.
7. Lawrence, P. R., and Lorsch, J. W. *Organization and Environment*. Homewood, Illinois: R. D. Irvin Inc., 1969, p. 3.
8. Drucker, P. F. *The Age of Discontinuity*. New York: Harper and Row, 1969, p. 41.
9. Ibid, p. 15.
10. Reilly, M. Occupational therapy can be one of the great ideas of 20th-century medicine. *Am J Occup Ther 16*:1–9, 1962.
11. Dubos, R. *The Mirage of Health*. New York: Harper, 1959.
12. Lawrence, P. R. and Lorsch, J. W. *Organization and Environment*. p. 14.
13. Dubos, R. *So Human an Animal*. New York: Charles Scribners Sons, 1968, p. 27.
14. Freidson, E. *Professional Dominance*. pp. 5–6.
15. Drucker, P. F. *The Age of Discontinuity*. pp. 52–53.
16. Freidson, E. *Professional Dominance*. pp. 91–93.

22

1973 Eleanor Clarke Slagle Lecture

Academic Occupational Therapy:
A *Career Specialty*

Alice C. Jantzen, PhD, OTR

I would like to express my appreciation to you as colleagues for the accolade of being selected as the sixteenth recipient of the Eleanor Clarke Slagle Lecture Award of our Association. In particular, I would like to thank the therapists who nominated me and also the many therapists with whom I have been associated during my professional life in the area of occupational therapy education.

Having free choice in the selection of a topic for the lecture and one year to work on the assignment does create some dilemmas, as I am sure any student would understand. Throughout this past year I remained convinced that I should talk with you today about the area of occupational therapy which is of prime concern to me and the one that I know best—that of occupational therapy education.

The booklet "Chicago . . . Occupational Therapy Beginnings," by Beatrice Wade and Barbara Loomis, came to my attention recently, and I am pleased that they provided me with some ideas that make my presentation on this topic especially appropriate for a conference being held in Chicago. To quote, "a significant portion of occupational therapy education history occurred here, in Chicago, with the pioneer efforts of Eleanor Clarke Slagle." Further, "the . . . Lectureship was established in 1955 by AOTA to honor the contributions of Mrs. Slagle to occupational therapy education, to the profession and to the professional organization."[1]

Some of my Slagle predecessors have expressed their concerns about education. Ruth Brunyate Wiemer talked about clinical education; Mary Reilly presented "A Theoretical Basis for Planned Change in Professional Education"; Gail Fidler spoke about the teaching–learning process involved in education for professions; while Wilma West has written on graduate education, and in the 1960s, under her leadership, our Association carried out an ambitious curriculum study project.[2, 3, 4, 5, 6] I plan to talk about occupational therapy education from a somewhat different point of view. I would like to have you consider academic occupational therapy as a career specialty in our field, grounded in the basic bodies of knowledge required of clinical specialties, but requiring additional knowledge for competent performance in the academic setting.

Perhaps before I launch into the topic of academic occupational therapy it might be well to present my concept of what is meant by the term *specialization*.

The practice of occupational therapy is the heart of our field—the delivery of our particular kind of health care services to patients or clients is the reason for the existence of occupational therapy. In the practice setting, the different types of patients we work with demand that we become specialized in the knowledge required to provide effective service—psychiatric, physical disabilities, developmental—thus, we become clinical specialists. But there is another concept of specialization that needs to be clearly acknowledged. This is that the knowledge gained in clinical specialty areas is implemented in different types of career roles. These career roles—all of them essential to

Originally published 1974 in *American Journal of Occupational Therapy, 28,* 73–81.

occupational therapy—include expert practitioner, program supervisor, researcher, and educator. And the last three require a second set of specialized competencies in addition to clinical expertise. Thus, to return to my topic of academic occupational therapy, I propose that the educational component is both a necessary and essential part of our total field of endeavor and that competent performance as a university faculty member requires both clinical knowledge and additional knowledge and skills specific to this career role. The recent upheavals throughout higher education and the many and diverse changes which are occurring at this time demand that we give consideration to our educational activities. Since I feel qualified to talk from my own experience, some of my presentation will be autobiographical. However, I believe that the concerns I shall express are not unique to me, but are shared by all of us in this area of our field.

Establishment of a Program

Fifteen years ago I accepted a position at the University of Florida with the responsibility to initiate an undergraduate curriculum and simultaneously, to establish an occupational therapy service program in the yet-to-be-opened teaching hospital. There were pluses and minuses in the situation, as is true of most situations. On the minus side there was no student awareness of the field; thus, prospective students were nonexistent. Persons in the Health Center and university professed almost no knowledge as to what role occupational therapy played in health care services. At the time there were only about 25 occupational therapists working in Florida, most of them located in the central and southern parts of the state, and there was thus little opportunity to provide reference points for understanding of our field. There were no clinical training centers within an 800-mile radius of the university, and most of the therapists in the southeastern region had never been involved in training students. In essence, I found myself moving into a community in which it would be necessary to carve out and establish the role of occupational therapy in health care delivery, thereby justifying the validity of establishing the educational program.

In some ways no knowledge turned out to be a plus, since I was not confronted with a traditional mind-set about occupational therapy, but largely with lack of information. To be on board in a new venture was also on the plus side—a newly established Health Center complex, designed to house all medical and health related disciplines, in a state that had not previously trained its own health professionals. The administrative structure was such that we were housed, along with six other academic programs, in a separate College of Health Related Professions. A further plus was the inclusion of the teaching hospital as an integral part of the Health Center. In order for the academic and service programs to be in concert with each other, the chairman of each academic department was appointed as the director of the corollary service in the hospital. Another plus was the fact that the Health Center was located on the main campus of the University of Florida, a large university composed of 15 colleges with a multiplicity of departments and course offerings.

Thus, 15 years ago I saw the setting as having much to offer occupational therapy education. Further, I was most fortunate in being able to recruit five occupational therapists—Genevieve Jonas Widmoyer, Miriam Thralls, Grace Straw, Reba Anderson, Karen Rasmussen Rusnak—who were willing to join in a pioneering adventure of starting a curriculum and a clinical service program simultaneously.

The essentials for an accredited curriculum tend to foster the idea that our programs should preferably be based in universities with medical schools attached. Such universities usually also have many doctoral level programs, as illustrated by the fact that the University of Florida offers 255 possible majors for a doctoral degree. While there are certain advantages to such a setting, over the years I have learned that in the present stage of development of occupational therapy education, these settings are not without concurrent penalty for us. University administrations tend to reward post-baccalaureate professional programs, such as medicine and law, and those departments which offer Ph.D. programs. In fact, the cost accounting for teaching at the different levels varies, and not in our favor. Furthermore, our programs are inclined to be considered very small operations. For example, while our enrollment figures seem reasonable to us, in terms of numbers we are working with only three-tenths of one percent of the total number of students in our university. Thus the visibility of our program is difficult to achieve; and visibility is the determinant in the long run of staffing and funding for the program. Programs in colleges and universities where the primary emphasis is on undergraduate students are frequently in a far better position than we to be recognized and rewarded for their endeavors.

Also, I have recently learned that the advantages which led to the decision that all university academic operations be on the same campus resulted in the University of Florida being today one of the three most complex university administrative structures in the nation.

While the heart of the activity of a university occurs at the academic departmental level, there are usually many layers and levels of administrative activities which affect departmental operation, ranging on our campus from academic affairs, to finance and accounting, sponsored research, contracts and grants, and the registrar's office. On the other side, a university has numerous supportive services and resources which can be very helpful in our activities. These include the computer center, teaching resources laboratories, testing and counseling bureaus, student health services, and the financial aid office. A multiuniversity also has a multiplicity of elective course offerings available to our students. At the same time the numerous faculties in such a university provide a major challenge to us when we seek to make course and curriculum changes. In the same way, graduate programs, such as ours, which must work through the graduate school of a university can have a more difficult time than is true in colleges and universities that do not set this requirement.

At the time I accepted the position as chairman I was quite naive about the complexities of university administration, but I must admit that today I enjoy the challenge of making us both visible and academically respectable as an educational program. However, the job is not easy, and each year the pressure seems to increase rather than diminish. Further, with changes in the demands for membership in the university community, changes in the university administrative thinking in terms of accountability, time-shortened curricula, and the like, changes in the life demands made on students, as well as increased knowledge of the learning process and of methods of education, the task of providing quality education for occupational therapy students has become increasingly complex in these years.

In order to clarify for you my views about academic occupational therapy, I shall talk further about faculty, about students, and about our common point of reference, the curriculum.

Faculty Responsibilities

First, some thoughts about occupational therapy faculty, our specialized job demands, and the resultant need for specialized credentials to meet these responsibilities. On our campus, faculty activity is cost accounted into eight categories. I intend to talk about three of these—teaching, service, and research.

Let me talk first about our teaching responsibilities. "That *some* kind of preparation for college teaching is helpful there can be little doubt. But what kind?"[7] The Commission on Undergraduate Education in the Biological Sciences has issued a series of helpful monographs. One, concerned with the preparation of college teachers, categorized the activities and competencies of teachers under six headings. The dimensions are "content mastery," which includes the generally held idea "that one must know something in order to teach it, and that the teacher's information should be up to date"; "the ability to organize a domain of knowledge, to design and plan a course, to establish instructional objectives"; effective presentation skills—the "management of learning"; "personal interaction with students," which includes four paramount characteristics, accessibility, authenticity, possession of useful knowledge, such as how to register for next term, and the ability to relate to students; "ability to rigorously evaluate one's own teaching effectiveness"; and "professionalism" . . . those qualities which differentiate a scholar from an instructor.[7]

While in my view the above six dimensions should apply for both academic and clinical teachers, the locus of our work—the university, the classroom and the laboratory—makes different demands upon our teaching skills. We even have a different jargon, as was pointed up recently by a new faculty member, an experienced clinical teacher, who remarked after attending her first departmental faculty meeting that she hardly understood a thing we were talking about. Just as we, early in our occupational therapy education, received some orientation to medical technology, so, too, faculty members need an orientation to academic terminology.

In occupational therapy education, our faculty activity reports frequently look all right in terms of classroom teaching—student credit hours generated or time devoted to classroom contact. However, our faculty efforts at clinical teaching, a concept well accepted in medical and dental schools, have not yet really been recognized by university administrators. Occupational therapy education programs have been part of colleges and universities since World War II, but our clinical practice requirement seems to be a long way from being accepted as a university responsibility. The one program that led the way in implementing a plan for solving this was the University of Illinois under the leadership of Beatrice Wade. Yet, when deans and administrators seek to find how many faculty are necessary for an academic program, they continue to look to the average number, four or five, needed just for classroom teaching, and to ignore the educational staff of about 17 persons at Illinois.

Next, let me talk about faculty responsibilities for service. This component of a faculty member's role includes the university expectation that we serve on a variety of university committees and not just focus on departmental or college committees. In addition, we are expected to be active in service to the community outside the university confines, be it local, state, regional, or national community. At times I have heard people grumble in AOTA that educators seem to be overrepresented in state and national organizations. This is not merely for self-seeking aggrandizement as some might perceive; it is viewed by the university as one of our inherent responsibilities as faculty members. So too, we are expected to be active in a wide variety of local community service organizations and to serve as consultants to various groups and facilities. In other words, we are expected to communicate our portion of the university's storehouse of knowledge.

Next, let me discuss the research responsibilities of faculty. We tend to think the time spent for research is limited to undertaking a formal research project and following it through to conclusion. This is an erroneous assumption. As Van der Kloot says, "Time allocated for research almost invariably also includes time spent in the library, at seminars, talking with colleagues, and at scientific meetings. If I were to stop research tomorrow, all the activities mentioned must still be done, or else I would soon lose touch with my field and all effectiveness as a teacher."[8] So, faculty must devote research time to simply keeping up with their areas of knowledge.

According to Van der Kloot, "The view that the university is solely responsible for teaching, merely as an extension of the high school, is one of the most potentially disastrous ideas circulating in our society. The university has traditionally been responsible for teaching, for research, and for the preservation of knowledge. The tradition evolved because each activity feeds on the others. Any attempt to evaluate how well the job is being done by measuring only one parameter is bound to be incredibly misleading."[8]

To clarify faculty activity further there is a final comment that is worth making. The university is rightly considered a storehouse of knowledge, but the storehouse is not the libraries as some might think. The storehouse in each university is the heads of a few hundred professors who constantly keep up-to-date on their areas of specialized interests and who share this knowledge with colleagues and consumers. The university "can be understood only when the role of professor in processing, ordering, and storing information is taken into account and when we realize that the pressure for increasing faculty size comes from the exploding supply of information."[8]

When we consider that the field of occupational therapy reaches out in so many directions and that we present ourselves, in totality, as a field dealing with a myriad of problems, of people ranging in age from infants to elderly, it is apparent that our curricula are grossly understaffed to accomplish the true dimensions of responsibility of university faculty members. In essence, in terms of accountability for faculty time, some of us have been too naive in our knowledge of a university, how it functions, and what it considers important in terms of faculty effort. We, I believe, have therefore been unnecessarily penalizing ourselves and, in fact, the field of occupational therapy, by not paying sufficient attention to university concerns not only for teaching, but also for service, research, and the preservation and expansion of knowledge.

Faculty Credentials

An understanding of the multiple responsibilities of a faculty member in a university leads to identification of the credentials required for faculty status. Since ours is an applied field with the aim of education to prepare practitioners, we ourselves generally require the candidates have a period of work experience as practitioners. When seeking faculty members, we, in addition, usually look for persons with competence in specialized areas of practice, such as pediatric or psychiatric occupational therapy.

Whether we support the idea or not, universities no longer consider that competence in the doing, as demonstrated by performance as practitioners, is sufficient for faculty status. We are expected to be more than clinicians and teachers, we are expected to be scholars, and to contribute to knowledge. Thus, universities generally require that faculty candidates have earned the highest degree available in their particular discipline. For us presently that is a master's degree. The fact that most of us with graduate degrees have them in other fields points to the realization that in terms of knowledge areas we do not yet provide the necessary spectrum of options for our own field. Faculty members, in addition, need specialized skills for college teaching and to know how to design strategies for implementing research activities compatible with their interests. They also, as scholars, need to write for publication since the only way, other than by casual conversation, that they can be judged as to their development of specialized knowledge is by having the opportunity to read the results of their explorations. Thus, today we must pay realistic attention to university demands for specialized credentials for faculty.

Students

Now for some comments about today's students. I shall discuss the explosion in numbers of students seeking admission to programs, some of the developmental issues that today's students face as individuals, their potential for becoming helping professionals, and the interaction inherent in communications between students and faculty.

Fifteen years ago we were looking for students, and in 1959 found three willing persons and started our academic program. For several years we had essentially open enrollment, accepting all students who met the admission requirements of the university. It shortly became apparent that many students were interested in majoring in occupational therapy, but 10 years ago it was somewhat like a voice crying in the wilderness to suggest that at a national level we should focus not on student recruitment but on expanding consumer awareness of the services occupational therapy offers.

Today, academic programs are flooded with applicants. Why are so many of today's students selecting occupational therapy as a major? I wish I had a ready answer. Some of it is undoubtedly due to society's shift from a technological imagination to a social imagination; some due to the recent so-called glut of persons prepared in other fields who cannot find jobs. In any event, we as faculty and clinicians are communicating some positive and rewarding behaviors and attitudes which cause students to wish to join our ranks. Having talked with several thousands of prospective students over the years what I find especially encouraging is their lively concern for the ills of man and of society and their wish to bring about some improvement in the human condition.

In terms of providing a quality education, those programs which are able to limit enrollment, on the basis of available resources, are fortunate. For the past few years we have had three to four academically qualified applicants for each place in the class, a situation which results in our being confronted with a process of selecting which students to admit. Some attempts have been made to find criteria for selection in addition to placement scores and grade point averages. Unfortunately, we as yet do not have other measures which have been proven valid, reliable, and defensible, and the knowledge that seemingly all other helping professions are having the same difficulty is small comfort. The fact is today we must justify the exclusion of many qualified students from the program. How to handle pressure from parents, politicians, administrators, and other health professionals has therefore become an important element of an occupational therapy educator's role.

Next I shall comment about what today's students are like. I shall limit my remarks to those of typical undergraduate age—late teens and early twenties. I do this not only because it is the age group with which I am most familiar, but also because nationally most of our students are enrolled in undergraduate programs.

Today's college students are dealing with many shifts in values and standards in our society. Need we remind ourselves that this includes occupational therapy students. In our day we were guided by the indoctrination of an established set of values, moral, social and religious, that were geared to the premise that, although changes might occur, they would not be substantial, radical, or continuing. We expected the world we faced upon graduation to represent a milieu perpetuating the best of the past, and the stable endurance of the present. How wrong we were. College students of the 70s are facing the crucial need of a hierarchy of new values to guide them through the turmoil and crises of continuing changes.[9] On campuses many of the rules and regulations for student conduct have been eliminated, and a wide range of situations requiring personal decisions now confront today's undergraduates. Even as recently as five or six years ago such choices were largely deferred because of university strictures or were even nonexistent. Situations range from how to live in co-ed dormitories, to communal living arrangements, the drug scene, the "pill," and abortion. We as faculty need to be aware that our students are dealing with such concerns in their personal lives. Fortunately, most of today's occupational therapy students have lively and healthy character structures and seem able to handle decision-making in terms of their personal lives in an effective and mature fashion.

In considering the potential for professional development of today's undergraduate students, we find them to be a very bright and questioning group of young people. While they are ready to learn the necessary skills and techniques, they, along with their fellow students in the university, are ready to question the relevancy of what we teach in terms of both present and future performance demands. In essence, they wish to know not only "how to do," but "why" it is done that way. Fortunately, they are also generally effective in interpersonal relationships, and for us not only a challenge, but fun to work with.

In our roles as faculty some of the learning that took us so long to achieve we can shorten for them by communicating our present knowledge, pointing out uncharted areas demanding solutions, and directing them toward other areas of knowledge which may provide some of the answers they seek. We depend on them to keep the field alive and lively and by their performance as practitioners, to realize some of our dreams, hopes, and visions for the field. They depend on our experience, the knowledge we have gained, to guide them into becoming competent and confident occupational therapists. So far as I am concerned, that is what the role of educator is all about.

All effective educators fully expect some students to outdistance them in their performance and accomplishments. As educators we derive satisfaction from this. While grades are an important measure of competence, especially for undergraduate students, they need and merit positive reinforcement in still other ways which will indicate to them that they are on the right track toward achieving excellence. Frequently, I am afraid, we tend to focus on the student with problems and neglect to consider that the competent and capable student deserves equal, if not more, attention. Student-faculty interaction is, fortunately, a two-way street, and we as faculty do receive some measure of positive reinforcement from students and graduates. Some we get from teacher evaluations at the end of each quarter. Some from reports on the calibre of performance of our graduates at clinical affiliation centers. We derive satisfaction from a view of the accomplishments of graduates and also from incidental remarks, such as "Whatever you're doing, keep it up!" Such feedback makes it possible for faculty each year to pick themselves up off the floor of exhaustion after working with the presently enrolled classes and have the courage to start all over again each September with a new class of beginning students.

Curriculum

I would like now to talk some about curriculum both at the basic professional level and also as advanced education. While I shall not discuss assistant level education, I believe that some of my remarks could reasonably apply to such curricula.

In 1958 I had some ideas which I attempted to incorporate into the curriculum. These were a balance in course offerings between human biology and behavioral sciences, a design of so-called occupational therapy theory courses to emphasize evaluation and treatment principles in the two broad areas of physical and psychological dysfunction, and the inclusion as early as possible of clinical experience concurrent with didactic courses—that we term practicum. When the accreditation team arrived in 1960, we were informed that we met the essentials, but in a rather different pattern than was then usual. As one survey team member said, the plan was too revolutionary and probably would not work. When one is responsible for another person's education such a remark can be rather upsetting, but we derived comfort from the knowledge that the same kinds of remarks had been made to the College of Medicine faculty by their survey team. In retrospect, I am happy to say that the curriculum has worked, and very well when judged in terms of the performance of Florida graduates.

During the past 15 years, my ideas about curriculum design have evolved so that today I see curriculum in the following context. A curriculum is more than just a listing of general education courses, prerequisite courses and required courses in a major. A curriculum should have both an underlying philosophy and a specific identifiable design of the sequencing and patterning of course offerings.

I see two primary factors as determinants of the design. The first is an awareness that the educational objectives of an occupational therapy program include all three components in the taxonomy of objectives: the cognitive domain, the affective domain, and the psychomotor domain. The second major determinant of curriculum design is the awareness that the curriculum needs to be planned in a developmental frame of reference. This developmental focus determines both the sequencing and patterning of courses and also creates a necessary awareness of the developmental process occurring in the students themselves.

Let me first talk further about the three domains in the taxonomy of educational objectives. A group of college examiners interested in achievement testing developed a system of classifying the goals of the educational process by the types of responses specified as desired outcomes of education. They found that most objectives could be placed into one of three major classifications or domains: cognitive objectives, emphasizing recall of knowledge and the development of intellectual abilities and skills; affective objectives which include interests, attitudes, appreciations, values, and emotional sets of biases; and psychomotor objectives which emphasize motor skill, manipulation of material and objects, or acts which require neuromuscular coordination.[10, 11]

The practice of occupational therapy clearly emphasizes all three areas. When one reviews the essentials of an accredited curriculum it is evident that all three domains of educational objectives are included. It appears that occupational therapy is a prime example of an academic program whose goal is the development of learning in all three areas. I submit that the entire curriculum should be carefully planned and thoughtfully designed to meet the goals of cognitive, affective, and psychomotor learning required for occupational therapy practice.

In considering the developmental frame of a curriculum, just as Lela Llorens presents occupational therapy practice as facilitating growth and development of patients in seven defined areas necessary for effective performance, so too, we as faculty propose education as facilitating growth and development of students in the cognitive, affective, and motor skill areas of learning necessary for professional performance. "The development of a professional self-conception" according to Lortie, "involves a complicated chain of perceptions, skills, values and interactions. In this process, a professional identity is forged which is believable both to the individual and to others."[12] Vollmer and Mills state that, "You . . . have to go through an extended period of socialization . . . until you finally develop a psychological and social commitment to a professional career," and further, that "this period of socialization certainly includes formal training."[13] It seems essential, then, in designing academic programs that we keep clearly in mind that this time span is the beginning set in the development of the professional self-concept of an occupational therapist. To have education truly serve as a facilitating process in the growth and development of a professional occupational therapist requires that we consider not only students from a developmental frame of reference, but also all curricular components, the learning experiences, from a developmental frame of reference. This latter requires that we look cross-sectionally at all course offerings—what learning experiences should be offered concurrently; and that we should also look longitudinally to determine the sequencing of learning experiences.

Let me now attempt, by some illustrations, to clarify for you what I mean by curriculum design. When we accept a new class of juniors each fall, we know that in general they are about 20 years of age and that for most of them their major activity since about age five, three-fourths of their life span, has been to go to school. Most of their formal education to date has focused on the cognitive domain of learning, ranging from the three R's through English, physical science, humanities, biology and the like. As occupational therapy faculty we seek to continue their cognitive learning in content areas germane to our field. We strive to have them be well grounded in selected basic areas of human biology; in behavioral science; in the pathology, deviations and disorders to which human beings are subject. We also seek to ensure that they acquire sufficient motor skill in some of the tools of occupational therapy, those environmental things that we use in the treatment process.

Simultaneously, we wish to encourage affective learning in order that they become competent, helping health professionals. The affective domain is not only the hardest to communicate, but it is the area that students most resist. We seek to have them know who they are—to understand themselves, to know how others affect them, including patients who "look very different," fellow students, authority figures, and of equal importance, to help them understand how they affect others. How does one communicate to a student whose own reward system almost exclusively emphasizes high academic achievement that more is needed both as a clinician and a staff member than proof of A's in anatomy, neurology, skills, and the like? I am suggesting that it both can and has been done successfully and that we do it in our roles as educators working with students. Topics such as interpersonal and interprofessional relationships, group dynamics, and the like are built into the program and accomplished by how each course is structured and scheduled. We also seek to have students explore these affective dimensions through the kinds of questions asked on tests, by the reports—written and oral—we require, by term paper assignments, and by how we structure discussion groups.

Now for some examples of the developmental approach to curriculum design. We start off where they are and expand their knowledge of what is normal in the human condition, thus, courses in anatomy and growth and development. They also learn to observe normal social behavior among a wide range of the population; in community day care centers, nursery schools, boys' clubs, girl scout troops, the hamburger joints and pizza parlors adolescents frequent, adults at work and at play in a variety of settings, and the healthy elderly in their struggles and pleasures found in this business of living in today's society. Simultaneously, other components of the curriculum begin—that of learning necessary skills of occupational therapists—ranging from such content as weaving, woodworking, and leathercraft, to activity analysis, chart reading and reporting, and use of a medical library.

From these bases we move into providing students with knowledge of the abnormal—pathology, neurology, delayed development, with some emphasis given to the sociocultural overlay as an essential factor of concern in identifying physical or behavioral pathology and its effect upon possible remediation of a disorder. In subsequent terms we move to their learning the specific evaluation and treatment procedures which we use in working with people with physical or psychosocial problems. It has been our experience, using a developmental frame, that some topics which might come first in the ordering of chapters in a textbook or in a course outline, can be better presented with meaning to the students at the end of the course or of the program. It is not that we arbitrarily turn programs topsy-turvy, but the sequencing of topics needs to be planned thoughtfully in order to achieve the best learning.

Throughout the entire program students participate in part-time field work, ranging from observations in the normal workaday settings, as described earlier, to practicum assignments in the available clinical settings which surround the program. As they move along and gain knowledge in the content areas of the courses they are taking, they are concurrently expected to become participants in the activities of a clinician to whom they are assigned. Since we wish students to establish a professional identity, for practicum assignments we consider it essential that this in-process occupational therapist—one still learning to become a professional—must have a qualified occupational therapist to serve as role model in the assigned setting. We are also interested in their learning all the facets of the practitioners' jobs, so it is not necessary that the supervising therapist always be with a patient, as students are hopefully not learning to become patients. Thus, our felt need for faculty who are knowledgeable about the total curriculum and who can serve primarily as clinical educators, role-modeling for students what occupational therapists do in our familiar settings. Furthermore, we consider that the student, still attempting to determine what occupational therapy is all about, cannot realistically assess the role of occupational therapy in locations where none exist. Thus, we feel the need for additional faculty to explore, while at the same time sharing this experience with students, our potential roles in school programs for high-risk first graders, in camps for diabetic children, in crisis intervention centers, health programs for migrant workers, or in a work evaluation unit for hard-core unemployed.

Students themselves consistently tell us that the practicum, this part-time clinical experience component of the program, is one of the most meaningful experiences for them in the curriculum. It provides a "try-out" opportunity to help them determine if the role of occupational therapist suits their personal frames of reference, and also provides them with the reasons to concentrate on learning the content of the standard type courses.

Advanced Education

Up to now I have focused my remarks about curriculum design on the undergraduate basic professional level of occupational therapy education. I think, however, that these same considerations need to be given to advanced education in occupational therapy. The cognitive, affective, and motor skill areas of learning, and their interweaving, need to be considered as does the developmental frame of the course offerings and of the students enrolled. At this point it also seems important to reiterate some of my earlier comments as to how I perceive specialization in occupational therapy, since it directly affects my concept of advanced, graduate education for our field. Occupational therapy clinical specialties are grounded in the specialized problems of the different types of patients with whom we work. Career specialties in occupational therapy define the settings and types of positions in which we apply this specialized competence—teacher, practitioner or administrator.

Ten or 15 years ago, and when I did my several stints in graduate school, I saw the rationale for us in occupational therapy to earn graduate degrees as primarily that of education for competence in career specialty areas of teacher or administrator. After conversations with colleagues in charge of doctoral level programs, I have become more recently aware that our graduate programs in occupational therapy can be designed to evolve the body of knowledge needed for our field. Graduate education should therefore primarily focus on expanded knowledge in the clinical areas of occupational therapy. These can be classified developmentally, such as problems of children, adolescents, adults, or aged; or according to type of insult to the persons we seek to help, biological or psychological. The information needed as administrator, consultant, teacher, or researcher can be gained by means of electives in the program and integrated with the expanded occupational therapy content.

Colleagues in clinical psychology, speech pathology, and medical anthropology have made clear for me that faculty and adventuresome graduate students in their disciplines started together in search of new insights and a clear-cut identification and expansion of the body of knowledge specific to their fields. As time passed much was learned, old shibboleths disproved and dropped, new directions charted, and today these fields have achieved a status and are making contributions that far outdistance their original roles. Occupational therapy needs to be infused with the same adventuresome spirit as has occurred in other fields.

According to Ethridge and McSweeney, "the acquisition of knowledge through research, and the subsequent dissemination of this knowledge through publication . . . establishes the basic literature so necessary for the acceptance of occupational therapy as a profession."[14] Since research is an inherent job responsibility of university faculty members, I suggest that occupational therapy faculty should take leadership in the research activities for our profession. Further, I suggest that we who are university faculty members should begin to demand that university administration support us in these endeavors. Although our graduate program is just beginning its second year

I can guarantee that there is an excitement in working with enthusiastic colleagues and graduate students, each seeking to achieve excellence in a particular specialized area of occupational therapy. Parenthetically, I am sure that our present shortage of qualified faculty could be readily alleviated if clinicians were to perceive that this is the type of interaction in which we are engaged.

It is here that we must begin to think of academic occupational therapy as a career specialty area in the field, no less than academic medicine, academic sociology, psychology, and the like. A combination of the clinician's insight and the academician's discipline, as demanded by his environment, can serve to move the field to take its rightful place among others in the university setting. And this academic status will result in an enhancement of our contributions in the practice setting.

Summary

In summary, I have talked with you about occupational therapy education. First off, I identified my own frame of reference in order that you might understand the points of view I have about this phase of occupational therapy. I discussed briefly universities and colleges, their complexities and differences and how these affect an occupational therapy curriculum. Next I gave some information on what are considered by universities to be inherent responsibilities of faculty and some of the consequent qualifications that are considered necessary today for faculty status. I then provided some perceptions about today's students; pressures that they are dealing with, the qualifications of those presently entering the field, as well as dilemmas surrounding the explosion in numbers of prospective students. Following that, I gave some of my views concerning curriculum design—the necessity for considered sequencing and patterning of courses in terms of areas of learning, and in terms of the developmental process of both the students and of the educational objectives. Finally, I discussed advanced education in occupational therapy, a definition of what such education means to me, and suggestions as to how we can foster and develop this phase of the field.

I trust that my remarks will point out for you that, while I consider, as I said earlier, that the heart of occupational therapy is the practice of our field, the educational component, those of us who work in this career role, and our endeavors, are both necessary and essential to the totality of occupational therapy.

References

1. Loomis B, Wade BD: Chicago . . . Occupational Therapy Beginnings: Hull House. The Henry B Favill School of Occupations and Eleanor Clarke Slagle. Chicago, Curriculum in Occup Ther, Univ of Ill, 1973

2. Brunyate RW: Powerful levers in little common things. In Am Occup Ther Assn, The Eleanor Clarke Slagle Lectures 1955–1972. Dubuque, Kendall Hunt, pp 29–48, 1973

3. Reilly M: A Theoretical Basis for Planned Change in Professional Education, University of California at Los Angeles, unpublished doctoral dissertation, 1959

4. Fidler GS: Learning as a growth process: A conceptual framework for professional education. In Am Occup Ther Assn, The Eleanor Clarke Slagle Lectures 1955–1972. Dubuque, Kendall Hunt, pp 137–153, 1973

5. West WL: The present status of graduate education in occupational therapy. Am J Occup Ther 12: 291–292, 299, 1958

6. Am Occup Ther Assn: Curriculum Study, 16 volumes. New York, Am Occup Ther Assn, 1963, mimeographed

7. Dean DS: Preservice Preparation of College Biology Teachers: A Search for a Better Way. Washington, Commission on Undergraduate Education in the Biological Sciences, pp 16, 17, 20, 22, 1970

8. Van der Kloot WG: Comments on financing education. In Anlyan WG et al: The Future of Medical Education. Durham, Duke Univ Press, pp 191–192, 1973

9. Bowes N: The development of human values for the college graduate of the '70's. Bedford, June 1973, unpublished college commencement address

10. Bloom BS et al: Taxonomy of Educational Objectives. The Classification of Educational Goals, Handbook I: Cognitive Domain. New York, David McKay, pp 4, 7, 1956

11. Krathwohl DR, Bloom BS, Masia BB: Taxonomy of Educational Objectives, The Classification of Educational Goals, Handbook II: Affective Domain. New York, David McKay, p 7, 1964
12. Lortie DC: Laymen to lawmen: Law school, careers and professional socialization. In Vollmer HM, Mills DL (eds): Professionalization. Englewood Cliffs, Prentice-Hall, p 98, 1966
13. Vollmer HM, Mills DL (eds): Professionalization. Englewood Cliffs, Prentice-Hall, pp 88, 98, 1966
14. Ethridge DA, McSweeney M: Research in Occupational Therapy. Dubuque, Kendall Hunt, p 1, 1971

23

1974 Eleanor Clarke Slagle Lecture

Occupational Therapy:
Realization to Activation
Mary R. Fiorentino, MusB, OTR, FAOTA

Today I find myself standing before you in this honorable position feeling humble, yet privileged. It is with the deepest appreciation that I acknowledge all those who gave me the support, the assistance, and the contribution to my knowledge, to enable me to be in this position this afternoon.

It was very difficult to select a topic which I felt could contribute to the ongoing growth of the profession as it relates to service in the habilitation and rehabilitation of children. In doing so I knew it was necessary to go back in time and return to the lower levels of my own professional development, and to proceed with the sequential maturation that eventually brought me to this "standing position."

In narrowing down the broad spectrum of topics, a review of previous Eleanor Clarke Slagle Lectures revealed that both Lela Llorens and our President Jerry Johnson very aptly expressed two of my major concerns. Lela Llorens presented "a conceptual model for understanding the knowledge that presently supports the practice of occupational therapy with a discussion of how and where occupational therapy fits into the scheme of human development."[1] Jerry Johnson presented, "The success and perhaps survival of occupational therapy may well depend upon our ability to clearly identify our product and services, to determine where we can best provide these services, to obtain adequate sources of support for occupational therapy services, and to insure that we have experienced, competent personnel to provide these services."[2]

In the global overview of occupational therapy, these concerns continue to be of major importance. Does the occupational therapist fit into a developmental scheme, beginning as a neophyte in her profession and progressing to a therapist with special skills, competence, and a secure feeling about her basic knowledge? If so, what is the scheme? As a profession, are we able to identify and define this scheme from both an academic as well as a clinical viewpoint? Can we provide competent, professional therapists, therapists who are ready to provide services that will meet the demands of health care as we know it today? Are we ready to be challenged by the ongoing advances being made in medicine and research and changes in health care brought about by federal and state regulations? Finally, can we deal with the nebulous definition and role of occupational therapy as it is understood by third-party payees?

Therefore, from my vantage point, I made the decision to follow the theme: The growth and development of pediatric occupational therapy, and the pediatric developmental therapist, or occupational therapist, as they relate to the habilitation and rehabilitation of the physically handicapped child. I would like to explain how this growth and development can evolve, how it can be accomplished in a manner similar to the maturation of a child who is initially at the apedal level, who advances through the quadrupedal level, and finally reaches the highest level of control and skill, that is, the standing position, or bipedal level. I shall not delve into any fancy philosophy. I will

Originally published 1975 in *American Journal of Occupational Therapy, 29*, 15–21.

173

attempt to deal with the facts as they have unfolded over the years during my own levels of development evolving from "realization to activation."

The parallel to be drawn between a child's development in all spheres and an adult's development into a highly professional, skilled, competent therapist has many striking similarities. Also, many of the axioms or principles we use from the neurosciences, or more specifically the maturation of the nervous system, have their corollary in the educational development of the occupational therapist.

Let us compare the development of the occupational therapist with the development of the young child. We know now that the infant with an intact nervous system is born with all of the primitive reflexes and reactions. These are basic and necessary in order to have higher skills occur as integration and maturation proceed. We also know that an infant begins at the lowest level of development, the apedal level. He is born with many mechanisms for survival. He has all of the basic senses, cells, and systems of a normal infant's central nervous system (CNS) plus a full potential for learning and maturing. The amount of sensory input received into this nervous system, that is, how the infant is stimulated and handled, will eventually determine his ultimate potential. It is at this early age that the infant's CNS is the most pliable and capable of learning the fastest. Researchers today believe that it takes up to 21 years before the CNS is completely myelinated and matured; however, learning does continue within this system for many years.[3]

Initially, the infant relies on his mother for care, for proper or adequate stimulation, and for integration of the feedback resulting from *his* handling of the stimuli. Although he is essentially unable to sustain his own life without assistance, he learns to manipulate his environment by his behavior. The quality and quantity of these stimuli, their reinforcement, and their meaning to him as an organism will have a profound effect on his future development. As stated by Kaluger and Kolson,[4] "Each child develops a neural pattern for learning which includes organizing the cerebral functions and structures involved in the learning process to perform in sensory input, associative functions and motor output." They go on to explain further that integrating basic reactions and reflexes through use of a complex combination of cerebral processes for input, decoding, encoding, and output functions enables the child to progress to a purposeful responding, conceptualizing individual.

A child in the first several months of life has no mobility, cannot explore his environment, and must have experiences brought to him. He is fed, bathed, dressed, loved, spoken to, played with . . . all his senses are stimulated. There is constant change occurring and, if the stimuli are purposeful and meaningful, the child learns. The constant demands placed on the nervous system through all types of stimulation create the basic learning processes necessary to meet the requirement of future development and behavior.

Correlating this concept with a person entering a school of occupational therapy reveals that this individual has many of the same potentials and needs. A student must be provided with all experiences and exposures to ensure that he or she has a base upon which to develop a future as a therapist. The climate of a university allows for assimilation of material at a more rapid pace, but only if that material is presented in a manner that is meaningful, and allows for participation of the individual. It has been proved through animal and human studies that when there is deprivation of sensory stimuli there is no learning. Only when there is active participation does the individual learn more quickly and forget less.

Just as the basic mechanisms for learning and potential are altered if the newborn infant has CNS damage, so the basic education of an occupational therapist can be compromised if the material is not meaningful because it is outdated, or it is irrelevant to clinical advances. If the material is recognized by the student as not having observable application, the result is poorly understood information and inferior application of this knowledge to other situations in a generalized manner. The student or the infant then approaches his next level of development, the affiliation or quadrupedal level, ill-prepared to respond to a new set of stimuli, those that require a greater expertise from him.

At the quadrupedal level the child is ready for mobilization. The student should be ready to synthesize academic knowledge, explore new ideas, learn independently, develop interests, and make each experience as meaningful as possible to have the learning process continue. Therapeutic output will reflect the basic input received during the academic years. If basic courses have been appropriate, if basic preparation has been sufficient, then the student will take advantage of the meaningful experiences of the clinical centers. If the basic preparation has been meaningful, but the affiliation has not given the opportunity to explore, create, problem-solve, and learn, then sensory deprivation will predominate and learning will diminish. The student will continue to need the maturation and integration gained through experience to become a competent, self-sufficient individual performing at the highest level of development.

If there is lack of sensory input into a normal system, abnormal development will be manifest as a functional deficit during the life of the organism. Research tells us that each new learning experience, if properly reinforced, may cause a change in the nervous system to such an extent that behavior can be modified or even permanently changed. Therefore, the quadrupedal individual, infant or student, begins to mobilize and explore his environment, creating new experiences, changing his behavioral patterns while continuing to build up blocks of learning so that further integration can occur. Sequentially, he begins to prepare himself for the next higher level of development.

In the ongoing process of growth and development, the young child reaches standing and walking positions by the end of the first year. Much learning and maturation has occurred during this time; however, he has only basic motor movements and perceptions. The capacities of the adult evolve to meet the requirements of his natural environment. The extent to which these capacities are developed from birth and the rate at which they mature thereafter will depend upon the demands of the postnatal environment.

We know that in the learning process and in the maturation of the nervous system, the infant "perceives" through sensory stimuli into this system. This calls for a response that, in turn, creates new sensations which are immediately fed back into the CNS. Through repetition of an act, the response is "engrammed" into the system and a pattern of behavior is developed. Not until he utilizes this pattern over and over again will the response be an ingrained or semiautomatic, learned response, well integrated into this nervous system.

Thus, the CNS of the child by one year of age has integrated many primitive reactions and has developed higher reactions which enable him to reach the bipedal level. This has occurred through the learning process of perception, then repetition, then active participation. The child has undergone the learning process in all areas of behavior. He is beginning to reach out into his environment, extending his exploration for new fields of learning. He is becoming more independent in his decision-making, constantly changing and adding to the information which he has in order to develop higher cognitive skills necessary to cope with his adult environment.

In like manner, the "infant" therapist has basic knowledge at her command. She has perceived, repeated, and utilized this knowledge in preparation for achieving the higher level of development. At this point, he or she must now synthesize and act according to the dictates of this knowledge, problem-solve, make independent decisions, and continue the learning process. All of these actions require higher cognitive skills of behavior. If there has not been a "lesion" created somewhere along in the process of development, the new therapist will evolve into a competent, self-sustaining individual. He or she will be secure in their knowledge of the role of the occupational therapist and in their definition of occupational therapy as an essential discipline in the health fields. The idea of competent, skilled therapists solves the problem of establishing professionalism. Just as one cannot superimpose fine motor activities on a cerebral-palsied child who has no head or trunk control, one cannot superimpose professionalism on people ill-prepared to perform.

I would like now to discuss the role of occupational therapy in a pediatric setting as it relates to rehabilitation of the physically handicapped child. Let us go back down the road to when I started my professional career as a new therapist, full of enthusiasm and idealism about curing the ills of children. As would be expected, I felt that I had some competence and professionalism, but had no idea that, in reality, I was on the apedal level of development. Many events, problems, and frustrations have occurred over these many years to bring me to the bipedal level of development. It should not be necessary to say that, even at my age, I still have some dendritic, collateral growth left in my nervous system to continue to learn and to change according to the dictates of health care with these children. Similarly, our profession still can learn and change.

In the 1950s, when I started my career, the rehabilitative movement was predominant. As stated by Anne Mosey "During the period of 1942 to 1960, perhaps the most significant event influencing occupational therapy was the growth of the rehabilitation movement."[5] She considered the major catalyst for this growth to be the number of returning disabled World War II veterans and the failures of established institutions, the family, school, and organized medicine, to meet their needs. Together with other professional groups, occupational therapy jumped on the bandwagon first and then decided what our role would be in this rehabilitation process. We borrowed, begged, and maybe stole to supplement our armamentarium. The main therapeutic measures in the area of adult physical disabilities were activities of daily living (ADL) training, prosthetic and orthotic expertise, maybe some vocational training along with muscle strengthening and range of motion exercises accomplished mainly through the use of crafts. The latter were also used for diversional and "busy work" activities. These same treatment goals and these same craft modalities were used for children. In many instances, occupational therapy sessions were, in reality, all diversional in nature.

As an unsuspecting therapist starting her career, I had to apply these goals, methods, and modalities to all types of physical disabilities. If you will recall, I said that the therapist at this level of development does not have the expertise to generalize from her academic and brief clinical experiences. Therefore, can she really know what she is doing? Can she know where she is going? Can she know who she is, especially when she realizes that no one knows what occupational therapy is? What she hears is the label of "busy work" or "play ladies." On occasion we received a direct referral for ADL training, or to improve hand-eye coordination, or some type of order to supplement physical therapy in strengthening the upper extremities. Less frequently but more appropriately, we received referrals for upper extremity prosthetic training.

Can you remember when you received a referral requesting ADL training for a severe quadriplegic cerebral-palsied child? How successful were we? We know now that the abnormal patterns laid down during maturation of the CNS are the only patterns that can be elicited, especially on voluntary movement. Sensory input is abnormal; integration is abnormal; motor output is abnormal; sensory feedback into the CNS is abnormal. The child is still dominated by primitive reflexes and/or abnormal tone and he can move only in these stereotyped patterns. In the realm of emotional and psychosocial areas of behavior, we were seeing adverse reactions because of the child's frustration at his inability to succeed. He knew cognitively what he wanted to do, but could not work out the concept, the process of the task. Under these circumstances, what tools did we have to determine how to cope with this problem? "None." Where did we go for assistance? "Nowhere." The only conclusion was frustration! Frustration, not only for the therapist, but also for the child and his parents who were expected to carry out the therapist's directives.

At this time, in the fifties, therapeutic media and goals of treatment could be equated to the apedal level of development. I said previously that the infant is born with tremendous potential for development and learning, and that how he is stimulated and handled will determine the realization of this potential.

What is the quality of this stimulus when crafts are the only treatment modality? What is the meaningful experience to the child? Will it have a profound effect on his future development? Crafts were and are nonmeaningful to a child's function. There was and is no scientific basis underlying their use.[6] In addition, and perhaps even more damaging, the visual image created by these crafts as a treatment modality, and the inability of the therapist, many times, to give a convincing rationale for their underlying value, other than diversional, certainly was not and is not worth the cost to the professionalism of occupational therapy.

It was at this point that I "jumped" into my second stage of development, the quadrupedal level. My experience had not been a meaningful one. I had explored, tried to create, problem-solved; but sensory deprivation was setting in. It was necessary for me to mobilize if I was to provide quality treatment. Also, it was necessary for me to mobilize so that the role of occupational therapy could be accepted as a professional service to the rehabilitation of children.

Self-analysis was important at this point. I asked myself, "Who am I?" "What am I doing?" "Where am I going?"

Who am I? A qualified registered therapist with a certain body of knowledge and experience. What am I doing? Attempting to use this body of knowledge and experience to rehabilitate handicapped children in all areas of behavior to the best of my ability. Where am I going? I didn't know! Frustration and failure in accomplishing the goals of treatment pertinent to the needs of the children were obvious. Added to this frustration was an awareness of the lack of knowledge and acceptance of the profession as a necessary adjunct in the rehabilitation process.

As a consequence, it was imperative that I make a change or forego the pleasure of being an occupational therapist. The choice was clear. To make a change and mobilize into the next higher level of my development, it was necessary to deviate from the established protocol; change the working definition of occupational therapy; change the concept of occupational therapy; and, of utmost importance, alter the modalities.

One definition of the word "change" is to alter, implying the making of some partial change, as in appearance, but usually preserving the identity. Change was necessary to establish the professionalism of occupational therapy. Gross states, "As any occupation approaches professional status, there occur important internal structural changes and changes in the relation of the practitioners to society at large. A useful way of discussing these changes is by reference to the criteria of professionalization; the unstandardized product, degree of personality involvement of the professional, wide knowledge of a specialized technique, sense of obligation (to one's art), sense of group identity, and significance of the occupational service to society."[7]

Herein lies a basic professional concept for occupational therapy. If change is to occur within the organization to meet the standards of professionalism, the primary alteration must be made in the basic formation of a conceptual framework from which an individual can synthesize and then expand his knowledge. Explicit criteria that set standards of performance emanating from this basic conceptual model must be met. In this way a continuous spiral of behavior can be produced to meet and maintain these standards of ethics, group identity, personal obligation, and quality of service. In my estimation, many of these criteria were not manifested in an acceptable manner for recognition. Therefore, change had to come about secure in the knowledge that the identity must remain, that the personal characteristics of the professional must not be lost.

The next decision was to determine how to bring about this change in therapeutic modalities and goals of treatment. Therefore, I asked myself the questions, "What is important in this child's life? What does he need in his process of development to make him a functioning individual capable of coping with the problems of his environment?" Having made this decision, I then attempted to reach the professional stature of an accepted, scientifically based profession.

In his developmental process, important facets in any child's life are gross and fine motor skills, perception, and specific developmental stimulation. These are the concerns of occupational therapy. The therapist attempts to bring the child up to, or close to, his age level, with a thorough understanding of his emotional and social development.

How is he to gain these skills? I felt that the only way was to treat the problem directly and not through a diversional activity such as leather lacing, or weaving. The body of knowledge and expertise the occupational therapist has at her command are far too important in preparing a child to cope with his environment to be relegated to the realm of relaxation with craft activities. This is a basic concept that I feel is essential if we are to be considered a professional discipline.

The first step in the process of my development from apedal to quadrupedal integration went from "realization to activation" of the problems revolving around the needs of the children. The second step was to determine methods to give a child these skills. Through the process of integration of learning, higher levels were attained and I was closer to the bipedal level of development.

In the process of establishing the bipedal level, or the cognitive level of the adult, it was necessary to synthesize all the learning of the two previous levels; therefore, extended exploration into the tools and methods of treatment to professionalize the role of occupational therapy was carried out. This meant standardized evaluations, as much as possible; media which were meaningful to the needs of the child; technical expertise with a knowledgeable background; and, last but not least, the courage of my convictions to carry through these changes in spite of criticism by my peers.

In the areas of gross and fine motor development, we cannot accept, as a goal of treatment, functional use of the hands without first attaining stability of everything to which the hand is attached. Development is cephalo-caudal, proximal-distal, medial-lateral, gross to fine. This is how treatment should progress if we are to give children their maximal functional potential. Also, we should place our emphasis on normal, developmental sequences of CNS development; for example, learning on a subcortical basis, followed by cortical, voluntary learning, finally reaching the stage of spontaneous, automatic movements.

To reach this process in a meaningful manner, it was necessary to change to techniques of treatment that revolved around the sequential maturation of the CNS and that also emphasized the normal growth and development of the child. To give meaning to the use of these techniques and to provide the secure knowledge and competency to justify these techniques, it was necessary to learn the basic concepts of neurophysiology which were believed to underlie these methods of treatment. In this way I knew that I was not working in a vacuum; I knew that I could confront any physician and justify the "means to an end." This was not a simple task. I was told at one time that it would take 20 years to nurture and develop the "germ" of an idea, and it has taken that long.

Based upon this process of developmental learning, children, such as the cerebral palsied or others with a neuromuscular dysfunction, have benefitted from this treatment to a much greater extent than ever previously attained. Significant changes have been noted in their abilities, resulting in improved function. Many times when basic gross motor movements and then higher motor development have been attained, the child has sufficient fine motor control to begin voluntarily to function by feeding himself, removing his socks and shoes, or playing with toys. At this point, *he* is beginning to manipulate his environment, rather than allowing the environment to manipulate him.

In the process of attaining a goal of treatment, such as feeding, we cannot look at just the skilled act and feel that this is where the role of the occupational therapist begins. We know that the child cannot feed himself if he does not have at least some measure of head, trunk, and arm control. We know also that if the asymmetrical tonic neck or symmetrical tonic neck reflexes are dominating his nervous system with resulting interference of higher motor skills, he cannot perform this skilled act.

The inhibition and/or facilitation of these preparatory mechanisms are a part of the total functional skill. We, as occupational therapists, must have the knowledge, skill, confidence, and security *to treat the total child*. Why should we expect the physical therapist to "prepare" the child and then the occupational therapist merely to teach the child a given skill? First of all, we might find ourselves out of a job; with basic stability the child might function spontaneously. Second, the concept of upper extremities for the occupational therapist and lower extremities for the physical therapist is outdated. You cannot divide the child into parts, especially if you treat developmentally. It is more than the sum of all the parts which leads to the total normal organism; it is the integration of the parts. Therefore, let us break down our defenses and integrate our efforts, making the child our focus, and not permit personal prejudices and preconceived ideas to interfere with what we are all interested in: "The Child."

Two other major areas of treatment for the occupational therapist in pediatric rehabilitation should be: (1) Enhancing perceptual-motor and visual-motor integration; and (2) stimulating children who have lags in their growth and development. I will not proceed through the same process of paralleling development from apedal to bipedal, or from realization to activation, since both were similar to the development of the motor program. Suffice it to say that both of these programs are important in total functioning of any child. They must be included in any pediatric program.

Other rehabilitative goals specific to varying diagnoses are indicated in the area of pediatric-physical disabilities; however, the therapist must decide what is most important in meeting the goals set for her patients. The therapist must have the security and confidence to substantiate these goals and the competence in the methods used to reach them. It is not possible to be all things to all people. For this reason it may be necessary to select fewer major goals of treatment rather than attempting to encompass the gamut of defined goals of occupational therapy.

In the judgment of this writer, the occupational therapist in a pediatric setting should utilize her expertise for the development of the child in all areas of behavior. Hopefully, this should lead to an integrated functioning individual capable of reaching his maximum potential. Let us remember that a handicapped child is a child first, and then is a child with a handicap.

I should like to read a few statements from an article published in *Scientific American*. "It is obvious that the organism with fully developed and integrated sensory and motor capacities is better prepared to deal with its environment than is one who is lacking in development of these abilities. Beyond the coordination of input and output, however, additional skills are necessary for the higher organism to be successful in its world." The author continues, "The basic concepts of action and reaction, cause and effect, behavior and its consequences—which must be acquired through experience with the environment—are the building blocks upon which the organism's continuing understanding of his world will depend."[8]

Once we have gained the depth of knowledge necessary to substantiate with confidence our definition of occupational therapy and the role of the occupational therapist, and once we have decided and identified the means through which we can give our services as a professional service, then and only then will we be able to say that we have reached the highest level of development. Occupational therapy has undergone the same process of learning and development as the young child; but it has not reached its fullest potential. Cognitively we realize this; but we need to activate the realizations to meet the changing world of medicine, the controls of government, the demands of professionalism, and the obligations of competency *if we are to survive.*

In summary, the process of the growth and development of occupational therapy and the occupational therapist was compared to the growth and development of the infant from apedal to bipedal levels. A similar comparison was made of the methods of treatment and the modalities used to reach the highest level of development. Neurological maturation and integration must occur in the infant if he is to reach his highest level of development and to be able to function in his environment. Similar sequential maturation must occur from the student level to that of the skilled therapist if he or she is to become a competent professional. An overview of the course of occupational therapy revealed the necessity to mobilize from "realization to activation" so that the role of occupational therapy can be accepted as a professional adjunct in the rehabilitation of the child.

Acknowledgments

The author wishes to express appreciation for the contributions and assistance given by Constance Harasymiw, OTR, and Karen Stonesifer, MS, OTR, of my staff; Patrick J. Fazzari, MD, Josephine Moore, PhD, Ann Grady, OTR, Elnora Gilfoyle, OTR, Paula Habecker, OTR; and my mother and sister.

References

1. Llorens, LA: Facilitating growth and development: The promise of occupational therapy. The Eleanor Clarke Slagle Lectures. Dubuque, Kendall/Hunt Pub. Co., 1973, p 192
2. Johnson, JA: Occupational therapy: A model for the future. The Eleanor Clarke Slagle Lectures. Dubuque, Kendall/Hunt Pub. Co., 1973, p 229
3. Moore, JC: Neuroanatomy Simplified. Dubuque, Kendall/Hunt Pub. Co., 1969, pp 89–95
4. Kaluger, G., Kolson, CJ: Reading and Learning Disabilities. Columbus, Chas. E. Merrill Pub. Co., 1969, pp 29–30
5. Mosey, AC: Occupational therapy—A historical perspective: Involvement in the rehabilitation movement—1942–1960. Am J Occup Ther 25: 234–236, 1971
6. Moore, JC: Are we halfbreeds? (Editorial) Am J Occup Ther 17: 200, 1963
7. Gross, E: Professionalization. Englewood, Prentice-Hall, Inc., 1906, p 9
8. "The Nature and Nurture of Behavior." Readings from *Scientific American*. San Francisco, W. H. Freeman and Co., 1972, p 83

24

1975 Eleanor Clarke Slagle Lecture

Behavior, Bias, and the Limbic System

Josephine C. Moore, OTR, PhD

Human and animal behavior has always fascinated me. In my early years, Freud, Adler, Jung, Erickson, and others seemed to suggest the most plausible basis for understanding human behavior. However, during the 1930s and 1940s, scientific disciplines began to study behavior from a different perspective. Biochemistry, endocrinology, and neurophysiology studied behavior in relation to biochemical individuality, the function of enzyme deficiencies, and genetic defects and stimulation studies of the brain. In psychology, a number of individuals broke away from the Freudian school of thought in order to investigate behavior in relation to group interaction and environmental manipulation. Studies were extended into such areas as architectural design, color phenomena, crowding of populations, the effects of sensory deprivation, and other areas too numerous to mention. A number of neuroanatomists began to take a renewed interest in the organism they were studying, especially in regard to the functional implications of various systems, instead of just their structural and mechanical aspects. Paralleling this upsurge of interest in behavior, another group decided to study animals in an entirely new light. These scientists, who called themselves ethologists, realized that animals living in their own environment behaved quite differently from animals confined to a laboratory or an enclosed area. Therefore, the ethologists went out into the field in order to study animals in their natural habitat. By the 1960s a great deal of new and fascinating information had been accumulated from all of these different scientific disciplines concerning animal behavior. Because of my interest in this area, I began to look at man's nervous system, and especially the limbic system, in an entirely new way. Animal research seemed to provide a great deal of insight into the complexities of the limbic system in relation to man's behavioral mechanisms. Where is the limbic system in the brain, and what are the principal functions of this area?

The Location of the Limbic System

Picture a target with a gray bull's eye and several alternating white and gray bands surrounding the central area (Figure 24.1). The gray areas represent the location of specific groups of nerve cell bodies. The white areas represent the fiber connections between these gray areas. In actual numbers, the target has only three gray areas with two white ones interposed. The first gray area, or the bull's eye, represents the diencephalon or the thalamus, the next gray area represents the basal ganglia, while the outermost area represents the cerebral cortex. These concentric circles graphically depict the basic pattern of the gray and white matter of the brain. The lower parts of the nervous system—that is, the brain stem, cerebellum, and the spinal cord—have been removed in order to use this target concept to understand the structural and functional aspects of the brain in relation to the limbic system.

Originally published 1976 in *American Journal of Occupational Therapy, 30,* 11–19.

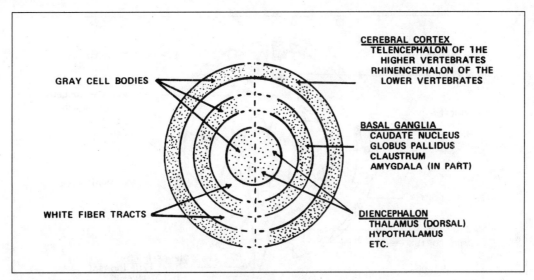

Figure 24.1. Target concept of the brain (brain stem removed).

Returning again to the target concept, the bull's eye represents some of the oldest evolutionary areas of the brain. The intermediate gray band represents the younger structures, while the most recent phylogenetically evolved area is located on the periphery. The same sequential pattern, from central to peripheral, also illustrates the functional hierarchy of the brain. As the newer and more peripheral structures develop, there is a tendency for these areas to control and regulate, to some extent, the older centers. Yet, due to the numerous white fiber tracts interconnecting all of these centers, the entire nervous system functions as a total unit.

The target illustration also aids in understanding the names of each of these gray areas. As previously mentioned, the central gray area is called the diencephalon or the thalamus. Diencephalon means "through brain." This implies that almost all of the information received by one's senses, from any part of the body, must pass through this area. The diencephalon integrates and modifies this information before relaying it to surrounding structures. In addition, numerous components of the motor pathways of the nervous system are influenced by this area. Last, but not least, is the fact that part of this area is the master controller of the endocrine system and the autonomic nervous system. Thus the term diencephalon identifies some of the basic functions of this central gray area. But how about the other term, the thalamus? This word means a "bridal chamber." Perhaps the forefathers of anatomy chuckled when they applied this term to this centrally located part of the brain. After all, this area is hidden away in a rather secluded and relatively safe location. Maybe these anatomists were also thinking about the synapses that occur here, and the importance of this center in relation to homeostatic mechanisms in the preservation of the species. Nevertheless, the term thalamus is a rather apt word for remembering the location of this area.

The next gray circle surrounding the thalamus is known as the basal ganglia. During early development of the brain, the ganglion, meaning a mass of gray cell bodies, was located at the base of the brain, hence the term basal ganglia. As the brain matured these cells divided into several distinctive groups and migrated upward in a circular fashion to partially surround the diencephalon (Figure 24.2). The basal banglia were destined to become regulatory centers for many stereotyped reflexes, for sensorimotor functions, for some aspects of visceral behavior, and for a multitude of other functions too numerous to mention.

The outer layer of gray matter represents the cerebral cortex or the bark of the brain. However, if one examines the brain of many of the lower vertebrates, having only a minimal amount of cortex, this outer gray ring represents the rhinencephalon or smell brain (Figure 24.1). The rhinencephalon is the oldest part of the cerebral cortex. As the higher vertebrates developed, this older cortical area was displaced medially and was

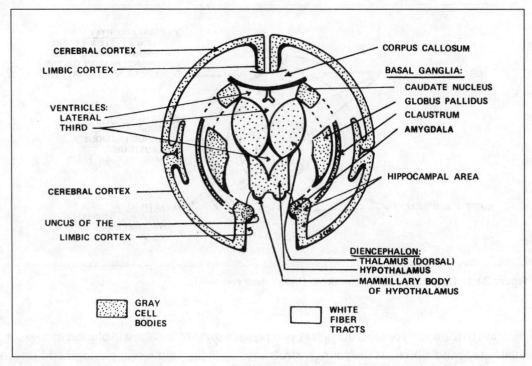

Figure 24.2. Modified target concept showing white and gray areas comprising the major structures of the brain.

eventually buried in a deeper location as additional cortex was added (Figure 24.2). In man, the exposed surface of the brain is still called the cerebral cortex, but the rhinencephalic cortex, which lies hidden from view, is now called the limbic cortex (Figure 24.2). What is the reason for this change in terminology? It is because this area of man's cortex is no longer concerned only with the sense of smell and survival mechanisms. As can be seen later, many other functions were incorporated into this area. However, the word *limbic* is a descriptive term, meaning border or the outside edge of a structure. If one examines the medial view of the human brain, the limbic cortex forms an almost complete ring or border of gray matter around all of the deeper structures of the brain (Figure 24.3).

This target concept is acceptable for understanding the very basic structural relationships of the brain, but it is limited when discussing different systems of the brain. What is a system in comparison to a structure? The easiest way to explain this is to compare the word nerve or neuron with the term nervous system. A nerve is a structural entity consisting of a neuronal cell body and all of the processes, whereas the term nervous system refers to all of the neurons and their processes, which function as a total unit and make up the entire nervous system. In other words, the term system denotes numerous components incorporated into one functional unit. In the same way the limbic lobe or limbic cortex is a limited structural area, while the limbic system comprises parts of the old and new cerebral cortex, as well as parts of the basal ganglia, thalamus, midbrain, reticular formation, autonomic nervous system, and on and on. It is not my intention to list in detail all of the structural and functional components of this system as volumes have been written on this subject. Rather, it is more important to understand a few concepts about this system. The *first concept* is that the limbic system ties together or integrates the newest cortical or cognitive centers of the brain with the older sensorimotor systems and the primitive visceral and reticular structures of the nervous system (1–5). The *second concept* is that several of the major structures which comprise man's limbic system evolved from the rhinencephalic cortex or the small brain of lower vertebrates (5–8).

In lower animals the small brain is the most prominent structure of the entire nervous system. In these animals it is regarded as the area which is primarily responsible for controlling and regulating instinctual drives and survival mechanisms. As the brain of the higher vertebrates evolved, the smell brain diminished in size in comparison to the newer evolutionary structures. However, the function of this area remains as a primary means of survival for the animal kingdom. For example, the sense of smell is necessary for hunting, for locating sources of food and water, and for tracking down distant prey. It is also used to recognize members of one's own group as opposed to those of the same species belonging to another group. It is important for knowing the boundaries of one's territory, finding a den or shelter after a hunt, or for following others during migration. And naturally, smell is one of the primary senses used for procreation of the species. Smell also enables the animal to react defensively or offensively when threatened because this primitive cortical area has a direct influence upon the animal's autonomic nervous system. Thus many of the behavioral instincts of the lower and higher vertebrates are incorporated into this area of the brain.[5,6,7,8] Even though man's limbic system is much more complex than the animals', man still retains many of the behavioral instincts of the other forms of animal life (5–10). One of nature's basic laws is to retain and enhance behavioral traits which have proved to be effective survival mechanisms, especially those which have assured the preservation of the species. Therefore, the basic functions of man's limbic system are similar, with some exceptions, to that of the higher vertebrates. Let us look at these functions and identify their relationship to behavioral mechanisms.

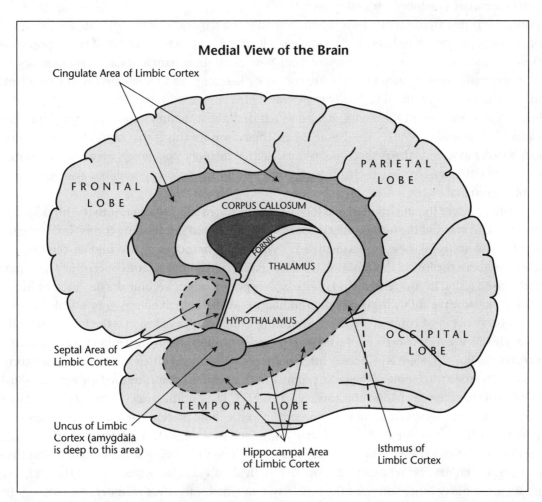

Figure 24.3. Major structures comprising the limbic cortex (brain stem and cerebellum removed).

Limbic System Functions

Perhaps the simplest way to understand the functions of the limbic system is to use the mnemonic word "M-O-V-E." The limbic system is believed to "move" or drive us so that we can survive as individuals and as a species.

M . . . of the word "move" stands for **m**emory.
O . . . stands for **o**lfaction or the sense of smell.
V . . . refers to **v**isceral or autonomic nervous system functions.
E . . . represents the **e**motional components of behavior.

First, let us look at the limbic system in relation to memory. Part of the limbic system appears to be involved with the organism's ability to have instinctual or genetic memory, as well as short and long-term memory. This does not imply that all memory is confined to the limbic system. Rather, parts of this system appear to contain vital centers through which information must be processed or retrieved in order that the entire nervous system can utilize memory for survival (1–3, 6, 7).

For example, in the medial aspect of the temporal lobe there is an area, known as the hippocampal formation, which is involved in one's ability to have new memory (1, 3, 11) (Figure 24.3). Two theories have been proposed concerning how this area functions in learning. One theory is that new information has to be processed through this center before it can be retained as memory. The other theory is that this area helps provide recall of memory, that is, this area is part of a memory retrieval system.

If this structure is destroyed on one side, the individual has a temporary loss of the ability to remember new information. Usually the person recovers and is capable of learning new facts. However, if the opposite side is subsequently lost, the individual is unable to learn anything new. Both short-term and long-term memory are permanently lost. Emotional memory, such as swearing, crying, or laughing, and basic defensive mechanisms usually remain and may, in fact, be enhanced or greatly exaggerated (1, 11).

A similar lesion at the base of the diencephalon, which destroys structures known as the mammillary bodies, may also cause this same syndrome (1, 11) (Figure 24.2). The reason for this is that both of these centers are relay stations along a major route or pathway that is necessary for either memory storage or retrieval of information. Therefore, destruction of either area interrupts circuitry, not only within the limbic system, but also between it and the newer areas of the cerebral cortex.

There is another area of the medial temporal lobe which is located slightly anterior to the hippocampal formation (Figure 24.3). This area and the surrounding tissue (the amygdala and surrounding cortex) can be destroyed unilaterally due to CVA (cerebral vascular accident) involving small branches of the middle cerebral artery. The interesting feature about the loss of this area is that no real predictions can be made concerning the behavior of an individual who has a lesion in this center (1, 11, 12, 13). One person might become docile. Another may be overly aggressive. Some may lose the ability to visually discriminate between different objects or be unable to recognize any object at all. Probably the most common syndrome resulting from the type of lesion is the loss of the ability to recognize people. There are several reasons for the behavioral variations seen following this kind of brain damage. One is that this area of the limbic system is intricately interconnected with several different cortical and subcortical structures which are concerned with some of the more primitive behavioral mechanisms used for survival—such as fear, anger and submissiveness, and visual and olfactory recognition (1, 11). Another reason depends upon the exact location of the lesion, such as a relatively small lesion occurring in the more posterior and lateral structures of this center, as opposed to a larger lesion encompassing many adjacent structures (1, 3, 11). The third reason concerns individual differences, such as one's basic inherited personality, one's biochemical individuality, and the environmental influences which have been impressed upon each individual's nervous system (1, 3, 11, 13, 14, 15).

Though there are many other lesions of the limbic system which can affect memory, perhaps the most interesting one is Korsakoff's syndrome (1, 11). This syndrome can occur in chronic alcoholics, but it may also result from tumors of the 3rd ventricle or from CVAs (cerebral vascular accidents) in this area (Figure 24.2). Actually, several areas of the limbic system can be involved in this syndrome, especially if this results from long-term degenerative changes. However, the most common site is in the medial part of the thalamus. Following a loss of this area, these individuals are unable to retain new information, and may not be able to give a true history of past events. And even though suffering severe intellectual impairment, these people may retain the ability to spin fascinating tales which may be emotionally charged and thus extremely convincing to the listener. However, within a relatively short time these individuals are unable to repeat the story and begin making up new tales.

The olfactory system is next. Though this sense is more important for survival of quadrupeds, it continues to play an important, though not well-defined, role in modern man. The olfactory system has direct pathways into the limbic system and has numerous indirect connections with the hypothalamic centers, which control the autonomic nervous system and the endocrine system (Figures 24.2 and 24.3). It is also connected with the reticular formation, which functions as a mechanism for alerting the entire cerebral cortex (1, 2, 3, 11). One can understand why the smell of a sizzling steak or the scent of a freshly baked pie can cause saliva and digestive juices to be secreted and make a person feel hungry. Certain smells can also trigger off emotionally charged memories which may be accompanied by visceral responses such as an increase or decrease in heart rate, respiration, sweating, or dilation of the pupils. For example, the odor of burning pine logs may remind one of pleasurable events surrounding a wonderful camping trip. This person may become relaxed and drift into a dreamy state recalling past memories. Another individual might be aroused because the pine odor reminds him of a fire which destroyed a home. Thus, odor can be an effective stimulus for bringing back rather specific memories, alerting individuals, or calming them down. It can also be used to stimulate digestion and enhance taste sensations. The reason is that the sense of taste and smell and their central connections in the nervous system are intricately associated with one another as well as with the limbic and autonomic nervous system.

Certain smells also play a very important role in man's sexuality. Many of these odors are believed to be more effective as stimulants if they are perceived on a subcortical or limbic level rather than at the level of cortical awareness. It is no wonder that the perfume and soap industries of the world have made billions of dollars a year catering to these behavioral mechanisms.

Lesions of the olfactory bulb and tract are not very common in man. When they do occur, especially if only one side is involved, they may not be noticed by the individual. However, there is one interesting area on the medial part of the anterior temporal lobe, called the uncus, which can be involved in irritative lesions and does present some rather specific symptoms having to do with olfaction (Figures 24.2 and 24.3). This area of the limbic system helps to integrate olfactory and visual sensations with emotional memories. A tumor or irritative lesion in this area can cause an individual to smell putrid odors which are not present in the atmosphere. This sensation may be accompanied by visual hallucinations associated with the unpleasant smell. As the lesion spreads, the person may have a focal seizure or "uncinate fit" following the sensation of the odor. Fortunately, this type of seizure tends to remain localized within the limbic system—it does not spread to the cerebral cortex. Thus the person usually remains conscious, even though he may not be aware of the seizure per se (1, 3, 11).

The next major limbic system function concerns the visceral components of behavior. It is now known that everything we do, that is, all behavior, is colored by concurrent changes taking place within our autonomic or visceral nervous system. This in turn modifies all future behavior. Thus the limbic system is believed to help integrate and coordinate visceral responses with cognitive, emotional, and sensorimotor behavior. In this way, the normal system maintains a homeostatic balance in favor of pleasurable rewards and away from painful or nonrewarding stimuli (3 5, 7 9).

However, there are occasions when this homeostatic balance goes astray. This is usually the result of excessive physical or emotional stress which is put upon a nervous system, which is unable to cope with these stresses (13, 16, 17). The resultant behavioral patterns which develop are many and varied and depend upon multiple factors. But usually the limbic system reacts with the most basic survival instinct known to mankind and this is fear (4, 5, 9, 13,

18–21). Once this behavioral mechanism is aroused, the entire nervous system is alerted, especially those areas of the autonomic nervous system which control our fight or flight response. If this arousal mechanism is allowed to continue for a long period of time, it may begin to dominate the other systems of the body. Homeostasis is lost, and eventually the entire nervous system can exhaust itself. Man has been trying to cope with this problem for ages. He has used a variety of methods to treat this syndrome, such as witchcraft, prefrontal lobotomies, electroshock and insulin therapy, psychotherapy, and more recently, drug therapy and biofeedback training. Unfortunately, no one method has been successful, or probably ever will be, for all individuals concerned. This is because of man's individual genetic and biochemical differences as well as his multiple and highly variable relationships with his environment (9, 13–15).

In the final analysis, no two nervous systems function alike, and this is especially true in regard to each individual's limbic system. Not only have each of us inherited our behavioral traits from different genetic pools, but no two of us have experienced the same environmental stresses. Because of this we have learned to cope differently. Therefore, the behavioral mechanisms of each person are biased by one's individual emotional needs, in spite of the fact that all humans share certain basic limbic drives (4, 9, 10, 12–17).

This brings us to **E** of the word M-O-V-E, or our emotional tone or drives. These drives have long been referred to as the "3 Fs," that is, the feeding, fighting, and reproductive drives. Many believe today that these three basic drives are genetically endowed—that is, they are inherited (6–9, 16).

Probably the most important of all of the limbic system mechanisms, if one can rank any facet of survival as more important than any other, is found under **E**, the emotional drive. This is the feeding drive. Actually, this drive for sustenance consists of two very fundamental and slightly different components. The first and most important is simply called love or TLC (tender loving care). The second component is food. Food, of course, is rather vital for survival but it appears to be less necessary than the need for love (9).

In lower animal terminology, love is defined somewhat differently than for man. Basically, however, it consists of the same principal components, such as the need to be touched and fondled, to be communicated with and accepted. It now appears that the genetic drive for TLC must be fulfilled, to some unknown degree, in order to assure survival. Also, TLC is believed to be the primary drive of gregarious animals. It is not believed to be directly linked to the productive drive per se. Rather, reproduction results only if this first drive is adequately fulfilled (5, 7, 9).

Research is also showing that this drive "to love and to be loved," to belong, to be accepted, may be the very foundation upon which many higher animals, including man, strive "to be"; upon which some of their territoriality may be based; and upon which survival of normal individuals is assured or lost. Indeed, this drive may be the very reason for standards, laws or codes of behavior, and biases which are found within and among the societies of all gregarious creatures. This drive for love, if adequately met, assures survival of the individual, the family, and the society (4, 5, 7, 9, 16, 18–21).

Thus the limbic system appears to be the seat of our ability to have memory, emotions, genetic drives, and pre-endowed standards of behavior. Just as important, of course, is the fact that this system is strongly influenced by the environment. Interaction with the environment continually shapes, modifies and biases our memory, behavior, and emotional tone in relation to everything we do at any given moment.

This continual modification or change of one's behavioral mechanism is not just the result of learned behavior. A great deal of it is probably due to the fact that much of the sensory information received from the environment is handled or taken care of by the nervous system at a subliminal or subcortical level (3, 9, 22). In fact, much of our early learning is believed to be primarily subcortical, that is, we do not have to think about our basic actions and reactions. The nervous system functions adequately for us on the lower emotional, autonomic, and sensorimotor reflexive levels of behavior. In fact, memory circuits are formed in these lower centers long before cortical control is fully developed and integrated into the limbic and subcortical centers (1–3). Likewise, since man is an emotional animal, he continues to function on this level throughout life, especially when he encounters either positively or negatively charged situations, such as love or fear. Man's nervous system is also genetically endowed or biased to gravitate toward rewards and away from that which is threatening. Likewise, as the nervous system matures, man, and the animal, quickly learns to reinforce or bias his drives toward pleasurable events, especially if he has received a normal amount of sensory stimuli from the environmental surroundings (3, 16, 22).

This biasing or reinforcement of the behavioral drives may be accomplished primarily at the limbic or emotional level of the nervous system. One of the most fascinating features of the limbic system is the complexity of the fiber connections of this area, not only with adjacent structures but within the confines of the system itself. It has long been known that electrical stimulation of the limbic system causes long-lasting after discharges—that is, a single stimulus can cause this system to continue to reverberate for a relatively long period of time after removal of the stimulus (11). This is not surprising if one examines the intricate connections of this system. In comparison to other areas of the nervous system, this center has a multitude of pathways which are circular in nature, that is, they feed back to themselves. Many of these are also reciprocal. Thus stimulation of any one area not only feeds to other areas of this system, but in turn these feed back both directly and indirectly into the same area which was initially stimulated. It has taken anatomists years to unravel the complexities of this reverberating circuitry, and even today many of these are not completely understood. In spite of this, man has experienced the reverberating nature of this system and has unknowingly used this circuitry for emotional learning. For example, following a stressful situation, these reverberating circuits may cause the entire episode, or particular aspects of the event, to keep coming back into the mind, over and over again. The event will continue to reverberate until it is resolved or forgotten. Likewise, a few notes of a song may be heard, and throughout the day the entire tune keeps repeating itself in one's mind. Undoubtedly the reverberating nature of this system is what enables the brain to learn, and store, emotionally charged memories much more rapidly and usually more permanently than nonemotional memory. This is also believed to be one of the reasons why emotional language, such as swearing, singing, crying, and laughing, is usually preserved when a cerebral vascular accident destroys either our cortical language center or its pathways within the nervous system.

Man and the Animal

We have discussed man and the animal in relation to the limbic system and behavioral mechanisms. Man, of course, is rather different from other species. Therefore, is it fair to compare him with animals, especially since he is endowed with a generous amount of cerebral cortex and has the most complex nervous system known to mankind? After all, doesn't man need to use all of this gray matter for learning erudite things he believes he must know in order to interact with and survive in this modern world? Yes, in some respects this makes man different. He is also different in that he seems to have lost some of the ability to function at a limbic or emotional level, that is he appears to use his intellectual pursuits to override his own needs as well as the needs of others. Could it be that man has not lost his emotional tone or ability to relate to others, but instead he is fearful of developing some kind of oral or anal complex? Perhaps he has also brainwashed himself into believing that he will be dominated by his reproductive or sex drives instead of his primary drive for love. It is my belief that man could eliminate some of his biases and fears by studying the animal, not just intellectually, but also on an emotional or on a limbic level. If he did this, he might begin to see why he behaves as he does, almost instinctively, to various situations he encounters in life. He might even learn more effective, and perhaps simpler and more direct, ways of coping with life without fearing himself or his fellow man.

It is interesting to note that man has associated himself with the animal long before the dawn of history. He has shared his home, affection, and some of his livelihood with four-footed creatures, such as the canines and the felines, down through the ages. These animals were not always used as beasts of burden, sources of food or for protection. Rather the animal as a pet probably enabled man to relate on a limbic level to a creature which readily understands and accepts him for what he is. The animal usually offers unlimited affection in return for a friendly word, a morsel of food, and perhaps some shelter. This enables man to unleash his intellectual drive and express his primary emotional need for love and understanding without the fear of being challenged, dominated, or questioned. Just as important, of course, is the fact that primitive man learned from and understood many of his own behavioral mechanisms and drives from his close association with animals. For example, according to the Indian legend of the Sioux Nation, the wolf was considered as a brother and a teacher. The Indian and the wolf lived together in harmony, sharing the same territory. It is said that they did not fear one another and even helped each other survive, especially if one were wounded, trapped, or lost. Modern man, on the contrary, somehow drifted away from having respect for and a mutual understanding of his four-footed friends. He came to consider animals as beasts of prey, unlimited sources of food or economic wealth, or as threats to his very existence. It is true that man continued to keep animals as pets, but intellectually he divorced himself from them. He denied that their behavior and drives were in any way related to his basic needs. He became so biased that he even failed to use any of his senses to recognize the similarities between himself and what he called "the lowly creatures." This may have been the time when man began to lose a great deal of his ability to comprehend himself, his environment, and especially the animals which resided in it. Fortunately, in the last several decades, man has begun to reverse his opinions. He is taking a new look at himself and his fellow creatures especially in relation to his surroundings, his evolutionary heritage, individual differences, and emotional drives. Man knows, for example, that he is not the only animal with the capability of learning a language and communicating this to his offspring or to others. He knows that he shares the ability to use tools with many of the higher vertebrates, and that this ability can be taught to others. Likewise, man is not the only beast having emotional needs such as the drive for love, touching, acceptance, communication, and understanding. His reactions are now known to be very similar to that of the animal, especially when this need is threatened or fails to be adequately provided throughout the entire life span of the animal (4, 5, 7, 8). Likewise, man recognizes the need to form bonding pairs, family units, and social groups. He is just beginning to comprehend why he has territorial needs, and how he can cope with this kind of behavioral mechanism. He is understanding why there are and have to be natural laws which regulate societies of gregarious animals, such as rules and standards of conduct which govern the behavior of all of the members and demands that individuals accept certain responsibilities if they wish to survive as individuals, as a family unit, and as a society.

Perhaps, through an indepth study of animal societies, man will gain additional insight and understanding concerning the differences between the emotional needs of the sexes. It is well known that the female and the male are genetically, biologically, and socially different from each other. It is theorized that, because of innate biochemical differences, the limbic or behavioral patterns of male and female are substantially different from one another throughout life (4, 7, 12, 14, 15, 17). Research in many scientific fields indicates that, among gregarious animals including man, the female of the species instinctively looks to the male for protection, security, and leadership (4, 7, 9, 10, 14, 16–21). This facet of behavior has never implied, either biologically, phylogenetically, or ontogenetically that the female is inferior to the male. It does say that she is different and has different needs and drives in relation to the opposite sex. This may explain why long ago the females of the human race recognized the need for and established many of the health care fields such as our own and numerous others, and why they have continued to be a major contributor and energy source behind societies which care for the needs of others. Also, it may explain why many of these "care organizations" have experienced rather turbulent histories trying to gain recognition and equality with fields that were established by and have been dominated by the opposite sex. If the male of the species does not or cannot fully recognize and understand the needs which the female recognizes, then it becomes rather difficult for the female to gain recognition, let alone equality, in those areas in which the male has less interest or limbic drive. Likewise, when intellectual beliefs are impressed upon these basic genetic differences, then it begins to look, especially from a man's point of view, and perhaps eventually the woman's, as if the female is the inferior individual. Is it not more accurate to say that the environment creates a feeling of insecurity, not inferiority, in the female of the species? It is well known that the female is neither inferior nor superior. Rather she is different, just as the male is different. Each sex has different drives in relation to one another. Likewise, each sex looks at and experiences the environment from a different biochemical and genetic perspective. This could be expressed as follows: the male drive is more concerned with the conquest of nature, while the female's is to nurture nature. However, both sexes have the same drive to be nurtured. All of these are of equal importance and are essential in the emotional preservation of the species. Animal societies recognize these differences and accept them for what they are. But the human primate has a tendency to forget or ignore them, because of his need to use his cortical gray matter for intellectual pursuits. Also, humans may be different, in that they have a built-in excuse for not understanding others on an intellectual level. It is theorized that the nervous system may not be capable of cortically comprehending that which it has not personally experienced. By the time the nervous system reaches maturity the intellectual brain is believed to be biased toward that which it can readily understand, and away from that which is different, strange, or unknown. It is no wonder then that man appears to be the only species among the higher vertebrates of the animal kingdom who sometimes fails to comprehend his fellow creatures and seems to spend a great deal of intellectual energy denying his emotional needs and forever defending his own biased views, instead of listening to the needs of others.

Conclusion

In conclusion, it is my biased belief that humans need to understand their emotional or limbic brain before they attempt to comprehend their complex intellectual brain. Humans should pause several times each day during their busy lives to observe, study, and interact with a family of canines, felines, or other gregarious animals so that they can begin to understand themselves. It is only in recent times that man has allowed himself to see the similarities which exist between humans, the higher vertebrates, and the environment. Also I feel that man can learn more from observing the animal, rather than his own complex species, because the animal presents a simplified, non-threatening, and rather rewarding model for comprehending behavioral mechanisms.

Through this avenue of understanding behavior, we might begin to take a second look at some of the comments we hear about our profession. Perhaps one of the most common remarks is that many of our treatment techniques are successful merely because we have the ability to motivate people. The intended implication is that no matter what we do, the individual seems to improve because of the motivation factor. Is this really what is being said? If it is, then the person is admitting that he or she has never listened to us with an unbiased mind. Also, it implies that the individual has failed to read the literature which substantiates many of our treatment techniques. Another implication might be that we, along with many other professions, need additional scientific research to verify some of our techniques. Actually, this remark could mean many things, but in reality the speaker is not listening to what he or she has said. It is a well-known fact that treatment of any kind may fail unless the individual being treated is motivated and has faith in those who are helping him. Thus a person who makes this kind of remark does not realize that he or she is actually giving us one of the highest compliments known to mankind. In effect, the person is defensively saying . . . "How in blazes can you motivate a person to do something when I can't?" Little does the individual know that certain kinds of motivation—or what might be called motivation at a limbic level—are of the utmost importance when working with those who need help. The ultimate expression of all of our limbic drives is the need "to be" . . . to be loved, to be understood, to be wanted and accepted for what we are, or just the need "to be." Unfortunately, this drive is an extremely intangible entity to measure and, of course, man must measure everything he does before he can accept anything as fact. Also, it is rather difficult to measure how quickly this drive "to be" can be lost or shaken when one is confronted with disease, injury, mental illness, loneliness, fear, loss of loved ones, radical changes in life, or any factor which upsets the routine of living. Persons who are not able to perceive the feelings of individuals who have lost some of this drive "to be" may not be able to understand others who have this perceptual ability. This initial lack of insight may also prevent these individuals from being able to comprehend the techniques which we utilize in patient treatment. Because of these factors, our profession and others like us may never win many accolades or be understood and recognized as equals in the health community. However, this should never deter us from utilizing treatment techniques which we feel are appropriate for the individual needs of each person. Above all, we should continue to perfect our perceptual abilities which enable us to relate to others on a limbic level instead of functioning entirely at the level of a biased intellectual.

References

1. Barr, ML: *The Human Nervous System,* second edition, New York, Harper & Row, 1974
2. Eccles JC: *The Understanding of the Brain,* New York, McGraw Hill Book Company, 1973
3. Williams PL, Warwick R: *Functional Neuroanatomy of Man,* Philadelphia, WB Saunders Company, 1975
4. Smythies JR: *Brain Mechanisms and Behavior,* New York, Academic Press, 1966
5. Barnett SA: *Instinct and Intelligence, Behavior of Animals and Man,* New Jersey, Prentice-Hall, Inc., 1967
6. Beritashvili IS (JS Beritoff): *Vertebrate Memory Characteristics and Origin,* New York, Plenum Press, 1971
7. Hinde, RA: *Biological Basis of Human Social Behavior,* New York, McGraw-Hill Book Company, 1974
8. Sarnet HB, Netsky MG: *Evolution of the Nervous System,* New York, Oxford University Press, 1974
9. Harlow HF: *Learning to Love,* New York, Jason Aronson, 1974
10. Goodall JVL: *In the Shadow of Man,* Boston, Houghton Mifflin Company, 1971
11. Willis Jr. WD, Grossman RG: *Medical Neurobiology,* St. Louis, CV Mosby Co, 1973
12. Valenstein ES: *Brain Control,* New York, John Wiley & Sons, 1973
13. Snyder HS: *Madness and the Brain,* New York, McGraw-Hill Book Company, 1974
14. Williams R: *Biochemical Individuality: The Basis for the Genetrotrophic Concept,* Austin, University of Texas Press, 1969
15. Levine S: Sex difference in the brain (April 1966). In *The Nature and Nurture of Behavior.* Readings from *Scientific American,* San Francisco, WH Freeman & Co., 1966
16. Dubos R: *So Human an Animal,* New York, Charles Scribner's Sons, 1968
17. Selye H: *Stress Without Distress,* Philadelphia, JB Lippincott, 1974
18. Lorenz K: *On Aggression,* New York, Harcourt, Brace & World, Inc., 1963
19. Ardrey R: *The Territorial Imperative,* New York, Dell Publishing Company, 1966
20. Mech D: *The Wolf,* New York, Natural History Press, 1970
21. Mowat F: *Never Cry Wolf,* New York, Little, Brown & Company, 1963
22. Moore JC: *Concepts from the Neurobehavioral Sciences,* Dubuque, IA, Kendall/Hunt Publishing Company, 1973

25

Touch With Care or a Caring Touch?

A. Joy Huss, MS, OTR, RPT, FAOTA

For 18 years my career as an occupational therapist has been predicated and developed on the premise that sensory input can influence motor output if used appropriately. As I studied the literature, worked with and observed patients, students, and colleagues, and had been a patient as well, I have come to an additional conclusion—the theme of this presentation. Since effective sensory input includes handling or touching the client, what implications does touch have in our culture, in the framework of occupational therapy, and as individuals? As I informally surveyed colleagues and students, I have been surprised to find that approximately 60 percent indicate that they are personally uncomfortable touching clients. Some have even expressed feelings of fear. Why? Is this necessary? If touching is therapeutic, how can we learn to be comfortable with it? What implications does this have for our educational curricula and for continuing education? Is touching applicable not only in physical dysfunction but also in psychosocial dysfunction? Are touching (handling) with care and a caring touch mutually exclusive or inclusive? Is touch to be used indiscriminately, or are there some possible guidelines? What is the neurophysiological rationale?

Review of the Literature

The neurobiological literature indicates that, first, the skin and the nervous system are derived from the same germ layer, the ectoderm, which provides a critical link between the two. Second, there are basically two major avenues for reception of touch/tactile information (1–3). Various terms have been used to differentiate between the two types of information. In the strict sense, touch is described as the spinothalamic system—protopathic, primitive, or protective—and is carried primarily in the ventral half of the spinal cord. Tactile information is described as the lemniscal system—epicritic, discriminative, or exploratory—and is carried principally in the dorsal half of the spinal cord. The sense of touch is older, whereas the tactile sense is newer phylogenetically and ontogenetically. Both provide us with information regarding the environment, although each may be processed differently and have different effects on higher centers. Until the touch system is integrated within the functioning of the central nervous system, the tactile system apparently cannot function adequately (4). Tactile areas, especially the lips, index finger, and thumb, have the largest cortical representation both sensorially and motorically. Because the nervous system functions holistically, final interactions of the touch/tactile inputs have effects on the autonomic, reticular, and limbic systems, thus having a profound effect on emotional drives. Moore, in the 1975 Slagle Lectureship, spoke of the need for Tender Loving Care (TLC) as a basic primary drive of the limbic system for survival (5). One of the important components of TLC is touch/tactile input.

Originally published 1977 in *American Journal of Occupational Therapy, 31,* 11–18.

Developmentally, touch is one of the first systems to myelinate and thus become functional. The fetus will begin to respond to touch at about eight weeks gestation. In utero, the skin is constantly stimulated by the amniotic fluid and the touch/pressure of the womb. There is tremendous stimulation of this sense during birth. Leboyer has been concerned with providing soothing input to tactual and other systems with his method of *Birth Without Violence* (6). After birth, the baby experiences the environment through touch: by being handled, by clothes, surfaces, objects, and by experiencing himself. It is through this system that the infant gathers information about his body and his external environmental relationships (7). Studies have shown that, without appropriate touch/handling, the infant will not thrive normally even though nourishment and other needs are attended to carefully (8). Does this not speak to the need of the nervous system for meaningful tactual input?

Does this need not stay with us throughout life? Our vocabulary reflects this need with a multitude of references to touch: "keep in touch," "handle with care," "I am touched," "I feel . . . ," "how does it feel?" "it feels like . . . ," and an experience is "touching." We use such expressions as "being tactful," "rubbing someone the wrong way," "we all need certain strokes," someone has a "soft touch," or "human touch," or is "touchy," and we speak of the need for "tangible" evidence. In addition, many adjectives such as rough, smooth, tender, and painful would have no meaning without previous tactual experience.

Frank (9) indicates that, because the tactual system is one of the first functional systems, the infant uses this as a primary mode of communication. As other systems (auditory, visual, and kinesthetic) mature, they gradually supercede the tactual mode, leading eventually to symbolic communication. The individual learns the taboos of tactual experience through satisfaction and conflict so that eventually the child inhibits touching and operates on a symbolic level. This is said to lead to ego development. Frank further states that: "Since living in a symbolic world of ideas and concepts is a most difficult and subtle achievement, denial or deprivation of primary tactile experiences may be revealed as crucial in the development of personalities and character structure, and also in the configuration of a culture."[9] (p. 230)

Initial tactual experiences assist in the development of internal homeostasis. Without internal homeostasis, there will not be an adequate awareness of the external world; thus there arises an inability to shift from tactual dependency to linguistic-symbolic communication. Therefore, with early deprivation we see not only the physical manifestations of speech retardation, learning disabilities, and other gross disturbances, but also emotional and affective problems such as schizophrenia (8, 9).

Tactual contacts begin to diminish at about ages five to six in our culture, with the evasion or denial of touch directed more strongly toward the male. The desire to touch and be touched suddenly increases at puberty, first between members of the same sex and then heterosexually. However, in our adult culture, it is reserved primarily for that most intense of human experiences, the sexual process (8–12). Frank indicates that, in this sexual form of interpersonal communication, the primary mode of tactile communication is reinstated "provided the individuals have not lost the capacity for communication with the self through tactile experiences."[9] (p. 233)

We learn the boundaries for tactual communication culturally. These boundaries vary from culture to culture. Those of Anglo-Saxon origin, especially the English and German, are relatively nontactual. Those of Latin, Russian, Black, Jewish, and primitive cultures are highly tactile peoples. People in the United States are generally considered nontactile (7–16). There are even laws that legislate against touching. Within these cultural groups there will be individual variations that appear to be somewhat dependent on one's experiences within child rearing practices. The need for tactual input is there, however, and may be one explanation for the plethora of pets found in the American culture. Touching and being touched by a pet is acceptable when human touch interaction is denied.

The American culture tends to substitute verbal interaction for body contact with specific distances delineated for various types of communication. Hall has found these verbal interaction distances to be up to 1.5 feet for intimacy; 1.5 to 4 feet for personal subject matter; 4 to 12 feet for nonpersonal, social information; and 12 feet or more for public disclosures (8, 11, 12, 17). It is much easier to talk with an individual or a small group than with a larger one because of the greater distance involved and the smaller amount and kind of feedback received as distance increases.

Goffman (18), however, indicates that middle class Americans are handling one another all the time, if we keep our eyes open to see it. Handling punctuates communication at times when there can only be one meaning received. Thus, the context is all important. It is also involved with status (10, 13). For example, it is all right for an adult to touch a young child and for a doctor to touch a patient (high status to touch low status). However, it is generally not acceptable for the patient to reach for the doctor. A group of therapists recently said to me that it was all right to touch the patient, but it was not all right to touch others. In the psychoanalytical tradition it is even taboo for the doctor to touch the patient.

The fact that touching goes on all around us and is ignored indicates our attitude toward it. We equate tactual contact with sex unless it is perfectly clear there is no connection. Thus we use it sparingly to express warmth, affection, understanding, and acceptance. Contact tends to be perfunctory between individuals of the same sex, between parents and their grown children, and in medicine, including the occupational, physical, and speech therapies. The touch is often mechanical and without feeling for fear of revealing too much of oneself or of being misinterpreted, especially if that contact occurs on any part of the body other than the upper extremities. Unless involved in lovemaking, most of us tend to be disembodied, with our bodies disappearing from our experience. We suffer from "skin hunger" (10, p. 139) as children, as adolescents, and throughout the adult years. Fortunately, child-rearing practices are changing with breast feeding, child backpacks, and the use of cradles on the increase. Rocking chair use by adults is also on the increase, but that form of tactual input, important as it is, is still an impersonal one because it involves only one person. Encounter groups are positive attempts to help us get in touch with our bodies and those of others through various experiential activities.

Perhaps the elderly in our society are deprived the most because of impersonal care in nursing homes and the loss of loved ones. Their distance receptors of vision and hearing decrease in functional capacity; thus limiting experiential capability. These disabilities, compounded by the lack of meaningful touch with others, make their isolation even more acute. The elderly cling to those possessions that can be handled or that evoke memories of lost contact.

A recent, informal survey of 12 individuals in a comprehensive retirement home included the following questions. What is your most valuable possession? Why? The group consisted of eight women and four men; three are still married (two men, one woman), five are widows, two are widowers, and two are single women. Their status includes six in fair to very good health, two who are ambulatory with cardiac problems, three with cataracts, one with emphysema, and three in wheelchairs either because of rheumatoid arthritis, multiple sclerosis, or brain stem, cerebellar involvement.

I found their responses quite revealing. The single women responded with "my health," because it permitted them to do the things they wanted to, which included enjoying their friends. One of the married men also indicated his health. His wife was quite ill and I felt it significant that he did not respond to the question until about two hours later, after he had been to visit his wife. He was not asked "why."

One of the men, a minister, replied "my Faith because I have built my life on it and it keeps me going." The lady with multiple sclerosis gave a dual answer. "My husband because I love him the most, and my Bible because it is my hope and inspiration." This woman is quite dependent on her husband for care as the only movement she has is in her right hand.

Of the nine people whose spouses or children or both are still living, six responded that their most valuable possession was their spouse or their children. Their words were different but the basic reason for this was that they are "a part of me, make me feel needed and wanted, and are there if I need help."

One lady's response to the question was her diamond ring because her husband gave it to her. A widower replied "The picture of my wife. I loved her very dearly." Finally, one widow with two married daughters said, "If we had a fire I'd grab the picture of my husband and two girls because it can't be replaced."

All of the responses are expressions of a loving, reciprocal relationship that, in one form or another, includes touch, although the word "touch" was never used. Money and other material possessions as such were not mentioned.

As Americans we have tended to make a distinction between mind and body. The products of the mind, which rely heavily on the distance receptors, are considered clean, trustworthy, and good. Conversely, those products of the body, which depend on touch, taste, and smell, are considered unworthy—even bad. Some have said that the current sexual revolution will change our tactual habits. But touching is even more basic than sex as a primary drive. Until there is a change in early contact experiences between parent and child, it will be difficult, but not impossible, to change adult behavior (10).

Other cultures and eras placed a great emphasis on touch for healing, destruction, power, or the transference of a life force. Primitive cultures construe the use of touch as magical in curing both mental and physical illness. Many of history's great healers cured their patients by a "laying on of the hands." Galen, Mesmer, Greatrakes the Stroaker, and others in the early history of European medicine wrote of the healing powers of touch. Why then did the strong taboo regarding touch found in the psychoanalytical tradition emerge? Mintz (19) provided us with some historical insight. She thought one of the reasons for the taboo might be that Freud developed his theories during the Victorian era, which, in contrast to the Elizabethan era, was one of sexual prudery with a strong emphasis on the products of the mind. Freud and his associates probably had a strong desire to dissociate themselves from magic and religion in order to be established as scientists. Freud originally used stroking, hypnosis, and therapeutic massage in his practice. However, since he and his associates were viewed as sexual perverts because of their practices, it became important to avoid any contact with the patient no matter how neutral its intent. Although external circumstances at least played a role in the establishment of the taboo, two basic principles of the traditional psychoanalytic approach do seem to contraindicate touching: the rule of abstinence; transference should occur with minimal influence by the real personality of the therapist.

Many contemporary therapists have moved away from the traditional principles of psychotherapy. A review of their tenets finds a variety of attitudes toward touching ranging from nontouch to somewhat mechanical use of tactual input; to the use of contact as a natural part of the relationship; and to its use as a means of knowing through feeling. The literature is replete with the controversy—space not permitting, the reader is referred directly to the literature (8, 16, 19–38).

The nursing literature has been the most productive in providing controlled studies on the effects of touch (20, 39–41); theoretical concepts (42–44); guidelines for the use of touch in a variety of settings (17, 45–48); and student reactions (20, 46, 49).

Generally, it has been found that the areas most often touched are the patient's forehead, shoulder, and hand. McCorkle's (40) study on seriously ill patients indicated a significant difference between those patients who are touched and those who are not touched during verbal interaction. Ninety-three percent of the experimental group (those who were touched) versus 70 percent of the control group (those who were not touched) responded positively to the interaction. The analysis indicated that, although the patient may be unaware of the touch, he seems to be more aware of the nurse's concern, interest, and caring when touch is used.

Aguilera's controlled study in a psychiatric setting showed that the use of touch "resulted in increased verbal interaction, rapport, and approach behavior"[20] (p. 13), especially with the schizophrenic patients. Since the patient population was relatively small and some variables were not controlled, she suggests further study. She does not suggest that touch be used indiscriminately, but that the judicious use of touch may be one means of nonverbal communication with psychiatric patients.

Krieger's (39) research indicates that there is a significant change ($p > .001$) in hemoglobin values as a result of therapeutic touch. Research with plants and animals, where understanding by the recipient is not a factor, has shown significant changes in enzymes when therapeutic touch is used (50). So there is more to touch than just the emotional aspect of being accepted and cared for by someone who understands.

Burnside (45) and Preston (47) directed their interests toward the geriatric population with chronic brain syndrome. The basic premises of these studies are that:

1. In a regressed patient the inability to communicate has led to isolation;
2. Unless repeated contact is made with him he will continue to withdraw;
3. With a nonintact nervous system there is difficulty with the registration, retention, and recall of information;
4. Since tactual input has the characteristic of a conditioned response learned very early in life, the ability to use this system appears to remain viable (47).

Burnside's (45) goals were to:

1. Decrease inappropriate behaviors such as babbling, withdrawal, hallucinations, exhibitionism, and refusing to make eye contact;
2. Encourage appropriate behaviors such as laughing, smiling, spontaneous behavior, expression of negative feelings, display of affection, and tenderness;
3. Develop an awareness of clothes, food, and other people through eye contact and touching.

Touch was the primary method used to reach a small group of six patients. She used an Indian handshake at the beginning and end of each session; a hand on the shoulder when speaking to them; simple hand games; dancing; and other contact activities. And what were the results? The patients began touching each other and the group leader; there was an increase in appropriate verbal communication and eye contact; and they began to respond to music. She noted that they like polkas the best! I believe Ruesch's statement is most apropos. "Nonverbal language takes on prime importance in situations where words fail completely."[51] (pp. 189, 190)

For some time we have heard that under stress there is a tendency for the individual to regress. This has been said in regard to reflex activity when the primitive reflexes reappear, to emotional reactions, and to behavior patterns of the mentally ill and geriatric populations. Can you, from your own professional experience, think of other instances in which this supposition has been used? The scientific literature supports this premise (8, 14, 17, 18, 20, 30, 42, 43, 46, 52–54). Under stress the individual reverts to an earlier, more primitive method of coping, which at some point has been successful. This occurs whether we are healthy or ill physically, mentally, or emotionally. Since the nervous system acts holistically, and ultimately controls our physical, mental, and emotional states, stress can affect any or all three areas of function. Just as we need food, water, and sleep for physical survival, we have a constant emotional need for comfort, reassurance, and security. These needs are particularly active when there is increased stress. The need for body contact, which signifies being loved, comforted, accepted, and protected, can be affected by illness, anger, anxiety, and depression. Due to cultural influences body contact may be seen by the individual as unavailable, inappropriate, or childish, and therefore, he tries to conceal his need or seeks satisfaction through sex. However, if the person's sexual activity is looked at carefully, it may be seen that being held is really what is being sought (53, 54). Could this be one explanation for the increased popularity of massage parlors? It has been suggested that one reason people depend on drugs may be because they do not receive enough body contact, which is the first tranquilizer we experience (14).

Implications

If touch is as therapeutic and necessary for homeostasis as the literature appears to indicate, then what are the implications for us as therapists? How can we learn to use a caring touch? How do we learn to give and receive it comfortably?

At this point in the history of occupational therapy there is a great deal of emphasis on the sensorimotor treatment approaches of Ayres, Rood, Bobath, Knott, and Brunnstrom in both physical and psychosocial dysfunction. All of these include, to some degree, handling of the patient. As I taught these approaches to students and clinicians, I have become aware of those who learned the mechanics of application but were unable to use the approaches effectively. It is not uncommon to have therapists to students able to discuss the basic principles and, on paper, plan good programs. Yet, when provided with the opportunity to "lay on the hands," they sit back and wait for someone else to do it. I have also observed those who perform the treatment in a perfunctory way. They do not use their tactual sense to perceive the changes or lack of change in the patient and thus modify their approach accordingly. For a long time I wondered why this was so.

In other areas of occupational therapy, such as general medicine and surgery, orthopedics, geriatrics, psychiatry, and education, how is touch used, and is there a place for the caring touch? Based on my own professional and personal experience, I reply to that question with an unequivocal "yes," there is a place for the caring touch.

During my own hospitalizations, I became very sensitive to the difference between perfunctory touch and a caring touch, and their effect on my homeostasis. During a one-month stay two years ago, I was the recipient of physical and occupational therapy as well as the care of many nurses, aides, and physicians. I became aware of the fact that most communication was carried on in the 4- to 12-foot social distance range. When it was necessary to be close, the nonverbal message was still, for the most part, that of the greater distance. When touch was necessary, it was mechanical and gave no message of caring. Instead, it was a job to be performed. Being on complete bed rest and knowing that they really did not know what the problem was or how to treat it, I became acutely aware of the effects of sensory-tactual-deprivation. My salvation was one aide and the occupational therapist who were comfortable within the intimate and personal zones and whose hands conveyed a caring touch. They were the only two I perceived as caring for me as a total person and not just another problem occupying a bed. I was experiencing what Dominian (43) calls the "anxiety of disintegration," since my body refused to perform its daily tasks. At such times, physical contact is of great importance.

During my last hospitalization for surgery, I was able to compare the effect on my psyche by an intern who had not yet learned the caring touch, with the effect created by my primary physician who had learned it. I was distressed by the intern who invaded my intimate space with indifference. He appeared to be very uncomfortable. When the surgeon came to see me the day after surgery, he approached the bed, placed his hand on my knee, and asked how I was doing. I knew immediately that he cared about me as a human being. "The behavior of caring can elicit the feeling of caring."[30] (p. 173)

It has been observed that most patients coming out of anesthesia or some other unconscious state first begin their reorientation through tactual exploration. They reach for the bed rails or the nearest person and hold on tenaciously (42). My own experience was no exception. I shall be forever grateful for the presence of three people whose touch conveyed "I care." It is interesting to note that these three were not a part of the hospital staff but were two occupational therapy students and a retired nurse. The entire staff, with the exception of my surgeon, were quite distant throughout my hospital stay. I find this rather frightening.

Professionally, I have been aware of the number of individuals of all ages who have demonstrated the anxiety of disintegration and in one way or another reached out for understanding and acceptance. Does anyone hear their cries, or has the medical machine grown so large and impersonal that it zeros in on the specific problem, ignoring the broader aspects of the total human being? Occupational therapists have said that they treat the total person, that mind and body cannot be separated. And yet we, too, get caught up in the specialization process and concentrate on the problem presented by the patient. The educational process encourages this with compartmental learning. We may talk about the necessity of total care, the acceptance of the individual and the use of therapeutic touch, but our actions reinforce the cultural taboo regarding touch. Goffman (18) has said that touching can occur in an acceptable way when there is a medical perspective, but we still find that practitioners are uncomfortable using it. Following discussions about the effects of touch, students and colleagues have said to me, "Intellectually I can understand the importance of touch, but how can I learn to use it when my culture says no?" That question haunts me.

It is obvious from the literature and my own experiences that talking about it may be necessary, but talk alone is not sufficient. There must be experiential learning to reinforce it. I am also convinced that we must first experience it with our peers and understanding instructors who can help us sort out our feelings. Second, we must experience it with those in distress and be able to discuss it with a clinician who understands.

Touching involves risk. It is a form of nonverbal communication and, therefore, may be misunderstood by one or both parties involved. It invades intimate space and may be a threat. If we are not in tune with ourselves and the one we touch, it may be inappropriate. However, non-touch may be just as devastating at a time when words are insufficient or cannot be processed appropriately because of disintegration of the individual.

Some of us have had to learn to use therapeutic touch the hard way. Some use it and are not aware of the fact until someone points it out to them. Some perhaps assume that it "goes along with the job" and give it no thought, while others unconsciously fight it and wonder why they are so tense. There have been individuals who have told me that the kind of treatment I do is physical therapy, not occupational therapy, because I handle the patients. Could this possibly be an unconscious reaction to their own discomfort in touching and being touched by others? At the other end of the continuum, there are some therapists who experience an energy flow between themselves and the clients as they work with them.

How, then, can we learn to use touch appropriately? It is not feasible for all of us to participate in encounter groups. For those who do, it can be a very rewarding experience. What can we, as educators and clinicians, do to help our students, colleagues, and ourselves tune in to this vital form of communication?

I believe it is important first to be aware of our own use of and feelings toward nonverbal communication before we can use touch effectively with others. There are many techniques from Gestalt therapy and the Encounter movement that can be used either individually or in small groups. Books, such as *Joy* by Schutz (16), *Awareness* by Stevens (37), and *Sense Relaxation* by Gunther (55), can be very helpful in providing direction in experiential activities.

I would like to share with you some of the activities that I have found helpful. One very simple way to begin to look at your own feelings is to take time to write your name as slowly as you can. When you are finished, reflect on what you felt while doing this. Can you correlate your feelings with some of the reactions you have seen in your clients? One student said to me, "Now I can really understand the frustrations of the patient when he has to concentrate consciously on every movement he makes! No wonder he feels frustrated!"

A period of time spent relating with others without verbal communication can be very revealing. We tend to conceal ourselves behind the use of words, but when forced to communicate without them, we have to share our feelings and thoughts through body language. This can be very difficult for some, enjoyable and easy for others. But again, whatever your reactions, consider them thoughtfully and relate them to your experiences with clients.

There are many people who find it difficult to make contact with others. "Small talk" is threatening. ("How do I make a meaningful contact?" "What do I do or say?") For some it is easier to withdraw, saying "I don't care," and then live with the agony of loneliness. Others may overreact, becoming boastful or boorish, to cover up their insecurity. All of this may occur quite subconsciously.

One technique that helps to alert us to the conflict of being alone and together is called *Feeling Space* (16). The group sits close together. For five minutes, with eyes closed and hands outstretched, they feel the space all around themselves. They are instructed to feel their reactions to this space and to the contact made with others. Do they prefer to stay in the empty space and resent any intrusion of it by others? Do they feel uncomfortable when invading the space of others? Do they enjoy the touch contact? Do they seek it out or withdraw from it? What are the reactions of those around them? This is followed by a discussion of those feelings.

Similar but more generalized feelings about a total group awareness of others as human beings and one's role in a group can be experienced by milling around the room with eyes closed. There should be no verbal communication. When people meet they explore each other for however long and in whatever way they wish. Discussion follows the experience.

The blind walk is extremely helpful in awakening one's senses, and becoming aware of one's dependence on others, and one's reactions to touching and being touched. The participants pair up with someone they trust. One is blindfolded. They are not allowed to communicate verbally. It is the responsibility of the sighted partner to provide an opportunity for as many varied experiences as possible, including the senses of taste, touch, smell, and movement, as well as to provide for the safety of his partner. The blindfolded person is instructed to experience his environment and to identify those individuals with whom he comes into contact. At the end of the allotted time, 30 minutes or longer, they trade places. The immediate reaction upon reconvening is a flood of verbiage. Some have found it extremely difficult not to talk during the experience. They find that their senses of touch and smell are extremely important in orienting themselves and that touch is very meaningful in relating to others, developing trust, and a sense of caring, as well as being necessary for communication with their partner. This can then lead to a discussion of the use of touch with their clients.

These are only a few of the many experiential activities that might be helpful. You are urged to explore further.

In our educational process, sensitivity to the effects of touch could be incorporated into many different courses, and the earlier it is begun the better. The faculty, as a group, should first explore their own feelings through experiential activities. It would not only make us better instructors but also better coworkers, since we would be able to sense the feelings and reactions of ourselves and others. The experiential activities could then be incorporated into courses such as kinesiology, neuroanatomy, evaluation procedures, growth and development, physical and psychosocial dysfunction treatment theories, group process, community relations, and administration-supervision. As clinicians explore and become comfortable with a caring touch, it could then be incorporated into the students' field work assignments as well.

To assist the clinicians in their development, this course material could be included in many of the existing continuing education workshops. State associations could sponsor workshops for this purpose. Finally, we can also learn from our clients once we are tuned in to observe our behavior and theirs.

Conclusion

I believe that a concerted effort on our part could make a difference in our own lives and in the lives of those with whom we live and work. If we, as occupational therapists, would begin to use touch in a caring manner, in time we could make a difference in our culture.

Occupational therapists have the necessary academic background in the biological and behavioral sciences to be cognizant of the implications of a caring touch. What we need is an awareness of our feelings as human beings. We need to experience the touch that releases the energy that can refresh, regenerate, and revitalize us whether we are well or ill. "In the hands of a person who understands, touch can sometimes be as effective as drugs or surgery." (55, p. 112).

We must learn that touch can be an effective means of nonverbal communication as long as it is acceptable to the touchee and the toucher, together with the understanding that it has a unique meaning to those involved (20).

I urge you to not only review some of the literature, but, more importantly, to experience the caring touch.

"Reach out and touch
Somebody's hand
Make this world
A better place if you can." (56)

References

1. Barr ML: *The Human Nervous System,* 2nd ed. New York: Harper and Row, 1974
2. Noback CR, Demarest RJ: *The Human Nervous System—Basic Principles of Neurobiology,* New York: McGraw-Hill Book Company, 1975
3. Williams PL, Warwick R: *Functional Neuroanatomy of Man,* Philadelphia: W. B. Saunders Company, 1975
4. Ayres AJ: *Sensory Integration and Learning Disorders,* Los Angeles: Western Psychological Services Corporation, 1972
5. Moore JC: Behavior, bias, and the limbic system. *Am J Occup Ther* 30:11–19, 1976
6. Leboyer F: *Birth Without Violence,* New York: Alfred A. Knopf, 1975

7. Gibson JJ: *The Senses Considered as Perceptual Systems,* Boston: Houghton Mifflin Company, 1966

8. Montagu A: *Touching—the Human Significance of the Skin,* New York: Columbia University Press, 1971

9. Frank LK: Tactile communication. *Genet Psychol Monogr* 56:209–255, 1957

10. Davis F: *Inside Intuition,* New York: The New American Library, Inc., 1973

11. Hall ET: *The Silent Language,* Garden City, New York: Anchor Press/Doubleday, 1959

12. Hall ET: *The Hidden Dimension,* Garden City, New York: Doubleday & Company, Inc., 1966

13. Gorney R: *The Human Agenda,* New York: Simon & Schuster, 1972

14. Jourard SM: An exploratory study of body accessibility. *Br J Soc-Clin Psychol* 5:221–231, 1966

15. Lomranz J et al: Communicative patterns of self-disclosure and touching behavior. *J Psychol* 88(2d half):223–227, 1974

16. Schutz WC: *Joy—Expanding Human Awareness,* New York: Grove Press Inc., 1967

17. Durr CA: Hands that help—but how? *Nurs Forum* 10:392–400, 1971

18. Goffman E. *Relations in Public,* New York: Basic Books, Inc., 1971

19. Mintz EE: Touch and the psychoanalytic tradition. *Psychoanal Rev* 56:365–376, 1969

20. Aguilera D: Relationship between physical contact and verbal interaction between nurses and patients. *J Psychiatr Nurs* 5:5–21, 1967

21. Burton A, Heller L: The touching of the body. *Psychoanal Rev* 51:122–134, 1964

22. Carvell P: The loving touch. In *Man and Woman. The Encyclopedia of Adult Relationship,* Vol. 1. London: Greystone Press, 1970

23. DeThomaso MT: "Touch power" and the screen of loneliness. *Perspect Psychiatr Care* 9:112–118, 1971

24. Fromm-Reichman F: *Principles of Intensive Psychotherapy,* Chicago: University of Chicago Press, 1950

25. Horner A: To touch—or not to touch. *Voices* 4:26–28, 1968

26. Linden JI: On expressing physical affection to a patient. *Voices* 4:34–38, 1968

27. Lowen A: *The Betrayal of the Body,* New York: Macmillan, 1966

28. Mercer LS: Touch: comfort or threat? *Perspect Psychiatr Care* 4:20–25, 1966

29. O'Hearne JJ: How can we reach patients most effectively? *Int J Group Psychother* 22:446–454, 1972

30. Pattison J: Effects of touch on self-exploration and the therapeutic relationship. *J Consult Clin Psychol* 40:170–175, 1973

31. Perls FS, Hefferline RF, Goodman P: *Gestalt Therapy,* New York: Dell Publishing Company, 1965

32. Rogers CR, Stevens B et al: *Person to Person—The Problem of Being Human,* New York: Real People Press, 1967

33. Rogers CR: *On Encounter Groups,* New York: Harper & Row, 1970

34. Seagull AA: Doctor don't touch me, I'd love it! *Voices* 4:86–90, 1968

35. Searles H: Transference psychosis in the psychotherapy of schizophrenia. In *Collected Papers on Schizophrenia,* New York: International Universities Press, 1965

36. Spotnitz H: Touch countertransference in group psychotherapy. *Int J Group Psychother* 22:455–463, 1972

37. Stevens JO: *Awareness: Exploring, Experimenting, Experiencing,* New York: Bantam Books, 1971

38. Warkentin J, Taylor JE: Physical contact in multiple therapy with a schizophrenic patient. *Voices* 4:58–61, 1968

39. Krieger D: Therapeutic touch: the imprimatur of nursing. *Am J Nurs* 75:784–787, 1975

40. McCorkle R: Effects of touch on seriously ill patients. *Nurs Res* 23:125–132, 1974

41. Rubin R: The maternal touch. *Nurs Outlook* 11:828–831, 1963

42. Barnett K: A theoretical construct of the concepts of touch as they relate to nursing. *Nurs Res* 21:102–110, 1972

43. Dominian J: The psychological significance of touch. *Nurs Times* 67:896–898, 1971

44. Luckman J: What patient's actions tell you about their feelings, fears and needs. *Nursing* 5:54–61, 1975

45. Burnside IM: Caring for the aged: touching is talking. *Am J Nurs* 73:2060–2063, 1973

46. Johnson BS: The meaning of touch in nursing. *Nurs Outlook* 13:59–60, 1965

47. Preston T: Caring for the aged: when words fail. *Am J Nurs* 73:2064–2066, 1973

48. Riehl J, Chambers J: Better salvage for the stroke victim. *Nursing* 6:24–31, 1976

49. Amacher NJ: Touch is a way of caring—and a way of communicating with an aphasic patient. *Am J Nursing* 73:852–854, 1973

50. Grad B: Some biological effects of the laying on of hands; A review of experiments with animals and plants. *Human Dimensions,* 52:27–38, 1975

51. Ruesch J, Kees W: *Nonverbal Communication,* Berkeley: University of California Press, 1956
52. Barthol RP, Ku ND: Regression under stress to first learned behavior. *J Abnorm Soc Psychol* 59:135–136, 1959
53. Hollender MH: The need or wish to be held. *Arch Gen Psychiatry* 22:445–453, 1970
54. Hollender MH et al: Correlates of the desire to be held in women. *J Psychosom Res* 14:387–390, 1970
55. Gunther B: *Sense Relaxation—Below Your Mind,* New York: Macmillan, 1968
56. Ashford N, Simpson V: *Reach Out and Touch (Somebody's Hand),* Hollywood, CA: Jobete Music Company, 1970

1978 Eleanor Clarke Slagle Lecture

Toward a Science of Adaptive Responses

Lorna Jean King, OTR, FAOTA

An "asset almost peculiar to occupational therapists is their high tolerance for puzzlement, confusion and frustration." (1) Ten years ago this was the opinion of Dr. J. S. Bockoven, one of our profession's most vocal admirers. Today one might argue about the tolerance, but who could dispute the puzzlement, confusion and frustration as we look back on a good many years of effort to define practice, to structure theory, and to build philosophies of occupational therapy.

Need for a Comprehensive Theory

And, as we look toward an era of increasing specialization, we are soberly aware that, without a unifying theory to insure cohesiveness, specialization could easily become fragmentation. In fact, back at the time when the profession's definition began "Occupational therapy is any activity, mental or physical, . . . " (2), recreation, art, music, and dance all fell under the rubric of occupational therapy. The responsibility for the fact that these modality-based specialties have become separate professions can be assigned in large measure to the lack of unifying theory.

It seems readily apparent that splintering into small professions results in watering-down of job development effectiveness, the scattering of progressively scarcer financial resources for education, and the loss of political "clout." The economics of the health care delivery system will not indefinitely support professional proliferation and duplication of effort. To allow future specialization to result in further fragmentation might well be suicidal. Therefore, we need a framework that will give specialists the bond of a common structure.

We must also cope with the fact that today's consumers, far more sophisticated than in the past, expect to understand what they are paying for. They will no longer accept "on faith" what they are told. This underscores the need for a coherent theoretical model understandable, not just to the professional initiate, but also to the consumer. We may develop complex theories, but, in order to be really useful, they will need to be based on a straightforward structure that can be widely understood, and is clearly related to the client's life functions.

Difficulties in Constructing a Science of Occupation

As a prelude to an attempt to identify a usable theoretical framework, let us look at the roots of some of our difficulties in achieving a science of occupation. One of the difficulties is related to the fact that occupational therapy was born of common sense; and common sense is, by definition, "what everyone knows." Everyone knows that it is a good thing to keep busy. There is the old proverb, "The devil finds mischief for idle hands." Carlyle said it with

---

Originally published 1978 in *American Journal of Occupational Therapy, 32*, 429–437.
Please note that there was no Eleanor Clarke Slagle Lecture in 1977.

great feeling, "An endless significance lies in work; in idleness alone is there perpetual despair." (3) One must reach far down on the evolutionary ladder to find organisms that are not active, that simply exist. Occupation, or employment, or activity, is quite literally bred in our bones. Occupational therapy, then, deals with purposeful behavior—with people *doing*. But isn't this what people are engaged in during most of their waking hours? It is hard to see what is significant about such a commonplace fact of life, and that is precisely the problem, or one of them—something so ever present is hard to grasp conceptually. Whitehead is credited with saying that the more familiar something is to us, the more difficult it is to subject it to scientific inquiry (4). As a commonplace example, consider how many eons must have gone by before Man even thought to wonder about the nothingness that surrounded him. A great many more eons probably passed before Man realized that it was *not* nothingness, and named it atmosphere. I am suggesting, then, that the very universality of the filling or occupying of time with purposeful behavior has made it difficult to form concepts that would help us to construct a theory or science of occupation.

Who has not had the experience of trying to explain occupational therapy to someone, only to realize that people think they know all about it because, of course, they have *experienced* occupation and activity. They are thinking about it in everyday terms, and the therapist is, hopefully, thinking about it scientifically and analytically. So, although words are exchanged, frequently no communication takes place.

Another problem in constructing models is the difficulty that therapists sometimes have in communicating with each other because of the many levels on which purposeful behavior can be organized. One can talk about the effects of activity on the biochemistry of cells, or about its place as an essential component of neurodevelopment. Purposeful behavior is also basic to cognitive processes; and on the still broader scale of cultural anthropology, an individual's role in the cultural milieu can be thought of as determining purposeful behavior. Conversely, behavior may determine cultural roles. So, whether one looks at biochemical Man, psychological Man, social, economic or ecological Man, purposeful behavior is inextricably woven into the total fabric of human function. However, if one therapist looks at occupation solely in terms of its psychological implications, while another looks only at the cognitive issues, and a third describes chiefly the neurophysiological consequences, a situation results much like that of the blind men examining the elephant. One described the leg, another the ear, and another the trunk. Finally, they were convinced that they could not possibly be talking about the same creature. Certainly an outsider would be hard-pressed to find a principle unifying work simplification, sensory integration, hand splints, and acceptable outlets for aggression, to name just a few of the topics with which therapists may be concerned.

Naturally, attempts have been made to deal with this disparity of viewpoints. Development frameworks are appropriate for many clients, but are not particularly helpful with the normally developed adult who is suddenly faced with trauma or disabling disease. Other models deal with occupation in terms of chronic conditions or the sequelae of disease—a rehabilitative context. These are not readily applicable to developmental problems or acute, as contrasted with chronic, conditions. Few models that I am aware of have spelled out what it is that is peculiar to occupational therapy as contrasted with physical therapy or vocational counseling, for example. What *is* that factor which makes occupational therapy so uniquely valuable that, as Dr. Reilly says, if the profession were to disappear tomorrow, it would have to be quickly reinvented? (5)

General systems theory teaches that systems share common features, that large inclusive systems tend to recapitulate the features found in more specific units. As Laszlo says, "A system in one perspective is a subsystem in another." (6) It seems, then, that our task in finding a theoretical frame for occupational therapy is to identify a level of system that is not so specific as to shut out some of our areas of specialization, nor yet so general as to include a great many more areas than are applicable.

In short, in order to satisfy the profession's current needs, a theory or science of occupational therapy should provide:

1. A unifying concept that will apply to all areas of specialization;
2. A framework that will clearly distinguish occupational therapy theory and techniques from those of other disciplines;

3. A model that is readily explainable to other professionals and to consumers; and
4. A theory that is adequate for scientific elaboration and refinement.

Adaptation as a Unifying Concept

While mulling over some of these considerations, I read Konrad Lorenz's recent book, *Behind the Mirror: A Search for a Natural History of Human Knowledge* (7). Lorenz deals essentially with the evolutionary and individual processes of adaptation that are involved in Man's active acquisition of knowledge and techniques. I was struck with the implications of his work for occupational therapy. Then Kielhofner and Burke's recent review of the ideological history of occupational therapy (8) drew my attention to Dr. Ayres' phrase, "eliciting an adaptive response" (9), which seemed a succinct and accurate description of what an occupational therapist does. I was at this time going over the occupational therapy literature, and suddenly the words *adaptation* and *adaptive* seemed to leap out from almost every page. In fact, few of our professional articles fail to mention adaptation, regardless of the author's specialty or point of view. I was struck, like Cortez, with "a wild surmise" (10); could the *adaptive process* be an adequate synthesizing principle for our profession? Is it too nebulous a concept to be useful? Surely it is too simple an idea—or is it? Has its very familiarity, like that of the word *occupation*, blinded us to its true significance?

Certainly the words *adaptation* and *adaptive* are well known to us. We advertise on bumper stickers that occupational therapists are adaptive; we have large investments in adaptive equipment; and assumptions about adaptation are implicit in our literature. Adolph Meyer began his treatise on "The Philosophy of Occupation Therapy," in 1922, by defining disease and health in terms of adaptation (11). But I have not found evidence that we have rigorously analyzed the concept or used it consciously to explain our functions in any broad sense. Perhaps it is time that some of our implicit assumptions about adaptation be made explicit. Only when these assumptions are articulated can their validity be examined through research.

At the outset we must distinguish between adaptation as an evolutionary concept and the process of individual adaptation. Evolutionary adaptation refers to changes in the structure or function of an organism or any of its parts that result from the process of natural selection (12). Natural selection, in turn, is the process by which a differential survival advantage is transmitted to successive generations. The process of evolutionary adaptation is very slow, requiring at the minimum hundreds of thousands of years for significant changes in form or function to occur.

Individual adaptation refers to adjustments made by the individual that primarily enhance personal rather than species survival, and secondarily contribute to actualization of personal potential. Tinbergen says, "Adaptedness is a certain relationship between the environment and what the organism must do to meet it." (13)

The idea of using adaptation as a model in a health-related profession is reinforced by Dr. Rene Dubos in his book, *Man Adapting* (14). He says "states of health or disease are the expressions of the success or failure experienced by the organism in its efforts to respond adaptively to environmental challenges."

Rappaport, the general systems theorist, says "Science is clearly a systematized search for simplicity." He adds, "Seek simplicity, and distrust it." (15) I would invite you, then, to keep a healthy skepticism as we explore the concept, a relatively simple one, that the adaptive process constitutes the core of occupational therapy theory, and that specific attributes of adaptation are also the significant and characteristic attributes of occupational therapy. This will make explicit and specific and testable some of our heretofore unexamined assumptions.

Characteristics of the Adaptive Process

Initially, let us discuss four specific features of individual, as opposed to evolutionary, adaptation. The *first* characteristic of adaptation is that it demands of the individual a positive role. The adapting person is defined as "adjusting himself to different conditions or environments." (12) In doing this he is acting, not being acted upon. An adaptive response cannot be imposed, it must be actively created. To quote Nobel prize–winning ethologist Tinbergen again, "Living things do not move passively through the physical processes of the environment; they do something against it." (13) Active participation of the client in the treatment process has long been recognized as characteristic of occupational therapy.

Alexei Leontiev, Chairman of the Psychology Faculty of the University of Moscow, reminds us that "Even seemingly simple human functions develop as an interaction between sensory stimulation from the environment and the *person's own activity*." (16) (Italics by this author)

Even unprofitable or maladaptive adjustments to change are actively entered into. Withdrawal, for example, which is often considered a negative condition, is actually an active response sometimes appropriate, sometimes maladaptive.

Secondly, adaptation is called forth by the demands of the environment. The challenge of something the individual needs or wants to do—obstructed by change or deficit in the self or the environment—calls forth a specific adaptive response. We could say that occupational therapy consists of structuring the surroundings, materials, and especially the demands, of the environment in such a way as to call forth a specific adaptive response. Another way of saying this is that occupational therapy uses the demands of tasks or other goal-oriented activities in a specially structured environment to trigger the unfolding of a need adaptation.

Among the healing sciences, occupational therapy is unique in its utilization of the demands of the real-life environment. An adaptive response cannot truly be said to have occurred until the individual consistently carries it out in the course of ordinary activities. Thus an amputee may practice opening the hook of the prosthesis over and over, but has not truly adapted to it until the prosthesis is used habitually in a daily routine. The occupational therapist uses this knowledge by providing the amputee with many real-life activities in which to use the prosthesis. The therapist knows that pure exercise, no matter how repetitive, often does not generalize into daily activities, and therefore fails to be adaptive.

This brings us to the *third* characteristic of the adaptive response, namely that it is usually most efficiently organized subcortically, and, in fact, often can *only* be organized below the conscious level. Conscious attention to a task or an object permits the subconscious centers to integrate and organize a response. Dr. Yerxa, in her 1966 Slagle Lecture (17), gave an example that can hardly be improved upon. She said, "A year ago I helped evaluate a brain damaged client's function. She was asked to open her hand. No response occurred, except that she was obviously trying. Next she was moved passively into finger extension while the therapist demonstrated the desired movement. This time the client responded with increased finger flexion. In frustration she cried, 'I know, I know.' Finally she was offered a cup of water. As the cup was perceived, her fingers opened almost miraculously to grasp it." It would be hard to overemphasize the importance of the therapist's using his or her cognitive powers to structure situations that will elicit a subcortical adaptive response from the client. We tend to rely too much on the client's cognitive processes.

Another example of the importance of subcortical adaptive learning is less familiar to the therapist, but popular with the sports enthusiast. It is to be found in such concepts as "inner tennis." Gallweg, author of *The Inner Game of Tennis* (18), says, "There is a far more natural and effective process for learning and doing almost anything than most of us realize. It is similar to the process we all used but soon forgot as we learned to walk and talk. It uses the so-called unconscious mind more than the deliberate "self-conscious" mind, the spinal and mid-brain areas of the nervous system more than the cerebral cortex. This process doesn't have to be learned, we already know it. All that is needed is to unlearn those habits which interfere with it, and then to just *let it happen*." This approach recognizes the frequently *dis*organizing effects of analyzing consciously what should be automatic sequences of movement.

I stress this point because it is another essential reason why occupational therapists use purposeful activity instead of exercise: namely, that tasks, including crafts, or other goal-directed activities, such as play (where the goal is fun), focus attention on the object or outcome, and leave the organizing of the sensory input and motor output to the subcortical centers where it is handled most efficiently and adaptively. I am suggesting, then, that the distinguishing characteristic of occupational therapy, derived from a similar truth about adaptation, is that *there is always a double motivation:* first, the motivation of the activity itself—catching the ball, creating the vase, making the bed; and the second motivation, recovering from illness, maintaining health, preventing disability—in short, adapting. Now no *animal* recognizes the need to "adapt." It sets out to do something specific—escape a pursuer, or find food. The immediate objective provides the motivation. Adaptation is a secondary and unrecognized goal. But in dealing with humans we need to recognize that the double motivation of therapeutic activity may or may not need to be brought to the client's awareness, depending on age, cognitive function, and so forth. The therapist should see to it, however, that other professionals and the client's family are made aware of *both* motivations, and of how the direct motivation of the activity subserves the indirect, but *primary* motive of therapy.

The implications of the foregoing definitions of the nature of occupational therapy practice are important in light of certain current problems. As mentioned earlier, the profession has been concerned with role definition—how to delimit the boundaries that separate our practice from that of physical therapy or other professions. In a recent report of an American Occupational Therapy Foundation board meeting, to which Washington area therapists were invited, concern was expressed about occupational therapists "infringing on" exercise, the territory of physical therapy (19). And well may we be concerned, for it is *our* professional identity that will be diluted by this infringement, not theirs. Obviously all disciplines that are working with a client should work together cooperatively, but it seems equally obvious that it is uneconomic if there is duplication of function. Exercise has its important place, so also does purposeful activity as a producer of adaptive responses, and this latter is the realm of the occupational therapist. We need to be able to explain in terms of the principles outlined above why purposeful behavior can elicit adaptive responses that exercise alone cannot. Defining our role in this way will be much more satisfactory than the old way of dividing the patient in the middle and giving the top half to the occupational therapist and the bottom half to the physical therapist.

The *fourth* characteristic of the adaptive response is that it is self-reinforcing. In animal behavior the reward for successful mastery of environmental demand is survival, and the penalty for failure is death. In humans the results are seldom so immediate and stark. Nevertheless, mastery of environmental demand is a powerful reinforcer and Maslow lists the drive to master the surroundings as one of Man's innate needs (20). Mastery of one demand is rewarding and serves as a stimulus for attention to the next necessary response at a higher level of challenge. This is the genius of occupational therapy—that, as the old adage has it, "nothing succeeds like success." As the occupational therapist plans and structures successful efforts, each success serves as a spur to a greater effort. Exercise, psychotherapy, behavior modification are all means to an end. But with purposeful activity, the activity itself is an end, as well as being a means to a larger end, therapy or adaptation, hence the double motivation mentioned before.

To summarize the thesis thus far, I am implying that the essential purpose of occupational therapy is to stimulate and guide the adaptive processes through which an individual may best survive and develop. I have suggested that the basic characteristics of occupational therapy derive from the corresponding elements of adaptation; *first,* that it is an active response; *second,* that it is evoked by the specific environmental demands of needs, tasks and goals; *third,* that it is most efficiently organized below the level of consciousness, with conscious attention being directed to objects or tasks; and *fourth,* that it is self-reinforcing, with each successful adaptation serving as a stimulus for tackling the next more complex environmental challenge.

Having tried to identify the basic characteristics of the adaptive process from which the significant features of occupational therapy derive, let us look at some familiar aspects or categories of practice in the light of adaptation, and also at the adaptive process as an organizing principle in two newer or less familiar areas of practice.

In broad general terms we can divide individual adaptation, on the one hand, into the phase that is synonymous with developmental learning, and, on the other hand, the process of adjusting to change or stress.

Developmental Learning as an Adaptive Process

The organizing of sensory input into information, and the subsequent integration of an appropriate motor response, is a continuous adaptive process. As mentioned earlier, Leontiev suggests that human functions consist of the interaction of sensory input and individual activity. For example, we learn to see by seeing. The visual figure-ground skills of a child raised in the green leafy lights and shadows of the jungle will be different from those of the child raised in the clear light and great vistas of the Navajo reservation. Each child begins with similar, basic visual equipment, but the process of learning to see in each environment is a process of adaptation in which available stimuli, combined with active sorting and filing, produce patterned vision.

There are a number of theoretical frames for considering the adaptive processes of early childhood, and the occupational therapy profession can be proud of the several outstanding developmental theorists among its ranks. It is not the intention here to recapitulate developmental theories, but to emphasize the fact that "eliciting an adaptive response," in Dr. Ayres' apt phrase, is, in essence, eliciting goal-directed or purposeful behavior. This may be as basic as enticing an infant to lift its head to look at a toy, or more complex, such as suggesting to a child that he shovel sand into a wheelbarrow to trundle across the playground to a sand box. The child's goal is playing with the sand; the therapist's goal is stimulating co-contraction, heavy work patterns, and so forth, in the service of integrating and organizing sensory input and motor behavior.

The role of the occupational therapist in stimulating this sequence of integration and response appears deceptively simple to the consumer who cannot be expected to understand, without explanation, that it takes considerable knowledge and professional finesse to know which adaptive response is needed and to provide the proper setting and stimuli for a given action at the opportune moment when the individual's development makes it possible for him to make a successful response.

We have been considering the well-known field of developmental learning in children. However, it is not only in childhood that one must organize sensory data and respond appropriately. This process goes on throughout life. Afferent, or incoming impulses, particularly those characterized as proprioceptive feedback, play a crucial role in sensory integrative processes in adults as well as in children. The key concept is that sensory input is the raw material for adaptation at *any* age. If developmental adaptation does not take place normally in childhood, the adult will show various disabilities ranging, as an example, from mild motor planning problems to severe disabilities such as process schizophrenia. Recent studies, suggesting that the adult brain is relatively plastic, give some hope that even in adulthood developmental adaptations can be facilitated.

The role of sensory data in the adult has been strikingly illuminated in the last 25 years by a large number of sensory deprivation studies, which have, as a matter of fact, strengthened the theoretical base for sensory integration theory. However, the critical relationship between these studies and the health of the average citizen is just beginning to be appreciated. As an example, consider the scenario for an all too familiar tragedy that goes something like this. An elderly man, in somewhat precarious health, must undergo major surgery. As a precaution, he is kept somewhat longer than usual in the intensive care unit. When he is moved to a room, he is kept very quiet, sedated, curtains drawn, and visitors restricted. Somewhere between the third and fifth day, post-surgery, the nurse's notes show that the patient appears to be confused and disoriented. The following day he is hallucinating and has to be restrained because he is trying to get out of bed. There are no family members who are willing to care for him in his apparently deranged state, so he is transferred to a nursing home where he continues in a state of relative sensory deprivation, and his mental and physical condition deteriorates rapidly.

The tragedy is that this kind of occurrence is often preventable. And in the instances where confusion or disorientation occur in spite of precautions, it is important to note that it is often reversible if suitable sensory input is provided. Lipowski, whose studies (21) suggest the reversibility of deprivation-caused psychiatric symptoms, also warns that around age 55 vulnerability to the effects of sensory deprivation increases quite sharply. Thus it is apparent that it is not just the very old who are at risk.

It is also important to note that the effects of deprivation are cumulative, and that the more sensory modes that are understimulated, the faster confusion and disorientation result. One of Lipowski's most significant findings appears to be that immobilization is the most disabling form of deprivation, and that, if added to other sensory losses, is very likely to produce psychiatric symptoms in the vulnerable.

In terms of the emphasis of this discussion on adaptation, we may think of confusion and disorientation as *dis*-adaptation—failure of organization and response. Hallucinatory and delusional phenomena, on the other hand, represent *mal*-adaptation; the sensory data is organized, but incorrectly, and therefore, of course, the response seems inappropriate. So-called unpatterned stimuli are as bad or worse than complete absence of stimuli. "White noise," such as the constant hum of a motor, is an auditory example, while the test pattern on a television set is an instance from the visual domain. Kornfeld, Zimberg, and Malm, in a paper on psychiatric complications of open heart surgery (22), report that "The patient might first experience an illusion involving, for example, sounds arising from the air conditioning vent or the reflection of light from the plastic oxygen tent. Many experience a rocking or floating sensation. These phenomena were often not reported to the staff and could then develop into hallucinatory phenomena and associated paranoid ideation." Kornfeld and his group confirm the harmful effects of immobilization, noting that many patients interviewed after recovery remembered as one of their chief discomforts not being able to move. Let us emphasize again that *sensory input is the raw material for adaptation*. Without adequate sensory data, the individual's adaptive capacity is greatly curtailed.

Motivational loss is another aspect of hospital-induced sensory deprivation that is of critical importance in rehabilitation or therapy. Zubek, in a report on electroencephalographic correlates of sensory deprivation (23), reports that not only were alpha frequencies progressively decreased during 14-day deprivation experiments, but this was also accompanied by severe motivational losses. The abnormal encephalograms persisted for a week after the subjects returned to normal living conditions, *but the motivational losses lasted even longer*. These findings have profound implications for all medical personnel who are trying to motivate patients toward independence. Perhaps the cart has been ahead of the horse! Perhaps the first thing to do is to provide sensory stimulation, particularly of the proprioceptors, through whatever degree of mobility is possible. Then motivation for independent behavior might follow more quickly and spontaneously.

I am indebted to Lillian Hoyle Parent for discussing with me some of the material on sensory deprivation, and, as she points out in her recent helpful summary of the deprivation studies (24), occupational therapists are better prepared than any other health care professionals to make use of this information. A dozen exciting research projects come readily to mind in reference to hospital-induced deprivation. For example, a control group receiving the usual post-operative care could be compared with an experimental group receiving systematic meaningful sensory stimulation under an occupational therapist's supervision. Comparisons could be made of number of hospital days post-surgery, incidence of complications, and amounts of pain and sleep medications.

We have suggested that sensory input and motor output are the essentials of individual adaptation as seen in the familiar field of developmental learning, and we have looked at the less familiar concept of sensory deprivation as a prime factor in *dis*-adaptation or *mal*-adaptation.

Therapeutic Adaptation to Change or Stress

The *second* general category of adaptive response is adaptation to change or stress. One aspect of response to change is represented by a very active current field of specialization in occupational therapy, namely the field of physical disabilities. This field concerns itself with the individual's adaptation to physical change.

Changes within the person can be of many kinds; what they have in common is they demand that the individual alter habitual responses. Arthritis, heart disease, amputations, spinal cord injuries, stroke, blindness are a few examples. The use of adaptive equipment, work simplification, splinting, development of strength and skill in residual body segments are among the adaptive considerations in this area of practice. Sometimes the acquiring of appropriate adaptive responses may actually be a matter of survival, as with the cardiac client. More often adaptation means the possibility of actualizing potential that would otherwise be wasted.

While the concepts of adapting to physical change are very familiar to us as therapists, we have had less direct experience with the relatively new field of adaptation as it relates to stress medicine. The role of activity in adapting to or coping with stress is an old idea whose scientific time has come. Dr. Hans Selye, who is considered the "father" of stress medicine, comments, "The existence of physical and mental strain, the manifold interactions between somatic and psychic reactions, as well as the importance of defensive-adaptive responses, had all been more or less clearly recognized since time immemorial. But stress did not become meaningful to me until I found that it could be dissected by modern research methods and that individual tangible components of the stress response could be identified in chemical and physical terms." (25) Dr. Selye called this stress response the "general adaptation syndrome." Today few literate people are unaware of the fact he demonstrated: that any stimulus which appears to pose a threat to survival elicits a response that includes the secretion of the cortico-steroids which prepare the body for a fight or flight reaction. The heightened blood pressure, pulse, and respiration that follow a danger signal had a distinct survival value when the appropriate reaction was running, or climbing, or hand-to-hand combat. In our present culture, running, climbing, or fighting are seldom considered appropriate responses, and threats are often perceived as long continued, like the danger of losing one's job, or the daily stress of driving through rush-hour traffic. There are well-known stress diseases such as ulcers, high blood pressure, and heart disease, to mention the most common, that follow chronic stimulation of cortico-steroid secretion. The current vogue for jogging, marathon running, and other strenuous sports owes part of its very real usefulness as a health maintenance measure to the fact that exercise metabolizes and renders harmless the stress hormones that otherwise might accumulate and cause permanent damage to the body.

What is not so often considered is the effect of either subtle or overt stress on an already over-taxed system. A person who is already feeling ill is told he must enter the hospital. Whether it is for surgery or for tests, or for nursing care, everything about the experience spells danger: the strangeness, the uncertainty, the painful or uncomfortable procedures, but most of all the feeling of helplessness. Stress hormones are poured into a system that not only is already reacting to the stress of illness, but also has few opportunities for activity that might help to metabolize and dissipate the cortico-steroids. Stress hormones can make the sick person sicker and can retard recovery.

It is often assumed that *rest* is what is needed in the hospital, but, as Dr. Selye points out, unless the organism is completely exhausted, activity of some sort is much more appropriate to stress dissipation than too much rest. Many years ago an occupational therapist frequently stopped into a hospital room and made available purposeful, goal-directed activities that allowed the patient an adaptive response to stress. If we had known then what we know now, we might have called it *stress management* or *stress reduction therapy*. Instead, someone used the word *diversional*, with the result that the whole area of human needs has been virtually abandoned, and the word *diversional* has become the equivalent of profanity. In fairness we must point out that few third-party reimbursement agents are willing to pay for something labeled *diversional*.

To turn to another aspect of this subject, before the stress hormones and their physiological effects had been identified by Dr. Selye, we often spoke of *tension*, and in the mental health field were able to recognize the usefulness of activity, even though the reasons were vague. Dr. Roy Grinker writes of the treatment of *battle fatigue* or *war neuroses* (26) and says, "In their free time physical activities are encouraged in order to dissipate accumulated tensions. Enforced idleness and rest are bad therapy for these states." Later he comments, "The patients are busy the whole day with physical and mental activities and various aspects of occupational therapy."

The high hopes held for the usefulness of the psychotropic drugs led to the serious curtailment of other forms of treatment such as those described by Grinker. Now that there is widespread disillusionment with the major tranquilizers, which seem to cause almost as many problems as they solve, perhaps the efficacy of what might be called *adaptational therapy* will be rediscovered.

The psychiatric disorders provide excellent examples of the interrelatedness of the various aspects of the adaptive process. In some instances, as in autism or in process schizophrenia, we are probably dealing with inadequate developmental adaptive learning and the attendant severe problems in perception and communication. These problems inevitably produce stress and the concomitant physical changes produced by the stress hormones. These, in turn, probably further derange the sensory-integrative processes. Many of the symptoms seen in the psychoses represent either disadaptations or maladaptive behavior. As the therapist is able to facilitate adaptive development, that is, sensory integration, coping behaviors improve. Activity also helps to metabolize stress hormones and thus increases the client's feeling of well-being. Though basic biochemical causes may ultimately be found for some of the major psychoses, there will probably always be a need for facilitating adaptive or coping skills in a society that seems increasingly stressful.

Psychologists Gal and Lazarus, it seems to me, have made the strongest case of activity as an adaptive response to stress. Their article, "The Role of Activity in Anticipating and Confronting Stressful Situations" (27), spells out the physiological correlation of activity with the reduction, or metabolism, of the stress hormones. They point out that while activity which is related to the cause of the stress is best, yet activity of any kind is better than none. Their useful analysis of the literature concludes with these words: "Regardless of the interpretation, it seems quite evident that activity during stressful periods play a significant role in regulating emotional states. We are inclined to interpret activity as being a principal factor in coping with stress. As has been repeatedly argued by Lazarus a person may alter his/her psychological and physiological stress reactions in a given situation simply by taking action. In turn this will affect his/her appraisal of the situation, thereby ultimately altering the stress reaction."

To summarize, we may divide adaptation in response to change or stress into three major components of concern to the occupational therapist:

1. adaptation to physical change (which includes a component of adaptation to stress because the physical changes are in themselves stressors); 2. adaptation to the stress of hospitalization or acute illness; 3. adaptation to reduce stress reactions in psychiatric conditions.

We have engaged in a lengthy exploration of stress and adaptation because it seems that in the foreseeable future coping with or adapting to stress is going to be one of the major health challenges facing humanity. Toffler, in his book *Future Shock* (28), makes a good case for the thesis that the extremely rapid rate of change in almost all of our cultural institutions is a significant cause of stress for large segments of humanity, certainly including our own. Ethologist Tinbergen warns, "The amounts of strain now imposed on the individual may well overstretch man's capabilities to adjust." (13) If it is true that stress is a major health problem for modern man, and if, as Gal and Lazarus propose, activity is of major importance in stress adaptation, then occupational therapy has a major role to play in health maintenance and disease prevention as well as in health restoration.

One of my colleagues (Roene Shortsleeve) once drew a cartoon that expressed this rather well. She drew a bearded figure in the white robes of a prophet. In his hand was a placard which read, "The world is NOT coming to an end; therefore, you had better come to occupational therapy and learn to cope."

Conclusion

I have attempted to demonstrate in this paper that the adaptive process can provide a theoretical framework for occupational therapy that meets the criteria suggested at the outset: that it can be applied to all the specialty areas as a unifying concept; that it will differentiate occupational therapy from other professions; that it is readily explainable to other professionals and to consumers; and that it is adequate in depth to allow for scientific elaboration and refinement.

The adaptive process is probably not the only tenable model for occupational therapy. If this paper spurs others to articulate a more suitable theory, it will have served its purpose.

Toffler, in concluding *Future Shock,* comments that, as yet, there is no science of adaptation. Is it too ambitious to suggest that occupational therapists are uniquely prepared to begin constructing *a science of adaptive responses?* It is a challenge worthy of our best.

References

1. Bockoven JS: Challenge of the new clinical approaches. *Am J Occup Ther* 22: 24, 1968
2. Dunton WR: *Prescribing Occupational Therapy,* Springfield, IL: Charles C Thomas, 1947
3. Carlyle T: *Past and Present,* Boston: Houghton Mifflin, 1965, p. 196
4. Thayer L: Communications systems. In *The Relevance of General Systems Theory,* E Laszlo, Editor. New York: Braziller, 1972, p. 96
5. Reilly M: The educational process. *Am J Occup Ther* 23: 300, 1969
6. Laszlo E: *The Systems View of the World,* New York: Braziller, 1972, p. 14
7. Lorenz K: *Behind the Mirror: A Search for a Natural History of Human Knowledge,* New York: Harcourt Brace Jovanovich, 1977
8. Kielhofner G, Burke JP: Occupational therapy after 60 years; An account of changing identity and knowledge. *Am J Occup Ther* 31: 657–689, 1977
9. Ayres AJ: *Southern California Sensory Integration Tests Manual,* Los Angeles: Western Psychological Services, 1972
10. Keats J: On first looking into Chapman's Homer. In *Century Readings in English Literature,* JW Cunliffe, Editor. New York: The Century Company, 1920, p. 639
11. Meyer A: The philosophy of occupation therapy. *Arch Occup Ther* 1: 1–10, 1922
12. Stein J (Editor): *Random House Dictionary of the English Language,* Unabridged. New York: Random House, 1966
13. Tinbergen N, Hall E: A conversation with Nobel prize winner Niko Tinbergen. *Psychol Today,* March 1974, pp. 66, 74
14. Dubos R: *Man Adapting,* New Haven: Yale University Press, 1965, p. xvii
15. Rappaport A: The search for simplicity. In *The Relevance of General Systems Theory,* E Laszlo, Editor. New York: Braziller, 1972, pp. 18, 30
16. Leontiev AN, cited by Cole M, Cole S: Three giants of Soviet psychology, conversations and sketches. *Psychol Today* 10: 94, 1971
17. Yerxa E: Authentic occupational therapy. *Am J Occup Ther* 21: 2, 1967
18. Gallweg WT: *The Inner Game of Tennis,* New York: Random House, 1974, p. 13
19. The Foundation. *Am J Occup Ther* 31: 114, 1978
20. Maslow AH, Murphy G (Editors): *Maturation and Personality,* New York: Harpers, 1954
21. Lipowski ZJ: Delirium, clouding of consciousness and confusion. *J Nerv Ment Dis* 145: 227–255, 1967
22. Kornfeld DS, Zimberg S, Malm JR: Psychiatric complications of open-heart surgery. *New Engl J Med* 273: 287–292, 1965
23. Zubek JP: Electroencephalographic changes during and after 14 days of perceptual deprivation. *Science* 139: 490–492, 1963
24. Parent LH: Effects of a low-stimulus environment on behavior. *Am J Occup Ther* 32: 19–25, 1978
25. Selye H: *The Stress of Life,* New York: McGraw-Hill, 1956, p 263
26. Grinker R: *Men Under Stress,* 2nd edition, New York: McGraw-Hill, 1962, pp. 30, 218
27. Gal R, Lazarus RS: The role of activity in anticipating and confronting stressful situations. *J Human Stress* 4: 4–20, 1975
28. Toffler A: *Future Shock,* New York: Random House, 1970

27

1979 Eleanor Clarke Slagle Lecture

Remember?

L. Irene Hollis, OTR, FAOTA

Being named an Eleanor Clarke Slagle lecturer brings many problems, especially for someone who is about to retire. The delight in being named for this high honor is tempered by the reality of the responsibility involved. Choosing a topic for the lecture is especially difficult. From the moment the letter from the President of the Association arrives with the news that you have been selected—asking whether you will accept—your mind races along trying to choose a topic that will be of general interest.

As most of you know, my last 15 professional years have been involved in hand rehabilitation. The 20 before that had been much more diversified. I went into occupational therapy in 1944 after nine years of teaching home economics. One might say that Lorna Jean King, last year's Slagle lecturer, and I are "late bloomers" since she, also, has had about 35 years of experience. Checking back over the list of recipients of the Slagle award I found that June Sokolov, who gave the second Slagle Lecture in 1956, had only nine years of experience in occupational therapy when named to the honor. Josephine Moore, the 1975 lecturer, had 11. The average number of years of experience of the 21 lecturers, so far, was 19.

During the period of time that I was struggling to decide on a topic for my Lecture, I was on one of my numerous flights to or from a city where I had been teaching. I was reading the magazine supplied at each seat and enjoyed an article entitled "Memory" reprinted from the August 1978 issue of *Fortune Magazine*. This helped me decide on the topic. I had been considering the idea of how important one's professional roots are and how much one is indebted to the people who have been influential through the years. In 1675 Sir Isaac Newton said: "If I have seen further . . . it is by standing on the shoulders of giants." It has been my good fortune to have many giants in our profession to boost me along the way. If you will indulge me, I would like to relate some of the meaningful memories I have accumulated these 35 years. It is said that one remembers things better and longer if they are pleasant, so the memories I relate will be the ones that brought pleasure. In general, my years in occupational therapy have been exciting and fulfilling, and I only hope that those of you who are young in the field will get as much satisfaction from your work as I did. My enthusiasm still runs high.

In 1944 I was happily teaching high school home economics only 30 miles from a large Army hospital in central Texas. World War II was raging. There was an announcement in the local paper asking for volunteers to help thread looms in the Occupational Therapy Department of this Army hospital. Since I had studied weaving in my home economics textiles courses, I drove over each Saturday to help out. Clinics were open six days a week then, and, in some instances, seven days a week in the psychiatric sections. While threading looms, I observed the other activities going on in the clinic and was quite intrigued. When the therapists informed me that the Army was setting up some war emergency courses to help relieve the shortage of occupational therapists, I applied and was accepted.

Originally published 1979 in *American Journal of Occupational Therapy, 33*, 493–499.

There were 30 Army hospitals at that time and all of them were in need of staff. Mrs. Winifred Kahmann, a lively lady who had been an occupational therapist since 1917, was recruited to set up the War Emergency Courses. Six hundred carefully selected students with degrees in related subjects were enrolled in seven schools of occupational therapy over the next several years. I was sent to the University of Southern California where I had my initial encounter with Los Angeles smog. Margaret Rood was head of the occupational therapy program at U.S.C., and that was an encounter of quite a different kind—a very exciting one. She and Mrs. Kahmann saw to it that we were well indoctrinated as to what occupational therapy was all about. A good foundation was laid and a good dose of enthusiasm for O.T. was given. I was in the first class, starting July 1944, and as far as I know I am the only person with a certificate in occupational therapy from one of those abbreviated, but intensive, courses who has been selected as an Eleanor Clarke Slagle lecturer.

I returned to Texas from California and had two enjoyable years working at the amputee center where I had been a volunteer. Several thousand soldiers were being treated there, so that I worked with many patients who had lost one or more extremities. Nothing can make one appreciate the marvelous instruments—the human hands—more than working with patients who have lost one or both. Could this have had an influence on the direction of my interests in later years so that I was led to work in the special area of hand rehabilitation?

In 1946 the amputee center was closed and I was sent to San Antonio to work at Brooke Army Hospital in the physical disabilities section. At that time, the occupational therapists in Army hospitals were civilians, classified as subprofessionals. The War Department, at Mrs. Kahmann's insistence, requested that Civil Service reclassify occupational therapists to professional status. This was done!

In 1947, through Mrs. Kahmann's influence and a resultant Act of Congress, commissions were granted occupational therapists in the Army. Since it was optional, I chose to remain a civilian, and had five memorable years there at Brooke.

Soon after I arrived, Virginia (Ginny) Bond Scardina came. She had been at the University of Southern California working on her master's degree and was all fired up. In her inimitable fashion she organized an in-service training program for the staff. She assigned topics and we studied hard to be prepared to present our material to our co-workers. There was a large staff with unequal knowledge bases so that this program was beneficial to all of us. Ginny's leadership ability assured its success.

During my years at Brooke the burn unit was set up in the section where I had a clinic. Before that we had treated the few burn patients on the wards. If they had survived severe injuries, they were among the most difficult patients with whom to work. There had been no way to control infections until the introduction of antibiotics in the late 1940s. The odor around a badly burned patient before the advent of antibiotics is a memory I cannot erase. It was always a difficult decision for me to make regarding whether I would go to see such a patient before lunch and ruin my appetite, or go after I had eaten and lose my lunch. The management of the burn patient has undergone numerous changes through the years, but nothing else has had the impact of antibiotics. It was a welcome change.

Another challenge that came about while I was at Brooke Army Hospital was to pioneer in setting up a cerebral palsy treatment unit for dependents of Armed Forces personnel. San Antonio in the late 1940s had no facility for treatment of these children. One of the medical residents who wanted a pediatric residency in the Army approached me to work with him on such a project. None of us knew how far-reaching this project would be. Dr. George Deaver, a consultant from New York, came to speak to the staff, and he arranged for me to visit various facilities in the New York area. As a civilian attached to the Army, I could get time off, but it was at my own expense that I flew up to the big city to start learning the necessary details of how to set up a cerebral palsy treatment program.

With the help of a talented aide and several volunteers, we soon had the essential equipment constructed, space was made available, and patients were waiting to be treated. The Army extended the use of the facility to Air Force personnel in the vicinity as well as to the children of civilian employees on the bases. We had an active half-day program underway quite soon. A physical therapist who had been working at the Kabat Kaiser Institute in the Washington area came to Brooke to do her two-week reserve duty. Sharing her experiences with the early neuromuscular facilitation concepts, which were associated with the Institute where she had worked, helped us in handling some of our more difficult patients. We managed to have her two-week stay extended to more than a month. This was a marvelous learning experience. I studied hard, returned to New York to take a course offered by United Cerebral Palsy, and was active in the State Crippled Children's Society. Although the cerebral palsy treatment program was only on a half-time basis, it was very engrossing, and for more than two years I made a special effort to be an effective therapist with this group, in addition to carrying on the regular treatment program.

Before I conclude the discussion of my years with the Army program, I would like to pay tribute to Col. Ruth A. Robinson, whom I was fortunate to get to know since she came to Brooke soon after I arrived. The Army hospitals had very liberal budgets and plentiful supplies for occupational therapy. We even had sterling silver for our patients to use. But Col. Robinson taught us all to use the supplies judiciously. Her favorite statement: "Remember, this is the taxpayers' money," has influenced me through the years. True, we should have a budget for equipment and supplies in our work, but we should never overestimate the need for expensive equipment and supplies since they are not necessarily indicative of a good treatment program.

After I left the Army program, working with polio patients was my next challenge. As you may recall, it was through Franklin D. Roosevelt, himself a victim of polio, and his influential friends that the Warm Springs, Georgia, treatment center for poliomyelitis was organized. The annual March of Dimes brought in funds to use for research, for payment for treatment, and for stipends that were made available to doctors, nurses, occupational and physical therapists, and social workers so that they could attend courses where special training prepared them for work with polio patients. I applied for the Georgia Warm Springs course, was accepted, and began in October 1952. There was an epidemic of poliomyelitis in the world then, and the hospital was full. Patients came from all over the United States and from many foreign countries. Therapists and doctors from other countries came to take the course, also.

The first three months of the course were devoted to acute care, and the second three months to functional training. Again, my good fortune held and I was exposed to some excellent instructors. The polio virus usually affects only the anterior horn cells in the spinal column, so patients with poliomyelitis had intact sensation and very discrete muscle involvement. In order to work effectively with these patients, one needed detailed knowledge of anatomy and kinesiology, refined muscle testing techniques, and, in addition, ability to relate to these people in a way that helped them adjust to their period of restricted activity. Protection of the affected parts was considered most important during the acute phase. The temptations the patients had to carry on with functional activities, even though such activities called for abuse of the involved muscles and substitution patterns that were detrimental, required stern discipline by the therapist. In so many areas of treatment we urge patients to become more functionally independent, but in treating the acute polio patient, much of our emphasis was on the curtailment of physical activity. Supportive and protective devices were applied to restrict undesirable motion. The psychological impact was devastating, so that every therapeutic skill was recruited.

I was asked to serve as instructor in the post-graduate courses at Warm Springs and stayed on after completing my six months of training. The upper extremity was mainly the responsibility of the occupational therapists, so that teaching these units was fun. After two years, I moved back to Texas to work with respiratory polio patients in Houston. Warm Springs did not accept patients who required breathing aids, so that this was an added dimension to the problem. I became accustomed to working with patients who slept in an iron lung or on a rocking bed and were made mobile by donning chest respirators so that they could come to occupational therapy in wheelchairs. This group was wonderful to work with, and taxed every bit of ingenuity one could muster. John Gardner's book, *No Easy Victories*, describes so well the way I felt when working with these severely involved patients and the way I feel about occupational therapy today. "What could be more satisfying than to be engaged in work in which every capacity or talent one may have is needed, every lesson one may have learned is used, every value one cares about is furthered?" (1, p. 32)

Fortunately, the Salk vaccine was perfected during the years I worked at Warm Springs. The intensive public effort to vaccinate everyone paid off and polio is now a rarity. However, the recent outbreak in an Amish community in Pennsylvania is cause for renewed concern and effort toward prevention.

By late 1956, the vaccine had polio under control so that the acute need for therapists in that specialty area waned. I then moved to the Houston Veterans Hospital and had a small clinic where hand cases were treated: fractures, and other types of trauma, peripheral nerve problems, and numerous quadriplegic patients. All my experience to date was made use of in this particular setting.

I had been there a year when AOTA announced that a grant-financed position was being established for a Field Consultant in Physical Disabilities. That was just the job I wanted and that was just the job I got! AOTA offices were in New York during that period and Marjorie Fish was the executive director. Establishing that new service would have been impossible without her able guidance. Helen Willard and Wilma West, as presidents of AOTA during those years, gave their support and assistance. Many other therapists helped me, also. My sincere thanks go to all of them for their willingness to advise and consult along with me. Frequently, I merely served as a means of getting the ones who wanted help in touch with therapists who could supply the needed guidance.

The entire United States was my territory, and I was presented with an enormous range of problems within the field of physical disabilities in occupational therapy. Many of the problems we have today are the same ones that we had when I was a consultant. I doubt that the profession will ever be problem-free. Again Gardner's *No Easy Victories* offers the premise that problems serve to stimulate and spark us toward our best performances. A life with no problems would be so dull that an intelligent person would go out and set up a situation that would provide him or her with a problem—a challenge. That, according to Gardner, is why people play golf or other sports. Artificial problems sought out by the bored person do not call upon one's full resources, though. The problems in occupational therapy certainly do. They "interest the whole mind, the aggregate nature of man more continuously and more deeply." (1, p. 32) Isn't it consoling to think that all our problems might be quite therapeutic for us!

I had taken this job as consultant for three years and stayed on for five. At the end of those five years I felt somewhat drained, and I took a year off to go to Europe. What a rejuvenating year that was! I had promised myself that I was on a vacation, but was tempted from time to time to look in on some interesting occupational therapy programs. My first three months were spent in the deep snows of southern Switzerland, in the French-speaking section. Friends of mine had a cerebral palsy treatment center in a small Swiss village where I was. They used Bobath methods in their treatment program, and it was all I could do to keep from becoming involved. How I wished I could have known about some of their interesting concepts during the years I had worked with children with cerebral palsy. Instead of working in the therapy sessions, I volunteered to mend and sew for them. That gave me more freedom to take off on a beautiful sunny day to ride the lift to the top of a ski area nearby. Needless to say, I rode the lift back down the mountain, too. I tried skiing, but since I was 50 that year, my better judgment made me give up the idea because I was afraid I would break a leg.

When I returned to the United States I went to the AOTA offices to check on positions available in North Carolina. During my five years of consulting I had gone to nearly all of the states and had selected the Chapel Hill–Durham area as a favored location. I could hardly believe it, but there was an opening in Chapel Hill for a therapist to work with a hand surgeon. That sounded pretty good to me. So my start in hand rehabilitation was not a premeditated move on my part, but an act of fate. It does illustrate that, with our broad basic preparation in occupational therapy, if, in the drama of our professional lives, the casting director should put us in one particular role or another, we can perform adequately. At times we may be fortunate and have preparation meet opportunity. This role in hand rehabilitation suited me as an individual and suited my talents, I grew in it, and it continued to provide challenges for 15 years. The flexibility made possible by our broad humanistic base in occupational therapy enables us to build up into peaks of professional excellence or into specializing at times. The base should not be ignored, even though attention might be temporarily focused on the elegant points of the peaks.

In 1958, Carlotta Welles had an article in *The American Journal of Occupational Therapy* with the intriguing title "DaVinci is Dead! The Case for Specialization." She stated that Leonardo daVinci had been dead for more than 400 years and that he was possibly the "last single individual to possess a significant portion of existing knowledge." (2, p. 289) Today there is so much to be known about such a wide variety of subjects. The quantity of published information rapidly increases: libraries keep expanding; information is put on microfilm in order to consolidate it for storage. Ideas used to outlive people. Now people often outlive ideas. There is a proliferation of new ideas—some good and some bad. Keep in mind the questions that T. S. Eliot asked in his poem *The Rock*, "Where is the wisdom we lost in knowledge? Where is the knowledge we have lost in information?" (3, p. 81) What we need is a good system to filter this mass of information so as to capture the knowledge that will be beneficial and to screen again to help select those things that will make us wise, at least in one area of concern.

Acquisition of new knowledge might well rank below the formulation of a new attitude toward, or a better understanding of, old knowledge. Many so-called specialties in occupational therapy are nothing more than a special arrangement of things that are already familiar to us, or a reorganization of our services to meet the needs of a specific group. How often I have found this to be true in my own career. In the first issue of the Physical Disabilities Specialty Section *Newsletter* last summer, there was an open letter from Louise Elfant expressing her concern about the danger of overspecialization. She feared that one might sometimes trade off treating the whole person for treating the parts more effectively. This, in my opinion, will not happen if one remembers to consider what the illness or trauma means to the patient. The therapist's special competence must be combined with compassion at all times. An extremity with a slight residual deformity might well serve, but a warped and crippled mind or personality can never be useful. Helping the patient put an injury or illness into proper perspective is fundamental to occupational therapy. We would be remiss in our responsibilities if we neglected this important aspect of treatment, even though we might be concentrating on a particular segment. We know full well that patients must become involved and rehabilitate themselves. This is impossible unless we help them understand and adjust to their conditions.

Being a clinician has been my way of functioning as an occupational therapist. We clinicians are on the front line and are more often than not the ones from whom the public formulates an image of our profession. This is quite a responsibility and one that I have never taken lightly. Flexner, when addressing a national conference on social work in 1915, stated the criteria by which a profession could be identified (4). He also developed the thesis that what matters most is professional spirit. He thought that trades carried on with such spirit might rise toward the professional level. Conversely, accepted professions might sink toward the trade level if people within the group lose such a spirit. That really emphasizes the importance of the role of the clinician and the spirit in which the duties of the clinician are carried out.

Rather than thinking of myself as a specialist, I prefer to rank myself as a master clinician. There have been numerous suggestions through the years favoring the use of such a designated title, and I find it rather pleasing to the ear and to the ego. One does not become a master of anything without putting forth some concentrated effort in the right direction. One needs to become more deeply committed and to make an effort toward acquiring definitive knowledge in the particular sphere selected. As Martha Moersch quoted (from Richard L. Kenyon) in her summary of the Curriculum Revision Study in 1966, ". . . academic training is the base for founding a professional career and it is the quality of growth thereafter that builds the professional." (5, p. 57) Continuing education as a means of growth, whether it be by reading extensively, by attending workshops and courses, or by communicating with others personally must be an active ongoing process. One statement that sticks in my mind is that continuing education is active exercise, not massage. An accumulation of intellectual facts is of little value. One must absorb the material and have a change in attitudes and behavior in order to grow. Every single day one should give oneself a chance to be a good occupational therapist—the very best! In anticipation of an unusual problem a patient might present, therapists should be confident of their ability to deal with that problem. If they feel inadequate, they should make a concerted effort to read a ready reference or call in a consultant to help them solve the problem—to grow professionally. A patient or client will more likely be impressed by the honesty of the therapist who admits to an inadequacy and demonstrates a desire to get help than to have the therapist attempt treatment in an area in which the therapist lacks competence. All of us have had times when we needed to turn to someone for advice. The less experienced the therapist is, the more important it is to be working in a clinic under supervision. Help is readily available then. Getting out on one's own too soon or going into a specialty area of practice prematurely may put one in a compromising situation and arrest professional development. One should give serious consideration to these matters as one embarks upon a career.

As I said in my introductory remarks, being named the Eleanor Clarke Slagle lecturer is quite an honor. I have never aspired to national acclaim. My main goal has been to work with patients to help them improve and to help them assume responsibility for caring for themselves. I have never felt guilty about working in a medical setting. Much of what I do is preventive in nature, even though it might be categorized as secondary rather than primary prevention. The medical setting enabled me to save energy and time since case-finding was simplified. The people who needed my services were gathered in one spot. I always did enough community work to let it be known what my program entailed, and at the Hand Rehabilitation Center I could take direct self-referrals. In this way, people could come to a convenient location to have services rendered. I was comfortable in this environment and I am sure that helped me to be productive.

All I did was "to do the common things uncommonly well," as some advertisement has said. That is what brought success. May I give an example of how only one aspect of treatment was developed with some measure of success?

When there is edema in the hand, we know that reducing it is of primary concern. The small joints of the fingers cannot tolerate the presence of this scar-producing fluid in and around the soft tissues that surround these compact joints. Limited motion results and the stiffness that follows can turn an otherwise delicate instrument like the hand into a clumsy tool.

Through the years we have had an opportunity to study the effectiveness of a variety of ways in which edema reduction routines have been carried out in both occupational and physical therapy. Methods of monitoring the size of the hand such as water displacement, as suggested by Dr. Paul Brand (personal communication), as well as circumferential measurements by tape or ring size, have enabled us to determine the effects of various treatment approaches. Massage, heat, cold, whirlpool, application of the Jobst intermittent pressure unit, active exercise, exercise in elevation, elevation alone, and a variation on string wrapping have been among the approaches evaluated. Some patients reacted adversely to massage and the same was true of the Jobst unit or other approaches.

If we found that any one of these modalities led to an increase in volume, it was discontinued in favor of one or more of the other more effective techniques. As a general rule, we found that warm whirlpool was most often detrimental but active exercise in an elevated position was most effective in edema reduction. Sanding projects positioned at or above shoulder level, cord knotting similarly placed, and leather lacing with a long strip of lacing are ideal occupational therapy projects. Close supervision is essential to get the correct routine established. The combination of fine motion of the fingers that involves use of the intrinsic muscles of the hand as well as movement of the entire arm so as to get active involvement of forearm and upper arm muscles will bring the best results. The contraction of the muscles is what gets the pumping action started to mobilize the fluid, and the elevated position facilitates flow from distal to proximal areas of the arm.

During waking hours, rather than have the patient place the arm in a sling, which would encourage inactivity of the arm muscles, we found that it was far better to teach the patient to elevate the hand above the head frequently, using his or her own muscle power; to rest the hand on top of the head, up on an elevated surface or door frame; as well as to use a cane or crutch to position the hand at the desired level. Most patients watch television for several hours daily throughout their convalescent period. One speaker I recall suggested that the patient should be instructed to raise the arm toward the ceiling each time a commercial came on. Actively making a fist and relaxing it while the hand is in elevation during these numerous times works wonders to control edema. What a simple approach to a complicated problem!

All of us are aware of fluid accumulation during sleeping hours. Eyes get puffy, fingers feel stiff upon awakening, and some time is required to mobilize the so-called normal hand. Think how much more difficult it is to mobilize the hand when one has any pathology. We tried various things to help keep edema out of the hand while the patient is in bed. One was a special sling into which the arm could be strapped. It held the hand elevated with the elbow flexed and the forearm in a vertical position. Bunk beds in our center facilitated hanging the sling since it could be attached to the upper bunk, but I.V. stands, hat racks, or constructed L-shaped frames with one section to slip in under the mattress could be provided for home use.

Another item suggested for night use was some type of external pressure. The company that makes the intermittent pressure unit also makes custom-fitted gloves from two-way stretch fabric. These gloves are fine but they are expensive and it takes some time to order and have them delivered. Since I am so cost conscious I found that used surgical gloves, which were available to us free of charge from the nearby hospital, sufficed. Too, the Thrift Shop had stretch nylon gloves at a minimal cost. The colors of the gloves did not matter since they were to be worn at night, and if only one of a pair was available, that was fine, also. A patient usually needs only one. If my supply of gloves consisted only of those for the left hand and my patient had an injured right hand, I would turn the glove wrongside out. This proved to be fortuitous since the seam on the outside made it more comfortable for the patient. Necessity is truly the mother of invention. A word of caution here: do not put a glove that fits too snugly on the edematous hand since circulation might be impaired. Always try the glove for at least 30 minutes, then remove it to check on the circulation in the fingertips.

Another way to provide external pressure is to make a Temper-foam sandwich splint. Two pieces of Temper-foam, a NASA by-product, can be used next to the hand and heavy cardboard can be put outside, top, and bottom. The splint can be strapped together around the hand. This type of external pressure is excellent for use with any hand with the combined problem of edema and a tendency toward flexion contracture. The hemiplegic's hand responds well since this splint reduces edema as well as holding the fingers in extension. It also provides neutral warmth which, according to Miss Rood, encourages relaxation.

I have gone into some detail in discussing this aspect of treatment to point out how unsophisticated these methods are, but how very effective. Occupational therapy is commonplace and unsophisticated often, and therapists are frequently apologetic about this aspect. Instead, we should take pride in our use of the ordinary and commonplace to bring about desired results when more sophisticated modalities have failed. I take frank delight in being innovative.

None of us has any idea what the world, and specifically occupational therapy, will be like in 2020 AD. About that time a beginning therapist of today will have reached my age. Remarkable changes have taken place during my time—television, jet airplanes, credit cards, computers, synthetic fabrics, frozen foods, drug abuse problems of great proportions, Medicare, too many people, Blue Cross–Blue Shield, Velcro, transplantations, space travel, holography, bio-plastics, antibiotics—the list could go on and on. Some of these things affected me and my profession directly—others indirectly—but the shocks came in small, adaptive doses. We were hardly aware of how important each one was.

The young will more than likely face as many or more changes in their lifetimes. Their opportunities will be cleverly disguised with seemingly insoluble problems. I only hope that we can all help them to grow and handle their futures. In my senescence—notice that I am avoiding the use of the term senility—I want to volunteer my efforts along the way.

In conclusion, I would like to quote an excerpt from a poem written by another occupational therapist, Edward Dunning. This appeared in the December 1973 *AJOT:*

> . . . *We've better things to do than reruns of old projects,*
> *Better scripts to write than catalog the past*
> *Or lose the present by condemning it.*
> *You've got a future to invent! How about it?* (6, p. 472)

References

1. Gardner JW: *No Easy Victories,* New York: Harper & Row, 1968

2. Welles C: DaVinci is dead! The case for specialization. *Am J Occup Ther* 12: 289, 1958

3. Eliot TS: *The Wasteland and Other Poems,* New York: Harvest Books, 1934

4. Flexner A: Is social work a profession? In *Proceedings of the National Conference of Charities and Correction,* Chicago: Hildmann Printing Co., 1915

5. Moersch M: Implications of the occupational therapy curriculum study. In *Proceedings of Final Conference,* New York: American Occupational Therapy Association, 1966; Quote from Kenyon RL: Designing professional education. *Chem Eng News,* 1966

6. Dunning RE: Vibrations on two instruments. *Am J Occup Ther* 27: 472, 1973

28

The 1970s: Discussion Questions and Learning Activities

The Lectures

Finn, G. L. (1972). The occupational therapist in prevention programs (1971 Eleanor Clarke Slagle Lecture). *American Journal of Occupational Therapy, 26,* 59–66.

Johnson, J. A. (1973). Occupational therapy: A model for the future (1972 Eleanor Clarke Slagle Lecture). *American Journal of Occupational Therapy, 27,* 1–7.

Jantzen, A. C. (1974). Academic occupational therapy: A career specialty (1973 Eleanor Clarke Slagle Lecture). *American Journal of Occupational Therapy, 28,* 73–81.

Fiorentino, M. R. (1975). Occupational therapy: Realization to activation (1974 Eleanor Clarke Slagle Lecture). *American Journal of Occupational Therapy, 29,* 15–21.

Moore, J. C. (1976). Behavior, bias, and the limbic system (1975 Eleanor Clarke Slagle Lecture). *American Journal of Occupational Therapy, 30,* 11–19.

Huss, A. J. (1977). Touch with care or a caring touch? (1976 Eleanor Clarke Slagle Lecture). *American Journal of Occupational Therapy, 31,* 11–18.

King, L. J. (1978). Toward a science of adaptive responses (1978 Eleanor Clarke Slagle Lecture). *American Journal of Occupational Therapy, 32,* 429–437.

Hollis, L. I. (1979). Remember? (1979 Eleanor Clarke Slagle Lecture). *American Journal of Occupational Therapy, 33,* 493–499.

Learning Activities

1. Investigate the occupational profile of most Americans in the 1970s. Some useful bibliographical references to explore appear in Appendix B.
   - What was the average family size?
   - What was the average salary? What were some typical jobs?
   - What did homes cost?
   - What were the clothing styles of the decade?
   - What was significant about the popular culture of the decade (e.g., music, film, books)?

2. If you have access to a complete collection of the *American Journal of Occupational Therapy,* scan the table of contents for each issue. What were some common topics? Can you identify any patterns in these topics? How do these relate to the messages of each Eleanor Clarke Slagle Lecture?

3. Try to summarize each Eleanor Clarke Slagle Lecture in a sentence that captures the main theme. Complete the sentence "This lecture was about. . . ."

4. Consider each lecture. Are there common threads among them that you identify? Are there any common themes that emerge when you consider these lectures together?

5. Review the biography of each lecturer of this decade (see Appendix A). Read some of the other work by the lecturer to gain an insight to the reasons why each one received this honor.

6. Consider what was happening in the history of the occupational therapy profession at the time of each Eleanor Clarke Slagle Lecture. Appendix C provides some useful bibliographical references for the history of the profession in the United States, and Appendix D has references for the global history of the profession.

7. Review what each president of the American Occupational Therapy Association presented as his or her vision for the profession at the time of each Eleanor Clarke Slagle Lecture. (A list of these presidents appears in Appendix E.) How do the lectures relate to these visions? The presidents addressed the profession through several forums, including columns in the *American Journal of Occupational Therapy,* such as "President's Address," "Nationally Speaking," and "The Issue Is."

8. Review each lecture in light of the *Centennial Vision.* What themes of the *Vision* stand out the most? What additional insights into the *Vision* do the lecturers offer?

Discussion Questions

1. Geraldine Finn's 1971 Eleanor Clarke Slagle Lecture expanded on Wilma West's 1967 Eleanor Clarke Slagle Lecture regarding health promotion. Finn proposed that occupational therapists move into the arena of public health as "health agents." How did Finn back up her argument of moving toward becoming health agents? What must occupational therapists do in this role?

2. Finn discussed many issues to be considered in the development of prevention programs, including education. What are some things the occupational therapist must possess in order to work in health promotion and prevention? Do you see these being addressed in entry-level or continuing education today?

3. Identify and explain the 5 elements in the decision-making process for developing strategies for the profession's future as identified by Jerry Johnson. Do you believe these elements are useful for developing the profession's future? How?

4. At the beginning of her lecture, Johnson spoke of needing to be concerned with the interrelationships and interrelatedness of occupational therapy with other professions. Do occupational therapists currently depend on other professions to keep going? If so, in what ways?

5. Alice Jantzen argued that academic education should be considered a career specialization. What are the bases of her argument, and what are your reactions to this argument? Would the same bases she used for supporting academic specialization serve to support clinical specialization (e.g., hand therapy)?

6. How, or in what ways, have the "storehouses of knowledge" Jantzen spoke of grown or changed in occupational therapy since 1973?

7. What do you think Mary Fiorentino meant by the statement, "Together with other professional groups, occupational therapy jumped on the bandwagon first and then decided what our role would be in this rehabilitation process. We borrowed, begged, and maybe stole to supplement our armamentarium"? Give examples that illustrate her point, and discuss how this relates to the notion of "professionalism."

8. Fiorentino stated, "The concept of upper extremities for the occupational therapist and lower extremities for the physical therapist is outdated." More than 30 years later, do you see evidence of this? Where?

9. What were 3 of the most important concepts about the limbic system Josephine Moore wanted the profession to understand? How are these related to the practice of occupational therapy?

10. In the last sentence of her lecture, Moore stated, "We should continue to perfect our perceptual abilities, which enable us to relate to others on a limbic level, instead of functioning entirely at the level of a biased intellectual." What do you think she meant by this? How would this statement influence occupational therapy? Is this a concept you think is considered in today's practice?

11. Joy Huss stated that 5 dimensions place the person in a position of either needing or rejecting touch: physiological make-up, culture, functional performance, safety/risk, and education. Choose 2 of these dimensions, and explain how they place the person in such a dichotomous position.

12. Discuss how you think Huss's choice of topic for the Eleanor Clarke Slagle Lecture fits in the legacy of these lectures so far. Does she build on any identified themes?

13. Lorna Jean King suggested that occupational therapy was in need of an "integrating theory." Does occupational therapy have such a unifying theoretical framework today? What is it or what could it be?

14. How did King define "purposeful activity" and its use in practice? How does this compare to other Eleanor Clarke Slagle lecturers or other writers in the field?

15. What are your thoughts regarding Irene Hollis's statement that specializing in any particular area of occupational therapy practice could detract from the holistic nature of the profession? Provide scholarly support for your position.

16. Hollis stated that occupational therapy is "commonplace and unsophisticated." Explain what she meant by this and how this characteristic strengthens or weakens occupational therapy's professional image.

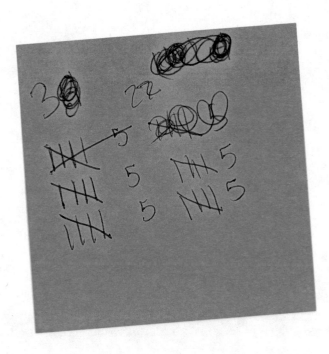

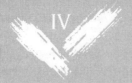

THE 1980s
Professional Identity

29

Historical Context of the 1980s

Around the World

The 1980s dawned much like the 1970s: pockets of terrorism, civil war and international confrontations around the world, and the United States and Soviet Union engaging in the chess game of the Cold War. By the end of the decade, however, great change loomed on the horizon.

In September 1980, Iraqi troops laid siege to several Iranian oil refineries after years of border skirmishes. Taking advantage of the distraction, on April 4 the United States attempted to rescue the 53 hostages still captive in Iran, but mechanical problems and a sandstorm thwarted the effort, which almost ended in total disaster. The rescuers retreated with eight casualties, and the hostages remained captive for nearly three more months during which time the Iraq–Iran conflict grew into outright war. The hostages were finally released the following January after 444 days of captivity when the United States promised to release certain Iranian funds. Iran–Iraq hostilities persisted and by 1983 had spread to the Persian Gulf. This bloody war continued until 1986, when a tenuous peace agreement was reached.

A few months later, news broke that the United States had been covertly aiding Iran by supplying arms and aircraft parts in hopes of gaining assistance from moderates in Iran in the release of U.S. hostages in Lebanon. This news ultimately ended in a congressional investigation that embroiled several members of President Ronald Reagan's Cabinet. Later these Cabinet members claimed the alliance with Iran was necessary to avoid further Soviet incursion in the area. The situation elsewhere in the Middle East remained heated throughout the decade. Reports of military attacks and counterattacks became overshadowed by nearly daily reports of terrorist bombings in Israel, Palestine, and Lebanon.

Soviet troops invaded Afghanistan in late December 1979 and set up a Communist government after anti-Communist Muslim guerillas killed the president. The United States covertly supplied Afghan guerrilla forces with arms to resist the Soviet occupation throughout the decade. After Mikhail Gorbachev became general secretary of the Soviet Communist Party in 1985 and called for sweeping economic changes in the Soviet Union, negotiations were initiated to resolve the situation in Afghanistan. However, it was not until 1988, after dramatic reforms in the Soviet economy, that Soviet forces finally left Afghanistan, leaving a puppet government in place. The United States continued its covert support of Muslim rebels in an effort to oust the government well into the 1990s.

Historians characterize the 1980s as the era of crumbling socialist governments, and indeed the decade featured dramatic changes in nearly all countries that were behind the Iron Curtain. In 1980, for example, Polish shipyard workers went on strike to protest the cost of living. To do so, they organized the first independent labor union, Solidarity, in a socialist country. This union became one of the main forces in ending 40 years of strict Communist rule in Poland in 1989. Worldwide recession caused similar movements in Hungary, Romania, Czechoslovakia, Bulgaria, and the Baltic Republics (Estonia, Latvia, and Lithuania). Most dramatic, though, were the changes within the Soviet Union, where partial transfer of power to democratically elected legislatures resulted in the naming of Secretary Gorbachev to the post of president and, by the end of the decade, the election of a parliament with opposition leaders.

One event in China in 1989 seemed to presage dramatic changes to follow in the next decade. University students had been staging pro-democracy protests in large cities for several years. In January 1989, students began congregating daily at Beijing's Tiananmen Square and took over the square in May. They remained there until June, protesting the abuses of government officials. On June 6, the Chinese government sent in troops, who fired into the crowd, killing hundreds. The troops eventually executed the leaders of the student movement despite appeals from Western governments. The U.S. Congress imposed sanctions on China, but President George H. W. Bush secretly sent an emissary to meet with Chinese officials and waived congressional sanctions.

As the world paid attention to the dramatic events in China and the changes taking place in the Soviet bloc countries, the Cold War continued through numerous covert actions by the superpowers in Latin America, usually involving the United States tacitly or covertly supporting governments and Soviets supporting rebels. Nicaragua, where a government with a socialist bent had been established after a bloody civil war, was a notable exception. In 1985, President Reagan wanted to support an insurgent movement, the "Contras," but the U.S. Congress voted to prevent the President from supplying anything but "nonlethal" aid. By 1987, it was clear that Reagan had failed to obey Congress and had covertly distributed nearly $48 million, profit from secret arms sales to Iran, to the Nicaraguan Contras. International scandal grew when it was discovered that the United States had allied itself with Panamanian dictator Manuel Noriega to carry out the "Iran–Contra" deal. By 1989, Noriega, a well-known drug trafficker, had lost U.S. favor and, after a quick U.S. invasion of Panama in December of that year, was extradited to the United States to face criminal charges.

In the United States

After the Vietnam War and the Watergate scandal, there was a deepening economic insecurity for much of the population. This was coupled with environmental deterioration and a growing culture of violence and family disarray, including divorce, abandonment, and abuse. Voters stayed away from the polls in large numbers, declaring their alienation from the political system through their nonparticipation. A citizenry disillusioned with politics turned its attention to entertainment, gossip, and myriad self-help schemes. Whereas protest marches were nearly an everyday occurrence in the 1970s, their frequency dropped dramatically in the 1980s. Inflation had increased to the double digits. The death of former Beatle John Lennon and the wounding of President Reagan in 1980 called attention to the increase in handgun violence, which by 1980 resulted in an average of 29 deaths a day.

During his presidency, Reagan increased military spending to support his Strategic Defense Initiative, which called for the deployment of satellites in space that could destroy incoming nuclear missiles. The Soviet Union viewed this as an escalation of the arms race. Reagan's plan came to be known as "Star Wars" and represented a stumbling block to disarmament of the United States and Soviet Union. It was not long after the severe popularity blow dealt to Reagan by the Iran–Contra affair and the instability of the Soviet economy that Reagan and Gorbachev signed an agreement in 1987 to eliminate medium-range intermediate nuclear weapons in both superpower arsenals. However, "Star Wars" was a boost to the space program, and NASA initiated several projects. A particularly sad event that marked the decade was the explosion of the space shuttle Challenger in 1986 after several successful missions. All seven astronauts on board were killed.

The 1980s saw the beginning of the U.S. government's war on drugs. Marijuana and cocaine had been pouring into the United States from Latin America for years. In 1982, it was estimated that more than 25 million Americans smoked marijuana, spending $24 billion on this controlled substance. By 1983, crystallized cocaine, known as crack, had been introduced to the country, and 3 years later nearly 75 metric tons of Colombian cocaine had flooded into the United States a year. Adolescents and young adults became the most frequent users, the crime rate increased, and health emergencies multiplied.

One of the most significant stories of the 1980s by far was the awakening of the United States and the world to the reality of acquired immune deficiency syndrome (AIDS). In 1981, San Francisco and New York City physicians reported a growing number of deaths among gay men. By the end of the year, reports included deaths of drug addicts using contaminated needles and of people given blood transfusions. By early 1987, more than 32,000 Americans had been diagnosed with AIDS, and nearly 60% had died. In that year the Federal Drug Administration finally approved azidothymidine (commonly known as AZT) for the treatment of AIDS. Although the drug did not cure the disease, it extended lives and relieved many of its symptoms. However, by the end of the decade, AIDS-related deaths continued to escalate around the world, reaching epidemic proportions in parts of Africa and Asia.

This decade saw several legislative changes related to the lives of people with disabilities. In 1980, Congress passed the Civil Rights of Institutionalized Persons Act (P.L. 96–416), which authorized the U.S. Justice Department to file civil suits on behalf of residents of institutions whose rights were being violated. That year, Congress also passed several Social Security amendments (P.L. 96–265) designed to address work disincentives within the Social Security Disability Insurance and Supplemental Security Income programs. The trend during President Reagan's tenure was to threaten to revoke various aspects of the Rehabilitation Act of 1973 (P.L. 93–112) and the Education for All Handicapped Children Act of 1975 (P.L. 94–142). Disability rights advocates responded with an intensive lobbying effort and a grassroots campaign. After three years, the Reagan Administration abandoned its attempts to revoke or amend the regulations but succeeded in terminating the Social Security benefits of hundreds of thousands of disabled recipients.

A variety of groups, including the Alliance of Social Security Disability Recipients and the Ad Hoc Committee on Social Security Disability, sprung up to fight these terminations, claiming they were an effort to reduce the federal budget and did not reflect any improvement in the condition of those being terminated. Several people with disabilities, in despair over the loss of their benefits, committed suicide. Finally, in 1984, Congress passed the Social Security Disability Reform Act (P.L. 98–460) in response to the complaints of hundreds of thousands of people whose Social Security disability benefits had been terminated. The law required that payment of benefits and health insurance coverage continue for terminated recipients until they had exhausted their appeals. In addition, it required that decisions by the Social Security Administration to terminate benefits be made only on the basis of "the weight of the evidence" in a particular recipient's case.

A series of landmark cases known as the Baby Doe cases involved the rights of children with disabilities. In 1982, the parents of "Baby Jane Doe" were advised by their doctors in Bloomington, Indiana, to deny a surgical procedure to unblock the newborn's esophagus because the baby had Down syndrome. Although disability rights activists tried to intervene, Baby Doe starved to death before legal action could be taken. The case prompted the Reagan Administration to issue regulations calling for the creation of "Baby Doe squads," or ethics review groups, to safeguard the civil rights of newborns with disabilities. Two years later a similar case involving an infant who had been denied necessary medical care because of her disability resulted in litigation before the U.S. Supreme Court in *Bowen v. American Hospital Association*. This litigation resulted in passage of the Child Abuse Prevention and Treatment Act Amendments of 1984 (P.L. 98–457).

In spite of the legal battles surrounding health benefits, advances in accessibility for improved participation in society of people with disabilities did take place during this decade. In 1982, the Telecommunications for the Disabled Act (P.L. 97–410) mandated telephone access for deaf and hard-of-hearing people at important public places, such as hospitals and police stations. It also mandated that all coin-operated phones be hearing aid–compatible by January 1985. In addition, it called for state subsidies for production and distribution of telecommunications devices for the deaf (TDDs, more commonly referred to as TTYs).

In 1985, the U.S. Supreme Court ruled in *City Cleburne v. Cleburne Living Center* that localities cannot use zoning laws to prohibit group homes for people with developmental disabilities from opening in residential areas solely because its residents had disabilities. In 1986, the Voting Accessibility for the Elderly and Handicapped Act (P.L. 98–435) required that all polling places in federal elections be accessible for elderly people and people with disabilities. Some advances in accessibility were hard won, however. In 1983, a grassroots organization called American Disabled for Accessible Public Transit (ADAPT) was organized in Denver, Colorado. For the next seven years, ADAPT conducted a civil disobedience campaign against the American Public Transit Association and various local public transit authorities to protest the lack of accessible public transportation.

By 1986, the National Council on the Handicapped issued a report outlining the legal status of Americans with disabilities, documenting the existence of discrimination, and citing the need for federal civil rights legislation. Such legislation was called for by many advocacy groups and introduced in several forms to Congress over the years but would not be passed until 1990 as the Americans With Disabilities Act.

30

1980 Eleanor Clarke Slagle Lecture

Occupational Therapists Put Care in the Health System

Carolyn Manville Baum, MA, OTR, FAOTA

I address you today with a sense of pride and great thanks for your recognition for this most singular honor. I am also thankful for the opportunity to have experienced the year of growth the responsibility of this honor imposed.

I hope to share with you my perspective of occupational therapy and its position in the health system. Occupational therapists' tremendous commitment to Man and to his ability to shape his destiny through activity and accomplishment puts us in a very favorable position because we provide a service that the health care system is reorganizing to assure it is delivered. Our responsibility as a profession is to implement a broader perspective of health care delivery—one that places its values on individuals as they accept the responsibility for their own health status.

To accomplish this task, I want to lead you through a process of assessment, recognition, and strategy development. For my framework, I will use the process each of us uses daily in our service delivery.

The Referral Has Been Received

"The health care system must be directed at improving the health of the American people by encouraging health, providing constructive behavior and improving the effectiveness of our medical care system" (1, p. iii). This mandate (our referral) came from President Jimmy Carter in his introductory remarks in the Department of Health, Education, and Welfare's publication *Health and United States*, 1978 (1).

The Problems Requiring Management. 1. High quality health care at a reasonable cost is often inaccessible. 2. Health care is beyond the means of many. 3. The system is focusing on hospital acute care rather than ambulatory and preventive care. 4. Technology has been exploited. 5. There is poor distribution of medical personnel. 6. Human beings are not allowed to control their own health status (2).

The Goal. Organize and humanize the system.

Requested Service. Develop a plan for implementation to effect change as quickly and as simply as possible.

To meet this challenge our profession must develop a plan—thus we need a "treatment plan."

We always perform an assessment before establishing a plan. Only when we have a sense of the total picture can we have vision. The health care system is very complex and involves many characters. Our first process, that of assessment, involves seeking to understand each of the characters and their contributions to the current health care dilemma.

Originally published 1980 in *American Journal of Occupational Therapy, 34,* 505–516.

The Characters

I. The consumer. As a framework for the consumer, I have chosen the work of Hadley Cantril (3). He describes humanistic characteristics that must be considered by Man in relating to Man. Man requires that his survival needs be satisfied and wants security in physical and psychological meaning to provide orientation and integration through time. Security protects gains made and allows Man to look to the future. It is also important to have enough order or certainty in life to enable Man to judge with some accuracy what will or will not occur. Human beings have the capacity to make choices. People perceive only what is relative to their choices and make choices accordingly. Humans require the freedom to exercise the choices they are capable of making. Humans must know they are valued by others. The individual must have values and beliefs to which he or she can commit himself with some certainty (3).

These are the humans who get sick, have accidents, and appear at the door of the health care system. They are in jeopardy of losing control of themselves and they are afraid. As professionals we must recognize their tremendous vulnerability and offer them services in which they have choices and control.

To describe the consumer, I would say: . . . some are saved, . . . some are used, . . . some are passive, . . . some want control, . . . some are sick, . . . some are well, . . . some are disabled, . . . some are crocks. Yet ALL are HUMAN and ALL are INDIVIDUALS.

Consumers feel that health care has become a right. The current situation is governed by a "more is better" attitude—that is, more resources, more facilities, more manpower, more of what it will take to provide what "I" need with no thought to how the services will be paid for. Human life is considered priceless and no amount of money is too much to devote to "my" life (4).

II. The federal government. The federal government is a multibillion-dollar operation organized to protect the consumer at the expense of the consumer. Federal involvement in health care began in 1907 when the Hygienic Laboratory was formed to work toward the eradication of public health problems in food and water. From this laboratory, the National Institutes of Health (NIH) were developed. The NIH is the biomedical research center of the country. It houses 11 institutes that study specific diseases and organ systems. The NIH is the main support of the majority of medical teaching institutions. Medical schools' dependence on federal subsidies encourages specialization and emphasizes technology as the answer to health problems (4). The public health service no longer focuses on health promotion and disease prevention.

The following represents the major dates that led to the current federal regulation of health care.

- 1935—The Social Security Act of 1935 put the federal government in the health business. It gave grant-in-aid to states to provide Maternal and Child Health Assistance and Assistance to Crippled Children. It has led now to more than 1,000 specialized programs.
- 1940—The start of third party reimbursement—basically so that hospitals and doctors would be assured of being paid.
- 1943—The start of Health Manpower training, with grants to educational institutions to prepare manpower.
- 1946—Hill–Burton construction grants were initiated and to date have totalled more than 4 billion dollars.
- 1959—Government employees were given health insurance.
- 1960—Medical schools were having difficulty surviving so that the government provided support through manpower funds, thus increasing revenue to the schools.
- 1965—Medicare and Medicaid provided help to the poor and elderly to obtain health service.

As expenditures for health care increased so did the government's concern, and eventually its involvement shifted from purely contributory to regulatory. The major controls placed on the health industry today are:

The Occupational Safety and Health Act (OSHA) enacted in 1970 was designed to protect the worker in the work environment. It has provided some protection, but it has also increased costs.

The Professional Standards Review Organization (PSRO) initiated in 1972 also had a humanistic goal—to assure that appropriate care was given to individuals by qualified professionals. This program has had a major impact on delivery of services by imposing control, restricting access to care, and increasing costs.

In 1974, the National Health Planning Resource Act (HSA) presented in law the concept that health care is a "right." Its impact has been on the control of capital expenditures, and the creation of a political football game with providers and consumers on opposing teams. The government serves as referee, and occasionally can be accused of making poor calls on the plays.

The transition from public health promotion and disease prevention to a high technological mode has been influenced by the federal government in the following ways:
- The sponsorship of high technology biomedical research
- The sponsorship of programs to produce specialization
- Money for training nearly 200 health professionals
- The construction of facilities.

III. The physician. Early health care was concerned with the individual. Public health and prevention were emphasized and dominated most thinking until the early 1900s. Until that time, the state of medicine was primitive and lacked a scientific base. Also, health problems were primarily a result of poor sanitation, poor living conditions, and contaminated water.

Health care has changed because medicine has become a scientific discipline as well as a political force. Specialist societies were formed for scientific and educational purposes. Most physicians initially were general practitioners, but focused on a specialty part time. A particularly strong influence for change in medicine was the publication of the Flexner report in 1904, where the disparities in the quality of education and the standards of performance in teaching institutions were exposed. This led to the development of medicine as a science.

Physicians are generally trained to think science and to think "sick." Most are dedicated to saving life at all costs. Few are oriented to the humanities and social sciences. The profession requires a tremendous time commitment to ensure competence.

The physician is the person each of us turns to for guidance and direction when we have a health problem. Physicians are in powerful positions and play a critical role in the delivery of care and in any changes in health care delivery.

IV. Medical school. Medical schools for the most part continue to separate the art and the science of medicine. They remain elite and do not use community resources for health delivery. The schools continue to prepare specialists and do not emphasize the social and behavioral sciences.

V. The health care administrator. This individual is taught to be decisive and in control, and the measurement of his or her performance is best described by the following "want ad" for a health facility administrator:

Wanted: *Health Facility Administrator*

The position requires a person with the ability to maintain an average occupancy rate of at least 96% on medical/surgical nursing units, 63% on ICU/CCU units, and 63% on obstetrics units, while scheduling all emergency surgical patients and, on the average, 21 out of the 100 medical patients each week. No more than 5 scheduled patients out of every 1,000 can be cancelled and no more than 15 out of 1,000 ICU/CCU patients, 5 out of 1,000 OB patients, or 10 out of 1,000 emergency patients can be turned away.

In addition, the person in this position is responsible for allocating nurses to each of these nursing units (1) so that an average of 5.0 hours of nursing care is maintained for each patient each day, (2) so that registered nurses, licensed practical nurses, and aides are assigned to each unit to utilize their skills fully, (3) so that the nurses' individual work stretches with or without 3-day weekends, and (4) so that quality nursing care is provided.

Applicants must have knowledge or skill in setting up systems for physicians to control patient placement in appropriate levels of care, and to control medical necessity of patient services (5).

These are the people who run our systems and our resources for implementing our concepts. They manage a complex system and are rarely trained or oriented in the concepts of human service delivery.

VI. Allied health professionals. This group in general is striving for professional status and is very competitive in the health services market place. The knowledge base of most allied health professionals has grown to the point that they seek recognition as independent health practitioners. The skills of the allied health professional are rarely used fully to support the delivery system. In our assessment process I will look in depth at one of the allied health professional characters; namely, occupational therapists.

Our profession started with the basic premise that Man has control over his health status by having control over his use of time, body and mind. In the early 1900s, when our profession was conceived, society did not have specific knowledge in biochemistry, neurology, or behavior. Modern medical science was in its infancy when the original paradigm of occupational therapy was developed. By today's standards, the body of knowledge was minute and, although research had begun to be a part of medicine, it was greatly limited. In the second half of the 19th century, the bacterial origin of many infectious diseases had been demonstrated. This led to the concept of asepsis, which made surgical management a possibility. From World War I to World War II, progress in medical science quickened. The sulfonamides were introduced in 1934, and penicillin was discovered in the 1930s. After WW II, the antibiotic era came into its own. A by-product of this era was the realization by the American people of the impact of research on the creation of knowledge. As a result, the public's expectations about medicine changed dramatically (6).

Occupational therapy was initially associated with and today continues to be a profession closely allied with medicine. We are not a medical model profession but we do have a medical base. The scientific inquiry in medicine as a science has had a major impact on our profession. Rather than take an active role in the scientific inquiry, we have relied on the work of others to provide direction to our principles. Thus by not directly addressing the concepts of activity and its impact on the nervous systems, behavior, or the cardiovascular system, we have not based our principles on the scientific movement.

We must do more than speak about our theories. We must develop a rage for knowledge and document our principles as a scientific discipline.

In 1969, the President of AOTA (Ruth Brunyate Wiemer) challenged the profession to address questions that would document the relationship between
- Deprivation or affluence of play and teenage aggression
- Deprivation of work or enforced retirement and the onset of illness after age 65
- The lack of work and recreation and the apathy of the slow learner
- The inescapable uselessness of the terminally ill and longevity (7).

Do we wish to continue to talk about the effect of activity or do we wish to do something about it? Now 11 years later, if we want to make a mark in both the humanistic and scientific movements, we must address questions like these and support the people who ask them.

As a profession we are not to date unlike the Bakhtiari Tribe of Persia. This is a nomadic tribe of goat herders who daily move their entire tribe to new grazing land. They have taught us that a group cannot refine a culture on the move. The Bakhtiari life has changed very little since 10,000 B.C. They have only the simple technology that can be carried on daily journeys. The simplicity is not romantic, it is a matter of survival (8). In applying this analogy to Occupational Therapy, I have to ask the question, when are we going to stop following the grazing trail and develop the technology to plant our own fields?

As a profession we have seen our nearly singular roles in vocational rehabilitation, basic living skills, and use of activity come and go. Other professions have implemented what initially were our roles, but we have survived! This means that the health care system is looking to us for a special emphasis on health care delivery. We must internalize this positive concept of us. I think we can develop a fertile strain that will allow our fields to be very fruitful. We have something very unique to harvest. We must master our own product, understand it, and use that understanding to mold the living environment.

Within our profession there are many capable people in education and clinical practice yet we have difficulty developing a master plan for and getting started on a program to define our practice in scientific terms. I want to share with you my perspective of a conflict that I think has our profession at a standstill and is preventing us from developing our "fertile strain."

Our professional organization, the American Occupational Therapy Association (AOTA), has supported the development and continuance of a structured pluralism with education and practice being separate in structure and function. Two prevailing thoughts have developed out of this relationship.

The first thought is:

Because occupational therapy educators do not practice clinical occupational therapy, they do not have the knowledge, attitude, or skill to produce students trained in current practice.

Since the middle 1960s, therapists in clinical practice have been working their way into the changing health system. To do this required the following eight activities:

- Acquire third party reimbursement
- Establish collaborative working relationships with other professionals involved in direct service
- Define practice standards for professional review
- Establish cost effective services
- Identify patient populations and develop services to support program implementation
- Develop treatment methodologies that can be included in short term care facilities
- Establish networks for referral of the patient to long term or community services to obtain maximum benefit for occupational therapy
- Design activities and intervention that support the theory of occupational therapy.

Treatment interventions have been established by practitioners to provide remediation to impaired areas of function as well as to promote healthful behaviors. For us to gain identity as a scientific discipline each area of function must be supported by research supplied from the basic sciences.

Some of the fields that relate to *motor and sensory-integrative function* are neuropathophysiology, neurology, anatomy, physiology, neurophysiology, neuroanatomy, chemistry, and physics. Some of the fields that relate to *cognitive, psychological and social function* are psychology, sociology, psychopathology, and chemistry.

I think therapists in practice have stimulated their own growth by graduate study in areas to support understanding of function—not exclusively relying on advanced occupational therapy education to provide it, possibly because occupational therapy educators are not publishing information to answer the basic questions needed to be answered about the body systems' ability to respond to the demands required to function in these areas. The professional dialogue for practitioners is primarily with others in clinical practice through publications and continuing education experiences. Because of this I believe practitioners have adopted the following notion:

Because occupational therapy educators do not practice clinical occupational therapy, they do not have the knowledge, attitude or skill to produce students trained in current practice.

Now I will describe the second thought that has developed.

The practitioner is ignoring his or her responsibilities and compromising the field of occupational therapy by collaborating with other professionals and not demonstrating occupational therapy as an independent health profession.

In 1977, a report of the Ad Hoc Committee on Education was submitted to the Executive Board of the AOTA and eventually published in *The American Journal of Occupational Therapy* (9). The stated purpose was to raise issues that influenced our attempt to become a fully recognized profession. I will present the education description directly from the Ad Hoc Committee Report.

Issues in Education

I. Faculty characteristics and responsibilities. Faculty are operating autonomously with minimal involvement with university missions, which undermines efforts to continue association with these institutions.

Faculty generally give up patient treatment and remove themselves from the practice of occupational therapy.

Faculty engage in repetitive and time-consuming requirements for accreditation that deprive faculty of valuable time, some of which might be spent in research, scholarly activities and other endeavors, expected of all university faculty members.

II. Faculty shortage. There is a serious shortage of qualified faculty members at every academic level. The Association efforts and resources are focused on baccalaureate and associate degree entry-level preparation and exclude resources to clinical specialization and graduate education.

III. Multiple entry routes leading to certification as an OTR. Our multiple entry points serve to support the thesis that occupational therapy is a semi-profession or a technical profession. The value of our educational preparation is negated by multiple entry routes that do not rely upon a liberal arts base. "The processes of acquiring and assuming the knowledge . . . unique to occupational therapy, are seldom the priorities of our educational programs, ..."

IV. Lack of research. "The lack of research related to hypotheses supporting our theoretical foundations, treatment modalities, and modes of intervention seriously impedes all aspects of education and practice."

V. External influences and forces. "Actions and decisions made by external agencies continue to have a negative influence and impact on our development." Examples cited are the limitation of funding of health programs, especially at the post-baccalaureate level, and the control that the American Medical Association has over our education programs.

VI. AOTA member readiness to decide on semiprofessional or professional status. The committee reported that members do not focus in either education or practice upon those functions and behaviors that are traditionally identified with the status of a profession. The authors state the following behaviors are necessary by the membership to reach professional status.

1. Willingness and responsibility for diagnosing problems;
2. Providing service without referral from physician;
3. Working without physician supervision or members of other disciplines;
4. Conducting one's own professional assessment;
5. Accepting the necessity for research to substantiate or refute the principles upon which treatment is based (9).

This completes the description of the Ad Hoc Committee on Education Report.

Thus we have documentation of the pervasiveness of the second idea:

The practitioner is ignoring his or her responsibilities and compromising the field of occupational therapy by collaborating with other professionals and not demonstrating occupational therapy as an independent health profession.

I have now described those six I think are the main characters in the health system and described in depth my perception of the character of occupational therapy. From these descriptions, I perceive that the entire system is in conflict. Each character has its own values, knowledge, structure, and personality.

This causes the system, which should be a team of specialists organizing to develop a network of interactions, to be at a stalemate resulting in power struggles and strained communications.

The patient is frequently the victim of the isolation caused by this poor communication. The definition of a closed system is that the system is isolated from its environment and the final state is determined by the initial conditions. Certainly the health system is made up of many closed systems (10). The patients unfortunately become a closed system also because they have no mechanism for being in a dynamic state with their environment and in control of their own status.

The prejudices harbored by each of the characters in the health system seek to maintain the independent status of each character rather than focusing on the individual human being who is paying for the service to change his or her health status.

I have now completed the assessment process of our plan. I see three separate problems that the profession has to address to meet its responsibilities in organizing and humanizing the health care system:

The three problems are:

- A perceived conflict between occupational therapy practice and occupational therapy education, to actually destroy what I perceive as myths
- A focus on health services delivered within the acute care model
- The health system's lack of orientation toward the human being.

Now that we have completed the assessment by looking at the characters and identifying the problems, let us take each problem one at a time and develop our treatment plan.

Treatment Plan

Problem I. A Perceived Conflict Between OT Practice: OT Education

GOAL: *Resolve the conflict between practice and education.* It is important that our profession reduce the social distance between education and practice and move from pluralistic positions into one of integration. We need a link between education and practice with the purpose of further developing occupational therapy as a scientific discipline. This focus will remove the need for maintaining the conflict and move us toward integration and further away from fragmentation—thus, we will destroy the myths.

In investigating methods to resolve the conflict, I went to C. P. Snow's lecture on "Two Cultures." Snow perceives that there is conflict between the scientist—who believes that literary intellectuals are totally lacking in foresight, peculiarly unconcerned with humanity—and the nonscientist—who has a rooted impression that the scientist is shallowly optimistic and unaware of man's condition (11). I wondered whether occupational therapy housed any scientists, so I found myself engulfed in *The Search,* also by C. P. Snow, a novel that describes the scientist through a number of behaviors ranging from unending curiosity to the need to understand things even if they can't be controlled (12). It became clear to me that the educational preparation of the occupational therapist does not encourage the scientist.

For the profession to ascend, we will need to produce true professionals who are skilled in inventing, inferring, and analyzing, and who can communicate with basic researchers in a collaborative relationship to investigate areas of our clinical practice as well. We must prepare professionals who possess the humanistic qualities to relate to an individual who requires our service. Since these qualities are not mutually exclusive, the educational preparation of the occupational therapist must develop both qualities.

As I became more aware of the lack of basic scientists in our profession, I explored ways to approach the production and distribution of knowledge.

According to Machlup, a profession must be responsible for producing two types of knowledge: 1. internal knowledge, which answers questions to measure the effectiveness of our service—this knowledge is developed by daily dialogue with each other and through our newspapers and journal—2. new knowledge that assists society in expanding its understanding (13). I believe the profession must contribute societal knowledge in the following areas:

1. The activity process and activity's effect on the human body.
2. The process of adaptation and its effect on the human body.
3. The process of integration of human function through activity and adaptation.

To produce discoveries through inventing, inferring, analyzing, or evaluating is not enough (13, p. 30). For discoveries to be valuable, they must be conveyed. Knowledge is produced in three basic ways, all under the general category of research.

- *Research* is defined as a systematic intensive study directed toward fuller knowledge of the subject studied.
- *Basic research* is directed toward the increase of knowledge. It is research where the primary aim of the investigation is a fuller understanding of the subject under study rather than the practical application thereof.
- *Applied research* creates directly applicable knowledge. The researcher looks for results which promise to be of ultimate use in practice.
- *Development* is the systematic use of scientific knowledge directed toward the production of useful materials, systems methods or process (13, pp. 146–147).

Within the profession two of these three types of research can and are being accomplished—applied research and development. Our greatest lack is in basic research. To do basic research requires a scientist with not only the scientific approach, but also the scientific background. I do not know of a profession that performs basic research entirely for themselves—certainly medicine does not—and I do not know why we should continue to struggle with the idea of performing our own basic research to the detriment of our educational process.

I propose that educators and clinicians formulate collaborative relationships with social scientists to address the social, cognitive, and psychological aspects of function and with biological scientists to address the motor and sensory integrative aspects of function.

A research team should inspire a collaborative relationship between the occupational therapy educator, the basic scientist, and the clinician or clinicians. The occupational therapy educators must assume the role of coordinator and facilitator of research projects. The clinician should function as a clinical scientist who logs observation and inferences, and communicates with the educator who can organize teams to design and implement research to answer pertinent questions.

One reason these research teams have not yet developed is that educators and practitioners have not been interested in addressing common questions. The stability and then the ascent of our profession depends on the establishment of common goals for research and a commitment on the part of the educator and the clinician to collaborate on research questions of interest to both. By including the appropriate basic science researchers the gap in the basic sciences on the part of both the educator and the clinician can be narrowed so that questions can be addressed as they relate to the human body and mind and its response to activity.

We can no longer afford to destroy each other with words and lack of action. The profession must make a commitment to action using a team collaborating for the outcome of producing internal knowledge for the benefit of our patients and societal knowledge for the benefit of mankind. We must develop the skill and accept the responsibility to critically analyze our work and not react defensively to criticism but realize that criticism will help the profession grow.

We must recognize that too few of us have the skills or resources to do basic scientific research. However, it has to be done if we are to attain a credible status with the public in the subject areas we do know—that of adaptation and integration. I predict that, through the experience of collaborative relationship with the basic scientist, many of us will develop the skills necessary not only to do the basic research ourselves, but also to teach these skills to others within our profession. I think we would then attract more students interested in a scientific discipline. We also would have greater strength as a profession in relating to other groups who are infringing on our territory because we would have a strong theory base for our service delivery. Our confidence would be strong knowing that we are the profession to deliver our services—this would be built into our images of ourselves as professionals. The issues from the practice arena and the issues from the education arena would all be given a tremendous boost and be closer to resolution if the credibility of our profession was housed in research methodologies that are strong. It is important for clinicians and educators to recognize the extreme pressures facing each group as each works to gain a stable position within the health system. Perhaps we can all feel that we are approaching the problems together. It is critical that we channel our energy away from conflict and into research. I believe funding for research would be forthcoming from the government for coordinated projects that demonstrate a link with the basic sciences.

Time is a problem for all of us. However, well designed and funded research projects should provide resources to support the clinician and educator in research activities. We have to organize and order our priorities to accomplish basic research for the sake of professional stability. Looking outside the profession, I find that similar conflicts between education and practice are not uncommon. Survival of the profession is an issue whether one is from the university structure or a clinical facility. The missing link in destroying this conflict is collaborative research with a commitment to the growth of our profession. Some persons might not agree that the social or biological scientist must enter the picture, but I am now convinced that the skills and attitude of those individuals are critical for the process to proceed.

Now we must develop a treatment plan for the second problem.

Problem II. The Health Services Delivery Primarily Within the Acute Care Model

GOAL: *Expand the delivery of occupational therapy service from the acute care model of service.* Hospitals initially were a shelter for the socially unfit whether due to severe disability, mental illness, or indigence. The hospital was set apart from the medical community. This was the population served when occupational therapy was initiated as a profession. Private patients were not treated in hospitals until the turn of the century. Insurance did not pay for hospital care until the 1930s and then for only a few. Not until the late 1950s was there a major breakthrough in third party reimbursement. Social forces and the scientific revolution have produced many changes in hospital care. These forces have grown so strong coupled with government regulations and escalating costs that a new organizational structure for hospital systems has been mandated. Hospitals are being forced to become more and more responsive to community health needs, and more accountable to the community for their performance (14).

The economic forces of high cost, capital equipment obsolescence, cost containment directives, reimbursement, and government control are generating pressure on hospitals to share services within a geographic area.

The social forces of population shifts to the cities while health resources move to the suburbs, the push for consumer rights, the increase in the elderly and chronic disease population coupled with a declining birth rate have forced consideration of role modifications in hospitals.

Political forces of government involvement, more pressures to achieve regionalization, cost containment, and the requirement for quality control ensure more comprehensive services. We can expect to see an alteration in the thinking of institutions that will yield a more effective and accessible delivery of care for consumers (15). This means for occupational therapy that we can assist our institutions in their survival while expanding our services into a community model that supports the basic concepts of our profession.

We have many hospital-based occupational therapy programs currently functioning within the community model of occupational therapy service delivery. Two that we can use as models are Memorial Hospital in Sarasota, Florida, directed by Louise Sampson, OTR, and Research Medical Center, Kansas City, Missouri, directed by Sharon East, OTR, and Gloria Scammahorn, OTR. Both programs are in community hospitals of 600 to 700 beds.

At Memorial Hospital, the occupational therapy department contracts with the county school system, Head Start, the Public Health Department, the Home Care Team, the Guidance Center, two extended care facilities, and an outpatient rehabilitation center. Groundwork has been laid for the community's outpatient dialysis unit. Future programs include a private facility for the mentally retarded, day care centers, service programs for the elderly, and a hospice.

At Research Medical Center, the occupational therapy department contracts with schools, nursing homes, and small rural community hospitals. Future programs include industry and home health services.

I asked each of these program directors to respond to the following questions: How do you view outreach in terms of your philosophy of Occupational Therapy practice?

Louise Sampson: *I believe that a hospital-based program is the most effective way to provide "outreach" occupational therapy services. If services are planned and accomplished properly, we do not have to remain a "medical model" and can serve the expressed needs of the community. I feel that the solid base has many advantages including decreasing the fragmentation and isolation of therapists, being cost effective with full utilization of staff and equipment providing more flexible opportunities for professional growth and a general consistency otherwise unavailable* (16).

Sharon East/Gloria Scammahorn: *The outreach concept has certainly facilitated the growth and expansion of occupational therapy into new markets. Our association with a medical center has been an important aspect to the success of occupational therapy's involvement in outreach. Had there been no association with the medical center, I feel certain occupational therapy's efforts would have been stifled early on.*

The whole outreach approach has provided so much stimulation and remotivation for the staff involved that regardless of the outcome the experience for the staff has been well worth all the effort. That is not to say that we're not concerned with the outcome—we still maintain the same standards and quality of care for the outreach contracts as we do for the patients at our facility (17).

The outreach concept provides a stability for services that promotes creativity. It also will assure the continuance of our profession in modern economic times. It expands occupational therapy concepts into a community model with the hospital functioning as the base unit. It reduces the fragmentation and isolation of therapists, it is cost effective, it fully uses staff and equipment, and it promotes professional growth. It allows therapists with specialized skills to use their skill to fill contract hours using their expertise. It also allows facilities that otherwise would not have occupational therapy to obtain the services to fulfill needs.

Public Law 93-641 of 1974, the Health Planning and Resource Development Act, establishes the following priorities for national attention:

1. The provision of primary care services for medically underserved populations, especially those in rural or economically depressed areas.
2. The development of multi-institutional systems for consideration of institutional health services.
3. The development of medical group practices, especially those services that are appropriately coordinated or integrated with institutional health services and health maintenance (18).

Occupational therapists, we have a mandate: break down those walls. We have been accustomed to patients coming to us—we have to go to them. Let us establish occupational therapy as a viable community service implementing the basic philosophy of our profession and help our hospitals survive in the process. The challenge is here now—let us respond and further develop our profession in the process.

Now we will develop our treatment plan for problem three.

Problem III. The Health System Is Not Oriented Toward the Human Being

GOAL: *Develop human oriented programs encouraging man to explore his potential in producing a change in his own health status.* The human that enters the health system has little knowledge of this situation and the health professional little of the individual's situation. We are nothing more than a bystander in the life of that individual until a relationship is formed.

Our service delivery is initiated by assessment with a resulting relationship that has the potential of making impact on that individual.

It would be difficult to expect an individual to be at home in a sterile and unfamiliar environment that has produced chaos. The individual must establish some control over the forces of chaos. In establishing control the client demonstrates a variety of behaviors, either by an internal mental operation or by external activity (19). Occupational therapists have the skills, attitude, and knowledge to provide the relationship and the structure through activity to introduce meaning to that individual and thus give him control.

In *Anatomy of an Illness,* Norman Cousins tells of a personal experience with Pablo Casals that had a profound impact on him. I want to share it with you because it so poignantly expresses activity and its ability to produce meaning in the human.

I learned that a highly developed purpose and a will to live are among the prime raw materials of human existence. I became convinced that these materials may well represent the most potent force within human reach. . . . About Pablo Casals.

I met him for the first time at his home in Puerto Rico just a few weeks before his ninetieth birthday. I was fascinated by his daily routine. About 8 A.M. his lovely young wife Marta would help him to start the day. His various infirmities made it difficult for him to dress himself. Judging from his difficulty in walking and from the way he held his arms, I guessed he was suffering from rheumatoid arthritis. His emphysema was evident in his labored breathing. He came into the living room on Marta's arm. He was badly stooped. His head was pitched forward and he walked with a shuffle. His hands were swollen and his fingers were clenched.

Even before going to the breakfast table, Don Pablo went to the piano—which, I learned, was a daily ritual. He arranged himself with some difficulty on the piano bench, then with discernible effort raised his swollen and clenched fingers above the keyboard.

I was not prepared for the miracle that was about to happen. The fingers slowly unlocked and reached toward the keys like the buds of a plant toward the sunlight. His back straightened. He seemed to breathe more freely. Now his fingers settled on the keys. Then came the opening bars of Bach's Wohltemperierte Klavier, *played with great sensitivity and control. I had forgotten that Don Pablo had achieved proficiency on several musical instruments before he took up the cello. He hummed as he played, then said that Bach spoke to him here—and he placed his hand over his heart.*

Then he plunged into a Brahms concerto and his fingers, now agile and powerful, raced across the keyboard with dazzling speed. His entire body seemed fused with the music: it was no longer still and shrunken but supple and graceful and completely freed of its arthritic coils.

Having finished his piece, he stood up by himself, far straighter and taller than when he had come into the room. He walked to the breakfast table with no trace of a shuffle, ate heartily, talked animatedly, finished the meal, then went for a walk on the beach.

After an hour or so, he came back to the house and worked on his correspondence until lunch. Then he napped. When he arose, the stoop and the shuffle and the clenched hands were back again. . . . As before, he stretched his arms in front of him and extended his fingers. Then the spine straightened and his fingers, hands and arms were in sublime coordination as they responded to the demands of his brain for the controlled beauty of movement and tone. Any cellist thirty years his junior would have been proud to have such extraordinary physical command.

Twice in one day, I had seen the miracle. A man almost ninety, beset with the infirmities of old age, was able to cast off his afflictions, at least temporarily, because he knew he had something of overriding importance to do. There was no mystery about the way it worked, for it happened every day. Creativity for Pablo Casals was the source of his own cortisone. It is doubtful whether any anti-inflammatory medication he would have taken would have been as powerful or as safe as the substances produced by the interaction of his mind and body. . . . He was caught up in his own creativity, in his own desire to accomplish a specific purpose, and the effect was both genuine and observable (20).[1]

We all can recount of patients with strong wills. With the introduction of activity, we too have seen miracles.

As a profession, occupational therapy harnesses will and gives the individual control through activity. That is human, that is care. We are respected by physicians and the health care system for that caring, perhaps because we have a strong background in the physical and biological dimensions of life, as well as the psychological and social. Most importantly we have respect for the human and the unknown. This is empathy.

Brian Hall describes empathy as:

The capacity for one person to enter imaginatively into the sphere of consciousness of another, to feel the specific contour of another experience, to allow one's imagination to risk entering the inner experiencing process of another. (19, p. 162)

---

[1]*Excerpt reprinted from* Anatomy of an Illness, *by Norman Cousins, with the permission of the publisher, W. W. Norton & Company, Inc., New York, New York. Copyright © 1979 by W. W. Norton & Company, Inc.*

Through our professional relationships we reach out and with empathy show that we care hoping that from this caring that the person will find his or her own strength.

The humanistic approach to patient care is the initial reason most health professionals entered their respective careers. Each of us is supposed to remember why we entered the human services system rather than have coursework that would intensify our commitment to the human being by the introduction of theories of humaneness, motivation, and values. I would like to see our curricula increase their program content in the area of values and motivation.

There are other groups of professionals, especially medical sociologists, who are trying to work their way *into* the health system to effect change from within. They desire the position that fields such as occupational therapy hold—that of a primary service, professionally recognized by physicians and reimbursed by third party payment—because we are in the position to implement a total concept of health, a concept of caring. Also we are a recognized part of the health delivery system.

Those who do understand and support the humanism of health delivery must exert their control and influence in shaping the system in that direction. Health programs must be designed that support the patient's need to have control of his life, especially while he is receiving health care. Clinical studies can be designed by occupational therapists relating to the outcome of care when the individual has control over his environment and is valued for his contribution to his care as opposed to giving up control.

A growing body of evidence indicates there are limits to what medicine can be expected to accomplish. There are still many unknowns. There is still healing, there is still coping, and there is still the individual who must survive with dignity.

The major chronic conditions must be dealt with and outside the strict medical model. Improvements in these conditions require significant changes in personal life style, habits, and environmental conditions.

Roger M. Battistella, in his essay "The Future of Primary Health Services," states:

A strong foundation of simple and inexpensive services, for the treatment of routine illness and the care of illness apart from the relief of suffering, is essential.

The importance of personalized relationships for the treatment of illness in which psychological and physical factors are heavily interconnected, the necessity to influence life styles in the management of chronic illness, and the compelling obligations for the humane care of the incurable long-term ill and dying indicates that the relationship between the patient and the health professional displaced by progress in scientific medicine has to be restored. . . . (21, pp. 315–316)

We must move prevention *into* the curative model as we contribute our skills and performance to the population served by the medical care system.

A humanistic health care system is possible—the possibility, however, requires much out of each professional, which decreases the probability. Occupational therapists have unique skills and a tremendous commitment to Man and his abilities. We must show great confidence in implementing our concepts of caring.

I have now presented strategies for three problems the profession must address.

By directing professional energies toward solving these problems we will:

- Develop our services as scientific discipline, thus gain a stronger position with a strong professional identity
- Increase the dialogue of educators and clinicians toward common goals
- Expand the acute care model of service to include an ambulatory and health prevention model
- Extend occupational therapy manpower by expanding services into intercity and rural delivery through multi-hospital systems
- Assist the individual in gaining control over his health status by having control of his environment and engaging in activity.

I want to share with you a very important thought of Bronowski's, from *The Ascent of Man.*

Man is a singular creature. He has a set of gifts which make him unique among the animals so that, unlike them, he is not a figure in the landscape. He is a shaper of the landscape. . . . His imagination, his reason, his emotional subtlety and toughness, make it possible for him not to accept the environment, but to change it (8, p. 19).

This thought is true for us. It is true for each patient or client we serve. Are we a profession that supports change? I believe so.

Another quote from Bronowski:

We are all afraid—for our confidence, for the future, for the world. That is the nature of the human imagination. Yet every man, every civilization, has gone forward because of its engagement with what it has set itself to do. The personal commitment of a man to his skills, the intellectual commitment and the emotional commitment working together as one, has made the Ascent of Man. (8, p. 438)

As a profession and as professionals, let us put our resources, intelligence, and emotional commitment together and work diligently toward the ascent of our profession. The health care system, the clients we serve, and each of us individually will benefit from our commitment.

References

1. *Health and United States,* U.S. Department of Health, Education, and Welfare, Public Health Service, Health Resource Administration, 1978, p iii
2. Brown JHU: *The Health Care Dilemma,* New York: Human Sciences Press, 1978, pp 10–12
3. Cantril H: *Challenges of Humanistic Psychology,* New York: McGraw-Hill, 1967, pp 14–16
4. Battistella RM, Rundell TG: *Health Care Policy in a Changing Environment,* Berkeley: McCutcheon, 1978, pp xv–vxiii
5. Warner DM, Holloway DC: *Decision Making and Control for Health Administration,* Ann Arbor: Health Administration Press, 1978, pp 337–378
6. Glaser RJ: Some Thoughts of Medical Education and Medical Care, Health Manpower Education and Distribution, The Carnegie Commission Report, The Dedication Proceedings, Oct. 12, 13, 14, 1977, pp 65–66
7. Weimer R: *Educational Aspects of The Changing Role of Occupational Therapy,* Committee on Basic Professional Education Educational Forum, Oct. 31, 1969, "O.T." Community Health Alienation vs. Non-alienation, p 9
8. Bronowski J: *The Ascent of Man,* Boston: Little, Brown and Company, 1973, pp 62–64
9. Ad Hoc Committee on Education (Nationally Speaking) Issues in Education. *Am J Occup Ther* 32: 355–358, 1978
10. Von Bertalanffy L: *General Systems Theory,* New York: George Brazier, 1963, p 39
11. Snow CP: *The Two Cultures and a Second Look,* Cambridge: University Press, 1964, p 5
12. Snow CP: *The Search,* New York: Charles Scribner and Sons, 1968, p 49
13. Machlup F: *The Production and Distribution of Knowledge in the United States,* Princeton: Princeton University Press, 1962, p 122
14. Sheps CG: Trends in hospital care. In *Multi Hospital Systems: Strategies for Organization and Management,* Germantown, MD: Aspen Systems Press, 1980, pp 3–4
15. Brown M: Current trends in cooperative ventures. In *Multi Hospital Systems: Strategies for Organization and Management,* Germantown, MD: Aspen Systems Press, 1980, pp 14–19
16. Sampson L: Written Interview with Carolyn Baum, January 1980
17. East S, Scammahorn G, Conery W: Written Interview with Carolyn Baum, January 1980
18. Brown M: Sharing: An overview. In *Multi Hospital Systems: Strategies for Organization and Management,* Germantown, MD: Aspen Systems Press, 1980, pp 96–97
19. Hall BP: *The Development of Consciousness A Confluent Theory of Values,* New York, Paulistic Press, 1976, p 83
20. Cousins N: *Illness as Perceived by the Patient,* Toronto: W. W. Norton and Company, 1979, pp 72–75
21. Battistella RM, Rundell TG: *Health Care Policy in a Changing Environment,* Berkeley: McCutcheon, 1978, pp 315–31

31

1981 Eleanor Clarke Slagle Lecture

Occupational Therapy Revisited:
A *Paraphrastic* Journey

Robert K. Bing, EdD, OTR, FAOTA

I wish to dedicate the 1981 Eleanor Clarke Slagle Lectureship:

To my parents, who provided me with those cumulative experiences and values that inevitably led me to the decision to become an occupational therapist;

To a very great woman, Beatrice D. Wade, OTR, FAOTA, who has been my valued teacher and beloved mentor for more than 30 years;

To my cherished colleagues, Lillian Hoyle Parent and Jay Cantwell, both occupational therapists, who constantly stimulate me and insist on a high level of constructive activity;

To Charles H. Christiansen, OTR, whose personal and professional qualities and insistence on excellence from himself and others assure me of the future of occupational therapy.

Without the examples, teachings, guidance, counseling, and friendship of these individuals, I could never have achieved this exalted opportunity. Try as one might, it is impossible to recount the evolution of occupational therapy so that it resembles the cliff-hanging biographies of Butch Cassidy and the Sundance Kid. Masters and Johnson, as well as Kinsey, who took years to amass their stories, had something going for them that does not exist for us. Somewhat puckishly I was tempted to entitle this paper, *Everything You've Ever Wanted to Know About Occupational Therapy, But Were Afraid to Ask.* That would not have been altogether misleading. Because of my part German heritage, and true to that cultural bias and tendency, I thought I should take us back to the Thirty Years' War and bring everyone up to date. After all, it is important territory occupational therapy has won and lost.

The title, *Occupational Therapy Revisited: A Paraphrastic Journey,* prevailed because this paper is a tour to what should be familiar historical landmarks and progenitors. For some of us, it will renew old friendships and acquaintances. For others, it will be a second-hand account of certain ancestors, not unlike those stories that emanate from grandmothers. For some, it will only be like an endurance of those pictures that inevitably get projected on the screen by vacationers returning home.

Because of the relative youthfulness of those of us in practice (most have entered within the past decade), now seems the time to critically examine our ancestral roots and subsequent grafts to determine the nature of the present and to offer some speculations about why we (and the profession) developed as we did through several generations. This is not *the* history of occupational therapy nor of the Association that supports our endeavors. Nor is it *a* history like someone else might well find it. It is *not* a detailed, definitive account of how we multiplied, divided, and invaded several areas of medicine and health care. It is *one person's* way of telling the story of who we are and citing some lessons to be learned. That is important! After several months of

Originally published 1981 in *American Journal of Occupational Therapy, 35,* 499–518.

submergence just off the coast of Texas (as my colleagues in Galveston will attest), I have at long last come up for air and am ready to declare my findings.

This is a statement of how an idea, born in a philosophical movement, became activated through *the good works of men and women* who inalterably believed in the ideal that those who are sick and handicapped can regain, retain, and attain some semblance of function within the fundamental limitations of the human organism and the expectations of the society in which all must exist: that this may occur through the most obvious means of all—*one's reorganization through occupation, through activity, through leisure, and through rest.*

This journey about occupational therapy, its evolution and development, presents vexation: one must accept a fair number of ambiguities, something some today consider a fundamental problem in occupational therapy; a more than reasonable amount of astonishment; and a certain degree of messiness, closely akin to what is created by the beginner in fingerpainting. What can it all mean? What was taking place at the time? Will the patient recover? Most significantly, does it make any difference? To answer these and related questions I wanted to conduct some scholarly research that could be equally interesting, helpful, and valuable to students, occupational therapy assistants, occupational therapists, and others who are interested in our profession. This is how I interpret the intent of the originators of the Eleanor Clarke Slagle Lectureship.

Such an historical presentation should be long enough to say something, yet short enough to be tolerated.

To give you some idea of the continuing dilemma I encountered these past several months in preparing the lecture and in limiting its scope and length, I wrote:

There once was an historian named Dan,
Whose prose no one could scan,
When, once, asked about it,
He said, "I don't doubt it,
Because I try to cram as many facts and dates into each sentence as I possibly can.

Significant Landmarks

Let us start this paraphrastic journey and take note of some significant landmarks along the way—those recurring patterns and themes of the past 200 years that give us today's relevance:

1. There is an inextricable union of the mind and the body; the employment of activity or occupation must be based on this precept, which is unique to occupational therapy.
2. Activity, inherently, contains modes the patient may employ to gain understanding of and ascendancy over one's feelings, actions, and thoughts: these modes include the habits of attention and interest; the perceived usefulness of occupation; creative expression; the processes of learning; the acquisition of skill; and evidence of accomplishment.
3. Activity provides a balance between the practical and intellectual components of experience; therefore, a wide variety of activities must be accessible to meet human objectives for work, leisure, and rest.
4. One's approach to the patient is as significant to treatment and rehabilitation as is the selection and utilization of an activity.
5. Essential elements of occupational therapy practice are continuous observation, experimentation, empiricism, and analysis.
6. An appreciation of the pain that accompanies any illness or disability; a strong desire to reduce or remove it; a gentle firmness; and a knowledge of the patient's needs are fundamental characteristics of the provider of therapeutic occupations.
7. Therapeutic processes and modes of treatment are synonymous with the processes of learning and methods of education.
8. The patient is the product of his or her own efforts, not the article made nor the activity accomplished.

A Theory of Experience

We could go back to the Garden of Eden to begin this story, if time permitted, since occupational therapy could well have started in that idyllic spot. Dr. Dunton, one of the founders of the 20th century movement, insisted that those fig leaves had to have been crocheted by Eve, who was trying to get over her troubles. They had something to do with her being beholden to Adam and his rib. We will unfortunately pass over all of that and begin the modern epoch with a brief description of what was taking place in Europe approximately 200 years ago.

It was the *Age of Enlightenment,* or, as some prefer, the *Age of Reason.* The roots of 20th century occupational therapy are visible in the empiricism of John Locke, an English philosopher and physician, who fostered confidence in human reason and human freedom; in Etienne de Condillac, a French philosopher, who advanced the dualism of body and mind; and in Pierre Cabanis, a French physician and theorist, who offered an explanation of the importance of the moral and social sciences in perfecting the art of medicine. These three, together with others, popularized the new ideas. Indeed, it was the *best of times,* a clear demarcation in the emergence of the modern world.

If one were to combine the thoughts of these three, one would arrive at a *theory of experience.* John Locke, in his famous *Essay Concerning Human Understanding,* published in 1690 (1), examines the nature of the human mind and the processes by which it learns about and comes to know the world. When born, the human is a blank tablet (tabula rasa). Because of an innate ability to receive sensations from the outside world, the human can assimilate and organize impressions. As contact with the environment stimulates the senses and causes impressions, the mind receives and organizes these into ideas and concepts. Since the human mind does not already contain innate ideas, all must come from without (2, p. 287).

There is a second source for the accumulation of experience, according to Locke. It is the mind itself: ". . . the perception of the operations of our own mind, . . . (such as) thinking, doubting, believing, reasoning, knowing, . . . this source of ideas every man has wholly within himself." (see 3, p. 74) Locke strongly held that the body and mind exist as real entities and they interact. He spent a great deal of time developing his perspective. He spoke of the aim of education as the process of knowing and learning through experience and in striving toward happiness. Ideally, he contended, one should work toward a sound mind in a healthy body. To achieve this ideal, Locke advocated physical exercise as a hardening process, and an exposure to a wide variety of sensations from the physical and social worlds.

Condillac was Locke's apologist. He tried to simplify Locke's fundamental theory by arguing that all conscious experiences are the result of passive sensations; these sensations are the raw materials from which one forms complex and interrelated ideas. Learning is the noting of incomplete ideas, considering each separately, combining them into relationships, and ordering them. This process results in retaining the strongest degrees of association. Condillac asserted: "Then we shall grasp (ideas) easily and clearly and shall understand their origins entirely." (see 3, p. 7)

Elsewhere in his writings Condillac presented his thoughts on analysis. One cannot have the proper conception of a thing until one is in a position to analyze it. "To analyze," claimed Condillac, "is nothing more than to observe in successive order the qualities of an object, . . . the simultaneous order in which they exist." (4, p. 17)

The third philosopher, Pierre Cabanis, tended to apply medicine to philosophy and philosophy to medicine. Cabanis considered illness and its impact upon the formulation of values and ideas. Through the social sciences, which emerged in the *Age of Enlightenment,* he explained *moral* as a psychological phenomenon on a physiological base. He concluded that moral impressions can have both physiological and pathological results. At last, there was a rational explanation for the psychological production of disease in which the so-called moral (emotional) passions play a significant part (see 5, pp. 37–38). Cabanis contributed a socially based theoretical explanation of human experience that became the cornerstone for the moral management of the insane.

Age of Enlightenment and Moral Treatment

Moral treatment of the insane was one result of the *Age of Enlightenment.* It sprang from the fundamental attitudes of the day: a set of principles that govern humanity and society; faith in the ability of the human to reason; and the supreme belief in the individual. The rapid changes caused by this new philosophy advanced the disappearance of the notion that the insane were possessed of the devil. Mental diseases became legitimate concerns of humanitarians and physicians. The discontinuance of the idea that crime, sin, and vice were at the core of insanity brought forth humane treatment. Up to this time the insane had been housed and handled no differently than were criminals or paupers—often in chains.

Two men of the 18th century working in different countries, and unknown to each other, initiated the moral treatment movement. "No two men could possibly have been chosen out of all Europe at that time of whom it could be said more truly that they were cradled, and nursed, and educated among widely differing social, political, religious influences. . . ." (6, pp. 24–25) Philippe Pinel was a child of the French Revolution, a physician, a scholar, and a philosopher. He is described as ". . . far exceeding the bounds of pure humanitarianism . . . to encompass the goals of a naturalist, . . . a reformer, a clinician, . . . and, above all, a philosopher." (7, *Intro*) William Tuke was a devout member of the Society of Friends (Quakers).

Philippe Pinel: Physician–Reformer

Whenever Philippe Pinel's name comes up in a conversation among health professionals, he is immediately mentioned as the *striker of the chains* at two French hospitals. His efforts and contributions go way beyond that reformational act. As a physician, he began his most serious work in 1792 as superintendent of Bicêtre, the asylum for incurable males in Paris.

As a natural scientist, Pinel achieved exceptional skill in the observation of human behavior and the bringing of ". . . some order into the chaos of . . . treatment methods by means of critical and objective investigations." (5, p. 42) Pinel says this about himself: *Desirous of better information, I resolved for myself the facts that were presented to my attention; and forgetting the empty honours of my titular distinction as a physician, I viewed the scene that was opened to me with the eye of common sense and unprejudiced observation.* (8, p. 109) From his own experience, he urged that observations ". . . be the basis upon which (one) should decide what opinions to believe." (see 9, pp. 74–75) Throughout his work, he held constantly before him his own motto of independent thought: "Chercher à èviter toute illusion, toute prèvention, toute opinion adoptèe sur parole" (to seek to avoid all illusion, all prejudice, all opinion taken on authority; see 10, pp. 8–9).

Pinel's descriptions of the mentally deranged provide insight into his own compassionate nature. For him, the loss of reason was the most calamitous of human afflictions. The ability to reason principally separates the human from other living forms. Because of mental illness, the human's ". . . character is always perverted, sometimes annihilated. His thoughts and actions are diverted. . . . His personal liberty is at length taken from him. . . . To this melancholy train of symptoms, if not early and judiciously treated . . . a state of the most abject degradation sooner or later succeeds." (8, pp. xv–xvii)

What Pinel entitled *revolution morale,* or moral revolution, is the ultimate insight of the insane into the delusional and absurd nature of their experiences (7, p. 256). This, to him, was the basis for treatment. Some historians believe that he was stating that moral treatment is synonymous with the humane approach. His own writings do not bear this out. Pinel believed that each patient must be critically observed and analyzed; then treatment should commence. "To apply the principles of moral treatment, with undiscriminating uniformity, would be . . . ridiculous and unadviseable." (8, p. 66) The moral method is well reasoned and carefully planned for the individual patient.

According to Pinel, moral management is a maintained continuity of approach; a predictable routine, infused with vigor by personnel who inspire confidence. Moreover, moral treatment calls for a constant, observed study of patient behavior and performance. It includes a gentle, but firm approach. Each patient is given as much liberty within the institution as he or she can tolerate. The approach is designed to give the patient a feeling of security as well as a respect for authority. Pinel asserted: "The atmosphere should be the same as in a family where the parents are quite strict. To establish this relationship, the doctor must convince the patient that he wishes to help him and that recovery is a real possibility." (see 9, p. 76)

Occupations figured prominently in Pinel's conception of moral treatment. He used activities to take the patients' thoughts away from their emotional problems and to develop their abilities. He considered literature and music as effective in altering patients' emotions. Physical exercise and work should be part of every institution's fundamental program and be employed in accord with individual tastes. He concluded: "The (occupations) method is primarily designed and intended to reach man at his best which . . . means human understanding, intelligence, and insight." (see 3, pp. 63–64)

The concept of *moral treatment* belongs solely to Philippe Pinel. His fundamental belief was that its purpose is to restore the patient to himself, ". . . to use the patient's own emotions to balance his emotional excesses." (see 9, p. 76) Truly, Pinel and his efforts, rooted in the *Age of Enlightenment,* mark the beginning of the modern epoch in the care of the mentally ill.

William Tuke: Philanthropist–Humanitarian

Across the channel, in England, things were astir at the same time. King George III, who was giving the American colonies fits, was himself in similar trouble. In 1788 it became public knowledge that the King was seized with mania. Questions arose about his fitness to continue ruling. Nevertheless, public sentiment was on his side. For the first time, insanity and its treatment formed a topic of public discussion: "The subject had been brought out of concealment in a way which defeated the conspiracy of silence." (see 11, p. 42) This being the *Age of Enlightenment,* the public openly sympathized with the sufferer; there was no condemnation. No one suggested that the King was being visited by the Devil, or that he was being punished for his sins.

The Society of Friends, derisively called *Quakers,* originated in 17th century England and became one of the most distinctive movements of Puritanism: "They arose out of the religious unrest of England . . . and stood for a radical kind of reform within Christendom which contrasted sharply with Protestant, Anglican and Roman patterns alike." (12, p. 118) George Fox, founder of the Society, discovered ". . . the spirit of the living Christ and knew that it was an experience open to all men. 'This was the true light that lighteth every man that cometh into the world!' " (13, p. 1)

William Tuke, a devout Quaker, wealthy merchant, and renowned philanthropist, was made aware of the deplorable conditions in the insane asylum in York, England. There were tales of extreme neglect and possible cruelty. He was an unusual man, not given to listening to sensational reports and acting rashly (14, p. 12). In true Quaker fashion Tuke presented a concern at a Friend's Quarterly Meeting in the spring of 1792—that an institution for the insane be established in York under the direction of the Society. At first, he was met with considerable resistance by those who believed that there were too few mentally ill Quakers, and that no one would want them concentrated in such a lovely, quiet locale (15, p. 58).

The York Retreat

Initially, Tuke was disheartened; yet, he pressed on, and within 6 months *The Retreat for Persons* afflicted with *Disorders of the Mind,* or simply, *The Retreat* came into being. Up until then the term *Retreat* had never been applied to an asylum. Tuke's daughter-in-law suggested the term to convey the Quaker belief that such an institution may be ". . . a place in which the unhappy might obtain refuge; a quiet haven in which (one) . . . might find a means of reparation or of safety." (16, p. 20) The cornerstone simply stated the purpose of the institution: "The charity or love of friends executed this work in the cause of humanity." (15, p. 19)

William Tuke became the superintendent. Thomas Fowler, an unusually open-minded man, was appointed visiting physician. After a trial-and-error period, they came to believe that moral treatment methods were preferable to those involving restraint and use of harsh drugs. The new approach was a product of Tuke's humanitarianism and Fowler's empiricism.

Several fundamental principles became evident within a short time. The approach was primarily one of kindness and consideration. The patients were not thought to be devoid of reason, feeling, and honor. The social environment was to be as nearly like that of a family as possible, with an atmosphere of religious sentiment and moral feeling (16, p. 35).

Tuke and Fowler strongly believed that most insane people retain a considerable amount of self-command. Upon admission, the patient was informed that treatment depended largely upon one's own conduct. Employment in various occupations was expected as a way for the patient to maintain control over his or her disorder. As Tuke reported: ". . . regular employment is perhaps the most efficacious; and those kinds of employment . . . to be preferred . . . are accompanied by considerable bodily action." (16, p. 156) The staff endeavored to gain the patient's confidence and esteem, to arrest the attention and fix it upon objects opposite to any illusion the patient might have. The fundamental purpose of employment and recreation was to facilitate the regaining of the *habit of attention,* as Tuke called it. Various learning exercises were used, such as mathematical problems, to help the patient gain ascendancy over faulty habits of attention.

Tuke and Fowler determined that "indolence has a natural tendency to weaken the mind, and to induce ennui and discontent. . . ." (16, pp. 180–181) A wide range of occupations and amusements was available. Patients not engaged in useful occupations were allowed to read, draw, or play various games. Tea parties, walks, and visitations away from the institution were planned regularly in preparation for the patients' returning home. All activities were closely analyzed through observation in order to individualize patients' needs.

The pioneer work of William Tuke and his son, Samuel, who wrote the definitive treatise on *The Retreat,* opened a new chapter in the history of the care of the insane in England. Mild management methods, infused with kindness, and building self-esteem through the judicious use of occupations, resulted in the excitation and elicitation of superior, human motives. Patients recovered, left *The Retreat,* and rarely needed to return for further care. The entire regimen was carefully patterned ". . . to accord (patients) the dignity and status of sick human beings." (17, p. 687)

Moral Treatment Expansion

As soon as Pinel's major work on moral treatment (1801) and Samuel Tuke's description of *The Retreat* were published (1813), there was a rush toward implementing many reforms in other hospitals, particularly in England and the United States. In both countries occupations were introduced as an integral part of moral treatment (18, pp. 83–84). Some unusual experiments were undertaken by Sir William Charles Ellis, a physician, who became the superintendent of a pauper lunatic asylum. The mainstay of his asylum management was useful occupations. He moved well ahead of mere amusements and "introduced a gainful employment of patients on a large scale and even had them taught a trade." (19, p. 62) Ellis and his wife undertook other reforms. She organized the women patients into groups under the supervision of a *workwoman* to make useful and fancy articles.

Another Ellis innovation was the development of what would eventually be called *halfway houses*. Keenly aware of environmental and social influences on insanity, Ellis suggested ". . . after-care houses and night hospitals as a stepping stone from the asylum to the world by which . . . the length of patients' stay would be reduced and in many cases the cure completed. . . ." (17, p. 871) He insisted that convalescing patients should go out and mix with the world before discharge. His proposals were made in the 1830s!

In the United States, few public and private asylums existed in the post-Revolutionary era; however, institutional reforms were needed. Any recounting of this period must include two very important individuals and their work: Benjamin Rush and Dorothea Lynde Dix. Their efforts did not overlap; they did not know one another; nor was one influenced by the other. Just as in the cases of Pinel and Tuke, no two individuals this side of the Atlantic could have been more unlike one another in background, education, or experience. Nevertheless, each recognized the hapless plights of the institutionalized insane and set out to alleviate dire conditions and the inauguration of moral treatment, including occupations and exercise.

Benjamin Rush: Father of American Psychiatry

Benjamin Rush, often referred to as the *father of American psychiatry*, was a Philadelphia physician in the latter half of the 1700s. Through his training in Europe and several visits there, he adopted many of Pinel's practices; however, Rush did not adopt moral principles until later. As a member of the staff of Pennsylvania Hospital, he was placed in charge of a separate section set aside for the insane, the first hospital in America to reserve such a section. He was appalled by the conditions and he appealed to the staff and the public for change. Change did come and humane treatment was instituted. Rush saw to it that "certain employments be devised for such of the deranged people as are capable of working. . . ." (see 20, p. 257) This approach was based upon his philosophical stance that man, by his very nature, is meant to be active; "Even in paradise (Garden of Eden) he was employed in the health and pleasant exercises of cultivating a garden. Happiness, consisting in folded arms, and in pensive contemplation . . . by the side of brooks, never had any existence, except in the brains of mad poets, and love-sick girls and boys." (21, pp. 115–116)

In his major writing, *Medical Inquiries and Observations Upon the Diseases of the Mind*, Rush clearly differentiates between goal-directed activity and aimless exercise: "Labour has several advantages over exercise, in being not only more stimulating, but more endurable in its effects; . . . it is calculated to arrest wrong habits of action, and to restore such as regular and natural. . . ." (21, pp. 224–225)

Dorothea Lynde Dix: Humanitarian–Reformer

Dorothea Lynde Dix, a reform-minded humanitarian during the middle 1800s, vehemently pressed for improved conditions of the insane who were incarcerated in jails and almshouses. She presented a number of *Memorials* to state legislatures, believing that the public had an obligation to care for such individuals. By 1848 numerous states had responded to her efforts, and she decided to tackle a more formidable object—the Federal government. Dix envisioned the sale of public lands to finance the building of a federal system of hospitals for the indigent blind, deaf and mute, as well as the insane. For 6 years she wheedled and cajoled members of the Congress. Finally, in 1854, the bill was ready for President Franklin Pierce's signature. He was a close friend of Miss Dix and she felt highly confident of the outcome. The President vetoed the bill claiming unconstitutionality: ". . . every human weakness or sorrow would take advantage of this bill if it became law. . . . It endangers states' rights." (see 22, p. 20) Through her contacts with physicians in several states, Miss Dix embraced moral treatment as the most humane method. She strongly advocated ". . . decent care, quiet, affection and normal activity (as) the only medicine for the insane." (see 22, p. 11)

United States: Individual Treatment, Occupations, Education

The Quakers brought moral treatment to the United States as part of their intellectual and religious luggage. Through published accounts about *The Retreat* in York, some private asylums were established in which moral principles were practiced. A number of public institutions altered their programs to include individualized treatment, occupations, and education. Those patients who had remained for years unimproved and listless, even on the verge of apathy ". . . are seen in encouraging instances, when transferred to attendants who have more disposition to attend to them, . . . to waken (them) from their torpor, to become animated, active and even industrious. . . ." (23, pp. 487–488)

Moral management also was taking on a new facet: the influence of a sane mind upon the insane mind. Those who daily attended the sick were to impress upon the insane the influences of their own character, designed to specifically improve the patients' behavior. Personnel must possess a number of traits: observational skills to see the "... actual condition of the patient's mind ... and a faculty of clear insight. ..." (23, p. 489) Other traits: "... seeing that which is passing in the minds of (patients). ... Add to this a firm will, the faculty of self-control, a sympathizing distress at moral pain, a strong desire to remove it. ..." (23, p. 489)

Arguments appeared in the literature relative to the moral use of firmness and gentleness. Strong cases were made for both extremes; however, it took two alienists (the precursor to psychiatrist), John Bucknill and D. Hack Tuke, grandson of Samuel Tuke, in 1858 to settle the dispute: "The truth, as usual, lies between; and the (individual) who aims at success in the moral treatment of the insane must be ready to be all things to all men, if by any means he might save some" (23, p. 500). They elaborate on their thesis by stating: "With self-reliance, ... it requires widely different manifestations, to repress excitement, to stimulate inertia, to check the vicious, to comfort the depressed, to direct the erring, to support the weak, to supplant every variety of erroneous opinion, to resist every kind of perverted feeling, and to check every form of pernicious conduct." (23, p. 500)

Bucknill and Tuke also wrote that moral treatment included the gaining of the patient's confidence, fixing his or her attention on interesting and wholesome objects of thought, diverting the mind from introspection, and loosening the hold on concentrated emotion. They explain: "For (these) purposes useful occupation is far superior to any form of amusement. The higher the purpose, and the more appellant the nature of the occupation ... the more likely it is to draw him from the contemplation of self-wretchedness, and effect the triumph of moral influences." (23, p. 493)

The next step in institutional occupations emphasized education. Those occupations that require a process of learning and thought were determined far preferable, from a curative point of view, than those that require none. "Moral treatment is as wide as that of education; ... it is education applied to the field of mental phenomena. ..." (23, p. 501) Therefore, it was not unusual to find specific mental activities included with occupations. The purpose was to educate the individual in order to provide him or her with "the power of controlling his feelings, and his thoughts, and his actions." (24, pp. 166–167)

With continued experience, a number of alienists decided that occupations and amusements also could serve as a prophylactic against insanity. One interesting prescription for the return and maintenance of sanity was: "... rest in bed, occupation, exercise and amusements." (25, p. 14) D. Hack Tuke declared: "If idleness is a curse to the sane, it is the parent of mischief and ennui to the insane, especially to the pubescent and adolescent." (26, p. 1315) He urges that the same approach be taken with the sane and the insane: "Employment, Nature's universal law of health, alike for body and mind, is specially beneficial, ... seeing that it displaces ideas by new and healthy thoughts, revives familiar habits of daily activity, restores (and maintains) self-respect while it promotes the general bodily health." (26, p. 1315)

Decline of Moral Treatment

Moral management and treatment by occupations reached its zenith in the United States just before the outbreak of the War Between the States (Civil War). Corporate, private asylums continued to expand their efforts. State- and public-supported institutions withdrew their programs, so that by the last quarter of the 19th century, virtually no moral treatment was taking place.

Several reasons for this decline and eventual disappearance can be identified, including a nation at war with itself. Bockhoven cites others: 1. the founders of the U.S. movement retired and died, leaving no disciples or successors; 2. the rapidly increasing influx of foreign-born and poor patients greatly overtaxed existing facilities and required more institutions to be built with diminished tax support; 3. racial and religious prejudices on the part of the alienists, beginning to be called psychiatrists, reduced interest in treatment and cure; and 4. state legislatures became increasingly more interested in less costly custodial care (27, pp. 20–25).

Essentially, there was no place in the public institutions for moral treatment. "The inferior physical plants and facilities, poorly trained and insufficient staff, . . . and, worst of all, overcrowding, prohibited any attempts to practice moral management." (28, p. 128) A belief emerged that many insane were incurable. One eminent psychiatrist stated: "I have come to the conclusion that when a man becomes insane, he is about used up for this world." (29, p. 155) Such pessimism was predominant for a century in this country. Custodial care had come to stay for a very long time.

As we shall see next, moral principles and practices emerged in the early years of the 20th century through the efforts of individuals, then by a group who founded an organization dedicated to those principles. This group, in collaboration with others, established a definition and fundamental principles that have carried over through several generations of specifically educated practitioners of occupational therapy.

Once again, as with Pinel and Tuke, Rush and Dix, the individuals who founded and pioneered the 20th century occupational therapy movement could not have been more diverse in their backgrounds, experience, and education. They included a nurse, two architects, a physician, a social worker, and a teacher.

Susan Tracy: Occupational Nurse

Susan Tracy was this century's first proponent of occupations for invalids. A trained nurse, she initiated instruction in activities to student nurses as early as 1905 as part of their expanding responsibilities. She also developed the term *occupational nurses* to signify specialization (30, p. 401). By 1912 she decided to devote all her energies to patient activities and she distinguished herself by applying moral treatment principles to acute conditions. As Tracy stated, "The application of this most rational remedy to ordinary, everyday sick people, as found in the general hospital, is almost unknown." (31, p. 386) She strongly claimed that remedial treatments "are classified according to their physiological effects as stimulants, sedatives, anesthetics . . . , etc. Certain occupations possess like properties." (31, p. 386) The physician may select stimulating occupations, such as watercoloring and paper folding; or sedative occupations such as knitting, weaving, basketry.

Throughout Tracy's many years of work she employed experimentation and observation to enhance her practice. Her carefully worded writings provide ample evidence of her intense desire to bring scientific principles to the application of invalid occupations. In 1918 she published a remarkable research paper on 25 mental tests derived from occupations; for example, by instructing the patient in using a piece of leather and a pencil, "require him to make a line of dots at equal distances around the margin and at uniform distances from the edge. This constitutes a test of *Judgment* in estimating distances." (32, p. 15) Continuing with the same piece of leather, the patient is instructed to punch a hole at each dot. "In order to do this he must consider the two sides of leather, the two parts of his tool and bring these together thus making a *Simple Coordination* test." (32, p. 16) Other tests in the fabrication of the leather purse include *Aesthetic Coordination and Rhythm, Differentiation of Form and Size, Purposeful Relation*. In all 25 tests, she stressed a completed, useful and "not unbeautiful" object.

Tracy's other writings state the value and usefulness of discarded materials to successful ward work (33, p. 62). She also emphasized high quality workmanship: "It is now believed that what is worth doing at all is worth doing well, and that practical, well-made articles have a greater therapeutic value than a useless, poorly made article." (34, p. 198) A premium is placed upon originality and the ". . . adoption of the occupation to the condition and natural tastes of the patient." (35, p. 63) Further, she believes that ". . . the patient is the product, not the article that he makes." (see 33, p. 59)

Tracy's major work, *Studies in Invalid Occupation,* published in 1918 (36), is a revealing compendium of her observations and experiences with different kinds of patients, for instance: "the child of poverty and the child of wealth, the impatient boy, grandmother, the business man."

By 1921, Susan Tracy had adopted the term *occupation therapy* originally coined by William Rush Dunton, Jr., and defined it and differentiated it from vocational training. She felt this was necessary because of the arising confusion between the two concepts following World War I. She wrote: "What is occupation? The treatment of disease by occupation. . . . The aim of occupation is to get the man well; that of vocational training is to provide him with a job. Any well man will look for a job, but the sick man is looking for health." (37, p. 120)

Throughout all of her writings she stated that nothing is ". . . too small to be pressed into the service of resourceful mind and trained hands toward . . . the establishment of a healthy mind in a healthy body." (33, p. 57)

George Barton: Re-education of Convalescents

George Edward Barton, by profession an architect, contracted tuberculosis in his adult life. This plagued him for the remainder of his years. His constant struggle led him into a life of service to the physically handicapped. Out of his own personal concerns came the establishment of Consolation House, an early prototype of a rehabilitation center. He was an effective speaker and writer, often given to hyperbole; he gained his point with the listening or reading public.

Barton's central themes were hospitals and their responsibility to the discharged patient; the conditions the discharged patient faces; the need to return to employment; occupations and re-education of convalescents. These were intense concerns to him because of his own health problems.

His first published article, derived from a speech given to a group of nurses, points out a weakness he perceived in hospitals: "We discharge from them not efficients, but inefficients. An individual leaves almost any of our institutions only to become a burden upon his family, his friends, the associated charities, or upon another institution." (38, p. 328) In the same article, he warms to his subject: "I say to discharge a patient from the hospital, with his fracture healed, to be sure, but to a devastated home, to an empty desk and to no obvious sustaining employment, is to send him out to a world cold and bleak. . . ." (38, p. 329) His solution: ". . . occupation would shorten convalescence and improve the condition of many patients." (38, p. 329) He ended his oration with a rallying cry: ". . . it is time for humanity to cease regarding the hospital as a door closing upon a life which is past and to regard it henceforth as a door opening upon a life which is to come." (38, p. 330)

Barton established Consolation House in Clifton Springs, New York. Those referred to his institution underwent a thorough review, including a social and medical history, and a consideration of one's education, training, experience, successes, and failures. Barton believed that "By considering these in relation to the condition (the patient) must presumably or inevitably be in for the remainder of his life, we can find some form of occupation for which he will be fitted. . . ." (39, p. 336) He claimed that Consolation House was "getting down to our social difficulties." (39, p. 337)

By 1915, Barton had adopted Dunton's term, *occupation therapy,* but preferred the adjectival form: occupational therapy. He declared: "If there is an occupational disease, why not an occupational therapy?" (40, p. 139) He expansively stated: "The first thing to be done . . . is for occupational therapy to provide an occupation which will produce *a similar therapeutic effect to that of every drug in materia medica.* An exercise for each separate organ, joint, and muscle of the human body. An exercise? An occupation! An occupation? A useful occupation! Then (occupational therapy) can fill the doctor's prescriptions . . . written in the terms of materia medica." (40, p. 139) He even advocated a laxative by *occupation.*

Re-education entered Barton's terminology with the aftermath of World War I. He viewed hospitals as taking on a mission different from that previously adopted. A hospital should become ". . . a re-educational institution through which to put the waste products of society *back and into the right place."* (40, p. 139) Using alliteration, he declared: ". . . by a catalystic concatenation of contiguous circumstances we were forced to realize that when all is said and done, what the sick man really needed and wanted most was the restoration of his ability to work, to live independently and to make money." (41, p. 320)

Barton's major contribution to the re-emergence of moral treatment was the awakening of physical re-construction and re-education through the employment of occupations. Convalescence, to him, was a critical time for the inclusion of something to do. Activity ". . . clarifies and strengthens the mind by increasing and maintaining interest in wholesome thought to the exclusion of morbid thought . . . and a proper occupation . . . during conva-lescence may be made the basis of the corollary of a new life upon recovery. . . . I mean *a job, a better job, or a job done better* than it was before." (42, p. 309) With Susan Tracy, Barton held that the major consideration of occupations ". . . should be devoted to the therapeutic and education effects, not to the value of the possible product." (43, p. 36)

William Rush Dunton, Jr.: Judicious Regimen of Activity

Of the founders of the 20th century movement, William Rush Dunton, Jr., was the most prolific writer and the most influential. He published in excess of 120 books and articles related to occupational therapy and rehabilitation; served as president of the National Society for the Promotion of Occupational Therapy; and, for 21 years, was editor of the official journal. As a physician, he spent his professional career treating psychiatric patients in an institutional setting. Key to his treatment methods is occupational therapy, a term he coined to differentiate aimless amusements from those occupations definitely prescribed for their therapeutic benefits. Before embarking on what he called *a judicious regimen of activity,* he read the works of Tuke and Pinel, as well as the efforts of significant alienists of the 19th century.

From his readings and from observations of patients in Sheppard Asylum, a Quaker institution in Towson, Mary-land, Dunton concluded that the acutely ill are generally not amenable to occupations or recreation. The acutely ill exhibit a weakened power of attention. Occupations at this time would be fatiguing and harmful. The prevailing prescription is ". . . to let the patient alone, meanwhile improve (his) condition, restore and revivify exhausted men-tal and physical forces. . . ." (44, p. 19) Later, activities should be selected that use energies not needed for physical restoration. Stimulating attention and directing the thoughts of the patient in regular and healthful paths would ensure an early release from the hospital. Dunton developed a wide variety of activities from knitting and crochet-ing to printing and the repair of dynamos, in order to gain the attention and interest, as well as to meet the needs, of all patients.

Dunton's proclivities for history and research led him to extensive readings and experimentations—all related to the human, his need for work, leisure, rest, and sleep; the causal factors of mental aberrations; various cures of mental illness. Each excursion brought him back to *a judicious regimen of activity* as the treatment of choice, regard-less of whether the patient was mentally or physically ill. He became more and more convinced that attention and interest in one's work and play are as efficacious, if not more so, than the many and varied other medications avail-able. He stated it this way: "It has been found that a patient makes more rapid progress if his attention is concen-trated upon what he is making and he derives stimulating pleasure in its performance." (45, p. 19)

At the second annual meeting of the National Society for the Promotion of Occupational Therapy (AOTA) in 1918, Dunton unveiled his nine cardinal rules to guide the emerging practice of occupational therapy, and to ensure that the new discipline would gain acceptance as a medical entity: 1. Any activity in which the patient engages should have as its objective a cure. 2. It should be interesting; 3. have a useful purpose other than merely to gain the patient's attention and interest; and 4. preferably lead to an increase in knowledge on the patient's part. 5. Curative activity should preferably be carried on with others, such as in a group. 6. The occupational therapist should make a careful study of the patient in order to know his or her needs and attempt to meet as many as possible through activity. 7. The therapist should stop the patient in his or her work before reaching a point of fatigue; and 8. encour-agement should be genuinely given whenever indicated. Finally, 9. work is much to be preferred over idleness, even when the end product of the patient's labor is of a poor quality or is useless (46, pp. 26–27).

The major purposes of occupation in the case of the mentally ill were outlined in Dunton's first book (47, pp. 24–26). The primary objective is to divert the attention either from unpleasant subjects, as is true with the depressed patient; or from day-dreaming or mental ruminations, as in the case of the patient suffering from dementia praecox (schizophrenia)—that is, to divert the attention to one main subject.

Another purpose of occupation is to re-educate—to train the patient in developing mental processes through "... educating the hands, eyes, muscles, just as is done in the developing child." (47, p. 25) Fostering an interest in hobbies is a third purpose. Hobbies serve as present, as well as future, safety valves and render a recurrence of mental illness less likely. A final purpose may be to instruct the patient in a craft until he or she has enough proficiency to take pride in his or her work. However, Dunton did note that "While this is proper, I fear ... specialism is apt to cause a narrowing of one's mental outlook.... The individual with a knowledge of many things has more interest in the world in general." (47, p. 26)

Dunton continued to write and publish his observations, each one elaborating on a previous one. His texts became required reading for students preparing for practice. Even in his 90s, well beyond retirement from practice, he maintained an interest in our profession and continued to offer counsel.

Eleanor Clarke Slagle: Founder–Pioneer

Eleanor Clarke Slagle qualifies as both a founder and a pioneer. She was at the birth of the Association in 1917. Before that time she had received part of her education in social work and had completed one of the early Special Courses in Curative Occupations and Recreation at the Chicago School of Civics and Philanthropy. Following this, she taught in two courses for attendants of the insane; directed the occupations program at Henry Phipps Clinic, Johns Hopkins Hospital, Baltimore, under Dr. Adolf Meyer; returned to Chicago to become the Superintendent of Occupational Therapy at Hull House. Later, Mrs. Slagle moved to New York where she pioneered in developing occupational therapy in the State Department of Mental Hygiene. In addition, she served with high distinction in every elective office of the American Occupational Therapy Association, including President (1919–1920) and as a paid Executive Secretary for 14 years (see 48, pp. 122–125); (see 49, pp. 473–474); (50, p. 18); (see 51).

She found occupational therapy to be "... an awkward term ..." but felt "... it has been well defined as a form of remedial treatment consisting of various types of activities ... which either contribute to or hasten recovery from disease or injury ... carried on under medical supervision and that it be *consciously* motivated." Further, she emphasized that occupational therapy must be "a *consciously* planned progressive program of *rest, play, occupation and exercise....*" (52, p. 289) In addition, she explained it is "... an effort toward normalizing the lives of countless thousands who are mentally ill, ... the normal mechanism of a fairly well balanced day." (53, p. 14) She enjoyed quoting C. Charles Burlingame, a prominent psychiatrist of her day: " 'What is an occupational therapist? She is that newer medical specialist who takes the joy out of invalidism. She is the medical specialist who carries us over the dangerous period between acute illness and return to the world of men and women as a useful member of society.' " (52, pp. 290–291)

Slagle placed considerable emphasis upon the personality factor of the therapist: "... the proper balance of qualities, proper physical expression, a kindly voice, gentleness, patience, ability and seeming vision, adaptability ... to meet the particular needs of the individual patient in all things.... Personality plus character also covers an ability to be honest and firm, with infinite kindness...." (54, p. 13)

The issue would constantly arise about the use of handicrafts as a therapeutic measure in the machine age. Her response is a classic: "... handicrafts are so generally used, not only because they are so diverse, covering a field from the most elementary to the highest grade of ability; but also, and greatly to the point, because their development is based on primitive impulses. They offer the means of contact with the patient that no other medium does or can offer. Encouragement of creative impulses also may lead to the development of large interests outside oneself and certainly leads to social contact, an important consideration with any sick or convalescent patient." (52, pp. 292–293)

Habit training was first attempted at Rochester (New York) State Hospital in 1901. Slagle adopted the basic principles and developed a far greater perspective and use among mental patients who had been hospitalized from 5 to 20 years and who had steadily regressed. The fundamental plan was ". . . to arrange a twenty four hour schedule . . . in which physicians, nurses, attendants and occupational therapeutists play a part. . . ." (54, p. 13) It was a re-education program designed to overcome some disorganized habits, to modify others and construct new ones, with the goal that habit reaction will lead toward the restoration and maintenance of health. "In habit training, we show clearly an academic philosophy factor . . . that is, the necessity of requiring attention, of building on the habit of attention—attention thus becomes application, voluntary and, in time, agreeable." (54, p. 14)

The purposes of habit training were two-fold: the reclamation and rehabilitation of the patient, with the eventual goal of discharge or parole; and, if this was not reasonable, to assist the patient in becoming less of an institutional problem, that is, less destructive and untidy.

A typical habit training schedule called for the patients to arise in the morning at 6:00, wash, toilet, brush teeth, and air beds; then breakfast; return to ward and make beds, sweep; then classwork for 2 hours, which consisted of a variety of simple crafts and marching exercises. After lunch, there was a rest period; continued classwork and outdoor exercises, folk dancing, and lawn games. Following supper, there was music and dancing on the ward, followed by toileting, washing, brushing the teeth, and preparing for bed (55, p. 29).

Once the patient had received maximum benefit from habit training, he or she was ready to progress through three phases of occupational therapy. The first was what Slagle called *the kindergarten group*. "We must show the ways and means of stimulating the special senses. The employment of color, music, simple exercises, games and storytelling along with occupations, the gentle ways and means . . . (used) in educating the child are equally important in reeducating the adult. . . ." (54, p. 14) Occupations were graded from the simple to the complex.

The next phase was *ward classes in occupational therapy* ". . . graded to the limit of accomplishment of individual patients." (56, p. 100) When able to tolerate it, the patient joined in group activities. The third and final phase was the *occupational center*. "This promotes opportunities for the more advanced projects . . . (a) complete change in environment; . . . comparative freedom; . . . actual responsibilities placed upon patients; the stimulation of seeing work produced; . . . all these carry forward the readjustment of patients." (56, p. 102)

This founder, this pioneer, this distinguished member of our profession provided a summary of her own accomplishments and philosophy by stating: "Of the highest value to patients is the psychological fact that the patient is working for himself. . . . Occupational Therapy recognizes the significance of the mental attitude which the sick person takes toward his illness and attempts to make that attitude more wholesome by providing activities adapted to the capacity of the individual patient and calculated to divert his attention from his own problems." (54, p. 290) Further, she declared: "It is directed activity, and differs from all other forms of treatment in that it is given in increasing doses as the patient improves." (see 57, p. 3)

Adolph Meyer: Philosophy of Occupational Therapy

Dr. Adolph Meyer is cited in this account of the evolution of occupational therapy because of his outstanding support and because his approach to clinical psychiatry was entirely consistent with the emerging occupational therapy movement.

Adolph Meyer, a Swiss physician, immigrated to the United States in 1892 and accepted a position initially as pathologist at the Eastern Illinois Hospital for the Insane in Kankakee. Over the next 14 years he held various positions in the United States and became professor of psychiatry at Johns Hopkins University in 1910. Throughout this period he developed the fundamentals of what was to become the psychobiological approach to psychiatry, a term he coined to indicate that the human is an indivisible unit of study, rather than a composite of symptoms. "Psychobiology starts not from a mind and a body or from elements, but from the fact that we deal with biologically organized units and groups and their functioning . . . the 'he's' and 'she's' of our experience—the bodies we find in action. . . ." (58, p. 263) Meyer took strong issue with those in medicine: ". . . who wish to reduce everything to physics and chemistry, or to anatomy, or to physiology, and within that to neurology. . . ." (58, p. 262) His enlightened point of view is that one can only be studied as a total being in action and that this ". . . whole person represents an integrate of hierarchically arranged functions." (see 59, p. 1317)

His common sense approach to the problems of psychiatry was his keynote: "The main thing is that your point of reference should always be life itself. . . . I put my emphasis upon specificity. . . . As long as there is life there are positive assets—action, choice, hope, not in the imagination but in a clear understanding of the situation, goals and possibilities. . . . To see life as it is, to tend toward objectivity is one of the fundamentals of my philosophy, my attitude, my preference. It is something that I would recommend if it can be kept free of making itself a pest to self and to others." (see 60, pp. vi–xi)

From the very beginning of his work in Illinois, he was concerned with meaningful activity. In time, it became the fundamental issue in treatment. "I thought primarily of occupation therapy," he stated, "of getting the patient to do things and getting things going which did not work but which could work with proper straightening out." (see 60, p. 45) In a report to the Governor of the State of Illinois in 1895, Meyer wrote: "Occupation is, with good right, the most essential side of hygienic treatment of most insane patients." (see 60, p. 59)

By 1921, Meyer had become Professor of Psychiatry at Johns Hopkins University in Baltimore, and had had extensive experiences with others, such as William Rush Dunton, Jr., Eleanor Clarke Slagle, and Henrietta Price, leaders in the occupational therapy movement. At the Fifth Annual Meeting of the National Society for the Promotion of Occupational Therapy in Baltimore, October 1921, Meyer brought together his fundamental concepts of psychobiology to produce his paper, *The Philosophy of Occupational Therapy*. Through time, this has become a classic in the occupational therapy literature. It bears study by all of us.

Psychobiology is clearly visible in his statement that ". . . the newer conceptions of *mental problems* (are) *problems of living,* and not merely diseases of a structural and toxic nature. . . ." (61, p. 4) The indivisibility and integration of the human are cited in this manner: "Our conception of man is that of an organism that maintains and balances itself in the world of reality and actuality by being in active life and active use. . . ." (61, p. 5)

Because of the nature of his paper, *The Philosophy of Occupational Therapy,* Meyer emphasized occupation, time, and the productive use of energy. Interwoven are the elements of psychobiology. He stated: "The whole of human organization has its shape in a kind of rhythm. . . . There are many . . . rhythms which we must be attuned to: the larger rhythms of night and day, of sleep and waking hours . . . and finally the big four—work and play and rest and sleep, which our organism must be able to balance even under difficulty. The only way to attain balance in all this is actual doing, actual practice, a program of wholesome living is the basis of wholesome feeling and thinking and fancy and interests." (61, p. 6)

According to Meyer, a fundamental issue in the treatment of the mentally ill is ". . . the proper use of time in some helpful and gratifying activity. . . ." (61, p. 1) He expands on this precept by stating: "There is in all this a development of the *valuation of time and work,* which is not accidental. It is part of the great espousal of the *values of reality and actuality* rather than of mere thinking and reasoning. . . ." (61, p. 4) The introduction of activity is ". . . in giving opportunities rather than prescriptions. There must be opportunities to work, opportunities to do and to plan and create, and to learn to use material. . . . It is not a question of specific prescriptions, but of opportunities . . . to adapt opportunities." (61, p. 7) He concluded his philosophic essay by returning once again to time and occupations: "The great feature of man is his new sense of time, with foresight built on a sound view of the past and present. Man learns to organize time and he does it in terms of doing things, and one of the many things he does between eating, drinking and . . . the flights fancy and aspiration, we call work and occupation." (61, pp. 9–10)

Near the end of his working life, Meyer summed up his major efforts. He wrote of dealing with individuals and groups from the viewpoints of *good sense;* of *science,* ". . . with the smallest numbers of assumptions for search and research. . . ."; of *philosophy;* and of *religion,* ". . . as a way of trust and dependabilities in life." (see 62, p. 100)

Occupational Therapy Definitions and Principles

As the founders and pioneers were experimenting with and writing their concepts, a definition of occupational therapy was emerging. It is remarkable that so early in the formation of the 20th century movement, a definition could be developed and stand for several decades and several generations of occupational therapists. Many of us were required in school to immortalize it through needlepoint, embroidery, and even printing.

H. A. Pattison, M.D., medical officer of the National Tuberculous Association, advanced his view at the annual conference of the National Society for the Promotion of Occupational Therapy in Chicago, September 1919. It was also adopted by the Federal Board of Vocational Education: "Occupational Therapy may be defined as any activity, mental or physical, definitely prescribed and guided for the distinct purpose of contributing to and hastening recovery from disease or injury." (63, p. 21) Twenty-two years later, in 1931, John S. Coulter, M.D., and Henrietta McNary, OTR, added one phrase: ". . . and assisting the social and institutional adjustment of individuals requiring long and indefinite periods of hospitalization." (see 64, p. 19) This was inserted in order to recognize occupational therapy's involvement in chronicity.

By 1925, a committee, made up of four physicians including William Rush Dunton, compiled an outline for lectures to medical students and physicians (65, pp. 277–292). Though their document never received the official imprimature of the AOTA, it nevertheless served for several years as a guide for practice (see 66, p. 347). Fifteen principles were enunciated: "Occupational therapy is a method of training the sick or injured by means of instruction and employment in productive occupation; . . . to arouse interest, courage, confidence; to exercise mind and body in . . . activity; to overcome disability; and to re-establish capacity for industrial and social usefulness." (65, p. 280) Application called for as much system and precision as other forms of treatment; activity was to be prescribed, administered, and supervised under constant medical advice. Individual patient needs were paramount.

The outline stressed that "employment in groups is . . . advisable because it provides exercise in social adaptation and stimulating influence of example and comment. . . ." (65, p. 280) In selecting an activity, the patient's interests and capabilities were to be considered and as strength and capability increased, the occupation was to be altered, regulated, and graded accordingly because "The only reliable measure of the treatment is the effect on the patient." (65, p. 280)

Inferior workmanship could be tolerated, depending upon the patient's condition, but there should be consideration of ". . . standards worthy of entirely normal persons . . . for proper mental stimulation." (65, p. 281) Articles made were to be useful and attractive, and meaningful tasks requiring healthful exercise of mind and body provided the greatest satisfaction. "Novelty, variety, individuality, and utility of the products enhance the value of an occupation as a treatment measure." (65, p. 281) While quality, quantity, and the salability of articles made could be of benefit, these should not take precedence over the treatment objectives. As adjuncts to occupations, physical exercise, games, and music were considered beneficial and fell into two main categories: gymnastics and calisthenics, recreation and play.

One last principle spoke of the qualities of the occupational therapist: ". . . good craftsmanship, and ability to instruct are essential qualifications; . . . understanding, sincere interest in the patient, and an optimistic, cheerful outlook and manner are equally essential." (65, p. 281)

Occupational Therapy's Second Generation

The die was cast. Practice rapidly expanded in a phenomenal number of settings following the establishment of the founders' principles and definition. A *second generation* of therapists emerged during the late 1920s and the 1930s. They were the practitioners and educators who elaborated, codified, and applied the initial theory upon which present-day practice is based. A chronicle of their efforts would offer a highly valuable and valued study in itself. The names of Louis Haas, Mary Alice Coombs, Winifred Kahmann, Henrietta McNary, Harriet Robeson, Marjorie Taylor, and Helen Willard would figure prominently in such an account.

For the purpose of *this history,* a composite of these and others is drawn into one individual who exemplifies the spirit and deeds of the *second generation* of occupational therapists—those whose efforts are lasting and ensure our present and future education and practice.

Understandably, it would be a woman. She would devote her professional career to either teaching, practicing, or administering. Quite possibly she would combine two or more of these. She would acquire an expertise in one area of practice, such as the mentally ill.

Her belief in the treatment of the total patient would guide her thoughts and actions. Occupational therapy, she would declare, "since its founding has concerned itself with the basic tenet—the treatment of the total patient. This approach is unique to occupational therapy among the . . . health disciplines. . . . There has always existed a strong component concerned with the behavior of the physically ill or disabled, as well as the mentally sick; with the entirety of man and his functioning as a patient. This occupational therapy concept," she would continue, "prevented (as has occurred in medical practice) an undesired separation of the psychiatric therapist from those who develop knowledge and skills centered in the treatment of the physically disabled." (67, p. 1) Stated another way, "The major emphasis in occupational therapy is not the body *as such* but the individual *as such.* The therapist's background is strongly weighted in an understanding of personality adjustment and reactions to social situations; . . . and in the patients' attitudes toward an adjustment to acute and chronic disabilities." (68, p. 9)

At some point in her work, she would be asked to serve as a consultant to one or more medical facilities, possibly a state hospital system. In time, she would produce a report and re-state her definition of occupational therapy. It might well go this way: "The goal of all treatment in a modern mental hospital is the physical, social and economic rehabilitation of the patient. . . . The accepted function (of occupational therapy) . . . is the scientific utilization of mental and physical activities for the purpose of raising the patient to the highest level of integration; to assist him in making his initial adjustment to the hospital; to sustain him while his body responds to physical treatment and his mind to psychotherapy; or to assist him in making a satisfactory adjustment to chronic illness." (69, p. 24)

In the report she would also call for an atmosphere as normal as possible, where a patient could be encouraged to respond in as normal a manner as possible: a balanced program of work and play, with flexibility to meet individual needs: "There must be organized a succession of steps through which the patient will be gradually led to his highest level of integration. . . . At each level . . . the patient experiences a feeling of success and self-respect. One cannot overemphasize the importance of careful planning . . . in order that there be a systematic progression up this ladder of integration." (69, p. 24)

In another context, supportive care, as a vital concern to the therapist, would also be described, particularly in the care of the physically disabled: "To name only a few of its treatment objectives, occupational therapy may function as a diagnostic evaluative instrument; as corrective treatment; . . . or a design for effecting prevocational evaluation. Incorporated in each . . . is a treatment phase referred to as supportive care. This is a most fundamental and yet less definitive and indeed the least spectacular element of the total rehabilitory program. In supportive care, the occupational therapist (is concerned) with the behavioural factors which have and will affect the patient's response to the rehabilitation program. . . ." Convincingly, she would say: ". . . it can be said with conviction that successful rehabilitation can be effected only when the patient has attained a true state of rehabilitation 'readiness.' " (70)

Not just a woman of words, she would find one or more ways to activate her philosophy. She might well become active with a group of former patients and assist in organizing an association of and for individuals who have been hospitalized—for instance, the mentally ill. Such an endeavor would be the first of a kind. Through such an experience, she would conclude: "One difficulty which presented itself again and again was the need to instill in these (former) patients a philosophy toward their own rehabilitation; . . . an organized effort beyond the hospital which would offer special training, guidance and professional evaluation of their potentials." (71, p. 3)

This would lead her to even greater endeavors on behalf of a whole category of patients. As an example, she would find that the 1920 Federal Vocational Rehabilitation Act excluded former psychiatric patients. In the manner of Dorothea Lynde Dix, whom she probably emulated, she would wage a relentless battle to right such a wrong. By enlisting the assistance of physicians' associations and veterans' groups she would see the legislation change. As part of her campaign she would write: "The former mental patient, in his struggle for economic rehabilitation, incurs the burden imposed on the physically handicapped 'plus' the stigmatization based on the popular misconception of mental disease. He must cast aside self-pity or the idea that the world owes him a living. The world does owe him understanding and guidance." (72, p. 114) Finally, amendments to Public Law 113 were passed and signed by President Franklin Roosevelt. Psychiatric patients could now qualify for the benefits of the vocational rehabilitation act.

With such efforts the therapist's personal beliefs about emotional illness become even more strongly felt: "The majority of mentally ill are (sick) through no fault of their own . . . any more than one who has contracted a physical illness. Persons suffering from mental disease are generally ill as a result of an accumulation of unsuccessful efforts . . . to adjust to his environment." (72, p. 83)

Two continuing concerns of all occupational therapists would be commented upon: the qualifications of the therapist and the use of media. One is as significant as the other. "The personality of the therapist," she would say, "must command respect, admiration, hope and confidence, . . . for no therapy is better than the therapist who directs it." (72, p. 83) Therapeutic media have a number of inherent qualities, such as providing a vehicle for objectively recording patient performance, and, for the patient, affording opportunities for ". . . creative expression and evidence of accomplishment. The therapist should have a wide variety of activities (available) in accordance with the interests, aptitudes, and mental state of the patient. A craft track mind has no place in preparing such a program," she would state (72, p. 103).

The accumulation of experiences as a clinician, and educator, or an administrator, or possibly a combination of these, would lead this *therapist of the second generation* to arrive at a new definition of occupational therapy. It would precede by several years an altered definition by the national organization. It would incorporate the social and behavioral sciences, with a diminished emphasis upon medicine. Human development would appear for the first time as a focus for the treatment of physical and psychosocial dysfunction. She would declare: "Occupational therapy's function is to provide skilled assistance in influencing human objectives; its approach is inextricably conjoined with the behavioral factors involved. It is interested in how the process of growth and development is modified by hospitalization, chronic illness or a permanent handicap." (73, p. 2)

This re-focus was quite explainable and understandable to her since occupational therapy, and its ancestral emphasis, has always been the totality of the human organism. She would say, "It was inevitable, therefore, that there evolve an ever increasing emphasis in occupational therapy . . . a greater understanding of the part that the developmental process plays in the preventive and therapeutic factors of this form of treatment." (74, p. 3)

The foregoing has been a descriptive composite of a whole generation of therapists and assistants. The composite is actually the story of one individual; her observations alone have been cited. That individual is *Miss Beatrice D. Wade, OTR, FAOTA.*

The story is far from finished. Without a doubt, someone sometime will chronicle the lives and works of those who are still making contributions from that era to the present generation. Among them are Marjorie Fish, Virginia Kilburn, Mary Reilly, Ruth Robinson, Clare Spackman, Ruth Brunyate Wiemer, Carlotta Welles, and Wilma West. Each one, together with many others, continues to serve us well as clarifiers and definers of reasonable and reasoned alternatives. As counselors, they confirm old values and clearly point out *new directions* as well as our faithfulness or infidelity to those timeless principles established by our professional ancestors.

Lessons From Our History

The history of occupational therapy is the most neglected aspect of our professional endeavors. Seemingly, *old values* are least considered when charting *new directions*. On occasion we have been accused of taking leave of our historical senses. More to the point is that we have no historical sense. The problem primarily lies in not taking the time to assiduously locate our profession's diggings, to excavate what is relevant, and, then, to learn from what has been unearthed.

Archival materials from the past 200 years have been abundantly used in the development of this paper. Location and excavation has been difficult at times; however, it is reassuring to note that records and accounts still exist that are extremely relevant to today's endeavors. Lessons can be learned and they must. May I encourage each of you to determine for yourself what you have learned from this paraphrastic journey to our profession's diggings. To assist in this endeavor, may I cite a few lessons I have gained.

Mind and Body Inextricably Conjoined

No less than our professional ancestors, we must refuse to accept any alternative to the belief in the wholeness of the human—that the mind and body are inextricably conjoined. Illness, treatment, and the return to a healthful state simultaneously affect the physiological and emotional processes. Indeed, should these processes ever become separated, then occupational therapy would be of no value. The patient has died!

The Natural Science of the Human

The inextricable union of the human leads to another lesson. The science fundamental to our practice is the natural science of the human. No amount of neurophysiology, psychology, sociology, or child development alone can determine the differential diagnosis, treatment, or prognosis of the patient undergoing occupational therapy. The current trend toward specialization, with its varying emphases upon one or another science, to the neglect of other human sciences, and indeed to the neglect of other nonscientific aspects of occupational therapy, borders on superstition and mythology. It is the continuous acquisition and scientific synthesis of the ingredients of the human organism and its surround that guarantees authentic occupational therapy.

The Human Organism's Involvement in Tasks

Occupational therapy is the only major health profession whose focus centers upon the *total* human organism's involvement in tasks—a making or doing. In spite of the many grafts we have effected, our roots remain in the subsoil of the *art,* the *craft:* a paradigm of the total activity of the human. Just as those who have come before us, we think of ourselves and others fundamentally as makers, as users, as doers, as tools. We look at: ". . . craft as a way in which man may create and cross a bridge within himself and center himself in his own essential unity." (75, p. vii) The procedures one goes through in rearranging and reassembling the basic elements in art or craft operate upon and within the doer: ". . . his material modifies him as he modifies it, in proportion to his openness, his awareness of the exchange that is taking place." (75, p. x)

The Differentiation of Occupational Therapy

Any definition, any description, any differentiation between ourselves and other health providers must have as its major theme occupation and leisure. Without it, we become a blurred copy, a xerography of a host of others.

Without the dynamics of human motion inherent in purposeful activity, we become quasi-physical therapists. Without the interaction between human objects and the objects of work and leisure, we become quasi-social workers, psychologists, or nurses. Without the demonstrated and proven interrelationships between healthful, normal growth and development, activity, and the pathology of illness and disabling conditions, we become quasi-physicians and psychiatrists.

The more we intermingle our fundamental philosophy and our treatment techniques with others, the more we intermarry, the more likely we will become enfeebled, the more likely we will degenerate, the more likely we will eventually disappear. Though speaking in another context, the Durants offer a lesson we must accept: "All strong characters and peoples are race conscious and are instinctively averse to marriage outside their own . . . group." (76, p. 26)

A Refusal to Accept the Common Verdict

As Hugh Sidey has noted, "History is a marvelous collection of stories about men and women who refuse to accept the common verdict that certain achievements (are) impossible." (77, p. 18) The history of occupational therapy is the story of the ideals, deeds, hopes, and works of *individuals*. Changes and advancements came from those who eliminated inhumaneness, which prevented or discouraged the sick and disabled from achieving their potential. These same individuals were willing to assume the care and responsibility for those *who were not highly valued by the society:* the mentally ill and retarded, the severely disabled—all those defined as "non-producing, . . . an economic burden." (65, p. 277)

In numerous places and on countless occasions these same individuals were derided, hated, or, at best, ignored, because they pressed for change in the human condition. Yet, they persevered, knowing there was nothing innately unusual about themselves or what they wished to achieve. Few ever saw their names inscribed on monuments.

They were a *cast* quite diverse in character, and largely obscured because of the immensity of the saga being enacted. A few received *speaking parts*, primarily through reporting their own clinical findings. Only very few were singled out to be stars. None ever became members of the *audience*, passively observing events. All were *actors*.

The very same can be said of the present occupational therapy generation. We are actors, not observers. We continue to willingly strive on behalf of those who are not highly valued by the society. We refuse to see this as a burden. Rather, we perceive it as an obligation, as an opportunity, as a way of life.

Legacy of Experience

Too often we are disposed to think that those lessons another generation learned do not apply to the present generation. We should be remindful that there are two ways to learn: by our own experience and from those who have made discoveries, regardless of how long ago they were made. The experience of others is a magnificent heritage, and the more we learn from them, the less time we waste in the present, proving what already has been proved.

Those of us who are teachers and clinicians have a special obligation to pass on the legacy of experience, the knowledge of timeless principles and practices that do not change merely because times change.

Who They Were, What They Did

The legacy of experience suggests one more lesson. So often we are caught up in our daily activities we tend to forget what it is we owe those who came before us. All probably agree that each occupational therapy generation seemingly acquires a sense of self-sufficiency. It is true that we of the present occupy the positions that once were filled by others.

It is, however, of great import that we realize we are influenced by those who came before us more than we can truly know. Who they were and what they did has immeasurable bearing upon what we are and what we do. No generation is capable of isolating itself from its past. The past, plus what we are and what we do, greatly assists in fashioning our future.

The archives, the portraits and photographs, the published accounts, the personal memorabilia and scrapbooks are records of considerable moment. At the least, they are a profound reminder of the possibility that someday, someone may be looking back and may be wondering who we were and what we did.

Conclusion

It is altogether fitting and proper to conclude this lecture with the observations of two former Presidents of the Association, Mr. Thomas B. Kidner and Mrs. Eleanor Clarke Slagle. In 1930, Mr. Kidner offered a personal impression of the state of occupational therapy at the annual meeting of the Connecticut Occupational Therapy Society. In part, he said: "May we, therefore, look on occupational therapy—with increased faith as the years go by—as a natural means of aiding in the restoration of the sick and disabled to health and working capacity (which means happiness) because it appeals to all our human attributes." (57, p. 11)

Mrs. Slagle, a year after she retired in 1937, made this observation: "The story of the profession of occupational therapy will never be fully told, nor will that of the patients who have so abundantly appreciated the opportunities of the service. There has been no fanciful crusading 'for the cause'; it has meant that a few have perhaps borne many burdens, but in the slow process that make permanent things of great value, it can be said that there is a fine body of professional workers, experienced and well trained, coming forward and being welcomed to a really great human service, that of helping to show the way to the person with large disabilities to make the best of his incomplete self." (78, p. 382) Finally, in an editorial "From the Heart," she concluded: "The integrity of your profession is in your hands. I bid you all Godspeed in your work." (79, p. 345)

Acknowledgments

A study of this nature and scope is not possible without the valuable and valued assistance of numerous individuals and sources. I wish to recognize the incomparable services provided by the staffs of the Moody Medical Library, The University of Texas Medical Branch at Galveston; the Quine Library, University of Illinois at the Medical Center, Chicago; the McGoogan Library of Medicine, University of Nebraska Medical Center, Omaha; and the Archives, Shapiro Developmental Center (Eastern Illinois State Hospital), Kankakee.

Lillian Hoyle Parent, OTR, was unusually helpful in locating obscure documents for me. The prior research of Kathryn Reed, OTR, greatly facilitated my search. William C. Levin, MD, President, The University of Texas Medical Branch, was most generous with his support and consistent encouragement.

Several reviewers' comments helped to improve the manuscript: John G. Bruhn, PhD, a medical sociologist, Dean, The University of Texas School of Allied Health Sciences, Galveston; Chester R. Burns, MD, PhD, an historian, The Institute for Medical Humanities, The University of Texas Medical Branch, Galveston; and four occupational therapists: James L. Cantwell, PhD; Charles H. Christiansen, EdD, of The University of Texas School of Allied Health Sciences, Galveston; Suzanne Hooker, DipOT, Western Australian Institute of Technology, Shenton Park, Western Australia; and Lillian Hoyle Parent, MA, College of Associated Health Professions, University of Illinois at the Medical Center, Chicago. Eleanor Porter, Managing Editor, *Texas Reports on Biology and Medicine,* was a valuable advisor.

Others who provided invaluable help with ideas, documents, memorabilia, and personal remembrances were Shirley H. Carr, OTR, Tuskegee Institute; Barbara Loomis, OTR, University of Illinois at the Medical Center; Margaret Mirenda, OTR, Mount Mary College; Beatrice D. Wade, OTR, Professor Emeritus, University of Illinois at the Medical Center; and Kay B. Hudgens, OTR, Archivist, Shapiro Developmental Center, Kankakee, Illinois.

Two members of the AOTA staff were extremely helpful: James Garibaldi and Mardy Hicks. Betty Cox also provided needed assistance. Three members of the Learning Resource Center, The University of Texas School of Allied Health Sciences, Galveston, accomplished the highly effective visual presentation: Randall Rogers, W. Gregory Hunicutt, and Judy Hargett. I am indebted to them. Other individuals must be mentioned: Daniel L. Creson, MD, PhD, offered his counsel and unqualified support throughout this endeavor; Lucille M. Burnworth typed several drafts and the final copy of the paper; Adele Jaco offered valuable clerical assistance; Laura Reed and Judy Grace, both occupational therapists, provided creative assistance at a much needed time. All personify the finest meanings of *friends.*

Finally, I wish to recognize Frances Sawyer, COTA, and the Board of Directors, The Texas Occupational Therapy Association, Inc., who placed my name in nomination for this exalted honor. My gratitude to them is immeasurable.

References

1. Locke J: *An Essay Concerning Human Understanding* (Two Volumes), New York: Dover Press, 1690 on p. 307F

2. Frost SE: *Basic Teachings of the Great Philosophers,* New York: Barnes and Noble, Inc., 1942

3. Riese W: *The Legacy of Philippe Pinel: An Inquiry into Thought on Mental Alienation,* New York: Springer Publishing Co., 1969

4. Condillac EB de: *Oeuvres Philosophiques de Condillac,* Paris: Presse Universataires de France, 1947

5. Ackerknecht EH: *A Short History of Psychiatry,* New York: Hafner Publishing Co., 1968

6. Tuke DH: *A Dictionary of Psychological Medicine* (Vol One), Philadelphia: P Blakiston, Son & Co., 1892

7. Pinel P: *Traité Médico-Philosophique sur 'Alienation Mentale,* Paris: Richard, Caille & Rover, 1801

8. Pinel P: *A Treatise on Insanity in Which Are Contained the Principles of a New and More Practical Nosology of Maniacal Disorders,* Translated by DD Davis, London: Cadell & Davis, 1806 (Facsimile published by Hafner Publishing Co., New York, 1962)

9. Mackler B: *Philippe Pinel: Unchainer of the Insane,* New York: Franklin Watts, Inc., 1968

10. Folsom CF: *Diseases of the Mind: Notes on the Early Management, European and American Progress,* Boston: A. Williams & Co., Publishers, 1877

11. Jones K: *Lunacy, Law, and Conscience: 1744–1845: The Social History of Care of the Insane,* London: Routledge & Kegan Paul, Ltd., 1955

12. Dillenberger J, Welch C: *Protestant Christianity: Interpreted Through Its Development,* New York: Charles Scribner's Sons, 1954

13. Philadelphia Yearly Meeting of the Religious Society of Friends: *Faith and Practice,* Philadelphia: Philadelphia Yearly Meeting, 1972

14. Tuke DH: *Reform in the Treatment of the Insane. Early History of the Retreat, York; Its Objects and Influence,* London, J & A Churchill, 1872

15. Tuke DH: *Reform in the Treatment of the Insane: An Early History of the Retreat, York: Its Objects and Influence,* London: J & A Churchill, 1892

16. Tuke S: *Description of The Retreat, An Institution Near York for Insane Persons of the Society of Friends: Containing an Account of Its Origins and Progress, The Modes of Treatment, and a Statement of Cases,* York, England: Alexander, 1813

17. Hunter R, Macalpine I: *Three Hundred Years of Psychiatry, 1535–1860: A History Presented in Selected English Texts,* London: Oxford University Press, 1963

18. Connolly J: *The Treatment of the Insane Without Mechanical Restraints,* London: Smith, Elder & Co., 1856 (Facsimile copy published by Dawson's of Pall Mall, London, 1973, with introduction by R Hunter, and I Macalpine)

19. Ellis WC: *A Treatise on the Nature, Symptoms, Causes, and Treatment of Insanity,* London: Holdsworth, 1838

20. Goodman N: *Benjamin Rush: Physician and Citizen, 1746–1813,* Philadelphia: University of Pennsylvania Press, 1934

21. Rush B: *Medical Inquiries and Observations Upon the Diseases of the Mind* (4th Edition), Philadelphia: J Grigg, 1830

22. Buckmaster H: *Women Who Shaped History,* New York: Macmillan Pub. C., 1966

23. Bucknill JC, Tuke, DH: *A Manual of Psychological Medicine,* New York: Hafner Pub. Co., 1968 (Facsimile of 1858 Edition)

24. Barlow J: *Man's Power Over Himself to Prevent or Control Insanity,* London: William Pickering, 1843

25. Skultans V: *Madness and Morals: Ideas on Insanity in the Nineteenth Century,* London: Routledge & Kegan Paul, 1975

26. Tuke DH: *A Dictionary of Psychological Medicine: Volume Two,* Philadelphia: P Blakiston, Son & Co., 1892

27. Bockhoven JS: *Moral Treatment in American Psychiatry,* New York: Springer Publishing Co., Inc., 1963

28. Dain N: *Concepts of Insanity in the United States, 1789–1865,* New Brunswick, NJ: Rutgers University Press, 1964

29. Deutsch A: *The Mentally Ill in America: A History of Their Care and Treatment from Colonial Times* (2nd Edition). New York: Columbia University Press, 1949

30. Tracy SE: The development of occupational therapy in the Grace Hospital, Detroit, Michigan. *Trained Nurse Hosp Rev* 66:5, May 1921

31. Tracy SE: The place of invalid occupations in the general hospital. *Modern Hosp* 2:5, June 1914

32. Tracy SE: Twenty-five suggested mental tests derived from invalid occupations. *Maryland Psychiatr Q* 8, 1918

33. Barrows M: Susan E. Tracy, RN: *Maryland Psychiatr Q* 6, 1916–1917

34. Tracy SE: Treatment of disease by employment at St. Elizabeths Hospital. *Modern Hosp* 20:2, February 1923

35. Parsons SE: Miss Tracy's work in general hospitals. *Maryland Psychiatr Q* 6, 1916–1917

36. Tracy SE: *Studies in Invalid Occupation,* Boston: Witcomb and Barrows, 1918

37. Tracy SE: Power versus money in occupation therapy. *Trained Nurse Hosp Rev* 66:2, February 1921

38. Barton GE: A view of invalid occupation. *Trained Nurse Hosp Rev* 52:6, June 1914

39. Barton GE: Occupational nursing. *Trained Nurse Hosp Rev* 54:6, June 1915

40. Barton GE: Occupational therapy. *Trained Nurse Hosp Rev* 54:3, March 1915

41. Barton GE: The existing hospital system and reconstruction. *Trained Nurse Hosp Rev* 69:4, October 1922

42. Barton GE: What occupational therapy may mean to nursing. *Trained Nurse Hosp Rev* 64:4, April 1920

43. Barton GE: *Re-education: An Analysis of the Institutional System of the United States,* Boston: Houghton Mifflin Co., 1917

44. Sheppard Asylum: *Third Annual Report of the Sheppard Asylum,* Towson, MD, 1895

45. Dunton WR: The relationship of occupational therapy and physical therapy. *Arch Phys Ther* 16, January 1935

46. Dunton WR: The Principles of Occupational Therapy. *Proceedings of the National Society for the Promotion of Occupational Therapy: Second Annual Meeting,* Catonsville, MD: Spring Grove State Hospital, 1918

47. Dunton WR: *Occupation Therapy: A Manual for Nurses,* Philadelphia: WB Saunders, 1915

48. Komora PO: Eleanor Clarke Slagle. *Ment Hyg* 27:1, January 1943

49. Pollock HM: In memoriam: Eleanor Clarke Slagle, 1876–1942. *Am J Psychiatr* 99:3, November 1942

50. American Occupational Therapy Association: *Then and Now, 1917–1967,* New York: American Occupational Therapy Association, 1967

51. Loomis B, Wade BD: *Chicago . . . Occupational Therapy Beginnings: Hull House, The Henry B. Favill School of Occupations and Eleanor Clarke Slagle.*

52. Slagle EC: Occupational therapy: Recent methods and advances in the United States. *Occup Ther Rehab* 13:5, October 1934

53. Slagle EC: History of the development of occupation for the insane. *Maryland Psychiatr Q* 4, May 1914

54. Slagle EC: Training aides for mental patients. *Arch Occup Ther* 1:1, February 1922

55. Slagle EC, Robeson HA: *Syllabus for Training of Nurses in Occupational Therapy,* Utica, NY: State Hospital Press, date unknown

56. Slagle EC: A year's development of occupational therapy in New York State Hospitals. *Modern Hosp* 22:1, January 1924

57. Kidner TB: Occupational therapy, its development, scope and possibilities. *Occup Ther Rehab* 10:1, February 1931

58. Meyer A: The psychological point of view. In *Classics in American Psychiatry,* JP Brady, Editor, St. Louis: Warren H Green, Inc., 1975 (Also, In *The Problems of Mental Health,* M Bentley, EV Cowdey, Editors, New York: McGraw-Hill, 1934)

59. Arieti S: *American Handbook of Psychiatry* (Vol Two), New York: Basic Books, Inc., Publishers, 1959

60. Lief A: *The Commonsense Psychiatry of Dr. Adolf Meyer: Fifty-two Selected Papers,* Edited with Biographical Narrative, New York: McGraw-Hill Book Co., 1948

61. Meyer A: The philosophy of occupation therapy. *Arch Occup Ther* 1:1, February 1922 (Also in *Am J Occup Ther* 31(10):639–642, 1977)

62. Meyer A: The rise to the person and the concept of wholes or integrates. *Am J Psychiatr* 100, April 1944

63. Pattison HA: The trend of occupational therapy for the tuberculous. *Arch Occup Ther* 1(1), February 1922

64. Coulter JS, McNary H: Necessity of medical supervision in occupational therapy. *Occup Ther Rehab* 10(1), February 1931

65. An outline of lectures on occupational therapy to medical students and physicians. *Occup Ther Rehab* 4(4), August 1925

66. Elwood, ES: The National Board of Medical Examiners and medical education, and the possible effect of the Board's program on the spread of occupational therapy. *Occup Ther Rehab* 6(5), October 1927

67. Wade BD: Occupational Therapy: A History of Its Practice in the Psychiatric Field. Unpublished paper presented at 51st Annual Conference, American Occupational Therapy Association, Boston, October 19, 1967

68. Advisory Committee in Occupational Therapy: The Basic Philosophy and Function of Occupational Therapy. *University of Illinois Faculty—Alumni Newsletter of the Chicago Professional Colleges.* 6:4, January 1951

69. Wade BD: A survey of occupational and industrial therapy in the Illinois state hospitals. *Illinois Psychiatr* 2(1), March 1942

70. Wade BD: Supportive care. *Bull Rehab Inst Chicago,* date unknown

71. Wade BD: Supportive care. *Bull Rehab* Rehabilitation of the Mentally Ill. Unpublished paper presented to the Department of Public Welfare, State of Minnesota, June 26, 1958

72. Willard HS, Spackman CS: *Principles of Occupational Therapy* (First Edition), Philadelphia: JB Lippincott Co., 1947

73. Wade BD: The Development of Clinically Oriented Education in Occupational Therapy: The Illinois Plan. Unpublished paper presented at 49th Annual Conference, American Occupational Therapy Association, Miami, November 2, 1965

74. Wade BD: Introduction. *The Preparation of Occupational Therapy Students for Functioning with Aging Persons and in Comprehensive Health Care Programs: A Manual for Educators,* Chicago: University of Illinois at the Medical Center, 1969

75. Dooling EM: *A Way of Working,* Garden City, NY: Anchor Press/Doubleday, 1979

76. Durant W, Durant A: *The Lessons of History,* New York: Simon and Schuster, 1968

77. Sidey H: The presidency. *Time* 116(22), December 1, 1980

78. Slagle EC: Occupational therapy. *Trained Nurse Hosp Rev* 100(4), April 1938

79. Slagle EC: Editorial: From the heart. *Occup Ther Rehab* 16(5), October 1937

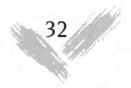

32

1983 Eleanor Clarke Slagle Lecture

Clinical Reasoning:
The Ethics, Science, and Art

Joan C. Rogers, PhD, OTR, FAOTA

As I join the roster of Eleanor Clarke Slagle lecturers, I am keenly aware of the privilege and responsibility of being so honored by my professional colleagues. Since my selection for the award was based on a recognition of a synthesis of skills in occupational therapy practice, education, and research, it seemed fitting for me to pursue a topic that would in some way enable me to reflect this synthesis. Thus, in developing the theme of clinical reasoning, I have taken a practice issue, studied it from an educational perspective, and formulated a conceptual framework for guiding the development of a clinical science of occupational therapy.

A therapist, employed at a regional rehabilitation center, extracts cues from the records of acute hospitals, to judge the rehabilitation potential of patients referred for admission. Another therapist, working with persons with mental retardation, selects a treatment approach based on task analysis to teach self-care skills. A third therapist, serving on a geriatric assessment team, uses scores on a mental status examination and performance ratings in daily living activities to estimate patients' ability to continue living alone in their homes. A fourth therapist reviews patients' progress in manual dexterity to formulate a recommendation for or against hand surgery. These four therapists are using their clinical reasoning skills to collect and transform data about patients into decisions that have critical implications for the quality of life of their patients.

If we questioned the therapists about their decisions, each would probably comment on their potential fallibility. Some patients, denied occupational therapy because of a perceived lack of potential for rehabilitation, would make substantial gains in functional skills if intervention were initiated. Some patients with mental retardation will not benefit from the task breakdown approach to self-care training. Some geriatric patients admitted for institutional living could have been supported adequately in the community. Some patients undergoing hand surgery will lose functional abilities. The possibility of error in our clinical judgments and the potential ensuing negative consequences urge us to develop ways of improving our assessment and treatment decisions.

Despite the obvious importance of clinical judgment in the occupational therapy process, little attention has been given to explicating the thinking that guides practice. My research, albeit with a small number of occupational therapists, suggests that our cognitive processes are regarded as intuitive and ineffable. For example, when therapists were asked how they arrived at their treatment decisions, they commonly responded by saying, "I have never really thought about it." or "I don't know how I reached that conclusion. I just know." Cognitive activity constitutes the heart of the clinical enterprise. Our failure to study the process of knowing and understanding that underlies practice precludes an adequate description of clinical reasoning. This in turn prevents the development of a methodology for systematically improving it and for teaching it.

Originally published 1983 in *American Journal of Occupational Therapy, 37*, 601–616.
Please note that there was no Eleanor Clarke Slagle Lecture in 1982.

I intend to explore here the reasoning process through which we learn about patients so that we may help them through engagement in occupation. I will construct an intellectual device for viewing clinical reasoning from the perspective of the basic questions the therapist seeks to answer through clinical inquiry. The scientific, ethical, and artistic dimensions of clinical reasoning will be elucidated as these questions are explored. The device will be useful for directing and appraising our thoughts about treating patients and for developing a clinical science of occupational therapy. In developing my thoughts, I have relied on the basic scheme of clinical judgment presented by Pellegrino (1) for medicine and have adapted it to the occupational therapy process.

The Goal of Clinical Reasoning

The goal of the clinical reasoning process has an impact on each of the steps taken to achieve the goal. Hence, an appreciation of this goal provides insight on the whole process.

Patients come to occupational therapy when they, their physicians, family members, or caregivers perceive that they are not adequately performing their daily activities. Performance in self-care, work, and leisure occupations has been compromised because of the consequences of disease, trauma, abnormal development, age-related changes, or environmental restrictions. The disruptions in occupational functions are characteristically severe and enduring as opposed to transitory. To regain a former level of performance, maintain the current level, or achieve a more optimal one, the patient enlists the aid of the therapist. The therapist's task, therefore, is to select a right therapeutic action for the patient (1). In other words, the goal of clinical reasoning is a treatment recommendation issued in the interests of a particular patient. Decision making is highly individualized.

The occupational therapy treatment plan details what a particular patient should do to enhance occupational role performance. The therapeutic action must be the right action for this individual. This implies that it must be as congruent as possible with the patient's concept of the "good life." Treatment should be in concert with the patient's needs, goals, life style, and personal and cultural values. A therapeutic program that is right for one patient is not necessarily right for another. The ultimate question we, as clinicians, are challenged to answer is: What, among the many things that could be done for this patient, ought to be done? This is an ethical question. It involves a judgment to which facts contribute but that must be decided by weighing values. A salient criterion of an ethical action is its agreement with the patient's valued goals. The clinical reasoning process terminates in an ethical decision, rather than in a scientific one, and the ethical nature of the goal of clinical reasoning projects itself over the entire sequence.

Ethical decisions regarding treatment are not made in isolation from scientific knowledge. The patient comes to the therapist for expert advice regarding adaptation to chronic dysfunction. The factual basis for decision making is provided by the therapist. When therapists set out to solve clinical problems, they are confronted with an unknown—the patient. Scientific methodologies are used to learn about the patient. Once the patient's condition is adequately understood, scientific and empirical knowledge is applied in the efforts to enhance occupational status. Although ethical considerations can override scientific ones, they do not displace the need to secure a scientific opinion.

Clinical Questions

To ascertain the right action for each patient, clinical inquiry focuses on three questions: What is the patient's current status in occupational role performance? What could be done to enhance the patient's performance? And what ought to be done to enhance occupational competence? These are the fundamental questions that I previously alluded to as guiding the clinical process. Each question will be considered first in terms of the knowledge needed to answer it, and, subsequently, in terms of the cognitive processes used to obtain the knowledge.

What Is the Patient's Status?

The first question to be considered is the assessment question: What is the patient's occupational status? The occupational therapy assessment is a concise and accurate summary of a patient's occupational role performance that arises from an investigation of the patient. The occupational therapy assessment tells us what we need to know about the patient to plan a sound intervention or prevention program. To serve this function, the assessment includes several features: it indicates what is wrong with the patient, it indicates the patient's strengths, and it indicates the patient's motivation for occupation.

The word *assessment* is preferable to the terms *diagnosis* or *problem definition* for the evaluation of occupational status because it has a much broader meaning. Diagnosis and problem definition connote the identification of pathological, abnormal, dysfunctional, or problematic processes or states. To assess means to rate the value of property for the purpose of taxation. The word *assessment,* then, with its emphasis on the evaluation of the worth of something, is an appropriate term to apply to the process of collecting information to resolve clinical problems and to the statement that summarizes the results of that process. Occupational therapy is concerned with helping disabled persons to adapt to chronic disability more effectively. This may be accomplished by enhancing abilities as well as by remediating or reducing dysfunction. The occupational therapy assessment serves as the end point of evaluation and the starting point for treatment planning. To serve this pivotal function, the assessment must specify both assets and liabilities. Thus, diagnosis, or the determination of what is wrong with the patient, is only a part of the assessment.

Knowledge. The assessment process usually begins with diagnosis, since knowledge of dysfunction tells us what is wrong and requires correction or amelioration. The therapist seeks to ascertain the specific problems the patient is having in performing self-care, work, and leisure occupations. Disruptions in occupational role are commonly of two major types: an inability to perform socially defined age-appropriate tasks and an inability to coordinate these tasks effectively in daily life. To the extent that a person has disruptions in occupational role, or impairments that we can predict will result in such disruptions, that person is an appropriate candidate for occupational therapy. The occupational therapy diagnosis clearly articulates the disruption in occupational role that is of concern for treatment. For example, we might state that Tom Smith is totally dependent in hygiene and dressing and requires physical assistance with feeding. This diagnosis indicates that these are the major problems at this time.

The occupational therapy diagnosis has a temporal quality. Participation in daily living tasks may change over the course of an illness or other disorder. For example, as Tom Smith gains competence in self-care, the diagnosis may switch to dysfunctions in home management. Similarly, as an individual matures and needs and interests change, the occupational therapy diagnosis changes, and intervention is refocused. Thus, the range of problems that comprise the occupational therapy diagnosis is broad and variable, and the diagnosis may change over time.

Often, the occupational therapy diagnosis indicates not only the disruption in occupational role, but also the suspected cause or causes for this disruption. This is the etiological component of the diagnostic statement and it offers an explanation of why the individual behaves or fails to behave in some way.

The most prevalent perspective for defining the etiology of occupational role dysfunctions is based on the biopsychosocial model. This enables us to pinpoint the causes of performance dysfunctions in terms of biological, psychological, and social variables. For example, we might state that Ida Cox cannot dress herself because she has contractures in her upper extremities, thus attributing the cause to a biological variable. Or, we might suggest that she cannot dress herself because of a memory problem, thus attributing the cause to a psychological variable. Or, we might conclude that the reason she is unable to dress herself is because she cannot reach her clothes from a wheelchair. In this case, the dressing dysfunction is attributed to the interaction of a biological variable, motor impairment, and a social variable, the man-made environment. Such attributions allow us to plan appropriate treatment. We can plan to remediate the contracture or memory deficit or to circumvent their effects on performance. We can remove the architectural barriers.

An occupational therapy diagnosis stemming from the biopsychosocial model is so specific that it is applicable to only one patient. For instance, an occupational therapy diagnosis might state: Homemaking disability secondary to a lack of endurance for shopping to procure groceries, and postural instability in negotiating the stairs to the laundry facilities in the basement; ability is complicated by blurred vision in both eyes as a consequence of cataracts. Such a diagnosis is unlikely to be appropriate for more than one patient. Although the diagnostic statement is highly descriptive, it is also highly prescriptive. For example, the above diagnosis suggests such interventions as: employing homemaker services, scheduling and performing activities in such a way as to control fatigue, using good light with no glare, and using mobility aids or environmental supports.

In addition to a description of what the patient cannot do and why, the occupational therapy assessment includes a description of what the patient can do and how well it can be done. Although the problem is diagnosed, it is the person who is assessed. The need to acknowledge positive factors was well expressed by the little boy who reacted to the scolding he received about his report card by saying, "Daddy, I think your eyes need fixing. You only saw the D and not the four As." Knowing a person's problems or deficits tells us little about his or her strengths. The image of the patient drawn from problem behaviors is distorted. It needs to be supplemented with snapshots of the patient's occupational competencies and strengths to enable the therapist to construct a fair and valid impression of the patient.

The assessment of occupational competence requires a wide-angled lens. Occupational performance emerges from a complex network of transactions between the internal characteristics of the individual and the external properties of the surrounding environment. Just as features of a particular situation may account for a limitation of ability, so they may also allow the expression of ability. The qualities of the environment are important enablers of human performance. You cannot swim without water or play tennis without a partner. Both the physical and the social environments influence the patient's ability to occupy time productively. To assess occupational competence, the therapist evaluates the people, places, and objects associated with the patient's occupational endeavors to determine the extent to which they support occupation.

The final requirement of the occupational therapy assessment is to summarize the patient's motivation to engage in occupation. Who among us has never pondered over the patients with excellent potential who fail to achieve and those with intractable conditions who surpass all expectations. We cannot understand the patient without an appreciation of the way in which the urge toward competence has been habitually satisfied. The ontogenetic aspects of occupation have critical implications for recovery and growth. The patient's history of occupation informs us whether the present dysfunction is extenuated by a pattern of adaptive behavior or augmented by a career of maladaptive behavior. The patient's mastery of the environment is documented in occupational achievement, while exploration of the environment is recorded in the use of time. Since time is occupied by doing things of value, the patient's use of time provides insight into the varieties of occupations that are meaningful to him or her. The patient's past is reviewed to shed light on how occupational behavior is organized and to lend perspective to activities that are important and incidental to the life plan.

Historical assessment is directed toward a deeper understanding of the patient's occupational nature. The normative sequence of occupational endeavors begins in childhood play and self-care. Participation in arts and crafts, games, academics, chores, and part-time work are added to the repertoire through young adulthood. Productive occupation in the form of employment predominates in adulthood. This often changes to leisure pursuits during later maturity. The therapist thus captures the development and balance of self-care, work, and leisure occupations in studying the sequence of pre-school, school age, worker, and retiree roles.

The yield of the occupational therapy assessment is a model of the patient that describes and explains his or her unique functioning in occupation. The model superimposes current functional abilities on disabilities, and relates these to environmental demands and to past performance. It is from this comprehensive model of the patient that future capacity is predicted and treatment goals are recommended.

Process. Having described the requirements of the occupational therapy assessment, I will now turn to the cognitive processes used to formulate it. What is involved in clinical inquiry? How do we go about the task of constructing a model of the patient? The approach used here for looking at the cognitive processes that undergird practice reflects on information-processing view of cognition. The human mind is thus conceptualized as a computer that has certain information processing capabilities. It can do some things better than others and uses certain labor-saving strategies to overcome its limitations. A primary limitation of the human mind is its small capacity for short-term or working memory. Because of this limitation, data must be selected judiciously, processed serially, and managed through simplifying strategies (2). In assessment, the clinician has as intake to the information-processing system cues gathered from the patient or about the patient. The output is the conclusions summarized in the occupational therapy assessment. The conversion of intake data to output conclusions is a critical feature of clinical reasoning.

The therapist begins the assessment by choosing a plan for studying the patient. We say to ourselves, "Of all things that I could consider about this patient, what am I going to think about?" We typically respond to this question by constructing an image of the patient from the pre-assessment data and use this image to direct our plan. Our pre-assessment image tells us what to include and what to exclude as we observe the patient. Thus, the first labor-saving device the therapist uses is to limit the parameters within which the patient will be studied.

The pre-assessment image of the patient is derived from the conceptual frame of reference or postulate system of the therapist. A conceptual frame of reference represents a therapist's unique view of occupational therapy. It consists of facts derived from research studies, empirical generalizations drawn from experience, theories and models accepted by the therapist, and principles of practice obtained from instructors and colleagues. My frame of reference represents what I believe about occupational therapy practice. A frame of reference operates largely as a nonconscious ideology in forming the pre-assessment image. The therapist links his or her frame of reference with the pre-assessment data to construct an image of the patient that furnishes the outline for the clinical investigation.

Two salient pre-assessment factors are the medical diagnosis and age. By knowing even these elementary facts, we can predict certain things about a patient. For example, if we know that a patient's dominant arm has been amputated, we can anticipate problems in manual dexterity and bilateral coordination. If, in addition, we know that the patient is 6 years of age, rather than 76, we can expect to direct treatment toward habilitation of hand skills as opposed to rehabilitation.

The pre-assessment image of the patient is used to generate a series of testable working hypotheses. The therapist reasons that, if a particular hypothesis is valid, then it should follow that such and such will be found in further study of the case. For example, a therapist learns from the occupational therapy referral that the patient is a 40-year-old woman with depression. The therapist reasons that, if this patient is depressed, she is likely to be disheveled, to have a low level of involvement in activities, and to concentrate on events associated with negative affect. In other words, by knowing that the patient is depressed, the therapist is able to view the patient as a representative of the class of depressed patients, and, thus, hypothesizes that she will exhibit characteristics of depression. The therapist then sets out to perform the procedures needed to substantiate the hypothesis.

Up to this point, the reasoning process is essentially deductive in nature. The therapist recalls some general postulates from memory and applies them to a specific patient. The open-ended question of what is wrong with the patient has now been refined to a set of better-defined problems for exploration and resolution.

The working hypotheses provide a plan for acquiring cues from the patient to test the hypotheses. A cue is any bit of information that guides or directs the assessment (3). Cues arise from the observational process that employs three general types of data-gathering methodologies: testing or measurement; questioning, including history taking and interviewing; and observation. Accurate clinical decisions are dependent on the collection of good cues. Two tests of the goodness of cues are reliability and validity.

Cues can be used to test the working hypotheses developed from deductive reasoning. By comparing each cue to the working hypotheses, sense may be made of the data. The therapist reasons, "This is what I expect to find, now what do I find?" A cue may be interpreted as confirming a hypothesis, disconfirming a hypothesis, or noncontributory to a hypothesis. Thus, as information is collected about the patient, the therapist decides repeatedly whether or not a finding is related to the patient's problems. Confidence in each hypothesis increases or decreases, based on the interpretation of additional data. Extensive case data are reduced by eliminating, or holding in reserve, data that do not appear significant. Hypothesis testing is thus another of the mind's strategies for simplifying data management. Hypotheses direct the collection of data and determine how they are organized and filed in memory. This organization prevents the mind from becoming overloaded with irrelevant facts and assists the therapist in retrieving information from memory.

Cues may also be combined to formulate new hypotheses. As cues are collected to test the validity of the deduced hypotheses, some cues may not fit well. Some of the performance problems we had expected to find will not be found, and others that we had not anticipated will become manifest. Our thinking begins to move from the classical, textbook picture of the disorder, to the disorder as it is uniquely manifested in this patient. The reasoning process now becomes inductive, with problem definition induced from empirical study of the patient, rather than deduced from the therapist's frame of reference. Additional cues may then be collected to test the inductively derived hypotheses. Clinical reasoning proceeds by developing hypotheses that pull together several inferences into a broader pattern or model of the patient.

After gleaning a clear perception of the patient's problems, the therapist then begins to search for cues indicative of the health of the patient as avidly as the search was conducted to identify dysfunction. Inductive reasoning and hypothesis testing are the basic processes through which the clinician assesses the patient's competencies, motivation for occupational achievement, and the environments in which the patient operates or will operate. These kinds of data are highly personal and hence are less likely to be deduced from knowledge of disease or disorder.

Data collection cannot continue indefinitely, and at some point the therapist decides that adequate information has been collected. How much data constitutes adequate data is dependent on the ethical consequences of an error in judgment (2, 4). A recommendation to institutionalize a patient because he or she is unable to look after his or her self-care needs would require more evidence than that required for the prescription of a rocker knife. Regardless of how many data are collected, however, the data base remains incomplete. The data base represents only a sampling of the patient's behavior. The therapist's task is to use this incomplete information to make a judicious decision. Decision making takes place under conditions of uncertainty.

Throughout the process of data collection, the therapist's pre-assessment image of the patient has been revised and elaborated, based on the accumulated cues. Once cue collection is stopped and no new information is being generated, hypothesis testing also ceases. The clinical reasoning of the therapist now resembles the dialectical process in which the therapist argues or defends the interpretation of the data in much the same way as a lawyer pleads a case in court. Does the patient have a dressing problem that is of concern? Is the cause of the patient's performance difficulties visual-perceptual problems? Is the mental status of the patient adequate for self-care? The evidence supporting or opposing each alternative is weighed with the objective of rendering one explanation more cogent than another. Inferences that are compatible are retained and others are rejected or modified as contradictions appear. Through the dialectical process the model of the individual patient is polished and repolished. In this way, the therapist arrives at a cohesive conception of the patient, and, having grasped the whole, re-interprets the parts in the light of this understanding. Once a holistic picture of the patient has been devised, the function of the assessment moves from model building to decision making.

What Are the Available Options?

The second of the three general questions guiding clinical inquiry is the therapeutic question: What can be done for this patient? Having proposed a model of the patient's occupational status, we then begin to explore the actions that could be taken to enhance occupational role performance. The intent is to generate a list of the treatment options available for the problems and assets presented by this patient. For example, suppose a patient's problems in self-care were attributed to hemiplegia subsequent to a cerebral vascular accident. To treat this problem, we might consider a neurological approach aimed at regaining controlled action in the involved arm, or a rehabilitative approach aimed at training the uninvolved arm to perform skilled activities, or a combination of these approaches. The aim, at this stage of clinical reasoning, is to foster an awareness of the range and kind of treatment possibilities. In effect, the therapist uses the model of the patient to construct a theory of practice for the patient.

Knowledge. The therapist's consideration of what could be done includes a review of the relative effectiveness of each treatment approach. If a particular treatment option is initiated, what results can be expected, and how long will it take to achieve them? Any hazards associated with the various treatments, or with no treatment, are evaluated in the light of the potential benefits.

Decision making concerning the appropriate action can approach certitude if the deleterious effects of a disorder without treatment are known, and if there is substantial evidence of how these effects can be altered by a particular treatment. We know, for instance, that if joints are not moved, contractures develop and the joints become immobile. Thus, movement becomes the scientifically acceptable treatment for preventing contractures.

For most occupational therapy approaches or procedures, however, the scientific evidence is not definitive. Rarely are the outcomes of research so specific that they allow us to know with 100 percent accuracy what will happen. Scientific findings generally emerge as probabilities rather than as certainties. They may, for example, tell us that 95 percent of the patients with right hemiplegia receiving self-care training will become independent in self-care. But when we apply this finding to Edith Jones, we do so with the recognition that her chances of becoming independent remain 50-50. The response of a patient to treatment cannot be predicted with certitude. Scientific knowledge can improve our chances of making accurate technical decisions but it cannot assure this. When the scientific evidence is inconclusive, the therapist has considerable leeway in devising treatment recommendations.

In the absence of scientific knowledge about the effectiveness of treatment options, clinicians rely on knowledge gleaned from their own clinical experience or from the experiences of others. Knowledge derived from practice rather than research indicates what works but may not indicate what works best.

Process. To draw up a list of the patient's treatment options, the therapist searches memory for relevant scientific and practice knowledge. Clinical experiences are stored and classified in memory and retrieved as needed for application to new patients. Each time a therapist treats a patient, a clinical experiment is performed in which the objective is to replicate a successful outcome of a past experiment (5). As a first step in reproducing the experiment, the therapist mentally reviews previous patients whose occupational status resembled the patient at hand. Although no two patients are exactly alike, the therapist assembles a subgroup of patients who are most similar to the patient under study (6). Treatment is selected for the new patient by analyzing and comparing the therapeutic actions and outcomes of the patients in the reference group. If there is a high degree of similarity between the patient being treated and previous patients, the therapist will select a treatment that is highly replicative. If the similarity is low, or if previous treatment was not very effective, the therapist will propose a treatment that is more inventive.

The cognitive process involved in the selection of treatment is again that of dialectical reasoning. The therapist argues one treatment option against another without recourse to new clinical data. The process of enumerating the patient's treatment alternatives relies heavily on the content of long-term memory. The more clinical experience therapists have, the more empirical data are available to guide decision making. It is impossible for therapists to consider a treatment with which they have no familiarity. Similarly, clinicians cannot debate the scientific merits of one procedure over another, unless the procedure has been scientifically investigated and the research has been assimilated.

What Ought to Be Done?

The third and final question to be considered is the ethical question: What ought to be done to enhance occupational competence? Simply because a goal appears technically feasible for the patient does not mean that it should be set as a goal. And, simply because a treatment approach can be initiated does not imply that it should be instituted. We must avoid confusing action that can be taken with action that ought to be taken. From an ethical standpoint, decisive action must take the patient's valued goals into account. It must conform to the patient's definition of health, accomplishment, and the "good life."

Knowledge. Ethical principles arise from reflection on the nature of humanity and human dignity. Respect for individuals requires that each individual be regarded as autonomous. Each individual has a definite pattern and characteristic style for mastering the environment in the pursuit of occupational competence. The life plan is guided by personal and cultural values. Values give meaning and direction to one's life by inciting future goals and sustaining involvement in activity.

The concept of respect for the individual implies that the occupational therapy treatment plan should not interfere with the patient's intentions for recovery. To develop an appropriate plan, the patient's values are distilled from the thematic continuity of the assessment of occupational status and taken into account in the review of technically feasible treatment options. When there is a range of possibilities for treatment goals and substantial lack of certitude concerning the technical merits of treatment alternatives, the therapist has considerable latitude in shaping recommendations. Expert advice is based more on opinion than fact. Ethical decision making requires the therapist to search for an understanding of the patient's life rather than to make an evaluation of it. This understanding facilitates the selection of options to be discussed with the patient.

The goal of the clinical encounter is to devise a therapeutic plan that preserves the patient's values and represents a mutual understanding between the therapist and patient. Occupational therapy involves habit training and often requires major restructuring of the way in which personal values are to be satisfied. If habits are to be developed, patients must choose the objects and processes that they want to master in occupational therapy. Worthwhile achievement is the end product of personally deliberated decision making. Occupational achievement begins with the choice to develop one's capabilities. It is the patient who restores, maintains, and enhances occupational performance. The patient, not the therapist, is the agent of change. The patient's active participation is required not only in determining and prioritizing the goals of treatment, but also in deciding on the methods to be used to achieve the goals. As a result of assuming personal responsibility for treatment decisions, the patient emerges from the assessment with an increased sense of self-determination and control, and a sense of commitment to accomplishing planned goals. In the capacity of expert advisor, the therapist guides patients through the decision-making process, and helps them fuse the intellectual and emotional aspects of decision making into choices that are right for them.

It cannot be assumed that the goals selected by a patient for himself or herself will match those the therapist would select. Each may have a different view of the "good life." Because most persons with quadriplegia secondary to a spinal cord lesion at the level of the 6th and 7th cervical vertebrae can relearn dressing skills, the therapist may reason that Tim Robbins should work toward this goal. However, Tim may conclude that he would prefer to spend his limited energy relearning how to manage his home computer.

When the therapist and patient have different goals, the potential for conflict is high, and the resolution of conflict can easily be tipped in favor of the therapist's view. Two factors contribute significantly to the therapist holding the balance of power (1). First, the therapist has the knowledge and skills to alleviate the problems facing the patient. The patient is thus dependent on the therapist for help. Second, the patient's position of dependency is compounded by the patient's vulnerability. As a result of disease or other disorders, patients sustain insults to functions regarded as integral to human life and living. The very fact that they need help may diminish their sense of autonomy. Adaptive functioning in basic life tasks, such as eating and dressing, may be impeded. Patients may even be unable to express their own values or make rational choices. Such impairments place a patient's moral agency at risk, and often make it easy to take advantage of the patient's right to control his or her life.

Process. The methods used to answer ethical questions differ from those used in science. While scientific questions are answered by accumulating data and testing hypotheses, ethical questions are resolved by coming to grips with values and making value judgments (7). To empower the patient to act as his or her own moral agent, the therapist provides the patient with the knowledge needed to participate effectively in decision making. The patient's choice must not only be autonomous, it must also be informed. Patients are not adequately informed to make choices, unless they can anticipate the results of their choices. The ethical and scientific dimensions of clinical reasoning are closely intermingled. The therapist presents the possible options for treatment, projects the outcomes of each option, explains how the outcomes are achieved, and outlines a time sequence for goal attainment. Together the therapist and patient consider each recommendation and evaluate the consequences of each alternative in terms of the patient's occupational potential and goals. If necessary, the therapist tempers unrealistic expectations, corrects inaccurate information, and points out any inconsistencies in rationalization. In effect, the therapist assists the patient in imagining what might occur, if treatment is to be undertaken or rejected. The strength of arguments for one action over another is assessed by dialectic. Greater weight is assigned a position according to the importance it holds for the patient. The selection of treatment becomes more difficult as the merits of one action over other actions become more ambiguous. The therapist makes known his or her preferences for the patient's treatment as well as the rationale for this decision. The patient ends the deliberation by making a choice.

Once the patient has determined the course of action, the therapist supports or confirms the decision. The therapist captures the persuasive elements of the dialectical argument, and uses them to instill in the patient a belief that treatment X is the best course of action and should be undertaken. At the same time, the therapist strives to bolster the patient's belief that he or she can carry out the treatment and achieve the goals. The reasoning process ends, therefore, in persuasive rhetoric, which we call "motivating the patient." In situations where therapists judge that they cannot lend support to the patient's choice, responsibility for providing occupational therapy services is terminated.

The therapist is privileged to help the patient select from the available opportunities those that are to be brought to fruition. As the patient executes and fulfills his or her choice, the therapist learns about the healing power of occupation. Occupational choice rekindles the will to live, and mobilizes the mind to discipline the body, in enacting the creative processes associated with reversing disability. The subtle wisdom of participation in self-initiated and self-directed occupation becomes apparent as confidence is rebuilt and hope is restored. Choices are not confined to the outset of treatment. Assessment and planning are on-going processes and there are repeated occasions to consider if treatment should be continued, terminated, modified, or supplemented.

This discussion of the ethical dimension of clinical reasoning has been based on three cogent assumptions: 1. that patients can serve as their own moral agents; 2. that the patient's choice is the ultimate one, and 3. that the therapist acts independently. None of these conditions may be met in a particular situation, which introduces further complications into the already complex process of ethical decision making. Surrogates may substitute for patients in the planning process because patients are too young, too impaired mentally, or too emotionally disturbed to participate in decision making. The rights of family members and the values and resources of society may limit the choices patients can make. The conjoint decision of therapist and patient may be modified or set aside by the health care team. These are vital issues that cannot be avoided in clinical decisions.

In summary, the data collected in clinical inquiry play three roles in clinical reasoning. First, clinical data are used to describe the patient's occupational status. This description includes an indication of the patient's adaptive skills, performance dysfunctions and their presumed causes, and competency motivation. Second, clinical data are used to conjure up a group of patients who have an occupational status and history comparable to the patient under consideration. These patients serve as a reference group for the identification of treatment options and prediction of treatment outcomes. Third, clinical data are used to identify therapeutic options appropriate to the specific needs of the patient, and to recommend a course of action consistent with the patient's values. As the clinical reasoning process moves from an assessment of occupational status, to a review of treatment options, to a selection of the right action, the scientific mode of reasoning gives way to nonscientific intellectual processes. Choosing a course of action involves many value considerations. The closer we come to making a clinical judgment, the less use is made of facts and hypothesis testing, and the more reliance is placed on the dialectical process, opinion, and persuasion.

Perfecting Clinical Inquiry

Now that what is involved in clinical study has been considered, it seems appropriate to ponder how our habits of inquiry can be improved. My suggestions are intended to be directional rather than comprehensive.

Model of the Patient

The therapist's understanding of the patient is highly dependent on the development of a model of the patient. It is pertinent to point out that studies conducted with counseling professionals have consistently supported the value of inductive theory building for practice, as opposed to the application of deductive theory. McArthur (8), for example, found that psychologists who applied existing theories in a doctrinary fashion turned out to be the poorest appraisers of personality. The critical element in devising a model of the patient is meticulous attention to the cues obtained from the patient. The ability to use assessment-related data to develop hypotheses is a vital professional skill.

Although hypotheses have adaptive value for organizing and managing data, they represent strong conceptual biases. In collecting and interpreting data, we have a tendency to overlook evidence that does not support our hypotheses. This is accompanied by an inclination to overemphasize positive evidence. In other words, we are psychologically prone to confirm our ideas and feel less compelled to refute them (4, 9). Agnew and Pyke (10) drew a salient comparison between the blindness imposed by hypotheses and that generated by love. They commented: "The rejection of a theory once accepted is like the rejection of a girlfriend or boyfriend once loved—it takes more than a bit of negative evidence. In fact, the rest of the community can shake their collective heads in amazement at your blindness, your utter failure to recognize the glaring array of differences between your picture of the girl or boy, and the data." (p. 128) The rigid application of a conceptual bias emerged as a major concern in my study of occupational therapists' thinking (11). The medical diagnosis was used to formulate the pre-assessment image of the patient and that image remained stable, even in the face of cues portending a revision.

Once cognizant of the pitfalls involved in hypothesis use, the therapist can initiate steps to avoid them. Obtaining a second opinion through consultation is one method commonly used to check the validity of one's interpretation. Consultants should perform their own assessments without reference to the patient's data base. Objectivity will be destroyed if consultants read reports or participate in discussions about the patient before conducting their own evaluations. The consultant's final opinion, however, should be based on the total available data (5).

A fixed data collection schedule is another mechanism used to prevent premature closure of hypothesis generation. The Occupational Therapy Uniform Evaluation Checklist (12) is an example of a fixed data collection schedule. It specifies the boundaries of occupational therapy practice and lists the variables to be reviewed for assessment. The Checklist forces the therapist to examine occupational performance from a panoramic view rather than microscopically. In so doing, it fosters the search for information that might suggest hypotheses the therapist might not otherwise have entertained. Adherence to a fixed routine assures the therapist that observations will be conducted that afford a fair and adequate opportunity to disprove as well as to confirm favorite hypotheses (13).

Research on the assessment process suggests that practitioners' "favorite" hypotheses concentrate on the dysfunctional aspects of patient performance (14, 15). We seem to be more interested in exploring why Alice Thompson falls so often than in ascertaining why she maintains her balance for so long. This preoccupation with problematic behaviors probably stems from the fact that they are the reason for the patient's referral to occupational therapy and constitute the focus of interventive efforts. Our first response to the question concerning the patient's occupational status is that it is dysfunctional. Our image of the patient changes as we collect additional cues and make adjustments in the initial picture. However, once our thoughts are anchored in dysfunction, it becomes difficult to switch our focus and too few modifications may be made in the image (16). Wright and Fletcher (14) point out that the perception of strengths and weaknesses as a unit, that is, as belonging to one person, requires the therapist to integrate two dissimilar qualities and that such synthesis is difficult. The same rationale may also be used to explain why practitioners are prone to see more pathology in their patients than the patients themselves perceive. Patients live with disability and adapt to it. Professionals regard disability as something to be eliminated. From this vantage point it is hard for professionals to see how disability can have any positive implications. Unfortunately, an emphasis on negative perceptions results in a skewed image of the patient. Dysfunctions are overestimated and abilities are underestimated (14).

Research also indicates that practitioners are more likely to hypothesize that a patient's problems are caused by factors within the patient as opposed to factors in the patient's physical and social milieu (14, 15). For instance, we are more apt to attribute a patient's distress to an inability to deal with authority figures than to an unreasonable supervisor. One reason for this tendency is that we generally have a clearer picture of patients than we do of the situations in which they live, work, and play. We generally see patients in health care settings and rarely sample their behaviors in natural settings. Thus, the patient's environment has a quality of vagueness about it compared to the patient, who appears more real. Another explanation for our neglect of the environment is that it is often impossible or very difficult to change the environment. Even if the patient's supervisor is irrational, the patient still has to learn to manage the situation or to find another job. Nevertheless, it should be recognized that our "clinic-bound" view of the patient may lead us to ignore or underestimate impediments to occupational performance residing in the environment. Furthermore, since patients often attribute their difficulties to situations rather than to themselves, there is a potential conflict between the therapist's and patient's perceptions of causation. The validity of the patient's causal attribution should not be dismissed lightly by the therapist because patients are attuned to situational exigencies by their struggle for occupational competence.

Recognizing the distortion that may occur because of the exploration of hypotheses oriented toward dysfunction rather than function, and emphasis on the person as opposed to the environment, the therapist can take steps to countermand these biases. The data collection schedule can be arranged to include both assets and liabilities for every aspect of occupational performance evaluated. Since a patient's self-perceptions of competence are as important for participation in activity as is competence itself, the checklist should also highlight the patient's subjective impressions of occupational status. The schedule can also be extended to include the physical and social environments. These additions will serve to remind us of the significance of these variables for occupation and to foster the habit of routinely evaluating them.

Integration of Data

The challenge presented to the mind by the occupational therapy assessment is intensified by the need to integrate the wide variety of information gathered about the patient. Although we may isolate aspects of human functioning for the purposes of data management, humans function as unities or wholes. Competence requires the individual to function as an integrated organism, with the physical, mental, emotional, and social dimensions of occupational behavior interacting with the surrounding human and nonhuman environment. The selection of treatment proceeds from a holistic conception of the patient. If the therapist is to manage the array of complex clinical data required to understand occupational behavior, a simplifying strategy is needed to ward off chaos in the information processing capabilities of the human mind. Clinical judgments are not made on the basis of one or two test scores. And, although the statistical integration of clinical data may be possible in some situations, it is impractical in most. We need a labor-saving device to assist the mind in integrating data. General systems theory provides such assistance.

According to the systems metaphor, data are framed in terms of relationships between systems and systems are ordered hierarchically based on increasing levels of complexity. In the assessment of a patient with a traumatic spinal cord injury, for example, we would look at the effects of disorder on other biological systems, such as the musculoskeletal and integumentary. At the same time, the rules of systems hierarchy would direct our attention to factors in the psychological system, such as competency motivation, which will strongly influence the recovery of the biological system as well as the social re-integration of the patient. Although the assessment checklist is useful for reminding us of the spectrum of occupational performance, general systems theory provides rules for organizing the list so that the assessment data can be meaningfully related and stored in memory.

Occupational Therapy Assessment

Once an occupational therapy assessment has been made, viable therapeutic approaches are selected. The selection of treatment rests on a comparison between the patient under consideration and similar patients previously treated. Thus, the effective application of treatment requires that patients be accurately identified and grouped together according to characteristics that are salient for occupation. If the results of a clinical experiment are to be replicated, we must begin with a patient who closely resembles those used in the original experiment.

At the present time, occupational therapy has no meaningful way of systematically describing occupational role performance and of differentiating homogeneous subgroups based on occupational characteristics. The medical diagnosis is inadequate for delineating the diverse levels of occupational performance that occur in patients with the same diagnosis. It also lacks utility for identifying the similar levels of occupational performance that occur in patients with different medical diagnoses. Occupational therapy lacks a standardized way of classifying the functional disabilities that result from disease and other disorders. In the absence of an agreed upon system for thinking about, remembering, and expressing our clinical observations, each therapist develops his or her own idiosyncratic system for describing occupational performance. To the extent that these informal descriptions facilitate a comparison of patients, based on salient occupational characteristics, the inferences resulting from the comparison will be valid. However, until a systematic scheme for describing and organizing clinical data is developed, we will not be able to communicate meaningfully with each other, either in informal exchanges in the clinic, or in more scientific dialogue in our journals.

Selection of Treatment

We have seen that a treatment recommendation is largely based on the therapist's recall of similar cases. Some memories are more easily recalled than others (6). We are more likely to think of patients treated recently than those treated in the past. It is easier to remember patients who are seen frequently than those treated less often. Exceptional cases, either of success or failure, make strong impressions. Inferences gleaned from patients who happen to come to mind are likely to be less accurate than those derived from systematic analysis. Although we can all recount our brilliant successes, how many of us know what our batting average is? How good are we as judges of occupational potential? By keeping a score of the accuracy of our clinical predictions, our judgmental abilities can be improved. Checking our initial predictions against discharge data is something that can be readily incorporated into the clinic routine. Did the patient accomplish what I predicted he or she would? If not, why not? Since the ultimate test of treatment is what happens after discharge, mechanisms should also be sought for testing the accuracy of our discharge predictions with follow-up data.

A common error made by therapists in arriving at a clinical judgment is to assume that the patient is like oneself (17). This assumption enables us to know the patient through ourselves. In using the self as a referent, one rationalizes, "I will treat the patient as I would wish to be treated if I were in this situation." This kind of reasoning risks denying the validity of the patient's values. The therapist ascribes meaning to the patient's situation according to his or her own criteria. The patient is presented with a decision, rather than a list of options, and the choice of occupation is denied. Respect for the individual implies giving the patient the same opportunity to express and achieve what the patient sees as worthwhile as one would desire for oneself. We must be sensitive to the human spirit and curb the offering of pseudo choices of activity that have little meaning for the patient.

Instrumentation

The validity of clinical reasoning is grounded in the collection of good cues. This is a critical point to consider as we concentrate our energies on developing assessment instruments for practice. The nature of the phenomena we are interested in evaluating dictates the appropriate kind of instrumentation. As clinicians, our primary interest lies in evaluating performance in self-care, work, and leisure occupations. Our concern is with the ability to do and that doing is observable. You do not need to infer that I can dress from my grip strength, or mental acuity. You can observe my ability. Performance is not an abstract construct as is intelligence, anxiety, or sensory integration. We can see performance. Furthermore, we know that performance in occupation depends on the environment or situation as much as it does on the patient. Recognizing the interplay between the patient and the environment leaves us with two fundamental ways of evaluating occupational performance. First, we can go into the environments where our patients live, work, play, and observe their performance. Second, we can simulate the occupational environments of our patients by providing test stimuli, such as beds, chairs, games, arts and crafts, and work and collect a series of behavior samples in our clinics. In this case, the validity of our evaluation depends on how well we approximate the places where function is to occur.

There is inherently little uniformity in the occupational environments of our patients and, if we try to establish that uniformity, we will obscure the validity of our evaluation. The strength of occupational therapy assessment lies not in placing patients in contrived and standardized situations and recording their responses, but rather, in observing them in real life settings and evaluating their adaptive competence. Thus, development of occupational therapy instrumentation depends on a conceptualization of the task environment, since this constitutes the test stimulus that evokes behavior. Our description of occupational behavior will be incomplete until we can mesh it with a description of the task environment.

The Art

Our exploration of the intellectual technology of clinical reasoning has focused on the scientific and ethical aspects. We have not considered the art except by implication and innuendo. In the peroration, I return to the therapist who says, "I don't know how I know, I just know that I know." While the scientific dimension of clinical reasoning is directed toward specifying the correct treatment from a technical standpoint, and the ethical dimension is geared toward selecting the treatment that meets the patient's criteria of right occupational role performance, the artistic dimension pursues excellence in achieving a right action—and it does this in the face of individuality, indeterminacy, and complexity (6). Artistry involves the orchestration of broad strategies for grappling effectively with the uncertainties inherent in clinical practice.

Skill in Thinking

Artistry is knowing as it is revealed in our actions (6). It is exhibited in knowing what to do and how to do it, rather than in knowing about something. In the early stages of acquiring a skill, such as dressing or piano playing, our actions are slow and clumsy. We have to think a lot about what we are doing and we make a lot of errors. But as skill develops, our actions become smooth, flexible, and spontaneous, and our thinking becomes automatic. We get a feel for the skill and that feeling allows us to repeat our performance. You know how to touch the piano keys to play a Mozart piano concerto, and your artistry is apparent in your music. If you were to describe your "knowing how to" play the piano, you would find this difficult, if not impossible, just as someone else would find it difficult to acquire the skill of piano playing by following your instructions.

Clinical reasoning may be viewed as a skill akin to piano playing. The skill consists of reducing the ambiguities inherent in clinical practice to manageable risks, and by so doing, enabling the formulation of prudent decisions (6). In each clinical transaction, the therapist is challenged to apply the theories and techniques of occupational therapy to a particular patient. Our textbooks inform us of the implications of blindness, hemiplegia, and age-related changes, but the hiatus between theory and practice becomes readily apparent when 90-year-old John Green, accompanied by his loving wife and devoted daughter, stands before us with hemiplegia, blindness, and the beginning signs of brain failure. Who among us has not experienced the gap between what we learned in school and what we need to know in the clinic.

Clinical problems are not neat. They are messy and complex. Everything that could be known about the patient is not known and much of the data collected are flawed and imperfect. Clinical problems deal with the uniqueness of patients rather than with their similarities. And, as Gordon Allport (18) reminds us, uniqueness is not equivalent to the sum of the ways in which a person deviates from the hypothetical average human. Unlike the simple cause and effect problems associated with basic science, clinical problems involve a complex interplay of multiple variables, the effects of which are largely unpredictable. The outcomes of occupational therapy treatment cannot be guaranteed. Clinical problems change as patients progress and regress and as the occupational opportunities provided by the environment fluctuate.

No one can provide "cookbook" recipes for dealing with situations in which uniqueness, uncertainty, complexity, and instability are the chief characteristics. There are no formulas or algorithms that tell us how to use the interneuronal processes associated with perception, memory, reasoning, and argument. In the clinical situation, the therapist is under pressure to act and to act now. One cannot interrupt an assessment to go to the library and read up on a critical point. In handling the uncertainties contained in clinical practice, therapists rely on their accumulated experience, conceptual and judgmental heuristics, intuition, and insight to "apply their knowledge" and make clinical judgments. In spite of defective data and incomplete information, artistic inquiry enables the therapist to make prudent decisions and to know why a treatment will work for a particular patient.

The artistry of clinical reasoning is exhibited in the craftsmanship with which the therapist executes the series of steps that culminates in a clinical decision. It is expressed in the interpersonal skills through which the therapist invites involvement in decision making, builds trust, explains treatment alternatives, and offers encouragement. Artistry manifests itself in the adeptness with which the therapist gathers cues: by selecting questions, probing for information not volunteered, clarifying discrepancies, administering tests, and observing performance. The degree of perfection with which the data to be processed are obtained influences the reliability and validity of the data, and hence sets limits on the quality of the final judgment. The art extends to grouping cues effectively, recognizing patterns, and depositing in memory organized reference images. The knowing derived from perceptual acuity, such as that needed to discern spasticity and achievement motivation, is also contained in the art of clinical reasoning. Linking the model of the patient with the appropriate memory structures to build a theory of practice for the patient requires considerable acumen. Artistic insight reaches its peak in combining evidence and opinion to support arguments convincingly, thus bringing closure to the decision-making process. Although each of these processes is difficult to master in and of itself, getting them coordinated and "on line" so that one can think "on one's feet" is an even vaster task.

Experts and Novices

The automation of clinical reasoning is not merely a matter of thinking faster. Experts think differently from novices. Because of the limited capacity of short-term memory, the human mind can only consider five to nine units of information at a time (16). This is why we find it difficult to remember telephone numbers. If I asked you to remember 9 1 9 9 6 6 2 4 5 1, chances are you would have forgotten the number long before you arrived at a telephone to dial it. However, if you knew that the area code for Chapel Hill is 919, and that all university numbers begin with the prefix 966, it is likely that you would have remembered the number 919-966-2451 correctly. Memory is aided by organizing and chunking information into larger units. By chunking telephone digits into familiar patterns, the number of units to be remembered is reduced and falls within the capacity of working memory.

Evidence is accumulating that expert and novice problem solvers differ in their use of problem-solving strategies, such as chunking (19). The expert sees and stores cues in patterns and configurations, whereas the novice records individual cues. Experts chunk data into larger information units than novices do. The expert creates memory structures by classifying data according to how they are to be applied in practice. The novice's memory structures, on the other hand, arise from features more peripheral to functional usage. The novice relies on conceptual principles to get things out of memory. The expert retrieves knowledge on the basis of situational cues as well as on conceptual stimuli. As the reasoning process unfolds, experts monitor their own thinking and understanding, which enables them to curtail errors and omissions. The ability to think faster is thus a result of thinking more efficiently, more functionally, and more critically.

Simply because our knowledge is in our action does not mean that we cannot think about it. When skill breaks down, and we strike a discordant note, drop a stitch, or fall off a bicycle, we step back, slow down our pace, and reflect on our actions. In clinical reasoning, skill breakdown occurs when clinical data are incongruous with our expectations and experience. Artistic inquiry is spurred by perplexity. As long as we are assessing patients whom we perceive as highly similar to those we have treated in the past, the clinical encounter presents no challenges, our intuitive understanding of the situation remains tacit. However, when we are no longer able to see things as we previously saw them, or do things as we previously did them, our curiosity is engaged, our anxiety is aroused, and we become inquisitive practitioners.

Expert clinicians are those who are competent in action and, simultaneously, reflect on this action to learn from it (6). They create opportunities for introspection by critically examining their reasoning to disclose bias and inconsistency. Artistic inquiry is also initiated through reframing, that is, by looking at the clinical situation from a new perspective. For example, a therapist might reason, "What would happen if this patient with low back pain were treated by diverting attention from back pain to pleasurable activity, instead of with exercises to improve body mechanics."

As thinking becomes less automatic and more conscious, through self-criticism and reframing, it also becomes more accessible to explanation. Although our explanations and descriptions of clinical reasoning may never be complete, they can become progressively more adequate through reflection, and the artistic dimension can be better understood. The conversion of our practice into theory revolves around a cycle of concrete experience, reflective thinking, conceptual integration, and active experimentation.

In conclusion, the clinician functions as a scientist, ethicist, and artist. The scientific, ethical, and artistic dimensions of clinical reasoning are inextricably intertwined, and each strand is needed to strengthen the line of thought leading to understanding. Without science, clinical inquiry is not systematic; without ethics, it is not responsible; without art, it is not convincing. The intentions and potentials of chronically disabled patients are difficult to discern, but a therapist of understanding will elicit them, and use them to help patients discover health within themselves.

Acknowledgments

Sincere appreciation is expressed to the following individuals for their critical review of the ideas presented in this paper: Anne Blakeney, David Hollingsworth, Teena Snow, and Joyce Sparling.

References

1. Pellegrino ED, Thomasma DC: *A Philosophical Basis of Medical Practice,* New York: Oxford University Press, 1981
2. Scriven M: Clinical judgment. In *Clinical Judgment: A Critical Appraisal,* HT Engelhardt, SF Spicker, B Towers, Editors. Dordrecht, Holland: D. Reidel Publishing Co., 1979, pp 3–16
3. Cutler P: *Problem Solving in Clinical Medicine: From Data to Diagnosis,* New York: Basic Books, Inc., 1979
4. Sober E: The art of science of clinical judgment: An informational approach. In *Clinical Judgment: A Critical Appraisal,* HT Engelhardt, SF Spicker, B Towers, Editors. Dordrecht, Holland: D. Reidel Publishing Co., 1979, pp 29–44
5. Feinstein AR: Scientific methodology in clinical medicine, III. The evaluation of therapeutic response. *Ann Intern Med* 61: 944–966, 1964
6. Schön DA: *The Reflective Practitioner: How Professionals Think in Action,* New York: Basic Books, Inc., 1983
7. Brody H: *Ethical Decisions in Medicine,* Boston: Little, Brown, and Co., 1981
8. McArthur C: Analyzing the clinical process. *J Counseling Psychol* 1: 203–208, 1954
9. Koester GA: A study of diagnostic reasoning. *Educ Psychol Measurement* 14: 473–486, 1954

10. Agnew NM, Pyke SW: *The Science Game,* Englewood Cliffs, NJ: Prentice-Hall, 1969

11. Rogers JC, Masagatani G: Clinical reasoning of occupational therapists during the initial assessment of physically disabled patients. *Occup Ther Res* 2: 195–219, 1982

12. Shriver D, Mitcham M, Schwartzberg S, Ranucci M: Uniform occupational therapy evaluation checklist. In *Reference Manual of the Official Documents of The American Occupational Therapy Association,* Rockville, MD: American Occupational Therapy Association, 1983

13. Elstein AS, Shulman LS, Sprafka SA: *Problem Solving: An Analysis of Clinical Reasoning,* Cambridge, MA: Harvard University Press, 1978

14. Wright BA, Fletcher BL: Uncovering hidden resources; A challenge in assessment. *Prof Psychol* 13: 229–235, 1982

15. Bateson CD, O'Quin K, Pych V: An attribution theory analysis of trained helpers' inferences about clients' needs. In *Basic Processes in Helping Relationships,* TA Wills, Editor. New York: Academic Press, 1982, pp 59–80

16. Matlin M: *Cognition,* New York: Holt, Rinehart and Winston, 1983

17. Sarbin TR, Taft R, Bailey DE: *Clinical Inference and Cognitive Theory,* New York: Holt, Rinehart and Winston, 1960

18. Allport GW: *Pattern and Growth in Personality,* New York: Holt, Rinehart, and Winston, 1961

19. Feltovich PJ: Expertise: reorganizing and refining knowledge for use. *Professional Education Researcher Notes,* December 1982/January 1983, pp 5–9

33

1984 Eleanor Clarke Slagle Lecture

Transformation of a Profession

Elnora M. Gilfoyle, DSc, OTR, FAOTA

During the past few decades occupational therapy has been in a state of identity crisis where the reality of occupational therapy and its proper place within health care systems is being questioned. Our profession must also question its value system, dimensions of practice, and educational requirements. In examining our place within health care systems, the profession must consider the current biomedical model, future trends for medicine, and the renaissance of the feminist movement. Our crisis should be recognized as a necessary impetus for the evolution that is under way. This crisis is our opportunity, not our pathology (1, p. 25).

Occupational therapy is in a period of transformation, a period of paradigm shift, which is a shift in ways of thinking about old concepts. Paradigm shifts are similar to upward spirals that transform perceptions of the present into new perspectives. During a paradigm shift, an evolution takes place, a move from one form of unity through a phase of disunity and on to reintegration at a higher level (2, p. 28). The disunity phase of an identity crisis can become positive in an emerging culture by shifting perspectives from static structures to perceptions of dynamic change. When we view evolution from the perspective of dynamic change, crisis becomes transformation (1, p. 71).

For example, as we question our philosophical base from a perspective of dynamic change, crisis over therapeutic media and methods will lead to new perspectives of *occupation* and *occupational*. As we question our allegiance to medicine, new perspectives regarding practice dimensions will be transformed from the medical model to a model of healthfulness where patients influence their own state of health. As we question competencies needed to enter professional practice, requirements and organization of our educational process will be transformed to prepare independent health professionals. Occupational therapy's paradigm shift, as a transformation process, will evolve into new understandings of the value of occupation and the patients' occupational process in promoting their own health. Our practices and education will be organized around our evolving value system.

Our present transformation is dramatic and stressful because the rate of change in society is too rapid for us to have time to react. Our current transformation is not just a paradigm change of occupational therapy, but a crisis of multiple dimensions. Occupational therapy is involved in a crisis affecting our professionals, profession, culture, health care systems, communities, states, nation, and world.

Through this transformation period, if occupational therapists operate within a closed system, we are doomed to regress. If we enlarge our awareness to include social, economic, and political factors; admit new information from a variety of sources; and take advantage of the capacity to integrate past and present perceptions and concepts, we will leap forward. Although dramatic and stressful, crisis can bring about a positive evolution in which we come to a new understanding of the present.

Originally published 1984 in *American Journal of Occupational Therapy, 38,* 575–584.

Transformation directs itself to the present and the future; however, occupational therapy's history cannot be ignored. To view our present as if there were no past would make a caricature of our profession. Our present achievements are not a museum of finished products but an ongoing progress that is three-fold: past, present, and future integrated into the upward spiral of our profession's evolution (3, p. 20).

To prepare for this upward spiral, we need a new recognition of some of the values we previously discarded. Two such values are the idea of patients' "doing" as the occupational process and our mission to provide services for severely and chronically disabled. We need to re-examine those conceptual models and professional principles that dominate our present, such as our allegiance to the biomedical model, physical disabilities and psychosocial disorders as a framework for education and practice, and principles of media and methods based on activity as an extrinsic force. We need to prepare ourselves for changes that go beyond educational readjustments that are based on physical and psychosocial disabilities and acute care. We need to go beyond the debate over particular theoretical orientations and models of practice to show how occupational therapists' attitudes and behaviors reflect a value system that underlies our culture. Also, we must acknowledge that our current changes are manifestations of a much broader cultural transformation that includes the impact of the feminist movement, transition from medical care to holistic health, and change from institutional care to self-care, and of an adjustment of our allegiance to rational knowledge to include the value of intuitive knowledge (2, p. 42). Through integration and examination of occupational therapy's past, present, and future, our profession's activities will show a constant flow of transformation and change.

In our past, conflict and struggle brought about important progress in our scientific foundations. Scientific progress will continue to be an essential part of the dynamics of change. However, research and science are not the only sources for paradigm change. Cultural aspects of our professional nature will also provide impetus for the profession's evolution. Additionally, social, economic, and political environments external to occupational therapy have boundless capacities for influencing our transformation. Among the many factors that affect change, three merit attention:

1. The shift in our values, dimensions of practice, and educational focus that forms the reality of occupational therapy;
2. The decline of our allegiance to the biomedical model; and
3. The slow, reluctant, but inevitable decline of patriarchy (2, p. 30).

Value System

Occupational therapy's reality lies in its culture. Culture is a synthesis of the objective and subjective contributions that make us a profession. Culture integrates our activities and behaviors, and provides a sense of direction for our practice. Culture has a powerful influence on what we do as occupational therapists because it is the driving force behind the development and success of our profession. Central to occupational therapy's culture is the science and art of the occupational process that facilitates meaning and order in the lives of persons with disabilities. Our culture, based on the use of occupation, includes the basic concepts and beliefs of our profession. Thus, values underlie our culture and form the heart of our profession.

In our day-to-day practices, "choices must be made and values are an indispensable guide in making them" (4, p. 22). Values become the essence of occupational therapy's philosophy because they describe what we do along with what is unique about our profession. Occupational therapy's values are reflected in the professions' belief in a person's ability to influence his or her own state of health through the use of occupation. Our value system emerges from our rational knowledge of occupation and our intuitive knowledge of the purposefulness of the occupational process. Because our profession's values have profound influence on what we do, they must be a matter of great concern for our profession and Association (4, p. 22).

During our transformation, our value system will change; however, we must not let external demands dictate those changes. Rather, *we should change because we continue to seek the truth of our values*. Professional values grow from the search for truth, and during our transformation we must act on the values of our history, and we must continue to seek the meaning and truth of our present (5, p. 211).

Occupational therapy had its roots in the belief that the health of individuals could be influenced by "the use of muscles and mind together in games, exercise and handicraft as well as in work" (6, p. 3). During the 1920s, Meyer's philosophy of occupational therapy proclaimed that human beings could maintain and balance themselves by being in active life and use. Meyer stated that the use humans make of themselves gives the ultimate stamp to their being (7).

Our early ideas of occupation and action were modified by the demands of both World Wars I and II, with wounded soldiers needing rehabilitation (8). Following the impact of the World Wars, occupational therapists' patient population changed and increased. Our early belief in games, exercise, handicrafts, and work (9, 10) evolved into beliefs in constructive activities, activities of daily living, work simplification, and training in the use of adaptive equipment, and prosthetic and orthotic devices. During the 1950s and 1960s our culture was based on sensorimotor rehabilitation techniques for physical dysfunction that were borrowed from physical therapy and on the concept of the therapeutic use of self in the treatment of psychiatric disorders, which was borrowed from psychology. In the 1960s and 1970s the idea of purposeful activity emerged. The value of activity was based on a neurobehavioral or an occupational behavior orientation, or on the biopsychosocial model underlying our practice (6, pp. 4–6). During the past decade, the concept of adaptation as the unifying theory for occupational therapy began to appear in our literature (11, 12).

Recently, our Association adopted an official statement that proclaims our philosophy and directs our practice (13). In the statement our belief in activity is presented:

- Including its interpersonal and environmental components
- As a means to prevent and mediate dysfunction
- As a means to elicit adaptation
- As having intrinsic and therapeutic purpose.

We offered this philosophy to describe our belief system and to declare what we do that makes us unique. However, in our day-to-day practices, occupational therapists frequently find themselves without convincing responses. Our proclaimed philosophy does not appear to provide us with a certainty about the sense of direction for our practices. Our literature communicates an internal debate: We have supported our values in activity, but have questioned the efficacy and credibility of activity as a therapeutic medium.

We, in occupational therapy, suffer from a pervasive uncertainty about our values, an uncertainty that undermines our commitment and leadership. Uncertainty about our therapeutic media and methods along with the interrelatedness of our science and art are central to our identity crisis. Therefore, our uncertainty must be recognized as an opportunity for us to transform traditional knowledge of activity into new perspectives of occupation and occupational. To maintain our upward spiral, our profession must re-examine the scientific view and value system that has been the basis of present concepts regarding activity and focus on future concepts based on a science of occupation and an art of purposefulness.

Re-examination of past concepts of occupation and a patient's action, together with integration of past ideas with our present concepts of activity, will direct our paradigm shift. Our paradigm shift will transform our concepts of purposeful activity into new dimensions of the concepts of occupation and occupational.

In 1909, C. Floyd Haveland said, "The therapeutic value of occupation for the insane is axiomatic and is based upon sound psychological laws" (8, p. 8). Treatment by means of occupation was termed *humane treatment* or *ergo-therapy* or *moral treatment* or *habit training* (8, pp. 6–7). In 1914, the term *occupational therapy* was first used by George Barton at a conference of hospital workers in Massachusetts. The term ran like a contagion, and earlier terms were dropped (14). By 1917, the objectives of the Association were formed, and statements of principles adopted occupational therapy as a method of treatment by means of purposeful occupation (8, p. 8).

Although the term *occupational* has been used since the early 1900s, we have not defined it. We have instead discussed terms such as activity, work, play, self-care, and most recently, human occupations, but we have neglected to examine the concept of occupational. Through re-examination of our early ideas, a value system based on the dimension of occupational will emerge.

Occupational is defined as a process of action in which a person is the action agent or the "doer." Our philosophy will be based on occupation as action with the events of the environment and occupational as the action process. Values of "doing" or "action," and the "doer" or "action agent" are the integrating force that will bring the science and art of the therapeutic purposefulness of occupation into focus.

Values are not rules of conduct, but concepts that group together certain modes of behavior (4, p. 14). Therefore, occupational therapists' scientific activities generate values that unite our practice and practitioners. Values provide unity and become the unifying force in our philosophy.

Our profession has been pleading for a generic or unifying theory. However, we must realize that unity may not mean a single theory, but rather a system of theories. Because theories are approximations of reality, occupational therapy needs a variety of scientific theorems, because each would be valid for a specific range of phenomena (2, p. 10). There cannot be a unified or universal description of occupational therapy in a single closed theory. During our transformation, we must not expend our resources developing a generic or single theory of occupational therapy, rather we must synthesize our concepts into a unifying system of values.

In the science of occupation no concept or belief can be considered final; concepts have been made and will be remade with new ideas becoming part of a broader understanding. Thus, the science of occupational therapy becomes an endless process of analysis. Also, although science analyzes experiences, scientific analysis does not provide the total picture of the world of therapy. It provides the materials for the picture. Human imagination synthesizes the materials to provide a more coherent picture of the world. Thus, through scientific activity and human imagination, the value system of occupational therapy will evolve (15).

Imagination is the common quality in both science and art. In science, imagination organizes experiences into concepts, and in art imagination allows us to enter into human experiences (5, pp. 18–20). Science offers explanations and rational knowledge, whereas art carries an awareness or intuitive knowledge. Science of therapy is a creation to explain, and the art of therapy is a creation to relate, one where the patient receives and recreates in his or her own image.

Therapeutic art is not an external giving by the therapist; it is an internal receiving by the patient. *It is through internal receiving that occupational experiences become purposeful*. Through science, the therapeutic value of occupation can be predicted and explained, but purposefulness of an occupational process cannot be measured and explained through research. Thus, the purposefulness of occupation will always remain as our art.

Society judges occupational therapists by the outcomes of our activities and behaviors. Therefore, our day-to-day practices must reflect our value system. Our lifelong learning process must also be designed to facilitate learning of and belief in our values. Study of values continually clarifies the power of our profession, and at the same time recognizes that the profession and society are in a continual interactive process. As occupational therapists we can view ourselves as professionals, freely controlling our own practice, or as adaptive therapists "at the beck and call of others" (16, p. 20).

A system of values is our key to professionalism. Without a value system we will continue to be dependent on others. Conformity, the need for external approval and reliance on directions from others, characterizes an adaptive therapist. Independence, creativity, and self-directiveness characterize an integrated professional.

As an independent profession we must promote an integrative approach to our practice. Occupational therapists who argue against the effectiveness of activity are being forced to be adaptive. Arguments against the use of activity have appeared in our literature. West (17) has summarized these arguments:

1. Length of stay in acute settings is insufficient to show progress through activities.

2. There is pressure from physicians, administrators, and third-party payers to demonstrate cost-effective and objective measurable improvements.
3. Use of activities jeopardizes reimbursements.
4. Requirements for quality assurance reduce the use of crafts for substitutions that are reliable standardizations.
5. Crafts can be negative reinforcers to a patient who has lost skills.
6. Use of activities limits practice in the area of physical dysfunction.
7. Activities may be too complex for many of our low functioning patients (p. 16).

These arguments are worthy of our attention, but we must also be aware that they reflect the reality of external forces, the profession's conformity to external approval, reliance on directions from others, and our need for survival and immediate recognition. Arguments presented also subscribe to a narrow perspective of activity. Through transformation, a broader perspective of occupation and occupational will emerge, and declaration of our value system will promote an integrative approach to practice.

Scientific knowledge of occupational therapy is not a notebook of facts about occupation or therapy; rather, our rational knowledge is an imaginative arrangement of concepts that are a creation of the human mind. Our scientific knowledge is a responsibility for the integrity of what we are, primarily of what it is we value. Our values come from our experiences, from testing what does and does not work; values are modified through the development of our profession and the environment and culture of our time. As occupational therapists, we cannot maintain our professional integrity if we let others direct our values while we continue to live out of a "ragbag of morals that come from past beliefs" (3, p. 436).

Dimensions of Practice

Within the changing milieu of the 1980s, there are two environments for which occupational therapy must focus its actions, medical and educational. Medical and educational arenas will have a direct impact on the dimensions of our practice. Occupational therapy's allegiance to the medical model has historic roots dating back to our beginnings. Our need for acceptance and survival within the medical world, our orientation to short-term gains, and society's acceptance of patriarchal authority have been major factors in our development as an allied medical field. However, legislation in the 1970s delineated one aspect of occupational therapy services as an education-related service, not a medical service (18). The term *related service* has had important influences upon the changing concepts of our profession and the implementation of educational services. Introduction of the term *related service* has been a major impetus for change in both definition and concept of occupational therapy and education.

Implementation of related services has been a problem for our traditionally endowed public education systems and our medically based practitioners. Factors that present problems within educational systems include:
1. Occupational therapy services have traditionally been available from medical systems and therefore should not be offered through educational systems.
2. Educational personnel have neither been trained nor do they consider themselves qualified to deliver related services. School personnel should not supervise and have legal responsibilities for occupational therapists.
3. Problems of interagency coordination have too often been compounded with traditional health agencies refusing to assume responsibility for health care services that are now defined as educationally related.
4. Services are costly, which puts pressure on local school budgets that have been only partially funded by federal reimbursements. Thus, the ratio of therapist to students has been too large to provide services.

These factors are real. Thus, it is not surprising that educational systems have tried to protect their limited resources by searching for appropriate limits on related services. Educational organizations have tried to do this by attempting to define various services as not being educationally related at all; that is, they claimed that occupational therapy provided care to persons with conditions not educationally related but medically related.

Education's attempt to limit related services led to critical judicial decisions. Most notable was the expansion of the term *education* to encompass those self-care areas important for children with handicaps. Federal courts emphasized that education for handicapped children may be directed to achievement of "self-sufficiency or to some degree of self-care" (19, Connecticut, 1977). Thus, basic skills such as eating, walking, talking, and dressing, which come easily to nonhandicapped children, represent a high level of educational gains for some children. In effect, education is no longer defined as what schools have traditionally done; rather, education may include programs that have the capacity "to equip a child with the tools needed in life" (19, *Fialowski vs. Shapp,* Pennsylvania, 1975). As summarized in the Delaware Supreme Court in 1980: ". . . education is concerned with much more than simply the 3 R's—the definition would include instruction to teach one to dress oneself, toilet training, eating skills and other self-help skills" (19, p. 26). The net result is that federal laws, expanded by federal court decisions, have adopted broad definitions of both "education" and "relatedness," and as such the laws have defined occupational therapy as an education-related service. Efforts to limit the extent of related services run counter to legal precedent. In fact, the major limitation to the concept of "relatedness" is not in the law or courts, not in regulations or policies, not with educational administrators, but within ourselves. Occupational therapists' concept of related services appears limited to direct treatment programs. Our need to hang on to our traditional medical model service delivery patterns not only presents education with questions of our medical relationships, but introduces a further dilemma with our own professional identity.

Educators and occupational therapists continue to argue that the specific services provided by and described as occupational therapy should be properly considered medical in nature and thus should be delivered in medical settings. However, medical services is a specific legal term in P.L. 94–142, the Education for All Handicapped Children Act. Despite common usage of the word *medical,* the law defines medical as only those services "provided by a licensed physician." Thus, any service that is education-related and provided by a nonphysician is not a medical service under P.L. 94–142.

Although most handicapped conditions served by an occupational therapist can be described as medical in their origin, the effect and amelioration of the conditions are often educational, particularly under the broad concept of education. Thus, related services such as occupational therapy are an educational responsibility.

Through our transformation, occupational therapy services will continue to expand within educational systems. Federal courts and federal laws will continue to mandate related services. Educational and health care systems will need to collaborate in programs for children and youth. The concept of occupational therapy as an education-related service will be accepted by our professionals, the profession, our Association, and society.

Expanding related services within public school systems will inevitably tax existing resources. However, as a legal and, perhaps even more important, as a practical matter, efforts to limit related services seem destined to fail. Public schools are becoming a lead agency in services for handicapped children and youth; thus efforts to minimize legal interpretations of related services run counter to expanding concepts of education entitlement. Our energies must be expended in optimizing interagency cooperation, developing more efficient service delivery systems, reallocating funds and staffing resources, and generating additional resources whenever possible. Regardless of the direction of the future, legal, political, economic, professional, and organizational issues will influence our transformation. By recognizing both external and internal issues and by identifying strategies, we can influence our own future.

One of the major external forces to affect education-related services of occupational therapy will be the future of health care delivery systems. Because health care industries will influence our services, we must identify issues related to health so our profession can develop appropriate strategies for action.

Health care, now the third largest category of the gross national product, represents more than $2 billion a year in costs (1). Health care has become too large, too complex, and too expensive for our practices to depend on traditional or conventional systems of providing services for persons with special needs. Health care professionals can no longer practice solo; solo practices of the past decades are too expensive. Health care services depend on collaborative efforts. Health care and educational agencies will collaboratively service children and youth, and health care and community agencies will service adults. Also, occupational therapists will find themselves practicing and providing services in collaboration with a variety of professionals.

In 1980, federal, state, and local public funds represented approximately 65 percent of medical payment, with 30 percent coming from third-party providers such as insurance companies. Less than 5 percent of health costs come from private individuals. Thus, third parties and taxpayers pay for medical care. Although the majority of the health care dollar goes to hospitals, physicians continue to decide how the dollar will be spent. However, as we move to a system of prospective payment, one that gives the hospital an economic incentive to be more efficient and less expensive in its management of patients, the incentives for physicians and health care providers may be in direct opposition to the incentives of hospitals. Prospective payment will influence the concept of acute medical care within medical establishments, and a transition to personal responsibility or self-care and home health programs will occur. Transition from institutional care to self-care will have a direct impact on service delivery patterns of occupational therapists.

Predictions for delivery modalities for the upcoming decade include:

1. Increased outpatient care
2. Increased home health services as an alternative to hospital care
3. Increased quality and quantity of long-term care for the severe and chronically disabled
4. Increased sensitivity to physical and emotional suffering of the aged
5. An increase in multi-institutional systems that provide cost-effective services and enhance use of personnel
6. Increased interaction and cooperation among systems, with increased competition for personnel, new markets, and access to capital and technology.

If these predictions prove correct, five assumptions seem appropriate for the delivery of occupational therapy services:

1. Occupational therapy will continue to be practiced through organizational structures with increased pressures to make these organizations cost effective.
2. New and more effective communicative networks must be developed to ensure continuity of care among the various health professionals.
3. Demands for interagency collaboration will be imperative.
4. Power and political issues operating within health and educational organizations will increase rather than decrease.
5. New service delivery patterns involving consultation and monitoring, and collaborative programming will be imperative.

Our literature suggests that many occupational therapists are frustrated because management concepts are not being used in practice and because students are not being taught management concepts and skills. Occupational therapists will have to learn skills associated with effective consultation, supervision, leadership, and communication. It is not enough to learn the theory and practice of occupational therapy. Obviously a problem occurs; predictions for the future suggest multidisciplinary interagency collaboration, which requires management, consultation, communication, and leadership skills. Our literature suggests we are not providing these skills for our practitioners. Thus, occupational therapy curricula must modify traditional approaches to course content to prepare professionals for the changing health care systems.

Educational Focus

The nature of our education determines essential aspects of occupational therapy practices. Attempts for paradigm change or transformation must include changes in our educational focus and certification requirements. Accreditation with the American Medical Association has established a link between medicine and occupational therapy, and this link has dominated our educational system ever since. The biomedical model's influence on education is reflected in our academic and fieldwork divisions of physical dysfunction (treatment of the body), psychosocial dysfunction (healing of the mind), and pediatric and geriatric age groups (facilitation of development). We promote an artificial division within our profession by educator's attention to a particular age group or to the body or mind. Certification to practice ensures successful mastery of knowledge of physical dysfunction and psychosocial dysfunction, not the ability to promote a patient's care of self and meaningful life through the use of occupation. Our educators must begin to base curricula on our value system of occupation and the occupational process, and on the science of occupation and the art of purposefulness. We must also address our allegiance to holistic and ecological concepts of health, and our relationship to education. In addition, management, leadership, and consultation skills need to be included in our curricula.

Transformation of our educational focus, together with our reexamination of concepts, will provide impetus to solve our identity crisis. Along with these activities, we must also examine our entry-level requirements for professional practice. Currently our entry-level requirements are inadequate for dealing with the major problems of our times and predicted demands for future practices. Predicted increases in home health practices, transition from medical to holistic health care, declaration of our profession as an education-related service, new dimensions of service delivery, and an increase in our scientific activities are but a few of the many aspects of transformation that need to be addressed by our entry-level preparation and requirements.

Decisions and recommendations related to our educational focus and requirements must be based on careful study, but they must begin immediately. Transformation of our profession is underway; our emerging culture with its new perspectives must be reflected in our educational preparation processes. Official bodies of our Association, particularly the Commission on Education, Executive Board, and Representative Assembly, must recognize the crisis in our education preparation and determine resolutions.

Occupational therapy reality will include transformations of our value system, dimensions of practice, and educational focus. Crisis of our reality will evolve into new perspectives of our profession. Although our paradigm shift occurs within, society's decline of allegiance to the biomedical model and to patriarchal authority have significance to occupational therapy's practice within health care systems.

Decline of Patriarchy

In *The Aquarian Conspiracy*, Ferguson proclaimed: "The power of women is the powderkeg of our time" (1, p. 221). Feminism has become a major force in our culture. Because 95 percent of our professionals are women, it is imminent that the women's movement shall play a pivotal role in the transformation of occupational therapy. A renaissance of feminist ideals is creating new images of women and men. New modes of thinking and value systems are emerging. Role shifts and sharing of responsibilities are bringing about far-reaching changes in society's attitudes and behaviors. Our culture has been based on the belief that self-assertive behavior is ideal for men and submissive behavior is expected from women. Self-assertion was manifested through power, control, and domination of others. Competitive behaviors characteristic of self-assertion have been highly regarded and promoted in our society. Women have been expected to be submissive and to fulfill the needs of others, and to perform those services that make life more comfortable. Society has expected women to "create the atmosphere for the competitors to succeed" (2, p. 45).

In the past, science and technology have been based on the belief of male supremacy and dominance. Medical societies in particular have not respected women's contributions to science and technology; rather, the culture of medicine has expected women to provide the caring, not the knowledge to understand the cure or the process to heal. Masculine supremacy has led to a medical high-tech dissonance. We are going from forced masculine technology to a balancing of "high tech/high touch." As Naisbitt (20) pointed out, high-tech dissonance is being transformed to balance with high touch. High tech/high touch is part of the balancing of feminist and masculine values. With this balancing, more respect for women's contributions to medicine, health, and education will occur. The allied health fields, dominated by women, will be recognized not as allied but as independent health professions.

Transformation to an integrative power of technology and touch within medicine will further shake the foundations of occupational therapy.

Decline of Allegiance to the Biomedical Model

As medicine transforms to be in keeping with society's demands, our allegiance to the current biomedical model will decline. Modern scientific medicine has been based on a biomedical model that views the body as a machine. Disease, illness, and handicapping conditions represent malfunctions of the body machine's mechanisms. Only the physician knows how to correct malfunctioning, because he or she has been the one with scientific knowledge and technology. Authority and responsibility have been delegated to the physician who intervened and fixed the machine. Society has been spellbound by the mystique of medicine (2, p. 158).

Americans are losing faith in medical establishments and physicians because the increase in medical costs far exceeds the effectiveness of care. Although human life expectancy has increased and many types of illnesses have been controlled, the health of our population has not improved. For example, there are increases in learning disabilities, child and adult abuse, mental illnesses, and suicide among youths. Medicine's dependence on high technology has increased problems of health, with biomedical interventions having little impact on the health of entire populations (2, p. 138).

Current medical therapy is based on principles of intervention. The medical profession has relied on outside forces such as drugs and surgery without viewing the patient as a responsible individual who has a healing potential within and who can initiate the process of getting well (2, p. 152). Principles of intervention have also dominated the practice of occupational therapy. For example, we have based our philosophy and research on the outside force of activity or the effects of adaptive equipment or devices. Although these are important, we must not forget the values that are inherent to our profession: the patient's intrinsic motivation to "do" and the "doing" aspect of healing.

Transformation of the biomedical model is underway with the paradigm shift based on an awareness of the "essential interrelatedness and interdependence of all phenomena—physical, biological, psychological, social, and cultural" (2, p. 265). Concepts of prevention, relationships of physical and social environments, and the interplay of body, mind, and environment in the healing process are beginning to influence medicine. Medicine's paradigm shift is opening up new areas in search of a health orientation. Medical science now acknowledges that the art of healing is essential to all health care. With new emphasis on the human aspects of health, there will be an increased move from the medical establishment (institution) to personal responsibility (self-care and home health).

Occupational therapy has been a profession that has based its values on a paradigm of wellness. We consider patients active participants in their own care. We believe people are able to influence their own health and recognize the interplay of body, mind, and environment. With transformation of the biomedical model to a holistic health model, our profession must proclaim these values and communicate our philosophy. Medicine and society are catching up with us, but we must not let them pass us by.

Summary

Professional evolution includes a period of disunity, a phase when old values and concepts are being examined, and new perspectives emerge. Disunity can be a positive impetus for dynamic change. Transformation provides a higher level reintegration through which new understanding and progress unfold. Occupational therapy's transformation is now; it is time for careful analysis and creative synthesis.

Transformation is a three-fold process of integration of past, present, and future into an upward spiral of professional development. Transformation is a constant flow of activities influenced by both internal and external factors. Although there are multidimensions that influence occupational therapy's transformation, three major components are inherent in the profession's paradigm shift: (1) society's decline in patriarchal authority;

(2) decline in allegiance to a biomedical model; and (3) shift in values, dimensions of practice, and education that form the reality of occupational therapy.

Transformation of our profession will be a paradigm shift:

- In our value system of purposeful activity to a new perspective of occupation and occupational
- In our quest to develop a unifying theory for recognition of the unifying force of values
- In our concepts and theories to include the science of occupation and the art of purposefulness
- From total allegiance to scientific knowledge to include intuitive knowledge
- From being an allied medical field to an independent health profession that is both educationally and medically related
- From a biomedical model to a paradigm of wellness
- In balancing of feminine and masculine values of human nature
- In organizing educational curricula and entry-level requirements that reflect our value system and predicted practice dimensions.

As Naisbitt said, "We are living in the time of parenthesis, the time between eras" (20, p. 249). Occupational therapy has not left the past behind, but it has not quite embraced the future either. Thus, our profession is in a time of parenthesis that brings us many uncertainties. Uncertainties, however, can be our opportunity. We need only make use of the challenge and possibilities that are part of our dynamic present. Transformation is a time to direct our own future. "We stand on the brink of a new age, the age of an open world, a time of renewal when a fresh release of spiritual energy in the world culture may unleash new possibilities. The sum of all our days is just our beginning" (1, p. 42).

We have reached our turning point. We have the means to solve our crisis and continue our transition to higher dimensions. However, we must *choose* to do so.

References

1. Ferguson M: *The Aquarian Conspiracy: Personal and Social Transformation in the 1980's.* Los Angeles: JP Tarcher, Inc., 1980
2. Capra F: *The Turning Point: Science, Society, and the Rising Culture.* Toronto: Bantam Books, 1983
3. Bronowski J: *The Ascent of Man.* Boston: Little, Brown & Co., 1973
4. Deal TE, Kennedy AA: *Corporate Cultures: The Rites and Rituals of Corporate Life.* Reading, MA: Addison-Wesley Pub. Co., 1982
5. Bronowski J: *A Sense of the Future.* Cambridge, MA: MIT Press, 1977
6. Hopkins H, Smith H: *Willard and Spackman's Occupational Therapy,* 6th Edition. Philadelphia: JB Lippincott, 1983
7. Meyer A: The Philosophy of Occupational Therapy. *Archives of Occupational Therapy* 1(1): 1–10, 1922
8. Kidner TB: *Occupational Therapy, The Science of Prescribed Work for Invalids.* Stuttgart, Germany: W Kohlhanne, 1930
9. Slagle EC: Training aids for mental patients. *Archives of Occupational Therapy* 1(1): 1–10, 1922
10. Hall HJ, Back M: *Handicraft for the Handicapped.* New York: Moffact, Yard & Co., 1916
11. King LJ: Toward a science of adaptive responses. *Am J Occup Ther* 32: 429–430, 1978
12. Gilfoyle E, Grady A, Moore J: *Children Adapt.* Thorofare, NJ: Charles B. Slack, 1980, Chapter 3
13. The Philosophical Base of Occupational Therapy. American Occupational Therapy Association Resolution #531, April 1979
14. Barton GE: *Teaching the Sick: A Manual of Occupational Therapy and Re-education.* Philadelphia: W. B. Saunders, 1914, p 4
15. Bronowski J: *The Visionary Eye: Essays in the Arts, Literature and Science.* PE Ariotti, Editor. Cambridge, MA: MIT Press, 1978, pp 20,21,31
16. Hall Bryan P: *The Development of Consciousness: A Confluent Theory of Values.* New York: Paulast Press, 1976, p 20
17. West W: A reaffirmed philosophy and practice of occupational therapy for the 1980's. *Am J Occup Ther* 38:15–23, 1984
18. Education for All Handicapped Children Act, 1975, P.L. 94-142, *Federal Register,* Tuesday, Aug. 23, 1977, Sec. 121A 13
19. Related services and medical services requirements under current legal standards. *Focus* 1(2), 1981. Reprinted in Information Packet, Occupational Therapy in the School Systems. Rockville, MD: AOTA, 1982, pp 25–29
20. Naisbitt J: *Megatrends.* New York: Warner Books, 1982, Chapter 2

34

1985 Eleanor Clarke Slagle Lecture

A Monistic or a Pluralistic Approach to Professional Identity?

Anne Cronin Mosey, PhD, OTR, FAOTA

In my review of occupational therapy literature, professional identity seems to be one of our major areas of concern. Who are we, how do we define ourselves, what are we about? The issue of professional identity is important. Without a collective sense of self we cannot effectively deal with other factors, both internal and external, that do and will continue to influence our practice.

Professions can take one of two approaches to their identity: monistic or pluralistic (1, 2). Borrowing from philosophy and taking some liberties (3), these terms are defined as follows.

Monism is the belief that there is one basic principle that is the essence of reality: that all processes, structures, concepts, and theories can be reduced to one governing principle.

Pluralism is the belief that there is more than one basic principle: that everything cannot be reduced to a single principle.

Translated into a language more common to us, monism is the attempt to define occupational therapy by one of its elements or a facet of an element: for example, a philosophical statement, a legitimate tool, or a particular frame of reference. The element selected is viewed as the basic principle that governs all other elements. Because there is only one basic principle, a monistic approach to professional identity tends to be relatively static.

On the other hand, a pluralistic approach suggests a broader perspective. Pluralists feel that all elements of the profession must be taken into consideration. The whole can only be defined by all of its parts. Moreover, it should be defined in such a way that the ever-changing nature of the profession can be easily accommodated.

As a guide to where this presentation is going, I will

- Briefly outline the elements of a profession,
- Describe and assess a monistic approach to professional identity,
- Discuss some factors that lead to the consideration of a pluralistic approach, and
- Outline the rationale for the nature of a pluralistic identity.

My preference is pluralism, lest anyone think I intend to be totally unbiased here.

The Elements of a Profession

The term *elements* refers to those components that constitute the substance of a profession (4–8). Thus, any group that describes itself as a profession has the following elements.

Originally published 1985 in *American Journal of Occupational Therapy, 39,* 504–509.

A Set of Philosophical Assumptions

This is a collection of beliefs about the nature of the individual, the relationship of individuals with their environment, and the goals of the profession. Philosophical assumptions are identified, developed, and analyzed through philosophical inquiry, not, it should be noted, through empirical research.

A Code of Ethics

This is a statement of various principles of human conduct. This code outlines the responsibilities and privileges of members of a profession in relationship to society, their clients, and each other.

A Body of Knowledge

This is a collection of various theories that serve as the scientific foundation for practice. Theory, as used here, refers to a description of a set of events. It is concerned with predicting how and under what circumstances these events occur and how they relate to each other.

The body of knowledge of a profession is made up of theories that are a) selected from a variety of sources because they have specific relevance to practice and b) developed by the profession.

As mentioned, the goals of a profession are outlined in its philosophical assumptions, whereas a profession's body of knowledge describes the means for reaching these goals.

Domain of Concern

This is a statement of those areas of human experience in which a profession has expertise and offers assistance to others. In occupational therapy these areas are often described as being made up of occupational performances (e.g., activities of daily living, family interactions, play/recreation, and work) and of performance components (e.g., cognitive, psychological, and motor functions; sensory integration; and social interaction).

Aspects of Practice

This is a statement of the sequence of events whereby members of a profession assist clients in problem identification and resolution. In occupational therapy, these aspects include screening, formal evaluation, intervention, and termination. All of these interactions include communication and documentation.

Legitimate Tools

These are the vehicles that practitioners in a given profession use to assist clients. The legitimate tools of occupational therapy are not well defined. This issue is addressed later.

A Linking Structure

This is a framework whereby theories are restructured into a form that makes them applicable to practice (9–15). Professions need a linking structure because the only function of a theory is to predict relationships. No action is suggested or recommended. Theories do not answer the questions of how they should be applied, when they should be applied, relative to whom, and so forth. Linking structures answer these questions and thus provide the practitioner with a guide for action. The linking structure we have in occupational therapy is usually labeled a "frame of reference." We have a number of frames of reference, each of which addresses different components of our domain of concern. They help us identify what we should evaluate for and how to go about the process of evaluation, goal setting, and intervention.

Practice

This is the application of one or more linking structures (in our case, frames of reference) to meet the particular needs of each patient. This is what we do in the clinic, school, community, or wherever we choose to make use of our knowledge and skills.

Empirical Research

This is the study of people, things, and events through observation. It may be qualitative or quantitative in nature. The major types of empirical research in occupational therapy are a) evaluative, which determines the effectiveness of our various frames of reference, and b) theoretical, which develops and tests theories that are, or may become, part of our body of knowledge. These are two very different types of research that provide us with different kinds of information (16).

The elements outlined earlier are common to all professions. A profession without an ethical code, for example, would never be allowed to practice, at least not in our society; a profession without a set of philosophical assumptions, although a changing one, would be without direction.

Professions are complex and are made up of many elements. What is the best way, then, to go about the process of establishing professional identity? We are back to the major question raised earlier. Which is more prudent, a monistic or pluralistic approach?

A Monistic Approach

Some of the monistic approaches that have been suggested for occupational therapy are Human Growth and Development (17), Purposeful Activity (18, 19), Occupational Behavior (20), Adaptive Responses (21), the Ecological Systems Model (22), and Human Occupation (23). As mentioned, a monistic approach proposes that one of the profession's elements, or a facet of an element, serves, or ought to serve, as primary. This element becomes the principle that governs all other elements. Structurally, a monistic approach usually takes the form of a comprehensive theory. As used in the context of a profession, a comprehensive theory is a grand theory with broad parameters (24–26). One element, or a facet of an element, serves as the nucleus of the theory. A select number of concepts and postulates are derived from this nucleus and form the substance of the theory.

The following four assumptions are made about a theory: First, a comprehensive theory, when adequately stated, contains all the important content of the subordinate elements. Second, its structure allows it to serve as a guide to practice; no linking structure is necessary. The theory provides sufficient information for evaluation, goal setting, and intervention, regardless of a client's particular areas of function and dysfunction. Third, the theory is the sole valid focus of a profession's research endeavors. Fourth, a comprehensive theory gives a profession a unified identity.

Proponents of the various monistic approaches listed have each, in one way or another, recommended the development of a comprehensive theory. However, each has suggested a different theory, with a different element or concept as the nucleus.

Aside from the conflict inherent in so many different suggested monistic approaches, the idea of a single comprehensive theory raises the following critical issues.

1. A comprehensive theory tends to be exclusionary. Important aspects of a profession's practice may not be included. For example, if we decided that human growth and development should be the core concept of our comprehensive theory, how would we fit into that theory such things as dealing with diminished range of motion or edema? Moreover, who should decide what will be included and what will be excluded?

2. A comprehensive theory usually has a strong philosophical overtone (23, 27). The profession's body of knowledge and philosophical assumptions are often so intertwined that it is difficult to determine what is a theoretical statement and what is a statement of belief. Thus, scholarly activities may be difficult to pursue. For example, should one use the tools of empirical research or the tools of philosophical inquiry?

3. When a profession opts for a comprehensive theory, its members are placed in a constricted position. The comprehensive theory becomes so central and requires such a degree of loyalty that creative, divergent, and/or independent thinking may not be encouraged or even tolerated.

To give a historical example, if we had decided that our comprehensive theory ought to be based on the nuclear concepts of play and work, would Ayres' ideas about sensory integration have been accepted, both as part of our body of knowledge and as one of our frames of reference? Research undertakings are usually considered appropriate only when they are concerned with the elaboration or refinement of the comprehensive theory or its application in practice (28, 29). Research designed to test the validity of the theory is rarely suggested; in fact, it may not be considered.

4. A comprehensive theory, when well articulated, tends to be rigid; and by extension, the profession ascribing to that theory does also. The needs of society, new knowledge, and new ideas tend to be ignored. It is difficult to alter a comprehensive theory: if you add a new concept or postulate, the whole theory may need to be altered, which is a difficult task.

5. Occupational therapy is a diverse profession. We assist people in all age groups and who have difficulties in many areas of function. A comprehensive theory may simplify to the point that the diversity and the richness of our body of knowledge, domain of concern, and practice may be lost.

6. In simplification, a comprehensive theory may become so nebulous that it inhibits research. Global and ill-defined concepts (e.g., adaptive responses and purposeful activity) are difficult to operationalize. Only when a concept can be reduced to the level of a variable is the validity of a theory or the effectiveness of intervention based on that theory able to be determined.

7. Further, in simplification, a comprehensive theory may become so vague that it offers little guidance for practice. For example, the comprehensive theory of Human Occupation describes the individual as being an "open system," influencing and being influenced by external stimuli. The individual responds to external stimuli, receives feedback, alters his or her behavior, gets more feedback, and the cycle continues. When all goes well, the patient becomes a more functional individual. The problem here is what external stimuli? When a therapist assists an individual who has an eating disorder (as opposed to an individual with third-degree burns), what external stimuli should the therapist make available? Does Human Occupation provide this information? Does any proposed comprehensive theory provide this information?

8. A comprehensive theory that is not exclusionary, takes into consideration the diversity of the profession, and is not simplistic has to be complex. In its complexity, it may become so intricate and labyrinthine that it is incomprehensible to any but the most dedicated scholars. Unless we have a comprehensive theory that is easily understood by all therapists, theory may become disconnected from practice. Not a happy situation to contemplate. We may indeed return to the time when it was acceptable to say, "My approach is eclectic." Such a statement is often an expression of considerable uncertainty about the theoretical bases for one's practice.

9. Finally, as mentioned, one of the major functions of a comprehensive theory is to give unity to a profession. If the deficits outlined earlier are not avoided, a comprehensive theory may provide an illusion of a unified identity but would serve no practical purpose.

A monistic identity, then, has many pitfalls. With that in mind, a pluralistic approach is another possibility. The following describes some of the factors that led me to consider such an approach. It is, if you will, a wandering in that direction.

Wanderings

The history of our profession has been used to substantiate most of the various monistic approaches identified earlier. That is a little hard to take. When history is used to support very disparate ideas, questions must be asked. We seem to have the idea that the original members of our profession were all of one mind about what occupational therapy ought to be. What their collective beliefs were, if there ever was such an agreement, differs according to who is writing the history. There are many individuals currently engaged in the study of our history. Hopefully, their efforts will provide more accurate information about our past.

The understanding and appreciation of our history is important. However, to use it to substantiate a number of different ideas of what we are or ought to be is a questionable practice. In addition, the year 1917 is a long time ago. The knowledge, beliefs, and issues of that time are not the same as those of 1985.

Another factor that leads me to consider a pluralistic approach is an issue raised by Rogers (30). She suggested that one of our major philosophical questions is whether the goal of the profession should be the enhancement of occupational performances or the development of performance components. She implied that it had to be one or the other; that a choice needed to be made. Why must we make such a choice? Multiple goals for the profession may provide needed flexibility.

A third reason to consider pluralism is related to our lack of a common vocabulary. Everyone has their own definition for a particular term, has no definition at all, or uses the same term to label very different concepts. An example is the term *model*. It is used in several different ways in our literature. I have identified at least five, most of which are not clearly defined. In addition, the term is sometimes modified. Thus, we have conceptual models, theoretical models, practice models, and probably some I missed (22, 27, 31).

Let me give a few more examples. There are also no agreed-upon definitions for "theory," "frame of reference," or "taxonomy." Hypothesis may refer to a conjecture or a postulate stated in operational terms. Philosophical assumptions are rarely differentiated from theoretical statements. And I could continue . . . the lack of a common vocabulary could mean many things: a disregard for adequate definitions, an attempt to label each idea as new, or a lack of interest in communicating with each other.

Another factor in the consideration of a pluralistic identity was a review of other professions. Those who, in the past, embraced a monistic approach seemed to experience difficulties. The classical example is psychiatry. From approximately the early 1950s until the late 1960s, psychiatry on the whole had one comprehensive theory: psychoanalysis. This theory was used to explain all problems in mental health—from psychosis to marital discord. Every problem was made to fit into the theory. Psychoanalysis, with or without some modification, was the treatment of choice. However, many people were unable or unwilling to engage in this type of treatment. Also, for many of those who did, the treatment was not effective. Society turned to other sources for help: behaviorism, various types of self-help and encounter groups, and psychopharmacology. Thus, psychiatry lost a good deal of credibility, patients, and money.

The fifth situation that prompted me to consider a pluralistic approach is the difficulty we have in designating and defining our legitimate tools (32–35). "Purposeful activity" has received the most attention. Yet, it has been defined so broadly that it includes just about everything and so narrowly that it includes little that we actually do. Then there are those who suggest that we change the label of purposeful activity to "occupation." Our literature is replete both with attempts to define purposeful activity and documentation that we use other modalities for intervention (2, 36, 37). There are no criteria for determining what is and what is not a legitimate tool for occupational therapy.

Finally, I suggest a pluralistic approach based on the observation of everyday practice. What occupational therapists actually do is very diverse. There does not seem to be any one unifying element. It could be that we have had a pluralistic identity for some time; that such a decision was made long ago in action but was never recognized or clearly stated. Therefore, the limitations of a monistic approach and the factors just outlined seem to suggest consideration of pluralism.

A Pluralistic Approach

A pluralistic approach to professional identity is based on the belief that no one principle or element can define a profession, that each part is distinct and different. There are several characteristics of a profession that support a pluralistic approach. Some of the major ones follow.

First, all elements of a profession are of equal importance. One is in no way subordinate to another. The tools of a profession, for example, are of no greater or lesser importance than the theories that underlie their application.

Second, it is the content of each profession's elements that differentiates one from another (38). The collective content of each profession is unique in its totality, not in its parts. In illustration, we share part of our body of knowledge with other professions, such as human growth and development; we also share some of our philosophical assumptions, such as belief in the holistic nature of the individual. Early childhood educators use activities as one of their major tools. The content of a given profession, its beliefs, knowledge, and skills, is unique only because members of that profession have mastered it in its totality. Members of other professions and the average person may understand parts, but not the whole.

Third, the contents of elements change over time; there are both additions and deletions. And there will be change. Professions evolve to take advantage of new knowledge, new ideas, and beliefs and to meet society's ever-changing needs. For example, the original members of the profession did not fabricate splints. No one mentioned learning disabilities when I was in school. Our understanding of the brain is changing daily. This fluid and constant state of flux is good and necessary. Without such modifications, a profession would stagnate, wither, and become part of the past. We are not what we were ten years ago nor are we what we will be ten years from now.

Finally, and related to the last point, professions are rarely of one piece. Incompatibilities of elements and content of elements are legion. For example, our recognized body of knowledge does not include theories regarding the properties of heat. Yet, some occupational therapists use heat as one of their therapeutic modalities. Analytic frames of reference are not really congruent with frames of reference based on learning theories. A profession usually attempts to bring unity to the contents of its elements. But just as all of the elements are apparently in symmetry, another change comes along that must be integrated.

To reiterate, all elements of a profession are of equal importance, professions are unique only in their totality, they are in a continual state of change, and there is always likely to be incompatibility between elements and within elements. Because of these characteristics, a pluralistic approach to professional identity may be more in accord with reality.

The structure for articulation of a pluralistic identity must be loosely organized. Rather than the composition of theory, which by definition is closely knit, a taxonomy is proposed. As used here, taxonomy refers to schema for classifying and ordering a set of phenomena. There are, of course, many different kinds of taxonomies. I recommend a cluster taxonomy in which groupings are formed based on similarity of defined characteristics. The groupings suggested for a pluralistic identity are the elements of the profession. In other words, each element would be clearly defined, and under that major heading the content of each element would be outlined. Thus, for example, we would clearly define what we meant by a philosophical assumption and then list our various philosophical assumptions. The same would be done for our ethical code, frames of reference, and so forth. With such a schema, the content of each element is apparent. Incongruencies can be readily identified. Content can easily be added or deleted as circumstances dictate. Our identity would be all of our elements. And, as their content changes over time, our identity is modified.

The structure for articulation of a pluralistic identity may seem too simple, too plain. No mystery at all. But perhaps that is as it should be. There really is no need to pretend complexity and enigmas where there are none. A straightforward statement of who we are may serve us best.

A pluralistic identity gives us freedom to grow and progress. It gives us the opportunity to engage in practice and scholarly pursuits unencumbered by tradition, authority, or ideology. More specifically, it allows us to

- Analyze critically our philosophical assumptions,
- Select and/or develop new theories,
- Make changes in our domain of concern,
- Consider alternative legitimate tools, and
- Formulate more definitive and additional frames of reference.

A pluralistic identity may not be comfortable for everyone. It is certainly not a panacea, nor is it meant to be. But perhaps such an identity would prepare us to meet the needs of those who seek our help. Perhap it can enable us to deal effectively with internal and external factors that will always influence our practice.

Acknowledgments

The author thanks Estelle Breines, MA, OTR, FAOTA; Wendy Colman, PhD, OTR; Francia de Beer, MA, OTR; and Brena Manoly, PhD, OTR, for providing assistance in the preparation of this paper.

References

1. Gilfoyle EM: Eleanor Clarke Slagle lectureship, 1984: Transformation of a profession. *Am J Occup Ther* 38:575–584, 1984
2. Llorens LA: Changing balance: Environment and individual. *Am J Occup Ther* 38:29–34, 1984
3. *The Random House Dictionary of the English Language,* J Stein, Editor. New York: Random House, 1966
4. *Education for the Profession of Medicine, Law, Theology and Social Work,* EC Hughes, Editor. New York: McGraw-Hill, 1973
5. McGlothlin W: *The Professional Schools.* New York: The Center for Applied Research in Education, 1964
6. Mosey AC: *Occupational Therapy: Configuration of a Profession.* New York: Raven, 1981
7. Popper KP: *Objective Knowledge: An Evolutionary Approach.* London: Oxford Univ Press, 1972
8. Schein EH: *Professional Education.* New York: McGraw-Hill, 1972
9. Cassidy HG: *The Sciences and the Arts: A New Alliance.* New York: Harper, 1962
10. Ford D, Urban H: *Systems Psychotherapy.* New York: Wiley, 1963
11. Hilgard E, Bower G: *Theories of Learning.* New York: Appleton-Century-Crofts, 1975
12. Marx M, Hillix W: *Systems and Theories in Psychology.* New York: McGraw-Hill, 1963
13. Nagel E: *The Structure of Science.* New York: Harcourt, Brace & World, 1961
14. Pittinger OE, Gooding CT: *Learning Theories in Educational Practice.* New York: Wiley, 1971
15. Snelbecher GE: *Learning Theory, Instructional Theory and Psycho-Educational Design.* New York: McGraw-Hill, 1974
16. Llorens LA, Gillette NP: Nationally speaking—The challenge for research in a practice profession. *Am J Occup Ther* 39:143–145, 1985
17. Llorens LA: *Application of Developmental Theory for Health and Rehabilitation.* Rockville, MD: AOTA, 1976
18. Fidler GS: From crafts to competency. *Am J Occup Ther* 35:567–573, 1981
19. Huss AJ: From kinesiology to adaptation. *Am J Occup Ther* 35:574–580, 1981
20. Reilly M: A psychiatric occupational therapy program as a teaching model. *Am J Occup Ther* 20:61–67, 1966
21. King LJ: Eleanor Clarke Slagle lectureship, 1978: Towards a science of adaptive responses. *Am J Occup Ther* 32:429–437, 1978
22. Howe MC, Briggs AK: Ecological systems model for occupational therapy. *Am J Occup Ther* 36:322–327, 1982
23. Kielhofner G: *Health Through Occupation: Theory and Practice in Occupational Therapy.* Philadelphia: Davis, 1983
24. Merton RK: *Social Theory and Social Structure.* Glencoe, IL: Free Press, 1968
25. Mills CE: *The Sociological Imagination.* New York: Oxford Univ Press, 1967
26. Williamson GG: A heritage of activity: Development of theory. *Am J Occup Ther* 36:716–722, 1982
27. Sundstrom C: In search of erudition: The evolution of a philosophical base for occupational practice in the army. *Occup Ther Ment Health* 3:7–13, 1983
28. Yerxa EJ: Research priorities. *Am J Occup Ther* 37:699, 1983
29. Christiansen CH: Editorial: Towards resolution of crises: Research requisites of occupational therapy. *Occup Ther J Res* 1:115–124, 1981
30. Rogers JC: The spirit of independence: The evolution of a philosophy. *Am J Occup Ther* 36:709–715, 1982
31. Reed KL: Understanding theory: The first step in learning about research. *Am J Occup Ther* 38:677–682, 1984
32. Breines E: The issue is—An attempt to define purposeful activities. *Am J Occup Ther* 38:543–544, 1984
33. Hinojosa J, Sabari J, Rosenfeld MS: Purposeful activities. *Am J Occup Ther* 37:805–806, 1983
34. Lyons BG: The issue is—Purposeful versus human activity. *Am J Occup Ther* 37:493–495, 1983
35. West WL: A reaffirmed philosophy and practice of occupational therapy for the 1980s. *Am J Occup Ther* 38:15–23, 1984
36. Bissell JC, Mailloux Z: The use of crafts in occupational therapy for the physically disabled. *Am J Occup Ther* 35:369–374, 1981
37. English C, Karch M, Silverman P, Walker S: The issue is—On the role of the occupational therapist in physical disabilities. *Am J Occup Ther* 36:199–202, 1982
38. *The Body of Knowledge Unique to the Profession of Education.* Washington, DC: Pi Lambda Theta, 1966

1986 Eleanor Clarke Slagle Lecture

Tools of Practice:
Heritage or Baggage?

Kathlyn L. Reed, PhD, OTR/L, FAOTA

Over the years, occupational therapists have adopted or adapted numerous media and methods. The list is so long it staggers the imagination. Yet explanations for the changing practice scene are rare. Few therapists seem to know *why* media come and go or even *when* or *how* various media or methods became part of the occupational therapy tool kit. Why do occupational therapists drop some media or methods like so much excess baggage? Is occupational therapy losing its heritage or keeping up with the times?

The question of heritage first occurred to me during Mary Fiorentino's Slagle Lecture (Fiorentino, 1975). She said she used no arts and crafts in her clinic, implying that such media were no longer useful in the treatment tool kit of occupational therapists. Many people applauded her pronouncement as if occupational therapy finally had shed its 19th century image and joined the 20th century. Her denunciation of arts and crafts set me thinking. Why did arts and crafts become a medium of occupational therapy in the first place? What about other media and methods, such as sanding blocks or work-related programs? Discussions with colleagues produced few answers except that arts and crafts had always been taught since the days of the founders. Therefore, I decided to investigate the literature, historical documents, and old photographs to find some answers.

The objective of this article is to suggest reasons why certain media and methods have evolved as the treatment of choice in occupational therapy in a particular period of time. Likewise, a discussion of why certain media and methods fall into disfavor is relevant.

Definition of Media and Methods

A *medium* is an intervening mechanism through which a force acts or an effect is produced (Morris, 1981). In therapy the medium is the means by which the therapeutic effect is transmitted. A sanding block, a weaving loom, a vestibular board, and a large plastic ball are all media or means by which the therapeutic effect of occupational therapy is activated. Of course, the same objects can be used for other purposes not related to the therapeutic effect of occupational therapy.

Methods are the manner of performing an act or operation: a procedure or technique (*Dorland's*, 1985). In therapy the methods constitute the steps, sequence, or approach used to activate the therapeutic effect of a medium. Examples include one-handed techniques, joint protection, work simplification, and activity configuration. Thus, media and methods are two sides of the same coin. Media provide the means, and methods provide the manner through which the therapeutic effect of occupational therapy is achieved.

Definitions describe but do not determine what will become a therapeutic medium or method. To discover how an object or approach becomes identified as having therapeutic potential, one must look outside a dictionary.

Originally published 1986 in *American Journal of Occupational Therapy, 40,* 597–605.

Analysis of media and methods over several years has suggested to me that there are eight primary factors that account for which media and methods are selected or discarded from the occupational therapy tool kit. These factors are cultural, social, economic, political, technological, theoretical, historical, and research (Christiansen, 1981; Cynkin, 1979; Di Sante, 1978; English, 1975; Jantzen, 1964; Johnson, 1983; Kielhofner, 1985; Kielhofner & Burke, 1983).

Factors in Selecting and Discarding Media and Methods

Culture is the most pervasive but hidden factor in the selection of media and methods in occupational therapy practice (Cynkin, 1979; Kielhofner, 1985). Occupational therapy was organized around the concept of improving people's abilities to deal with their daily lives. Therefore, it is logical that activities, occupations, or daily living tasks would be selected and used as media and methods. The activities, occupations, and daily living tasks are determined by the culture in which a person lives. A simple example is eating utensils. In Western culture the knife, fork, and spoon are used, but in Eastern culture chopsticks are used to get food from the serving vessel to the mouth. Thus, an occupational therapy clinic in America likely will contain eating utensils that resemble knives, forks, and spoons, but an occupational therapy clinic in Japan likely will contain chopsticks or adaptations of chopsticks.

The social factor is more conspicuous than the cultural (Cynkin, 1979; Kielhofner, 1985). Media and methods are subject to social acceptance or nonacceptance, which often is influenced by marketing and advertising strategies and changing values. The marketing strategies and changing values in turn create fads or trends that influence purchasing decisions. An example is the ongoing issue of whether handmade or machine-made products are superior in quality and value. Is there a difference in the warmth provided by a sweater made of the same yarn when one is handmade and the other made by machine? Probably not. Why then would a person pay more for one than the other? Because social factors, such as perceived value, enter the picture.

The economic factor affects the selection or discarding of media because some media cost more to use and may or may not be reimbursable by third-party insurance. Building a 16-foot boat could be a very therapeutic occupational activity, but the cost is a little high for many therapists' budgets and probably not reimbursable through most health insurance plans.

The impact of political factors on media and methods has been well documented. Diversional methods of occupational therapy have been ruled out of reimbursable services for many years. More recently there have been disputes over the use of occupational therapy for people with hip replacements or sensory integrative dysfunction.

Technological factors can have a dramatic impact on the media and methods of occupational therapy. Perhaps the best example is the change that has occurred in splinting with the advent of plastics. Originally splints were made from plaster reinforced with wire. The process was tedious, and the product subject to frequent breakdown. Then came plastics, but they had to be heated at high temperatures and tended to become brittle with age. The advent of low-temperature plastics allowed a splint to be made in a few minutes in a small frying pan. Splints from this material last for many months without noticeable change in molecular structure.

Some media and methods develop directly from a given theoretical model. An example is the use of vestibular boards, which is a direct application of the sensory integration model. When a medium or method is associated only with one theoretical model, it is easy to determine the origin. However, some media and methods can be used within a variety of theoretical models, and thus identification becomes more difficult. Cooking, for example, can be viewed as essential to nutrition, a pleasurable reward, a social activity, a paid vocation, a leisure skill, or an educational task. How many theoretical models encompass cooking as a medium and method?

The historical factor influences media and methods because some media and methods have been associated with occupational therapy from the earliest records and their origin is now obscure. For example, the use of the bicycle jigsaw can be traced back to occupational therapy clinics in 1918, but the trail is difficult to follow beyond that point. Who built the first bicycle jigsaw, and what was the original therapeutic objective?

Finally, research influences the selection and discarding of media and methods. For example, the research on building muscle strength led to the concept of progressive resistive exercise, which in turn led to the development or adaptation of media that can be modified to provide increased resistance. Many floor looms were modified in the 1950s and 1960s to provide increased resistance to shoulder, arm, hand, and leg muscles.

These factors can be explained further in a set of assumptions about their effect on the selection and discarding of media and methods in occupational therapy. The 14 assumptions can be stated as follows:

1. Media and methods become tools of occupational therapy through one or more of the eight factors.
2. Media and methods disappear from the tool kit of occupational therapy because of one or more of the eight factors.
3. The factors may operate to change the selection or discarding of media and methods singly or, more often, in combination.
4. Occupational therapists should understand the effects of the eight factors on the media and methods used in occupational therapy practice. (See Table 35.1 for a list of subfactors under the factors.)
5. Media and methods are selected from the dominant existing culture.
6. The sociocultural meaning of a medium and its methods may change over time and be used for a different reason or be discarded.
7. When the sociocultural rationale for a medium or method is lost or changed, the medium may be used in therapy in ways that make little sense to patients or other health professionals.
8. Economic considerations affect the selection and discarding of media and methods and thus restrict their use if the price is too high or if the cost is not reimbursable.
9. Changes in political issues may restrict or facilitate both the selection and use of various media and methods in occupational therapy based on decisions to cover them under or to exclude them from health care programs.
10. Technology introduces new possibilities or modifies existing ones, allowing new media or methods to emerge.
11. Media and methods may be selected because they operationalize an existing theoretical model recognized by the profession.
12. A medium or method may be used in more than one model. Therefore, the therapist must know why a medium or method is being used and change the explanation when a new model is adopted.
13. Historical precedent is the least desirable justification for the existence and continued use of a medium or method but the easiest to explain.
14. Selection and use of media and methods based on research and study is the most professionally responsible approach to justifying the use of a medium or method but the most difficult to obtain.

To illustrate how the eight factors and 14 assumptions operate, I have selected three media and their methods from among the many possible choices. The three are arts and crafts, sanding blocks, and work-related programs. Arts and crafts will illustrate the cultural, social, technological, and historical factors; the sanding blocks will illustrate the theoretical and research factors; and work-related programs will illustrate the political and economic factors.

Arts and Crafts

The use of arts and crafts as media and methods in occupational therapy is directly attributable to the arts and crafts movement that was in full swing during the formative years of occupational therapy early in this century (Levine, in press-a, in press-b). The movement was designed as a cure for the social ills of a society struggling to deal with the impact of the Industrial Revolution. During the 1800s, Western civilization changed from an agrarian to a manufacturing economy; from a cottage industry to a mass production society; from a consumer-driven marketplace to a producer-driven marketplace; from a patronage system to an industrial wealth system; from pride

Table 35.1. Factors in the Selection and Use of Media and Methods

1. Cultural factor	**5. Technological factor**
Dominant culture	New invention
Subdominant culture	Modification of known invention
2. Social factor	**6. Theoretical factor**
Upper, middle, or lowerclass custom	Organismic philosophy
Fad or tradition	Mechanistic philosophy
3. Political factor	**7. Historical factor**
Family or extended family politics	Significant
Local community politics	Incidental
State or national politics	**8. Research factor**
4. Economic factor	Supports statements
Budget of department or hospital	Refutes statements
Reimbursement policies	

in workmanship to concern for profit; and from an ordered society of similar cultural backgrounds to a disordered society of many cultures and customs. These factors all played a role in the demise of moral treatment. The arts and crafts movement provided a means of revitalizing the ideas of moral treatment in a new rationale, which the founders and early leaders of occupational therapy were quick to understand. Thus, the arts and crafts movement is the missing link between moral treatment, which dominated the practice of medicine in the 1800s, and the treatment models to follow.

The arts and crafts movement began in England. The original philosophy was based on the "conviction that industrialization had brought with it the total destruction of 'purpose, sense and life' " (Naylor, 1971). Mechanical progress had been gained at the expense of human misery and the destruction of fundamental human values. Thus, the arts and crafts movement "was inspired by a crisis of conscience" (Naylor, 1971). Its motivations were social and moral, and its aesthetic values derived from the conviction that a society produces the art and architecture it deserves (Naylor, 1971). To that idea could be added the thought that society produces the life-style it deserves.

Many people contributed ideas and thoughts to the arts and crafts movement, and not all agreed as to their importance. Therefore, a summary of concepts must be general. The arts and crafts movement did the following:

- Advocated the simplification of life and ordering of daily activity as opposed to the overcomplicated or idle life (Borris, 1986; Kornwolf, 1972; Lears, 1981; Shi, 1985; Wagner, 1904);
- Valued the "craftsman" ideal, in which occupation was pursued at its own pace and not on a production schedule (Borris, 1986; Kornwolf, 1972; Lears, 1981);
- Valued the standard of craftsmanship that gave an honest day's work for an honest day's pay, rather than exploitation of the worker or cheating by the employee (Borris, 1986; Kornwolf, 1972; Naylor, 1971);
- Favored returning to the land and the home as a means of escaping the crowded, unhealthy, unnatural conditions of the city and factory (Lears, 1981; Shi, 1985);
- Ennobled the power of handwork as useful, important, a joy, and a pleasure, as opposed to mindless, repetitive activity on an assembly line, which was viewed as drudgery (Borris, 1986; Lears, 1981);
- Promoted an appreciation of performing the process and the inherent satisfaction or pride in doing or making a product, as opposed to concern only for sale and profit (Naylor, 1971);
- Encouraged respect for the inherent properties of materials and opposed any deception designed to make a material look like something it was not (Kornwolf, 1972);
- Considered functionalism and fitness of purpose the best guide to decoration, as opposed to ornamentation that served no purpose (Borris, 1986; Kornwolf, 1972);
- Believed that manual training of children would increase knowledge of moral aesthetics and improve work skills, as opposed to intellectual learning only (Borris, 1986; Lears, 1981);
- Valued the creative spirit in the artist and abhorred the mindless copying of designs (Borris, 1986);

- Attempted to improve the standards of taste and aesthetics, as opposed to allowing moral decay (Borris, 1986; Shi, 1985); and
- Viewed people as more than mere machines; human beings as having morals, values, and a sense of purpose (Kornwolf, 1972; Shi, 1985).

One early influence of the arts and crafts movement on occupational therapy came from Jane Addams. In 1900 she started the Hull House Labor Museum, because she wanted young people to see that the complicated machinery of the factory had evolved from the simple tools that their parents had used in the old country before immigrating to America. She wanted to interest young people in the older forms of industry so they would see "a dramatic representation of the inherited resources of their daily occupation" (Addams, 1945). The Labor Museum not only showed how spinning, weaving, pottery, and many other crafts were done, but also provided classes to teach people how to do the crafts. Addams admonished educators, saying that "educators have failed to adjust themselves to the fact that cities have become great centers of production and manufacture, and manual labor has been left without historic interpretation or imaginative uplift" (Addams, 1900, p. 236). Thus, when the training courses for attendants were started in 1907, in conjunction with the Chicago School of Civics and Philanthropy, there was a stress on the idea that occupation should be used as a means of education and that education was to substitute for custodial care of the mentally ill (*20th Biennial Report,* 1909).

In 1914, Eleanor Clarke Slagle started the Community Workshop under the auspices of the Illinois Society of Mental Hygiene. Its purpose was to serve as a clearinghouse for cases of doubtful insanity whom the courts considered as showing promise of a return to usefulness if given a proper environment and trade (Favill, 1917). The environment was the Hull House Labor Museum. In 1917 the Community Workshop became the Henry B. Favill School of Occupations. The following year, the first course in curative occupations and recreation was offered (*Special Courses,* 1917). Again the Labor Museum at Hull House served as the laboratory until the school was moved to the headquarters of the Illinois Society of Mental Hygiene in late 1919.

Another person to incorporate the ideas of the arts and crafts movement into treatment was Herbert J. Hall. In 1904 Hall began his studies of alternate treatments to the "rest cure" for neurasthenia. He was assisted by Jessie Luther, OTR, the first curator of the Hull House Labor Museum (Luther, 1902). Hall states that the "modern Arts and Crafts idea appealed very strongly, because of the growing interest in the movement and because of the clean, wholesome atmosphere which surrounds such work, and because of the many-sided appeal which such a work as the making of pottery, for instance, has to most educated minds" (Hall, 1905). Hall believed that faulty living was the cause of neurasthenia and that what was needed was a change in occupation and habits. Manual work based on the life of the artisan (craftsman ideal) was recommended itself because it was simple. The "simple life," he felt, was best for neurasthenics because it offered the least food for the nourishment of neurasthenia and provided a structure of normality. Today the person with neurasthenia would be classified as suffering from stress or burnout. The "simple life" would be called stress reduction, and the "craftsman ideal" would be called time management.

In 1906 Hall received a grant from the Procter Fund of Harvard University for $1,000 to "assist in the study of the treatment of neurasthenia by progressive and graded manual occupation." His study at Marblehead, Massachusetts, probably was the first grant-funded research project on the use of occupation as a means of treating patients. He reported that 59 of 100 patients improved, 27 were much improved, and 14 received no relief (Hall, 1910).

The arts and crafts philosophy was summarized in the "Philosophy of Occupation Therapy" by Adolf Meyer (1922). He said, "Our industrialism has created the false idea of success in *production* to the point of overproduction, bringing with it a kind of nausea to the worker and a delirium of the trader . . ."—in other words, loss of the craftsman ideal. Meyer said, "The man of today has lost the capacity and pride of workmanship and has substituted for it a measure in terms of money." In other words, there was a loss of respect for hand work. And he said that there is "a real pleasure in the use and activity of one's hands and muscles." In other words, one can find pride and satisfaction in performing and doing. Furthermore, "Our body is not merely so many pounds of flesh and bone figuring as a machine."

A final example of the influence of the arts and crafts movement on occupational therapy is the regional location of the arts and crafts societies that developed to organize the work of the arts and crafts movement. The three major areas of the country that responded to the arts and crafts movement were New England, Chicago and the Midwest, and the Pacific area (Clark, 1972). There is a strong correspondence between these three areas and the areas where there are large numbers of occupational therapists today.

The specific location of the societies also influenced occupational therapy. Thirteen states had at least one known arts and crafts society in 1904 (West, 1904). Of the 13, nine (69%) developed early programs in occupational therapy before 1920. All 13 states have occupational therapy programs today (West, 1904).

Considering its influence, what happened to the arts and crafts movement? It was overtaken by World War I. The rules of the game changed for many people. The war effort provided its own sense of purpose. Some industries did hire craftsmen to improve designs, and machine-made products did improve in quality. City life improved as sanitation efforts made inroads against the piles of garbage. The expanding population meant that machine manufacture was the only means of providing products for everyone. Hand production was just too slow and too expensive.

How did the changes influence occupational therapy? What factors were changing the role of the arts and crafts in practice? The cultural scene had shifted: Society was no longer struggling to adapt to city life, and the factory system had been integrated in the fabric of American life. The number of people living on the land would continue to decrease over the coming years. People had become used to the technological changes the factory had produced. Machine-made goods were acceptable and could be made in quantities unknown under the handmade system. Young therapists did not remember the arts and crafts movement and did not know what it represented. They only knew that arts and crafts always had been a part of occupational therapy's tool kit. Finally, a new philosophy was overtaking the profession. The humanistic ideas of the founding years were being challenged as unscientific and unmeasurable. The profession was being reformulated in such a manner that the arts and crafts philosophy made little sense. Not until the 1960s would the founding ideas resurface. Figure 35.1 illustrates the changing theory and philosophy of the arts and crafts ideology.

Sanding Blocks

Sanding blocks, or sandblocks, are a common sight in many occupational therapy clinics. Nearly all occupational therapists become acquainted with them during their education, and many have made sanding blocks. Yet, few can describe the origin and original purpose of the sanding block or trace the changes in thinking about their use over the years.

Figure 35.1. Relative influence of organismic and mechanistic models on occupational therapy practice.

Mechanistic	⟵	⟶	Organismic
1880			End of Model Treatment
1890			Rise of the Arts and
1900			Crafts Movement
1910	Flexner Report		
	Medical Schools Increase Science Study		
1920			
1930	Rise of the Orthopedics Model		
1940	Rise of the Biomedical Model		Rise of the Developmental Model
1950			
1960	Dominance of the Psychoanalytic Model		Rise of Systems Model
1970	Dominance of the Behaviorism Model		Return of Humanism
1980			
1990			

Table 35.2. Types of Sanding Blocks

1. Proximal sanding blocks (Abbott, 1957; *Photographs*, 1947)
2. Proximal interphalangeal sanding block (Abbott, 1957; *Photographs*, 1947)
3. Metacarpal phalangeal sanding blocks (Abbott, 1957; *Photographs*, 1947)
4. Distal sanding block (Abbott, 1957)
5. Opponens sanding block (Abbott, 1957)
6. Shoulder abduction sanding block ("Adapted," 1957; Bennett & Driver, 1957)
7. Spring squeeze sanding block (Gurney, 1959)
8. Grip sanding block (Hightower et al., 1963)
9. Reciprocal sanding device (Mathews, 1965)
10. Weighted sander or progressive resistive exercise sander (Svensson & Brennan, 1954)
11. Bilateral sander, horizontal or vertical handles (*Photographs*, 1947)
12. Wrist exercise sander (Blodgett, 1947)
13. Hemiplegia sander (Forbes, 1951)
14. Graduated sanding blocks—graduated straight handles or graduated round knob handles (*Photographs*, 1947)

Woodworking and sanding can be traced to the beginning of occupational therapy history. The initial use of sanding blocks, however, is unclear. The first mention of them appears in 1934 in an article by Henrietta McNary. In the same article, the first description of an adapted sanding block also appears. Its purpose was to improve opposition. The last article in our literature on a sanding block, a reciprocal sanding device, appears in 1965 (Mathews, 1965). In all, 14 different types of sanding blocks are presented. These are listed in Table 35.2.

The dates of the articles on sanding blocks coincide with the rise and fall of the orthopedic and kinesthetic treatment models of occupational therapy. The orthopedic model followed the arts and crafts model. It was concerned with muscle strengthening and range of motion. Stretching contractures, exercise, and physical tolerance also were included. These concepts form the basis of the objectives for which the sanding block was used. A summary of these purposes or objectives is found in Table 35.3.

The use of sanding blocks has not disappeared, but the theories underpinning their development and use have been superseded by the sensorimotor and sensory integration models. As a result some unusual uses of sanding blocks have surfaced. For example, one therapist was observed giving a patient a sanding block with no sandpaper and an incline plane made of formica. Because the patient did not want to make anything, the therapist explained that the purpose of the activity was bilateral exercise. In this example, the fundamental concepts of occupational therapy, performance through doing and the use of occupation toward some purpose, were overlooked or separated from the application. The medium of sanding blocks and the methods of setting up the activity to obtain selected objectives had been separated from the original concepts so the meaning and purpose of the activity were lost. The *motion* of sanding is a necessary but not sufficient part of the *activity* of sanding. The media, the methods, and the objective of an occupation must be consistent with each other. Three out of three—medium, method, and objective—must be the rule, not the exception.

Table 35.3. Purposes or Objectives of Sanding Blocks

Sanding blocks were adapted to provide the following:
1. Different hand grip position for active or passive stretching:
   a. Handles were added and enlarged.
   b. Holes or grooves were drilled or carved for finger and thumb placement.
   c. Straps were added to hold the hand in place.
   d. Gloves were used to position the hand.
   e. Construction was altered to provide a different grip than that normally used.
2. Dynamic exercise of wrist, elbow, or shoulder—usually range of motion
3. Increased grip strength of hand and fingers
4. Bilateral activity of the upper extremities
5. Reciprocal activity of the upper extremities
6. Improved trunk stability
7. Standing and physical tolerance

Sanding blocks illustrate the factors of theory and research. The many adaptations of the sanding block are based on the theoretical concepts of the orthopedic and kinesthetic treatment models, which stress positioning the body part in the desired pattern of motion and then encouraging that motion to stretch, strengthen, or increase the motion of a particular body part or parts. Research supported the concept that increased amounts of resistance applied to a given muscle group would strengthen the muscle group involved. This concept became known as progressive resistive exercise.

Work-Related Programs

Work-related programs were a part of the early ideology of occupational therapy. The term *work-related programs* is used to represent all efforts to enable people to engage in productive occupations through occupational therapy, whether the effort is aimed at vocational education, vocational guidance, prevocational evaluation and training, vocational training or retraining, vocational readiness, work hardening, work adjustment, or career education.

Hall was very interested in helping patients find an alternate occupation that would be less stressful and more suitable to the person's needs. The "work cure" was based on the assumption that by substituting or bringing about "by a gradual process the conditions of a normal life, a life of pleasant and progressive occupations, as different as possible from the previous life, a person could overcome the mental and nervous problems in his life" (Hall, 1905).

George E. Barton said he was going to "try to prove that the hours of idleness in convalescence could be filled with pastimes which would be useful not only to pass the time, but to prepare the person for remunerative labor later on to get a job, a better job, or to do a job better than it was before" (Barton, 1914). Consolation House was created to serve the needs of people who were learning to put their lives back together and who needed assistance to find an occupation suitable to their abilities but not limited by their disabilities.

Slagle had experience in assessing people's fitness for a job at the Community Workshop at Hull House. At the founding conference of occupational therapy in Clifton Springs, New York, she spoke of a family of five who had been supported by charities for many years. After one year at the Community Workshop, the family was self-sufficient (Dunton, 1917).

Thomas B. Kidner, Vocational Secretary to the Military Hospitals Commission in Ottawa, Canada, was well acquainted with the vocational side of occupational therapy. In June 1918, he was loaned by the Canadian government to the United States as a special adviser on rehabilitation to the Federal Board for Vocational Education (FBVE). The FBVE had been created the previous year to establish a federal-state program in vocational education. In 1918 it had been given the authority and responsibility for the vocational rehabilitation of veterans ("Editorial," 1922). Elizabeth G. Upham (later Davis), who had been instrumental in starting the occupational therapy course at Milwaukee Downer College, also joined the FBVE in 1918. She wrote two documents illustrating the role of occupational therapy with the disabled veteran (Upham, 1918a, 1918b) and recommended that the FBVE be given control of military patients as soon as possible in order to prepare them for adjustment to normal life (Davis, no date). Had her recommendation been accepted, occupational therapy's role in vocational preparation would have been larger than it has been. Both Kidner and Upham left the FBVE in 1919.

The medical department of the army also had a plan for the rehabilitation of disabled soldiers. It had created a system of orthopedic reconstruction hospitals that included vocational workshops and employment bureaus (Gritzer & Arluke, 1985). The dispute over who would do what came to the floor of the U.S. Senate in July 1918. The medical department of the Army was granted the exclusive right to all aspects of functional restoration and medical control over curative work. This action bound occupational therapy to medicine's domain. The FBVE on the other hand was given responsibility for vocational rehabilitation. The separation became more divided in 1920 when the Industrial Rehabilitation Act was passed without any coverage for medical services. Bulletin #57 of the FBVE makes it quite clear than any occupational work not related to the vocation for which the injured person is being trained is evidently given for its therapeutic value. Therapeutic use of work was viewed as part of the injured person's physical rehabilitation rather than vocational rehabilitation and therefore was not covered under the act ("Industrial Rehabilitation," 1920). Thus, occupational therapy was cut off from many of its work-related programs by a political compromise over which it ultimately had little control. Work-related programs were not reestablished until 1943 when the Vocational Rehabilitation Act was changed to include coverage for medical services (Lassiter, 1972). In 1954, the Vocational Rehabilitation Act was further modified to include coverage for the training of rehabilitation personnel, including occupational therapists. In addition there were monies for research and demonstration projects (Lassiter, 1972). Among the demonstration projects were prevocational evaluation and training centers in which occupational therapists played a significant role. However, by the 1960s these projects became too expensive to continue, and the role of occupational therapy in work-related programs again went into a period of decline. Finally in the 1980s the interest returned. A position paper was written and a grant was funded to increase occupational therapists' awareness of the role of occupational therapy in work-related programs. Some of the current interests are assessment of work potential and aptitude skills, physical capacities assessment and work hardening, job evaluation, work experience, career exploration and job seeking skills, independent living, and industrial consultation.

The level of occupational therapists' interest and opportunities in work-related programs has waxed and waned over the past 80 years. The fluctuations can be traced to politics and economics. When both were favorable or neutral, occupational therapists provided many examples of programs designed to help a person to gain or regain productive skills. However, when the politics and economics made it difficult for occupational therapists to provide such skill assessment and skill training, their activity in work-related programs decreased. The challenge will be to shape the political and economic factors in favor of occupational therapy if therapists want to maintain their role in helping people attain or regain productive skills.

Occupational Analysis

As illustrated thus far, the selection and discarding of media and methods in occupational therapy have not been accidental. Factors converge and diverge to increase or decrease the likelihood that a particular medium and its methods will be selected or discarded in the practice of occupational therapy. Culture sets the major parameters, but changes in society frequently alter the cultural set. Political and economic factors often work in combination. Political factors can be influenced by occupational therapists, but some events may occur over which therapists have little control. The results may be felt most keenly economically when reimbursement patterns result in changes in coverage of occupational therapy services. Technology may lead to dramatic changes in media or methods. Theoretical factors often introduce new media and methods into the treatment setting. Sometimes the new theory or model brings new media and methods with it; at other times just the explanation and the use of an existing medium or method changes. History often is used to explain the existence of media or methods when the origin has been lost through time. Research offers a better explanation for the use of media and methods but is more difficult to obtain.

All of these factors need to be considered when examining why certain media and methods appear in a clinic or practice setting. Can practicing occupational therapists explain why each medium or method is used in their practice setting? Is the explanation the best one, or is the explanation of history used by default? Perhaps a more systematic use of occupational or activity analysis should be promoted which includes the selection and discarding of factors as well as considerations such as range of motion, sensory stimulation, or amount of social interaction obtained.

Central to each of the factors are the concepts of interests and values. A culture, individuals, and professionals have interests and values. An interest is defined as a set that guides behavior in a certain direction or toward certain goals (Chaplin, 1975). A value is a social end or goal that is considered desirable to achieve (Chaplin, 1975).

In occupational therapy there seem to be three major areas to consider in interest and values. These are culture and society, the individual, and the profession. The eight factors that affect selection and discarding of media and methods can be organized under the cultural and social interest and values and professional interests and values.

Under the *cultural and social* area are the cultural, social, economic, political, and technological factors. Under the *professional* are the theoretical, historical, and research factors. Under the *individual* are factors that must be determined by assessment of each individual. These are the roles performed by the individual and the functional abilities, skills, and capacities of the individual. When the three areas of cultural–social, individual, and professional interests and values are considered, there should be less chance of using media and methods that are out-of-date in society, not meaningful to the individual, and of questionable use to the profession.

Summary

This article presents and illustrates the major factors that influence the selection and discarding of media and methods in occupational therapy. The eight factors are the cultural, social, economic, political, technological, theoretical, historical, and research factors. The factors may operate in various combinations or alone to influence the use of a specific medium or method in practice. Therapists are encouraged to know these eight factors and in particular to be familiar with (a) what media and methods occupational therapists use, (b) why occupational therapists use those media and methods, (c) from where the media and methods come, (d) with whom the media and methods should be used in treatment, (e) how the media and methods are used, (f) when the media and methods are used, and (g) how much of the medium or method should be used. Educators, in particular, need to teach why a medium or method is used as well as how. Researchers need to provide more information as to why certain media and methods became part of our tool kit. Practitioners would be wise to follow the statement, If you know how, be sure you know why and be sure the why is consistent with the philosophy of occupational therapy.

References

Abbott, M. (1957). *A syllabus of occupational therapy procedures and techniques as applied to orthopedic and neurological conditions.* New York: American Occupational Therapy Association.

Adapted sand block. Part I. (1957). *American Journal of Occupational Therapy, 11,* 198.

Addams, J. (1900). Social education of the industrial democracy. *Commons, 5,* 17–28.

Addams, J. (1945). *Twenty years at Hull House, with autobiographical notes.* New York: Macmillan.

Barton, G. E. (1914). A view of invalid occupation. *Trained Nurse & Hospital Review, 52,* 327–330.

Bennett, R. L., & Driver, M. (1957). The aims and methods of occupational therapy in the treatment of the after-effects of poliomyelitis. *American Journal of Occupational Therapy, 11,* 145–153.

Blodgett, M. L. (1947). Sanding for exercise. *American Journal of Occupational Therapy, 1,* 6.

Borris, E. (1986). *Art and labor: Ruskin, Morris, and the craftsman ideal in America.* Philadelphia, PA: Temple University Press.

Chaplin, J. P. (1975). *Dictionary of psychology* (2nd ed.). New York: Dell.

Christiansen, C. H. (1981). Editorial: Toward resolution of crisis: Research requisites in occupational therapy. *Occupational Therapy Journal of Research, 1,* 115–124.

Clark, R. J. (1972). *The arts and crafts movement in America: 1876–1916.* Princeton, NJ: Princeton University Press.

Cynkin, S. (1979). *Occupational therapy: Toward health through activities.* Boston: Little, Brown.

Davis, E. U. (no date). *Just another biography.* Unpublished manuscript.

Di Sante, E. (1978). Technology transfer: From space exploration to occupational therapy. *American Journal of Occupational Therapy, 32,* 171–174.

Dorland's illustrated medical dictionary (26th ed.). Philadelphia, PA: W. B. Saunders, p. 809, 1985.

Dunton, W. R. (1917). *The growing necessity for occupational therapy.* New York: Teachers College. (In AOTA Archives, Moody Library, Galveston, TX.)

Editorial: The sixth annual meeting. *Archives of Occupational Therapy, 1,* 419–427, 1922.

English, C. B. (1975). Computers and occupational therapy. *American Journal of Occupational Therapy, 29,* 43–47.

Favill, J. (1917). *Henry Baird Favill: 1860–1861.* Chicago: Rand McNally, p. 87.

Fiorentino, M. R. (1975). Occupational therapy: Realization to activation—1974 Eleanor Clarke Slagle lecture. *American Journal of Occupational Therapy, 29,* 15–21.

Forbes, E. S. (1951). Two devices for use in treating hemiplegics. *American Journal of Occupational Therapy, 5,* 49–51.

Gritzer, G., & Arluke, A. (1985). The making of rehabilitation: A political economy of medical specialization, 1890–1980. Berkeley, CA: University of California Press.

Gurney, G. W. (1959). Spring-squeeze sandblock. *American Journal of Occupational Therapy, 13,* 278.

Hall, H. J. (1905). The systematic use of work as a remedy in neurasthenia and allied conditions. *Boston Medical & Surgical Journal, 112,* 29–32.

Hall, H. J. (1910). Work-cure: A report of five years' experience at an institution devoted to the therapeutic application of manual work. *Journal of the American Medical Association, 54,* 12–14.

Hightower, M. D., et al. (1963). Grip sander. *American Journal of Occupational Therapy, 17,* 62–63.

Industrial rehabilitation—A statement of policies to be observed in the administration of the Industrial Rehabilitation Act. (1920). *FBVE Bulletin, 57.*

Jantzen, A. C. (1964). The role of research in occupational therapy. *Proceedings of the 1964 Annual Conference* (pp. 2–9). New York: American Occupational Therapy Association.

Johnson, J. A. (1983). The changing medical market-place as a context for the practice of occupational therapy. In G. Kielhofner (Ed.), *Health through occupation: Theory and practice in occupational therapy* (pp. 163–177). Philadelphia, PA: F. A. Davis.

Kielhofner, G. (Ed.). (1985). *A model of human occupation: Theory and application.* Baltimore, MD: Williams & Wilkins.

Kielhofner, G., & Burke, J. P. (1983). The evolution of knowledge and practice in occupational therapy: Past, present and future (pp. 3–54). In G. Kielhofner (Ed.), *Health through occupation: Theory and practice in occupational therapy.* Philadelphia, PA: F. A. Davis.

Kornwolf, J. D. (1972). *M. H. Baillie Scott and the arts and crafts movement.* Baltimore, MD: Johns Hopkins Press.

Lassiter, R. A. (1972). History of the rehabilitation movement in America. In J. G. Cull & R. E. Hardy (Eds.), *Vocational rehabilitation: Profession and process* (pp. 5–58). Springfield, IL: Charles C Thomas.

Lears, T. J. J. (1981). *No place of grace: Antimodernism and the transformation of American culture: 1880–1920.* New York: Pantheon.

Levine, R. E. (in press-a). Guest editorial: Historical research: Ordering the past to chart our future. *Occupational Therapy Journal of Research.*

Levine, R. E. (in press-b). The influence of the arts and crafts movement on the professional status of occupational therapy. In W. Coleman (Ed.), *Written history monograph.* Rockville, MD: American Occupational Therapy Association.

Luther, J. (1902). The labor museum at Hull House. *Commons, 7,* 1–13.

Mathews, T. (1965). Reciprocal sanding device. *American Journal of Occupational Therapy, 19,* 354–355.

McNary, H. (1934). Anatomical considerations and technique in using occupations as exercise for orthopedic disabilities: III. Wrist and fingers. *Occupational Therapy Rehabilitation, 13,* 24–29.

Meyer, A. (1922). Philosophy of occupational therapy. *Archives of Occupational Therapy, 1,* 1–10.

Morris, W. (Ed.). (1981). *American heritage dictionary of the English language.* Boston: Houghton Mifflin, p. 815.

Naylor, G. (1971). *The arts and crafts movement: A study of its sources, ideals and influence on design theory.* Cambridge, MA: MIT Press.

Photographs of occupational therapy adapted equipment as developed in Veterans Administration and Army hospitals. (1947). Washington, DC: Department of Medicine & Surgery, Veterans Administration.

Shi, D. E. (1985). *The simple life: Plain living and high thinking in American culture.* New York: Oxford University Press.

Special courses in curative occupations and recreation. (1917, December). Chicago: Chicago School of Civics and Philanthropy Special Bulletin.

Svensson, V. W., & Brennan, M. C. (1954). Adapted weighted resistive apparatus. *American Journal of Occupational Therapy, 8,* 13.

20th biennial report of the Board of Public Charities of the State of Illinois, July 1, 1906–June 30, 1908. Springfield, IL: Illinois State Journal Co., p. 58.

Upham, E. G. (1918a). Training of teachers for occupational therapy for the rehabilitation of disabled soldiers and sailors. *Federal Board for Vocational Education Bulletin, 6,* 1–76.

Upham, E. G. (1918b). Ward occupations in hospitals. *Federal Board for Vocational Education Bulletin, 25,* 1–57.

Wagner, C. (1904). *The simple life.* New York: Grosset & Dunlap.

West, M. (1904). The revival of handicrafts in America. *Bureau of Labor Bulletin, 55,* 1573–1622.

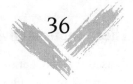

36

1987 Eleanor Clarke Slagle Lecture

Activity:
Occupational Therapy's Treatment Method

Claudia Kay Allen, MA, OTR, FAOTA

Difficulties in explaining the value of using activity as a treatment method have been with us from the beginning (Fields, 1911). During a testimonial dinner in tribute to Eleanor Clarke Slagle, Dr. Adolph Meyer (1937) struggled to explain the value of activity. He said, "I should like to voice adequately what so many of my patients have gained through Mrs. Slagle and her pupils and what it means for the sufferers, but also for the healthy . . . those with 'time on their hands' " (p. 6). Fifty years later, his explanation has a familiar ring, *keeping the patients busy*. Keeping the patients busy is a misleading phrase because it makes therapeutic activity sound easier to do and less important to the patient than it really is. A more accurate assessment of the value of therapeutic activities is required.

My goal is to provide a philosophical framework that can be used to explain and evaluate the use of activity as a treatment method for disabled people. The framework is analogous to a skeleton, offered with the expectation that muscles, nerves, and vital organs will need to be added later. The framework consists of a vocabulary with definitions and typologies to categorize terms.

As much as possible, the development of the framework adheres to several professional ideas. I use common dictionary definitions of terms while attempting to avoid the pitfall of talking just common sense. I cite social science references that suggest a philosophical approach to the study of activity, but try to avoid obfuscating jargon. A strict adherence to original social science references is not essential or even beneficial. The detection of tautologies and the special needs of occupational therapy's patient populations justify departures from the original sources. I am pursuing the ideal of creating a foundation for occupational therapy's unique view of activity with the notion that this foundation must correspond to the realities of clinical practice, including empirical investigation with control groups. Ideally, a philosophical foundation should fuse the splintered efforts currently existing between competing theories and produce a more efficient use of limited creative resources.

This lecture has a motto, borrowed from a research group that I have been working with in developing the typologies, which is "Things that appear simple, tend to get complicated, before they get simple again" (personal communication with M. Brinson, L. Cargill, M. A. Mayer, and E. L. Stone, February 1987). Two techniques to assist the reader through the complicated part will be followed. First, most of the line drawings that can be used to illustrate the cognitive levels can be found in a book I published in 1985; two new ones appear here. Second, an analogy to locations in the clinic will be used: During the last year, while therapists have been out working in their communities, I have been reorganizing the occupational therapy clinic. I have thrown some things away and brought in some new things. Mostly, I have relocated a lot of familiar supplies and tools, so it will be hard to find things for a while. Finally, I am not going to offer any guarantees about whether or not the reorganization of the clinic was worth the effort; we will have to wait and see how it works in practice.

Originally published 1987 in *American Journal of Occupational Therapy, 41*, 563–575.

Therapeutic Activity

The only branch of the social sciences that has used the concept of activity as a central focus of study is Soviet psychology. During the last few years, a lot of conceptual material has been translated into English, providing a rich resource of 60 years worth of conceptual experience and critical analysis. These translations allow us to profit from the Soviets' experience. Soviet psychology offers two approaches to the study of activity. One was developed by Vygotsky, and the other by Leontyev (Wertsch, 1979).

In recent years, a problem with Leontyev's theory of activity has been discovered (Kozulin, 1986). Leontyev used activity in two ways: as an explanatory principle and as a focus of study. This two-way usage is a familiar problem in 20th-century psychology, and what happens is the formation of a tautology. In effect, tautologies make people go around in theoretical circles. Earlier in this century, Vygotsky suggested a way out of the circle that has recently been rediscovered. Vygotsky suggested the need for an information processing system that serves as a mediator between the focus of study and the explanatory principles (Kozulin, 1986). I will use all three of Vygotsky's elements to develop a definition of therapeutic activity. Then I will turn to Leontyev's hierarchy to explain activity analysis.

Disability: A Focus of Study

The focus of this study is analogous to the first thing one sees upon entering the occupational therapy clinic. In this instance, it was a table that showed the wear and tear of ongoing debates and questions in occupational therapy: What is the difference between diversional and therapeutic activities? Should the art or science of practice be emphasized? Should entry level education stress technical or theoretical concepts? What should be done about the split between theory and practice? All of these questions can be traced to the acceptance of an assumption that there is a difference between applied and pure sciences, with pure sciences having higher academic status. Within the analogy, I have sent the old table and the associated questions to a museum; the assumption of a division between applied and pure sciences is obsolete. This decision is based on the philosophy of science espoused by Toulmin (1972), who described similar problem-solving processes in the applied and pure sciences. The traditional academic division between applied and pure science has misled academicians into seeking a theory based on pure science that addresses normal human activity. I think it is time to free occupational therapy from the yoke of this artificial division so that therapists can focus their attention on refining the quality of services delivered to disabled people.

Disability is the selected focus of study, analogous to bringing a new table into the clinic. A disability is the state or quality of being unable to function normally due to physical and/or cognitive loss, including prenatal loss. As defined by the federal government, disability is an "inability to engage in any substantial gainful activity by reason of a medically determinable physical or mental impairment which can be expected to last, or has lasted for a continuous period of not less than 12 months" (Dorland's, 1981, p. 384). A disability is a sequela to a disease or a disorder. A disease is "any deviation from or interruption of the normal structure or function of any part, organ, or symptom (or combination thereof) of the body that is manifested by a characteristic set of symptoms and signs whose etiology, pathology, and prognosis may be known or unknown" (Dorland's, 1981, p. 385). Information required by therapists to evaluate and treat the disability falls into the following categories:

- *Limitations*—Capabilities that have been taken away by a disease process.
- *Assets*—Capabilities that have been untouched by a disease process.
- *Capacity*—Present abilities plus the power to receive and develop new abilities. The new ability may be physical (neuromuscular) or cognitive (sensorimotor): (a) the physical "power or ability to hold, retain or contain" and (b) the "mental ability to receive, accomplish . . . or understand" (Dorland's, 1981, p. 213).
- *Competence*—The ability to produce a satisfactory result, as determined by prevailing social and historical conditions. Competence to manage one's own affairs is a legal determination.
- *Prognosis*—The expected change in severity as a consequence of medical treatment and/or the natural course of the disease.

- *Community support*—Adjustments made for disabled people by care givers to ensure safe and productive living within available social and historical conditions.

Therapists evaluate and treat disabilities. While the need to evaluate a lack of ability is readily explainable, the treatment of a lack of ability is harder to explain. Treatment is "the management and care of a patient for the purposes of combating disease or disorder" (Dorland's, 1981, p. 1388). The difficulty resides in explaining how disabilities can be combated. The medical dictionary can help clarify the deficiency. Occupational therapy is defined as "the use of any occupation for remedial purposes" (Dorland's, 1981, p. 1358). A remedy is "anything that cures, palliates, or prevents disease" (Dorland's, 1981, p. 1141). Palliative is "affording relief, but not cure" (Dorland's, 1981, p. 1389). While it is true that therapists are able to offer some remedies, there are many disabilities that are not remediable. A term that describes services provided for remediable and unremediable conditions, with criteria for terminating services, is required; compensation is recommended.

Compensatory treatment makes up for a deficit. Compensatory treatment may make up for a defect that is a consequence of a disease or disorder by making a change in capacity or community support. In the past, most treatment has been aimed at changing capacity by restoring functions or teaching new skills. By changing the patient's capacity, treatment uses the patient's assets to counteract the disease process. A change in the patient's capacity is a remedy, and remedies are treatment objectives that are consistent with acute medical care. The acute medical model has been so pervasive that it is often difficult for therapists to see other changes as a form of treatment. In addition, acute care remedies must be achievable within a short time. When services are extended beyond acute care, additional treatment objectives are required.

As patients make the transition into the community, therapists make recommendations about the type of community support required by residual limitations, with particular concern about hazardous functioning. Changes in capacity that require prolonged training or training in specific settings are part of community support. A number of changing social and historical conditions suggest a need for further development of community support services: the increasing number of elderly people with disabilities; the improved medical interventions that keep people alive but leave them with unremediable limitations; the shorter lengths of acute hospital stays with remediable and unremediable limitations at the time of discharge; the support for occupational therapy services delivered in the home; and the growing number of self-help groups. With community support, the change is initiated and sustained for the patient by care givers. By changing the community support, the treatment process evaluates the patient's limitations and recommends physical adjustments in the environment and designs training procedures. Community support aims at preventing complications, accidents, and injuries that are a risk to people living with a disability and at training people in living effectively in a specific setting.

With compensatory treatment, the ideal role of the therapist is to evaluate the disability with accuracy and precision in order to identify areas where a change in capacity or community support can be realistically achieved. Once the compensations have been made, there is no need to continue to provide occupational therapy services even though residual limitations continue to exist. Social responsibilities mandate that a line be drawn between those residual limitations that can be compensated for and those that cannot. Drawing the line will not be easy, because the process is apt to force confrontations with permanent or prolonged loss of abilities. A change in the state of the disability, for better or worse, is an indication for reevaluation for additional potential compensatory treatments. The unique treatment offered by occupational therapists is compensation for physical and cognitive disabilities.

Activity: The Explanatory Principle

Activity is the selected explanatory principle. Disability is understood within the context of doing an activity. Activity refers to the units of life that orient people to the world of objects (Leontyev, 1981). Human functioning is the process of engaging in purposeful motor actions within a context of material objects and people. The world of objects needs to be adjusted for or by people with a disability so that they can use their remaining functional abilities. Common adjustments are as follows:

- The range of activity is expanded by creating special tables, chairs, sidewalks, and doors for the physically disabled;
- Protection from getting lost is provided by locking doors or escorting the cognitively disabled;
- Once seated, the thoughts/movements required to manipulate material objects can be adjusted;
- And finally, when a product has been produced, the standards of performance can be adjusted to account for the disability.

Information required to clarify functioning in a world of material objects and people falls into the following categories:

1. *Definitions*—Words and categories that form a typology for determining the boundaries of functional activities that disabled people can do in the world of material objects and people.

   Several typologies will be suggested and should be evaluated according to

   a) Their exhaustiveness (Do the terms cover everything that might be done?) and

   b) Their mutual exclusiveness (Can distinctions between the terms be made?).

2. *Descriptions*—Statements or pictures that clarify the outward appearance of the way people with a disability do activities.

3. *Interpretations*—Clarifications of what is not immediately apparent (such as potential hazards in driving with a disability). Therapists evaluate the underlying reasons for (physical and/or cognitive) difficulties in doing activities that most people take for granted. The evaluation is an interpretation of the difficulty, which is explained to the patient, their loved ones, and other professionals.

4. *Expositions*—Detailed accounts of multiple relationships between definitions, descriptions, and interpretations required by therapists for the precise use of the information.

The ideal role of the therapist is to analyze the activity with accuracy and precision and identify areas where adjustments, necessitated by the limitations of the disability, can be made. The following section on activity analysis will expand on making adjustments.

Purpose: The Mediating Process

The advantages of describing an information processing system is an advance in twentieth-century psychology, and the work of Piaget is frequently cited in the occupational therapy literature. The difficulty that therapists encounter with most of the descriptions of an information processing system is that language is the identified mediator of thought. Therapists observe voluntary motor actions which may not require much thought, such as chewing food. An information processing system that guides voluntary motor actions is needed.

Within the clinical analogy, the information processing system is similar to bringing a disabled person into the clinic and giving the patient an activity to perform. The therapist gives directions, observes performance, and asks questions while trying to evaluate the patient's disability. The directions given introduce sensory cues. The performance observed is a voluntary motor action. The questions asked can clarify the patient's thoughts that guide the activity (see Figure 36.1).

Thoughts guide human activities. Information is processed for a reason. When humans do an activity it is for a purpose. All functional activities contain some degree of purpose, except in the comatose patient. Comatose patients can be guided through passive range of motion, and their reflexes can be elicited, yet these actions are initiated and sustained by the therapist. Voluntary motor actions that are initiated and/or sustained by conscious human beings are purposeful. In occupational therapy, purpose can be inferred from the degree of sensorimotor thought processed during a period of functioning. Different states of function can be evaluated by observing the sensory cues used to guide motor actions during a particular time period.

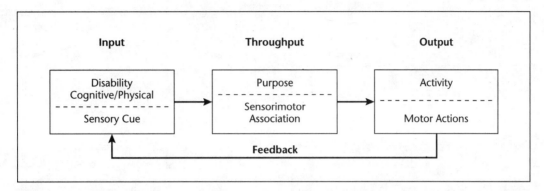

Figure 36.1. Information processing system.
Note. Purpose is inferred from the degree of sensorimotor thought processed during a state of function. Different functional states can be evaluated by observing the sensory cues used to guide motor actions.

Therapists observe many motoric purposes for doing an activity, such as moving because it feels good, or repeating an action because it is interesting. What is needed is a description of the degree of thought used to guide the different functional states. I have developed a scale of six cognitive levels to describe the qualitative differences between functional states. The cognitive levels are an ordinal description of functional states as delineated by the sensorimotor associations used to guide voluntary motor actions (Allen, 1982, 1985; Allen & Allen, 1987). These levels are used as guidelines for predicting the patient's ability to do familiar activities and to learn new ones and for determining the amount of care giver assistance needed. An overview of the levels follows. I'll start at the top with normal functional activity and show how purposes can be progressively removed by a disease process.

At Level 6, symbolic cues are used to formulate plans, producing reflection on performance. Purpose is a premeditated, reflective state, using symbols to anticipate and plan the future. Pauses to think, to consider several hypothetical possibilities, and to select a preferred course of action are observed (Allen, 1985, figure 2.18). Future events are anticipated, behavior is organized, and satisfactory results are produced independently (Allen, 1985, figure 2.20, figure 2.21). Verbal and written directions can be followed and the demonstration of a care giver or supervisor is not required (Allen, 1985, figure 3.2). *Anticipation* is the term used to describe the functional importance of symbols and signs. Unsatisfactory results can be foreseen and prevented, and meaningless activities can be avoided. Theoretically, Level 6 is designed to describe the capabilities of normal adults (80% of a control sample). Most of the social science information processing literature assumes that human beings are functioning at Level 6.

At Level 5, the relationships between material objects are associated with exploratory actions producing experimentation with the physical properties of objects. Purpose is an experimental state, testing the effects that motor actions have on material objects. The process is characterized by overt trial and error, using inductive reasoning to understand cause and effect. *Learning by doing or by being shown what to do* are the terms used to describe overt trial-and-error processes that generalize to other activities and environments (Allen, 1985, figure 2.15). Performance is not organized to plan for or anticipate future events (Allen, 1985, figure 2.16). Situations that require planning, organization, and deductive reasoning are not done effectively (Allen, 1985, figure 2.17); supervisory assistance to anticipate safety hazards is advised.

At Level 4, visible cues are associated with goal-directed actions, producing compliance with an established procedure. Purpose is a compliant state, following known procedures or procedures established by others to achieve a short-term goal. Purpose can also be a noncompliant state, refusing to follow established procedures. Established daily routines can be followed, but the reliance on visual cues can produce misinterpretations of reality (Allen, 1985, figure 2.10). Inattention to visible details can, but not always (figure 2.11). As Figure 36.2 shows,

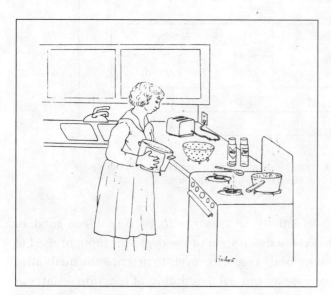

Figure 36.2. Unnoticed safety hazards.
Note. Hazards that may not be noticed by the person with Level 4 cognitive deficits can lead to accidents or injuries.

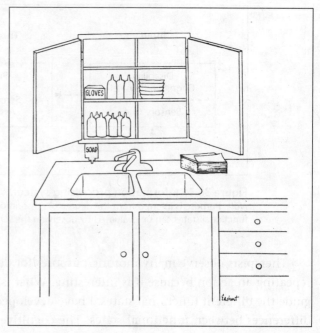

Figure 36.3. A specific setting for training.
Note. For persons with Level 4 cognitive deficits, training is situation specific and does not generalize to other settings.

inattention to the invisible properties of objects, such as heat, electricity, and chemical reactions, produces a lack of attention to hazards that necessitates daily, on-site supervision (see also Allen, 1985, figure 2). A limited capacity for learning is present (learning to put glue bottles away), but learning does not generalize to other environments or activities (putting the glue away in the room across the hall or putting away in general) (Allen, 1985, figure 3). *Training* is the term used to describe a limited capacity for learning that is situation specific; training does not generalize to other activities or environments (see Figure 36.3). Trained actions must be repeated many times, and many reminders are usually required before consistency is achieved.

At Level 3, tactile cues are associated with manual actions, producing an interesting result. Purpose is a chance state of interest in an immediate action. Actions are frequently repetitive and often seem inappropriate, pointless, or destructive to others (Allen, 1985, figure 2.6). Therapists must guide the patient's actions if a project is to be made (Allen, 1985, figure 3.6). At the end of the project, the patient may express surprise in seeing that he or she has made something. *Long-term repetitive training* is the term used to describe the ability to acquire a limited awareness of routine activities that are initiated, sustained, and/or terminated by care givers. Twenty-four-hour supervision is advised.

At Level 2, proprioceptive cues are related to postural actions to produce a sense of comfort or discomfort. The purpose is to produce or maintain a state of physical comfort. Postural actions can take on bizarre qualities (Allen, 1985, figure 2.4). Material objects in the external environment are largely ignored, but cooperation in doing some gross motor activities can usually be elicited (Allen, 1985, figure 2.5). *Discernment* is the term used to describe a limited ability to perceive the external environment and to recognize the external as separate or different from the self. Instructions in the use of neuromuscular functions are poorly followed and may be actively resisted. Twenty-four-hour nursing care is advised.

At Level 1, the person is conscious, but hardly aware of anything. Some cooperation with vital tasks, such as eating and drinking, can be obtained by using sharp commands. The command seems to have a subliminal registration that can be associated with an automatic action, and the purpose obtained is a temporal change in the state of arousal. *Arousal* is the term used to describe a limited ability to respond to external cues. Without external cues from care givers, the person stares into space, or, if agitated, engages in random actions. The distinction between the self and the external environment is blurred (Allen, 1982, 1985; Allen & Allen, 1987). Training is usually impossible or impractical and 24-hour nursing care is necessary.

The thoughts that guide purposeful actions are formed by associating a sensory cue with a motor action. The quality of thought is described by the mediating sensorimotor associations, and the assessment is an inference, drawn by the therapist, about what is going on in the patient's mind. The severity of the disability is observed while the person is in the process of doing an activity.

To evaluate the cognitive complexity of an activity, the same sensory cues and motor actions are used. Activity with mosiac tiles provides a good illustration: Manual actions and tactile cues are used to place tiles in a disorderly fashion at Level 3; compliance with visual cues and goal-directed actions required to do a checkerboard pattern occurs at Level 4; experimentation with colors and spacing can be explored to produce a diagonal pattern at Level 5; and a design of one's own can be imagined and planned at Level 6 (Allen, 1985, figure 3.12). The same patterns are apparent in a kind of needlepoint called "bargello" and in stringing beads (Allen, 1985, figure 10.8). Qualitative differences in the cognitive complexity of the activity can be objectively described and this information can be used to select activities that are appropriate for the individual's current cognitive ability.

If your patients are all functioning at Level 6, the notion that voluntary motor actions are mediated by sensorimotor associations is not critically important to the delivery of your services. But you should be aware of some terms that often indicate the presence of an undetected cognitive disability: *uncooperative, resistive, dependent, passive, manipulative, engaging in secondary gain, intrusive, egocentric, unrealistic, unmotivated,* or *not ready for rehabilitation.* These terms all connote a tendency to blame the patient for the presence of a cognitive disability. Obviously, this is unfair. What the patient will and will not do is based on the patient's ability to associate the sensory cues and motor actions that form a purpose. To put it simply, it is not that they won't; they can't. Therapists need to evaluate for a possible cognitive disability, and when a disability is detected, the difference between "won't" and "can't" needs to be explained to other care givers and the patient's family.

A definition of therapeutic activities can be suggested by combining the elements of disability, activity, and purpose. Therapeutic activities are used to evaluate and compensate for disabilities while recognizing the patient's functional purpose and reducing difficulties encountered in the activity.

Hierarchy for Activity Analysis

With a general definition of therapeutic activities in place, our attention can shift to developing the concept of activity as an explanatory principle. Activity as an explanatory principle is analogous to a reorganization of the supplies kept in the occupational therapy clinic. Over the years there has been a fair amount of disagreement about the supplies that ought to be kept in the clinic: crafts, prevocational equipment, activities of daily living, splints. There have been many recommendations to get rid of this or that activity. When it comes to activity analysis I will not recommend getting rid of anything, but I did reorganize the place.

Leontyev's (1978) hierarchy of activity analysis will be used, with modifications required to explain results produced by people with disabilities. Three levels of activity analysis are suggested: activities, actions, and operations. First, I will give an overview of Leontyev's hierarchy to provide a general impression; and, then, I will go back and define the terms for occupational therapy. Leontyev's levels are helpful in delineating how various occupational therapy theories have focused on different aspects of activity.

At the top of the hierarchy, activities tell us why something is done and give us the associated motivational concepts of personal sense and meaning. Occupational behavior/human occupation focuses on this level of analysis. Actions tell us what is done and give us the associated results. Sensory integration and cognitive disabilities focus on this level of analysis. Operations tell us how, when, and where something is done and give us the associated means and conditions. Physical disabilities focus on this level of analysis. Operations and actions are separated for theoretical and research purposes, but in real life, they are usually combined; task refers to their combination (Cole & Cole, 1979; Leontyev, 1978; Lyons, 1983; Wertsch, 1979, 1985).

Authors of papers, books, and research proposals have a tendency to emphasize one level of analysis over another. Authors need a selected emphasis because the subject matter of human activity is too vast to be managed all at once. When engaged in knowledge development, a selected focus of study is essential. Authors of research designs, treatment techniques, and theories must be granted the freedom to do an in-depth study at one level of analysis. Clinicians, on the other hand, cannot be granted that freedom because, in practice, clinicians must have answers to all of the questions posed by the levels of analysis: the *how, when, where* of operations; the *what* of actions; and the *why* of activities. Clinicians frequently draw from the work of several authors in identifying potential answers to those questions.

Occupational therapists start service delivery by evaluating the operations that the patient can and cannot do. Therefore, I have turned the Soviet psychology hierarchy upside down and have added key adjectives to modify the nouns. I am now talking about *feasible operations, satisfactory results* (the term *results* has replaced the term *actions*), and *desirable activities*. These changes have been made to clarify occupational therapy concerns.

Feasible Operations

Operations identify the specific circumstances: the means of carrying out the action and the condition in which the action is done (Leontyev, 1978). At the level of operations, the focus is on the steps required to produce a product. The materials, instruments, and tools used are considered, including the adapted equipment required by the disabled patient. The level of operations is the most specific level of activity analysis.

Experienced therapists have a huge amount of knowledge about the operations of disabled people, but this knowledge is not documented in the occupational therapy literature. This gap in the literature may explain the continued requirements for fieldwork experiences, and a major obstacle to filling in this gap resides in developing a typology to organize the information. During the last year, some progress in the development of a typology has been made (personal communication with M. Brinson, L. Cargill, M. A. Mayer, and E. L. Stone, November 1986).

Feasible operations answer three kinds of questions: how, when, and where. The question of how includes answers for how much pressure, strength, coordination, frequency, fluid measure, liquid measure, and number of objects required to do the activity. The question of when includes timing decisions about duration, sequence, and endurance. The question of where provides answers for range of motion, part/whole arrangements, sorting and bundling by classifying objects, and directionality, as in sanding with the grain of the wood.

Therapists evaluate the functional severity of disabilities while the patient is in the process of performing an operation. With physical disabilities, the patient may not have the neuromuscular strength, range of motion, or coordination to do the operation successfully. With cognitive disabilities, the patient may not form the sensorimotor judgments required to determine how much, how long, or where to put something. Therapists evaluate the patient's assets and limitations through observations of operations with the ultimate objective of identifying feasible operations. Feasible operations delineate the neuromuscular and sensorimotor characteristics of the activity in which successful performance can occur.

A review of the occupational therapy literature did not reveal any typologies resembling the categories for feasible operations; it can therefore be concluded that this is a new approach to activity analysis. The original reason for developing the typology was to increase the accuracy of interpreting the process of doing an operation. What is emerging is a different approach to evaluation. The identification of feasible operations starts by analyzing the activity and then looking to see if the patient can do it. Most occupational therapy evaluations work the other way around: first the therapist evaluates the patient; and, then, the therapist looks for an activity. While the outcome of a different approach is still uncertain, two optimistic objectives are being considered: one, to increase the reliability and validity of the therapist's interpretations of feasible operations, and two, to develop a shorter, and therefore more efficient, comprehensive evaluation checklist of potential operations.

Satisfactory Results

Once feasible operations have been identified, those operations can be organized into satisfactory results. A number of departures from Leontyev's description of actions are necessitated by the focus on disability and the identification of purpose as a mediator. As mentioned above, a distinction will be made between the patient's purpose for doing an action and the results of that action. To do this, a typology of efficient actions developed by Kotarbinski (1965) will be used to define results.

Purposeful actions produce a result. The effects of motor actions are events, and it is these events that therapists use to determine competence. The effect, or result, is always a change in something or a state of something. The advantage of focusing on results is that results can be objectively described and used to develop standards of performance. Historically, the separation between standards of performance and the value judgments of the therapist has been difficult to make. Therapists need standards of performance that can be used in any geographical area, and across diagnostic categories, to describe a disabled person's ability to produce a satisfactory result.

Four types of results have been defined by Kotarbinski (1965): constructive, destructive, preservative, and preventative. Constructive and destructive results are permanent in the sense that an object is changed from the initial stage to the final stage. Constructive and destructive results are observed after the patient has completed the process of making something or doing something.

A constructive result adds a property to an object, and a destructive result subtracts a property from an object. Constructive results include attaching objects (nailing, tying, gluing, and sewing), covering surfaces (spreading, wiping, painting, staining, and soaping), and combining objects (blending and stirring). The term destructive is a departure from common usage, but the clear differentiation between terms provided by subtracting a property justifies the departure. Destructive results include removing surface elements (sanding, filing, and polishing), reducing size (slicing, cutting, and shaving), altering form or shape (pressing, hitting, punching, and rolling). Most arts and crafts, as well as the activities of daily living and prevocational tasks, produce constructive or destructive results. Standards of performance in producing satisfactory results in these areas would help therapists make recommendations concerning the patient's ability to function in settings outside of the occupational therapy clinic.

There is a relationship between feasible operations and satisfactory results that can be illustrated as follows: Unsatisfactory sanding may be explained by problems with pressure, strength, rate, duration, endurance, or directionality. During an assessment process, the therapist's goal is to pinpoint the problem so that the operational barrier can be removed if possible.

At the time of discharge, therapists are often asked to predict the patient's ability to function in various community settings. Most of the concerns about a disabled person's ability to function in the community center around preventative and preservative results. Preventative and preservative results protect an object from unwanted change. Preventative and preservative results identify the basic requirements for safe living in the community.

Preventative results avoid a change in the property of an object from the beginning to the end of a period of time. Potential injuries to the self that need to be prevented include cuts, burns, falls, malnutrition, obesity, electric shocks, poisoning, medical complications, noncompliance with treatment, and allergic reactions. Potential damages to objects include spoilage, infestation, thefts, loss of money, the giving away of objects, hoarding, loss of an object of great value, or damages caused by stains, breakage, and fires. Annoyances to oneself and others include getting lost, misplacing objects, forgetting messages, leaving a mess, being involved in minor traffic accidents or violations, preparing food poorly, having body odors or an odd/dirty appearance, and getting bruises.

Preservative results maintain the properties of objects. Physical safety includes maintaining body temperature, weight, fluids, cleanliness, and emergency communications. Security from harm includes protecting furniture, clothing, utilities, appliances, and other housewares.

Preservative and preventative results require the anticipation of a need to protect or shield material objects and people from undesirable changes. Anticipation occurs at cognitive Level 6, but anticipation does not occur at the lower cognitive levels. A disabled person's inability to anticipate undesirable changes may be a major factor in discharge planning. Disabled people who do not recognize the need to engage in preventative and preservative results require protection in the community.

The contrast between the actions associated with constructive and destructive results, versus preventative and preservative results, is striking. The differences probably explain the difficulties therapists have in generalizing from clinical observations, where accidents, injuries, and damage must be minimized, to community functioning. Some of the gap might be bridged by focusing the therapist's observations on the patient's anticipation of, the response to, minor errors and mistakes that can be observed in clinical settings. A patient's purpose can produce an intentional or unintentional result; observations of responses to unintentional results may be helpful in predicting community functioning.

An overview of some distinctions between terms may be helpful. This classification of results is restricted to a process of changing an object or the state of that object. The agent of the action is a patient. The patient's purpose may produce intentional or unintentional results. The term *product* is used to describe the physical object; a product begins to exist when the result has been achieved. Prior to the achievement of the result, physical objects are referred to as materials. Instruments, tools, and supplies are external substances used during the process of transmitting power or pressure (Kotarbinski, 1965). The analysis of the efficient use of materials, instruments, or tools occurs at the level of operations. The intended product serves as a standard for evaluating the quality of the finished product.

In our clinics, the sample of the project can serve as a standard of performance. The sample is the intended result. To use the sample as a standard, the expectation that the disabled person produce a replica must be explicitly stated. This may be achieved by asking the patient if he or she can make the project look like the sample. The directions given and the questions asked during the process of producing the result influence the quality of the final product.

Defining the problem that will explain unsatisfactory results cannot be done accurately by looking at the results. Usually, there are several possible explanations for an unsatisfactory result. Accuracy is derived from observing the process of doing the activity at the level of operations. Questions asked and directions given by therapists are directed toward evaluating the problem and removing operational barriers. The therapist's perspective tends to emphasize operations. In contrast, family members, employers, and other health professionals tend to emphasize results. Therapists explain unsatisfactory results to other care givers by precisely defining the underlying operations that produced the results.

Desirable Activities

One of the merits of Soviet psychology is the recognition that desirable activities are derived from existing social conditions (Wertsch, 1979, 1985). Individual human activity is not simply a matter of personal choice and interest but is derived from a person's status in society and depends on social and historical conditions. For example, watching football as a leisure time activity is not only based on a person's interest in football but also depends on the availability of television sets and satellites. To extend this analogy, the availability of advanced technology has caused computers to be used in occupational therapy treatments.

Disabilities seen by therapists are often associated with seemingly deep and dramatic reductions in a person's social condition. The psychological adjustment to disability must extend beyond the individual's choices and interests; reorientation requires a restructuring of the patient's social relationships so that the patient can perform feasible operations and produce satisfactory results. In essence, many of the disabled people seen by therapists need assistance in objectively assessing their situation and determining a role within the available social conditions.

Finding an acceptable role is facilitated when people generate their own desires. Desirable activities have two effects: They create a personal sense or recognition of the disability in the patient and they reveal the social meaning of the implications of the disability to the patient. Personal sense as perceived by the individual is created during the process of doing an activity and after it is completed. Relevant cultural norms are added to a personal sense and clarify the meaning of a disability (Leontyev, 1978).

For evaluation purposes, therapists distinguish between assets, limitations, capacity, competence, and prognosis. These distinctions are often carried over into recommended treatment methods. The development of the patient's personal sense of the disability does not seem to include these distinctions. Assets and limitations, for example, are combined when patients learn to feed themselves while wearing a splint or move while in a wheelchair. It is more troublesome when cognitively disabled persons fail to recognize the presence of a disability. People functioning at Level 3 often fail to recognize a blatantly unsatisfactory result, such as a picture that is upside down. At Level 4, the unsatisfactory result may be recognized in a particular project, but the patient is unable to interpret the social meaning of slow performance or the social implications of insisting on idiosyncratic results. At Level 5, the social ramifications of ignoring established standards of performance may not be anticipated.

Because therapists use activity as a treatment method, they are in a position to see the social meaning of a disability and witness the formation of a personal sense of the disability. The tragedy is apparent. The social meaning of a disability frequently is that activities usually taken for granted are beyond the reach of the disabled person. The harsh reality is that the usual range of desirable activities is severely limited. Few feasible operations may be available, with few desirable activities. Those that are feasible may be rejected by patients, families, and society. Therapists use a tremendous amount of ingenuity to find desirable activities. They often succeed by looking for feasible operations and by making adjustments in the standards for satisfactory results, in the hope of coming up with an activity both legal and desirable. For these reasons, we cannot afford to discard any of our clinical supplies.

Treatment Hypothesis

Now it is time to see how all of these definitions look in practice, to begin to put some muscles on the bones of this skeleton and see what begins to emerge. If the terms are helpful, they should clarify our explanation for using activity as a treatment method with populations for whom treatment objectives are difficult to write.

For many years, therapists have used the remedial treatment hypothesis to explain the effectiveness of their treatment methods—which is [that] doing an activity produces an improvement in the patient's ability to function. An improvement in the patient's capacity was the required criterion for evaluating treatment effectiveness. Improved capacity is an acute, medical model treatment hypothesis that reflects years of hospital-based services.

The need to expand the treatment hypothesis seems to be more essential in some areas of practice than in others. Therapists working with hand injuries, for example, can rely on the remedial hypothesis because hand injuries have a good prognosis for an improvement in capacity. In addition, the simple cause-and-effect relationship between doing an activity and improving functional ability is relatively easy to document when changes in muscles and nerves are expected. When changes in capacity cannot be expected or cannot be explained by engaging in therapeutic activities, additional treatment objectives are required.

In recent years, problems with the remedial treatment hypothesis have been identified; one major difficulty lies in the need to recognize a poor prognosis. Another difficulty lies in the need to recognize alternative explanations besides therapeutic activities for a good prognosis. Progress in addressing these problems has been made by adopting position papers describing the roles and functions of occupational therapy in long-term care and with severely disabled persons (Rogers, 1983; Sabari, 1983). Treatment dilemmas continue to exist and will be examined to clarify the use of activity as a treatment method.

Three treatment dilemmas that require reformulation of treatment objectives can be identified. First, some acute disease processes have a good prognosis but have alternative explanations for improvement (i.e., medication effects, the natural healing process, and normal growth and development). Alternative explanations suggest that other factors, besides activity, account for improvement in capacity (Allen, 1982, 1985). The nagging question, implicit in the recognition of other causes of change is, if other factors produce the improvement in capabilities, why use activities as a treatment method? Diagnostic categories affected by this question include primary affective disorders, anxiety disorders, substance abuse, all pediatric conditions, head trauma, and cerebral vascular accidents. Studies of a change in capacity with these populations require a control group of people who are not receiving treatment aimed at changing capacity.

Second, some disease processes (e.g., Alzheimer's) that are characterized by a progressive loss of capabilities require a recognition of the loss and a realistic statement of what can and cannot be done. Third, the persistent limitations, such as those present with spinal cord injuries and schizophrenic disorders, require a recognition of the lack of medical knowledge to correct the disability and a realistic statement of what can and cannot be done to ease the difficulty of living with the disability. Additionally, long-lasting disabilities require criteria for terminating occupational therapy services. To demonstrate treatment effectiveness with these three populations, which constitute the majority of the patients seen by therapists, greater precision in explaining the importance of activity is required.

Alternative Explanations

The diagnostic category that I have selected to illustrate alternative explanations for improved capabilities is primary affective disorder. The prognosis is a return to normal functioning (Goodwin & Guze, 1985). The antidepressants improve the patient's functional abilities, and the degree of improvement can be described by using the cognitive levels as a repeated measure: Typically patients move from Level 4 (gravely disabled at admission) to Level 6 (a return to a normal level of function at discharge). With acute depressive episodes, activities can be used as an objective appraisal of medical interventions, answering such questions as, Are the medications working? Is the patient ready to be discharged yet? Can a longer stay be justified for utilization review? Can the patient protect her children from harm? Can the patient go back to work yet? When observations of activities are used to answer these questions, the need for reliable and valid evaluations becomes intense. Alternative explanations for changes in capacity suggest a need for precise evaluations.

The cognitive levels are being used as a repeated measure at different times of day and with many different activities. A therapist may be asked to make qualitative comparisons between polishing fingernails, sewing a pot holder, and typing a letter. The comparisons require precise definitions of task equivalence, a degree of specification known only to therapists with years of experience. With the typologies for feasible operations and satisfactory results, we hope to make the information available to new therapists. In doing so, we will need to develop a degree of specification in our literature that has been lacking. Specification has not been very popular in American occupational therapy; it is often ridiculed with labels such as the "cookbook approach." I think it is time to change that attitude. Accuracy, objectivity, and measures of change in capacity that may be influenced by other factors all require specification. It is time to become more accountable for what we evaluate and more responsible for what we recommend. Further refinements in activity analysis may help us sharpen our evaluation procedures and clarify the influence that other factors have on changes in capacity and community support.

Lifelong Disability

The use of activity to treat people with lifelong disabilities requires another perspective. The psychiatric diagnosis commonly associated with this prognosis is a schizophrenic disorder, but the recognition of the longevity of the problem is relatively recent (Mechanic, 1986). Because of the ambiguities and controversies surrounding the long-term care of patients with schizophrenic disorders, the value of activity as a treatment method is not clearly defined. I often find it helpful to examine the physical disabilities literature when rehabilitation for mental disorders is unclear. In this case, I selected spinal cord injuries; moving back and forth between physical and cognitive disabilities often helps gain perspective.

One statement in the spinal cord injury literature came as a surprise to me, namely, that the rehabilitation of spinal cord injury focuses on ADL and mobility. Our professional ideal suggests that therapists would go beyond the content of ADL. A further examination of the spinal cord literature revealed the limitations in therapist's current capacities to deal with this disorder. A lot of information delineating an association between level of lesion and enervated muscles is available. Guidelines for probable associations between level of lesion and ADL also exist (De Jong, Branch, & Corcoraw, 1984; Delgado, 1982; Rogers & Figone, 1979; Wilson, McKenzie, & Barber, 1974). Guidelines for other activities do not exist. The literature does not provide information that would help the therapist suggest other feasible operations and satisfactory results.

At this point, clinical experience seems to be essential to determine whether an operation is feasible for the patient with spinal cord injuries. That experience should be put to work to develop a list of feasible operations associated with levels of lesion. With such a list, therapists could evaluate any activity that might be desirable to a patient. In addition, the list of feasible operations should guide the therapist in reducing, or even better, eliminating operational barriers that impede satisfactory results. Used in this manner, activity analysis verifies the basic knowledge therapists need to facilitate engagement in desirable activities.

In examining the adjustment to spinal cord injury, Trieschmann (1980) suggested that the content of rehabilitation programs needs to be expanded to consider a "reason for getting out of bed in the morning." She was able to clarify this further by identifying the following three areas of functioning associated with a successful life:

- The prevention of medical complications and the utilization of activity of daily living and mobility skills.
- The maintenance of a stable living environment, including the social skills required to put nondisabled people at ease.
- The engagement in productive activity which is flexibly defined as vocational, avocational, educational, or voluntary.

Interviews with people who have had the disability for a long time suggest that adjustment is lifelong, but that the need for the presence of a therapist is not lifelong. Of interest to therapists is the fact that the people with spinal cord injuries who are the most productive do not express the loss in physical terms; the greatest loss is expressed as a loss in activity (Trieschmann, 1980).

Similar views of functioning occurred when Trieschmann's view of success was translated into the *Mission and Goal Statement* (1986) for the Los Angeles County Community Support System. Professionals, family members, and clients with severe and persistent mental disorders ratified the following summary of needs:

> The abilities and disabilities of the population both require attention when identifying needs. Problem areas for these individuals identify a need for services which prevent medical complications and promote the maintenance of a stable living environment. On the other hand, strengths identify a need for programs that provide a personal sense of belonging and a meaningful involvement in the community, that is, to find one's niche in life. (p. 2)

By listening to people with long-term disabilities, some conclusions about the value of activity can be drawn. Activity actualizes a person's strengths. Using their remaining abilities provides disabled people with a sense of belonging and establishes a meaningful involvement in the community. Activity ensures a place in life for people with lifelong disabilities.

The examination of lifelong disabilities reaffirms the human need to engage in desirable activities. Disabilities restrict the number of options, and the therapist's special knowledge is required to compensate by designing feasible operations with satisfactory results. Therapists help locate a realistic place in life but once the location is established, direct services can be discontinued.

Up until now, the need for special assistance has been easily recognized with physical disabilities, but harder to explain with cognitive disabilities. At the present time, Americans are spending a great deal of money on people with lifelong psychiatric disabilities. These people fall into a cycle of being picked up by the police, brought to the psychiatric hospital, sent to court, discharged to the street, picked up by a psychiatric emergency team, taken to a medical unit, discharged to a board and care, taken to a community mental health center, supported by social security insurance, moved to the street, moved to a warmer climate, picked up by the police, and so on. A stable placement for these people could save both anguish and money. Satisfying these patients' rights by maintaining stable placements for them should be an obligation for our democratic society (Dearth, Labenski, Mott, & Pellegrini, 1986).

To get cognitively disabled people to agree to stay in a given setting, desirable activities must be available. Occupational therapists can design activities that these people enjoy doing because many of them will stay if they like what they are doing. Many of these people want a job, but we know that many of them are functioning at Level 4 and cannot learn to meet the standards of performance set by a free enterprise system (although they can be trained to do a specific job). Supportive employment, a rehabilitation concept for people with developmental disabilities, might work for the psychiatric population. Supportive employment is lifelong and takes place in a real job setting under supervision. The therapist's knowledge of all three levels of activity analysis would be extremely helpful in training people in supportive employment: The job will have to be desirable to keep the cognitively disabled person there; the results will have to be satisfactory from the company's perspective; and the therapist will have to design a training program that uses feasible operations.

Progressive Decline

The value of activity in disorders characterized by progressive decline in capabilities requires a realistic appraisal of a tragic situation. With the dementias, such as Alzheimer's disease, the professional ideal is to help the patients use their remaining abilities for as long as possible. Activities that retain their feasibility the longest are those that the patients engaged in most frequently in the past; thus, a history of previous interests and participation is helpful. As the dementia progresses, there is a corresponding reduction in the cognitive level and satisfactory results.

The timing of restricted access to activities that the patient enjoys poses difficult questions: When should the patient stop driving, stop living alone, stop taking walks around the neighborhood, stop working in the kitchen, and stop using the bathroom alone, and when should the patient go to a nursing home? The discontinuation of activities is based on an assessment of potential hazards. When identifying undesirable results (i.e., results to be prevented) and desirable results (i.e., results to work for) a list of potential hazards and concerns relevant to the patient's preferred life-style must be prepared. A favored selection in our clinic is the preparation of macaroni and cheese because we can observe patients' ability to exercise safety in handling boiling water and hot food as well as to correctly time the cooking process, remember to turn off the stove, and to clean afterwards.

Progressive decline illustrates a primary emphasis on desirable and undesirable results. Compensatory treatment aims at recommending the associated community support required by the severity of the disability. The increased number of disabled people in the population as a whole suggests an increased demand for this aspect of occupational therapy services.

Suggested Treatment Hypothesis

I am summarizing this lecture by taking the philosophical concepts and making them simple once again. This is analogous to leaving the occupational therapy clinic and explaining the value of activity to other professionals and the general public. From the examination of the patient populations a refined treatment hypothesis can be suggested: Therapeutic activity compensates for disability by utilizing remaining capabilities to accomplish desirable activities with satisfactory results.

Occupational therapy is a service delivered to disabled people. Service delivery supports the use of remaining capabilities by minimizing operational barriers that, if left unattended, would impede the achievement of satisfactory results. Inactivity, or unsupervised activity, tends to exacerbate medical complications and produce additional injuries and/or disabilities not inherent in the underlying illness.

Desirable activities provide a sense of belonging and a meaningful involvement in the community. It is true that activity is valued by all people, but activity is especially important to disabled people because their opportunity to engage in successful activity is limited. That is why occupational therapists have always used activity as a treatment method, and why we will continue to do so.

References

Allen, C. K. (1982). Independence through activity: The practice of occupational therapy (psychiatry). *American Journal of Occupational Therapy, 36,* 731–739.

Allen, C. K. (1985). *Occupational therapy for psychiatric diseases: Measurement and management of cognitive disabilities.* Boston: Little, Brown.

Allen, C. K., & Allen, R. E. (1987). Cognitive disabilities: Measuring the social consequences of mental disorders. *Journal of Clinical Psychiatry, 48,* 185–190.

Cole, M., & Cole, S. (1979). *The mind: A personal account of Soviet psychology.* Cambridge, MA: Harvard University Press.

Dearth, N., Labenski, B. J., Mott, M. E., & Pellegrini, L. M. (1986). *Families helping families: Living with schizophrenia.* New York: Norton.

De Jong, G., Branch, L. G., & Corcoraw, P. J. (1984). Independent living outcomes in spinal cord injury: Multivariate analysis. *Archives of Physical Medicine & Rehabilitation, 65,* 66–73.

Delgado, C. (1982). Functional levels of quadriplegia. Downey, CA: Rancho Los Amigos Hospital.

Department of Mental Health, Los Angeles County, California. (1986). *Mission and Goal Statement.* (Available from author at 2415 West 6th Street, Los Angeles, CA 90057.)

Dorland's illustrated medical dictionary (26th ed.). (1981). Philadelphia: Saunders.

Fields, G. E. (1911). The effect of occupation upon the individual. *American Journal of Insanity, 68,* 103–109.

Goodwin, D. W., & Guze, S. B. (1985). *Psychiatric diagnosis* (3rd ed.). New York: Oxford University Press.

Kotarbinski, A. (1965). *Praxiology: An introduction to the science of efficient action.* New York: Pergamon Press.

Kozulin, A. (1986). The concept of activity in Soviet psychology: Vygotsky, his disciples and critics. *American Psychologist, 41,* 264–273.

Leontyev, A. N. (1978). *Activity, consciousness and personality.* Englewood Cliffs, NJ: Prentice Hall.

Leontyev, A. N. (1981). *Problems of the development of the mind.* Moscow, USSR: Progress Publishers.

Lyons, B. G. (1983). The Issue Is—Purposeful versus human activity. *American Journal of Occupational Therapy, 37,* 493–495.

Mechanic, D. (1986). The challenge of chronic mental illness: A retrospective and prospective view. *Hospital Community Psychiatry, 37,* 891–896.

Meyer, A. (1937, September 14). Address at testimonial in honor of Eleanor Clarke Slagle in Atlantic City. (Typescript). (Available from the Archives of the American Occupational Therapy Association, University of Texas–Medical Branch, Galveston, Texas 77550-2782.)

Rogers, J. C. (1983). Roles and functions of occupational therapy in long-term care: Occupational therapy and activity programs. *American Journal of Occupational Therapy, 37,* 807–810.

Rogers, J. C., & Figone, J. J. (1979). Psychosocial parameters in treating the person with quadriplegia. *American Journal of Occupational Therapy, 33,* 432–439.

Sabari, J. (1983). The roles and functions of occupational therapy services for the severely disabled. *American Journal of Occupational Therapy, 37,* 811.

Toulmin, S. (1972). *Human understanding: Volume 1.* Oxford: Clarendon Press.

Trieschmann, R. B. (1980). *Spinal cord injuries: Psychological, social and vocational adjustments.* New York: Pergamon Press.

Wertsch, J. V. (Ed.). (1979). *The concept of activity in Soviet psychology.* Armonk, NY: M. E. Sharpe, Inc.

Wertsch, J. V. (Ed.). (1985). *Culture, communication and cognition: Vygotskian perspectives.* New York: Cambridge University Press.

Wilson, D. J., McKenzie, M. D., & Barber, L. M. (1974). *Spinal cord injury, a treatment guide for occupational therapists.* Thorofare, NJ: Charles B. Slack.

37

1988 Eleanor Clarke Slagle Lecture

Occupational Therapy Knowledge:
From Practice to Theory

Anne Henderson, PhD, OTR

Theory building is requisite to the orderly production of knowledge in occupational therapy. Theory fosters both the development of articulated knowledge and the organization of knowledge for education and practice. This paper presents a point of view on theory development. I believe that the techniques used in occupational therapy practice are an important source for theory. Therefore, the focus of this paper is on technology and technological theory. Technology is a generic term, like science, used to include the whole of technical knowledge in a given practice profession. As used in this paper, technology includes both processes and products. Thus the technology of medicine includes processes such as surgery and products such as drugs.

Occupational therapy technology is our body of knowledge of assessment and intervention techniques. Occupational therapy practice includes a few technological products such as splints and adaptive equipment and many technological processes, such as activity group therapy, oral-motor treatment, and training in self-care.

The first topic of this paper is technology as one category of knowledge needed in occupational therapy practice. I will identify categories of professional knowledge and discuss the differences, characteristics, and uses of the various categories. This will allow further definition of technology and highlight its place in practice.

The second topic is the development of scientific technology. This will be discussed in the context of the development of knowledge and theory in general as well as in the context of the similarities and differences between science and technology.

The third part of the paper will focus on one specific area of occupational therapy technology, that of object manipulation, particularly in children with neurological disorders. I will present a history of the treatment of disorders of fine motor function in cerebral palsy and present some suggestions for the development of a technological theory.

Technology: A Category of Professional Knowledge

Categories of Professional Knowledge

There are many ways of categorizing the knowledge needed in professional practice. The one I have selected begins by classifying human knowledge into ordinary knowledge and specialized knowledge (Bunge, 1983a). Ordinary knowledge is knowledge that is generally accessible to everyone within a culture, it is what everybody knows. For the professional, I would also include knowledge gained in a liberal arts education, because this knowledge is accessible to everyone in higher education and is considered to be an essential foundation for professional education.

Originally published 1988 in *American Journal of Occupational Therapy, 42,* 567–576.

The second general category of human knowledge is specialized knowledge. Specialized knowledge is defined as knowledge one obtains because one seeks to enter a particular field or vocation (Bunge, 1983a). Specialized knowledge can also be divided into two broad areas. In occupational therapy, specialized knowledge can be divided into knowledge that is needed by health professionals and practitioners in general, and occupational therapy knowledge—knowledge that is peculiar to the practice of occupational therapy.

Generic health professional knowledge includes information about the administration of health programs, health policy, individuals, and social systems such as the family. Llorens (1984) identified such knowledge as that which is needed for occupational therapists to fill a broader role in health care.

Knowledge Specific to Occupational Therapy

For this discussion, I have identified three categories of occupational therapy knowledge: philosophy, technology, and science.

By philosophy, I mean our value system and the philosophical beliefs and assumptions that guide our practice. Our value system reflects our commitment to a holistic and humanistic practice. Our belief system includes our "commitment to the occupational nature of humans" (Kielhofner & Burke, 1983, p. 38) and to the importance of purposeful activity in recovery and adaptation. Generic frames of reference such as Occupational Behavior and the Model of Human Occupation "explain the overall philosophy of values and beliefs of occupational therapy" (Reed, 1984, p. 97).

Scientific knowledge, the knowledge on which we base our practice, includes knowledge from the founding sciences such as anatomy, physiology, and psychology that we have selected as relevant to our discipline as well as knowledge of the science of occupation, which we are in the process of developing.

Technology is the knowledge that tells us how to use purposeful activity to help our patients reach independent function. When we speak of occupational therapy practice we are often thinking of our technology. However, practice is based on more than technology. A practitioner must be knowledgeable in all the categories I have mentioned; he or she must possess knowledge common to health professionals, knowledge of professional values and beliefs, and scientific knowledge, as well as technology.

The classification I have presented was selected for two reasons: first, to allow me to stress the importance of each category of specialized knowledge; and second, as a basis for discussing differences between the various categories of knowledge.

Importance of Each Category of Professional Knowledge

I think we all agree that a therapist entering practice must have both knowledge specific to occupational therapy and knowledge of the health care systems in which our practice is set. I also think everyone agrees that sciences are an important foundation for practice, although we may not agree on what those sciences should be. However, I am not sure that we agree about the relative importance of philosophy and technology, and it appears to me that there is a lack of clarity about the role of each in guiding practice. Therefore, I will discuss these two categories in some detail.

Over the past 15 or more years many voices have been raised calling for a reaffirmation of the value of occupation in human well-being (e.g., Bing, 1981; Kielhofner & Burke, 1983; Reilly, 1962; West, 1984; Wiemer, 1979). I fully support the movement that called for the reestablishment of the philosophical principles on which occupational therapy was founded, making beliefs and assumptions about occupation central to occupational therapy practice. The efforts of scholars and writers have been successful and have resulted in the formal adoption of a philosophy by the American Occupational Therapy Association (1979, p. 785).

However, in my review of editorials and papers, I have found very little praise for the growth of occupational therapy technology, which to me appears to be phenomenal and a great source of professional pride. It is my impression that in their concern for the reestablishment of occupational therapy philosophy, writers have often—perhaps unintentionally—deemphasized or even disparaged technical knowledge.

Therefore, I wish to state my point of view: that occupational therapy technology is an essential part of our professional knowledge and is equal in importance to occupational therapy philosophy. Not more important, but as important. This is not a new concept (e.g., McGourty, 1986; Mosey, 1981, 1985; West, 1979), but it is one that deserves repeated emphasis. It has, perhaps, been most clearly stated in a paper published in 1983 by Tristram Engelhardt titled "Occupational Therapists as Technologists and Custodians of Meaning." In this paper, Engelhardt stressed the importance of occupational therapy's continual commitment to its original humanistic concerns for "the importance of patients as individuals and the significance of activity for health . . . including joy in performing physical tasks" (Engelhardt, 1983, p. 143). But Engelhardt also said that occupational therapists must be scientist-technologists, concerned with musculoskeletal, sensory motor, neurological, and intrapsychic states to help patients regain independent function. He states the following:

> It must be recognized that there need be no competition between a technical or scientific account of therapy, human function, and habits, and accounts in the spirit of Adolf Meyer. These must instead be seen to be complementary, as integral to two distinct but inseparable elements of the profession of occupational therapy. (Engelhardt, 1983, p. 144)

Both philosophy and technology are essential to the practice of occupational therapy because they serve different functions in guiding practice. Our beliefs and values tell us what we should do and technology tells us what we can do and how to do it (Bunge, 1983b, Vol. 7, p. 34). Our philosophical assumptions and humanistic values tell us about the meaning of occupation and our technology tells us about the application of occupation.

Why do I consider it important that we differentiate between categories of knowledge? After all, in practice all our specialized knowledge is used and intertwined in the daily decisions we make with our patients, and that is how it should be. I have, however, three reasons for highlighting the differences.

First, it is only by understanding that these are two separate domains of knowledge that we can place them in the proper perspective in practice and recognize that both philosophy and technology are essential to practice but that neither one can stand alone. If we rely too much on technical skills, treatment will be incomplete or inappropriate. If we rely too much on our philosophical assumptions, we may circumscribe practice and deny the patient the best treatment occupational therapy can offer.

Second, if students are to appreciate the importance of values and beliefs in practice professions, they must learn to differentiate philosophical concepts from technological concepts. Understanding the differences, they can learn how to ensure that their philosophy and technology are congruent and to use both in their clinical reasoning.

Third, this differentiation between philosophical frames of reference and technology has clarified for me some of the controversial issues in the profession and, perhaps, may help you to do so also.

Consider the controversy over specialization and the related issue of professional unity. Concern has been expressed that specialization fragments the profession (e.g., Gillette, 1967; Johnson, 1973; "Task force," 1974). The lack of a single unifying base has been held responsible for separate paths for clinical research and theory development and for a haphazard accumulation of knowledge and technique (Kielhofner & Burke, 1983, p. 43). The issue is resolved if we separate philosophy and technology. Gilfoyle suggested in her Slagle lecture that our professional unity lies in our philosophical heritage, that it is a system of values that potentially unites practice and practitioners (Gilfoyle, 1984).

In a discussion of the merits and pitfalls of specialization in occupational therapy, West (1979) wrote the following:

> All occupational therapists should be *both* generalists *and* specialists. We are *generalists* through the common bond of our use of occupation in the sense of purposeful activity for the general therapeutic effects it has on dysfunction and making possible a more productive and satisfying life. We are *specialists* in the use of occupation, still in the sense of purposeful activity, but now also age-appropriate and problem-oriented for its therapeutic effects in meeting needs of the particular client group served. (p. 46)

The controversy disappears when we say "both . . . and." We need both generic occupational therapy as expressed in models that, as Reed (1984) has indicated, explain overall philosophy of values and beliefs. And we need specialty occupational therapy as expressed in technological models appropriate to specific disability areas and practice settings. I believe we should continue to foster specialization and to provide both advanced education and recognition for specialty practice. At the same time we should ensure through basic education and professional dialogue that our fundamental values and beliefs permeate both our practice and the ways in which we communicate with those outside our profession.

One final difference between philosophy and technology: Our philosophical values and assumptions are enduring. Technology can, however, be expected to change. Science is constantly changing, and techniques grounded in science will also change.

Summary

In summary, I believe it is important that we give equal value to our assumptions and our techniques, but that we differentiate between the uses of philosophical knowledge and the uses of technical knowledge. We need to be unified in our fundamental assumptions, but diverse in our technical knowledge. We need to recognize that the characteristics of philosophical frames of reference and technical knowledge differ. Philosophical values are humanistic, holistic, generic, and relatively unchanging. Technical knowledge is pluralistic, relatively reductionist, diverse, and reflects changes that occur as a result of the evolution of science and theory. Understanding the differences should strengthen the place for each in our profession.

The Development of Scientific Technology

My discussion thus far has focused on the place of technology in occupational therapy practice. I now turn to a consideration of *scientific* technology and the ways in which it develops.

Scientific Technology

How does scientific technology differ from other technology? Occupational therapy, in common with other practice professions, includes a wide variety of treatment strategies that have been used successfully and handed down in practice, but that have not been validated through research. Such knowledge would be considered prescientific. Scientific technology is technology that has been shown to be successful through intervention research, that is, knowledge that has been tested by scientific methods (Bunge, 1983b, Vol. 7, p. 121).

Scientific technology differs from other technical knowledge in two ways. First, it must involve theory or general principles abstracted from knowledge of what works, and second, the principles must be shown to be successful in a high percentage of cases (Bunge, 1967b, Vol. 2, p. 128). There is no clear demarcation between scientific and prescientific technology. Rather, some technologies are more scientific than others.

All practice professions are a mix of scientific technology, technology based on cumulative experience, and the skilled observation and judgment of the practicing therapist. I think this will always be true for any profession dealing with the uncertain and unique nature of real-world problems. The goal of research is to increase the *proportion* of scientific technology in professional knowledge.

Technology and Science

Scientific technology differs from other technology, but it also differs from science. Those who write about technology make a clear differentiation between pure science, applied science, and technology (e.g., Bunge, 1983b; Feibleman, 1983; Jarvie, 1983), and I find their definitions useful in considering scientific technology and technological theory.

Pure science and applied science are both knowledge-producing systems. They differ in that the aim of pure science is merely to discover and describe natural laws, whereas the aim of applied science is useful knowledge. Applied science is therefore a bridge between pure science and technology (Bunge, 1983b).

Technology uses the scientific method. However, technology is not science. Science is "know that"; technology is "know how." Science tells us what is true and sometimes why technology is effective. Technology tells us what works in the world—what is effective (Jarvie, 1983). Scientific technology, then, differs from science in that although it uses the methods of science, its purpose and goals are not the same. It has been said that "whereas scientists, whether basic or applied, change things in order to know them, technologists study things in order to change them" (Bunge, 1983b, Vol. 7, p. 239).

How can we increase the scientific base for our technology? Central to the growth of scientific technology is the development of technological theory. It is instructive to first consider how scientific theory develops.

Approaches to Theory Development in Science

Two major approaches to the development of theory in science and applied science have been identified: the analytic method, which Reynolds (1971) has termed the "research then theory" method, and the synthetic method, which Reynolds calls the "theory then research" method. In actuality, elements of both analytic and synthetic approaches are needed in theory development. The differences lie in how one chooses to begin the process.

The analytic or "research first" approach begins with data. The process begins with the measurement and description of characteristics of small units or components of the phenomenon under study. The findings are then analyzed for the discovery of relationships between the components that have been identified. A conceptual pattern of the whole is built, and theoretical statements are developed from the patterns identified (Bunge, 1967a; Reynolds, 1971). Ayres's early research appears to follow this pattern. Sensory perceptual deficits in learning-disabled children were selected for study, tests were developed, the data were subjected to factor analysis, and the patterns that were found were formalized into sensory integration theory (Henderson, Llorens, Gilfoyle, Myers, & Prevel, 1974).

The synthetic or "theory first" approach begins with the development of a holistic theoretical structure. From this structure, a hypothesis is derived and tested in research. Either the hypothesis is accepted and the theory is supported or it is rejected and the theory is changed. This approach is characterized by the development of theory from a model of practice such as the Model of Human Occupation (Kielhofner, 1985) or Occupational Behavior (Rogers, 1983).

Each of these approaches has its weaknesses. The analytic method fails when data gathering is scattered and unrelated to any whole, and when research goes no further than the study of components in isolation. On the other hand, starting with a grand synthetic view has often proven to be unscientific (Bunge, 1967a, Vol. 1, p. 30) because the theoretical statements are too vague or general to be testable. Good theory development needs to be a process of both analysis and synthesis.

The "research then theory" strategy has characterized, and been the more successful in the development of, physical and biological sciences (Bunge, 1967a). Reynolds (1971), however, suggests that the "theory then research" strategy is more appropriate for the study of social phenomena because of their complexity. Since the study of occupation is grounded both in social science and in biological science, I would like to suggest that both approaches are needed in occupational therapy: the first to study phenomena resulting from biological disorders, and the second to study the meaning of occupation, or purposeful activity, in human existence.

Approaches to Theory Development in Technology

Technological theory differs from scientific theory. Scientific theory is designed to explain the world. Technological theory is made up of principles for action. Dickoff and his associates termed scientific theory as *situation relating,* or predictive, and technological theory as *situation producing,* or prescriptive (Dickoff, James, & Wiedenbach, 1968).

Although technological theory differs from scientific theory, approaches to their development are similar in some ways. A more synthetic approach would be to derive technological theory from scientific theory (e.g., Dickoff et al., 1968). A more analytic approach would be to abstract general principles from practical knowledge. The literature on technology suggests that technological theory develops both ways (Bunge, 1967b).

The derivation of technological theory from science is a theory-to-practice approach. The development of a science of occupation will yield knowledge from which technological theory can be derived. Practice models and philosophical frames of reference can be translated into a structure of theoretical statements that can generate testable hypotheses. These theory-to-practice approaches are important to the development of scientific knowledge in occupational therapy.

Technological theory is on firmer ground when it is based on scientific theory. Certainly, proposing a technological theory incongruent with known scientific knowledge would not be appropriate. However, although generating technological theory from science is ideal, it is often not practical. Scientific theory is seldom either pertinent or sufficiently developed to provide insights for needed action. Historically, many achievements in technology arose without science (Feibleman, 1983). For example, bridges were built before the physical sciences were developed. In my early practice, I made successful splints before the relevant neurophysiological and musculoskeletal knowledge was available to me. It is therefore most practical to approach theory development in more than one way.

The practice-to-theory approach would begin with the knowledge of what treatment strategies work. The knowledge of what works in practice settings would be enhanced if tested by intervention research. Research directed toward the validation of treatment strategies is directly useful to practice; however, I am suggesting that it can be more than that. I believe that such research can also provide the building blocks from which theory can be developed and tested.

I am not talking about grand theories encompassing the occupational therapy process, but rather of the building of small technological theories that will guide aspects of practice, that is, guide the use of specific techniques for specific disorders. For example, a small theory could be developed around the adaptation of habits, objects, or environment to make possible independence in self-care. I foresee that, as such theories are validated, relationships between theories will be discovered and more generic and parsimonious theory will be developed.

A third approach to theory building is somewhere between the approaches I have described. This approach begins with a discrete practice problem. The practitioner-theorist would go to the scientific literature to seek answers to the problem and develop a working theory from which treatment strategies would be derived. This is the approach that seems to be used the most and can be illustrated by an account of the development of a treatment approach.

Margaret Rood began with a practice problem, that of determining better ways of improving motor performance in children with cerebral palsy. Rood went to the scientific literature in neurophysiology and derived a rationale for a new technology, which she developed into practice-specific treatment techniques based upon that rationale. Such a treatment rationale provides a logical basis for intervention. However, Rood's approach, as well as the other neurophysiological approaches, falls short of being scientific because it has never been formally tested. Treatment rationales are seldom tested and are often not testable. To evolve into scientific technology, the rationale must be converted to sets of hypotheses, which are then systematically tested.

Summary

To summarize the second topic of this paper, let me say again that we have a wealth of time-tested technical knowledge in occupational therapy. The purpose of technological theory and research is to strengthen the scientific base of that knowledge. Three approaches to the development of technological theory are the theory-to-practice approach, the practice-to-theory approach, and an approach that combines the two. I believe that occupational therapy needs researchers following each of these approaches.

Object Manipulation in Cerebral Palsy

To illustrate the development of a specific technology and the ways in which its scientific base might be created, I present for your consideration techniques used to develop competency in the manipulation of objects by children with cerebral palsy.

It seems to me that it is particularly appropriate for occupational therapists to have the responsibility for the treatment of hand dysfunctions: first, because of our knowledge of the motor, perceptual, cognitive, and psychological components of hand use; and second, because hand function is basic to areas of occupation such as play and self-care. Moreover, hand dysfunction appears to me to be an area in which theory development has been neglected. It is an area ripe for applied research, research which I believe occupational therapists can do better than anyone else.

A comprehensive technological theory of the treatment of disorders of the hand would include all the performance components; however, I am limiting this account to one segment of treatment, that of motor functions of the hand, in which I include reach and carry, grasp and release, bilateral hand use, finger use, tool use, and in-hand manipulation (Exner, 1987). These basic functions required for object manipulation may be selectively disturbed by biological dysfunction.

I will begin with the presentation of a brief history of the treatment of basic hand dysfunction in children with cerebral palsy. My historical review will focus primarily on textbooks and early journals. Textbooks can provide clues to changes in technology and to continuity and discontinuity in the development of a technology. The early journals provide insight into our philosophical heritage in the treatment of hand dysfunction. I found this heritage first in my study of the early use of activity in the treatment of physical disabilities.

Early History of Treatment of Physical Disabilities

Occupational therapy for the restoration of physical function has its roots in the days when the profession was founded. A major impetus came from the need for rehabilitation of soldiers disabled in World War I (Baldwin, 1919; Dunton, 1919). The use of activities as exercise for the restoration of hand function was developed by reconstruction aides during and following the war. Mock (1918) describes occupational therapy's role as restoring usefulness, overcoming deformities, and teaching new functions to compensate for lost abilities.

The early use of activity in the restoration of physical function demonstrated the advantages of occupation for psychological as well as physical purposes (Woodside, 1971). Therapists sought to find activities that both provided the needed exercise and stimulated interest (Faulkes, 1924). Time was a valuable asset to therapy as patients spent the large part of the day in the craft shops (Green, 1922). The importance of occupational therapy was in the dual advantages of active voluntary muscle action and the work psychology provided by the production of articles.

The Treatment of Children With Cerebral Palsy

The first mention of the treatment of physical dysfunction in children was by Susan Tracy. In her book *Invalid Occupations,* published in 1910, Tracy discussed the treatment of hand deformities at the Industrial School for Crippled Children in Boston. She notes that clay modeling had been found useful for deformed hands, but her emphasis was on giving "one hand lessons" and on adaptive equipment such as clamps and vises to "supply the assistance given by the less active hand" (Tracy, 1910, p. 67).

Articles on occupational therapy for the restoration or development of physical function in children began to appear regularly in the latter half of the 1920s. Most of the work in pediatrics was designed to meet the activity needs of hospitalized children (Smith, 1927; Tracy, 1910), but by the late 1920s, occupational therapists were being employed not only in hospitals, but in schools for crippled children (e.g., Paisley, 1929; Smith, 1927) and in programs in curative workshops (Goodman, 1928; Graham, 1928). At this time, the treatment of cerebral palsy began to emerge, primarily for children with spastic hemiplegia (Graham, 1928; Paisley, 1929, 1930). The early emphasis was on correct hand posture and the stimulation of coordination in the use of the handicapped extremity by using toys, games, and craft activities. Treatment of cerebral palsy stressed voluntary effort, the importance of posture and postural support, and rhythm in activity (Paisley, 1931).

In 1937, bilateral activities such as bead stringing and rhythm toys were mentioned for the training of the spastic hand, as was the use of both hands in daily tasks of lifting objects, buttoning, tying, and typing (Johnson, 1937).

By 1940, cerebral palsy was clearly considered a specialization separate from orthopedics (Hurt, 1940). Different types of cerebral palsy were identified and differentially treated (Martin, 1939). The emphasis in treatment was now on training in self-care as well as on hand activities. Montessori boards were introduced for learning clothing fastenings, and techniques developed for feeding, hygiene, writing, and typing were described. Coordination of hand use was combined with self-care training. Primitive splinting and supported seating were introduced.

During the next two decades, the dual emphasis on fine motor skill and self-care skill continued and the technology expanded (Willard & Spackman, 1947, 1954). Practice was considered necessary for the acquisition of skill (Brunyate, 1949; James, 1951). This period saw, therefore, a development of adaptive equipment and toys both to facilitate self-care and to provide practice opportunities in the training of basic hand skills.

A major theoretical development was the identification of developmental factors in training in self-care and basic hand functions. The research of Gesell and his associates was used to chart normal development as a guide to treatment (Hadra, 1950a, 1950b). In 1957, Frantzen published a guide for the use of toys for the development of hand skills. The publication was based on a 3-year research study of 130 disabled children and 60 normal children. The development of skill was studied, and the arm and hand functions needed for the use of various toys were analyzed. The reported finding was that the order of the stages of development of hand functions was the same for the normal as for the disabled infants.

After this promising beginning, in the late 1950s the growth of technology for the treatment of motor functions of the hand virtually ceased. Textbooks continued to mention hand skills in cerebral palsy, but with decreased detail and emphasis (Willard & Spackman, 1963, 1971). Very few articles on hand skills were published in the 1960s and 1970s. We have no data on the degree to which therapists continued to incorporate manipulation skills in their cerebral palsy treatment repertoire, but it is probable that it was not universal or extensive. From personal experience, I know that treatment of hand functions was supplanted by perceptual training and gross motor activities in many clinical settings.

Factors Affecting the Treatment of Hand Functions in Cerebral Palsy

Why did the treatment of motor functions of the hand in children with cerebral palsy not continue? One reason for the discontinuation of a technology is that something has happened to make it unnecessary or obsolete. However, the recent resurgence of attention to motor functions of the hand in cerebral palsy makes this unlikely. Rather, it seems that the hiatus in the growth of this technology resulted from development in other areas of professional practice.

One change that occurred was in the use of assessment tools. The early developmental checklists for evaluating self-care and reach, grasp, and prehension were replaced in many clinics by the more formal assessments of development such as the Denver or Bayley tests. These had the advantage of being standardized and of providing an overall developmental profile, but the items were less useful for the independent assessment of the motor components of hand function.

A second factor was the development of technologies that competed with the technology directed toward the development of competency in hand functions in cerebral palsy. Three of these technologies were the treatment of perceptual motor, gross motor, and oral-motor dysfunctions.

The recognition that perceptual deficits can have a large impact on fine motor skill in some children with cerebral palsy led to the expansion of treatment to include perceptual motor training. In time, the focus on the perceptual component of skill supplanted the technologies directed toward the motor component. In a similar way, the development of oral-motor therapy changed the focus in feeding from hand skills and tool use to control of the lips, tongue, and jaw.

However, the technology that had the greatest impact on the treatment of cerebral palsy was gross motor therapy. The extent of its impact is shown in articles and in textbooks in which the term *motor development* includes only the development of postural and locomotor functions. Gross motor therapy was more than a competing technology. The treatment rationales on which it was based worked against the continued treatment of hand skills. The major theoretical streams that emerged during this period were the neurophysiological treatment approaches of Rood, Bobath, and others. These treatment approaches not only emphasized the development of automatic postural responses, but suggested that hand use should not be encouraged (Bobath, 1964). It was thought that hand functions would emerge naturally or more readily as a result of the development of postural stability.

The rationales of the neurophysiological approaches to treatment were based on a scientific theory of the peripheral control of movement. Neurophysiological theories have undergone considerable modification since the 1960s, and the newer concepts of the central control of movement show concepts of peripheral control to be neither appropriate nor adequate to the understanding of the motor functions of the hand ("Central Control," 1971). Furthermore, the motor tracts of the central nervous system have been reclassified into medial and lateral systems; the medial system is thought to be responsible for postural functions, and the lateral system for fine finger function (Brinkman & Kuypers, 1972; Kuypers, 1982; Lawrence & Kuypers, 1968a, 1968b).

A second source of treatment rationale was the developmental postulate that proximal skill develops before distal skill (Ayres, 1954; Stockmeyer, 1967). However, several recent research studies have failed to support this proximal-distal hypothesis (Fetters, Fernandez, & Cermak, 1988; Loria, 1978; Wilson, 1983).

I have cited these examples of treatment principles that were derived from science, and yet turned out to be wrong in respect to the hand, because of their negative impact on the development of technology for the improvement of object manipulation skills in cerebral palsy. However, I must point out that each of the competing technologies also had positive effects on practice with children with cerebral palsy.

In the last few years, attention has again been given to the object manipulation skills of children with cerebral palsy. Developmental hand dysfunction is being evaluated and treatment strategies are being designed (e.g., Boehme, 1988; Erhardt, 1982; Exner, in press; Peterson & Peterson, 1984). This can be the beginning of the development of a technological theory of competency in object manipulation in cerebral palsy. To foster this development, I suggest we do the following:

1. Describe and classify techniques currently used in practice for the development of object manipulation skills.
2. Conduct intervention research studies that compare different approaches to treatment of motor dysfunction in hand use.
3. Take the practice problem of object manipulation to science: to the neurophysiology of dual motor systems, to motor learning theory, and to the developmental psychology of motor skill.
4. Conduct research in normal and abnormal hand skill development and recovery of hand function, particularly beyond the first year of life.
5. Formulate and test general principles abstracted from the information gained. The theoretical statements should specify what works and with whom and under what conditions the procedures result in the expected outcomes.

Conclusion

I have used object manipulation as an example of a technology in occupational therapy. All areas of practice have an equal potential for theory development.

In the approach I have presented, it is the clinician who has the initial responsibility for theory development. Occupational therapy technology has its roots in the creativity of the individual practitioner who finds out what works or does not work in the real world of practice (Schön, 1983). The insightful, inventive practitioner uses his or her specialized knowledge together with skilled observation and clinical judgment to both evaluate and develop our technology.

However, something else is required of the clinician. The discovery of successful strategies must be communicated, and in writing, if it is to endure. Only then can the knowledge be used to build theory.

From the knowledge of the treatment strategies that clinicians have found to work, as well as from the findings of intervention research, the theorist can begin the process of developing, classifying, and abstracting general principles from the practice knowledge. From the conceptual pattern that emerges, theoretical statements can be made and tested. That theory, as it evolves, will further guide practice.

In conclusion, we must take pride in our wealth of technology even as we strive to improve it. We must recognize the importance of theory in the growth of professional knowledge. We must see theory building as something we *can* do, and each of us must accept responsibility for our part in theory development. The broader the base of participation in this process, the greater the potential for the growth of knowledge in occupational therapy.

Acknowledgments

I wish to express my appreciation to the American Occupational Therapy Association and to my colleagues who supported my nomination for this award. My appreciation also goes to the faculty and staff of the Department of Occupational Therapy of Boston University–Sargent College of Allied Health Professions for their support in the preparation of this paper, with special thanks to Sharon Cermak for her time and effort on my behalf.

References

American Occupational Therapy Association. (1979). [Minutes of] 1979 Representative Assembly—59th Annual Conference. *American Journal of Occupational Therapy, 33,* 781–813.

Ayres, A. J. (1954). Ontogenetic principles in the development of arm and hand functions. *American Journal of Occupational Therapy, 8,* 95–99, 121.

Baldwin, B. T. (1919). *Occupational therapy applied to restoration of movement* (Walter Reed Monograph). Washington, DC: Walter Reed General Hospital, Occupational Therapy Department.

Bing, R. K. (1981). Eleanor Clarke Slagle Lectureship—1981. Occupational therapy revisited: A paraphrastic journey. *American Journal of Occupational Therapy, 35,* 499–518.

Bobath, B. (1964). The facilitation of normal postural reactions and movements in the treatment of cerebral palsy. *Physiotherapy, 50,* 246–262.

Boehme, R. (1988). *Improving upper body control.* Tucson: Therapy Skill Builders.

Brinkman, J., & Kuypers, H. G. (1972). Cerebral control of contralateral and ipsilateral arm, hand and finger movements in the split-brain rhesus monkey. *Brain, 96,* 653–674.

Brunyate, R. (1949). Occupational therapy means freedom for parents. *The Crippled Child, 26,* 11–13.

Bunge, M. (1967a). *Scientific research* (Vol. 1). New York: Springer-Verlag.

Bunge, M. (1967b). *Scientific research* (Vol. 2). New York: Springer-Verlag.

Bunge, M. (1983a). *Treatise on basic philosophy* (Vol. 6). Dordrecht, Netherlands: D. Reidel.

Bunge, M. (1983b). *Treatise on basic philosophy* (Vol. 7, Part 2). Dordrecht, Netherlands: D. Reidel.

Central control of movement. (1971). *Neurosciences Research Program Bulletin, 9,* 1–59.

Dickoff, J., James, P., & Wiedenbach, E. (1968). Theory in a practice discipline. *Nursing Research, 17,* 415–435.

Dunton, W. R. (1919). *Reconstruction therapy.* Philadelphia: W. B. Saunders.

Engelhardt, H. T. (1983). Occupational therapists as technologists and custodians of meaning. In G. Kielhofner (Ed.), *Health through occupation* (pp. 139–145). Philadelphia: F. A. Davis.

Erhardt, R. P. (1982). Developmental hand dysfunction: Theory, assessment, treatment. Laurel, MD: RAMSCO.

Exner, C. (1987, April). *The development of in-hand manipulation.* Paper presented at the annual conference of the American Occupational Therapy Association, Indianapolis, IN.

Exner, C. (in press). Development of hand functions. In P. N. Clark & A. S. Allen (Eds.), *Occupational therapy for children* (2nd ed.). St. Louis: C. V. Mosby.

Faulkes, W. F. (1924). Restoration of the crippled. *Archives of Occupational Therapy, 3,* 113–116.

Feibleman, J. (1983). Pure science, applied science and technology: An attempt at definition. In C. Mitcham & R. Mackey (Eds.), *Philosophy and technology: Readings* (pp. 33–41). New York: The Free Press.

Fetters, L., Fernandez, B., & Cermak, S. (1988, June). *The relationship of proximal and distal control of movement during development.* Paper presented at the annual conference of the American Physical Therapy Association, Las Vegas, NV.

Frantzen, J. (1957). *Toys: The tools of children.* Chicago: National Society for Crippled Children and Adults.

Gilfoyle, E. M. (1984). The 1984 Eleanor Clarke Slagle Lectureship. Transformation of a profession, *American Journal of Occupational Therapy, 38,* 575–584.

Gillette, N. P. (1967). Changing methods in the treatment of psychosocial dysfunction. *American Journal of Occupational Therapy, 21,* 230–233.

Goodman, H. B. (1928). Corrective work for children. *Occupational Therapy and Rehabilitation, 7,* 181–188.

Graham, L. H. (1928). Occupational therapy with children. *Occupational Therapy and Rehabilitation, 7,* 245–248.

Green, N. (1922). Occupational therapy for orthopedic cases. *Archives of Occupational Therapy, 1,* 269–278.

Hadra, R. (1950a). Developmental factors in the cerebral palsied child, part 1. *The Crippled Child, 28,* 18–19, 29–30.

Hadra, R. (1950b). Developmental factors in the cerebral palsied child, part 2. *The Crippled Child, 30,* 22–23, 30.

Henderson, A., Llorens, L., Gilfoyle, E., Myers, C., & Prevel, S. (Eds.). (1974). *The development of sensory integrative theory and practice: A collection of the works of A. Jean Ayres.* Dubuque, IA: Kendall-Hunt.

Hurt, S. (1940). Occupational therapy in functional work. *Occupational Therapy and Rehabilitation, 19,* 163–168.

James, E. M. (1951). Occupational therapy for cerebral palsy. *British Journal of Physical Medicine, 14,* 149–154.

Jarvie, I. C. (1983). Technology and the structure of knowledge. In C. Mitcham & R. Mackey (Eds.), *Philosophy and technology: Readings* (pp. 54–61). New York: The Free Press.

Johnson, G. V. (1937). Occupational therapy for the spastic hand. *Occupational Therapy and Rehabilitation, 16,* 29–33.

Johnson, J. A. (1973). Occupational therapy: A model for the future. The 1972 Eleanor Clarke Slagle Lecture. *American Journal of Occupational Therapy, 27,* 1–7.

Kielhofner, G. (Ed.). (1985). *A model of human occupation.* Baltimore: Williams & Wilkins.

Kielhofner, G., & Burke, J. P. (1983). The evolution of knowledge and practice in occupational therapy: Past, present and future. In G. Kielhofner (Ed.), *Health through occupation* (pp. 3–54). Philadelphia: F. A. Davis.

Kuypers, H. G. (1982). A new look at the organization of the motor system. *Progress in Brain Research, 57,* 381–403.

Lawrence, D., & Kuypers, H. (1968a). The functional organization of the motor system in the monkey: I. The effect of bilateral pyramidal lesions. *Brain, 91,* 1–14.

Lawrence, D., & Kuypers, H. (1968b). The functional organization of the motor system in the monkey: II. The effects of lesions in the descending brain stem pathways. *Brain, 91,* 1–14.

Llorens, L. A. (1984). Changing balance: Environment and individual. *American Journal of Occupational Therapy, 38,* 29–34.

Loria, C. (1978). An analysis of the relationship between proximal and distal motor development. *Physical Therapy, 60,* 167–172.

Martin, E. F. (1939). Occupational therapy in a school for brain injuries. *Occupational Therapy and Rehabilitation, 18,* 185–190.

McGourty, L. K. (1986). Applying theory to practice: Fieldwork education. In *Occupational Therapy Education: Target 2000—Proceedings* (pp. 126–128). Rockville, MD: American Occupational Therapy Association.

Mock, H. E. (1918). Curative work. *Carry On, 1*(9), 12–15.

Mosey, A. C. (1981). *Occupational therapy: A configuration of a profession.* New York: Raven Press.

Mosey, A. C. (1985). A monistic or a pluralistic approach to professional identity? The 1985 Eleanor Clarke Slagle Lecture. *American Journal of Occupational Therapy, 39,* 504–509.

Paisley, S. A. (1929). Occupational therapy treatment for a group of spastic cases; children under twelve years of age. *Occupational Therapy and Rehabilitation, 8,* 83–92.

Paisley, S. A. (1930). From a therapist's notebook. *Occupational Therapy and Rehabilitation, 9,* 291–292.

Paisley, S. A. (1931). Fundamentals of occupational treatment in spastic paralysis. *Massachusetts Association for Occupational Therapy Bulletin, 5*(1).

Peterson, P., & Peterson, C. E. (1984). Bilateral hand skills in children with mild hemiplegia. *Physical and Occupational Therapy in Pediatrics, 4,* 77–87.

Reed, K. L. (1984). *Models of practice in occupational therapy.* Baltimore: Williams & Wilkins.

Reilly, M. (1962). Occupational therapy can be one of the great ideas of 20th century medicine. The 1961 Eleanor Clarke Slagle Lecture. *American Journal of Occupational Therapy, 16,* 1–9.

Reynolds, P. D. (1971). *Primer in theory construction.* New York: Bobbs-Merrill.

Rogers, J. C. (1983). The study of human occupation. In G. Kielhofner (Ed.), *Health through occupation* (pp. 93–124). Philadelphia: F. A. Davis.

Schön, D. A. (1983). *The reflective practitioner.* New York: Basic Books.

Smith, W. (1927). The relationship between the work of the occupational therapist and the academic teacher in a children's hospital or a school for crippled children. *Occupational Therapy and Rehabilitation, 6,* 187–188.

Stockmeyer, S. A. (1967). An interpretation of the approach of Rood to the treatment of neuromuscular dysfunction. *American Journal of Physical Medicine, 46,* 900–956.

Task Force on Target Populations. (1974). *American Journal of Occupational Therapy, 28,* 158–163.

Tracy, S. (1910). *Studies in invalid occupations.* Boston: Whitcomb & Barrows.

West, W. L. (1979). Professional unity. *American Journal of Occupational Therapy, 33,* 40–49.

West, W. L. (1984). A reaffirmed philosophy and practice of occupational therapy for the 1980s. *American Journal of Occupational Therapy, 38,* 15–23.

Wiemer, R. (1979). Traditional and nontraditional practice arenas. In *Occupational therapy: 2001 AD* (pp. 42–53). Rockville, MD: American Occupational Therapy Association.

Willard, H., & Spackman, C. (Eds.). (1947). *Occupational therapy.* Philadelphia: Lippincott.

Willard, H., & Spackman, C. (Eds.). (1954). *Occupational therapy* (2nd ed.). Philadelphia: Lippincott.

Willard, H., & Spackman, C. (Eds.). (1963). *Occupational therapy* (3rd ed.). Philadelphia: Lippincott.

Willard, H., & Spackman, C. (Eds.). (1971). *Occupational therapy* (4th ed.). Philadelphia: Lippincott.

Wilson, B. N. (1983). *Proximal and distal function in children with and without sensory integrative dysfunction: An E.M.G. study.* Unpublished master's thesis, Boston University, Boston.

Woodside, H. H. (1971). The development of occupational therapy 1910–1929. *American Journal of Occupational Therapy, 25,* 226–230.

38

1989 Eleanor Clarke Slagle Lecture

Neuroscience and Occupational Therapy:
Vital Connections
Shereen D. Farber, PhD, OTR, FAOTA

Occupational therapy practitioners have embraced concepts from diverse origins that are prerequisites for our theoretical foundations. The philosophical base of occupational therapy has evolved by weaving relevant views into technology (Henderson, 1988). During the last decade, we have witnessed a technological revolution in some of our foundation sciences, especially neurobiology, that has resulted in the modification of theories and methodology. The continuous integration of new neuroscientific concepts into occupational therapy theory and practice has thus become mandatory.

My clinical, research, and teaching experiences have led me to formulate the following hypothesis: In-depth knowledge of the neurosciences serves as a common denominator that can enhance our ability to interpret all aspects of human behavior. Because occupational therapy encompasses heterogeneous practice areas, three widely divergent practice disciplines are presented to test the hypothesis: Neuroimmunomodulation (the relationship that exists among several body systems, including the central nervous system [CNS], immune system, and endocrine system); organic bases of psychopathology (as they apply to schizophrenia specifically); and traumatic brain injury (particularly, factors that influence reorganization of the CNS after injury). Current neuroscientific findings in each of these areas are described along with associated treatment and research questions. A neurobiology curriculum philosophy is incorporated to present main concepts important to the lifelong neuroscientific education of occupational therapists.

Neuroimmunomodulation

Neuroimmunomodulation describes the developing interdisciplinary practice that investigates the relationships among participating body systems and associated basic sciences. The term is considered more inclusive than *psychoimmunology* or *neuroimmunology* (Pierpaoli & Maestroni, 1988). A functional knowledge of neuroimmunomodulation will assist occupational therapists in understanding how and why persons become ill. Therapists may then counsel patients to gradually modify maladaptive life-styles that contribute to either immunosuppression or overactive immune reactions.

Figure 38.1 presents a simplified overview designed to emphasize the overlapping of the endocrine, immune, and central nervous systems. These three systems may share common structures, receptors, regulatory methods, and substances (Blalock, Bost, & Smith, 1985). Bone marrow is the site of the precursor stem cells that give rise to immune cellular components (Pierpaoli, 1985). The two divergent cell lines situated in the bone marrow are the nonlymphoid and lymphoid stem cells (Cohen, 1988; Stein, 1986). The nonlymphoid stem cells differentiate into granulocytes and monocytes; monocytes further differentiate into macrophages, which are immunocompetent cells that secrete

Originally published 1989 in *American Journal of Occupational Therapy, 43,* 637–646.

interleukin-1 (IL-1) (Calabrese, Kling, & Gold, 1987; Farrar, Hill, Harel-Bellan, & Vinocour, 1987). IL-1 is known to facilitate the differentiation of the precursor lymphoid stem cell into B cells and T cells. B cells mature in the bone marrow and then migrate to a variety of lymphoid tissues such as lymph nodes, Peyer patches, spleen, appendix, and tonsils, thus becoming part of humoral immunity (circulating antibody–antigen reactions) (Calabrese et al., 1987). The cells migrate from the bone marrow to the thymus, where, under neuroendocrine influence, they subdivide into helper, killer, and effector cells. T cells are considered part of cell-mediated immunity (cell–antigen reaction). Helper T cells produce interleukin-2 and other mediators that facilitate B-cell maturation. Plasma cells arise from B cells and produce antibodies, also known as

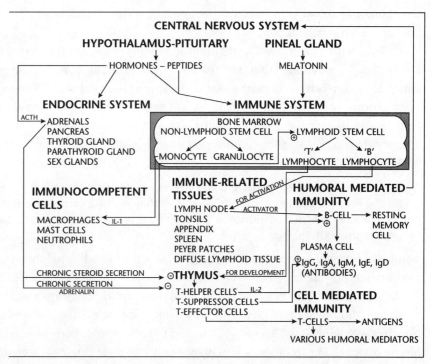

Figure 38.1. An overview of interactions between the immune, endocrine, and central nervous systems.
(ACTH = adrenocorticotropic hormone; IL-1 = inter-leukin-1; IL-2 = interleukin-2).

immunoglobulins. Each of these immunoglobulins has a specific function. Suppressor T cells can block the production and secretion of immunoglobulins (Calabrese et al., 1987). The many interactions of the immune system are quite complex and beyond the scope of this presentation. Simply stated, immune system components of a normal, healthy person are in delicate balance.

Various immune elements, as shown in Figure 1, can cross the blood–brain barrier and interact with the CNS. In turn, several CNS sites send regulatory messengers to interact with multiple body regions. Neuroendocrine products (peptides, hormones, releasing factors) from the hypothalamic–pituitary axis influence the function of the body's endocrine, immune, and nervous system structures. For example, consider the relationship between the pituitary gland and hypothalamus and the adrenal glands. Adrenocorticotropic hormone, when released into the circulatory system, stimulates the adrenal cortex to secrete corticosteroids (Blalock, 1988). Additionally, the posterior hypothalamus (the location of regulatory neurons for the sympathetic division of the autonomic nervous system) may stimulate the adrenal medulla to produce adrenalin. In small amounts, corticosteroids and adrenalin can be used to fight an acute stressful situation. In chronic situations, such as depression or long-term stress, corticosteroids, adrenalin, or both are known to suppress T-cell competency (Schleifer et al., 1984; Stein, 1986). This explains, in part, why our health is compromised when we experience chronic stress. The autonomic nervous system is known to innervate numerous immune-related structures, thus further influencing immune function (Bullock, 1987).

The pineal gland, located in the epithalamus, is said to participate in circadian fluctuations of hormones. Melatonin, one of its secretions, has been found to improve immune competency; chronic stress is said to reduce pineal function (Pierpaoli & Maestroni, 1988).

Opiate hormones (beta-endorphins and enkephalins) are produced in diverse places in the CNS. One known function of these natural opiates is to modulate pain perception (Pinchot, 1984). Moderate exercise releases endorphins and can produce a sense of well-being, whereas extreme exercise, such as overtraining and running in a marathon, may actually compromise the immune system (Mackinnon, 1989; Sforzo, 1988). "All things in moderation" appears to apply to exercise.

Patients with cancer have been taught to visualize their lymphocytes attacking cancerous cells located within their bodies. It was reported that those patients who used visualization to supplement chemotherapy survived longer than those who received chemotherapy alone (Simonton, Matthews-Simonton, & Creighton, 1978). Although these investigations contain important ideas, such as patients assuming responsibility for appropriate aspects of their treatment, serious flaws in the research designs of these imagery studies prevent the validation of imagery as a therapeutic modality (Laszlo, 1988). There is little evidence suggesting that patients can will their immune systems to kill cancer cells. After a complete review of Simonton et al.'s (1978) research, Laszlo said,

> It is easy to make lofty claims, but when lives and costs are at stake it is imperative that investigations be careful and follow the "rules." If anything, studies that are inadequately set up or are misinterpreted to make a point (no matter how well intentioned) ultimately serve only to undermine confidence rather than contribute to supportive strength. (p. 266)

Eventually, imagery may be considered a useful adjunct to traditional therapy for those with disturbances in immune function, but only after well-designed experimentation validates it as a legitimate modality.

Rabin, Ganguli, Cunnick, and Lysle (1988) suggested that in some cases of schizophrenia there may be an underlying autoimmune abnormality. This would suggest that components of the immune system attack the CNS as though it were an enemy. Recently, Stein and Nikolic (1989), both of whom are occupational therapists, reviewed the use of relaxation techniques in schizophrenia. In their single-subject study, the subject demonstrated marked improvement on a standardized state–trait anxiety inventory after relaxation therapy. A logical follow-up for Stein and Nikolic would be to collaborate with an immunologist on a prospective study. The investigators could conduct behavioral testing and collect blood samples to evaluate immune competency before and after relaxation therapy. Such a study would allow the immunologist to determine if there is a relationship between relaxation training and immune function in schizophrenia, while the occupational therapists could determine if immune function correlates with performance on the state–trait anxiety inventories. Such a collaboration has the potential to substantiate whether schizophrenia is at least in part an immune disorder.

Occupational therapists often use biofeedback and other methods of relaxation training in realistic environments rather than in an isolated laboratory. Once a patient masters the basic relaxation methods in a sensory controlled environment, the monitoring of his or her ability to perform functional activity in an occupationally relevant setting seems essential to facilitate a transition from laboratory performance to adaptive functioning in real-life situations.

As we age, we experience a decrease in immune system competency (Kelley et al., 1987; Solomon et al., 1988). It is encouraging to note that geriatric patients who have received relaxation training have improved T-cell competency (Kiecolt-Glaser, Glaser, & Williger, 1985). Many older people have not achieved a balance between health-promoting relaxation and unhealthy inactivity. Older people often become immobile, which may contribute to immune incompetency. Occupational therapists, who, by their training, consider all aspects of an older person's performance, can assist with planning the appropriate amounts and types of activity and environmental modifications to enhance occupationally relevant behavior.

Much work has been done to measure the immune competency of depressed patients. Persons with depression have been shown to have altered immune responses compared with normal control subjects (Schleifer et al., 1984). Conversely, emotional well-being can enhance immune function (Borysenko, 1982). As occupational therapists plan treatment programs, activities for both the mind and the body should be addressed. For example, moderate exercise, because it stimulates endorphins, can result in a sense of well-being.

The use of placebos is controversial; however, responses of numerous patients revealed that expectations affect their autonomic nervous system and body chemistry (Cousins, 1983). We must examine whether occupational therapists with positive, supportive attitudes influence patients in a manner that improves immune competency. We must also examine how therapists present treatment techniques. For example, one therapist declares to the patient, "I am going to try a new treatment technique. I have never done it before; I just learned it in a workshop last weekend and I am not sure I can do it correctly." Another, more confident, therapist says, "I am now going to use a treatment approach that is designed to help strengthen your arm muscles." The second therapist makes no promises but seems more likely to gain the patient's confidence and respect. It is possible that some of our modalities have a placebo effect; regardless, many physicians consider placebos to be a legitimate form of therapy.

Pearsall (1987) said that "superimmunity is the capacity to think and feel in ways that can protect us from disease, heal us when we are sick, and help us attain new levels of wellness . . . far beyond the mere absence of symptoms" (p. xi). We as occupational therapists, because of the nature of our holistic interaction with patients, are in a perfect position to foster the development of enhanced immunity. We can encourage patients to establish positive attitudes (empowerment) and reduce helplessness and hopelessness. This action might improve the patient's immune function.

The prevalence of AIDS should mandate that we be aware of the characteristics of those who are considered long-term AIDS survivors, that is, those who live longer than 3 years after their condition is diagnosed (Solomon, 1987). Fifty percent of persons diagnosed with AIDS live for 1 year or less. These statistics are changing with the widespread use of azidothymidine (AZT) and other new forms of therapy. Solomon, Temoshok, O'Leary, and Zich (1987) investigated the personal attitudes of long-surviving patients compared with those who succumbed rapidly. The long-term AIDS survivors

1. Had realistic attitudes, accepting their disease but believing in life
2. Possessed a fighting spirit
3. Modified their life-styles and left maladaptive situations
4. Were assertive
5. Attended to their personal needs
6. Talked freely about their illness
7. Assumed responsibility for their own health and considered themselves part of the treatment team
8. Helped others who had AIDS.

Solomon et al. (1987) proposed that further investigation of these attitudes and behaviors in AIDS survivors may yield some understanding of the mediators of relationships among cognitive, emotional, autonomic, and immunologic phenomena.

It is appropriate in concluding the section on neuroimmunomodulation to reflect on the philosophy espoused by Norman Cousins (1983) that we must focus on the possibilities of life instead of the limitations. Norman Cousins embodies the spirit of occupational therapy.

Organic Bases of Schizophrenia

During the last 100 years, various neurologists and neuroscientists, including Kraepelin, Alzheimer, Brodmann, Nissl, and Gaupp, theorized that mental illness was the result of brain pathology (Kraepelin, 1919). Unfortunately, these pioneers lacked the critical tools necessary to decipher the neuropathological substrata of mental conditions (Andreasen, 1988; Roberts & Crow, 1987). In the early 1900s, mental health personnel developed a classification system that separated mental disease into two categories: organic mental disease and functional mental disorders (Lishman, 1983). New technology has continuously evolved to examine both organic diseases and neurological conditions, whereas functional mental disorders were studied by Freud and his followers. The Freudians explored the wishes, intents, dreams, desires, and affects of their patients, thus providing valuable behavioral insights but yielding little understanding of the neuropathology involved in mental illness (Lishman, 1983). In the mid-1970s, a landmark study was conducted with the use of computerized tomography (CT) scanning to compare the ventricle size of schizophrenic subjects with that of control subjects (Johnstone, Crow, Frith, Husband, & Kreel, 1976). This experiment validated early pneumoencephalography investigations that suggested that at least one subgroup of schizophrenic persons had enlarged ventricles, fissures, sulci, and decreased amounts of cerebral cortex (Shelton et al., 1988). Conclusions of earlier pneumoencephalography studies were poorly received due to research and methodology flaws (Seidman, 1983). Many CT studies have been published subsequently, verifying the results of Johnstone et al. (1976) and demonstrating that the ventricle–brain ratio is not related to length of illness, race, or sex (Seidman, 1983; Shelton & Weinberger, 1986).

It is now a common assumption that the disturbances of thought and affect seen in schizophrenia are due to changes in brain morphology, metabolism, or neurochemistry (Hornykiewicz, 1986). This conclusion has been based on studies employing magnetic resonance imaging (MRI), positron emission transaxial tomography (PETT), CT scans, and electroencephalography, all of which allow continuous, noninvasive analyses of mental state (Seidman, 1983). Preliminary work with the PETT scan, a relatively new experimental tool, indicated that persons with schizophrenia demonstrated abnormal use and regulation of glucose, particularly in the frontal lobes and basal ganglia, and decreased neuronal activity. PETT scan researchers have postulated that there is a relationship between length of illness and impairment of glucose metabolism. Chronic schizophrenic persons also show decreased cerebral blood flow (Lichtigfeld, Sandyk, & Gillman, 1988).

Schizophrenia is unlikely to be a simple deficit in a given neurotransmitter. Problems in neuroregulation among various neurochemicals and receptors are more plausible in this heterogeneous syndrome. Researchers, using labeled chemicals in MRI studies, have described dopamine and noradrenalin abnormalities in the CNS of some schizophrenic persons. It is unclear whether the neurotransmitter pathology is an outcome of the condition or is secondary to treatment with various pharmacological agents (Hornykiewicz, 1986). Numerous investigators have examined the neurochemical correlates and brain dysfunction or atrophy in mental illness (Andreasen, 1988; Goetz & van Kammen, 1986; Lohr & Jeste, 1988; Stevens & Casanova, 1988). It is clear that we have much to learn about neurotransmitter interactions in both normal and abnormal populations. Deficits in inhibitory neurotransmitters can result in sensory overload or sensory saturation commonly seen in schizophrenia. Carol North, a psychiatrist and recovered schizophrenic, heard voices and saw visual interference patterns from the time she was 6 years of age. Her behavior often became more adaptive when environmental demands and stimulation were controlled. North (1989) presented vivid descriptions of her personal experiences and perceptions as a person with schizophrenia during periods of excessive multisensory stimulation.

Figure 38.2 depicts dichotic listening, a noninvasive tool used to assess one aspect of brain function. Dissimilar auditory stimuli are simultaneously delivered to both ears of a subject. The speech center is located in the left hemisphere in 95% of the population. When auditory stimuli are presented to the right ear, they project to the left hemisphere. Therefore, when a normal person's right ear is stimulated with a verbal stimulus, it would be more likely to register in the left cerebral hemisphere than if a nonverbal stimulus were presented to the same ear. Normal persons seem to be more generally attentive to verbal stimuli compared with nonverbal stimuli. In contrast, a subgroup of schizophrenic persons demonstrated a left ear advantage for verbal stimuli, thus suggesting that their speech center may be located in the right hemisphere.

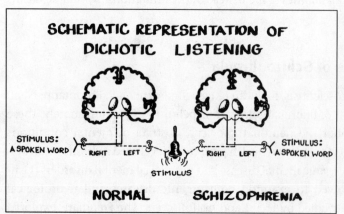

Figure 38.2. Dichotic listening in normal and schizophrenic persons.

Right cortical activation, improved speech comprehension, or both are even more pronounced in schizophrenia when paired stimuli are substituted for a simple verbal stimulus presented to the left ear or to one ear at a time (Green & Kotenko, 1980; Lishman, 1983). Occupational therapists need to be aware of their position in space around a schizophrenic patient and its potential effect on the patient's speech comprehension.

Investigators have identified the following sites of CNS damage in schizophrenia: (a) reticular formation, (b) vestibular system, (c) cerebellar vermis, (d) oculomotor system, (e) basal ganglia, (f) thalamus, (g) frontal cortex, (h) prefrontal cortex, (i) left hemisphere, (j) corpus callosum, (k) insular cortex, and (l) reversal of the normal left-right symmetries (Andreasen, 1988; Crosson & Hughes, 1987; Falkai & Bogerts, 1986; Golden, 1981; Hornykiewicz, 1986; Lishman, 1983; Lohr & Jeste, 1988; Ornitz, 1970; Patterson, 1987; Roberts & Crow, 1987; Stevens & Casanova, 1988). Patterson suggested that some persons with schizophrenia may suffer from an ontogenetic deficit in both the limbic and thalamic nuclei that can interfere with frontal lobe development. Schizophrenic patients are less able to create behavior on the basis of prior experience; hence, their behavior becomes progressively inappropriate.

The concept of positive and negative signs in neurological diseases was first presented by John Hughlings Jackson (Andreasen, 1988). Negative signs relate to a loss in function, whereas positive signs represent a distortion of function (Andreasen, 1988). The negative signs commonly reported in schizophrenia include decreases in affect, attention, ability to experience pleasure, emotional attachments, ability to initiate and persist in tasks, postural mechanisms, postrotatory nystagmus, and oculomotor responses. Schizophrenic persons with a predominance of negative signs tend to demonstrate enlarged ventricles (Andreasen, 1988). The positive signs in schizophrenia include hallucinations, perceptions of nonexistent sensations, sensory flooding or saturation, faulty neurointegration, and increased delta waves on an electroencephalogram (Andreasen, 1988; Lishman, 1983; Morihisha, Duffy, & Wyatt, 1983).

Because neuropathology has been documented in the CNS of numerous psychiatric patients, a neurorehabilitative approach may serve as a useful adjunct to traditional occupational therapy intervention designed to promote adaptive behavioral responses. King (1974), a pioneer in this area, used sensory integrative therapeutic intervention with the schizophrenic population. The following suggestions, summarized from the literature, may prove beneficial in a comprehensive treatment program in mental health:

1. Therapists should design the therapeutic environment with flexibility so that extraneous sensory stimulation can be minimized.
2. The occupational therapy profession must actively recruit more therapists to work in mental health, thus enabling us to reduce the size of the patients' treatment groups.
3. When using sensory input with a sensory saturated patient, the therapist should simplify the stimulus to a single sensory modality (unisensory modalities) instead of applying complex multisensory input (Farber, 1982). Ritvo (1969) found that autistic children showed improvement in the length of postrotatory nystagmus (an adaptive response) when they were tested in a darkened rather than a lighted room. Whereas the normal control subjects tolerated the combination of visual–vestibular input received during rotation in a lighted room, the autistic children produced marked reductions in postrotatory nystagmus under control conditions. Ritvo postulated that multisensory input may be overstimulating for the autistic child.
4. Relaxation training has been shown to improve the T-cell competency of older patients, and it enhanced performance on an anxiety–state–trait test in one single-subject study with a schizophrenic patient. Because one etiological theory of schizophrenia is autoimmune dysfunction, it seems logical that persons with schizophrenia might benefit from a regimen of relaxation activities.

In summary, the principles of neurorehabilitation may well complement the traditional psychiatric occupational therapy program. One might hypothesize that we are most likely to help psychiatric patients improve their functional performance when we address all aspects of their being, both mental and physical.

Traumatic Brain Injury

Plasticity refers to the integrated ability of the brain to remodel its connection in response to development, environmental changes, learning, stimulation, nutrition, and injury. The degree of plasticity that an organism possesses correlates inversely with its age (Cotman & Nieto-Sampedro, 1984; Lenn, 1987; Stein, Finger, & Hart, 1983). There are countless processes, substances, or factors that contribute to CNS plasticity. One example is *neurotrophic substances,* defined as factors, chemicals, hormones, and peptides that induce adaptive changes in the CNS by encouraging cells to respond to neurotransmitters. Nerve growth factor is one type of neurotrophic substance known to be released after an injury to specific cell types in the CNS (Hart, Chaimas, Moore, & Stein, 1978). It has been suggested that neurotrophic substances may be injected into a damaged brain at critical times to enhance recovery (Stein et al., 1983). After lesions, neurotrophic substances seem to be released to help in neural reorganization (Cotman, 1983; Cotman & Nieto-Sampedro, 1984; Skaper, Barbin, Longo, & Varon, 1982). Neurotrophic activity decreases with age, although diet, hormonal activity, and environmental conditions have positive effects on neurotrophic activity (Stein et al., 1983). *Neurotoxic substances* are also present in the brain and are capable of killing brain cells. Some neurotransmitters (e.g., dopamine) modify their molecular structure when exposed to ischemia by forming oxygen radicals, which are volatile molecules toxic to cells. The current medical treatment for ischemia may include the use of a class of drugs called oxygen radical scavengers.

Another plastic process is reactive synaptogenesis. When a target in the CNS suffers input deficits, it can receive substitute input from alternative sources. If one cell dies within a cell pool, the remaining cells can sprout and innervate the target; however, should the entire pathway be eradicated, reactive synaptogenesis cannot restore the connections. Scientists are unsure if reactive synaptogenesis always enhances functional behavior, but it does seem to be important in the brains of elderly persons, in persons with neurodegenerative disease, and in persons with minor traumatic brain injury (TBI) (Cotman & Anderson, 1988). *Synaptic turnover* is a normal housekeeping function in the CNS used to remove discontinued, nonfunctional synapses (Cotman & Nieto-Sampedro, 1984). The rate of synaptic turnover is also influenced by environment and aging (Cotman, 1985).

When a person suffers a TBI, a typical sequence of events occurs within the CNS. After the insult, the CNS goes into shock and synaptic activity is decreased. Cerebral edema results as cells die and dump their intracellular contents into the extracellular spaces. This action elevates intracranial pressure and compresses small blood vessels that deliver oxygenated blood. Edema makes ischemia worse, which in turn exacerbates edema by killing more cells. At this point, physicians often attempt to decrease the patient's CNS metabolic demands and intracranial pressure by administering barbiturates, reducing body temperature, or using osmotic agents (Trauner, 1986). Both neurotoxic and neurotrophic substances are released after injury (Skaper et al., 1982). Ultimately, the connections reorganize and progress can continue for decades (Stein et al., 1983). Persons with TBI may enjoy significant recovery, but they seem less tolerant of environmental perturbations or demands.

Another factor that influences the outcome of TBI is the rate of injury. Persons who have slow-growing lesions, such as tumors, demonstrate more plasticity but have persistent sequelae, whereas those who have acute injury generally show less plasticity, but sequelae do not persist as long (Joynt & Benton, 1964; Stein et al., 1983).

Environmental stimulation after the trauma is of great interest to occupational therapists. Unfortunately, the majority of studies in this area have been conducted with laboratory animals. One cannot generalize animal findings to human beings, but the results are of interest in the elucidation of potential mechanisms that may also occur in human brains. Whether or not an animal benefits from an enriched environment depends on the lesion site, the amount of environmental exposure, and the specific behavior being measured (Kelche, Dalrymple-Alford, & Will, 1987; Will, Rosenzweig, Bennett, Herbert, & Morimoto, 1977). Many environments housing patients with TBI are highly stimulatory with continuous multisensory input. I do not believe that this practice should be considered environmental enrichment or that sensory bombardment yields adaptive behavior in patients with TBI. Continuous contact with sensory input can also produce habituation. Occupational therapists should test the use of prescriptive environments that include sensory experiences, individualized for each patient to promote adaptive responses.

Brain cell transplants are one example of the technological revolution in neuroscience. Adrenal cell transplants have been conducted in patients with Parkinson disease at medical centers in Sweden, Mexico, China, and the United States. The brain has a degree of immunological privilege, so that when substances are placed within it, they grow relatively free of interference from the usual immunologic response. The advantages of brain cell transplants are that they

1. Can serve as endogenous sources of neurotransmitters in diseases where there is a transmitter deficit.
2. Induce an increase in plasticity and reorganization.
3. Cause a release of injury-induced trophic factors.
4. Promote new connections.

It is unclear whether brain cell transplants will facilitate long-term improvement in functional behavior. More work needs to be done with experimental models before behavioral outcomes are fully understood. In addition, although the brain does have some immunological privilege, cross-strain transplants do produce immunogenic activity leading to potential graft rejection. This finding raises the ethical, moral, and spiritual issue of how surgeons are to obtain viable transplant material for human beings. Genetic engineering offers us potential solutions to these problems. Occupational therapists may be routinely treating patients with brain cell transplants within the next two decades.

The major focus of my postdoctoral research was to determine if we could successfully transplant brain cells into a specific region of the brains of postischemic rats using a model of ischemia developed by Pulsinelli and Brierley (1979). Because ischemia produces a hostile cytotoxic environment, the scientific community believed that transplantation would not be successful. We hypothesized that if we delayed transplantation until the cytotoxicity stabilized, the transplanted cells would survive (Farber et al., 1988). Before we could transplant the brain cells, we had to demonstrate our ability to reproduce the model and determine baseline behavior. Figure 38.3 shows the performance of a normal rat and an ischemic rat in an open field maze, a test used to measure hippocampal function. The control and experimental animals were placed in a standardized open field maze box, and the following behaviors were quantified: (a) total number of squares entered; (b) location of squares (central or peripheral); and (c) number of rearing,

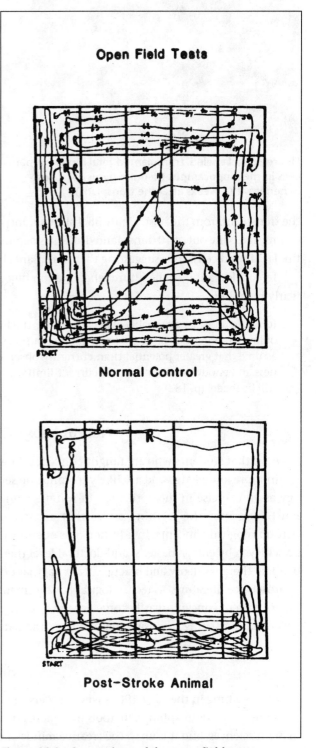

Open Field Tests

Normal Control

Post—Stroke Animal

Figure 38.3. Comparison of the open field maze performances of a control rat and a postischemic, nontransplanted rat.

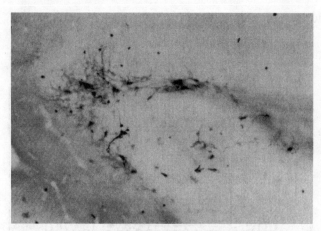

Figure 38.4. Labeled, transplanted fetal hippocampal cells in the hippocampus (dentate gyrus) of a post-ischemic rat (2 weeks after the transplant).

grooming, defecation, and urination episodes. Rats were tested at 1 and 2 weeks postischemia. Marked, statistically significant differences were noted between the postischemic rats and the control rats (Farber et al., 1986). The control animals explored the maze freely (both the center and peripheral squares), urinated and defecated infrequently, and reared and groomed frequently. The postischemic animals stayed in the periphery of the maze; perseverated, urinated, and defecated often (an indication of emotionality); and groomed infrequently. Postischemic rats also demonstrated tactile defensiveness.

At 2 weeks postischemia, the control and postischemic rats received labeled hippocampal cell transplants taken from fetal rats of the same strain. It was necessary to use a label on the transplanted cells to allow us to differentiate the transplant from the host. Figure 38.4 shows transplanted brain cells growing successfully in the brain of a postischemic rat. Nine out of 10 transplanted animals demonstrated successful transplants containing pyramidal and multipolar labeled cells, thus suggesting that transplants into focal regions of ischemically damaged brains are feasible.

In consideration of the future rehabilitation of patients with brain injury, the words of Lenn (1987) are particularly inspiring:

> It is difficult to set reasonable expectations for the brain damaged child without making self-fulfilling prophesies of limited potential. Since we know many examples of this type of error on the part of our predecessors, we can assume that greater potential than currently observed is possible. So our attitude must be critical open-mindedness and enough realism to know current limitations, combined with enough humility to accept that progress will be made. (p. 182)

Neurobiology Curriculum Philosophy

I believe that students who are taught conceptual neurobiology with direct application to occupational therapy retain more knowledge and are likely to continue self-study, compared with students who are taught neurobiology as an exercise in memorization of mindless minutiae. If we are to be effective in stimulating students, we must tune into the learning styles that are frequently used and employ a variety of methods to explain neurobiological concepts. In addition, it is essential that we develop a learning hierarchy of neuroscientific skills to be achieved by entry, master's, and doctoral level therapists so that we can better integrate neuroscience with occupational therapy theory and practice. It is vital that occupational therapists continue to explore the ever-evolving neuroscience literature. As technological advancements allow scientists to uncover new information, the modification of current concepts may become necessary. Occupational therapists should seek neuroscience mentors if help is needed in translating confusing methodology and data into meaningful information.

Summary

There was a time in the early 1900s when leaders in neuroscience had a collective intuitive understanding of brain mechanisms without appropriate tools to explore and elaborate concepts. We are now in a technological revolution in brain sciences, and it is up to the creative minds of occupational therapists to incorporate these new methodologies and discoveries into therapeutic advances. In 1902, Joseph Conrad said, "The mind of man is capable of anything because everything is in it, all of the past as well as all of the future" (p. 843).

Acknowledgments

I would like to express my appreciation to the American Occupational Therapy Association for this award. Thanks are also due to my family, friends, and colleagues, whose nurturance and encouragement have facilitated my personal and professional growth.

References

Andreasen, N. C. (1988). Brain imaging: Applications in psychiatry. *Science, 239,* 1381–1388.

Blalock, J. E., (1988). Immunologically-mediated pituitary adrenal activation. *Advances in Experimental Medical Biology, 245,* 217–223.

Blalock, J. E., Bost, K. L., & Smith, E. M. (1985). Neuroendocrine peptide hormones and their receptors in the immune system. *Journal of Neuroimmunology, 10,* 31–40.

Borysenko, J. Z. (1982). Behavioral-physiological factors in the development and management of cancer. *General Hospital Psychiatry, 4,* 69–72.

Bullock, K. (1987). The innervation of immune system tissues and organs. In C. W. Cotman, R. E. Brinton, A. Galaburda, & B. McEwen (Eds.), *The neuro-immune-endocrine connection* (pp. 33–47). New York: Raven Press.

Calabrese, J. R., Kling, M. A., & Gold, P. W. (1987). Alterations in immunocompetence during stress, bereavement, and depression: Focus on neuroendocrine regulation. *American Journal of Psychiatry, 144,* 1123–1134.

Cohen, J. J. (1988). The immune system: An overview. In E. Middleton, Jr., C. E. Reed, E. F. Ellis, N. F. Adkinson, Jr., & J. W. Yunginger (Eds.), *Allergy principles and practice* (pp. 3–12). St. Louis: C. V. Mosby.

Conrad, J. (1968). Heart of darkness. In J. Bartlett (Ed.), *Familiar quotations* (14th ed.) (p. 843). Boston: Little, Brown. (Original work published 1902)

Cotman, C. W. (1983). Effect of conditioning lesion on survival of transplants into rat hippocampus: Evidence for lesion induced growth factor. *Brain Research, 211,* 321–326.

Cotman, C. W. (1985). *Synaptic plasticity.* New York: Guilford Press.

Cotman, C. W., & Anderson, K. J. (1988). Synaptic plasticity and functional stabilization in the hippocampal formation: Possible role in Alzheimer's disease. In S. G. Waxman (Ed.), *Advances in neurology: Vol. 47. Functional recovery in neurological disease* (pp. 313–335). New York: Raven Press.

Cotman, C. W., & Nieto-Sampedro, M. (1984). Cell biology of synaptic plasticity. *Science, 225,* 1287–1294.

Cousins, N. (1983). *Human options.* New York: Berkley Books.

Crosson, B., & Hughes, C. W. (1987). Role of the thalamus in language: Is it related to schizophrenic thought disorders? *Schizophrenia Bulletin, 13,* 605–621.

Falkai, P., & Bogerts, B. (1986). Cell loss in the hippocampus of schizophrenics. *European Archives of Psychiatry and Neurological Science, 236,* 154–161.

Farber, S. D. (1982). *Neurorehabilitation: A multisensory approach.* Philadelphia: W. B. Saunders.

Farber, S. D., Murphy, S. H., Wells, D. G., Vietje, B. P., Wells, J., & Low, W. C. (1986). Experimental cerebral ischemia, tissue damage, and neuronal transplantation. *Society of Neuroscience Abstracts, 112,* 1287.

Farber, S. D., Onifer, S. M., Kaseda, Y., Murphy, S. H., Wells, D. G., Vietje, B. P., Wells, J., & Low, W. C. (1988). Neural transplantation of horseradish peroxidase-labeled hippocampal cell suspensions in an experimental model of cerebral ischemia. *Progress in Brain Research, 78,* 103–107.

Farrar, W. L., Hill, J. M., Harel-Bellan, A., & Vinocour, M. (1987). The immune logical brain. *Immunological Reviews, 100,* 361–378.

Goetz, K. L., & van Kammen, D. P. (1986). Computerized axial tomography scans and subtypes of schizophrenia. *Journal of Nervous and Mental Disease, 174,* 31–41.

Golden, C. J. (1981). Hemispheric asymmetries in schizophrenia. *Biological Psychiatry, 16,* 561–582.

Green, P., & Kotenko, V. (1980). Superior speech comprehension in schizophrenics under monaural versus binaural listening conditions. *Journal of Abnormal Psychiatry, 89,* 339–408.

Hart, T., Chaimas, N., Moore, R. Y., & Stein, D. G. (1978). Effects of nerve growth factor on behavioral recovery following caudate nucleus lesions in rats. *Brain Research Bulletin, 3,* 245–250.

Henderson, A. (1988). Occupational therapy knowledge: From practice to theory. 1988 Eleanor Clarke Slagle Lecture. *American Journal of Occupational Therapy, 42,* 567–576.

Hornykiewicz, O. (1986). Brain noradrenaline and schizophrenia. *Progress in Brain Research, 65,* 29–39.

Johnstone, E. C., Crow, T. J., Frith, C. D., Husband, J., & Kreel, L. (1976). Cerebral ventricular size and cognitive impairment in chronic schizophrenia. *Lancet, ii,* 924–926.

Joynt, R. J., & Benton, A. L. (1964). The memoir of Marc Dox on aphasia. *Neurology, 14,* 851–854.

Kelche, C., Dalrymple-Alford, J., & Will, B. (1987). Effects of post-operative environment on recovery of function after fimbria-fornix transection in the rat. *Physiology and Behavior, 40,* 731–736.

Kelley, K. W., Brief, S., Westly, H. J., Novakofski, J., Bechtel, P. J., Simon, J., & Walker, E. R. (1987). Hormonal regulation of the age-associated decline in immune function. *Annals of the New York Academy of Science, 496,* 91–97.

Kiecolt-Glaser, J. K., Glaser, R., & Williger, D. (1985). Psychosocial enhancement of immunocompetence in a geriatric population. *Health Psychology, 4,* 25–29.

King, L. J. (1974). A sensory-integrative approach to schizophrenia. *American Journal of Occupational Therapy, 28,* 529–536.

Kraepelin, E. (Ed.). (1919). *Dementia praecox and paraphrenia.* Edinburgh: Livingstone.

Laszlo, J. (Ed.). (1988). *Understanding cancer.* New York: Harper & Row.

Lenn, N. J. (1987). Neuroplasticity and the developing brain: Implications for therapy. *Pediatric Neuroscience, 13,* 176–183.

Lichtigfeld, F., Sandyk, R., & Gillman, M. (1988). New vistas in chronic schizophrenia. *International Journal of Neuroscience, 38,* 355–367.

Lishman, W. A. (1983). The apparatus of mind: Brain structure and function in mental disorders. *Psychosomatics, 24,* 699–703, 709–711, 714–720.

Lohr, J. B., & Jeste, D. V. (1988). Locus ceruleus morphometry in aging and in schizophrenia. *Acta Psychiatry Scandinavica, 77,* 689–697.

Mackinnon, L. T. (1989). Exercise and natural killer cells. What is the relationship? *Sports Medicine, 7,* 141–149.

Morihisha, J. M., Duffy, F. H., & Wyatt, R. J. (1983). Brain electrical activity mapping (BEAM) in schizophrenic patients. *Archives of General Psychiatry, 40,* 719–728.

North, C. S. (1989). *Welcome silence.* New York: Avon Books.

Ornitz, E. (1970). Vestibular dysfunction in schizophrenia and childhood autism. *Comprehensive Psychiatry, 11,* 159–173.

Patterson, T. (1987). Studies toward the subcortical pathogenesis of schizophrenia. *Schizophrenia Bulletin, 13,* 555–576.

Pearsall, P. (1987). *Superimmunity.* New York: Fawcett Gold Medal.

Pierpaoli, W. (1985). Immunoregulatory and morphostatic function of bone marrow-derived factors. In R. Guillemin, M. Cohn, & T. Melnechuk (Eds.), *Neural modulation of immunity* (pp. 205–237). New York: Raven Press.

Pierpaoli, W., & Maestroni, G.J.M. (1988). Neuroimmunomodulation: Some recent views and findings. *International Journal of Neuroscience, 39,* 165–175.

Pinchot, R. B. (Ed.). (1984). *The brain: Mystery of matter and mind.* New York: Torstar Books.

Pulsinelli, W. A., & Brierley, J. B. (1979). A new model of bilateral ischemia in the unanesthetized rat. *Stroke, 10,* 267–272.

Rabin, B. S., Ganguli, R., Cunnick, J., & Lysle, D. T. (1988). The central nervous system–immune system relationship. *Clinics in Laboratory Medicine, 8,* 253–268.

Ritvo, E. R. (1969). Decreased postrotatory nystagmus in early infantile autism. *Neurology, 19,* 653–658.

Roberts, G. W., & Crow, T. J. (1987). The neuropathology of schizophrenia—A progress report. *British Medical Bulletin, 43,* 599–615.

Schleifer, S. J., Keller, S. E., Meyerson, A. T., Raskin, M. J., David, K. L., & Stein, M. (1984). Lymphocyte function in major depressive disorder. *Archives of General Psychiatry, 41,* 484–486.

Seidman, L. J. (1983). Schizophrenia and brain dysfunction: An integration of recent neurodiagnostic findings. *Psychological Bulletin, 94,* 195–238.

Sforzo, G. A. (1988). Opioids and exercise: An update. *Sports Medicine, 7,* 109–124.

Shelton, R. C., Karson, C. N., Doran, A. R., Pickar, D., Bigelow, L. B., & Weinberger, D. R. (1988). Cerebral structural pathology in schizophrenia: Evidence for a selective prefrontal cortical deficit. *American Journal of Psychiatry, 145,* 154–163.

Shelton, R. C., & Weinberger, D. R. (1986). X-ray computerized tomography in schizophrenia: A review and synthesis. In H. A. Nasrallah & D. R. Weinberger (Eds.), *Handbook of schizophrenia, vol. 1: The neurology of schizophrenia* (pp. 207–250). Amsterdam: Elsevier.

Simonton, C. C., Matthews-Simonton, S., & Creighton, J. L. (Eds.). (1978). *Getting well again.* New York: Bantam Books.

Skaper, S., Barbin, G., Longo, F. M., & Varon, S. (1982). Brain injury causes a time-dependent increase in neuronotrophic activity at the lesion site. *Science, 217,* 860–861.

Solomon, G. F. (1987). Psychoneuroimmunologic approaches to AIDS. *Annals of the New York Academy of Science, 496,* 628–636.

Solomon, G. F., Fiatarone, M. A., Benton, D., Morley, J. E., Bloom, E., & Makinodan, T. (1988). Psychoimmunologic and endorphin function in the aged. *Annals of the New York Academy of Science, 521,* 43–57.

Solomon, G. F., Temoshok, L., O'Leary, A., & Zich, J. (1987). An intensive psychoimmunologic study of long-surviving persons with AIDS. *Annals of the New York Academy of Science, 496,* 647–655.

Stein, D. G., Finger, S., & Hart, T. (1983). Brain damage and recovery: Problems and perspectives. *Behavioral and Neural Biology, 37,* 185–222.

Stein, F., & Nikolic, S. (1989). Teaching stress management techniques to a schizophrenic patient. *American Journal of Occupational Therapy, 43,* 162–169.

Stein, M. (1986). A reconsideration of specificity in psychosomatic medicine: From olfaction to the lymphocyte. *Psychosomatic Medicine, 48,* 3–22.

Stevens, J. R., & Casanova, M. F. (1988). Is there a neuropathology of schizophrenia? *Biological Psychiatry, 24,* 123–128.

Trauner, D. A. (1986). Barbiturate therapy in acute brain injury. *Journal of Pediatrics, 109,* 742–746.

Will, B. E., Rosenzweig, M. R., Bennett, E. L., Herbert, M., & Morimoto, H. (1977). Relatively brief environment enrichment aids recovery of learning capacity and alters brain measures after post-weaning brain lesions in rats. *Journal of Comparative and Physiological Psychology, 91,* 33–50.

39

The 1980s: Discussion Questions and Learning Activities

The Lectures

Baum, C. M. (1980). Occupational therapists put care in the health system (1980 Eleanor Clarke Slagle Lecture). *American Journal of Occupational Therapy, 34*, 505–516.

Bing, R. K. (1981). Occupational therapy revisited: A paraphrastic journey (1981 Eleanor Clarke Slagle Lecture). *American Journal of Occupational Therapy, 35*, 499–518.

Rogers, J. C. (1983). Clinical reasoning: The ethics, science, and art (1983 Eleanor Clarke Slagle Lecture). *American Journal of Occupational Therapy, 37*, 601–616.

Gilfoyle, E. M. (1984). Transformation of a profession (1984 Eleanor Clarke Slagle Lecture). *American Journal of Occupational Therapy, 38*, 575–584.

Mosey, A. C. (1985). A monistic or a pluralistic approach to professional identity? (1985 Eleanor Clarke Slagle Lecture). *American Journal of Occupational Therapy, 39*, 504–509.

Reed, K. L. (1986). Tools of practice: Heritage or baggage? (1986 Eleanor Clarke Slagle Lecture). *American Journal of Occupational Therapy, 40*, 597–605.

Allen, C. K. (1987). Activity: Occupational therapy's treatment method (1987 Eleanor Clarke Slagle Lecture). *American Journal of Occupational Therapy, 41*, 563–575.

Henderson, A. (1988). Occupational therapy knowledge: From practice to theory (1988 Eleanor Clarke Slagle Lecture). *American Journal of Occupational Therapy, 42*, 567–576.

Farber, S. D. (1989). Neuroscience and occupational therapy: Vital connections (1989 Eleanor Clarke Slagle Lecture). *American Journal of Occupational Therapy, 43*, 637–646.

Learning Activities

1. Investigate the occupational profile of most Americans in the 1980s. Some useful bibliographical references to explore appear in Appendix B.
   - What was the average family size?
   - What was the average salary? What were some typical jobs?
   - What did homes cost?
   - What were the clothing styles of the decade?
   - What was significant about the popular culture of the decade (e.g., in music, film, books)?
2. If you have access to a complete collection of the *American Journal of Occupational Therapy,* scan the table of contents for each issue. What were some common topics? Can you identify any patterns in these topics? How do these relate to the messages of each Eleanor Clarke Slagle Lecture?
3. Try to summarize each Eleanor Clarke Slagle Lecture in a sentence that captures the main theme. Complete the sentence "This lecture was about. . . ."

4. Consider each lecture. Are there common threads among them that you identify? Are there any common themes that emerge when you consider these lectures together?

5. Review the biography of each lecturer of this decade (see Appendix A). Read some of the other work by the lecturer to gain an insight to the reasons why each one received this honor.

6. Consider what was happening in the history of the occupational therapy profession at the time of each Eleanor Clarke Slagle Lecture. Appendix C provides some useful bibliographical references for the history of the profession in the United States, and Appendix D has references for the global history of the profession.

7. Review what each president of the American Occupational Therapy Association presented as his or her vision for the profession at the time of each Eleanor Clarke Slagle Lecture. (A list of these presidents appears in Appendix E.) How do the lectures relate to these visions? The presidents addressed the profession through several forums, including columns in the *American Journal of Occupational Therapy*, such as "President's Address," "Nationally Speaking," and "The Issue Is."

8. Review each lecture in light of the *Centennial Vision*. What themes of the *Vision* stand out the most? What additional insights into the *Vision* do the lecturers offer?

Discussion Questions

1. At the beginning of her lecture, Carolyn Baum stated that "Our responsibility as a profession is to implement a broader perspective of health care delivery—one that places its values on individuals as they accept responsibility for their own health status." Explain three ways in which Baum supported occupational therapy doing this, making sure to include statements from the lecture. After explaining Baum's position on each of these, illustrate them with an example of your own, extending Baum's statement to your personal experience.

2. Baum stated, "The practitioner is ignoring his or her responsibilities and compromising the field of occupational therapy by collaborating with other professionals and not demonstrating occupational therapy as an independent health profession." Explain how Baum documented this statement. In what way do you think occupational therapy education can help develop independent health professionals?

3. According to Robert Bing, moral treatment had its rise and decline, and occupational therapy emerged to take its place. Do you see a decline that has occurred, is occurring, or might occur within occupational therapy over the course of its development (i.e., when was occupational therapy's heyday/decline)? What do you imagine would rise from occupational therapy if it were to decline?

4. As Bing explained, the originators of occupational therapy were not occupational therapists per se. How could the influence of other disciplines further a kind of "moral treatment" practiced in occupational therapy today?

5. Joan Rogers stressed the importance of the patient's involvement in his or her therapy and goal setting. She stated that "the goal of clinical reasoning is a treatment recommendation issued in the interests of a particular patient." If you were working in a setting where a coworker did not allow this autonomy in a client, how would you approach this therapist? Cite specific passages from Rogers's lecture to support your reasoning.

6. Rogers argued that, when therapists are asked why they decide to use a particular treatment method, they commonly reply, "I have never really thought about it" or "I don't know how I reached that conclusion, I just know." What can occupational therapists do to encourage others to be able to better respond to this question? How do you think the "typical" answer affects how other professions or the public view occupational therapy as a profession?

7. Elnora Gilfoyle stated, "We, in occupational therapy, suffer from a pervasive uncertainty about our values." In what way did Gilfoyle feel that occupational therapy's system of values has changed over the history of the profession? What is occupational therapy's value system today? Finally, why is it important or necessary to not have uncertainty about our values?

8. How did Gilfoyle explain the influence that cultural, economic, and political changes in the greater society have on the value system of occupational therapy? What present forces in society affect how occupational therapists view themselves, their clients, and their profession?

9. Explain how Anne Mosey characterized the difference between monism and pluralism. Give examples of these characteristics, and explain your own views or tendencies between these two positions.

10. At the very beginning of her lecture, Kathlyn Reed asked the question, "Is occupational therapy losing its heritage or keeping up with the times?" How do you respond to this question? When considering the media, in what ways is occupational therapy keeping up with the times? How is occupational therapy not keeping up with the times? Why is keeping up necessary? What evidence can you use to support your response?

11. Considering Reed's lecture, why (or why not) should the media, method, and objectives of occupational therapy be consistent with each other?

12. How did Claudia Allen relate "purpose" to the disease process? How can a therapist infer the purpose of the client?

13. What was Allen's definition of "action," and how did she support the notion that "activity is the explanatory principle" of occupational therapy?

14. Explain the differences Anne Henderson saw between "ordinary" and "specialized" knowledge. Give examples of each of these in your practice, and explain how each has contributed to the image others have of the profession.

15. Explain which methods philosophy and science use to develop theory, and which methods technology uses for the same purpose. Where does the theory come from, science or technology, that you most commonly use in practice? How does it help to know the difference?

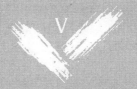

THE 1990s

Occupation Revisited

40

Historical Context of the 1990s

Around the World

A new world order emerged in the 1990s. The economic changes the Soviet Union had initiated in the 1980s signaled the fall of the Iron Curtain, and breakup and democratization movements swept the countries under its influence. After Hungary removed its border restrictions with Austria in 1989, thousands of East Germans escaped to the West, and mass demonstrations against the East Germany regime began. Official destruction of the Berlin Wall began in November 1989 and was completed less than a year later. In 1990, the economically beleaguered East Germans voted for reunification with West Germany. West Germany voted in a temporary tax to be paid by West German citizens and created investment stimulus packages for private industry in East Germany to make reunification work. However, the West German government quickly discovered that the state of the East German infrastructure was much worse than anticipated, and the economic drain placed on West Germany was almost more than it could bear. By 1994, the temporary tax had been extended twice. Also, because the conditions in the former East Germany had improved very little, there was a mass migration into the former West Germany, causing market shortages, higher unemployment, and housing crunches. This all added up to growing disillusionment with the reunification effort and resentment among both West and East Germans.

Following the Iran–Iraq War that lasted most of the 1980s, Iraq was extremely indebted to several Arab countries, including a $14 billion debt to Kuwait. Iraq hoped to repay its debts by raising the price of oil through Organization of the Petroleum Exporting Countries oil production cuts. Instead, Kuwait increased production, lowering prices, in an attempt to leverage a better resolution of their border dispute. In addition, Iraq charged that Kuwait had taken advantage of the Iran–Iraq War to drill for oil and build military outposts on Iraqi soil near Kuwait. Iraq also charged that it had performed a collective service for all Arabs by acting as a buffer against Iran and that therefore Kuwait and Saudi Arabia should negotiate or cancel Iraq's war debts. After Kuwait refused to negotiate, Iraqi forces invaded in 1990. The United Nations Security Council immediately voted to impose economic sanctions on Iraq. However, when Iraqi forces were amassed on the border with Saudi Arabia, United States President George H. W. Bush sent forces to the region. Because of popular opposition, the United States did not immediately launch an offensive action. Instead, together with several Arab states that had voted to oppose Iraq with military force, coalition forces began bombing Iraq in January 1991. After nearly 100,000 Iraqis were killed, about 100,000 Iraqi troops surrendered, and the remaining Iraqi forces retreated.

U.S. participation in these actions brought renewed animosity from radical factions in the area, and terrorist attacks on U.S. personnel escalated. A car bomb exploded in an underground parking garage at the World Trade Center in New York City in 1993, killing 6 and injuring more than 1,000. In 1996, a truck bomb exploded outside

U.S. military barracks, killing 19 American soldiers. The following year two U.S. embassies in Africa were bombed. The culprits of these bombings were to gain greater attention on September 11, 2001, with the destruction of the World Trade Center and the attack on the Pentagon.

The reforms Soviet President Mikhail Gorbachev had initiated in the mid-1980s had unleashed a democratic movement in almost all of the constituent republics of the Soviet Union. Gorbachev's two-tiered economic plan of reform and openness threw the Soviet Union into chaos as the different nationalities used their new freedoms to break away. The power of the central government was considerably weakened by these movements and in August 1991, a group of hard-line Communists organized a coup d'etat. They kidnapped Gorbachev and announced he would no longer be able to govern. The country went into an uproar. Massive protests were staged in most of the major cities of the Soviet Union. When the coup organizers tried to bring in the military to quell the protestors, the soldiers themselves rebelled, saying that they could not fire on their fellow countrymen. After three days of massive protest, the coup organizers surrendered. Gorbachev returned to the presidency but resigned effective the end of the year. By January 1992, by popular demand, the Soviet Union ceased to exist. In its place, a new entity was formed called the Commonwealth of Independent States, composed of most of the independent countries of the former Soviet Union. Each of these countries now has complete political independence, although they maintain economic ties for development. The collapse of the Soviet Union brought with it the closing of the Cold War.

The collapse of the Soviet Union brought chaos to many countries that had existed under its close influence. Most notably, Yugoslavia, itself a federation of smaller republics, fell apart in June 1991. Serbian president Slobodan Milosevic prevented Croatian leader Stipe Mesic from assuming the presidency, and Croatia and Slovenia seceded. The Yugoslav army moved into both republics. In July they left Slovenia but began ethnic cleansing in Croatia until January 1992, when a U.N.-supervised ceasefire took place. By this time, 25,000 people were dead. Macedonia declared independence in September 1991, although Greece requested that the country find a different name because Greece also had an area named Macedonia. Bosnia and Herzegovina seceded from Yugoslavia in April 1992.

The 1990s were also a decade of great change in South Africa. After more than 20 years of repressive rule, the White government was facing increasing internal and international pressures for change. Black South Africans had organized into a African National Congress (ANC) and began bringing weapons and guerillas into the country. Campaigns were launched in the United States and Great Britain against companies that did business in South Africa, causing many companies to disinvest and leave. Other foreign companies remained but agreed to abide by a code of conduct in their South African operations (e.g., move to equal pay for non-White people doing the same work as White people; employment and promotions based on ability, not on race). Facing increasing riots, in February 1990 the government released resistance leader Nelson Mandela, who had been held for 27 years in prison on charges of treason, in hopes he could help negotiate a political settlement between the Black and White populations. In March of the following year, South Africa's White population voted to give President F. W. de Klerk a mandate to end White-minority rule.

Finally, after the Berlin Wall fell and the Soviet Union collapsed, any substantive fears that some countries had about the possibility of a majority-led South Africa allying itself with the Soviet Union were gone. In 1994, Black people were admitted to the South African ballot booths, the ANC overwhelmingly won the majority of seats in the parliament, and Nelson Mandela was elected president.

Elsewhere on the African continent, President Juvenal Habyarimana of Rwanda, who had remained in power for more than 20 years, was facing rebel actions from the Rwandan Patriotic Front (RPF). In a move to discredit the rebels, in 1990 Habyarimana began ordering massacres of members of one ethnic group, the Tutsis, while blaming the massacres on another group, the Hutus, who acted against the government. This caused growing mistrust and resentment among members of these ethnic groups. By late March 1994, Hutu leaders were determined to slaughter massive numbers of Tutsis and Hutus who opposed Habyarimana. On April 6, the plane carrying Habyarimana was shot down, and a small group of his close associates executed the planned assassination. The Presidential Guard and other troops commanded by Colonel Théoneste Bagosora, backed by militia, murdered Hutu government officials and leaders of the political opposition, creating a vacuum in which Bagosora and his supporters could take control. Soldiers and militia also began systematically slaughtering Tutsis. Within hours, military officers and administrators far from the capital dispatched soldiers and militia to kill Tutsi and Hutu political leaders in their local areas. After months of warnings, rumors, and prior attacks, the violence struck panic among Rwandans and foreigners alike.

The rapidity of the first killings gave the impression of large numbers of assailants, but their impact resulted more from ruthlessness and organization than from great numbers. A U.N. expert evaluating population loss in Rwanda estimated that 800,000 Rwandans had died between April and July 1994. The RPF eventually was able to overcome the government and set up a new one. One of its most praised actions was the establishment of a unity and reconciliation commission as an avenue for people to express their feelings and to reflect on the past with a view to finding ways to build a united society.

In the United States

The issue of assisted suicide occupied American headlines for most of the 1990s, due in part to the actions of Dr. Jack Kevorkian. A retired pathologist, Kevorkian assisted a 54-year-old woman who had Alzheimer's disease to end her life in June 1990 and later helped at least 50 other people die. He repeatedly faced and was acquitted of criminal charges for his role in the deaths, all of which took place in Michigan. However, in late 1998, he crossed from passive to active euthanasia when he gave a man a lethal injection, rather than simply providing the man the means to kill himself, and videotaped the act for broadcast on national television, daring prosecutors to charge him with murder. They took him up on that dare, and in early 1999, Kevorkian was found guilty of second-degree murder and sentenced to 10 to 25 years in prison.

Attempts to legalize assisted suicide through voter initiative were defeated in Washington State in 1991 and in California in 1992. More than 20 state legislatures considered and defeated similar laws during the 1990s. In November 1994, Oregon became the first state to make assisted suicide legal. Its law, passed by a slim margin in a voter referendum, allows doctors to prescribe a lethal dose of drugs to terminally ill patients who meet certain qualifications. The law was blocked until 1997, when voters overwhelmingly ratified it and it went into effect. Most groups of medical professionals, including the American Medical Association, officially oppose assisted suicide.

Several events throughout the decade pointed to a growing sense of unrest in the United States. In 1991, a videotape of four White Los Angeles police officers beating and kicking Rodney King, a Black man, after a routine traffic stop made national headlines. In 1992, when the police officers were handed a verdict of not guilty, racial riots broke out in south central Los Angeles, leading to several days of looting and other violence. The riots left 55 people dead, more than 2,000 injured, and 1,100 buildings destroyed. The reality of unresolved racial tension in the country could not be denied.

In 1993, personnel from the Bureau of Alcohol, Tobacco, and Firearms (ATF) raided the Branch Davidian compound in Waco, Texas, after receiving reports that the cult group was illegally amassing weapons. The ATF's search warrant was executed in a "no-knock, dynamic entry" style attack on the community center, called Mount Carmel, a home shared by 130 men, women, and children. In the gunfight that resulted, six Davidians and four ATF agents were killed. When the ATF agents ran out of ammunition, they retreated from direct attack but kept the Davidians surrounded by armed forces. The siege was taken over by the FBI the next day and continued for 51 days. On April 19, claiming frustration over the Davidians' refusal to leave the building, the FBI used tanks to insert gas into Mount Carmel; a fire broke out, and 76 of the 85 people remaining in the center died. The tragedy fueled the growth of many clandestine militia groups throughout the United States that vowed to keep the federal government at check.

In 1995, Timothy McVeigh and Terry Nichols, two sympathizers with the clandestine militia ideology, carried out a terrorist attack that shook the nation. McVeigh had traveled to Waco, Texas, during the 1993 standoff between the Branch Davidians and federal agents and was said to have been angry about what he saw. On April 19, 1995, with the help of Nichols, McVeigh detonated a truck full of explosives outside the Alfred P. Murrah Federal Building in Oklahoma City, killing 168 people, including 8 federal marshals and 19 children. McVeigh and Nichols were charged and convicted for the bombing. McVeigh was executed by lethal injection in 2001.

The nation once again was shaken on April 20, 1999, when students Eric Harris and Dylan Klebold went on a shooting rampage at Columbine High School in Littleton, Colorado. They killed 12 students, 1 teacher, and themselves. Investigators later revealed that parents and authorities had overlooked many warning signals before the deadly shootout. This incident focused attention on the sense of isolation and alienation of students and brought to light the limited services that exist for this age group.

Political scandal seemed to be a mark of the decade. In 1990, Washington, DC, Mayor Marion Barry, Jr., was arrested by the FBI in a drug sting and later convicted of misdemeanor drug possession. In 1991, Supreme Court nominee Clarence Thomas was accused by Anita Hill of sexual harassment when she worked for him 10 years earlier. In 1994, questions of financial misdealing on the part of President Bill Clinton and his wife began to be investigated, leading to the Whitewater scandal.

By far, however, the greatest scandal was Clinton's admission in 1998 of an affair with White House intern Monica Lewinsky after denying it several times under oath. The House of Representatives convicted Clinton of perjury and obstruction of justice and moved for impeachment. The Senate later acquitted, but also censured, the president. In spite of this scandal, the president's approval rating with the public soared to an all-time high of nearly 76%.

As mentioned earlier, terrorism came to American soil for the first time in the 1990s. In February 1993, a car bomb explosion at the World Trade Center in New York City killed 6 people and injured more than 1,000 people. Investigations revealed a plot involving a self-exiled Egyptian fundamentalist Islamic, Sheik Omar Abdel-Rahman. In 1995, Abdel-Rahman and nine followers were found guilty. Abdel-Rahman's supporters threatened retaliation if he was extradited to Egypt on prior charges. Little did the American public imagine this event was a prelude to a much more dire terrorist attack in 2001.

The 1990s brought some landmark legislation with the potential of substantially changing the opportunities for social participation of people with disabilities. In 1990, the Education for All Handicapped Children Act was amended (P.L. 101–476) and renamed the Individuals With Disabilities Education Act, providing guarantees of inclusion for children in the public education system. That same year, President Bush signed the Americans With Disabilities Act (ADA) on the White House lawn, witnessed by thousands of disability rights activists. The law was the most sweeping disability rights legislation in history, for the first time bringing full legal citizenship to Americans with disabilities. Considered by many the civil rights act for people with disabilities, the ADA mandates that local, state, and federal governments and programs be accessible, that businesses with more than 15 employees make "reasonable accommodations" for workers with disabilities, and that public places such as restaurants and stores make "reasonable modifications" to ensure access for disabled members of the public. The act also mandates access in public transportation, communication, and other areas of public life.

With passage of the ADA, American Disabled for Accessible Public Transit (ADAPT) changed its name to American Disabled for Attendant Programs Today and shifted its focus to advocating for personal assistance services so people with disabilities can live in the community with real supports instead of nursing homes and other institutions. By 1990, about 2 million Americans were residing in nursing homes and other institutions because federal or state subsidies were available only to people living in such institutions. Noting that every state that received Medicaid must provide nursing home services and that community-based services were optional, ADAPT began drafting a bill in an attempt to fundamentally change the long-term-care system. This bill, the Medicaid Community Attendant Services and Supports Act (MiCASSA), was first introduced to Congress in 1997. MiCASSA proposed shifts in the proportion of Medicaid long-term-care dollars spent in community and institutional services. In addition, the bill proposed the development of a national program of community-based attendant services and supports for people with disabilities. There was legal precedence for the development of this bill. In 1995, the U.S. Court of Appeals for the Third Circuit ruled in *Helen L. v. Snider* that the continued publicly funded institutionalization of a disabled Pennsylvania woman in a nursing home, when not medically necessary and where the state could offer her the option of home care, was a violation of her rights under the ADA. MiCASSA was not passed in 1997 and has been reintroduced nearly every year since then.

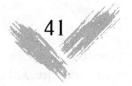

41

1990 Eleanor Clarke Slagle Lecture

Resilience and Human Adaptability:
Who Rises Above Adversity?

Susan B. Fine, MA, OTR, FAOTA

This Eleanor Clarke Slagle Lecture is a study of outcome—outcome that often defies the odds. It is a study of lives characterized by extraordinary hardships and remarkable abilities to move beyond them. It poses a core question: Who rises above adversity? It ventures beyond traditional concerns for pathology and vulnerability, beyond theoretical and statistical methods. In fact, its most valuable data come directly from the personal experiences of those confronted with chronic or terminal illness, physical and mental disabilities, abuse, impoverishment, the Holocaust, and other disasters. I have pursued many life narratives, not as a test of endurance in the face of human suffering (although it made for a more tearful year than most), not in search of heroes and heroines (although there were many), but in an effort to more fully understand factors that influence resilient responses. The voices of the resilient send a powerful message: Personal perceptions and responses to stressful life events are crucial elements of survival, recovery, and rehabilitation, often transcending the reality of the situation or the interventions of others. The inner life (affective and cognitive processes and content) holds the potential for transforming traumas into varying degrees of triumph. Ironically, these same phenomena are often ignored in the clinical reasoning and practice of many health professions, including our own.

Consequently, this paper is intended to heighten the reader's appreciation of the powerful interaction among a person's inner psychological life, his or her relationship to the surrounding world, and his or her emerging functional capacities. It pursues these themes by first providing an overview of theoretical constructs about the human response to adversity. Second, it focuses on extreme life events and the personal and social meaning ascribed to them. Third, it addresses the phenomenon of resilience and the means by which persons in extreme situations have coped. Implications for occupational therapy practice are then considered.

Overcoming Adversity: A Human Condition

The experience of adversity and the drive to rise above it are themes that characterize the human condition. The inevitability of life's trials and tribulations and the struggles between good and evil are evident in religious traditions, myths, the arts, and everyday conversation. Although adversity is ultimately a personal experience, in the bigger scheme of things it is faceless and timeless. We have grown up with both the ascendance of Cinderella and the failure of Icarus. We share such maxims as "It's always something" (Radner, 1989) or "You have to take the bad with the good." These universal themes attempt to guide us in matters of social order and disorder.

Originally published 1991 in *American Journal of Occupational Therapy, 45,* 493–503.

The Law of Disruption and Reintegration

There is also a professional literature devoted to understanding the human response to disruptions, the search for order and balance, and the consequences of prolonged imbalance. Although taxonomies and belief systems vary, a central theme, linked to Cannon's (1939) work in biology and physics, identifies a recurring cycle of disruption and reintegration as a natural and necessary part of one's growing capacities to adapt to internal and external change (Flach, 1988). In today's lexicon we speak of risk, stress, coping, competency, crisis theory, and biopsychosocial models. The past has been marked by a more disparate array of assumptions.

The relationship of stress to disease has been the highest priority among clinicians since Hippocratic times. Attempts at developing broader, systematic constructs have emerged from a number of disciplines. Psychoanalysis has given us ego mechanisms of defense as a metaphor for mental processes that handle crisis and threats. Freudian views emphasize a hierarchy of defenses that transform conflict-ridden impulses into more acceptable thoughts and actions. Ego psychology promotes reality-oriented, purposeful, conflict-free capacities (i.e., attention, perception, and memory) that are future-oriented and that render one capable of transforming situations rather than being transformed by them. In this formulation, adaptive functioning is seen as the relative use of coping capacities over defense mechanisms (Anthony & Cohler, 1987). The growth and cumulative effects of coping resources and skills over the life span are reflected in Erikson's (1963) classic developmental theories.

A behaviorist tradition also emerged with an early emphasis on the consequences of concrete problem solving. Today, as cognitive behaviorism, it is concerned with the cognitive components of coping skills and the Eriksonian belief that "successful coping promotes a sense of self-efficacy, which in turn, inspires more efforts at mastering difficult situations" (Moos & Schaefer, 1984, p. 6).

Endocrinologist Hans Selye (1978) assumed importance in the disruption–reintegration debate. Half a decade of work on stress and its hormonal and neurochemical correlates has had a great impact on professional and popular views of prevention and disease management. Selye's original emphasis on the singular importance of the stressful event itself has been mediated by a growing belief that the physical or psychological impact of any demand will vary depending on how we interpret the situation and how able we are to do something about it (Lazarus & Folkman, 1984).

Moos and Billings (1982) elaborated by organizing coping skills into three areas: appraisal-focused coping (i.e., efforts to understand and find meaning in a crisis), problem-focused coping (i.e., attempts to deal with the reality and consequences of the crisis and create a better situation), and emotion-focused coping (i.e., handling the feelings provoked by the crisis).

The cognitive appraisal process (how we interpret personal experiences) is central to a great deal of contemporary thought on coping. Stress itself has been defined as a "relationship between person and environment that is appraised by the person as taxing or exceeding his or her resources and endangering his or her well being" (Lazarus & Folkman, 1984, p. 19). Although social psychology traditionally emphasizes the role of external stressors and cognitive strategies (i.e., logical analysis, mental preparation, cognitive redefinition, and avoidance or denial), internal phenomena must not be ignored. Personal theories of reality about oneself and one's world, developed over time and generally outside of awareness, serve as a filter through which we perceive, interpret, and respond to experiences (Janoff-Bulman & Timko, 1987). Disturbing thoughts and memories can also heavily influence the appraisal process (Houston, 1987).

The credibility of the cognitive appraisal paradigm is enhanced by the newly integrated discipline of psychoneuroimmunology, which is "the study of the intricate interaction of consciousness (psycho), brain and central nervous system (neuro) and the body's defense against external infection and aberrant cell division (immunology)" (Pelletier & Herzing, 1988, p. 29). The impact of personal mood and attitudes on the immune system has opened new doors for researchers and clinicians. Studies have found that one's immune system benefits from confronting traumatic memories, looking at life optimistically, and living at a mildly hectic pace (Goleman, 1989). This line of thought will no doubt continue to provide us with newer and different hypotheses about the laws of disruption and reintegration.

For now, contemporary biopsychosocial formulations represent a robust model. Capacities to meet challenging demands and stand up to disruptions depend on inborn and acquired skills, the material and interpersonal resources in the environment, and the psychosocial capacities to handle anxieties that arise when one is performing various life tasks. Successful adaptation is dependent on the degree of fit among these factors. Although mastery is both developed and sustained by manageable challenges, challenges that are too demanding or too dangerous defeat resources for coping and reintegration (White, 1976).

And dangers there are! The law of disruption and reintegration does not promise, or always deliver, a rose garden. Life events continually test the durability of the balance we try to maintain.

Ordeals Beyond Our Control

There are life events that are experienced as traumatic because they are severe ordeals beyond our control. Under circumstances of predictable, moderate stress, persons call on conventional patterns and solve problems with characteristic resources and adaptive styles. But extreme situations and the stress accompanying them are not conventional. By their nature they are beyond the range of the predictable; previous experiences have not prepared us for them. How does one prepare for a spinal tumor, a brain injury, a schizophrenic episode, or a devastating earthquake? How does one comprehend Auschwitz or Dachau, where

> Dreams used to come in the brutal nights,
> Dreams crowding and violent
> Dreamt with body and soul,
> Of going home, of eating, of telling our story.
> Until quickly and quietly, came
> The dawn reveille:
> *Wstawàch.*
> And the heart cracked in the breast. (Levi, 1965, p. xi)

Extreme experiences such as these are characterized by a lack of conventional social structure, a loss of anchor in reality, and a lack of ability to predict or anticipate outcomes (Torrance, 1965). Although we associate such phenomena with the high drama of hostage situations, prolonged combat, or concentration camps, they may also define the experience of persons whose lives are linked with ours on a daily basis, that is, our patients. Perhaps we ourselves have endured trauma or the sudden onset of a life-threatening illness.

> Being full of strength and vigor one moment and virtually helpless the next . . . with all one's powers and faculties one moment and without them the next . . . such a change, such a suddenness, is difficult to comprehend and the mind casts about for explanations. (Sacks, 1984, p. 21)

There are those, like Lifton (1988), who view man "as a perpetual survivor . . . of 'holocausts' large and small, personal and collective, that define much of existence" (p. 12). Although the Holocaust was a horrifying reality, as a metaphor it illuminates many other ordeals, helping us to understand and negotiate them. The vivid words and images of those with illness and disability also reveal the deeper meaning of their experiences—meaning that defines the nature of their adaptive task and shapes the quality of their reintegration.

The Personal and Social Meaning of Trauma

There are many reasons to perceive extreme life events as threatening. The most stressful dimensions appear to be those that challenge personal assumptions about oneself and the structure of the world one lives in. Much of this is linked with the phenomenon of control: the ability (or the perceived ability) to change, predict, understand, or accept environmental transactions within a meaningful context (Potocki & Everly, 1989). The sense of being in control and the desire for such control are believed to be crucial aspects of personality affecting physical and mental health as well as recovery potential.

The perception of self, with its elements of body image, identity, and self-worth, were dominant themes in every narrative I encountered, whether the trauma occurred in Vietnam, Theresienstadt, a hospital in London, or a city in Arizona. The pervasive threat to, or loss of, identity was as potent a force as—and sometimes more significant than—any real threat to life and limb. The tattooed number on the arm of a concentration camp inmate had its counterpart in the history number on a hospital ID bracelet. As startling as this analogy may seem, in the eyes of the "number" it may well mean humiliation, a lack of personal validation, and varying degrees of dehumanization. Just as prisoners of war are stripped of rank, role, and place in their reference group, victims of fires suffer losses of important nonhuman anchors for personal identity (Rosenfeld, 1989). Stroke victims, made captive by their disease and an impersonal hospital environment, lose the ability and opportunity to act on their own behalf.

In losing one's identity, one must replace it with another. How one chooses the new altered self is no small task. "Feelings of fear, vulnerability . . . sadness over losses and weakness about not being able to control one's life or one's emotional reactions, contribute to feelings of defectiveness" (Marmar & Horowitz, 1988, p. 96). The impact of confinement, isolation, and perceptual distortions is described by neurologist Oliver Sacks following a near-death accident, serious leg injury, disturbing hospitalization, and role change from doctor to patient.

I was physiologically, in imagination, and feeling . . . a pygmy, a prisoner, a patient . . . without the faintest awareness. How could one know one had shrunk, if one's frame of reference itself shrunk? (1984, p. 157)

Experiences that reflect a loss of self-control are often a central issue in psychiatric disorders as well. It is evident in schizophrenia, for example, when unpredictable symptoms turn "sparkles of light into demon eyes" (McGrath, 1984) or when a partially observing ego is "aware enough to recognize the dangers of not being able to control what I'm doing or thinking" (a patient, personal communication, October 1989).

Psychological stress, induced by threats of loss of self or failure, is also highly dependent on social values and the person's acceptance of the culture's definitions of what is valuable. Finding a new self or coming to terms with the only self one has ever known is reflected in the mirror others place before us. There is humiliation and pain generated

by a gait to embarrass, to make children laugh, a clumsy countering locomotion . . . from only the most exacting, determined efforts to control. Inside my rolling head, behind my shocked, magnified eyeballs, my brain orders, with utmost precision, each awkward jerk of thigh, leg, foot. (Weaver, 1985, p. 43)

Jean Améry provides us with a powerful metaphor for thinking about a person's sense of his or her own body and place in the world when mastery and control of that body is violated through intentional political torture, abuse, or from the pain of illness and medical procedures.

He who has suffered torture can no longer feel at ease in the world. Faith in humanity—cracked by the first slap across the face, then demolished by torture, can never be recovered. (Améry, 1986, p. xiii)

There are, of course, many forms of torture. The torture that physical illness may bestow need not be limited to bodily discomfort or pain, but "visits upon [people] a disease of social relations no less real than the paralysis of the body" (Murphy, 1987, p. 4). Anthropologist John Murphy viewed his spinal tumor, growing paralysis, and confinement as an assault on his identity and a disruption of ties with others. In depicting his illness as an extended field visit to an unfamiliar culture, he identified a primal scene of sociology—the social confrontation of persons with significant flaws, where someone looks or acts differently and we are uncertain as to what to say or where to look. This robs the encounter of cultural guidelines, leaving those involved uncertain about what to expect and what to do. For Murphy, "it has the potential for social calamity" (p. 87).

This calamity is also experienced as being in limbo. Sacks (1984) viewed this as a by-product of his body agnosia and the empathic agnosia of his surgeon, who insisted that nothing was wrong. His disease and lack of a human foothold (i.e., adequate communication and validation) left Sacks with a sense of double nothingness. "Now doubly, I had no leg to stand on; unsupported, doubly" (p. 108). Kleinman (1988), in turn, characterized limbo, for those with chronic illness, as "the dangerous crossing of borders, the interminable waiting to exit and reenter normal everyday life . . . the perpetual uncertainty of whether one can return at all" (p. 181).

I heard this again and again: a common thread, a theme that plagued Holocaust survivors and Vietnam veterans as well as the physically and mentally disabled—the gulf between the self and others (family, friends, caregivers, society). Who will listen? Who will understand what we are experiencing? Who will believe where we have been and what we have endured? Who will validate us as we continue to deal with adversity and its imprints?

Resilience

For some, the imprints are so deeply etched that they succumb. Others endure under conditions that seem unsupportable to health. Redl's (1969) work with adolescents who have beat the odds inspired the concept of *ego resilience,* that is, the capacity to withstand pathogenic pressure, the ability to recover rapidly from a temporary collapse even without outside help, and the strength to bounce back to normal or even supernormal levels of functioning. Demos (1989) suggested that, in its most developed state, such buoyancy requires "an active stance, persistence, the application of a variety of skills and strategies over a wide range of situations and problems . . . [and] flexibility . . . to know when to use what" (p. 5).

The formal study of resilience emerged in epidemiological studies on susceptibility to heart disease over 25 years ago. It is only within the past 15 years, however, that more rigorous efforts have been made to extricate it from a disease model and focus instead on "good psychosocial capacities such as competence, coping, creativity, and confidence" (Anthony & Cohler, 1987, p. x). Although healthfulness remains a less-than-perfect body of knowledge, a variety of popular and scientific resources provide direction for the reader's ongoing investigation, including descriptions of personal experiences (Brown, 1990; Browne, Connors, & Stern, 1985; Cousins, 1979; Egendorf, 1986; Gill, 1988; Heller & Vogel, 1986; Miller, 1985; Minear, 1990; Nolan, 1987; Sheehan, 1982; Trillin, 1984), situational studies of combat (Elder & Clipp, 1988; Rahe & Genender, 1983), studies of disasters (Bolin & Trainer, 1978; Lifton & Olson, 1976) and illness (Cleveland, 1984; Cohen & Lazarus, 1973), studies of the invulnerable child (Anthony & Cohler, 1987; Dugan & Coles, 1989; Garmezy & Masten, 1986; Murphy & Moriarty, 1976), and longitudinal investigations of adaptation (Chess & Thomas, 1984; Vaillant, 1977; Werner & Smith, 1982).

Resilience has been chronicled in studies of famous men and women who were highly stressed and traumatized as children, among them, George Orwell, Charles Dickens, Anton Chekov, Kathe Kollowitz, Pablo Picasso, and Buster Keaton (Goertzel & Goertzel, 1962; Miller, 1990; Shengold, 1989). Resilience, however, is evident in all walks of life. What is less clear is how persons manage to marshal the necessary resources. What enabled young Ryan White, confronted with two life-threatening illnesses, humiliation, and rejection, to become so articulate a spokesman for AIDS? What contributed to the brutalized Central Park jogger's remarkable recovery and recent promotion in her highly competitive investment banking firm? These are questions whose answers have as many nuances as there are people and ordeals, for resilience is not all of one piece.

Resilience is made operational by cognitive and behavioral coping skills and the recruitment of social support. Lazarus and Folkman (1984) suggested that such skills do not come all at once. Rather, they are acquired through a developmental process—a process of selecting from available alternatives and having persons reinforce the skills that are necessary to make coping possible. Studies of vulnerability and competence in children and adolescents have provided valuable insight into some aspects of this multifaceted and shifting phenomenon. Theoretical models of stress resistance view the relationship between stress and personal attributes from several perspectives: as compensation (personal attributes help to improve adjustment when stress diminishes competence), as protection (personal traits interact with stress in predicting adjustment), or as a challenge (stressors enhance competence) (Garmezy, 1983). Dispositional attributes of the child, family cohesion and warmth, and the use of external support systems by parents and children are mechanisms that buffer stress and promote resilient responses. Temperament, sex, intellectual ability, humor, empathy, social problem-solving skills, social expressiveness, and an inner locus of control have been found to influence adaptation under adverse conditions (Garmezy, 1985). These phenomena, however, show variability over time and at different developmental periods (Werner & Smith, 1982) and are influenced by changing demands of the environment. Coping, for children and adults alike, reflects traitlike and situation-specific elements (Kahana, Kahana, Harel, & Rosner, 1988).

Resilience is often measured behaviorally on the basis of the person's competence and success in meeting society's expectations despite great obstacles. Internal indexes (thoughts and feelings) are often ignored, despite evidence that impressive social competence may well be heavily correlated with depression and anxiety (Miller, 1990; Peck, 1987). Clinicians and researchers are alerted to attend to the distinctions and interactions between adaptive behavior and emotional status. Resilience needs to be examined and understood from both perspectives.

Resilient Perspectives

Truly functional coping behavior has been characterized as not only lessening the immediate impact of stress, but also as maintaining a sense of self-worth and unity with the past and an anticipated future (Dimsdale, 1974). It involves two distinct tasks: a response to the requirements of the situation and a response to the feelings about the situation. Author Nancy Mairs (1986), struggling with multiple sclerosis, chronic depression, and agoraphobia, explained the process:

> Each gesture . . . carries a weight of uncertainty, demands significant attention: buttoning my shirt, changing a light bulb, walking down stairs. The minutiae of my life have had to assume dramatic proportions. If I could not . . . delight in them, they would likely drown me in rage and self-pity.
>
> Yet I am unwilling to forgo the adventurous life; the difficulty of it, even the pain, the . . . fear, and the sudden brief lift of spirit that graces . . . the pilgrimage. If I am to have it . . . I must change the terms by which it is lived. . . . I refine adventure, make it smaller and smaller . . . whether I am feeding fish flakes to my bettas . . . lying wide-eyed in the dark battling yet another bout of depression, cooking a chicken . . . [or] meeting a friend for lunch. . . . I am always having the adventures that are mine to have. (pp. 6–7)

Mairs accepted the challenge and altered her life-style in the face of unpredictable capacity while maintaining some semblance of control over her life through a commitment to scaled-down adventures. Even in the presence of many serious problems she demonstrated what Kobasa (1979) and colleagues have called *hardiness*. Hardiness is characterized by challenge, commitment, and control attributes. Challenge is expressed as a belief that change, rather than stability, is normal in life and is an incentive for growth rather than a threat to security. Control is expressed by feeling and acting as if one is influential rather then helpless. Influence is operationalized through the use of imagination, knowledge, skill, and choice. Commitment is a tendency to involve oneself rather then feel alienated from situations; it involves a generalized sense of purpose that allows one to find events, things, and people meaningful and to approach situations rather than avoid them.

In extraordinarily stressful situations (the ones that diminish social structure, connections with reality, and a sense of predictability), opportunities to operationalize commitment, control, and challenge orientations are greatly compromised. Nonetheless, cognitive and behavioral coping mechanisms and efforts to recruit social support emerge and find expression in the most remarkable ways. The personal perspectives of the persons whose anecdotes follow are a tribute to the resourcefulness of the human mind and spirit. Their thoughts, feelings, and actions reflect the true character of resilience.

Hope and the Will to Overcome

Hope and the will to overcome are evident in the poignant poetry of children who found comfort and inspiration in the resilience of nature while confined in a Czechoslovakian camp in 1944:

> The sun has made a veil of gold
> So lovely that my body aches.
> Above, the heavens shriek with blue
> Convinced I've smiled by some mistake.

The world's abloom and seems to smile.
I want to fly but where, how high?
If in barbed wire, things can bloom
Why couldn't I? I will not die! (Anonymous, in *I Never Saw Another Butterfly,* 1978, p. 52)

Hope and the will to overcome emerge in others as a fierce, sometimes raging will to live, that is, "the burning desire to tell, to bear witness" (Gill, 1988, p. 59), "to testifying on behalf of all those whose shadows will be bound to mine forever" (Wiesel, 1990, p. 15), "to live not for oneself, but to lament those who died [in Hiroshima]" (Tamiki, 1990, p. 30).

Affiliation and the Recruitment of Social Support

Acquiring a sense of belonging to a social group or, for that matter, to all of life, is a powerful way to sustain oneself in the face of death or other extremes. It may manifest itself by turning one's attention inward to memories and images of loved ones, by participating in an organized underground movement, or by devising a tap code to communicate through cell walls to other Vietnam prisoners of war. It also emerges through the collaboration of a therapist and a severely mentally ill woman who is struggling against great odds to restore a semblance of autonomy and self-respect:

> You believed in me . . . were willing to take a chance on my being able to handle an apartment when my family felt it would be a waste of money. We had hopes; I didn't want to let you down . . . and I haven't. (a patient, personal communication, 1989)

Finding Meaning and Purpose

The identification of purpose, or finding meaning in an ordeal, was described by Viktor Frankl (1984) as "the last of human freedoms"—choosing one's attitude in any given set of circumstances, having at least the power and the control over how you interpret and explain what happens to you. Individuals find meaning and purpose in many different ways. Some find it in an increased commitment to religion, a political ideal, or a social cause. Others find it by using intellect and creativity to combat devastating fear. Many concentration camp victims and prisoners of war played chess and built houses, nail by nail, in their mind's eye; one man prepared a full German–English dictionary on scraps of paper during his incarceration and published it after his release. Others claimed that even forced labor was sustaining.

Interestingly, despite confining, constraining situations with extremely limited resources, many sought to find meaning and retain interests, values and skills through focused, self-regulating activity. "The prisoners who fared the best in the long run were those who . . . could retain their personality system largely intact . . . where previous interests, values and skills could to some extent be carried on" (Hamburg, Coelho, & Adams, 1974, p. 413). In situational studies of combat, illness, and the anticipated death of family members, Gal and Lazarus (1975) reported reductions in anxiety and feelings of helplessness even when activities did not provide actual control over the situation. In contrast, the vulnerable were described by Eitinger as those who "felt completely helpless and passive, and had lost their ability to retain some sort of self-activity" (Hamburg et al., 1974, p. 413). Our continuing efforts to understand the complex role of occupation in remediating illness and maintaining health may be greatly enhanced through studies of the spontaneous behavior of those in stressful situations.

The Capacity to Step Back

Frankl's (1984) disgust with his own trivial preoccupations with survival found him, in fantasy, lecturing on the psychology of concentration camps. Both he and his troubles became the object of a psychoscientific study undertaken by himself that later contributed to the development of a school of psychotherapy. Frankl demonstrated the capacity to step back and, in so doing, preserved a part of himself from extraordinary degradation, pain, and loss. Functioning somewhat like a solution to a figure–ground problem, this process provides one with the option of ignoring aspects of the situation that are out of one's control. It may appear as a differential focus on the good, or it may be marked by a heightened capacity for observation, that is, a period of exalted receptivity when details of events, faces, words, or sensations are retained (Levi, 1987). This is evident in the writings of Wiesel (1990), Cousins (1979), Heller and Vogel (1986), Brown (1990), and Nolan (1987). None perceived themselves to be victims or survivors, but rather, witnesses to their own experience.

There Is More to Oneself Than Current Circumstance Suggests

The discovery of the new or real self is artfully reflected in Frank's (1988) study of embodiment—the experience and meaning of disability in American culture. She described a young woman born with quadrilateral limb deficiencies who stressed her assets instead of her deficits—her womanly figure (like Venus de Milo's) and her ability to write better with her stumps than with her artificial arms. Interestingly, her rehabilitation team viewed her refusal to use prosthetics as poor adaptation.

Dugan and Coles (1989), in turn, described a 6-year-old Black girl who was initiating school desegregation in New Orleans in the face of mobs, violence, and threats to her life. She hoped she would "get through one day and then another," and if she did, "it will be because there is more to me than I ever realized" (p. xiv).

Novel Applications of Problem-Solving Strategies

Coping involves creative and reflective behavior (White, 1976). Resilience is manifest in the ability to turn a familiar way of solving problems into a novel application, one that may save a life. When Sacks (1984) sustained his injury while mountain climbing alone, he was at great risk for dying of exposure. He reported that there came to his aid a kinetic melody, rhythm, and motor music. "Now, so to speak, I was musicked along" (p. 30). Remembrances of the Volga Boatmen's Song gave him the strength and rhythm to "row" himself along the ground for many hours until he found help.

Transforming Dross Into Gold

Vaillant's (1977) longitudinal study of the life and coping strategies of a group of Harvard graduates documented the way in which the mature ego mechanisms of altruism, humor, suppression, and sublimation function to transform disturbances into adaptive behavior, thus turning "dross into gold" (p. 16). This is, in part, the way the speechless, palsied Irish poet Christopher Nolan (1987) found his mellifluous voice:

> Fossilized for so long now, he was going to speak to anyone interested enough to listen. . . . Now he shared the same world as everyone else; he could choose how much to tell and craftily decide how much to hold back. His voice would be his written word. (p. 98)

The same mechanisms allowed comedian Buster Keaton to devote his life to making others laugh, while unable to laugh spontaneously himself (Miller, 1990). Long before Norman Cousins found health and fame in laughter and neuroscience linked it to our immune systems, humor was acknowledged to be one of the truly elegant defenses in the human repertoire (Lefcourt & Martin, 1986). "Like hope, humor permits one to bear and yet to focus upon what may be too terrible to be borne" (Vaillant, 1977, p. 386). This is precisely what ailing critic Anatole Broyard (1990) did when he quipped, "What a critically ill person needs above all is to be understood. Dying is a misunderstanding you have to get straightened out before you go" (p. 29).

Resilience is not a miraculous rescue. It can be a mere thread that wrestles itself to the surface of an otherwise despairing existence. It is reflected in the struggle of a 50-year-old chronically mentally ill woman who sustains her sense of altruism despite unrelenting suspiciousness, fear, and rigid thought processes. She is an ardent giver of small gifts, of greeting cards weeks before the actual event, and of postage stamps she hopes will acquire great value for the recipient's future grandchildren. The dignity and control she experiences in giving to others when she herself is in such great need allow her more comfort than she might otherwise have. It buffers her from the painful realization of how isolated and vulnerable she really is.

Hamburg et al. (1974) summarized the essence of survival under extreme duress by underscoring the importance of the maintenance of self-esteem, a sense of human dignity, a sense of group belonging, and a feeling of being useful to others.

How Durable Is Resilience?

Resilient responses to ordeals have phase-specific attributes. In the acute phase, energy is directed at minimizing the impact of the stress and stressor. In the reorganization phase, a new reality is faced and accepted in part or in whole. And then there is the rest of one's life. How durable is resilience? We know it is neither a single act nor a constant state. How and under what circumstances does it emerge, shift, or fail the person? Camus (as cited by Maquet, 1958) described its emergence: "In the depth of winter I finally learned that within me there lay an invincible summer." In contrast, Monette (1988) experienced its decline: "I used up all my optimism keeping my friend alive. Now that he's gone, the cup of my health is neither half full nor half empty. Just half" (p. 2).

The suicides of Primo Levi and Bruno Bettelheim prompt similar questions. Why did Levi, successful chemist and award-winning author who recorded his Holocaust experiences because there "were things that imperiously demanded to be told" (1987, p. 9), choose to die? Did cancer and the ill health of his mother chip away at the mission he had set for himself? Did a history of exemplary behavioral competence distract from the depression and anxiety that often accompany it? Did a major depression go untreated? What about Bettelheim? His essays bore witness to Nazi atrocities; his provocative style challenged a world he saw as too passive and naive. He enacted solutions to some of humanity's problems by developing therapeutic environments for severely disturbed children. Did retirement, physical ailments, or the loss of a familiar social network limit his ability to play out a meaningful life story? Did his resilience run out? Or was this last sorrowful act a measure of his need to be in control, exercising his own will, his way, while he could? He spoke prospectively of these issues in the introduction to *The Uses of Enchantment: The Meaning and Importance of Fairy Tales* (1977):

> If we hope to live not just from moment to moment, but in true consciousness of our existence, then our greatest need and most difficult achievement is to find meaning in our lives. . . . Many have lost the will to live, and have stopped trying, because such meaning has evaded them. An understanding of the meaning of one's life is not suddenly acquired at a particular age, not even when one has reached chronological maturity. (p. 3)

These anecdotes demonstrate the changing and highly personal nature of resilience, often attained at the cost of some degree of spontaneity and flexibility. This and the interplay among such factors as age, general health status, and changing roles and relationships may conspire to diminish the once raging will to live in some, while allowing others to continue to find meaning and commitment in changing life circumstances. Resilience appears to be less an enduring characteristic and more a process determined by the impact of particular life experiences on particular conceptions of one's own life history (Cohler, 1987), leading one, once again, to conclude that it is not so much what happens to people but how they interpret and explain it that makes a difference.

Integrating Personal Meaning, Behavior, and Reality: Implications for Practice

Who rises above adversity? Perhaps it is sufficient to say that human capacities can shrink, hibernate, and flourish under circumstances of extreme stress; the influence of personal perspective; and the people, places, and things in the environment. The lives I sampled in the course of this study heightened my appreciation for the richness of the coping process and the difficulties many face with the unrelenting demands of their illness and the ofttimes unresponsive health care system. Even a resilient outcome does not represent a simple linear trajectory. It often requires the empathic attention and skillful assistance of those, like us, who are empowered by training and, I hope, by inclination.

Ordeals Provide a Window of Opportunity

Physical and emotional disruptions, the circumstances that bring us and our consumers together, provide a window of opportunity. Timely and meaningful interventions can have a significant impact on the reintegration process. These interventions may involve us in multiple tasks, such as helping persons find meaning in their crises, helping them handle feelings provoked by their situation, helping them with the reality and consequences of their condition, and fostering the functional skills and behaviors that they will need to fulfill their potential. Unfortunately, individual needs and capacities do not necessarily run on the same time standard as that of third-party payers. Potential for resilience may be noted and nurtured, but not necessarily birthed in 6 inpatient days or 12 annual reimbursed outpatient visits. Illness, and certainly disability, is an ongoing process in which personal problems may constantly emerge to undermine technical control, social order, and individual mastery (Kleinman, 1988). The conflicts that arise among individual needs, professional values, and the system's priorities pose real challenges to those who need access before the window of opportunity is shut. We must examine our own role in perpetuating this dilemma. We must reevaluate and, in some instances, reframe, short- and long-term practice models. Additionally, we must educate colleagues, administrators, and insurers to the personal and financial impact of psychosocial factors on recovery and rehabilitation outcome in all areas of specialization.

Many Factors Influence Individual Response to Ordeals

Many intervening variables affect patients' major life changes on the one hand and illness outcome on the other. The good news is that those who rise above adversity do not belong to an exclusive club. It is not a closed system. However, some people are their own best facilitators, while others need help. Neither group should face its ordeals at the hands of caregivers and environments that induce more stress by diminishing humanistic contacts and links with reality, by neglecting the person's need to predict or anticipate outcomes, or by ignoring the inner elements of coping and competency behaviors. It is troubling to note how well many of our treatment centers fulfill the criteria for extremely stressful, negative life events.

The variability of resilience may come as bad news for some, because it does not permit a simple recipe for treatment. Instead, we must commit ourselves to understanding the complexities of personality, coping capacities, and environmental influences and use them to identify goals, interventions, and environments that are meaningful to a given person under a given set of circumstances.

Transforming Adversity Into Possibilities

Murphy (1987) reminded us that "there is a need for order in all humans that impels us to search for systematic coherence in both nature and society, and when we can find none, to invent it" (p. 33). Thoughts, feelings, and actions, influenced by neurobiology and environment, are the means by which our patients attempt to invent coherence and order that is acceptable to themselves and the outside world (White, 1976). The experiences documented in the present paper are testimony to how innovative and powerful human thoughts, feelings, and actions can be.

These capacities are also our most elegant professional tools for transforming adversity into possibilities, when we take the time to conceive of them as such. As always, Sacks (1984) captured the essence of this phenomenon best:

> Rehabilitation involves action, acts . . . [and] must be centered on the character of acts—and how to call them forth, when they have come apart, disintegrated, been "lost"—or "forgotten." (p. 182)

Calling forth the character of acts involves the therapist's understanding and using the patient's thoughts and feelings, collaborating with him or her, establishing trust, and reaching for the personal context that is partner to external reality and individual potentials for functional behavior.

Professional Entreaties

How well do we call forth the character of acts? I believe that as a group we are far more effective at defining reality and assessing and promoting performance then we are at assessing and making use of patients' views of themselves and their situation. Although our clinical prowess has grown greatly, we are too often committed only to present manifest performance. These snapshot approaches to capacity fail to reflect the unique adaptive style and potential of each person. If we are to enhance outcome, we must integrate the patients' experience of their condition and their preexisting patterns of self-regulating activity with our concerns and strategies for functional mobilization.

Kleinman (1988) proposed the use of clinical miniethnographic methods for acquiring a better picture, much like an anthropologist does in assessing a different culture. The ethnographer draws on knowledge of the context to make sense of behavior, allowing herself to sample the subject's experience. Occupational therapists are ethnographers of sorts. We have unique access to information about activities of everyday living and what it is like to live with an illness or disability. We need only to acknowledge and actualize it. But do we? Do we draw out the patient's perception of his or her situation? Or do we focus only on those aspects of function we can see, palpate, or measure?

Practice has changed dramatically over the past 30 years, as much a product of our growth and development as it is a measure of new knowledge and shifts in the health care system. We certainly have not been idle. It is therefore no surprise that we find ourselves pursuing the future with such vigor that we sometimes fail to look back to see if we have left something of value behind. I believe we are at great risk of leaving in our wake some of the most central and precious components of our practice—how people think and feel about themselves and the world in which they live. Evidence suggests that we may have already reframed the rehabilitation process to fit today's economy rather than to fit today's patients.

Our connections to the deeper personal experiences of our patients seem to be unduly mediated by professional objectivity, our personal reluctance to hear, and a narrow view of what belongs to a given area of specialization. Fleming (1989) identified the presence of practice dichotomies concerning the relative importance of the patient's personal phenomenological status and how best to relate to him or her. Although some therapists appear to use such information and their relationship in treatment, their ambivalence about acknowledging it relegates it to an underground practice and reflects troublesome conflicts in values. We must remind ourselves that psychosocial phenomena belong to everyone, irrespective of their diagnosis and health status. Practice that separates feelings from function and psychosocial from physical perpetuates disorder rather than fostering reintegration.

The profession's current efforts to examine the actuality of clinical reasoning show great promise for rescuing the person inside our patients and for allowing us to acknowledge the credibility of this element of clinical activity. Similarly, the study of resilient persons provides us with important opportunities to share their experience, rethink our beliefs about occupational therapy's domain of concern, and enrich the emerging science of occupation. Like the subjects of this paper, "each of us maintains a personal theory of reality, a coherent set of assumptions developed over time about ourselves and our world that organizes our experiences and understanding and directs our behavior" (Janoff-Bulman & Timko, 1987, p. 136). I believe that our responsiveness to the inner lives of others can add perspective to our professional assumptions and enhance our understanding of human performance capacity. In so doing, we will find ourselves far better able to help our patients refine their adventures, find meaning and purpose in their ordeals, discover there is more to themselves than current circumstance suggests, and transform the dross of their adversity into the gold of their accomplishments.

Epilogue

This is a work in progress. My purpose has been to examine the relevance of resilience to our practice. However, one person's efforts to orchestrate the chorus of resilient voices cannot do them justice. I urge the reader to explore this literature as well. It is likely to stimulate extraordinary personal and professional awakening. Moreover, it merits our collective thought and action, because the efforts of many are needed to give meaning to the hardships our patients endure and the difference occupational therapy can make.

Acknowledgments

I dedicate this lecture to three resilient women whose adaptive style and commitment to challenge have greatly enriched my personal and professional life: my mother, Elsie Babbitt; my mentor and friend, Gail Fidler; and my daughter, Deborah Fine. All three not only see the cup as half full, but strive to keep it overflowing for themselves and others.

References

Améry, J. (1986). *At the mind's limits: Contemplations by a surviror on Auschwitz and its realities.* New York: Schocken.

Anthony, E. J., & Cohler, B. J. (Eds.). (1987). *The invulnerable child.* New York: Guilford.

Bettelheim, B. (1977). *The uses of enchantment: The meaning and importance of fairy tales.* New York: Knopf.

Bolin, R., & Trainer, P. (1978). Modes of family recovery following disaster: A cross national study. In E. L. Quarantelli (Ed.), *Disaster theory and research* (pp. 233–247). London: Sage.

Brown, C. (1990). *Down all the days.* London: Mandarin.

Browne, S. E., Connors, D., & Stern, N. (1985). *With the power of each breath: A disabled women's anthology.* San Francisco: Cleis.

Broyard, A. (1990, April 1). Good books about being sick. *New York Times Book Review,* pp. 1, 28–30.

Cannon, W. (1939). *The wisdom of the body.* New York: Norton.

Chess, S., & Thomas, A. (1984). *Origins and evolution of behavior disorders: From infancy to early adult life.* New York: Brunner/Mazel.

Cleveland, M. (1984). Family adaptation to traumatic spinal cord injury: Response to crisis. In R. H. Moos (Ed.), *Coping with physical illness* (pp. 159–171). New York: Plenum.

Cohen, F., & Lazarus, R. S. (1973). Active coping processes, coping dispositions and recovery from surgery. *Psychosomatic Medicine, 35,* 375–389.

Cohler, B. J. (1987). Adversity, resilience and the study of lives. In E. J. Anthony & B. J. Cohler (Eds.), *The invulnerable child* (pp. 363–424). New York: Guilford.

Cousins, N. (1979). *Anatomy of an illness.* New York: Bantam.

Demos, E. V. (1989). Resiliency in infancy. In T. F. Dugan & R. Coles (Eds.), *The child in our times: Studies in the development of resiliency* (pp. 3–22). New York: Brunner/Mazel.

Dimsdale, J. E. (1974). The coping behavior of Nazi concentration camp survivors. *American Journal of Psychiatry, 131,* 792–797.

Dugan, T. F., & Coles, R. (1989). *The child in our times: Studies in the development of resiliency.* New York: Brunner/Mazel.

Egendorf, A. (1986). *Healing from the war: Trauma and transformation after Vietnam.* Boston: Shambhala.

Elder, G. H. Jr., & Clipp, E. C. (1988). Combat experience, comradeship and psychological health. In J. P. Wilson, Z. Harel, & B. Kahana (Eds.), *Human adaptation to extreme stress from the Holocaust to Vietnam* (pp. 131–154). New York: Plenum.

Erikson, E. (1963). *Childhood and society.* New York: Norton.

Flach, F. (1988). *Resilience: Discovering a new strength at times of stress.* New York: Fawcett Columbine.

Fleming, M. (1989). The therapist with the three-track mind. In *The AOTA Practice Symposium guide 1989* (pp. 70–73). Rockville, MD: American Occupational Therapy Association.

Frank, C. (1988). On embodiment: A case study of congenital limb deficiency in American culture. In M. Fine & A. Asch (Eds.), *Women with disabilities* (pp. 41–71). Philadelphia: Temple University Press.

Frankl, V. E. (1984). *Man's search for meaning.* New York: Washington Square Press.

Gal, R., & Lazarus, R. S. (1975, December). The role of activity in anticipating and confronting stressful situations. *Journal of Human Stress, 1,* 4–20.

Garmezy, N. (1983). Stressors of childhood. In N. Garmezy & M. Rutter (Eds.), *Stress, coping and development in children* (pp. 43–84). New York: McGraw-Hill.

Garmezy, N. (1985). Stress-resistant children: The search for protective factors. In J. E. Stevenson (Ed.), *Recent research in developmental psychopathology* (pp. 213–233). Elmsford, NY: Pergamon.

Garmezy, N., & Masten, A. S. (1986). Stress, competence and resilience: Common frontiers for therapist and psychopathologist. *Behavior Therapy, 17,* 500–521.

Gill, A. (1988). *The journey back from hell: An oral history—Conversations with concentration camp survivors.* New York: Morrow.

Goertzel, V., & Goertzel, M. G. (1962). *Cradles of eminence.* Boston: Little, Brown.

Goleman, D. (1989, April 20). Researchers find optimism helps body's defense system. *New York Times,* p. B15.

Hamburg, D. A., Coelho, G. V., & Adams, J. E. (1974). Coping and adaptation: Steps toward a synthesis of biological and social perspectives. In G. V. Coelho, D. A. Hamburg, & J. E. Adams (Eds.), *Coping and adaptation* (pp. 403–440). New York: Basic.

Heller, J., & Vogel, S. (1986). *No laughing matter.* New York: Avon.

Houston, B. K. (1987). Stress and coping. In C. R. Snyder & C. E. Ford (Eds.), *Coping with negative life events* (pp. 373–399). New York: Plenum.

I never saw another butterfly: Children's drawings and poems from Terezin Concentration Camp, 1942–1944. (1978). New York: Schocken Books.

Janoff-Bulman, R., & Timko, C. (1987). Coping with traumatic events: The role of denial in light of people's assumptive worlds. In C. R. Snyder & C. E. Ford (Eds.), *Coping with negative life events* (pp. 135–155). New York: Plenum.

Kahana, E., Kahana, B., Harel, Z., & Rosner, T. (1988). Coping with extreme trauma. In J. P. Wilson, Z. Harel, & B. Kahana (Eds.), *Human adaptation to extreme stress: From the Holocaust to Vietnam* (pp. 55–76). New York: Plenum.

Kleinman, A. (1988). *The illness narratives: Suffering, healing and the human condition.* New York: Basic.

Kobasa, S. C. (1979). Stressful life events, personality, and health: An inquiry into hardiness. *Journal of Personality and Social Psychology, 37,* 1–11.

Lazarus, R. S., & Folkman, S. (1984). *Stress, appraisal and coping.* New York: Springer.

Lefcourt, H. M., & Martin, R. A. (1986). *Humor and life stress: Antidote to adversity.* New York: Springer-Verlag.

Levi, P. (1965). *The reawakening.* New York: Collier.

Levi, P. (1987). *Moments of reprieve.* New York: Penguin.

Lifton, R. J. (1988). Understanding the traumatized self: Imagery, symbolization and transformation. In J. P. Wilson, Z. Harel, & B. Kahana (Eds.), *Human adaptation to extreme stress: From the Holocaust to Vietnam* (pp. 7–31), New York: Plenum.

Lifton, R. J., & Olson, E. (1976). The human meaning of total disaster. *Psychiatry, 39,* 1–17.

Mairs, N. (1986). *Plaintext: Deciphering a woman's life.* New York: Perennial Library.

Maquet, A. (1958). *Albert Camus: The invincible summer.* New York: Braziller.

Marmar, E. R., & Horowitz, M. J. (1988). Post traumatic stress disorder. In J. P. Wilson, Z. Harel, & D. Kahana (Eds.), *Human adaptation to extreme stress: From the Holocaust to Vietnam* (pp. 81–103). New York: Plenum.

McGrath, M. (1984). First person accounts: Where did I go? *Schizophrenia Bulletin, 10,* 638–640.

Miller, A. (1990). *The untouched key: Tracing childhood trauma in creativity and destructiveness.* New York: Doubleday.

Miller, V. (Ed.). (1985). *Despite this flesh: The disabled in stories and poems.* Austin, TX: University of Texas Press.

Minear, R. H. (Ed.). (1990). *Hiroshima: Three witnesses.* Princeton, NJ: Princeton University Press.

Monette, P. (1988). *Borrowed time: An AIDS memoir.* New York: Avon.

Moos, R., & Billings, A. (1982). Conceptualizing and measuring coping resources and processes. In L. Goldberger & S. Breznitz (Eds.), *Handbook of stress: Theoretical and clinical aspects* (pp. 212–220). New York: Macmillan.

Moos, R. H., & Schaefer, J. A. (1984). The crisis of physical illness: An overview and conceptual approach. In R. H. Moos (Ed.), *Coping with physical illness* (pp. 8–25). New York: Plenum.

Murphy, L. B., & Moriarty, A. (1976). *Vulnerability, coping and growth: From infancy to adolescence.* New Haven, CT: Yale University Press.

Murphy, R. F. (1987). *The body silent.* New York: Henry Holt.

Nolan, C. (1987). *Under the eye of the clock.* New York: Dell.

Peck, E. C. (1987). The traits of true invulnerability and posttraumatic stress in psychoanalyzed men of action. In E. J. Anthony & B. J. Cohler (Eds.), *The invulnerable child* (pp. 315–360). New York: Guilford.

Pelletier, K. R., & Herzing, D. L. (1988). Psychoneuroimmunology: Toward a mind–body model: A critical review. *Advances, 5,* 27–56.

Potocki, E. R., & Everly, G. S. Jr. (1989). Control and the human stress response. In G. S. Everly, Jr. (Ed.), *A clinical guide to the treatment of the human stress response* (pp. 119–136). New York: Plenum.

Radner, G. (1989). *It's always something.* New York: Simon & Schuster.

Rahe, R. H., & Genender, E. (1983). Adaptation to and recovery from captivity stress. *Military Medicine, 148,* 577–585.

Redl, F. (1969). Adolescents—Just how do they react? In G. Caplan & S. Lebovici (Eds.), *Adolescence: Psychosocial perspectives* (pp. 79–90). New York: Basic.

Rosenfeld, M. S. (1989). Occupational disruption and adaptation: A study of house fire victims. *American Journal of Occupational Therapy, 43,* 89–96.

Sacks, O. (1984). *A leg to stand on.* New York: Harper & Row.

Selye, H. (1978). *The stress of life* (2nd ed.). New York: McGraw-Hill.

Sheehan, S. (1982). *Is there no place on earth for me?* New York: Vintage.

Shengold, L. (1989). *The effects of childhood abuse and deprivation.* New Haven, CT: Yale University Press.

Tamiki, H. (1990). Summer flowers. In R. H. Minear (Ed.), *Hiroshima* (pp. 19–114). Princeton, NJ: Princeton University Press.

Torrance, E. P. (1965). *Constructive behavior: Stress, personality and mental health.* Belmont, CA: Wadsworth.

Trillin, A. S. (1984). Of dragons and garden peas: A cancer patient talks to doctors. In R. H. Moos (Ed.), *Coping with physical illness* (pp. 131–138). New York: Plenum.

Vaillant, G. E. (1977). *Adaptation to life.* Boston: Little, Brown.

Weaver, G. (1985). Finch the spastic speaks. In V. Miller (Ed.), *Despite this flesh: The disabled in stories and poems* (pp. 35–45). Austin, TX: University of Texas Press.

Werner, E. E., & Smith, R. S. (1982). *Vulnerable but invincible: A study of resilient children.* New York: McGraw-Hill.

White, R. W. (1976). Strategies of adaptation: An attempt at systematic description. In R. H. Moos (Ed.), *Human adaptation: Coping with life crises* (pp. 17–32). Lexington, MA: Heath.

Wiesel, E. (1990). *From the kingdom of memory: Reminiscences.* New York: Summit.

42

1993 Eleanor Clarke Slagle Lecture

Occupation Embedded in a Real Life:
Interweaving Occupational Science and Occupational Therapy

Florence Clark, PhD, OTR, FAOTA

Introduction

I address you with a sense of gratitude to my friends and colleagues in the profession for giving me the honor of joining the ranks of the Eleanor Clarke Slagle lecturers and to my profession for its ethical roots and its recognition of the centrality of occupation in the lives of people, a concept that inspires this lecture. Before I begin, I also wish to express my deep appreciation to Elinor Richardson and Penny Richardson. They were willing to tell their story "so that," as Penny put it, "something good could come out of all this." I will now begin with a brief story entitled "The Big A."

In July 1989, compact, trim, attractive, physically fit Professor Penny Richardson, Chair of the Higher Education Department in the University of Southern California School of Education, having taken a break from the teaching she had been doing in Hawaii, cooked a gourmet evening meal for her new friend Bill. She had just returned from a week-long kayak trip, a great adventure, and was enjoying regaling Bill with tales of mountainous swells and hair-raising experiences on the high seas. She had been with a wonderful group of people; they had been enjoying the stunning Hawaiian waterfalls, sleeping on the sand, having gourmet cookouts, "all that good outdoors Sierra Club stuff." Penny and Bill enjoyed their lavish meal, but in a sudden twist of events that night, Penny fainted and could not be revived. She was rushed to the hospital. Her head was shaven, holes were drilled in her skull, and subsequently she underwent several operations to alleviate the pressure caused by the bursting aneurysm, which she would later call the "Big A." She was 47 years old at the time, an independent, successful, academic woman, who had many friends and a rich professional life, who traveled widely, who had been a hiker, a skier, and a mountain climber. Nature encompasses not only the natural; in a moment it can disrupt our lives profoundly. Ironically, nature itself can bring about the unnatural.

Penny had been an acquaintance of mine before her trip to Hawaii. When she returned to the states, I decided to pursue a more intense friendship because, as an occupational therapist, I believed I might be able to help, and I was searching for an altruistic project that might distract me from the turmoil of my own life at the time. A second motive was that we were launching the occupational science project at the University of Southern California (USC) and I thought it would be helpful for me to be close to the recovery process of a woman who was dealing with the aftermath of a stroke as I took my place in the development of the new science. That Christmas, I received a Christmas letter from Penny which concluded with the following poem:

> I talk with a rasp
> I walk with a tilt
> I'm fed through a tube

Originally published 1993 in *American Journal of Occupational Therapy, 47,* 1067–1078.
Please note that there were no Eleanor Clarke Slagle Lectures in 1991 and 1992.

I eat applesauce by very small spoonfuls
I laugh with the best of them
. . . I love you all, Penny

She was in a skilled nursing facility at the time; it was 6 months after the aneurysm and she embraced a comic vision of her disability. At that time, she had no sense of what was to come when she would reenter the real world of human activity.

I am going to allow you to be privy to a dialogue of experience between Penny and me. The discourse, however, is not simply a conversation between friends, although certainly it was in part that. It emerged through our collaboration as life history ethnographers (Frank, 1979, 1984, 1986), interpreting her experience of disability over time from an occupational science standpoint, and as ethnomethodologists (Garfinkel, 1967) identifying the therapeutic process that emerged as I unexpectedly functioned as her occupational therapist while engaged in the research process. Research and therapy became intertwined. Was the study an applied scientific inquiry, the purpose of which was to apply the occupational science knowledge base to occupational therapy, or was it basic inquiry describing the relationship of childhood occupation to adult character and eventual recovery from stroke? I think you will agree, after hearing the story, that it was both.

I shall present the findings in the form of a narrative analysis. As I use this term, it means a story that emerges from qualitative research or historiography. Therefore, the complex set of events in the story will not be presented as unrelated episodes, but rather as linked by meaning, as a coherent story given plot by human feelings and intentions (Polkinghorne, 1988; Rosaldo, 1989; Sarbin, 1989). The creation of this story involved systematic procedures, the coding and analyzing of over 200 pages of transcriptions, representing approximately 20 hours of interview time. Penny brought to the project her experience of disability, her imagination, her gift with words, her humor, and her energy. I brought the occupational science standpoint and my experience as an occupational therapist. I present the story in what Bruner (1990b) would call broad but carefully selected strokes, without the kind of detail that could appear in a subsequent book. The Czechoslovakian author Milan Kundera (1991), in his book *Immortality*, stated that "Music taught the European not only a richness of feeling, but also the worship of his feelings and his feeling self." He then described "the violinist standing on the platform" who closes his eyes and plays the first two long notes. At that moment, Kundera wrote, "the listener also closes his eyes, feels his soul expanding in his breast, and says to himself, 'How beautiful' " (p. 204).

I think of the following story as a kind of musical composition, a symphony with three movements. You have just heard the prelude. The first movement is the *Allegro Spirituoso*, entitled "Childhood Occupation and the Building of Adult Character." It demonstrates how the occupational science framework evokes a particular kind of storytelling. Childhood occupation is related to adult character. Later, in the third movement, we find that telling the story this way contributed to Penny's recovery. The second movement, the *Grave*, entitled "The Big A—From This to That," shows that rehabilitation can be experienced by the survivor as a rite of passage in which a person is moved to disability status by experts and therapists and then abandoned. Finally, the last movement, the *Grande*, called "Nurturing the Human Spirit to Act," illustrates that storytelling and story making with survivors centered on the theme of occupation embedded in real life can be enormously therapeutic. It may constitute a powerful application of occupational science to occupational therapy. This complex and textured weave may be able to do what former Slagle lecturer Reilly (1962) called nurturing the human spirit to act. So prepare yourself; close your eyes, please; we are about to play the first note.

Allegro Spirituoso: Child Occupation and the Building of Adult Character

In occupational science we are interested in how people become independent, adapt to environmental demands, and achieve competency (Yerxa et al., 1989). I entered this project believing that childhood occupations sow the seeds of adult character. Ruddick and others (Ruddick, 1982) have argued that particular kinds of mindsets are shaped through everyday activity. I therefore suggested early in our ethnography that Penny tell me stories of her childhood occupations. What follows is a detailed description of her childhood, the importance of which will be evident in the story of her recovery.

Penny Richardson was born in Los Angeles on December 14, 1941, to Lloyd Richardson (affectionately called Bud) and Elinor Richardson. Later, the Richardsons had another child, her younger brother Steve. In Penny's view, her parents were very different kinds of people. Her dad "was kind of country style; he liked blue jeans; he was very down-home," a quiet man. Ultimately his career was in real estate, but Penny did not view him as particularly career-oriented. He cherished being on a farm, close to animals and to the rhythms of nature. Penny described her dad as having been "very low key, a Boy Scout leader," and "a gentle man." He had "a profound appreciation of people, whatever their walk of life," and he valued "keeping your word about things, steadiness, telling the truth, and following through on commitments." She admired him for having had the strength to do things that men at the time did not do, like cooking.

> He used to drive me to school every morning; he used to pick up both me and my girlfriends. . . . And when we would go to Easter Week in Balboa Island, he would always prepare stew for us one night. . . . Mr. Richardson's stew, that was a very favorite night of everybody. Oh great! Time for Mr. Richardson's stew!

Her mother Elinor continued with her career when her children were young in the 1940s and 1950s, a time when being a working mother was more unusual than it is now. Entering her profession as a teacher, Elinor soon became a school principal and went on to earn her doctorate in education. She was one of a group of educators who first brought educational television to the schools of Southern California. As in the case of her dad, Penny had a strong sense of what her mother valued: "being highly professional but also listening, being sensitive to others, caring, being a good leader."

At a very young age Penny began to write poems as a way of making sense of her world. For example, in third grade, she wrote the poem "Old Black Bull," which tells the story of a curly-haired city slicker who

> . . . on a farm had her first and worst alarm
> She went outside this very day,
> when the old black bull came out to play
> That city slicker began to scream and cry.
> If nobody saves me I will die. . . .

Eventually, the city slicker is rescued by a straight-haired country hick. This poem can be seen as reflecting a child's effort to deal with two worlds: the rural, down-home world of her father and the urban, professional world of her mother.

In 1946, when Penny was 5 years old, the family moved to Chancellor Farm in Whittier, California. Memories of Chancellor Farm are still particularly precious. These are preserved in a book of memorabilia with a bucking horse on the wooden cover that was carved by her grandfather. Penny edited this book as a child, complete with narratives and annotations so detailed they reveal how much the farm meant to her. In a map she made, she included the house, shed, orchard, the big pasture, and the little pasture as well as Sugar the horse, Cuddles the cat, Buck the horse, Valentine the cow, and so on. Her attention to detail was captured in the annotations of the pictures: "The trailer where we lived while the house was being built. Later, the clothesline was there, and west of the tree was pop's junk pile" (September 1946). Life on Chancellor Farm seemed to be filled with pastoral bliss; Penny celebrated it by writing songs and poems. At the age of 6, she was given her horse, Sugar. Another little girl, Judy Christmas, brought her horse Buck to board at the farm. Judy and Penny developed a deep friendship based on an imaginary world they created as a context for their adventures on their horses. They lived in imagined stories about hideouts and would play out their fantasies on horseback, romping in the meadows, negotiating the rocks in streams, setting out on co-conceived adventures. When I asked Penny what it was about horseback riding that she found so rewarding, she said,

> You have a certain independence. You can go places other people can't go. And it appeared courageous. I really enjoyed that time of my life with Judy creating stories which we read to each other on the phone.

By the time she was 8 years old, Penny had written six tablets full of stories about the "Big Bend Buckaroos," (BBBs for short), loosely based on a favorite radio show. Each story would have as its protagonist one of the eight

Big Bend Buckaroo gang members, each of whom Penny meticulously classified according to his or her nickname, surname, name of horse, breed of horse, color of horse, name of dog, breed of dog, color of dog, and so on, in a 9-in. × 16-in. matrix. The stories reflected Penny's preoccupation with confrontations between straight-haired country hicks and curly-haired city slickers; the heroic acts of animals who alternately save humans and die in the process; competition in horse shows, in which success must be handled graciously; and natural disasters that threaten the lives of the BBB gang members, who ultimately are survivors. Each book, interestingly, had the same form, 10 or 11 chapters of interlinked stories featuring different BBB members, followed by a neatly drawn and well-organized table of contents, and, at the end, annotated illustrations of story highlights.

Penny gave center stage to others with egalitarian fervor. Her stories celebrated plain people. Animals were major players in Penny's stories. It occurred to me that this childhood occupation of story making seems to reflect an emerging moral identity: beliefs about such polarities as justice and injustice, wisdom and folly, and honor and dishonor (see Sarbin, 1989).

In 1949, just 3 years after the house at Chancellor Farm had been completed, the family was forced to move because of an eminent domain seizure so that the Whittier Narrows Dam could be built. Just as Penny had dealt earlier in her childhood with the loss of her dog by writing a poem honoring Sparky, she again resorted to the childhood occupation of writing to cope with her experience of a new loss. One song ended with this chorus, which is sung to the melody of "Home on the Range."

> Now Chancellor's no more, no more playing galore
> Never more by the stream shall we roam
> It's a memory now and a good one and how
> For we still love our Chancellor home.

Memory in this song becomes a way of retrieving loss, but its existence is not quite enough to assuage Penny's pain and anger. The childhood occupation of writing became a way of venting anger when Penny, a desperate 8-year-old, wrote at the end of one of her stories: "P.S. I'll always hate the dam no matter if it saves thousands of lives. I hope it rots on top of the men who built it."

The family moved to East Whittier in 1949, where Penny felt like an outcast in third grade, then back to the country. But the Mill Street Bridge was washed away, and once again the family moved into downtown Whittier. Here, Penny began to rebuild her life, opening herself up to what city life would offer. She joined a Girl Scout troop and made friends, but stayed connected with the country life she still adored by riding her horse in local gymkhanas, where she won several prizes, and by going on camping trips with her family. At 14, upon graduation from Walter F. Dexter Junior High, she gave the graduation speech, entitled "If you make them, your *dreams* can come true."

From 1955 to 1959, Penny attended Whittier High School, where again occupation marked the memorable events. She did not make the drill team, she was elected to the Girls League Board, and she became editor of her high school newspaper, obviously a natural development of the literary thread in her life. She also joined the CAMYS, a girls' club, some of the members of which became lifelong friends.

She moved on from high school to Pomona College where she finally felt it "was OK to be me, to have a vocabulary of more than two-syllable words, to be literary and excited by ideas." This was also the setting in which she claimed she discovered boys, and they discovered her. Recycling her habit of organization, she kept a calendar of not only the number of dates she had, but also of how many times she had been kissed. She won the freshman creative writing prize at Pomona, earned her bachelor's degree in English Literature, and then went on to Harvard where she earned her master's degree. She taught public school for 5 years, returned to graduate school for a second master's degree in Television and Radio at Syracuse University, and ultimately, at the age of 35, earned her doctoral degree from Syracuse University in Instructional Technology, Educational Policy, and Curriculum. These years of graduate school were also punctuated by a 2-year stint in Lincoln, Nebraska, designing adult telecourses and finding out what the heartland was really about. Next, she took a position as Coordinator of Health, Education, and Welfare's (HEW) Lifelong Learning Project in the Carter Administration. In 1978, she joined the USC faculty of the School of Education; she received tenure in 1985 and became department chair in 1987. As chair she was invested in creating a sense of community, while doing a great deal of campus teaching. Embracing the philosophical stance of adult education, she believed that one should

> treat students with respect and create a kind of collaborative atmosphere for learning. . . . give them a chance to share experiences, because all adults have experiences. Heaven knows . . . not just the teacher telling, but the learners being equal participants.

She was appointed a residential faculty member in a Dean's Hall at USC and was known for throwing cookie parties. She also did consulting for companies such as Atlantic Richfield Company (ARCO), IBM, Encyclopaedia Britannica, and Polaroid Corporation that involved international travel and adventure. In midlife, Penny rediscovered the out-of-doors and went from being a typical woman "who didn't feel [she] should ever have to lift a hand or break a sweat" to getting "into the exciting new world of fitness" and recapturing the connection to nature that she had enjoyed in childhood occupations. She joined the Sierra Club and became absorbed in sports like skiing, mountain hiking, swimming, and, eventually, kayaking.

Grave: The Big A—From This to That

One evening, a middle-aged woman was admitted to the emergency room of a hospital in Hawaii after fainting. The man who brought her in had tried to revive her, to no avail. Shortly thereafter, she was diagnosed as having suffered a subarachnoid hemorrhage due to an aneurysm from the posterior inferior cerebellar artery. Apparently, prior to the infarct, she had had a fabulous week kayaking on the Na Pali coast of Kauai and had returned to Oahu in time for a gourmet meal with the man who admitted her to the hospital, apparently a friend. Her head was shaven, holes were drilled in her skull, and she later underwent several sessions of brain surgery.

Patients seem to materialize in emergency rooms as if they had no history. In the typical medical model, the work of health care practitioners is to fix patients physically, as a mechanic would a car, so that they can get back to functioning. First, the physicians do their part through surgery, medication, and other protocols. Then the nurses monitor progress, manage unexpected changes in the clinical picture, and generally create a climate of caring (Benner, 1984). At a certain point, the patient is moved on to rehabilitation. According to Kaufman (1988), the primary goal of all rehabilitation therapists working with stroke patients is " 'functional independence'—the ability of the patient to care for him or herself as fully as possible with or without assistive devices" (1988, p. 85). Kaufman stated that

> to be sure, physicians and therapists' goals are usually relevant and important to the patient, especially in the first few months following a stroke. However, as time passes, patients are ultimately engaged in a personal struggle for recovery. This goal is subjectively perceived and is not within the scope of physicians' or other providers' interventions. (p. 85)

Were Yerxa and her colleagues at USC (1989) worried that occupational therapy was heading in this direction when they warned that "acute care" was consuming "more and more resources, leaving less available for" occupational therapists to improve "the life opportunities of people with chronic disease and disability" (p. 2)? They described a health care system that seems "to have adopted an assembly line mentality," in which "occupational therapists are viewed as treatment machines and patients as products which can be displayed on a balance sheet" (p. 2). Penny remembered being wheeled down long corridors to rehabilitation where she would take her place in line with other victims, aimlessly sitting, until her turn came to be wheeled into the therapy room. She dutifully performed the routines they showed her; the therapy session ended, and she remembered once again being inserted into a line of wheelchairs to reexperience waiting her turn to be wheeled back to her room. She felt passive, disempowered, and not quite human, as therapists rushed around, caught up in their routine with no time to connect with the survivor as a person. She knew they were doing their best, but she felt resentful and angry. She was beginning to recognize that nature, fate, and social structures had intersected in such a way that she was now in a new slot, for, to some extent, identity is contingent on circumstance. Her hospital room walls were covered with cards she had received from friends, family, and loved ones, for which she was extremely grateful.

On the wall also was a schedule of USC Trojan football games, a symbol of her former life situation and a catalyst for connecting her physician to her personhood, as he was an avid Michigan State fan and she was a Trojan fan.

Also, the physician and her mother discovered their mutual love of golf, the outcome of which was greater rapport, a line of connectiveness scaffolded by common occupational interests. Yerxa et al. (1989) stated that people are "most true to their humanity when engaged in occupation" (p. 7).

Penny remembered the occupational and physical therapists as very helpful and caring people, although she had difficulty sorting out who was what. She thought everybody saw her as a miracle patient because she should have died, but did not. Overall, she remembered her hospital stay as a happy time, because the staff members were responsive, pleased with her progress, and encouraging. In fact, she truly remembered being the center of attention. At one point, she had a tube inserted through her mouth to her stomach; to communicate she had to write little notes.

Penny could hardly remember what she had done in the early phases of rehabilitation, as if they had been experienced as insignificant episodes, because they seemed to have no purpose. While she was in the hospital, she believed that one day she would be normal again, but she questioned the soundness of the therapeutic procedures. "It was just little stuff. It didn't make one feel tired, and it wasn't demanding."

She recounted an episode toward the end of her rehabilitation in the hospital when she vocally questioned whether she was making sufficient progress and got upset about it. "The therapists really knocked themselves out at that point. They got very positive, and started pushing me to walk on the parallel bars." Even then, however, she did not experience therapy as sufficiently demanding. What she had hoped for was that she would be able to set goals for herself so that she could have a sense of progress toward something and that the therapists, like personal coaches, would work with her to achieve them. Their obvious kindness, while very much appreciated, was not sufficient for one bent on complete recovery.

As time unfolded, Penny was discharged from inpatient rehabilitation and became an outpatient. Now she and her mother traveled several times a week in Los Angeles traffic so that she could participate in outpatient occupational and physical therapy. To stay committed, according to Mattingly (1991), Penny would have had to see how the treatment would move her into a future that she cared to gain. Penny viewed the sessions as disconnected from her project of recovery. If occupational therapy and physical therapy goals had been set by the therapists, she had not been cognizant of them. They would do things in therapy to her, but she was unable to reproduce those things on her own at home. She was unable to practice, to use her own initiative, to get well on her own time. Ultimately, she felt the therapists did not take responsibility for enabling her to do things on her own. They seemed quite happy just to send her off, and have her come back, in a seemingly neverending cycle without a forward-moving plot. At some point she was discharged, which gave her the sense that she had hit a plateau:

> I feel they abandoned me, and I feel that they did their thing. . . . but their thing was to do their things, not to help me do the things for myself. And so, in a sense, they kept control of the situation. I was not empowered to do it on my own. They did it with me and in a sense flunked me.

This part of Penny's story raises the question of the purpose of the concept of the plateau. What really is behind the statement that the survivor no longer can benefit from therapy? Is it a literal statement, or are the words used to conceal the reality that the patient has psychologically outgrown the rehabilitation context, can no longer tolerate it, and feels the urge to move on? Rather than relinquish control, the rehabilitation medical team makes the discharge decision, and the patient is now on her own, and must, at this arbitrary point, fend for herself. Or could the statement be a kind of code that actually serves third-party providers more than survivors?

Taylor (1970) and Crepeau (1993) likened certain hospital practices to ritual. After hearing a talk given by the anthropologist Alexander Moore, I realized that Penny's rehabilitation experience contained elements of a rite of passage as it is classically described in the anthropological literature (A. Moore, 1992). Rites of passage carry persons from one stage of life to the next and are thought of as having three phases: separation, transition, and reincorporation (A. Moore, 1992; Van Gennep, 1960). In the separation phase, the participant is separated from her old state. The transition phase is marked by the quality that Turner called "liminality" (1964, 1969). Moore described it as a state in which the participant is reduced "to his lowest common denominator" and most give up all the trappings of their former selves; "one is betwixt and between, neither what one was nor what one shall become" (A. Moore, 1992, p. 133). When this phase is completed, the participant begins the task of reentering the world from which she had been separated. Later, I discovered that Murphy and his colleagues had actually published papers that described not only the rehabilitation process, but the entire experience of disability as a kind of liminal state (Murphy, 1987; Murphy, Scheer, Murphy, & Mack, 1988).

Penny's description of her rehabilitation experience suggested that it had had a liminal quality. Her previous identity was not taken into account, except very superficially; she was stripped of her history; and she remained suspended in limbo until she was discharged and on her own. Then she had to focus on trying to reincorporate herself into the world from which she had been separated. The rehabilitation rite of passage seemed to have moved her along into the stage of her life in which she would live as a person with disability. Soon she realized that her disability was a barrier for others. Reincorporation meant going back to work at the university, but no longer being selected for off-campus courses; no longer participating in decision making because her department had been dissolved in her absence; and stoically observing some of her colleagues and friends gradually "wiggle" away.

In this new stage of her life, she felt she was being subjected to a lot of unintentional abuse. People ignored or made an outcast of her. She would sit in her office and nobody would come in, unlike before. People seemed embarrassed to interact with her and were without an etiquette for dealing with a person who had undergone this kind of transformation. Hardly anyone asked how she was, and if someone did, the answer was supposed to be "just fine." She stated: "Nobody really wanted to know. So the thing about 'laugh and the world laughs with you, cry and you cry alone,' I really know what that means."

One day she went to shop for a bathing suit at an outdoor equipment store she used to frequent and she had an important insight, "that occupations were important because they marked the new you versus the old you." There she was, poking through the racks of swimsuits, surrounded by ski and hiking equipment. Three years had transpired since the Big A. For a moment she flashed back to an earlier time when she had rented her skis for a ski weekend and backpacks for a mountain hike from this store. She thought; "Gosh, that used to be me. . . .Now my outdoor experience is lurching to take the trash out. I enjoy it, but it's all that I do." It was an emotion-ridden moment, and she began to cry wildly. The reaction presented itself suddenly: "There I was, sobbing my little heart out because I was in [the store] and I couldn't ski anymore." She had liked her old self just fine; but now she was struggling with "trying to be whatever I could of the old me, but becoming this new me if I had to."

Grande: Nurturing the Human Spirit to Act

At the time of the Big A, Elinor Richardson flew to Hawaii to be at her daughter's side; she had been living alone since 1970, when her husband Bud had died. Having had a successful career as an educator, she was now retired and had become a consultant in educational television. She also enjoyed a rich array of avocations and social activities. Among these, golf was her favorite. In one night's time, Elinor's life was radically changed. She worried that she would lose her daughter. Thomas Moore wrote that "all mothering . . . is made up of both affectionate caring and bitter emotional pain" (1992, p. 43). In Greek mythology, Demeter, the mother of Persephone who descends into darkness, symbolizes survival, "the profound maternal feeling in us for life, continuity, and fruitfulness" (T. Moore, 1992, p. 48). Nature and fate combined to reunite Penny and Elinor, and Elinor realized she would be taking on a new assignment: helping her daughter get well. She was the enduring presence who had known her daughter as an adventurous horseback rider and a member of an imaginary gang, the Big Bend Buckaroos. For 40 years, Elinor had saved the poems, stories, songs, and drawings that her literary and artistic child had produced, and had taken pride and delight in Penny's academic accomplishments as a mature woman. She, more than anyone else at the hospital that day, grasped the significance of what had happened, of the extent of damage and disruption. For the next 4 years, she would be with her daughter virtually every day. Inside, she knew her daughter had the spirit, if Penny could muster it, to move forward.

Elinor remembers the moment when Penny first wiggled a toe and when she choked on a piece of broccoli during a feeding session, an indicator that therapy should have begun with applesauce. By December 1989, Elinor had moved in with Penny, becoming her full-time caregiver. "It was very slow . . . steps backward instead of steps forward," Elinor said. One year later, Penny was eating whatever she wanted, was back to teaching, and was using a motorized scooter. A year after that, she could use a walker and was independent in all activities of daily living. Throughout this 2½-year period, Elinor also drove Penny to medical appointments and therapy sessions. "The individuals made an impression on me, but not the therapy that much."

Before her stroke, Penny would often have students over for cookie parties. Now Elinor assisted Penny in continuing this tradition. Penny said the following about these occasions. "We had afternoon cookie parties; we had evening cookie parties; we had out-in-the-lobby cookie parties; and it didn't matter; it always worked because there is something about sharing food in a home environment that works." This statement echoed the motif of Mr. Richardson's stew.

In the fall of 1992, Elinor and Penny bought and moved to a new townhome several blocks from campus. Just before that, in the spring of 1992, I was named the Eleanor Clarke Slagle Lecturer. In the fall I visited Penny at the new condo and invited her to collaborate with me on what I mistakenly thought would be limited to an ethnography of the relationship of her childhood occupations to her experience of recovery. Having been interested in developing my friendship with Penny, I had visited her many times over the course of her recovery. Informed by occupational science concepts, I had invited her to do activities that I thought would give her a sense of connection with her former self: a lecture by the sculptor J. Seward Johnson that celebrated ordinary activity as captured in art, an elegant lunch at the Four Seasons Hotel, a swim in a large 1940s vintage swimming pool in the women's gymnasium at USC, an occupational science symposium that featured the physicist Stephen Hawking as keynote speaker. I also encouraged her to attend lectures and social gatherings at which I would be present. As I had hoped, our friendship developed over time. When I invited her to collaborate on this project, she, a bit reluctantly, said yes, so that something good might come out of her awful experience.

We began our work on October 11, 1992, but, as the ethnography evolved, it soon became clear that I had begun to function as her occupational therapist, through encouraging her to tell her story and by helping her to imagine new possibilities. Nature had stripped Penny of many aspects of her old self, but fate had worked to assemble in her world people who were committed to helping and supporting her. Most individuals with disability probably do not develop to their full capacity because the development of human potential is, like identity, also contingent on circumstance. It is unlikely that most survivors of stroke possess the resources of an upper-middle-class family, have a retired mother positioned to dedicate her life to caregiving, and, on top of this, just happen to have a friend who is an occupational therapist. I began to view my role as similar to that of the coach of an elite athlete or ballet student, for, unlike most people who only develop a fraction of their ability, ballet dancers, Olympic athletes, and persons with disability must push themselves to the edge of their capacity and therefore need someone to coach them along the way. Perhaps, in part, it is because traditional occupational therapy is now so constricted by place and time, so decontextualized from the person's real life, that the statistics on independence of persons with disability are not more encouraging (Bergmann, Küthmann, Ungern-Sternberg, & Weimann, 1991; Cavazos, 1989; Dombovy, Sandok, & Basford, 1986; Howard, Till, Toole, Matthews, & Truscott, 1985; Kraus & Stoddard, 1991; Schaffer & Osberg, 1990).

I will now give a sort of coda of how occupational therapy unfolds when it is grounded in occupational science, and the progression through which I became a therapist–coach. This analysis can only capture the highlights of the process as they were interpreted by Penny, me, and our research assistant. Soon after we had begun the interview process, Penny realized that the sessions were therapeutic because they gave her a chance to reflect on her situation "with another person who has insights of her own into this, who is well-read, intelligent, and sympathetic . . . but not someone who pities me or just feels sorry for me or is trying to change me."

As time went on, Penny's view of how the sessions came to be therapeutic was further crystallized:

> One of the reasons I enjoy our conversations is because I put things into words. . . . and then they become intentions and I have this sort of an emerging plan towards things that I am going to do, that I just think up on the spot, and then I think about them afterwards and I think OK . . . yeah, get on with it, Penny.

At one point I asked her how I might approach teaching my colleagues how to do this form of occupational therapy. She responded by saying, "I think you can say, well [during clinical practice], pretend this is a research project and that you are going to take them [the survivors] through this exercise because it ends up being very therapeutic." Penny now saw our process as

> an investigation of my status and it gives me something interesting to think about. It has given me some new ways, all of which have had, the thing in common is that it has put me in charge, it has made me get to direct, conduct, if you like, my life.

We agreed that *recomposition,* modifying a term used by Bateson (1990), best captured what had been going on. The conversations were very free-flowing; they built one upon the next, and themes would emerge and then be recycled in modified forms in the next transcript, much as certain motifs unify the movements of a symphony in time. The discourse could be classified as Occupational Storytelling and Occupational Story Making.

Occupational Storytelling

Occupational science assumes that adult character and competence are shaped through childhood occupations (Clark et al., 1991; Primeau, Clark, & Pierce, 1989; Yerxa et al., 1989).

Another way of describing the process, based on the work of the French philosopher Foucault (cited in Rabinow, 1984), is to think of the self as formed, in part through its history of activities and conduct. It is not enough, he believed, to focus on the symbolic systems, the person is "constituted in real practices—historically analyzable practices" (p. 368). A crucial element of the recomposition process was to ground the work in Penny's occupational historicity. One interview had been focused almost entirely on tales of her childhood occupations and her experience in the world of adult activity. I have already presented much of the content of this interview in Movement 1, the *Allegro Spirituoso* of this paper. Interpretation of these stories gave me a feeling for Penny's spirit and a sense of her values. I came to respect her moral stances. Simply stated, I learned what she cared about, about the things that had always mattered in her life. Horseback riding symbolized independence and creativity; adventures with Judy Christmas, exciting opportunities for risk-taking; and the stories of Chancellor Farm, literary celebrations of nature, animals, and the cultural collisions of urban and pastoral life styles.

I was struck by how hard working, organized, and imaginative she had been as a child. She had not simply fantasized BBB episodes; she also took the time to write about them and nearly everything else of significance in her life. She had always been extraordinarily industrious, a person who, while free-spirited, also got an enormous amount accomplished. These were aspects of her character that now seemed dormant but which, I hoped, could be reawakened. It seemed that just after her stroke, she had needed to be totally invested in getting well, physically. Now she was ready to tackle other problems. In retrospect, I think when Penny told me the tales of her childhood, we were in the genre of what Mattingly (1991) called the storytelling facet of clinical reasoning, but, in this case, the stories were explicitly constructed around the theme of occupation. I therefore call this practice *occupational storytelling*. Every patient has important stories of childhood occupations that influence who they are today. Occupational storytelling is a means by which therapists better understand the spirit of the survivors with whom they work.

Occupational Story Making

The second type of clinical reasoning Mattingly (1991) described is story making, which involves the therapist and survivor creating stories that are enacted in the future, rather than telling them. I think it is fair to classify the second practice in this therapeutic approach as occupational story making. I knew that when Penny and I began the project, we would find ourselves in the middle of an unfolding story about her as an occupational being, but I had no idea how the subplots would evolve.

As it turns out, upon coding, I realized that this form of therapy departed from customary practice in that no mention was made of diagnostic categories, strengths or weaknesses, or assets or liabilities. Also, neither Penny nor I, nor both of us collaboratively, set goals for her. Instead, she identified the *problematiques* (a word borrowed from

Foucault; cited in Rabinow, p. 343) that were most disturbing in her life, and then she would search for and eventually enact solutions. For Foucault, problematiques are things in relation to which one feels threatened or endangered; they are not quite the same as bad things. He maintained that if things were dangerous, one would "always have something to do" (p. 343).

Through the interview process, Penny identified the overarching problematique in her life at the time: the moral imperative to fight against consignment to a disability role. Although she was now able to walk with a walker and was independent in activities of daily living, she was still fighting bouts of depression, the disclosure of which she believed threatened her social acceptability. She felt walled off, divided from the world of persons without disabilities, ignored, and disempowered. In one session she admitted that, like "Brer Rabbit he lay low," she was resorting to "hiding" as much as she could in the many work and social situations in which she felt threatened. Interestingly, before the Big A, she had been able to envision herself in the future as an active, nature-loving senior citizen, but she could no longer do this; she felt she had been "frozen over." It seemed that Penny was longing to move on by attacking this overarching problematique. She then broke it down into several more finely graded problematiques: a more manageable state in which she was able to invent solutions. The process by which she began to resolve two of these more finely graded problematiques is discussed below.

Problematique 1: How can I build an image of myself that bridges the old and the new me? After I had verbally painted some pictures to her of persons with disability who transcended stereotypes, Penny began to realize that she had the power to recompose her identity into one with which she would be comfortable; she simply did not have to allow herself to be slotted into the status of disabled, at least not entirely. In another interview, I drew parallels between aging and disability, giving Penny a sense of the ways in which disability overlapped with a process that we all undergo. On her own, she decided that one solution to this problematique would be to wean herself from the walker, which clanked and seemed to be a physical barrier to others; this solution inspired her to push herself to become competent using a cane. Recycling the motif of hiking (what Jackson [in press] would call recycling a theme of meaning), Penny began what she called "cane hiking." It occupied her every evening, and soon she was able to shed the clunky walker, a stigmatizing piece of orthopedic paraphernalia she had detested, for a cane. Initially, she was exceedingly proud of this accomplishment, but soon she needed to move on. The chrome cane with the orange rubber handle was a small, but still obvious, emblem of disability. In a conversation during which she told a dear friend of this milestone, the friend pointed out that in Britain the cane is a fashion accessory, and that she might like to take a trip to London (another occupation) to buy a cane at a shop in which the proprietor had gathered more than 13,000 canes. When Penny told me this story, I thought it was fabulous, and shared with her that Margaret Mead had used a cane and, as legend has it, would shake it at her students. Penny's friend, it turned out, had also mentioned that canes were wonderful because you could shake them at people.

This simple telephone conversation had a snowballing effect on our image-building process. The idea of the cane led us to play with the idea of building her new image around that of the British academic woman, as she continued to cane hike to further develop her ambulation. She now wanted to shop for clothes through which to embody this new image. In this way, the solutions to a problematique inspired new occupations. One day Penny called me ecstatically to tell me that she had forgotten both her walker and her cane on that day's shopping excursion, so she had taken the risk and walked without either all afternoon! To celebrate, we had an ice cream party, and several weeks later we went shopping in Los Angeles for an elegant British cane, the symbol of her new persona. She was no longer the person slinking around in the shadows. She was no longer hiding. She next moved on to the project of getting a driver's license. She contacted Rancho Los Amigos Medical Center and enrolled in the driving program. She described the occupational therapist as wonderful as they worked jointly on Penny's new project. Her brother Steve was delighted to take Penny for practice driving sessions in which she could perfect driving strategies she had begun to master in occupational therapy.

Problematique 2: How can I begin to take command in my world of social relationships when I feel so rejected? Interestingly, the process of image reconstruction inadvertently served as a partial solution to this problematique. During her cane hikes, Penny would encounter her neighbors who lived in the condominium complex. Just as she had once classified individuals as city slickers and country hicks, she divided condominium residents into those who were comfortable with her condition and those who were not. She then invented a kind of game of converting people into what she called "condo comrades" through handling discourse in a variety of clever, engaging, and humorous ways. This was her application of an idea that I had expressed, that wherever I went, I would search out the people who could be therapeutic for me. "Condo hiking" became a bridge to a world of social support and led to reincorporation into the social world from which the Big A had separated her.

Other solutions to this problematique led to an even richer round of occupations. The image of the British academic inspired Penny to buy a pair of season tickets to the opera. She had always loved opera and now planned to invite friends to join her in this occupation, which was a symbol of her past cultural situation and a medium through which she could give to others. She also decided to enroll in a gourmet cooking class and comically envisioned inviting friends to home-cooked gourmet meals: If they did not like the food, she would shake her cane at them. This was a particularly surprising solution since she had not been to a supermarket for nearly 4 years.

In summary, through occupational storytelling and occupational story making, Penny identified the problematiques of her immediate experience. To these she found solutions that resulted in engagement in a wide array of occupations; occupations that joined the old self and the new self that she was recomposing. We collaborated in the process: She had provided me with a sense of her historicity and identified the problematiques that were most pressing and their solutions. I helped her to do that by reminding her of her progress, making suggestions, probing her values, reflecting my interpretations of our discourse back to her, and listening in a way that conveyed my profound interest in her story. I also spent a good amount of time sharing my knowledge about the power of occupation in life recomposition, to give her a framework for how to use occupation in her recovery process. In the end, she moved into the world of activity, not as a disabled person lurching in the background, trying to be invisible, but as a slightly lame sort of British aristocrat in full command of her destiny. She had possessed her life in a new way.

Conclusion

I have presented results of work that is in the genre of interpretive occupational science. Donald Polkinghorne's book *Narrative Knowing and the Human Sciences,* along with his guidance, gave me the courage to develop a paper of this kind and provided an overall framework for this narrative interpretation. The methodology also combined elements of life history ethnography (Frank, 1979, 1984; Mandelbaum, 1973), ethnomethodology (Garfinkel, 1967), narrative analysis (Bruner, 1989, 1990a; Polkinghorne, 1988; Rosaldo, 1989) and the naturalistic approach used to study professional practice by Mattingly (1989) and Schön (1983). My colleague Michael Carlson and I (1991) suggested several years ago that innovative and unique methods would need to be developed to tackle the research questions posed by occupational science. I believe that the methodology used in the present study, which draws on the various qualitative approaches I have listed, is an example of one uniquely designed for occupational science inquiry.

My colleague, the anthropologist Gelya Frank, who pioneered use of the rich anthropological tradition of life history method with a woman who had a severe disability, in a dyadic context, wrote that the methods for which she is known can "offer images of the lives over time of persons with disabilities in their natural circumstances and settings, against which clinical practice can be reflected" (1984, p. 640). In another paper (Frank, 1979), she distinguished life histories from autobiographies. Unlike the latter, she pointed out, life history represents a collaboration of the investigator and the informant and reflects the consciousness of both. I believe that the method that Penny and I created for the present study also possesses these qualities that Frank described.

My mentor, Elizabeth J. Yerxa (1991), has presented compelling ethical and epistemological arguments for why qualitative methods are highly suited for occupational science. Her thinking is congruent with that of Geertz (1973), the renowned anthropologist, who stated that "Man is an animal suspended in webs of significance he himself has spun. I take culture to be one of those webs, and the analysis of it to be therefore not an experimental science in search of laws, but an interpretive one in search of meaning" (p. 5). If the concept of culture requires an interpretive science, so too does the narrower cultural construct of occupation.

This lecture has demonstrated how interpretive occupational science research speaks to practice, not by discovery of general laws or principles, but by providing thick descriptions of actual cases that practitioners can refer to as they submerge themselves in practice. I believe Penny Richardson's story can inform practice in the way that a series of relationships might inform a future decision about a mate. Just as we learn from each of the previous relationships, so too can we learn by collecting thickly described stories, grounded in an epistemology that respects subjectivity. Palmer (1987) has argued that all epistemologies end in a set of ethics: "Every way of knowing tends to become a way of living" (p. 22). He has written that objectivism "breeds intellectual habits" that "destroy a sense of community," making objects of one another and "the world to be manipulated for our own private ends" (p. 22). Unlike objectivism, which leans toward promoting competitive individualism, subjectivism, when handled sensitively, encourages friendship, rapport, and equality. Because I was her friend, Penny shared her story, and soon I became a sort of Judy Christmas in her adulthood. However, our stories were less about the BBBs—they were more directly about Penny Richardson as an occupational being.

In occupational science, occupations are defined as chunks of daily activity that fill the stream of time and can be named in the lexicon of the culture (Clark et al., 1991; Yerxa et al., 1989). As cultural phenomena they have been celebrated in the legacy of artists and craftsmen throughout history. Just as each civilization invented culturally specific occupations as solutions to their issues of lifestyle and survival, people place occupations within the framework of their lives. A crucial role for the occupational therapist, therefore, is to help survivors define their problematiques and find solutions. Occupational therapists cannot be expected to do detailed and time-consuming ethnographies in the clinic, but they can make occupational storytelling and occupational story making the core of their clinical reasoning as a way to nurture the human spirit to act.

Acknowledgments

I thank the Bureau of Maternal and Child Health, Department of Health and Human Services (Grant #MCJ 009048-10) for its support of this project. I also thank the American Occupational Therapy Foundation for its support of the AOTF Center for Scholarship and Research at the University of Southern California: The Relationship of Occupation to Adaptation and Its Implications for Occupational Therapy. I am deeply grateful to Shan-Pin Fanchiang, Bridget Larson, my friend Marian Karsjens, my daughter Sara Clark, and my husband John Wolcott for their unprecedented help and support. I also wish to express my deep appreciation to Penny Richardson and to Elinor Richardson. This lecture is dedicated to Elizabeth J. Yerxa, my mentor and the founder of occupational science.

Editor's Note

Penelope L. Richardson died of a second brain hemorrhage on August 1, 1993, 5 weeks after the presentation of the Eleanor Clarke Slagle Lecture.

References

Bateson, M. C. (1990). *Composing a life.* New York: Plume.

Benner, P. (1984). *From novice to expert: Excellence and power in clinical therapy practice.* Reading, MA: Addison-Wesley.

Bergmann, H., Küthmann, M., Ungern-Sternberg, A. V., & Weimann, V. G. (1991). Medical educational functional determinants of employment after stroke. *Journal of Neural Transmission, 33* (Suppl), 157–161.

Bruner, J. (1989). *Actual minds, possible worlds.* Cambridge, MA: Harvard University Press.

Bruner, J. (1990a). *Acts of meaning.* Cambridge, MA: Harvard University Press.

Bruner, J. (1990b). Unnamed lecture at conference entitled *The Notion of Knowing in the Social Sciences (Part II). Boundaries and Departures,* January 22, 1990, University of Southern California, Los Angeles.

Carlson, M., & Clark, F. A. (1991). The search for useful methodologies in occupational science. *American Journal of Occupational Therapy, 45,* 235–241.

Cavazos, L. F. (1989, March). *Chartbook on disability in the United States.* Prepared for U.S. Department of Education, Contract # HN 88011001. Washington, DC: National Institute on Disability and Rehabilitation Research.

Clark, F., Parham, D., Carlson, M. E., Frank, G., Jackson, J., Pierce, D., Wolfe, R. J., & Zemke, R. (1991). Occupational science: Academic innovation in the service of occupational therapy's future. *American Journal of Occupational Therapy, 45,* 300–310.

Crepeau, E. B. (1993). *Ritual and routine: An ethnographic study of geropsychiatric team meetings.* Paper presented at the Sixth Annual Occupational Science Symposium: Narrative and Action. University of Southern California, April 14, 1993. Los Angeles, CA.

Dombovy, M. L., Sandok, M. D., & Basford, J. R. (1986). Rehabilitation for stroke: A review. *Stroke, 17,* 363–369.

Frank, G. (1979). Finding the common denominator: A phenomenological critique of life history method. *Ethos, 7*(1), 68–93.

Frank, G. (1984). Life history model of adaptation to disability: The case of a congenital amputee. *Social Science Medicine, 19,* 639–645.

Frank, G. (1986). On embodiment: A case study of congenital limb deficiency in American culture. *Culture, Medicine, and Psychiatry, 10,* 189–219.

Garfinkel, H. (1967). *Studies in ethnomethodology.* Englewood Cliffs, NJ: Prentice-Hall.

Geertz, C. (1973). Thick description: Toward an interpretive theory of culture. In C. Geertz, *The interpretation of cultures.* New York: Basic.

Howard, G., Till, J. S., Toole, J. F., Matthews, C., & Truscott, B. L. (1985). Factors influencing return to work following cerebral infarction. *Journal of the American Medical Association, 253,* 226–232.

Jackson, J. (in press). Living a meaningful existence in old age. In F. Clark & R. Zemke (Eds.), *Occupational science: The first five years.* Philadelphia: F. A. Davis.

Kaufman, S. R. (1988). Stroke rehabilitation and the negotiation of identity. In S. Reinhartz & G. Rowles (Eds.), *Qualitative gerontology* (pp. 82–103). New York: Spring.

Kraus, L. E., & Stoddard, S. (1991, September). *Chartbook on work disability in the United States.* U.S. Department of Education, Contract # HN 89032001. Washington, DC: National Institute on Disability and Rehabilitation Research.

Kundera, M. (1991). *Immortality* (P. Kussi, Trans.). New York: Grove Weidenfeld.

Mandelbaum, D. G. (1973). The study of life history: Ghandi. *Current Anthropology, 14,* 177–206.

Mattingly, C. F. (1989). *Thinking with stories: Story and experience in a clinical practice.* Unpublished doctoral dissertation, Massachusetts Institute of Technology.

Mattingly, C. (1991). The narrative nature of clinical reasoning. *American Journal of Occupational Therapy, 45,* 998–1005.

Moore, A. (1992). *Cultural anthropology: The field study of human beings.* San Diego: Collegiate.

Moore, T. (1992). *Care of the soul. A guide for cultivating depth and sacredness in everyday life.* New York: Harper-Collins.

Murphy, R. F. (1987). *The body silent.* New York: Norton.

Murphy, R. F., Scheer, J., Murphy, Y., & Mack, R. (1988). Physical disability and social liminality: A study in the rituals of adversity. *Social Science and Medicine, 26*(2), 235–242.

Palmer, P. J. (1987, September/October). Community, conflict, and ways of knowing. *Change,* 20–25.

Polkinghorne, D. E. (1988). *Narrative knowing and the human sciences.* Albany, NY: State University of New York Press.

Primeau, L. A., Clark, F., & Pierce, D. (1989). Occupational science alone has looked upon occupation: Future applications of occupational science to the health care needs of parents and children. *Occupational Therapy in Health Care, 6*(4), 19–32.

Rabinow, P. (Ed.). (1984). *Foucault reader.* New York: Pantheon.

Reilly, M. (1962). Occupational therapy can be one of the great ideas of twentieth century medicine. The 1961 Eleanor Clarke Slagle Lecture. *American Journal of Occupational Therapy, 16,* 1–19.

Rosaldo, R. (1989). *Culture and truth.* Boston: Beacon.

Ruddick, S. (1982). Maternal thinking. In B. Thorne & M. Yalom (Eds.), *Rethinking the family: Some feminist questions* (pp. 76–94). New York: Longman.

Sarbin, T. R. (1989). Emotions as narrative employments. In M. J. Packer & R. B. Addison (Eds.), *Entering the circle: Hermeneutic investigation in psychology* (pp. 185–201). Albany, NY: State University of New York Press.

Schaffer, R. M., & Osberg, J. S. (1990). Return to work after stroke: Development of a predictive model. *Archives of Physical Medicine and Rehabilitation, 71,* 285–290.

Schön, D. A. (1983). *The reflective practitioner: How professionals think in action.* New York: Basic.

Taylor, C. (1970). *In horizontal orbit. Hospitals in the cult of efficiency.* New York: Holt, Rinehart & Winston.

Turner, V. (1964). Betwixt and between: The liminal period in rites of passage. Proceedings of the American Ethnological Society. Reprinted in W. Lessa & E. Vogt (Eds.). (1972). *Reader in comparative religion: An anthropological approach* (3rd ed., pp. 338–347). New York: Harper & Row.

Turner, V. (1969). *The retiral process: Structure and anti-structure.* Chicago: Aldine.

Van Gennep, A. (1960). *The rites of passage* (M. B. Vizedom & G. L. Caffee, Trans.). Chicago: Chicago University Press.

Yerxa, E. J. (1991). Seeking a relevant, ethical, and realistic way of knowing for occupational therapy. *American Journal of Occupational Therapy, 45,* 199–204.

Yerxa, E. J., Clark, F., Frank, G., Jackson, J., Parham, D., Pierce, D., Stein, C., & Zemke, R. (1989). An introduction to occupational science, A foundation for occupational therapy in the 21st century. In J. Johnson & E. J. Yerxa (Eds.), *Occupational science: The foundation for new models of practice* (pp. 1–18). New York: Haworth.

43

1994 Eleanor Clarke Slagle Lecture

Building Inclusive Community:
A *Challenge for Occupational Therapy*

Ann P. Grady, MA, OTR, FAOTA

Preparation of the Eleanor Clarke Slagle Lecture promotes reflection on the values and philosophy of occupational therapy. I chose the topic *Building Inclusive Community: A Challenge for Occupational Therapy* because it provided me with an opportunity to explore my own values and the values of the profession regarding inclusion of all persons into the community they choose and into the world community at large. The topic particularly led me to review my own work in adaptation theory developed with Elnora Gilfoyle (Gilfoyle, Grady, & Moore, 1990) in light of changes occurring or being promoted in society regarding opportunities for inclusion of all persons in all aspects of living. Ideas about inclusion; the meaning of community; the relationship between environment and community; the interaction between a person's past experience, present situation, and future hopes and dreams and its effect on the relationship that develops between an occupational therapist and a person seeking therapy services all became focal points for exploring our role in building inclusive community. The result has been some expansion of our understanding of the environment category of the spatiotemporal adaptation theory and exploration of the relationship between environment and community. In addition, exploring the concepts of the theory led to consideration of its relevance for enhancing our ability to plan with consumers of service who are creating or returning to their own community. Focal points for exploring the challenges related to building inclusive community include

- An understanding of the meaning of community building within a person's own environment and according to his or her choices.
- A review of current ideas about the nature of disability in relation to both philosophy and mandates for inclusion.
- An expansion of ideas about the role of environment in a person's adaptation to community living.
- A consideration of strategies for promoting choice and inclusion.

For as far back in time as we know, human beings have gathered together to share in daily living and use some form of symbols as means for communicating with each other, hence the building of community (Dance & Larson, 1972). To this day, we share meaning in our communities through symbols composed of pictures, words spoken in our own culturally determined language, and gestures or nonverbal expressions of our thoughts or feelings. Native Americans in the southwestern regions of our country choose to tell the stories of their community living and beliefs through petroglyphs, or rock art (Patterson-Rudolph, 1993). One expert in petroglyphs compared attempts at identifying subject matter and its significance to cloud watching in that no two people will interpret what they see in the same way. Petroglyphs were apparently not intended to represent words of a language as we know it, but instead were meant to convey more general concepts or global ideas about the society, such as ideas about religion, medicine, governance, art, war, and peace. An artist's rendition of petroglyphs

Originally published 1995 in *American Journal of Occupational Therapy, 49,* 300–310.

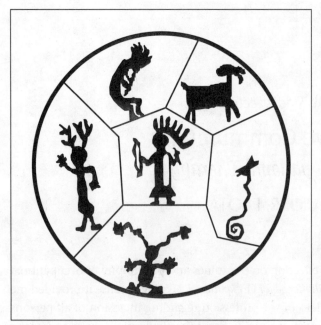

Figure 43.1. Circle of Friends petroglyph.
Note. Original metal sculpture by Kevin Smith, Golden, Colorado. Appears with permission of Kevin Smith.

titled "Circle of Friends" (see Figure 43.1) is chosen to represent ideas about community and inclusion that are central to the themes of this article. In rock art, spirals, concentric circles, and other geometric shapes are interpreted to be universal symbols used to convey conceptual ideas (Patterson, 1992). There are dozens of possible interpretations connected to each figure in the circle because rock art is interpreted not only according to the individual symbols present, but also by the figures that are combined in a panel, just like words in spoken language. For me, the Circle of Friends represents the encompassing nature of a community, whether it is the community that each of us constructs for ourselves or the larger environment in which we discover ourselves. The circle represents the wholeness of a community, and the figures relate to diversity that can exist within the community. Just as the circle is considered a symbol of inclusion and wholeness, the extension of the circle as a spiral is well known as a symbol of growth and continuity. Spirals frequently appear as symbols of continuity in Native American culture (Patterson, 1992). The spiral reflects evolution and renewal with growth emanating from continuous learning and new challenges. The spiral and its embedded circles will be used in this article to represent change and continuity.

Why is the idea of building inclusive community important to us as people and as occupational therapists? The idea is both profound and simple. Simply, we believe that people belong together regardless of real or perceived differences. All persons have the right to choose where they wish to live, work, learn, and play, and with whom they wish to spend time. On a deeper level, we believe that people belong together *because* of differences. There is a richness that characterizes a community constructed with appreciation for both differences and similarities among its members. The idea is not new, but as Winston Churchill said, "Men [and women] stumble over the truth from time to time, but most pick themselves up and hurry off as if nothing had happened" (McWilliams, 1994, p. 413).

The Nature of Community and Choice

Community provides a context for actualizing individual potential and experiencing oneness with others (McLaughlin & Davidson, 1985). The human condition yearns for a greater sense of connectedness, expressed as a need to reach out, deeply touch others, and throw off the pain and loneliness of separation. The term *community* encompasses *communication* and *unity*. Yankelovitch said that the community evokes in the individual the feeling that "here is where I belong—these are my people, I care for them, they care for me, I am part of them, I know what they expect from me and I from them, they share my concerns. I know this place, I am on familiar ground, I am at home" (1981, p. 224).

There are established communities such as towns, neighborhoods, schools, and workplaces, and there are personal communities we create for ourselves, which include family, friends, acquaintances, how and where we spend our time formally or informally, and the relationships we build over time. Our personal communities do not necessarily depend on specific location or specific time, although they are often embedded in established communities. Building inclusive community refers to both the larger, more formal community context and the smaller, informal community that a person identifies as a personal community. Ideas about diversity and inclusion in community in this article apply to all people, but we as occupational ther-apists have particular concerns for assuring choice in com-munity living for persons with disabilities and chronic health problems, as well as persons for whom disability and health issues can be prevented.

Personal community building begins at the center of the circle, where the person is embedded in family and close relationships (see Figure 43.2). Networks of informal support develop in the center of a personal community. Relationships grow because persons choose to be connected. The unique culture of personal community is created from family experience. Values are established: heritage, myths, and traditions are communicated. The foundation for build-ing personal community is established within the family.

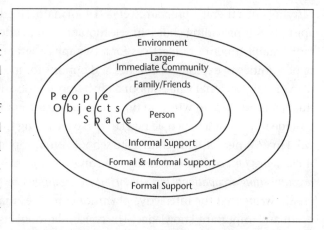

Figure 43.2. Personal community building.

> We all come from families. Families are big, small, extended, nuclear, multigenerational, with one parent, two par-ents, and grandparents. We live under one roof or many. A family can be as temporary as a few weeks, as perma-nent as forever. We become part of a family by birth, adoption, marriage, or from a desire for mutual support. Families are dynamic and are cultures unto themselves, with different values and unique ways of realizing dreams. Our families create neighborhoods, communities, states, and nations. (Shelton & Stepanek, 1994, p. 6)

For both children and adults, family provides a personal culture of embeddedness. Each person creates a com-munity of family culture in the broadest sense of the concept of community. Like all cultures, each culture we cre-ate within our community is based on our values and may differ substantially from another's uniquely consummated community. However the family is constituted, whether we judge it adequate or not according to our value system, a person is embedded in his or her family and that is our starting place for inclusion. *A challenge for occupational therapy practitioners is understanding each person's unique community, including its culture and the context in which it was formed.*

The concept of community is broadened to include relations with acquaintances, coworkers, and schoolmates as well as locations like neighborhoods, workplace, and town. The community circle includes both formal and infor-mal sources of support. The environment provides the context in which communities are formed. It is composed of persons, objects, and space—all of which can be combined for personal or formal community building. The envi-ronment generally provides formal support to persons in community. Community is not a static structure in the environment, but an ongoing process of interaction among persons, objects, and space. Community provides famil-iarity with daily interactions that reduces the uncertainty experienced in new and challenging situations and creates a sense of belonging.

A sense of belonging in a community provides the comfort and security needed to explore and use one's gifts. According to Maslow's hierarchy, belonging is an important component in the development of self-esteem. Building blocks to self-esteem include a sense of safety in one's immediate community, a sense of self-acceptance, identity, affiliation with others and a sense of competence and mission. In some instances, we seem to expect children and adults with disabilities to demonstrate a sense of self-esteem before they can be included in a typical classroom or work or living environment, forgetting that belonging to a typical community is the means by which a person devel-ops a sense of self (Kunc, 1994). *One of the challenges we often face is resolution of the conflict we have over the need for persons with disabilities to prove themselves capable before they are included in typical communities of their choice rather than creating opportunities for them to develop their capacities in their community with appropriate supports.*

Choice is a valued dimension of our community life. Choice means having alternatives from which to make a selection. As occupational therapists, we recognize the importance of choice in every person's pursuit of self-actual-ization, particularly as he or she fulfills occupational roles of daily living, work, school, and play and leisure. Choice in occupational therapy has traditionally meant that the person seeking services takes an active part in planning and carrying out a therapy program. Yerxa (1966) maintained that one of the most important roles an occupational therapist plays is providing choice in selection of therapeutic activities, interaction with the activities and, most important, establishment of objectives for a therapy program. Exercising choice in a therapeutic environment provides opportunities to explore capabilities and options for life outside the therapy setting. Making choices is another way of exploring personal values about daily living, relationships, roles, and the physical, psychological, social, and spiritual communities in which living needs to occur to pursue self-actualization. Making choices in therapy is only a prelude to the choices people need to make regarding their life in the community. How will I make a living? Where will I live? Where will my child go to school? What supports will I need to live fully in the community of my choice? *A challenge for occupational therapy practitioners is fostering choice that reflects their consumer's priorities for living and accomplishing occupational tasks, even if there are differences between them regarding values or perceptions of expertise.* Schön (1983) wrote that the interactive practitioner realizes that he or she is not the only one in the situation to have relevant and important knowledge. The consumer interacts by joining with a service provider to make sense of the situation and, by doing so, gains a sense of increased involvement and action—or choice.

Being part of a community provides opportunities for lifelong development. Persons with disabilities and their family members have a right to pursue and participate in all levels of their community, whether it is one they have known well or one they wish to build to accommodate new circumstances and fulfill new or old dreams. Each person creates a community of his or her own culture in the broadest sense of the concept. Like all cultures, each culture we create within our community is based in our values and may differ substantially from another's uniquely consummated community. Creating community opens doors to new cultural vistas with opportunities to cooperate with each other and participate in community activities. Inclusion in a community also means an end to loneliness and helplessness and the beginning of empowerment to fulfill dreams (McLaughlin & Davidson, 1985). Building inclusive communities with all persons provides opportunities for members of the community to experience different relationships. Each of us has the capacity for creating inclusive community through our work with individuals as well as our ability to influence society and its established institutions.

The Nature of Disability and Inclusion

A new sociopolitical environment is developing in which persons with disabilities are taking or creating social and political actions on their own behalf. Changing perceptions of disability and the histories of the civil rights movement in the 1960s and the women's rights movement in the 1970s resulted in substantial legislative action for disability rights. In his book *No Pity,* Shapiro (1993) chronicled the course of the disability rights movement in the United States. Shapiro stated that persons with disabilities insist simply on common respect and the opportunity to build bonds to their community as fully accepted participants in everyday life. In the past, disability was usually viewed as a medical problem with the expectation that, to be accepted, persons with disabilities needed to be as much like persons without disabilities as possible without regard for their own uniqueness. Now, persons with disabilities are thinking differently about themselves. Many no longer think of their physical or mental differences as a source of shame or something to overcome in order to be like others or inspire others. In *Flying Without Wings,* Beisser, who contracted polio as an adult, said "When I stopped struggling, working to change, and found means of accepting what I had already become, I discovered that changed me. Rather than feeling disabled and inadequate, I felt whole again" (1989, p. 169). Beisser views disability as a difference among people. Considering disability as a difference is in itself neutral and changes the way persons with disabilities view themselves and are viewed by others. For example, in the village of Chilmark on Martha's Vineyard Island in Massachusetts, more than half the residents in the 1800s were genetically deaf (Groce, 1985). All the people in the village were fluent in sign language. It has been reported that spoken and sign language were used simultaneously or, if a person who was deaf joined a speaking group, group members immediately started to use sign as well as speech. Deafness was not a disability in Chilmark. Disability is a dimension of diversity not unlike ethnic background, color, religious, or gender differences

(Shapiro, 1993). Differences do not necessarily equal limitations, but rather create opportunities for meaningful interaction (J. Snow, personal communication, 1994) as long as people are living together naturally.

Just as perceptions of disability are changing, so are the reasons that disability was so often seen as a limitation. The difference within the person is no longer viewed as the main problem; instead, the environment that cannot accommodate the person is considered responsible for society's failure to include persons with disabilities in the mainstream. Social considerations have led to a shift from the traditional medical view of disability to an interactional model that accounts for the relationship between person and environment. Gill (1987) summarized this shift in perspective as follows:

- According to the medical view, disability is considered a deficit or abnormality. In an interactional model, disability is a difference.
- In the medical view, being disabled is perceived as negative. In an interactional model, being disabled is in itself neutral.
- Medicine views disability as residing in the individual. In an interactional model, disability is derived from problems encountered during interaction between the individual and their environment.
- In medicine, the remedy for disability-related problems is cure or normalization of the individual. In an interactional model, the remedy for disability-related problems is a change in the environmental interaction.
- Finally, the medical view identifies the agent of remedy as the professional. An interactional model has proposed that the agent of remedy may be the individual, an advocate, or anyone who affects the arrangements between the individual and society.

The last interactional category in Gill's summary can have a significant effect on the roles for occupational therapists. The shift from a medical perspective to an environmental framework is not difficult for us to understand. Occupational therapists have always recognized that disability was not an illness that could be cured by medicine. *The challenge for us is to promote the interactive model for practice regardless of the venue of our practice. A concurrent challenge is to increase support for more practice venues in the community where engagement in real occupation takes place.*

Change in perception of disability has fostered the disability rights movement and legislative action. The disability rights movement has focused on the rights of persons with disabilities to be included in society according to the choices they make for themselves and their families. The rights movement could also be called an *inclusion* movement. Inclusion in community means that all persons regardless of differences participate in natural environments for living, learning, playing, working, resting, and recreating. For persons with disabilities, participation may be with specific support from others or with adaptations to the environment. According to Gill (1987), inclusion means removal of barriers to power, which results in a greater number of alternatives or choices.

Shapiro (1993) identified the 1960s as the beginning of the disability independent living movement started by Ed Roberts and other students at the University of California–Berkeley. The movement spread to include action in Washington, DC, that initiated funding for independent living. Groups of parents of children with disabilities began to form around the country at about the same time, primarily to provide support to other parents in the same situations. The groups were often connected to existing organizations like United Cerebral Palsy or the Easter Seal Society. Later, parent organizations would emerge as independent, social change groups.

The 1970s saw adoption of Section 504 of the Rehabilitation Act (Public Law 93–112) prohibiting discrimination on the basis of disability. But Section 504 was not implemented for nearly 5 years after its adoption and was implemented only after a group led by Roberts and others staged a sit-in at the Department of Health, Education and Welfare office in San Francisco. Besides succeeding in obtaining regulations for Section 504, the event in San Francisco created an awareness that linked groups of adults around the country in a civil rights movement. Also in the 1970s, Public Law 94–142 was adopted as the Education for All Handicapped Children Act (1975), mandating public education in the least restrictive environment for children with disabilities who were 5 years of age and older.

In the 1980s, support was provided for that act through the establishment of statewide parent information and advocacy centers in every state. The legislation was expanded to include infants and toddlers with passage of the Education for All Handicapped Children Act Amendments of 1986 (Public Law 99–457). With this expanded legislation for education came the components of family-centered care, or respect for a family's central role as decision maker for a child, or support for an adult, which is now considered best practice across the life span. Public Law 94–142 and Public Law 99–457 were combined and expanded in reauthorization as the Individuals With Disabilities Education Act of 1990 (IDEA) (Public Law 101–476). Meanwhile, the Technology-Related Assistance for Individuals With Disabilities Act (Public Law 100–407) (1988) began the process of changing policy and availability of assistive technology for persons with disabilities in all states. The legislative decade of the 1980s culminated with the Americans With Disabilities Act of 1990 (ADA) (Public Law 101–336). ADA encompasses ideology from all previous legislation by ensuring that the barriers to inclusion be eliminated for persons with disabilities. Although far-reaching disability rights legislation was officially adopted in the 1980s, we are still struggling with implementation of all the laws in the 1990s.

The disability rights movement and legislation has focused primarily on removing physical and legal barriers to inclusion. Legislative mandates serve the purpose of forcing inclusion. The spirit of inclusion only comes with attitude change supported by community preparation and relationship building. In a midwestern city, 9-year-old Amy, who has cerebral palsy, visited Santa Claus last year and had only one wish for Christmas—just one day in school when the kids did not tease her about her cerebral palsy. Clearly, Amy was present in school with her typical peers, and being there is a start. But she is not truly included since a community that accepts her for who she is has not been created. She needed a school community that gave her a sense of familiarity, caring, and belonging. She needed relationships that she could depend upon for support ("Disabled Girl Asks Santa," 1993). In another city, 14-year-old Kevin, who has Down's syndrome, has been with typical peers from the beginning of his school career. His inclusion has focused on preparation and relationship building that included Kevin along with the teachers and children in the building. When asked what it would be like if he was not included in typical school, he replied that he'd feel sad. "I like to be in school with my friends—I learn from them and they learn from me" (Kevin, personal communication, February 1993).

Inclusion is about relationships. Judith Snow, a consumer advocate in Canada, has said that the only real disability is having no relationships (personal communication, January 1994). Inclusion means participation. Inclusion in school is only the prelude to inclusion in life. Participation may require support not only in the traditional sense of personal assistance and adaptations, but also in terms of preparing the persons in the community to welcome differences into their community and help develop natural support systems. *A challenge for occupational therapy is development of programs that prepare persons and their families for life in the community while working to prepare the community and persons in it to welcome the gifts of diversity.* If we espouse the interactive model of disability, we can affect the arrangements between the individual and society and make unique contributions to the interactive model of change. We can assist with remediation of the person's physical or psychological problem to the extent that the manifestations of the problem can be changed. We can participate in modification of the person's environment so that it can accommodate the needs. We can assist with building community with the person or family in order to create a place for belonging that includes both the formal and informal sources of support. We can continue to promote inclusion as a value through our sociopolitical systems.

Building inclusive community sometimes requires change in value-based practices. The spiral (see Figure 43.3) serves as a model to illustrate that when we recognize differences in values, we may experience conflicts within ourselves or with others. If we cannot move beyond the downward spiral between values and differences, we will not be able to move beyond conflict. But if we move upward to change our perspective to one of appreciating differences, we can make a commitment to using differences in ways that productively build community. The spiral begins with a small, defined center focusing on personal values about differences. These values were established with past experience. As the spiral moves upward and widens, new experiences are included. The person uses past experience to respond to new situations. The response may be use of past behavior or of a new behavior that will modify old behaviors. For example, Bobbie wants to live alone in an apartment, but he cannot tie his shoes, button his shirt, prepare meals very well, or use the telephone to summon help. If your values about independence mean a person can only choose between doing everything alone or living in a segregated community, then Bobbie's proposal is different, causes conflict, and probably elicits a negative response. If you stay in a downward spiral of conflict between values and differences, you will continue to respond negatively to full inclusion for persons who cannot perform all tasks independently. But if you take an interactive view of disability, your perspective changes. You appreciate that Bobbie's disability resides in the community that cannot accommodate his differences.

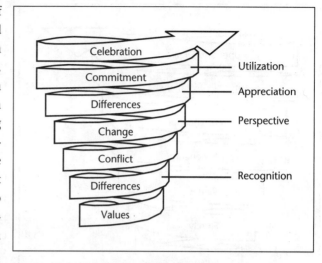

Figure 43.3. Celebrating diversity: Individual and society.

A change in perspective leads to modification of old behavior by new responses. A commitment to using rather than rejecting differences creates new possibilities for removing the barriers to inclusion. *The challenge for individual occupational therapists and the profession is making a commitment to inclusion in community for all persons with disabilities and chronic health problems.* The following values are proposed for occupational therapy:

- Every person has a right to be an integrated member of a community of choice.
- Every person has a right to active participation in decision making for self and family.
- Every person has a right to information and options as part of decision making.
- Every person has a right to choice of services delivered in natural environments in order to maximize success in occupational roles.

The Nature of Adaptation and Environment

To explore means for occupational therapists to meet the challenges of building inclusive community, I would like to turn to the spatiotemporal adaptation theory developed with my colleague Elnora Gilfoyle. The theory was developed when we were both involved in pediatric practice and education. During those years, pediatric occupational therapy and other disciplines focused knowledge development and research on typical child development as a means for designing programs for children who were not developing typically. Although the spatiotemporal adaptation theory articulated the importance of interaction between the child and the environment, it emphasized ways in which therapists could influence the child's development rather than ways in which the environment could be prepared to accommodate the child's function. In light of the shift from medical to interactive approach to disability, it seems appropriate to reexamine the categories of the theory, especially the environmental category of the model. The original categories in the theory included *movement, environment, adaptation,* and *spiraling continuum of development* (Gilfoyle et al., 1990).

In the theory, both development in children and ongoing functioning of adults is seen as a transactional process between a person and the environment; for example, movement provides a means for action and the environment presents a reason to act. The person influences and is influenced by the environment through a process of adaptation. According to Kegan, "adaptation is not just a process of coping or adjusting to events (of the environment) as they are, but an active process of increasingly organizing the relationship of self to the environment" (1982, p. 113). The relationship is transactional because persons organize themselves around events of the environment while

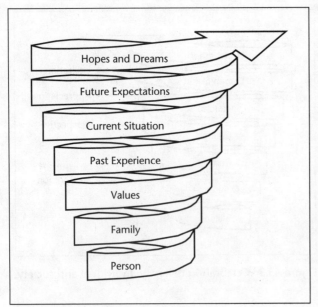

Figure 43.4. The person in life span.

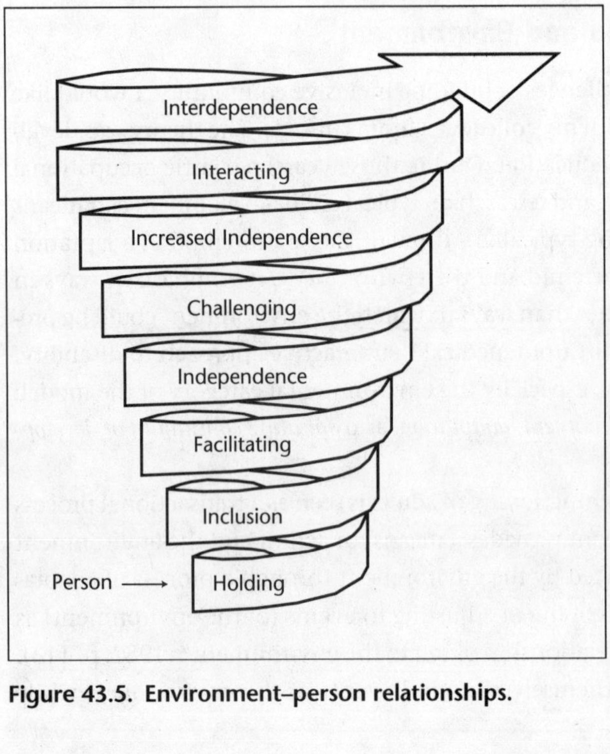

Figure 43.5. Environment–person relationships.

simultaneously organizing environmental events to meet their needs (Yerxa, 1992). Adaptation as a category of the theory is viewed as an ongoing process of change in behavior. The spiral again provides the model for the adaptation process (see Figure 43.4). Throughout the life span, a person uses past experience, including values established in early life, to adapt to current situations and prepare for future adaptations. Through adaptation, more complex behaviors evolve to respond to more extensive demands from the environment. If the demands of the current or future situations exceed the ability to adapt, the person may recall past behavior to respond until environmental events can be reorganized to elicit a higher level response. With adaptation as a process for organizing one's self and environment, interaction between person and environment sets up a system of relationships.

Environment as a category in the adaptation theory is all-inclusive. Environment represents the complete setting or surrounding in which a person lives, including self, other persons, objects, space, and relationships between all components in the environment (see Figure 43.2). According to Winnicott, a "good enough" (1965, p. 67) environment meets and challenges a person's need to grow and develop by adapting to stimulation from continually changing situations. Yerxa (1994) noted that persons need just the right challenge to make an adaptive response. Daloz said that

how readily we grow—indeed whether we grow at all—has a great deal to do with the nature of the world in which we transact our lives' business. To understand human development, we must understand the environment's part, how it confirms us, contradicts us and provides continuity. (1986, p. 68)

Environment–person relationships (see Figure 43.5) are conceptualized on a spiraling continuum from a *holding environment,* which promotes inclusion, to a *facilitating environment,* which promotes independence, to a *challenging environment,* which increases independence, to an *interactive environment,* which fosters interdependence. The holding environment begins in infancy and provides support through physical and psychological holding. Winnicott (1965) maintained that the holding environment is the context in which early development takes place. The infant experience can influence a lifetime. Kegan referred to holding as the "culture of embeddedness" (1982, p. 115), which means an environment that is for growth as well as for accumulating history and mythology. In the holding environment, the infant begins to acquire a culture based on values and traditions communicated during this phase. According to Kegan, there is no single holding environment in early life, but a succession of holding environments, a life history of embeddedness. Holding environments are psychosocial environments that hold us and let go of us. If the infant's experience is satisfactory, it becomes a reference point whenever holding or support is needed later in life. The holding environment promotes a sense of inclusion or belonging, which usually precedes movement away from sources of support and is vital for all persons' development of independence.

The facilitating environment motivates a person to move beyond a familiar setting and on to new challenges and independence. It provides just enough support for moving, literally or figuratively, into new situations.

The challenging environment focuses on separating the person from embeddedness in order to develop and test potential. Just the right amount of challenge is needed if the person is to make an adaptive response to the situation. Increased independence evolves from successful adaptation to challenges.

Finally, the interactive environment promotes interplay between person and environment by combining a sense of self with an appreciation for relationships with others. Interactive environment supports interdependence. Winnicott stated that independence is never absolute. The healthy person does not become isolated, but relates to the environment in such a way that person and environment can be considered interdependent. The different functions of environment and the spiraling sequence of relating to environment can be useful for helping persons identify the environment they need to seek or create for their own health and well-being.

The role of the therapist is construction of Winnicott's "good enough" environment (1965), depending on the person's adaptation needs (Letts et al., 1994). A new parent of a child with significant health problems may need a supportive holding environment to learn the special care that will be given at home. A teenager with a spinal cord injury may seek a facilitating environment when he decides to go to college. He may begin assembling the sources for assistance and adaptations he will need to live independently as well as the advocacy skills he will need to act on his own behalf. A woman recovering from a head injury may have regained considerable function in a rehabilitation setting, but may be fearful of being back in her community. She will need challenge to regain her independence, but with enough support and facilitation to ensure progressively successful adaptation. She may want to reconstruct the life she led before the accident, or she may construct a new community and need resources for her new life. An infant may literally require a supportive environment to learn sensorimotor skills or speech or to focus on learning through play. For all of us, gaining and maintaining a balanced interaction between self and environment is a work in progress. We often need to challenge ourselves if we wish to move ahead. Or we seek facilitation for new situations, or support in difficult times. A challenge for occupational therapy practitioners is development of skill in analyzing environments and helping consumers to identify the type of environmental milieu that will facilitate their adaptation process.

Interactive Strategies for Choice and Inclusion

The promise of occupational therapy lies in our ability to continuously combine the mandates put forth in the early tenets of our discipline with our constantly changing practice environments. Occupational therapy emerged from both community and medical models of practice, although our philosophy is more related to what we know as the community-based model because occupations are practiced in community settings. For decades we tended to practice more in institutions or specialized settings, usually trying to simulate real-life settings to prepare persons to live in their community. Some of our more visionary colleagues set the course toward a future that focused on community consultation models of service delivery. The founders and leaders in our profession have fostered the importance of providing services in a person's own setting and according to the person's own choices and priorities for gaining or regaining specific skills for living. Our philosophy from the beginning of our profession has included the value of choice, relevance, and active participation through engagement in meaningful occupations. Occupation provides a context for organizing one's self and one's environment, thus promoting the transactional process of adaptation within a community setting (Engelhardt, 1977; Gilfoyle et al., 1990; Grady, 1992, Meyer, 1922; Schwartz, 1992; Yerxa, 1966). Therapy programs are designed to prevent or remediate the effects of disability or health issues and promote independent living in the community through occupations such as self-care and daily care of others, ability to play independently or with other children, ability to learn as a child and engage in lifelong learning as an adult, ability to be engaged in meaningful work to make a living or for one's own satisfaction or both, ability to balance work and recreation, and ability to blend all occupational activity with rest. Although models for community service delivery have been promoted from within the profession, external mandates for change have also influenced expansion of our practice environments. The voices heard from our consumers, our colleagues, legislation at state and national levels, and rapidly changing payment systems direct us toward service delivery that focuses on consumers' priorities for goals and naturally occurring venues for activities. The new directions in practice allow us to combine our past experience and founders' mandates with the current realities of practice in ways that lead us to realize the future hopes and dreams of our consumers, ourselves as individuals, and the profession as a whole.

To build collaborative models of consumer-driven, community-based practice, we need to focus on a communication process that helps us understand other persons' unique culture and priorities for life occupations as well as meaning associated with past experiences, current situations, and hopes for the future. Recent developments in the field support a focus on communication that enhances a shift from medically focused to interactive models of practice in which the therapist serves as an agent of remedy to affect the arrangements between the individual and society. The use of narrative for storytelling has increased our understanding of a person's past and present experience. Reflective practice and clinical reasoning support our ability to gain insight into the interactive roles that can unfold between a therapist and a person seeking services. Ethnographic approaches to research have in general heightened our knowledge of persons living in their own environments (Clark, 1993; Mattingly & Fleming, 1994; Schön, 1983; Yerxa, 1994).

Therapist–consumer collaborative practice models mean that communication among the therapist, the person seeking services, the family members, and the close community members is critical. From the beginning, it is the relationships we build that are critical to our ability to collaborate effectively. Listening, talking, reflecting, informing, and demonstrating are all part of the ways we establish relationships. Human beings are uniquely constituted for giving and receiving information, making and sharing meaning. We have the capacity to use intrapersonal communication skills to explore the meaning of our own values and experiences, and interpersonal communication skills to link with another person's values and experiences. *Intrapersonal communication* refers to the creating, functioning, and evaluating of symbolic processes that operate within us. Such activities as thinking, reflecting, solving some problems, and talking with oneself are part of our unique intrapersonal communication system (Dance & Larson, 1972). Intrapersonal communication is active within us whenever meaning is attached to an internally or externally generated source of stimulation. Meaning associated with past events and current situations is deeply embedded in the intrapersonal system of both the persons seeking services and the service provider. Interpersonal communication serves to link us through verbal and nonverbal expression so that we can more explicitly share information and meaning. Through interpersonal communication, we can tell our stories; explore the meaning of relationships, events, and circumstances; reflect on similarities, differences, strengths, and challenges; and develop plans for working together toward future goals. Kegan said, "If you want to understand another person in some fundamental way, you must know where the person is in his or her evolution. You need to understand his or her underlying structure for making meaning" (1982, p. 113). The context in which we as therapists seek and receive the information shared by persons seeking services can enhance our communication and collaborative planning. A communication model of collaboration can be illustrated by the spiraling model of person in life span (see Figure 43.4). If we place spirals side by side and let one spiral represent the consultant therapist and the other represent a person seeking services, we can visualize the communication sequences that occur. Communication moves from intrapersonal reflection to interpersonal linking through listening and speaking (see Figure 43.6). A closer look at the circle representing past experience provides details that can be shared about the meaning embedded in values and culture of childhood, family, and personal community (see Figure 43.7). We can discuss past experiences in terms of activities and relationships with family and close friends, with personal community, and with the larger environment. Exploring the past provides insight into the values that have directed past choices and the types of environments that the person has experienced. Discussing the current situation (see Figures 43.8 and 43.9) in the same context allows the therapist to understand the extent and meaning of the change that has occurred in the person's life as well as the priorities

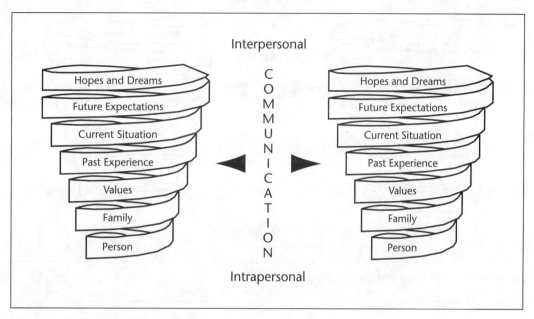

Figure 43.6. Linking past experiences.

and types of environments that need to be foremost in planning together. The persons can glean considerable information about the therapist's perspective on the current situation on the basis of past experience. The interpersonal linking increases understanding and promotes collaborative goal setting between person and therapist. As much as we have moved toward collaboration in family-centered and person-centered planning, we are still sometimes heard to say that we are having difficulty with a person receiving services accepting the goals we have set for their therapy. Interactive strategies mean that persons receiving services set the goals and therapists collaborate to design programs with them that will help address the goals. Information shared and the meaning it holds for both consumer and therapist provide the basis for collaboratively planning the future (see Figures 43.10 and 43.11). According to Schön (1983), there is gratification and anxiety for the reflective, interactive practitioner in becoming an active participant in a process of shared inquiry. For a therapist or consumer who wishes to move from traditional to reflective communication, there is the task of reshaping expectations for the relationship. But if we are to be agents of remedy in the arrangements between a person and the environment, we need to be able to share with and receive comprehensive information from the persons who are seeking choices for inclusion in their community.

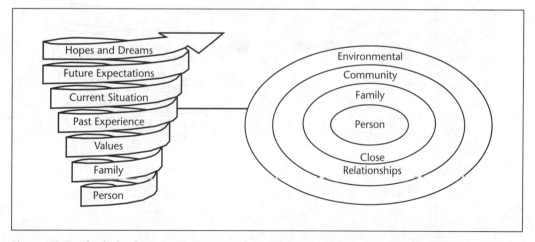

Figure 43.7. The link of past experience with personal community.

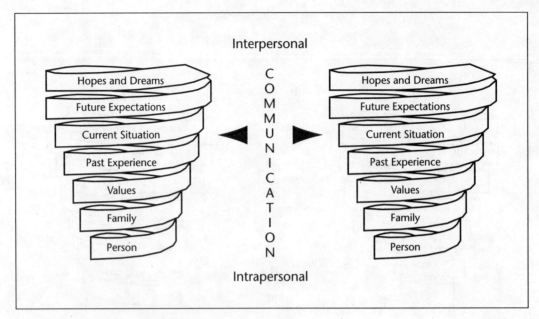

Figure 43.8. Linking current information.

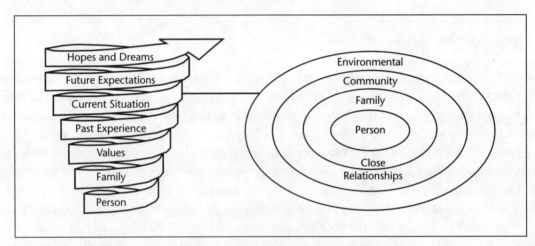

Figure 43.9. The link of current situation with personal community.

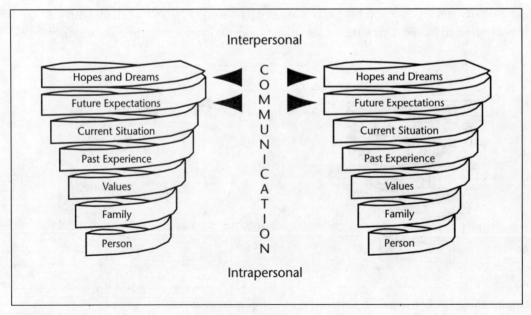

Figure 43.10. Exploring future possibilities.

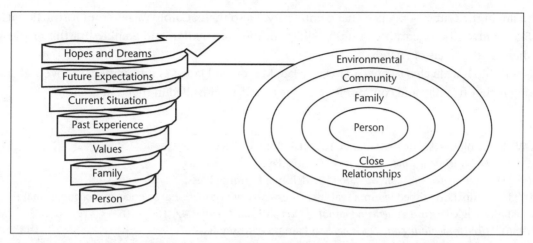

Figure 43.11. The link of hopes, dreams, and future expectations with personal community.

Summary

We have had an opportunity to focus on the challenges and opportunities for building inclusive community with the persons with whom we work in occupational therapy. We have gained understanding about the meaning of community and choice, reviewed current ideas about the nature of disability and mandates for inclusion, expanded ideas about environment and adaptation, considered strategies for promoting choice and inclusion, and related these concepts to the philosophy of occupational therapy. I had the extraordinary opportunity to explore my own values, past experience, current situation, and hopes for the future and I am forever changed by the experience. As Emily Brontë reflected, "I've dreamt in my life—dreams that have stayed with me ever after, and changed my ideas: they've gone through and through me, like wine through water, and altered the color of my mind" (cited in *The Quotable Woman,* 1991, p. 185). Leading the development of inclusive community is right for occupational therapy and we all have it in us to do it. The challenges before us are as follows:

1. Understanding each person's unique community, including its culture and the context in which it was formed.
2. Resolving the conflict we have over the need for persons with disabilities to prove themselves capable before being included in typical communities of choice rather than creating opportunities for developing capabilities in the community with appropriate supports.
3. Fostering choice that reflects a person's priorities for living and accomplishing occupational tasks, even when there are differences regarding values or perceptions of expertise.
4. Promoting the interactive model for practice, regardless of the venue of practice.
5. Increasing support for more practice venues in the community where engagement in real occupation takes place.
6. Developing programs that prepare people and their families for life in the community while working to prepare the community to welcome the gifts of diversity.
7. Making a commitment to inclusion in community for all persons.
8. Developing skill in analyzing environments and helping people identify the type of environmental milieu that will facilitate their adaptation process.

Acknowledgments

I thank Ellie Gilfoyle for leading the Eleanor Clarke Slagle nomination process and for a lifetime of creative collaboration; my colleagues who supported the nomination and by doing so offered focus for the topic; Lou Shannon for ongoing support and inspiration; my colleagues at The Children's Hospital for their support; Anita Wagner, Jackie Brand, and all the other parents who enlightened me with their perspectives and changed the course of my professional life; Betty Yerxa, whose philosophy and writings have influenced my thinking for many years; and my family, who are in the center of my personal community. I also thank Carol Wassell from Instructional Services at Colorado State University for creating beautiful slides for the presentation and graphics for this article and Diane Brians for drawing the Circle of Friends.

This lectureship is dedicated to my parents, the late Marion and James Grady, with deep love and appreciation for the strong focus on family and community that they lived and instilled in their children.

References

Americans With Disabilities Act of 1990 (Public Law 101–336) 42 U.S.C. § 12101.

Beisser, A. (1989). *Flying without wings*. New York: Doubleday.

Brontë, E. (1991). Cited in *The quotable woman*. Philadelphia: Running Press.

Clark, F. (1993). Occupation embedded in a real life: Interweaving occupational science and occupational therapy. 1993 Eleanor Clarke Slagle Lecture. *American Journal of Occupational Therapy, 47*, 1067–1078.

Daloz, L. (1986). *Effective mentoring and teaching*. San Francisco: Jossey-Bass.

Dance, F., & Larson, C. (1972). *Speech communication: Concepts and behavior*. New York: Holt, Rinehart, & Winston.

Disabled girl asks Santa to end teasing. (1993, December 14). *The Denver Post*, p. 1.

Education for All Handicapped Children Act of 1975 (Public Law 94–142).

Education of the Handicapped Act Amendments of 1986 (Public Law 99–457).

Engelhardt, H. (1977). Defining occupational therapy: The meaning of therapy and the virtues of occupation. *American Journal of Occupational Therapy, 31*, 666–672.

Gilfoyle, E., Grady, A., & Moore, J. (1990). *Children adapt* (2nd ed.). Thorofare, NJ: Slack.

Gill, C. (1987). A new social perspective on disability and its implication for rehabilitation. *Occupational Therapy in Health Care, 7*, 1.

Grady, A. (1992). Nationally Speaking—Occupation as vision. *American Journal of Occupational Therapy, 46*, 1062–1065.

Groce, N. (1985). *Everyone here spoke sign language: Hereditary deafness on Martha's Vineyard*. Cambridge, MA: Harvard University Press.

Individuals With Disabilities Education Act of 1990. (Public Law 101–476).

Kegan, R. (1982). *The evolving self*. Cambridge, MA: Harvard University Press.

Kunc, N. (1994). *The other side of therapy*. Port Alberni, BC: Axis Consultation and Training.

Letts, L., Law, M., Rigby, P., Cooper, B., Stewart, D., & Strong, S. (1994). Person–environment assessments in occupational therapy. *American Journal of Occupational Therapy, 48*, 608–618.

Mattingly, C., & Fleming, M. (1994). *Clinical reasoning: Forms of inquiry in a therapeutic practice*. Philadelphia: F. A. Davis.

Meyer, A. (1922). The philosophy of occupation therapy. *Archives of Occupational Therapy, 1*, 1.

McLaughlin, C., & Davidson, G. (1985). *Builders of the dawn*. Summertown, TN: Book Publishing.

McWilliams, P. (1994). *Do it again!* Los Angeles: Prelude.

Patterson, A. (1992). *Rock art symbols of the greater Southwest*. Boulder, CO: Johnson.

Patterson-Rudolph, C. (1993). *Petroglyphs and Pueblo myths of the Rio Grande* (2nd ed.). Albuquerque, NM: Avanyu.

Rehabilitation Act of 1973 (Public Law 93–112), 29 U.S.C. § 794.

Schön, D. (1983). *The reflective practitioner*. New York: Basic.

Schwartz, K. (1992). Occupational therapy and education: A shared vision. *American Journal of Occupational Therapy, 46*, 12–18.

Shapiro, J. (1993). *No pity*. New York: Times.

Shelton, T., & Stepanek, J. (1994). *Family-centered care for children needing specialized health and developmental services*. Bethesda, MD: Association for the Care of Children's Health.

Technology-Related Assistance for Individuals With Disabilities Act (Public Law 100-407) (1988).

Winnicott, D. (1965). *The maturational processes and the facilitating environment*. New York: International Universities Press.

Yankelovitch, D. (1981). *New rules*. New York: Random House.

Yerxa, E. (1966). 1966 Eleanor Clarke Slagle Lecture—Authentic occupational therapy. *American Journal of Occupational Therapy, 21*, 1–9.

Yerxa, E. (1992). Some implications of occupational therapy's history for its epistemology, values, and relation to medicine. *American Journal of Occupational Therapy, 46*, 79–83.

Yerxa, E. (1994). Dreams, dilemmas, and decisions for occupational therapy practice in a new millennium: An American perspective. *American Journal of Occupational Therapy, 48*, 586–589.

44

1995 Eleanor Clarke Slagle Lecture

Occupation:
Purposefulness and Meaningfulness as Therapeutic Mechanisms

Catherine A. Trombly, ScD, OTR/L, FAOTA

I chose the topic of *therapeutic occupation* because that was what attracted me to the profession, and it is the concept about which I have thought most. I became an occupational therapist because I liked arts and crafts and "medical things." When I was about 11 years old, my friend's sister came home with paintings and jewelry and other things she had made at college. She was enrolled in the occupational therapy program at the University of New Hampshire and told me she was preparing to work in a hospital using arts and crafts to help people get better. I decided then and there that that was the profession for me. So eventually I went to the university and enjoyed learning all those activities. Those were the days when a large proportion of the curriculum was devoted to developing knowledge and skill in crafts. We learned technique from artists and theory in our occupational therapy classes. We learned that activities were therapeutic because they were purposeful, that is, they demanded certain responses that might be deficient in people who had a disease or injury, and that by doing activities, people improved their skills and abilities. We learned how to adapt activities to change the demands as the person changed. We also learned that because the person got to choose from several activities that demanded similar responses, the chosen activity was meaningful and kept the person interested and working. These beliefs were based on anecdotal observations passed down from early occupational therapists.

These beliefs are still taught, but have hardly been researched. Current economic and scientific forces in our society require us to provide support for the hypothesis that engagement in purposeful and meaningful occupation improves impaired abilities or produces occupational functioning. It would be to our advantage also to discover *how* therapeutic occupation brings about those changes so that we can treat more effectively.

Because I have always felt the need to know more about what made occupation therapeutic, I took the opportunity of this lecture to attempt to sort out some concepts concerning therapeutic occupation for myself and to pull together evidence for whether and how occupation is therapeutic. My goal is to spark an explosion of research concerning therapeutic occupation.

If there is novelty in this lecture, to paraphrase White (1959), it lies in examining pieces that already lie before us, in seeing how to fit those pieces into a larger conceptual picture, and in determining what new pieces are needed to complete the picture.

Occupation

In the early days of occupational therapy, crafts were used as diversions, as general methods of recovery from disease and injury (Llorens, 1993; Slagle, 1914), and for their utilitarian value because products were produced that

---

Originally published 1995 in *American Journal of Occupational Therapy, 49*, 960–972.

could be sold (Haas, 1922). The purpose of the craft was to keep the patient occupied so that manic or depressive thoughts would be replaced (Dunton, 1914). Replacement happened because one cannot think about two things at once and occupation compelled attention. Believed prerequisite to the therapeutic value of the craft were the patient's feelings of interest and personal pride, which the instructor needed to instill if not evoked by the activity itself (Purdum, 1911). It was Susan Tracy who moved occupational therapy into the general hospital (Barrows, 1917; Editorial, 1929). She emphasized that the product was the patient, not the article he or she makes, and thereby changed the focus of occupation from a money-making enterprise to a specific therapeutic one (Barrows, 1917; Parsons, 1917). Occupation was primarily prescribed to remediate impairment (Barrows, 1917; Swaim, 1928), although there is a report that Tracy developed what we now call a *universal cuff* to enable persons to feed themselves (Cameron, 1917). By 1930, therapists were being invited to move beyond remediation to join the rehabilitation effort. The philosophy of rehabilitation is to focus not on what is lost, but on what capabilities remain, to prepare the person for return to the fullness of life's activities (Lowney, 1930). Occupation came to include activities of daily living (ADL) and prevocational training.

In the past several years papers have been written and several conferences held to discuss occupation, but consensus about what occupation is and is not continues to elude us. Nelson (1988) presented a detailed conceptualization of occupation in which he defined occupation as the relationship between occupational form and occupational performance. By *occupational form* he meant the task demands and environmental context. By *occupational performance* he meant the act of doing. According to his view, *therapeutic occupation* is the synthesis of an occupational form by the occupational therapist that either enables the patient to compensate to achieve a goal activity or produces an adaptive change in what Nelson called the person's developmental structure (1990). In this conceptualization, any voluntary activity a person does of *whatever complexity* is considered occupation as long as the occupational form of the activity has meaning from the person's point of view and the performance is based on a sense of purpose. According to this conceptualization, reaching for something of interest and preparing one's lunch are both occupations.

Occupation is limited to complex activity sequences by others. Clark and her colleagues (1991) defined occupation as "chunks of culturally and personally meaningful activity in which humans engage that can be named in the lexicon of the culture" (p. 301). By that they meant such things as doing one's job, dressing, cooking, and gardening. Christiansen and Baum, as reported by Christiansen (1991), defined *occupation* as all goal-oriented behavior related to daily living, including spiritual and sexual activities. In their view, the basic unit of occupation is activity. They defined *activity* as specific goal-oriented behavior directed toward the performance of a task. Bathing is an example of a task; filling the bathtub and washing one's self are examples of activities. They acknowledged that abilities are required to engage in activities and tasks, but did not seem to include this level in their characterization of occupation. *Occupation,* as defined by Clark and her colleagues and by Christiansen and Baum, seems to assume ability to perform. For those who treat patients with physical impairments, occupation thus defined is problematic because most of our patients cannot perform.

A Model of Practice for Physical Dysfunction

I want to suggest a different way of considering therapeutic occupation, but first I need to tell you how I view the practice of occupational therapy for adults with physical dysfunction and define some terms. I am limiting my examples to physical dysfunction because that is what I know best, although the ideas apply to many areas of practice. The model I am presenting is not my original idea. I think it has been used since the inception of the application of occupational therapy to this population, but I have named it the model of occupational functioning (Trombly, 1993). This model of practice parallels a certain conceptualization of occupational performance. This conceptualization of occupational performance is a descending hierarchy of roles, tasks, activities, abilities, and capacities (see Figure 44.1).

In the model of occupational functioning, the goal of occupational therapy is to develop a sense of competency and self-esteem. A competent person has sufficient resources to interact effectively with the physical or social environments and to meet the demands of a situation (White, 1959). A sense of competency is highly associated with feelings of self-efficacy (Abler & Fretz, 1988; Bandura, 1977), a belief that one is capable of accomplishing a goal. To be competent means to be able to satisfactorily engage in one's life roles (or to voluntarily reassign a role to another). The American Occupational Therapy Association (AOTA) (1994) categorized roles into the three performance areas of work, play and leisure, and activities of daily living. However, I prefer to categorize roles from the point of view of the person (Trombly, 1993)—for example, roles that relate to self-achievement or productivity; roles that are essentially self-enhancing or that add pleasure or joy to one's life; and roles that maintain the self, which in my view includes family preservation and home maintenance.

Any categorization, however, is deceptive in that it implies that particular roles can be unequivocally classified into one category or another. They cannot. A particular person may categorize one role as an achievement-productivity role, whereas someone else may classify the same role as an enhancement-recreational role. The example that comes quickest to mind is the role of shopper. For some persons shopping is recreation and adds joy to their lives; for others, shopping is a chore done simply to acquire the raw materials needed for living. The category depends upon the meaning that the role has for the person. This fact becomes readily apparent when we note the results of a study by Yerxa and Locker (1990). They examined how 15 subjects with spinal cord injury categorized their daily activities. They found that the same activity was often placed into different categories. For example, eating was categorized by different subjects as self-maintenance, rest, play, and "other."

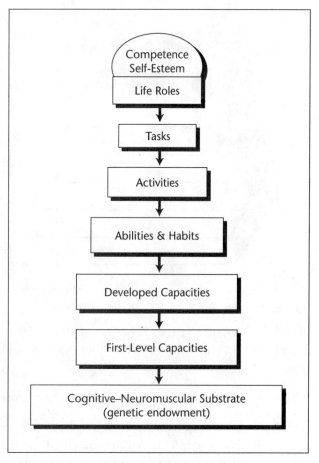

Figure 44.1. Conceptualization of occupational performance.

In order to engage satisfactorily in a life role, a person must be able to do the tasks and activities that make up that role within the natural context. Some tasks are essential to the role and must be mastered by whoever chooses the role. For example, the role of bus driver requires that the person be able to do the activity of steering the bus on a city street. Other roles are defined by the person so that the same role may be constituted in terms of different tasks by different persons. For example, one woman might consider the task of helping with homework an essential aspect of her mother role, whereas another, like the patient with chronic back pain interviewed by Nelson and Payton (1991), might consider roughhousing with her children as very important to that role. The patient, or a significant other, decides which roles the patient should work toward resuming. Furthermore, the person decides which tasks and activities constitute particular roles according to his or her values as well as sociocultural mores and expectations.

To go on with the description of the occupational functioning model, tasks are composed of *activities,* which are smaller units of behavior. For example, peeling a potato is an activity within the task of meal preparation. To continue further down the hierarchy, in order to be able to do a given activity, one has to have certain sensorimotor, cognitive, perceptual, emotional, and social abilities. *Abilities* are skills that one has developed through practice and that underlie many different activities—for example, eye–hand coordination. Abilities emanate from developed capacities that the person has gained through learning or maturation. *Developed capacities* are refinements, gained through maturation and learning, of biologically based capacities. Graded grasp to accommodate the size and shape

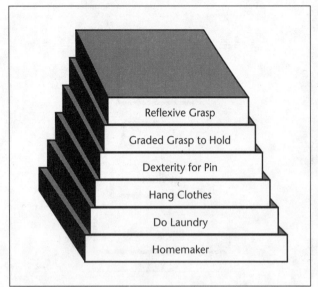

Figure 44.2. Nesting of levels of occupation.

of an object is an example of a developed capacity. Developed capacities depend upon first-level capacities. *First-level capacities* are reflex-based responses or subroutines that underlie voluntary movement and derive from a person's genetic endowment or spared organic substrate. For example, reflexive grasp and reflexive release, which underlie the higher capac-ity of graded grasp, are first-level capacities.

In this conceptualization, complex occupations, such as maintenance of one's clothes, have progressively simpler occupations nested within them (see Figure 44.2) (e.g., doing the laundry, hanging clothes on a clothesline, fastening the clothespin, grasping the clothespin). This nesting contributes to our quandary in characterizing what is, and what is not, occupation and in building a theory of therapeutic occupation. A second dimension that makes occupation difficult to define is time: occupations comprise a range of time from brief moments to the entire lifespan (Nelson, 1988; Yerxa et al., 1990). So not only does occupation have a vertical dimension, complexity, as I have just described, but it also has a horizontal dimension, time.

Another Look at Occupation

For me, one way to begin the characterization of occupation was to notice, in the process of thinking about the occupational functioning model, that in some situations we consider occupation as the goal to be learned and in other situations we consider occupation as the change agent. I have termed these *occupation-as-end* and *occupation-as-means*. I suggest this distinction because I think the goals and therapeutic processes of these two forms of occupation are different. Furthermore, there is historical basis for this separation because these two uses of occupation came into occupational therapy practice at different times. I equate the idea of occupation-as-end to the levels of activities, tasks, and roles in the occupational functioning model. At each of these levels, the person has a functional goal and tries to accomplish it by using what abilities and capacities heor she has. I think this is close to how Clark and others (1991) and Christiansen and Baum (Christiansen, 1991) defined occupation. Occupation-as-means, on the other hand, is *the therapy* used to bring about changes in impaired performance components. Occupation at this level often is limited to simple behaviors. Both occupation-as-end and occupation-as-means garner their therapeutic impact from the qualities of purposefulness and meaningfulness.

Purposefulness in Occupation-as-End

Occupation-as-end is purposeful by definition. According to many occupational therapy writers, purposeful occupation-as-end organizes a person's behavior, day, and life (Kielhofner, 1985, 1992; Meyer, 1922/1977; Slagle, 1914; Yerxa & Baum, 1986; Yerxa & Locker, 1990; Yerxa et al., 1990). Early occupational "workers" imposed purposeful occupation on persons who could not choose it for themselves; they were then able to act in more healthy ways (Slagle, 1914). Time-use studies indicate that people who are mentally able to envision goals distribute their awake time among occupational tasks and activities. The studies also indicate that this distribution is affected by age (McKinnon, 1992) or disability (Yerxa & Baum, 1986; Yerxa & Locker, 1990). For example, Yerxa and Baum found that the number of hours that community-living subjects with spinal cord injury devoted to particular occupations differed significantly from the number of hours their friends without disabilities devoted to those occupations. The subjects with spinal cord injury worked fewer hours and devoted more hours to occupations categorized as "other," which for some subjects included shopping, going to church, eating, or watching television. The problem with this study, for our purposes, is that subject-designated categories were used as the data. Subjects categorized the same occupation (e.g., eating) differently. Further research is needed concerning purposefulness in occupation-as-end. Time-use studies inform us that persons fill their time with activities and tasks that they can name and categorize. However, I found no studies in our literature on how occupation-as-end organizes persons' lives. One paradigm that might be fruitful is to examine how persons without mental illness, who are recently retired, in extreme circumstances such as in prison or lost in the wilderness, or even on extended lazy vacations try to impose organization on their lives by planning and carrying out purposeful occupations of various complexities.

Meaningfulness in Occupation-as-End

Occupation-as-end is not only purposeful but also meaningful because it is the performance of activities or tasks that a person sees as important. Only meaningful occupation remains in a person's life repertoire. Meaningfulness as a therapeutic aspect of occupation derives from our belief in the mind–body connection. The actions of the body are guided by the meaning ascribed to them by the mind (Bruner, 1990). Meaningfulness of occupation-as-end is based on a person's values that derive from family and cultural experiences. Meaningfulness also derives from a person's sense of the importance of participating in certain occupations or performing in a particular manner; or from the person's estimate of reward in terms of success or pleasure; or perhaps from a threat of bad consequences if the occupation is not engaged in.

Meaning is individual (Bruner, 1990) and although the occupational therapist can guess what may be meaningful based on a person's life history, he or she must verify with each patient that the particular occupation is meaningful to that person *now* and verify that the person sees a value in relearning it. The therapist cannot substitute his or her own values in selecting appropriate occupational goals for the patient. Two studies concerning differences in valuing between therapist and patient come to mind. In 1974, Taylor reported that the values attached to goals by 19 occupational therapists differed significantly from those of 44 patients with spinal cord injuries. The patients valued development of work tolerance most, followed by bladder and bowel control. They did not value ADL skills highly. The therapists valued development of adapted devices and ADL skills most and bowel and bladder control least. Chiou and Burnett (1985) surveyed 26 patients living at home after stroke to determine the relative importance of 15 ADL tasks to each of them. Then the researchers paired each patient with one or more of 10 visiting occupational therapists and physical therapists who were treating these patients, to form 29 pairs. Patients and therapists, independently, ranked the 15 items from not at all important to very important for the particular patient. Scores for each patient and therapist pair were correlated. Only one of the 29 pairs yielded a significant correlation, and that was only of moderate strength [.57]. These results seem to indicate that therapists were not good judges of the value ascribed by patients to particular ADL tasks.

The meaningfulness of occupation-as-end is so profound that people at least partially define life satisfaction in terms of competent role performance. For example, in the study by Yerxa and Baum (1986) of 15 subjects with spinal cord injuries and their 12 friends without disabilities, a significant, moderate correlation of $r = .44$ was found between satisfaction with performance in home management and overall life satisfaction. A slightly higher correlation of $r = .62$ was found between satisfaction with performance of community skills and overall life satisfaction. Bränholm and Fugl-Meyer (1992) surveyed 201 randomly selected 25- to 55-year-old northern Swedish persons without disabilities to determine what value they attached to certain roles in relation to their perceived level of life satisfaction. Roles associated with vocation, family life, leisure, and home maintenance correctly classified 62% to 78% of the subjects in terms of satisfaction with life. Smith, Kielhofner, and Watts (1986) studied 60 persons with a mean age of 78 years, half of whom were institutionalized, to determine the relationship between engagement in daily occupations and life satisfaction. They found that those subjects who were classified into the high satisfaction category engaged in recreation and work significantly more and in ADL and rest significantly less than those classified in the low satisfaction category.

Therapeutic Achievement of Occupation-as-End

I think that occupation-as-end is brought about by teaching the activity or task directly, using whatever abilities the patient has at his or her disposal or providing whatever adaptations are necessary. It is the Rehabilitative Approach (Trombly, 1995a) or skills training approach (Rogers, 1982). In this approach, occupations are analyzed to ensure that they are within the capabilities of the patient, but are not used to bring about change in those capabilities, per se. The patient learns, with the help of the therapist as teacher and as adaptor, of the task demands and context. In the therapeutic encounter, the therapist organizes the subtasks to be learned so that the person will succeed, provides the feedback to ensure successful outcome, and structures the practice to promote improved performance and learning. The purpose of the activity or task is readily apparent to the patient and, if the therapist has allowed patient goals to guide treatment, it is meaningful. Therapeutic principles for this approach derive from cognitive information processing and learning theories.

Occupation-as-Means

Occupation-as-means refers to occupation acting as the therapeutic change agent to remediate impaired abilities or capacities. Various arts, crafts, games, sports, exercise routines, and daily activities that are systematically selected and tailored to each person (Cynkin & Robinson, 1990) are examples of occupations-as-means. Occupation in this sense is equivalent to what is called *purposeful activity* (AOTA, 1993). Purposeful activity demands particular, more circumscribed responses than occupation-as-end.

The therapist analyzes the occupation to determine that it demands particular responses from the person and that the responses demanded are slightly more challenging than what the person can currently easily produce. The therapist provides the opportunity to engage in the potentially therapeutic occupation (Meyer, 1922/1977), and as the person makes the effort and succeeds, the particular impairment that the occupation-as-means was chosen to remediate is reduced.

Although occupation is provided, therapy may be absent. What makes occupation-as-means therapeutic? First, the activity must have a purpose or goal that makes a challenging demand, yet has a prospect for success. Second, it must have meaning and relevance to the person who is to change so that it motivates the will to learn and improve (Cynkin & Robinson, 1990). The therapeutic aspects of occupation used as a means to change impairments, then, are purposefulness and meaningfulness.

Purposefulness in Occupation-as-Means

Occupation-as-means is based on the assumption that the activity holds within itself a healing property that will change organic or behavioral impairments. We have further assumed that those inherent therapeutic aspects can be reliably identified through the activity analysis process (Llorens, 1986, 1993). However, if that assumption were true, therapists should fairly unanimously identify the inherent characteristic components of particular activities. But Tsai (1994), who surveyed 120 therapists experienced in the treatment of stroke, found poor consensus on the sensorimotor, cognitive-perceptual, or psychosocial components demanded by five particular activities that are commonly used in the treatment of patients who have had a stroke, such as stacking cones, putting on a shirt, and making a sandwich. Neistadt, McAuley, Zecha, and Shannon (1993) also reported discrepancies among therapists in identifying components required to do common activities.

Research Related to Purposefulness of Occupation-as-Means in the Motor Domain

When analyzing activities to remediate motor impairments, we have assumed that there are inherent aspects of an activity that elicit particular muscular responses. However, this assumption is not supported by electromyographic evidence. If the therapeutic benefit were inherent in the activity, then whenever any person did that activity, the effects should be similar from trial to trial and similar from person to person, especially in those with normal bio-mechanical and neuromuscular systems. However, a colleague and I completed an electromyographical study some years ago that examined the responses of hand muscles of 15 persons without disabilities when they were doing 16 different occupational therapy hand activities (Trombly & Cole, 1979). I had assumed in designing this study that if the goal was the same (e.g., "open this lock with this key"), and placement of objects was the same from subject to subject, and if each subject was positioned the same in relation to the objects (i.e., if the task demands were the same), then the same muscles would be used at similar levels by the various subjects. However, the results indicated that each subject used his or her own muscle activation pattern and amount of muscle activity. This finding was contrary to my expectations, but fully in agreement with predictions of Bernstein (1967).

Bernstein theorized that neuromuscular variability between trials is due to the redundancies in the muscu-loskeletal systems. Such redundancies allow the same goal to be accomplished effectively by a wide variety of muscle combinations and movement patterns (Horak, 1991; Morasso & Zaccaria, 1986; Newell & Corcos, 1993). Bernstein's ideas, and the evidence that supports them, contributed to the paradigm shift to the dynamical systems theory of motor control. The term *dynamical systems* refers to any area of concern in which order and pattern emerge from the interaction and cooperation of many systems (Hawking, 1988). Applied to motor behavior, dynamical systems refers to movement patterns that emerge from the interaction of multiple systems of the person and performance contexts to achieve a functional goal (see Figure 44.3) (Haugen & Mathiowetz, 1995; Mathiowetz & Haugen, 1994, 1995).

According to Bernstein's hypothesis, the central nervous system temporarily yokes muscles together to constrain the number of degrees of freedom to within its capability of control at the moment, given the current resources of the person and the particular demands of the context. This synergic coupling, or coordinative structure, forms as needed at the moment and then dissolves. The next time the person does the same thing, his or her muscles may be more warmed up, or there may be a slight difference in placement of task object in relation to the active limb, so a new coordinative structure evolves. That is, different muscles may be recruited, or the same muscles used before may be more or less active in order to accomplish the movement goal in the most efficient way. The motor goal is con-stant or invariant and requires a constant, invariant response, but this response can be fulfilled by a varying set of muscular contractions (Luria, 1973). The goal or purpose seems to organize the most efficient movement, given the constraints of person and context (see Figure 44.3).

What evidence is there that purpose organizes behav-ior? Motor commands issued to moving segments are not accessible to an experimenter and must be inferred from study of the limb trajectories that they ultimately produce (Jeannerod, 1988). Limb trajectories are recorded with instruments designed to track the spatial-temporal aspects of movement. Different spatial-temporal patterns, which are indicative of differences in movement organization, emerge for particular goals (Jeannerod, 1988). Movement organization can be detected from the shape of the veloc-ity profile (Georgopoulos, 1986; Kamm, Thelen, & Jensen, 1990) that changes depending on goal (Nelson, 1983). The goal of reaching to a large target that does not demand accuracy produces a unimodal and bell-shaped velocity profile. The goal of reaching precisely to a target, which requires accurate, guided movement, on the other hand, has a left-shifted velocity profile because more time is spent in deceleration than in acceleration.

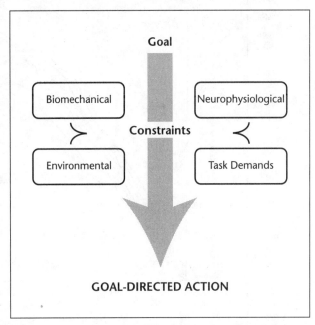

Figure 44.3. Dynamical systems theory of motor control hypothesizes that goal-directed action emerges from a synthesis of goal or purpose and personal and contextual constraints.

In 1987, Marteniuk, MacKenzie, Jeannerod, Athenes, and Dugas demonstrated for the first time the impact of goal on the organization of movement. They found that five university student subjects used a different movement organization when they reached for the same object for two different purposes. One goal was to pick up a 4-cm disk and place it in a slot; the other goal was to pick up the same disk and throw it into a basket. The task demands and the context were exactly the same. Only intent after the reach was different. The different purposes produced two different velocity profiles (see Figure 44.4), indicating different movement organizations, for the reaches to the disk. Reaches before placing the disk into a slot produced a left shift of velocity profile in which a significantly greater percentage of total reach time was spent in the deceleration phase and the acceleration phase was significantly shortened as compared to reaches before the throwing condition.

Mathiowetz (1991) tested whether the same motor organization was elicited when 20 subjects with multiple sclerosis performed functional tasks in natural, impoverished, partial, and simulated conditions. In one of the experiments, the subjects actually ate applesauce with a spoon in the natural condition; pretended to eat applesauce, with no applesauce, spoon, or dish present in the impoverished condition; pretended to eat applesauce with a dish and spoon, but no applesauce present in the partial condition; or did, in the simulated condition, the feeding subtest of the Jebsen–Taylor Hand Function Test (Jebsen, Taylor, Trieschmann, Trotter, & Howard, 1969) that requires the subject to pick up kidney beans with a spoon and transfer them to a can placed in front of him or her. The outcomes of each trial were described qualitatively in phase plane diagrams in which velocity is graphed against displacement. These should be replicable from trial to trial if the subject is using the same movement organization. However, the phase planes were judged, by experienced judges, to be different among the four conditions. Figure 44.5 depicts two trials of two conditions, the natural and the simulated, by one subject. The repeated trials are similar, but the two conditions are different. Because subjects produced unique phase planes for each condition, Mathiowetz concluded that subjects perceived each condition as an unique activity, having a different goal.

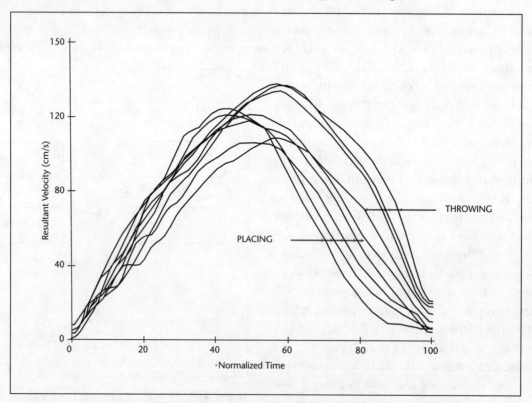

Figure 44.4. Velocity profiles for reaches to a 4-cm disk, after which the goal was to fit the disk into a slot or to throw it into a basket.
Note. From Marteniuk, R. G., MacKenzie, C. L., Jeannerod, M., Athenes, S., & Dugas, C. (1987). Constraints on human arm movement trajectories. *Canadian Journal of Psychology, 41*(3), 365–378. Used with permission.

In another test of differences in goal situation, Van der Weel, van der Meer, and Lee (1991) tested nine children of average intelligence, aged 3 to 7 years, who had right hemiparesis. They measured the children's range of supination and pronation movement when moving a drumstick back and forth in the frontal plane with the instruction "to move as far as you can" (the abstract condition). The children had previously experienced the full range of movement passively. Range was also measured when the children were told to use the same drumstick to "bang the drums" which were placed to require full range of motion (the concrete condition). Movement range was significantly greater ($t_8 = 6.75$, $p < .0001$) for the concrete task of banging the drums than for the abstract task, which had a vague goal.

Wu (Wu, 1993; Wu, Trombly, & Lin, 1994) investigated whether actually reaching for a pencil to write one's name, reaching the same distance for an imagined pencil, or reaching forward in a biomechanically similar way would produce different outcomes in terms of the organization of movement. In the sample of 37 college-aged subjects without disabilities, the materials-based occupation of reaching for an actual pencil elicited significantly different and more efficient organization of movement than imagery-based occupation of reaching for a pretend pencil or exercise. The reach was faster ($F_{2, 62} = 20.44$, $p < .001$) and straighter ($F_{2, 62} = 23.25$, $p < .001$), was more pre-planned ($F_{2, 62} = 22.13$, $p < .001$), and used less force ($F_{1, 62} = 6.13$, $p < .005$). The imagery-based occupation, on the other hand, produced a more guided, longer, and more convoluted path than did the exercise condition, probably because the goal was more vague in that condition.

Sietsema, Nelson, Mulder, Mervau-Scheidel, and White (1993) tested the effect of goal on overall active range of shoulder motion of 20 adults with brain injury. Each subject reached to a point 3 inches above the center of a table placed to require full forward reach. Each also reached the same distance to play a computer controlled game of flashing lights and sounds. Overall active range of motion was significantly greater as a result of the game than simply reaching to the more vague target ($t_{19} = 5.77$, $p < .001$).

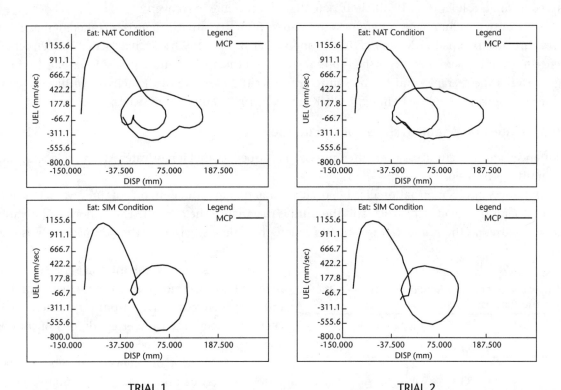

TRIAL 1   TRIAL 2

Figure 44.5. Phase planes (velocity × displacement) of two trials of two conditions (natural and simulated) by one normal subject.
Note. From Mathiowetz, V. G. (1991). *Informational support and functional motor performance.* Unpublished doctoral dissertation, University of Minnesota, Minneapolis. Used with permission.

At least in terms of motor responses, then, purpose does appear to organize behavior. Of course, much more study is required to verify this finding.

Meaningfulness in Occupation-as-Means

Whereas a meaningful occupation has purposefulness, strictly speaking, a purposeful activity may or may not be meaningful. Sharrott (1983) stated that the purpose of an action gives that action meaning. He may have been using *purpose* to denote the reason that a person does something, or the motive, rather than the goal of the action. I think that confounding these terms will impede research. The purpose is the goal, the expected end result. The meaning is the value that accomplishment of that goal has for the person. I have an anecdotal example of the separation between the two concepts. Some years back, my father had a right cerebrovascular accident with resultant hemiinattention. The occupational therapist gave him parquetry blocks to do. There were two purposes. One was the goal of the activity—to place all the blocks on the diagram. He understood the goal and tried to do what he was told. However, it had no meaning to him; he viewed this activity as a children's game and found it degrading. The therapeutic purpose, of course, was to improve his hemiinattention. That purpose had no meaning to him either; he did not think he had hemiinattention and did not get the connection between the child's game and the therapeutic goal.

What do we mean by *meaningful* and how does that quality of occupation-as-means affect behavioral responses? Meaning related to occupation-as-means may relate to basic values held by the person—similar to the way meaning is derived for occupation-as-end. However, meaning is probably generated from a less profound source when it applies to particular, circumscribed, time-limited activities used to promote some performance component. The meaningful aspect of occupation-as-means may be the emotional value that an interesting and creative experience offers the patient (Ayres, 1958). Or meaningfulness may stem from familiarity with the occupation, or its power to arouse positive associations, or the likelihood that completion of it will elicit approval from others who are respected and admired (Cynkin & Robinson, 1990), or its potential to contribute to recovery.

Although we often count on meaningfulness to emanate from the activity, there is no inherent meaningfulness quality in a particular occupation. Meaningfulness is individual. Bruner (1990) said that "action is interpretable only by reference to what the actor says he or she is up to" (p. 20). In therapy, meaningfulness is developed through an exchange between the therapist and the person to construct the meaning of the activity within the context of culture, life experiences, disability (Fleming, 1990; Kielhofner, 1992), and present needs.

Research Related to Meaningfulness of Occupation-as-Means

The importance of meaningfulness to us as therapists is that we believe that it motivates. What evidence is there that meaning motivates behavior?

Meaningfulness has been operationalized in occupational therapy studies in one of three ways. One is to offer a choice, another is to provide a product, and the third is to enhance the context. The response, motivation, has been operationalized as the number of repetitions or length of time engaged in the occupation or as the effort expended.

Table 44.1. Mean Number of Repetitions as a Result of Preference and Purpose in Assigned Tasks

Purpose	Task Assigned	
	Preferred	Nonpreferred
Yes	63	63
No	83	84

Note. Based on Bakshi, R., Bhambhani, Y., & Madill, H. (1991). The effects of task preference on performance during purposeful and nonpurposeful activities. *American Journal of Occupational Therapy, 45,* 912–916.

Choice. Bakshi, Bhambhani, and Madill (1991) studied 20 female college students who chose their most preferred and least preferred activity from eight offered activities. They completed each under conditions of purpose and nonpurpose, defined respectively as working on a product or not. There were no differences in number of repetitions performed between the preferred and nonpreferred occupation. Differences between product and no-product conditions were not significant due to high variability (see Table 44.1). On the other hand, LaMore and Nelson

(1993), in a more controlled study, did find a significant increase in repetitions (Z = 2.9, *p* < .01) when 22 adult subjects with mental disabilities were given a limited choice of which ceramic object to paint as compared with when they were told to paint a particular one.

Product. Thibodeaux and Ludwig (1988) tested whether performance time and heart rate (effort) would be significantly different when 15 occupational therapy students sanded a cutting board that they could keep as compared with when they sanded wood for no reason. Although the subjects reported enjoying the product-oriented activity significantly more and they worked longer at it, there was too much intersubject variability to detect significant differences between conditions (see Table 44.2).

Enhanced context. Riccio, Nelson, and Bush (1990) studied the effects of enhanced context. They tested the effect of imagery-based activity and exercise on the number of repetitions of 27 elderly nursing home residents when they reached up to pretend to pick apples and reached down to pretend to pick up coins versus when they simply reached up or down for exercise. There was a significant difference between the two conditions for the up direction (Z = 2.25, *p* = .012), indicating that pretending to pick apples was more motivating than exercise. The outcome for reaching down was in the same direction, but nonsignificant (Z = 1.60, *p* = .055), possibly because of a confounding effect of fatigue.

Lang, Nelson, and Bush (1992) tested the responses of 15 elderly nursing home residents under three conditions: materials-based activity, imagery-based activity, and exercise. In the materials-based condition, subjects actually kicked a red balloon. In the imagery-based condition, they pretended to kick a described balloon. In the exercise condition, they kicked as demonstrated. The number of repetitions associated with really kicking the balloon (54) was significantly greater ($F_{2, 28}$ = 6.62, *p* = .004) than those associated with imagining kicking the balloon (26) or kicking for exercise (18). This study was later replicated by DeKuiper, Nelson, and White (1993) on 28 elderly nursing home residents. Materials-based occupation produced significantly more repetitions than imagery-based occupation or rote exercise ($F_{2, 54}$ = 12.1, *p* < .001). In this study they also measured effort in terms of distance the foot was raised and speed of kick. There were no significant differences among the various contextual conditions for these variables (see Table 44.3).

A number of other researchers (Bloch, Smith, & Nelson, 1989; Kircher, 1984; Miller & Nelson, 1987; Steinbeck, 1986; Yoder, Nelson, & Smith, 1989) all demonstrated significantly greater numbers of repetitions or duration for what they termed purposeful versus nonpurposeful activity. The differences in the activities were actually differences in meaning in terms of context, not differences in purpose—the motoric purpose was the same: jump up and down or jump rope, stir dough for exercise or stir dough that will be made into cookies that the subjects could smell baking, squeeze a bulb to keep a ping-pong ball suspended in air or squeeze the same bulb for exercise. Some demonstrated significantly greater effort (heart rate) expended for the enhanced condition, but this was not a consistent finding (Bloch et al., 1989; Kircher, 1984; Steinbeck, 1986).

Meaningfulness, as operationalized by enhanced context, and possibly by choice, appears to motivate continued performance. However, more definitive research is needed. Additionally, basic research on what makes occupation-as-means meaningful and how best to operationalize this in both research and practice is needed.

Table 44.2. Effects of Product-Oriented and Non-Product-Oriented Activities

	Product	
Measures	Yes (Cutting Board)	No (Wood)
Preference	4.8	3.4*
Increased heart rate	13	17
Performance time	172	148

*p = .001.
Note. Based on Thibodeaux, C. S., & Ludwig, F. M. (1988). Intrinsic motivation in product-oriented and non-product-oriented activities. *American Journal of Occupational Therapy, 42,* 169–175.

Table 44.3. Average Effects of Materials-Based Occupation, Imagery-Based Occupation, and Rote Exercise

	Type of Occupation and Exercise		
Measures	Materials-Based	Imagery-Based	Rote
Repetitions to fatigue	127**	51	75
Distance foot lifted (cm)	29	31	26
Speed (cm/sec)	71	71	67

**p < .001.
Note. Based on DeKuiper, W. P., Nelson, D. L., & White, B. E. (1993). Materials-based occupation versus imagery-based occupation versus rote exercise: A replication and extension. *Occupational Therapy Journal of Research, 13,* 183–197.

Practice and Research

As occupational therapists we want our patients to achieve role competence. We use occupation-as-end and occupation-as-means now to achieve that. We need to document the successes of our current practices, but we also need to reconsider some of our practices. For example, practice based on an ascending hierarchical model has emphasized remediation of occupational components because it is assumed that lower level skills and abilities are prerequisite to higher level functioning. Although this assumption makes logical sense—persons who cannot lift their arms certainly cannot comb their hair in the usual way—practice has sometimes emphasized treatment to increase strength and other capacities and abilities to the exclusion of teaching functional skills. However, a thorough review of the literature on stroke rehabilitation (Wagenaar & Meijer, 1991a, 1991b) indicated that gains in component functions are small and do not automatically result in improved functional performance. When the results of several correlational studies were averaged together, the average correlation between motor impairment and ADL was .56 and between perceptual impairment and ADL was .58 (Trombly, 1995b). By squaring the r, the amount of variance of ADL accounted for by motor impairment was 31% (see Figure 44.6). Therefore, 69% of variance associated with ADL derives from other factors. Even if motor impairment were 100% remediated, would the patient be able to do ADL without specific training and adaptation? Studies are needed that compare skills training at the level of occupation-as-end with subskills training using occupation-as-means to effectively and efficiently achieve occupational functioning (Rogers, 1982).

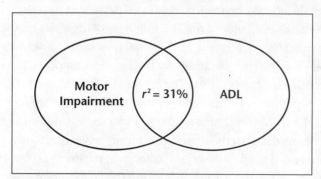

Figure 44.6. Pictorial description of r^2.

How the purposefulness and meaningfulness aspects of both levels of occupation contribute to the therapeutic effect need explication to guide practice. We need to study in more detail how purposefulness organizes behavior and meaningfulness motivates performance. The literature reviewed here is a beginning in this regard. Some of the studies reviewed indicated that the organization of motor behavior is different when the purposes or contexts are different, even if they are similar. This finding suggests that treatment in simulated contexts using simulated objects and simulated goals may not help a patient learn occupational performance for real life. Studies are needed to compare effectiveness of treatment with actual objects in natural contexts versus treatment with simulated objects in clinical settings. Follow-up studies of carryover of occupational performance from treatment center to home are also needed.

Those golden moments that we have all experienced as therapists probably came about when the patient succeeded in doing something that had great meaning to him or her. Sometimes we get complacent, though, and offer activities and occupations that we think ought to be meaningful to the person but are not really, or we offer a choice of activities from a selection in which none of the choices are meaningful. Much more attention needs to be applied to discovering the meaning of, or creating meaning for, therapeutic occupation. Methods to evaluate meaningfulness are needed both for research and practice. We need more well-controlled studies that test the effect of meaningfulness on perseverance and effort during therapy.

Conclusion

Occupational therapy was founded on the belief that engaging in occupation brought about mental and physical health. Over the years we have redefined health, for our purposes, as occupational performance having many levels of organization. In this context, occupation can be seen both as end and as means. In both dimensions, meaningfulness and purposefulness are key qualities. Purposefulness organizes and meaningfulness motivates. Purposeful occupation-as-end seems to organize time and a person's description of his life. Meaningful occupation-as-end motivates the person's participation in life. Purposeful occupation-as-means organizes behavioral responses, at least as far as motor responses are concerned. Meaningful occupation-as-means seems to motivate the person to persevere in his efforts long enough to achieve a therapeutic benefit. Research is needed to verify each of these hypotheses. I hope each occupational therapist will join me in taking responsibility to contribute to that effort.

Acknowledgments

Figures 44.1, 44.2, and 44.6, as well as all the slides in the original presentation, were prepared by Elizabeth (Boo) Murray, ScD, OTR, FAOTA, to whom I am very grateful. I further want to acknowledge the support and constructive critique of my colleagues in the Neurobehavioral Rehabilitation Research Center (NRRC), which is the American Occupational Therapy Association and American Occupational Therapy Foundation Center for Scholarship and Research at Boston University: Sharon Cermak, EdD, OTR, FAOTA; Wendy Coster, PhD, OTR, FAOTA; Anne Henderson, PhD, OTR, FAOTA; Karen Jacobs, EdD, OTR, FAOTA; Noomi Katz, PhD, OTR; Boo Murray, ScD, OTR, FAOTA; and Elsie Vergara, ScD, OTR, FAOTA.

References

Abler, R. R., & Fretz, B. R. (1988). Self-efficacy and competence in independent living among oldest old persons. *Journal of Gerontology: Social Sciences, 43,* S138–144.

American Occupational Therapy Association. (1993). Position Paper—Purposeful activity. *American Journal of Occupational Therapy, 47,* 1081–1082.

American Occupational Therapy Association. (1994). Uniform terminology for occupational therapy—third edition. *American Journal of Occupational Therapy, 48,* 1047–1054.

Ayres, A. J. (1958). Basic concepts of clinical practice in physical disabilities. *American Journal of Occupational Therapy, 12,* 300–302, 311.

Bakshi, R., Bhambhani, Y., & Madill, H. (1991). The effects of task preference on performance during purposeful and non-purposeful activities. *American Journal of Occupational Therapy, 45,* 912–916.

Bandura, A. (1977). Self-efficacy: Toward a unifying theory of behavior change. *Psychological Review, 84,* 191–215.

Barrows, M. (1917). Susan E. Tracy, R. N. *Maryland Psychiatric Quarterly, 6,* 57–62.

Bernstein, N. (1967). *The coordination and regulation of movements.* Elmsford, NY: Pergamon.

Bloch, M. W., Smith, D. A., & Nelson, D. L. (1989). Heart rate, activity, duration, and affect in added-purpose versus single-purpose jumping activities. *American Journal of Occupational Therapy, 43,* 25–30.

Bränholm, I-B., & Fugl-Meyer, A. R. (1992). Occupational role preferences and life satisfaction. *Occupational Therapy Journal of Research, 12,* 159–171.

Bruner, J. (1990). *Acts of Meaning.* Cambridge, MA: Harvard University Press.

Cameron, R. G. (1917). An interview with Miss Susan Tracy. *Maryland Psychiatric Quarterly, 4,* 65–66.

Chiou, I-I. L., & Burnett, C. N. (1985). Values of activities of daily living: A survey of stroke patients and their home therapists. *Physical Therapy, 65,* 901–906.

Christiansen, C. (1991). Occupational therapy intervention for life performance (pp. 1–43). In C. Christiansen & C. Baum (Eds.), *Occupational therapy: Overcoming human performance deficits.* Thorofare, NJ: Slack.

Clark, F., Parham, D., Carlson, M. E., Frank, G., Jackson, J., Pierce, D., Wolfe, R. J., & Zemke, R. (1991). Occupational science: Academic innovation in the service of occupational therapy's future. *American Journal of Occupational Therapy, 45,* 300–310.

Cynkin, S., & Robinson, J. M. (1990). *Occupational therapy and activities health: Toward health through activities.* Boston: Little, Brown.

DeKuiper, W. P., Nelson, D. L., & White, B. E. (1993). Materials-based occupation versus imagery-based occupation versus rote exercise: A replication and extension. *Occupational Therapy Journal of Research, 13,* 183–197.

Dunton, W. R., Jr. (1914). Roundtable. *Maryland Psychiatric Quarterly, 4,* 20–32.

Editorial. (1929). Susan E. Tracy. *Occupational Therapy and Rehabilitation, 8*, 63–66.

Fleming, M. (1990). Untitled invited paper presented at the American Occupational Therapy Foundation planning meeting for the Occupation Symposium, Boston, MA.

Georgopoulos, A. P. (1986). On reaching. *Annual Review of Neurosciences, 9*, 147–170.

Haas, L. J. (1922). Crafts adaptable to occupational needs: Their relative importance. *Archives of Occupational Therapy, 1*, 443–455.

Haugen, J. B., & Mathiowetz, V. (1995). Contemporary task-oriented approach. In C. A. Trombly (Ed.), *Occupational therapy for physical dysfunction* (4th ed.) (pp. 510–528). Baltimore: Williams & Wilkins.

Hawking, S. W. (1988). *A brief history of time: From the big bang to black holes.* New York: Bantam.

Horak, F. B. (1991). Assumptions underlying motor control for neurologic rehabilitation. In M. Lister (Ed.), *Contemporary management of motor control problems. Proceedings of the II STEP Conference* (pp. 11–27). Alexandria, VA: The Foundation for Physical Therapy.

Jeannerod, M. (1988). *The neural and behavioral organization of goal-directed movements.* Oxford: Clarendon.

Jebsen, R. H., Taylor, N., Trieschmann, R. B., Trotter, M., & Howard, L. A. (1969). An objective and standardized test of hand function. *Archives of Physical Medicine and Rehabilitation, 50*, 311–319.

Kamm, K., Thelen, E., & Jensen, J. L. (1990). A dynamical systems approach to motor development. *Physical Therapy, 70*, 763–775.

Kielhofner, G. (Ed.). (1985). *A Model of Human Occupation.* Baltimore: Williams & Wilkins.

Kielhofner, G. (1992). *Conceptual foundations of occupational therapy.* Philadelphia: F. A. Davis.

Kircher, M. A. (1984). Motivation as a factor of perceived exertion in purposeful versus nonpurposeful activity. *American Journal of Occupational Therapy, 38*, 165–170.

LaMore, K. L., & Nelson, D. L. (1993). The effects of options on performance of an art project in adults with mental disabilities. *American Journal of Occupational Therapy, 47*, 397–401.

Lang, E. M., Nelson, D. L., & Bush, M. A. (1992). Comparison of performance in materials-based occupation, imagery-based occupation, and rote exercise in nursing home residents. *American Journal of Occupational Therapy, 46*, 607–611.

Llorens, L. A. (1986). Activity analysis: Agreement among factors in a sensory processing model. *American Journal of Occupational Therapy, 40*, 103–110.

Llorens, L. A. (1993). Activity analysis: Agreement between participants and observers on perceived factors in occupation components. *Occupational Therapy Journal of Research, 13*, 198–211.

Lowney, M.E.P. (1930). The relationship between occupational therapy and rehabilitation. *Massachusetts Association for Occupational Therapy Bulletin, 4*(2), no pages.

Luria, A. R. (1973). *The working brain: An introduction to neuropsychology.* New York: Basic.

Marteniuk, R. G., MacKenzie, C. L., Jeannerod, M., Athenes, S., & Dugas, C. (1987). Constraints on human arm movement trajectories. *Canadian Journal of Psychology, 41*, 365–378.

Mathiowetz, V. G. (1991). *Informational support and functional motor performance.* Unpublished doctoral dissertation, University of Minnesota.

Mathiowetz, V., & Haugen, J. B. (1994). Motor behavior research: Implications for therapeutic approaches to central nervous system dysfunction. *American Journal of Occupational Therapy, 48*, 733–745.

Mathiowetz, V., & Haugen, J. B. (1995). Evaluation of motor behavior: Traditional and contemporary views. In C. A. Trombly (Ed.), *Occupational therapy for physical dysfunction* (4th ed., pp. 157–186). Baltimore: Williams & Wilkins.

McKinnon, A. L. (1992). Time use for self care, productivity, and leisure among elderly Canadians. *Canadian Journal of Occupational Therapy, 59*, 102–110.

Meyer, A. (1977). The philosophy of occupational therapy. *American Journal of Occupational Therapy, 31*, 639–642. (Reprinted from *Archives of Occupational Therapy, 1*, 1–10, 1922)

Miller, L., & Nelson, D. L. (1987). Dual-purpose activity versus single-purpose activity in terms of duration of task, exertion level, and affect. *Occupational Therapy in Mental Health, 1*, 55–67.

Morasso, P., & Zaccaria, R. (1986). Understanding human movement. *Experimental Brain Research, 15*, 145–157.

Neistadt, M. E., McAuley, D., Zecha, D., & Shannon, R. (1993). An analysis of a board game as a treatment activity. *American Journal of Occupational Therapy, 47*, 154–160.

Nelson, C. E., & Payton, O. D. (1991). A system for involving patients in program planning. *American Journal of Occupational Therapy, 45,* 753–755.

Nelson, D. L. (1988). Occupation: Form and performance. *American Journal of Occupational Therapy, 42,* 633–641.

Nelson, D. L. (1990). Untitled invited paper presented at the American Occupational Therapy Foundation planning meeting for the Occupation. Symposium, Boston, MA.

Nelson, W. L. (1983). Physical principles for economies of skilled movements. *Biological Cybernetics, 46,* 135–147.

Newell, K. M., & Corcos, D. M. (1993). Issues in variability and motor control. In K. M. Newell & D. M. Corcos (Eds.), *Variability and motor control* (pp. 1–12). Champaign, IL: Human Kinetics.

Parsons, S. E. (1917). Miss Tracy's work in general hospitals. *Maryland Psychiatric Quarterly, 6,* 63–64.

Purdum, H. D. (1911). The psycho-therapeutic value of occupation. *Maryland Psychiatric Quarterly, 1,* 35–36.

Riccio, C. M., Nelson, D. L., & Bush, M. A. (1990). Adding purpose to the repetitive exercise of elderly women through imagery. *American Journal of Occupational Therapy, 44,* 714–719.

Rogers, J. C. (1982). The spirit of independence: The evolution of a philosophy. *American Journal of Occupational Therapy, 36,* 709–715.

Sharrott, G. W. (1983). Occupational therapy's role in the client's creation and affirmation of meaning. In G. Kielhofner (Ed.), *Health through occupation: Theory and practice in occupational therapy.* Philadelphia: F. A. Davis.

Sietsema, J. M., Nelson, D. L., Mulder, R. M., Mervau-Scheidel, D., & White, B. E. (1993). The use of a game to promote arm reach in persons with traumatic brain injury. *American Journal of Occupational Therapy, 47,* 19–24.

Slagle, E. C. (1914). History of the development of occupation for the insane. *Maryland Psychiatric Quarterly, 4,* 14–20.

Smith, N. R., Kielhofner, G., & Watts, J. H. (1986). The relationships between volition, activity pattern, and life satisfaction in the elderly. *American Journal of Occupational Therapy, 40,* 278–283.

Steinbeck, T. M. (1986). Purposeful activity and performance. *American Journal of Occupational Therapy, 40,* 529–534.

Swaim, L. T. (1928). Does occupational work hasten recovery of the crippled? *Massachusetts Association of Occupational Therapy Bulletin, 2*(3), no pages.

Taylor, D. P. (1974). Treatment goals for quadriplegic and paraplegic patients. *American Journal of Occupational Therapy, 28,* 22–29.

Thibodeaux, C. S., & Ludwig, F. M. (1988). Intrinsic motivation in product-oriented and non-product oriented activities. *American Journal of Occupational Therapy, 42,* 169–175.

Trombly, C. (1993). Anticipating the future: Assessment of occupational function. *American Journal of Occupational Therapy, 47,* 253–257.

Trombly, C. (Ed.). (1995a). *Occupational therapy for physical dysfunction* (4th ed.). Baltimore: Williams & Wilkins.

Trombly, C. A. (1995b). *Relationships between motor and perceptual performance components and activities of daily living.* Unpublished paper, Boston University.

Trombly, C. A., & Cole, J. M. (1979). Electromyographic study of four hand muscles during selected activities. *American Journal of Occupational Therapy, 33,* 440–449.

Tsai, P-L. (1994). *Activity analysis and activity selection among occupational therapists: A survey.* Unpublished master's thesis, Boston University, Boston.

Van der Weel, F. R., van der Meer, A.L.H., & Lee, D. N. (1991). Effect of task on movement control in cerebral palsy: Implications for assessment and therapy. *Developmental Medicine and Child Neurology, 33,* 419–426.

Wagenaar, R. C., & Meijer, O. G. (1991a). Effects of stroke rehabilitation (1): A critical review of the literature. *Journal of Rehabilitation Sciences, 4,* 61–73.

Wagenaar, R. C., & Meijer, O. G. (1991b). Effects of stroke rehabilitation (2): A critical review of the literature. *Journal of Rehabilitation Sciences, 4,* 97–109.

White, R. W. (1959). Motivation reconsidered: The concept of competence. *Psychological Review, 66,* 297–333.

Wu, C-Y. (1993). *The relationship between occupational form and occupational performance: A kinematic perspective.* Unpublished master's thesis, Boston University.

Wu, C-Y., Trombly, C. A., & Lin, K.-C. (1994). The relationship between occupational form and occupational performance: A kinematic perspective. *American Journal of Occupational Therapy, 48,* 679–687.

Yerxa, E. J., & Baum, S. (1986). Engagement in daily occupations and life satisfaction among people with spinal cord injuries. *Occupational Therapy Journal of Research, 6,* 271–283.

Yerxa, E. J., Clark, F., Frank, G., Jackson, J., Parham, D., Pierce, D., Stein, C., & Zemke, R. (1990). An introduction to occupational science: A foundation for occupational therapy in the 21st century. *Occupational Therapy in Health Care, 6,* 1–32.

Yerxa, E., & Locker, S. (1990). Quality of time use by adults with spinal cord injuries. *American Journal of Occupational Therapy, 44,* 318–326.

Yoder, R. M., Nelson, D. L., & Smith, D. A. (1989). Added-purpose versus rote exercise in female nursing home residents. *American Journal of Occupational Therapy, 43,* 581–586.

45

1996 Eleanor Clarke Slagle Lecture

Why the Profession of Occupational Therapy Will Flourish in the 21st Century

David L. Nelson, PhD, OTR, FAOTA

Welcome to this celebration of our profession! Eighty-eight years ago, a young woman named Eleanor Clarke Slagle attended a course that explored the potentials of occupation as a therapeutic medium (Quiroga, 1995, chap. 1). Convinced of the power of occupation to enhance human life, Slagle went on to help found our profession. In her name, I am honored to present the 35th Eleanor Clarke Slagle Lecture.

Occupational therapy as a profession will flourish over the next century for the same reason that it has flourished over the past century. Real human beings needed therapeutic occupation in the days of Eleanor Clarke Slagle; they need therapeutic occupation in our times; and they will continue to need it beyond our days. Our service of occupational therapy is so sound because the idea of therapeutic occupation is so basic: The human being can attain enhanced health and quality of life by actively doing things that are personally meaningful and purposeful, in other words, through occupation. We are the profession uniquely devoted to helping persons help themselves through their own active efforts.

The Need for a Historical Perspective

To appreciate the core of occupational therapy and its importance for human health and quality of life over the next century, we need a macroscopic point of view. I am not referring to the immediate time frame of next year's health legislation in Congress, the year 2000, or even the year 2050. My time frame is approximately the year 2096, a good time for someone, certainly not me, to be summing up the second century of organized occupational therapy just as we are now in a position to sum up its first century.

What the 20th century teaches us is that apparently reliable trends on which people make predictions break down categorically in totally unforeseeable ways. Who in the progressive early 1900s could have predicted the horrors of World War I, the beginning of which was marked by soldiers on horseback and the end of which marked by mechanized trench warfare where combatants were at risk for instant death from distant unseen forces? Who could have predicted the Russian revolution; the worldwide economic depression; or the rise of fascism, genocide, and World War II with its unprecedented millions of dead, including civilians? Who could have predicted the nuclear terror of my generation or the rise of Pax Americana amidst the sudden, implosive collapse of the Soviet empire?

It will be at least as hard for us to predict the 21st century as it was for the first occupational therapists to predict the 20th century. We can do our best to extrapolate current trends into the future, but the trends that are visible now will break down categorically just as the optimistically progressive trends of 1900 broke down over the past

Originally published 1997 in *American Journal of Occupational Therapy, 51,* 11–24.

century. We will be surprised. Our descendants will be surprised. I put it this way because this is the larger context from which we should view the profession. Only those things will endure that are both fundamental to human nature and adaptable to a changing world. I believe that one of those things is occupational therapy.

The profession of occupational therapy was founded for one reason: To use occupation as a therapeutic method. The original articles of incorporation of the National Society for the Promotion of Occupational Therapy (1917) clearly stated the purposes of this new organization: "the advancement of occupation as a therapeutic measure," "the study of the effect of occupation on the human being," and "the scientific dispensation of this knowledge" (p. 1). It is important to note that the founders thought of occupation as a method, not just a goal. They believed that occupation could have therapeutic effects on the human being, and they wanted to document these effects through scientific research.

Mores have changed dramatically since the founding of our profession, and they will change in the future in ways that are unimaginable to us now. When we look at photographs of early occupational therapy (e.g., Howe & Schwartzberg, 1986), we see starched uniforms, serious and even stern facial expressions, military-like decorum, and highly structured crafts that required many sessions to complete. Those early photographs reflect a different era of America and of occupational therapy. It was a different culture, and the therapeutic occupations of those times reflected that culture. In like manner, occupational therapists 100 years from now will look back at the archives documenting today's occupational therapy and see quaintness in our dress, our mannerisms, and our speech. Yet, they will recognize their essential connectedness to us. Therapeutic occupations change with the times and with the culture, but the underlying idea of occupation as therapy remains constant.

Defining Occupation

Given our title as *occupational* therapists and given our reason for being, it is ironic that we have not spent much effort in defining occupation. This curious omission has been pointed out by advocates of occupation as therapy (e.g., Christiansen, 1990; Gilfoyle, 1984). Much of my work has focused on the definition of the term *occupation* (Nelson, 1988, 1994, 1996). Occupation is defined as the relationship between an *occupational form* and an *occupational performance* (see Figure 45.1). Occupational performance means the doing. Occupational form means the thing, or the format, that is done. For example, consider the occupation of a boy making potato pancakes (latkes) in December during the Jewish holiday of Hanukkah. His occupational form has physical features, such as the way those potatoes soak up oil and fry crispy on the outside, yet a little soggy on the inside. His occupational form also has sociocultural features, including its connection to his religious heritage and that the chef's hat he wears once belonged to his grandfather. The handle of the frying pan (part of the occupational form) elicits the occupational performance of grasping. Other aspects of his occupational performance include his speech, gaze, smile, and posture.

Occupational form and performance are objectively observable; we can see and analyze the boy's environment and movement patterns. But occupation also has subjective, experiential elements that are not directly observable. These subjective aspects of occupation are *meaning* and *purpose*. Meaning is the person's active interpretation of the occupational form. Meaning has to do with making sense of things perceptually; for example, the boy has a basic awareness that he is not too close to the fire. Meaning also has to do with interpreting the symbols in his occupational form, for example, the words of others and the idea of Hanukkah as a playful holiday. Meaning is also affective: The boy is having fun.

After meaning is present (i.e., the person makes sense of the occupational form), then purpose is possible. Purpose is the person's goal orientation; it is what the person wants or intends. For example, what does the boy making

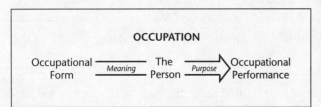

Figure 45.1. Occupation as the meaningful, purposeful occupational performance of a person in the context of an occupational form.

latkes want? Does he want to make his sister laugh? Does he want to make tasty latkes that he can douse with apple-sauce and eat or share with his family? Does he want to participate in a family tradition? At any given moment, a human being typically has multiple purposes—some immediate, such as wanting to hold onto the spatula, and some long term, such as wanting to belong within a family. It is characteristic of an occupational approach to consider both the immediate and the ultimate purposes of the person engaged in occupation.

Occupation influences the world around the person (see Figure 45.2). This influence is called *impact*. The human being is not just a passive respondent who is always under environmental control. The person can affect his or her own future occupational forms. The boy in the example actively changes his occupational form: The latkes are cooked and the kitchen is somewhat of a mess. The cooking occupation sets up the next occupation—eating.

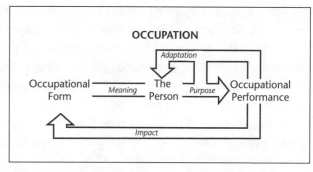

Figure 45.2. Occupation depicted with the occupational dynamics of impact and adaptation.

Another dynamic of occupation is that a person can literally change his or her own nature by engaging in occupation. This is called occupational *adaptation*. Active doing, or occupation, can lead to changes in sensorimotor abilities, cognitive abilities, and psychosocial abilities. As we do, so we become. For example, consider the occupation of a healthy 8-month-old boy playing peek-a-boo with his mother. The boy's occupational form includes a piece of cloth first placed over his face and later over his mother's face. By putting the cloth over her own face, the mother gives the boy an opportunity to have an impact through active occupational performance. He is rewarded by her smiling face and her animated talk when the cloth is removed. There is an established game that is present in the occupational form: Our culture makes available to us the game of peek-a-boo. The boy's occupational performance involves complex patterns of reaching, grasping, trunk rotation, posture, laughing, facial expression, and prespeech sounds. This occupational form is meaningful to the boy perceptually, symbolically, and affectively. He is full of purpose as he tries to reestablish eye contact with his mother by attempting to remove the cloth from her face. We can infer multiple sensorimotor adaptations, such as posture, reach, and grasp, but perhaps more importantly, there are cognitive and psychosocial adaptations. For example, the boy is learning the rules of reciprocal play. Additionally, object permanence is being established, and the boy is learning that important things, like mother, do not go away just because they cannot be seen temporarily.

Brief occupations such as these are the dynamics that while interacting with physiological maturation power human development. These brief occupations are nested within higher level occupations. Indeed, large roles in life are occupations that consist of thousands of brief occupations. For example, consider the reciprocal occupations of a father and daughter on a roller coaster at an amusement park. The man is smiling, however terrified. The girl raises her hands in adolescent bravado. For the girl, the roller-coaster ride is nested within a series of amusement park occupations over many years from the merry-go-round of her toddlerhood to the ultimate goal of going to the amusement park with friends, including boys (no parents needed, thank you). The ride on the roller coaster is also nested within all the summer and family vacations of the girl's life. Given past adaptations, she is ready to go on to new occupations and adventures. From the father's point of view, his daughter is an immediate part of his occupational form, but he would not be there on that screaming roller coaster with his 48-year-old vestibular system if it were not because this occupation is integrally connected to all the occupations of fatherhood. The artful interlocking of successive levels of a person's occupations, bound together by corresponding levels of purpose, connects the present moment to the life span. It would be just as reductionistic to ignore brief moments of occupation as it would be to ignore occupational roles that span decades. We cannot really understand the long-term occupations without understanding the short-term occupations that make them up and vice versa.

Occupational adaptation marks every age of the developing person. Consider the occupations of happy elderly newlyweds singing at a microphone. Their occupational form is the small town wedding celebration. In the basement hall of the American Legion with Old Glory in the background and long wooden tables decorated with balloons and banners, the newlyweds take their turn at the microphone. More than 200 people are present, including new in-laws getting to know each other, townspeople discussing their views on local events, young children racing through the aisles, and teenagers trying to sneak off to the parking lot. The occupational form of marriage means something profound to each marriage partner. Their purposes are both to sing a pretty good tune (pertaining to the immediate occupation) and to start a life together (pertaining to their long-term occupations). Growing beyond their recent roles as widow and widower, they adapt to new occupational roles. Occupational forms, the gifts of nature and of culture, not only sustain us, but also challenge us to engage in the continuous adaptations that constitute life.

A Conceptual Framework for Therapeutic Occupation

Given the power of occupation in healthy human development, it makes great sense to have founded a profession on the idea of occupation as therapy. We as a profession believe that a person can affect the quality of his or her life through occupation. We also believe that the person can be helped through this process by another person—an occupational therapist.

At the Medical College of Ohio, we advocate a Conceptual Framework for Therapeutic Occupation (CFTO; see Figure 45.3). The occupational therapist understands the potentials of various occupational forms and is willing to collaborate in synthesizing occupational forms that are meaningful and purposeful to the person. The occupational therapist hopes and predicts that the occupational form will be perceptually, symbolically, and emotionally meaningful to the person; that the occupational form and the meanings the person actively assigns to it will result in a multidimensional set of purposes (when therapy is best, the person is full of purpose); and that the person will engage in a voluntary occupational performance.

Consider the occupation of an older man who has had a stroke on the right side of his brain that led to left hemiparesis, perceptual problems, and left neglect. In the rehabilitation hospital, he was continuously told to do things with his left hand—"Use your left hand." "Look at your left hand." "Watch out for your left hand."—but he did not understand why until he hurt it in the spokes of his wheelchair. The man's therapeutic occupational adaptation occurs in the occupational therapy bathroom where he is given a comb in front of a mirror. Here the occupational form is full of salient cues for what is expected. Though there are many cues, the situation as a whole suggests a unified response: It is time to comb hair. The occupational form is immediately meaningful to him, words are really not necessary. He knows that the water should be turned on, so he independently does so. He

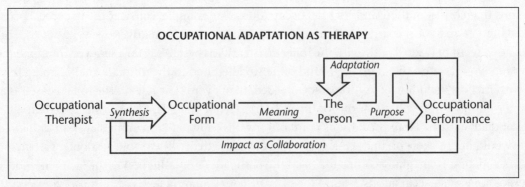

Figure 45.3. A Conceptual Framework for Therapeutic Occupation (for therapeutic adaptation). The occupational therapist collaboratively synthesizes an occupational form and makes a prediction concerning the person's meaning, purpose, occupational performance, and adaptation.

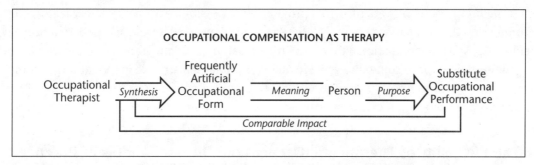

Figure 45.4. A Conceptual Framework for Therapeutic Occupation (for therapeutic compensation). The occupational therapist collaboratively synthesizes an occupational form (often somewhat atypical socioculturally). The resulting occupational performance substitutes for the typical way of doing things but leads to a comparable impact.

combs his hair in his accustomed way; that is, his left arm rises in synchrony and coordination with his right hand as he straightens his hair. Embedded in this occupation are left shoulder flexion and external rotation accompanied by elbow flexion with wrist, hand, and finger control. This coordinated pattern of movement takes place outside his visual range, hence guided by proprioceptive input. This occupation is an excellent intervention for his motor control, left neglect, and problems of body scheme. Of course, a single occupation does not result in dramatic gains, yet dramatic gains are impossible without a series of therapeutic occupations like this one.

Sometimes the person's problem is resistant to occupational adaptation. Hence, compensatory occupation is the goal (see Figure 45.4). In compensation, the therapist collaborates with the person in synthesizing an atypical or alternative occupational form. As always, the therapist hopes and predicts that the occupational form will be meaningful and purposeful. However, in compensation, the goal is to have a successful impact as a result of a substitute occupational performance or as a way around the problem.

Consider an older man who is holding his cafeteria tray with a myoelectric prosthesis. The prosthesis is an atypical part of an otherwise typical occupational form. However, the prosthesis has meaning to the man (he knows how to operate it), and it has purpose to him (he wants to operate it). The substitute occupational performance is that he contracts or relaxes the remaining segments of his upper arm muscles to control the device. The comparable impact is that the tray is held while he uses his dominant right hand to scoop the food. This is successful occupational compensation. Frequently, compensation depends on prior adaptations or learning how to use the compensatory device. In this example, the role of the occupational therapist was to help the man learn how to manipulate the prosthetic elbow and wrist joints and how to match his muscle contractions to the electronics of the prosthesis so that objects could be picked up without dropping or crushing them. Hence, adaptations led to successful compensations.

Occupational adaptation and adaptational compensation are different but dynamically interacting processes. Both depend on *occupational synthesis,* or design, of forms that are meaningful and purposeful to the person. Occupational synthesis is what we occupational therapists do for a living. Our specialty is to know about occupational forms in all their variety and to perceive the special capabilities of persons so that a therapeutic match can be made. Sometimes this involves highly naturalistic, everyday forms. But often, there is an element of simulation involved. Consider a boy with cerebral palsy whose occupational form involves virtual reality equipment and a new power wheelchair with an unfamiliar joystick. The meaningfulness and purposefulness of the occupational form to him can be inferred from his occupational performance: He manipulates the joystick in a sustained way and his gaze is set on the feedback device. His occupational adaptation is his learning how to operate the joystick that will control his wheelchair. This will provide him with compensatory mobility in the future.

The virtual reality in this example is "high tech," but we occupational therapists have always used virtual reality, or simulation, whether high tech or low. For example, the occupational therapy kitchen is a treatment area that simulates the homes of many patients while providing the possibility of special safety features and assistive devices. In some cases, the occupational therapy kitchen provides the ideal location; in others, a home visit would be more therapeutic. Much of occupational therapy clinical reasoning and program development depend on judgments about the suitability or unsuitability of simulated versus naturalistic occupational forms. Simulation can involve great creativity and technology, as with virtual reality or electronic work simulators. But the naturalistic occupational forms provided by our culture are the starting points for our ingenuity.

The Flexibility of Therapeutic Occupation: Diverse Models of Practice

Therapeutic occupation, the common core of occupational therapy, is a robust construct capable of accommodating many different approaches to intervention. Mosey (1970) introduced the term *theoretical frame of reference* to describe systematic guidelines for occupational therapy practice that are grounded in theoretical statements about the nature of the person and his or her relations to the world. Others, including Kielhofner (1992), have used the term *conceptual model of practice* to denote the diversity of theory-based approaches to occupational therapy.

My idea of model of practice has two main parts: (a) a theoretical base describing healthy and unhealthy occupation and (b) principles and techniques for occupational syntheses. The theoretical base draws from one or more disciplines. It is a coherent description of the potentials and pitfalls of human occupation, including the nature of the person, the role of occupational forms, the types of meanings and purposes experienced by the person, and the dynamics of successful and unsuccessful occupational performances. Basic research is cited as available. The second part of a model of practice provides principled yet practical guidelines for occupational syntheses that are consistent with the theoretical base. How does the therapist conduct occupational syntheses in the evaluation process? How does the therapist use occupational analysis in the goal-setting process? How does the therapist collaborate with the person in synthesizing occupational forms for adaptation or compensation? Applied research is cited as available.

There currently are many models of practice in occupational therapy. Some are more carefully worked out than others; all are works in progress. Consideration of selected occupational therapy models of practice from the past can enhance appreciation of today's diverse models of practice. In discussing these models, I will apply the same occupational terminology introduced earlier in this article (e.g., *occupational form, occupational performance*) to the diverse ideas expressed by various authors. I believe that this terminology provides a systematic way to compare and contrast occupational therapy models of practice.

Slagle's Habit Training Model of Practice

Slagle (1922) was a proponent of one of the first models of practice in occupational therapy. She drew from many different theoretical sources, including John Dewey's Chicago-school philosophy of pragmatism; William James's psychology of attention; Ruskin's arts-and-crafts movement; the Society of Friends's moral treatment; and Adolph Meyer's ideas about holism, mental hygiene, and use of time. Slagle theorized that habit reactions largely constitute the lives of most people. The healthy person engages each day in a rich succession of habit occupations—a balance of productive work, self-reliance, rest, and activation of what Slagle called the "play spirit" (p. 16). Underlying all habits is the necessity for attention; indeed attention itself is a habit that can be built.

Unlike the well-organized habits of healthy persons, the habits of persons with mental disorders are deteriorated and disorganized. Attention drifts restlessly and irrelevantly. Neither the joy of productivity nor the joy of play is experienced. Grandiosity on the one hand and passivity on the other are poor substitutes for actual occupation. Given this theoretical base of healthy and unhealthy occupation, what kinds of occupational syntheses are called for in the Slagle model of practice? The main occupational form that Slagle described was a 24-hour per-day schedule that provided a balance of self-care, physical exercises, work, and play (Kidner, 1930). Specifically noted were instructional periods for self-care (e.g., shoe lacing, teeth cleaning, toileting). Work occupations were to be individually graded from simple to complex. Stimulating music with clearly evident rhythm was recommended to accompany the physical exercises. Moving pictures, folk dancing, storytelling, and simple competitive games rounded out the day. After the basic habit occupations were attained, the patient could progress to the *occupational center,* also called the *curative workshop.* Here patients engaged daily in major crafts or preindustrial groups that required sustained attention over many sessions. The developmental structure of the discharged patient was enhanced by adaptations in the attentional mechanisms and habit reactions.

Baldwin's Model of Practice for the Restoration of Movement

Another early model of practice focused on different aspects of the developmental structure from those focused on by Slagle. Baldwin's (1919) model of practice was designed to restore movement abilities in young soldiers wounded in World War I and drew into occupational therapy concepts from kinesiology, biomechanics, and psychology. He detailed the relationships between various occupational forms and joint range of motion, strength, and endurance. He saw coordination as a high-level skill involving complex series of movements across several joints, and he believed that this high-level skill is inextricably linked to everyday occupations. Movement skill was viewed not just in terms of immediate learning but also in terms of what can be "transferred to another occasion or to other types of movements" (p. 7). Although he focused on the patient's motor abilities, Baldwin also cited "interest," "attention," "initiative," "inspiration," "optimism," and "cheerfulness" (pp. 6–9) as factors that affect the overall quality of the patient's occupations. Baldwin specifically identified social factors that typically inhibited the development of self-responsibility among disabled veterans, including the military's discouragement of the initiative typical of civilian life and the public's misdirected sympathy. Baldwin also considered the patient's intelligence and vocational aptitude when synthesizing therapeutic occupational forms.

Given this view of the person's developmental structure, the main guideline for occupational synthesis was to provide occupational forms that naturalistically challenge the identified problems of range, strength, endurance, and coordination. In Baldwin's (1919) own terms:

> Occupational therapy is based on the principle that the best type of remedial exercise is that which requires a series of specific voluntary movements involved in the ordinary trades and occupations, physical training, play, and the daily routine activities of life. (p. 5)

Occupational forms were analyzed in terms of their typical challenges for the purposes of grading from easy to hard and providing options to different patients, depending on their interests. The end-products, or the impacts, of the work were thought to enhance meaning and purpose; impact also provided direct feedback about the patient's progress. Baldwin favored the use of everyday occupational forms, including, but not restricted to, crafts. The advantages of naturalistic occupational forms were (a) the allowance for personal initiative, (b) the incentives provided for sustained effort, (c) the development of coordination, (d) the transfer of skills, and (e) the opportunity for membership in a social group of fellows working on parallel projects. Baldwin was a strong proponent of research that documented the effects of everyday occupational forms on motor abilities. Much of my research today (e.g., Nelson et al., 1996) investigates principles identified in Baldwin's model of practice that was described more than 75 years ago.

Other Early Models of Practice

It is important to realize that those who helped found the profession espoused different approaches to the use of therapeutic occupation. Each model of practice had its own conceptualization of healthy and unhealthy occupation, and each had its guidelines for synthesizing occupational forms. For example, Tracy (1910) presented a model for bedside occupations for hospitalized patients. The focus was on preventing the negative psychosocial consequences of bedrest so that the patient could be a full partner in his or her medical treatment. Synthesized occupational forms varied depending on the age of the patient, the nature of the disability, and interest. It is interesting to note that all three of the authors cited so far included calisthenics as a potentially valuable type of therapeutic occupation.

A fourth example of an early model of practice in occupational therapy is Hall's work cure for persons with what was then called neurasthenia. In a letter from Hall (1917) to William Rush Dunton, Hall expressed expertise in only one area of what he called therapeutic occupations. Is this not an early expression of specialization by model of practice while remaining cognizant of one's integral link to other models through the organizing framework of therapeutic occupations? Another early letter, however, makes clear that proponents of different models did not always accept or appreciate each other's differences. In a letter to Dunton, Barton (1916), the first president of the National Society for the Promotion of Occupational Therapy and an opponent of Hall's model of practice, expressed the hope that Hall "not put cyanide in our tea" (p. 2) to avenge his exclusion from the deliberations of the charter officers of the society. This facetious remark reflects an ongoing struggle among adherents of different approaches to the use of therapeutic occupation.

The Psychodynamic Model of Practice

How flexible is the concept of therapeutic occupation? Let us consider the change that accompanied American psychology and psychiatry in the 1930s and 1940s when the Freudians advocated a new and controversial view of the person. At that time, Fidler (1948), who has become one of the most influential leaders in the history of the profession, proposed the adoption of a psychodynamic approach in occupational therapy. How do dynamic theorists view the person and occupation, and given this viewpoint, what kinds of occupational forms are synthesized for therapy? In this model of practice, the most important meanings and purposes underlying occupation are unconscious reflections of biological drives. These powerful libidinal and aggressive impulses are theorized to be the products of psychosexual development in early childhood. With maturation, the ego defends itself against anxiety via a variety of unconscious mechanisms, some of which are relatively adaptive and some maladaptive.

Given this view of the occupational structure of the person, the early stages of occupational therapy involved a close, nonthreatening match between carefully selected occupational forms and individual personality. For example, the patient who is unconsciously aggressive is provided with clay to pound or with wood to cut, and the person who is compulsively neat is provided with an occupational form such as weaving, which requires much repetition and involves little waste. Over time, the therapist gradually introduces occupational forms that facilitate relatively mature defense mechanisms.

Humanistic Models of Practice

An illustration of how the profession can accommodate new models of practice can be seen in Fidler's ongoing developments. We can compare and contrast the Fidler and Fidler (1978) article, "Doing and Becoming: Purposeful Action and Self-Actualization," with the Fidler (1948) psychodynamically inspired article we have just discussed. The title of Fidler and Fidler's article indicates the sweeping changes occurring in the 1970s in American psychology and psychiatry. Humanism and existentialism were discovered and adopted as philosophical positions. Instead of conceptualizing the person as conflict laden due to unconscious drives, as in Freudianism, the humanist views the person as a consciously choosing, self-determining being with created values and interests. The person is looked on optimistically in terms of his or her ability to change self or to adapt via occupational performance. Self-actualization is viewed as a person's highest achievement.

The ideas of humanism have strongly influenced many leaders within the profession, including Reilly (1962), Yerxa (1967), and Kielhofner (1995). Kielhofner's Model of Human Occupation conceptualizes the person's occupations in terms of personal causation, values, interests, internalized roles, and habit patterns in addition to many different skills. Recently influenced by dynamic systems theory, Kielhofner currently emphasizes the volitional processes of attending, experiencing, and choosing, as well as the processes underlying changes in roles and habits. The person is the creator of a life story, a narrative. Given this viewpoint of the person, Kielhofner's occupational forms emphasize naturalistic options and the opportunity for success. Naturalistic options in the occupational form make choices with high levels of symbolic meaning possible. Intrinsic purpose in occupation is most highly valued. The occupational therapist's verbal responsiveness is also a critical aspect of the occupational form because the client and therapist collaboratively synthesize occupational forms. This model of practice has an optimistic viewpoint of the person's ability to adapt and take control of his or her own life, regardless of residual impairments.

The Sensory Integrative Model of Practice

Humanism was not the only great idea influencing Western civilization in the 1960s and 1970s. Another set of ideas with a profound effect on the development of occupational therapy models of practice has come through the advent of neuroscience. Consider Ayres's (1972) sensory integrative model. As with all the other occupational therapy models of practice we have and will discuss, most of the foundational ideas for sensory integration were taken from sources outside occupational therapy. Ayres conceptualized the person in neurological terms. The first words of her classic book were: "Learning is a function of the brain; learning disorders are assumed to reflect some deviation in neural function" (p. 1). In Ayres's original work, the brain is conceptualized phylogenetically and hierarchically, with higher level cognitive centers in the cerebrum that depend on lower level centers, especially those governing somatosensory input, including vestibular, tactile, and proprioceptive sensation. Ayres hypothesized that many children with learning disorders do not integrate somatosensory input with visual and auditory processing. She also hypothesized that children have an inner drive for mastery in occupation.

Given this conceptualization of the developmental structure, Ayres (1972) created some of the most fascinating occupational forms in the history of our profession: rolling and tumbling forms such as scooter boards and carpeted barrels that support or envelop the child while eliciting somatosensory meanings and bolsters, nets, and swings that hang from the ceiling and provide vestibular input in the occupational context of a game. These occupational forms that elicit whole-body occupational performances are prerequisites to the highly structured occupational forms of education, which assume adequate visual and auditory comprehension necessary for advanced cognition. Like humanistic models of practice, this neurologically based model of practice is optimistic about the person's ability to adapt via occupational performance.

Allen's Model of Cognitive Disabilities

A very different model of practice is also rooted in a neuroscientific conceptualization of the person. In Allen's (1985) model of cognitive disabilities, certain neurological disorders are considered intractable. Although the person's interests and sensorimotor abilities are considered, the focus of this model is on cognitive levels, which are viewed hierarchically from an unresponsive coma state to an advanced level of deductive reasoning. Given that progress from one cognitive level to the next cannot occur through occupation (but might occur in some disorders through the physiological healing of the brain), the emphasis in this model of practice is on evaluation and compensation. What kinds of occupational forms are used? The Allen Cognitive Levels test uses selected crafts (e.g., various forms of leather lacing) to challenge cognition. Crafts are readily recognizable in our society yet are not threatening in the way that many tests are. The materials provide definite structure across space and time, and the craft product (an impact) is an objective indicator of the quality of occupational performance. Hence, the occupational therapist can monitor changes along the cognitive dimension tested as the brain heals. In addition, the occupational therapist can synthesize compensatory occupational forms designed to match the patient's cognitive level. For example, the person who learns only by trial and error will need supervision for safety's sake in everyday occupational forms.

Toglia's Multicontext Approach to Perceptual Cognitive Impairments

An emerging model of practice that posits the adaptational capacity of persons with neurological impairment has been put forward by Toglia (1991). Drawing on knowledge from modern neuropsychology, Toglia hypothesized that metacognition and cognitive processing strategies can be enhanced through a variety of naturalistic occupational forms—a multicontext approach that uses everyday situations as the crux of therapy. Everyday situations from the supermarket to the bus line provide similar cognitive challenges yet provide sufficient variations for generalized learning to occur. Consistent with occupational therapy history, Toglia suggested that the everyday world of our communities can be the occupational therapist's clinic. As we encounter our everyday occupational forms, so we become.

Motor Control and Motor Learning Models of Practice

One of the fascinating events of the past 10 years has been the change in focus within the motor control models of practice. One way of describing this revolution is that theorists and therapists are focusing more on occupational synthesis. In the past, the emphasis was on the patient's physiology and movements (e.g., muscle tone, symmetry, isolation of movement patterns). While remaining sophisticated about the patient's physiology, therapists today are also becoming more sophisticated about the other half of the therapeutic equation: the occupational forms that the patient needs in order to engage in active occupational performance. Symbolic of this revolution is Trombly's (1995) Eleanor Clarke Slagle Lecture in which she cited research, theory, and practical experience in favor of occupational forms that are meaningful and purposeful to the person. Whether guided by the neurodevelopmental model of practice (Levit, 1995) or a contemporary approach drawing from dynamic systems theory (Mathiowetz & Haugen, 1995), therapists today are synthesizing naturalistic occupational forms of work, play, and self-care, with the active collaboration of the patient in the choice of those forms.

Selected Other Models of Practice

To suggest the tremendous range of potential applications of our core concept of therapeutic occupation, I will briefly mention a few of the many other occupational therapy models of practice. Occupational models of practice are being refined for persons with Alzheimer's disease and their caregivers (American Occupational Therapy Association [AOTA], 1994), and some models are being developed for the handwriting problems of schoolchildren (Amundson, 1992). Als's conceptualization of the premature infant is compatible with an occupational therapy model of practice geared toward both the emerging occupations of the infant and the occupations of parents (Vergara, 1993). A fourth area in which the special skills of occupational therapists are needed is hospice care (Pizzi, 1993), where meaningful and purposeful occupation is a reflection of the value placed on human life. Although these are but a few samples of the many areas in which therapeutic occupation is contributing to quality of life, my experience tells me that creative occupational therapy practitioners will continue to develop new models of practice that meet the real needs of real persons for therapeutic occupations—therapy by doing.

Beyond Direct Service Models

A commitment to the use of occupation as the method of occupational therapy does not commit us to direct service models as opposed to educational models or consultative models. The occupational therapist can play an essential and cost-effective role in the collaborative synthesis of occupational forms, even though the therapist will not be physically present when the person engages in the occupational form. Because the therapist has expertise in occupational forms—their physical and sociocultural complexity—he or she can advise the daughter of a woman with Alzheimer's disease about least restrictive environments (AOTA, 1994), a teacher or nurse about proper positioning (Dunn & Campbell, 1991), or the foreman of a workstation with a high rate of carpal tunnel syndrome about repetitive trauma disorders (AOTA, 1992). Such advice is a collaborative occupational synthesis. For the same reason, a truly occupational model of practice is used when the therapist advises patients with diseases of the hand about occupations in the home, at work, and at play (Kasch, 1990).

Occupational Therapy Models of Practice in the Future

What future roles will the occupational therapist play in the health care system? Readers 100 years from now will no doubt be aware of occupational therapy practice that we cannot dream of today. And I am sure that there will be an occupational therapy reader 100 years from today because of the fundamental power of occupation and its adaptability to new circumstances.

Independent Living Movement

One current trend that may well grow in the future is the independent living movement in which persons with disabilities see themselves as consumers of health care services. As consumers, they make decisions about their lives and rehabilitation with professional help but without the authoritarianism that sometimes accompanies the medical model. This approach is in tune with the principles of occupational therapy (AOTA, 1993; Yerxa, 1994). The problem is not to be thought of as lying in the consumers (their developmental structures), but in the everyday occupational forms they encounter, such as barriers to restaurants, workstations, and fields of play. Given this philosophy, the occupational therapist emphasizes collaborative occupational synthesis and compensatory strategies from ramps to robots and from social acceptance to political power. The consumer who takes control of his or her life within an insensitive society could not do better than to have an occupational therapist as an advocate.

Technology

The independent living movement dovetails nicely with another identifiable trend for the future: new technologies that promote successful and personally satisfying occupation. As Mann and Lane (1991) pointed out, the occupational therapist "can—and should—be the professional who takes responsibility for assembling the appropriate assistive technology team" (p. 26). The occupational therapist has the knowledge and experience to take a leadership role in working with the consumer in making the best possible match between the multiple factors in technologically oriented occupational forms and the multiple capacities of the consumer's developmental structure. We need to think of assistive devices as parts of the occupational forms that have meaning and purpose to the person, not as mechanical extensions of a mechanical person.

Wellness Models of Practice

Another trend is the move toward an increased emphasis on wellness, health promotion, and disease prevention. With the brave new world of capitation, managed care, primary care, efficacy, and efficiency, the health care system may at last get serious about wellness. Wellness pays. Nothing could be more positive for the profession of occupational therapy. Theorists within the profession have been preparing us for the advent of a health care system that emphasizes health as opposed to illness (Johnson, 1986; Rosenfeld, 1993). Occupational therapists working with persons who already have disabilities have long emphasized the importance of healthy occupational profiles and disease prevention to their patients, even though those efforts have not always been reimbursable. The wellness models of practice are in place and only await general funding.

Models for Public Health

Another role for the future of occupational therapy is in the solution of some of our society's chronic social and public health problems, such as drugs, violence, unprepared motherhood, unemployment, and homelessness. A problem of special interest for me is the development of an occupational therapy model of practice for the prevention of childhood obesity. Obesity has devastating lifelong consequences, with sensorimotor, cognitive, and psychosocial impairments and impoverished occupational patterns. A comprehensive model of therapeutic occupation needs to be tested for this major problem of public health. Occupational therapy leaders, such as Baum (1991), have found ways to fund occupational models of practice, even in a pessimistic sociopolitical environment where social programs are mistrusted. I call this America's 1990s regression to the social Darwinism of the 1890s. But sooner or later, the profession of Eleanor Clarke Slagle will provide occupational models of practice for homeless people with schizophrenia and occupational models of practice for persons in so-called nursing homes. (Let us call them homes for therapeutic occupation!) The mark of a great civilization is not its store of consumer goods but the meaningfulness and purposefulness of the everyday occupations of all its citizens.

Hospital-Based Models

I believe that occupational therapy will continue to play an essential role in the acute care hospital and in other medically related facilities from the rehabilitation hospital, to subacute sites, to extended care facilities, to the facilities of the future. It is true that hospitals are downsizing, and patients are being discharged more and more quickly. It is also true that the ideal health care system of the future will promote wellness as its highest goal. Nevertheless, people will continue to become ill; they will continue to go to the hospital, however downsized, for acute care. Many of these people will continue to need an occupational approach at one or more stages of their illness and recovery (Torrance, 1993). With increasing technology and quicker discharge, the need for therapeutic occupation increases, not decreases. Occupational therapists will be needed to work with patients in problem solving self-care occupations amidst the constraints of the tubes, monitors, and fixators; to activate patients at risk because of the deleterious effects of bedrest; to help patients and caregivers plan realistically for what the patients will do and for how the patients will live and care for themselves after discharge but before healing; and to assess patients' quality of life before and after hospitalization.

For an example of the importance of therapeutic occupation in an acute care setting, consider a 5-month-old girl born with a neuromuscular disease of unknown etiology. The disease is characterized by the total absence of many of the proximal muscles, including those responsible for respiration. Picture her with multiple intubations for respiration and nutrition and with life-support monitors. The occupational therapist carefully removes her from the crib and bounces her gently while talking to her in high-pitched, rhythmical tones. In response to this occupational form, the infant's adaptations are to learn to use the muscles controlling her vocal cords as she imitates the therapist; to learn to use the remaining muscles in her left arm as she grabs the therapist's keys; and most of all, to begin to learn that she too has a legitimate place in the human family. The therapist next places a piece of cloth playfully over the child's face, as in our prior example of the importance of peek-a-boo in healthy development. Like the healthy infant, this baby also removes the cloth and laughs. Despite the high technology setting, this baby also needs to encounter the occupational form of peek-a-boo in order to develop a sense of self and a sense of other. I believe that occupational models of practice will be needed for the acute care hospital for patients at all points on the life span as much as they are needed for community-based care.

Models of Practice and the Great Ideas of the 20th Century

Therapeutic occupation is a remarkably powerful yet flexible idea. Consider all the different philosophies and branches of science that have washed across the 20th century and that have become the theoretical bases of occupational therapy models of practice: the moral treatment initiated by members of the Society of Friends; the arts-and-crafts movement initiated by the British socialist Ruskin as an antidote to the negative effects of industrialism; the philosophy of pragmatism; the holistic medicine of Meyer; James's psychology of attention; principles of kinesiology and biomechanics; the dynamic theories of the Freudians, neo-Freudians, and ego psychologists; behaviorism and learning theory; developmental theory; humanism and existentialism; neuroscience and neuropsychology and their many schools; efficacy and competency theory; systems theory and dynamic systems theory; the social psychology of groups; ecological psychology; motor learning and motor control theories; cultural anthropology and ethnography; and narrative analysis. (For discussions of these topics and their influences on occupational therapy models of practice, see Breines, 1995; Christiansen & Baum, 1991; Kielhofner, 1992.) These schools of thought reflect many of the majestic ideas in the intellectual history of the 20th century. Even though every one of them originated from outside the occupational therapy profession, each has contributed essential theory to our models of practice. Across every model of practice, the core of therapeutic occupational synthesis can be identified: form, meaning, purpose, performance, evaluation, adaptation, and compensation. This robust flexibility at the core of our profession is the basis for my saying that therapeutic occupation will flourish in the 21st century.

Two Recommendations

Research

My first recommendation is research—research for occupational therapists conducted by occupational therapists and those who understand occupation as therapy. Our primary focus should be to examine the power of occupation as therapy. My vision for the 21st century is that occupational therapy will take its rightful place among the major professions in our society. The powers and complexities of occupation justify the sanctioning of a major profession. This will be especially true if the society of our descendants devotes increased attention to the actual occupations of daily life, to the meanings of life, and to the qualities of existence. Should there not be a Nobel prize for occupational therapy?

But to be a major force in research, we must examine our basic principles in highly systematic ways—ways that are accepted by the larger research community. If we do not examine the great ideas of occupational therapy, some other group will. For decades, occupational therapists have used common, everyday occupational forms and hands-on doing to enhance what Dunton (1945) called the "mental processes of reasoning or judgment or remembering" (p. 11). Recently, cognitive researchers, mainly psychologists, have developed a body of knowledge about the effects of subject-performed tasks (SPTs) on human cognition (e.g., Backman, 1985). The basic idea of SPTs is that hands-on doing, with its added sensory input and opportunity for feedback, is a greater cognitive stimulant than demonstration or other teaching techniques that do not involve hands-on experience. The problem is that the cognitive psychologists pursuing this line of research have not cited occupational therapy authors, who have advocated this principle since the beginning of the profession. Our problem here is that we have not done the research necessary to establish our special expertise in the area of hands-on doing, or occupation.

In like manner, we are only beginning to do the research that establishes our expertise in the area of occupationally embedded movement. Carr and Shepherd (1987) have written eloquently and at length about how everyday situations, such as a glass of water, can elicit therapeutic patterns of movement, such as a good hand path, in patients with neuromuscular disorders. However, these authors, neither of whom are occupational therapists, do not once cite occupational therapy or its history of using everyday occupational forms to promote therapeutic patterns of movement.

My point is that persons from other professions are coming late to the table and claiming credit for some of the great ideas of occupational therapy. These ideas deserve the most careful philosophical and scientific scrutiny. As occupational therapists, we need to own these ideas while enlightening other disciplines as to their usefulness.

Equally needed are basic research examining the nature of occupation and applied research examining models of practice. Academically respected quantitative and qualitative research methodologies should be used. One approach to research in occupational therapy is what I have called the experimental analysis of therapeutic occupation (Nelson, 1993). Here, occupational forms are contrasted to each other in terms of participants' occupational performances, impacts, adaptations, or reported meanings and purposes. A different approach, termed *occupational science,* has been proposed by Clark et al. (1991). These authors have recommended qualitative methods for studying the multiple dimensions of naturally occurring occupations. It is critical that the profession encourage different types of inquiry, at least until there is a broad consensus that a single type of inquiry satisfactorily deals with all the research problems of the profession. I predict that no such consensus will ever develop.

To support the research enterprise, funding will be essential. A specific goal of the AOTA should be the establishment of study sections specifically devoted to occupational therapy research in federal grants management agencies, as is the case with nursing. Only those with considerable knowledge of the profession of occupational therapy can appreciate and nurture the full potential of occupational therapy knowledge. In the interim, the AOTA and the American Occupational Therapy Foundation, which is to say all of us, should make special efforts to support research that is specifically occupational. A priority is the further development of doctoral programs devoted to the development of occupational therapy knowledge. More than anything else, a sound doctoral program is a socialization experience toward a new identity as a scholar in a particular field. Although scholars of diverse backgrounds have made great contributions to knowledge in occupational therapy, a true profession requires the intense engagement at its core, which is expected in doctoral programs devoted to the development of occupational therapy knowledge.

Occupation, Not the *A* Word

My second recommendation is for all of us to embrace and own the idea of occupation as therapy. Wilma West (1984) not only urged us to use the term *occupation* with pride, but also wrote that the term *occupation* "is infinitely more expressive and encompassing than 'purposeful activity' " (p. 22). Nothing is more important to this profession. We are called *occupational* therapists, and the essence of our profession is the use of occupation as a therapeutic method. In contrast, the term *activity* lacks the connotation of intentionality. The term *activity* denotes motion, for example, *volcanic activity, molecular activity*, and *gastric activity*, not occupation that is replete with meaning and purpose.

Another major problem with the use of the word *activity* is that we confuse the public. Slagle (1922) wrote about her "system of occupational analysis" (p. 16). Neither she nor we need to say activity analysis. If the essence of our profession is activity, then why are we not called activity therapists (Darnell & Heater, 1994)? We need to be able to explain occupation and things occupational to many different audiences from fellow professionals to payers, from persons with immaturities to persons with various disabilities, from journalists to the arts media, and from our students to ourselves. If we explain clearly that occupational therapy involves the active doing of things (occupations) for the sake of enhanced health, our public relations problem and our so-called identity problem will disappear immediately. We have the power to influence standard usage. There are more than 50,000 of us in this country and tens of thousands more in other English-speaking countries. If we are clear and forthright about the essential nature of our service—the use of occupation as method—then society will accommodate us. New words and new professions come into the language system all the time. This problem is entirely within our control.

Over time—keep in mind that we are talking about the next century—society and fellow health care professionals will adopt new terms that are related to what we call occupation. For example, since the founding of occupational therapy the terms *rehabilitation, allied health, deinstitutionalization, function, functional outcomes,* and *inclusion* have come into favor for very good reasons. As occupational therapists, we need to promote the good that is represented in these terms. Yet, we need to resist the temptation to redefine ourselves with every new trend in health care. We are not rehabilitation professionals—we are occupational therapists whose mission is much more basic and enduring than even the rehabilitation movement. Nor are we functional therapists or functional outcomes therapists. The term *function* is reflective of the mechanistic, business-oriented climate of these times. Automobiles function, toasters function, and livers function. Human occupation is far richer than the term *function* can possibly connote. In our era, every health professional from the surgeon to the dietitian must document so-called functional outcomes if they are going to be paid. What makes us unique is not that we document functional outcomes but that we use occupation as the method to achieve positive outcomes.

We are *occupational* therapists, and we are aptly named. Indeed we are named more aptly than many of the professions with which we work. We need to explain this clearly and assertively to the world, but a good starting point will be to explain this clearly and assertively to each other. Occupation as therapy is inclusive enough for all the occupational therapy models of practice. There is no reason to be afraid of cyanide in the tea.

Conclusion

To summarize, occupation is a powerful force in the development of the human being. The essence of our profession is the use of occupation as therapy whose core flexibly accommodates various past, present, and future models of practice drawn from historically important theories that originated outside the profession. I proposed a CFTO, including definitions of occupational form, occupational performance, developmental structure, meaning, purpose, impact, adaptation, compensation, and occupational synthesis. The CFTO highlights the core of therapeutic occupation across diverse models of practice and provides an analytical method for comparing and contrasting different models of practice.

Basic and applied research that investigate principles of occupation are necessary not only for the standing of the profession among other disciplines, but also for the sake of our own integrity. The ultimate statement of pride and confidence in the profession will be the full adoption of the term *occupation* in the language of the profession, with each occupational therapist taking personal responsibility for explaining to the world why we are called occupational therapists.

Acknowledgments

I thank all the colleagues, students, and loved ones who have contributed so much to the content and spirit of this lecture. My children, my sisters, and my mother say that they enjoyed being with us at the lecture.

This lecture included audiovisual themes that cannot be reproduced in article format; therefore, this article makes use of examples and explanations suited for the printed page as opposed to the lecture stage.

References

Allen, C. K. (1985). *Occupational therapy for psychiatric diseases: Measurement and management of cognitive disabilities.* Boston: Little, Brown.

American Occupational Therapy Association. (1992). Statement: Occupational therapy services in work practice. *American Journal of Occupational Therapy, 46,* 1086–1088.

American Occupational Therapy Association. (1993). Statement: The role of occupational therapy in the independent living movement. *American Journal of Occupational Therapy, 47,* 1079–1080.

American Occupational Therapy Association. (1994). Statement: Occupational therapy services for persons with Alzheimer's disease and other dementias. *American Journal of Occupational Therapy, 48,* 1029–1031.

Amundson, S. J. C. (1992). Handwriting: Evaluation and intervention in school settings. In J. Case-Smith & C. Pehoski (Eds.), *Development of hand skills in the child* (pp. 63–78). Rockville, MD: American Occupational Therapy Association.

Ayres, A. J. (1972). *Sensory integration and learning disorders.* Los Angeles: Western Psychological Services.

Backman, L. (1985). Further evidence for the lack of adult age differences on free recall of subject-performed tasks: The importance of motor action. *Human Learning, 3*(1), 53–69.

Baldwin, B. T. (1919). *Occupational therapy applied to restoration of movement.* Washington, DC: Commanding Officer and Surgeon General of the Army, Walter Reed General Hospital.

Barton, G. E. (1916, December 20). *Letter to W. R. Dunton, Jr.* (Available from the American Occupational Therapy Archives, Box 1, File 12, Wilma L. West Library, 4720 Montgomery Lane, Bethesda, MD 20814)

Baum, C. (1991). Professional issues in a changing environment. In C. Christiansen & C. Baum (Eds.), *Occupational therapy: Overcoming human performance deficits* (pp. 804–817). Thorofare, NJ: Slack.

Breines, E. B. (1995). Understanding 'occupation' as the founders did. *British Journal of Occupational Therapy, 58,* 458–460.

Carr, J. H., & Shepherd, R. B. (1987). A motor learning model for rehabilitation. In J. H. Carr & R. B. Shepherd (Eds.), *Movement science: Foundations for physical therapy in rehabilitation.* Rockville, MD: Aspen.

Christiansen, C. (1990). The perils of plurality. *Occupational Therapy Journal of Research, 10,* 259–265.

Christiansen, C., & Baum, C. (Eds.). (1991). *Occupational therapy: Overcoming human performance deficits.* Thorofare, NJ: Slack.

Clark, F. A., Parham, D., Carlson, M. E., Frank, G., Jackson, J., Pierce, D., Wolfe, R. J., & Zemke, R. (1991). Occupational science: Academic innovation in the service of occupational therapy's future. *American Journal of Occupational Therapy, 45,* 300–310.

Darnell, J. L., & Heater, S. L. (1994). The Issue Is—Occupational therapist or activity therapist—Which do you choose to be? *American Journal of Occupational Therapy, 48,* 467–468.

Dunn, W., & Campbell, P. H. (1991). Designing pediatric service provision. In W. Dunn (Ed.), *Pediatric occupational therapy* (pp. 139–159). Thorofare, NJ: Slack.

Dunton, W. R., Jr. (1945). *Prescribing occupational therapy* (2nd ed.). Springfield, IL: Charles C Thomas.

Fidler, G. S. (1948). Psychological evaluation of occupational therapy activities. *American Journal of Occupational Therapy, 2,* 284–287.

Fidler, G. S., & Fidler, J. W. (1978). Doing and becoming: Purposeful action and self-actualization. *American Journal of Occupational Therapy, 32,* 305–310.

Gilfoyle, E. M. (1984). Eleanor Clarke Slagle Lectureship, 1984: Transformation of a profession. *American Journal of Occupational Therapy, 38,* 575–584.

Hall, H. J. (1917, February 23). *Letter to W. R. Dunton, Jr.* (Available from the American Occupational Therapy Archives, Box 2, File 15, Wilma L. West Library, 4720 Montgomery Lane, Bethesda, MD 20814)

Howe, M. C., & Schwartzberg, S. L. (1986). *A functional approach to group work in occupational therapy.* Philadelphia: Lippincott.

Johnson, J. A. (1986). *Wellness: A context for living.* Thorofare, NJ: Slack.

Kasch, M. (1990). Acute hand injuries. In L. W. Pedretti & B. Zoltan (Eds.), *Occupational therapy practice skills for physical dysfunction* (pp. 477–506). St. Louis, MO: Mosby.

Kidner, T. B. (1930). *Occupational therapy: The science of prescribed work for invalids.* Stuttgart, Germany: Kohlhammer.

Kielhofner, G. (1992). *Conceptual foundations of occupational therapy.* Philadelphia: F. A. Davis.

Kielhofner, G. (1995). *A model of human occupation: Theory and application* (2nd ed.). Baltimore: Williams & Wilkins.

Levit, K. (1995). Neurodevelopmental (Bobath) treatment. In C. A. Trombly (Ed.), *Occupational therapy for physical dysfunction* (4th ed., pp. 446–462). Baltimore: Williams & Wilkins.

Mann, W. C., & Lane, J. P. (1991). *Assistive technology for persons with disabilities: The role of occupational therapy.* Rockville, MD: American Occupational Therapy Association.

Mathiowetz, V., & Haugen, J. B. (1995). Evaluation of motor behavior: Traditional and contemporary views. In C. A. Trombly (Ed.), *Occupational therapy for physical dysfunction* (4th ed., pp. 157–185). Baltimore: Williams & Wilkins.

Mosey, A. C. (1970). *Three frames of reference for mental health.* Thorofare, NJ: Slack.

National Society for the Promotion of Occupational Therapy. (1917, March 15). *Certificate of Incorporation of the National Society for the Promotion of Occupational Therapy.* (Incorporated in the District of Columbia and notarized by James A. Rolfe in Clifton Springs, New York)

Nelson, D. L. (1988). Occupation: Form and performance. *American Journal of Occupational Therapy, 42,* 633–641.

Nelson, D. L. (1993, June). The experimental analysis of therapeutic occupation. *Developmental Disabilities Special Interest Section Newsletter, 16*(2), 7–8.

Nelson, D. L. (1994). Occupational form, occupational performance, and therapeutic occupation. In C. B. Royeen (Ed.), *AOTA self-study series: The practice of the future: Putting occupation back into therapy, lesson 2* (pp. 9–48). Rockville, MD: American Occupational Therapy Association.

Nelson, D. L. (1996). Therapeutic occupation: A definition. *American Journal of Occupational Therapy, 50,* 775–782.

Nelson, D. L., Konosky, K., Fleharty, K., Webb, R., Newer, K., Hazboun, V. P., Fontane, C., & Licht, B. (1996). The effects of an occupationally embedded exercise on bilaterally assisted supination in persons with hemiplegia. *American Journal of Occupational Therapy, 50,* 639–646.

Pizzi, M. (1993). Environments of care: Hospice. In H. L. Hopkins & H. D. Smith (Eds.), *Willard and Spackman's occupational therapy* (8th ed., pp. 853–864). Philadelphia: Lippincott.

Quiroga, V.A.M. (1995). *Occupational therapy: The first 30 years, 1900–1930.* Bethesda, MD: American Occupational Therapy Association.

Reilly, M. (1962). Occupational therapy can be one of the great ideas of 20th century medicine. Eleanor Clarke Slagle Lecture. *American Journal of Occupational Therapy, 16,* 1–9.

Rosenfeld, M. S. (1993). *Wellness and lifestyle renewal.* Rockville, MD: American Occupational Therapy Association.

Slagle, E. C. (1922). Training aides for mental patients. *Archives of Occupational Therapy, 1,* 11–17.

Toglia, J. P. (1991). Generalization of treatment: A multicontext approach to cognitive perceptual impairment in adults with brain injury. *American Journal of Occupational Therapy, 45,* 505–516.

Torrance, M. (1993). Acute care occupational therapy. In H. L. Hopkins & H. D. Smith (Eds.), *Willard and Spackman's occupational therapy* (8th ed., pp. 771–783). Philadelphia: Lippincott.

Tracy, S. E. (1910). *Studies in invalid occupation: A manual for nurses and attendants.* Boston: Whitcomb & Barrows.

Trombly, C. A. (1995). Occupation: Purposefulness and meaningfulness as therapeutic mechanisms. 1995 Eleanor Clarke Slagle Lecture. *American Journal of Occupational Therapy, 49,* 960–972.

Vergara, E. (1993). *Foundations for practice in the neonatal intensive care unit and early intervention: A self-guided practice manual.* Rockville, MD: American Occupational Therapy Association.

West, W. L. (1984). A reaffirmed philosophy and practice of occupational therapy for the 1980s. *American Journal of Occupational Therapy, 38,* 15–23.

Yerxa, E. J. (1967). Authentic occupational therapy. 1966 Eleanor Clark Slagle Lecture. *American Journal of Occupational Therapy, 21,* 1–9.

Yerxa, E. J. (1994). Dreams, dilemmas, and decisions for occupational therapy practice in a new millennium: An American perspective. *American Journal of Occupational Therapy, 48,* 586–589.

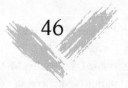

46

1998 Eleanor Clarke Slagle Lecture

Uniting Practice and Theory in an Occupational Framework

Anne G. Fisher, ScD, OTR

The roots of this lecture began years ago in the late 1960s, when I was an occupational therapy student. Occupational therapy was in the midst of what Kielhofner (1997) has termed the *mechanistic paradigm*. My physical dysfunction theory courses had a heavy focus on exercise and the neurophysiologic approaches of the Bobaths (Semans, 1967), Brunnstrom (1970), and especially Margaret Rood (as interpreted by Stockmeyer, 1967). While on my affiliations, I was guided by some of my supervisors to use weight lifting to strengthen the wrist extensors of clients with spinal cord injury. During my psychiatric affiliation, I was encouraged to give clients with unconscious hostility opportunities to act out their emotions through metal hammering. All of these clients did these activities whether they wanted to or not.

But there was another side to my early experiences. I remember vividly working with a young man who had quadriplegia as a result of a spinal cord injury. He was fascinated with electronics, and he wanted to explore the possibilities of being able to build electronic devices. I went to the local electronics store and bought a do-it-yourself radio kit filled with resistors, capacitors, circuit boards, and tiny nuts and bolts. I also bought solder and a soldering iron. Together, we worked on developing strategies he could use to manage the tools and materials. He had no active movement in his fingers, but because he wore wrist-driven flexor hinge splints, he was able to hold on to many of the objects. When he had difficulty, we worked together to create alternative strategies.

He built the radio, not I. And in the end, he had a radio he could listen to; he had the satisfaction that comes from accomplishment; and he had learned that he could develop for himself compensatory strategies when confronted with challenging circumstances. But that is not all he gained. As an indirect consequence of his participation in meaningful and purposeful activity, the muscles in his upper limbs became stronger, and his fine motor coordination improved. Although I regret that I do not remember this young man's name, I am grateful that he was included among the clients I worked with who have taught me the value of occupation as a therapeutic agent.

A few years later, I began working on a project with Lyla Spelbring. I remember Spelbring telling me about her philosophy of when occupational therapy practitioners should be involved with clients during the continuum of care that begins in the acute care phase and extends through discharge and into the community. Spelbring proposed that occupational therapy practitioners have an initial role in the early part of the acute care phase, addressing issues of self-care and the provision of assistive devices. Then, she said, we should let physical therapy take over to develop the clients' physical capacity. Only when the clients are strong enough to engage in occupation should we reenter and work with them during the latter part of their rehabilitation stays and as they transition back into the community.

Originally published 1998 in *American Journal of Occupational Therapy, 52*, 509–521.
Please note that there was no Eleanor Clarke Slagle Lecture in 1997.

Spelbring seemed to be saying that, throughout our involvement, our focus should be on enhancing occupational performance and not the remediation of underlying impairments. Her ideas felt radical, and with my own interest in neurophysiological techniques designed to remediate neuromotor impairments, I was not at all ready to hear the intent of her message. But still, I remember it, and now I realize she may have been right.

Soon thereafter, I went to graduate school. My master's thesis had to do with the effects of the inverted head position on alpha and gamma motor neuron activity in the upper extremity. Obviously, the mechanistic paradigm remained alive and well.

Catherine Trombly was my major advisor. Under her mentorship, I learned about, and came to value, the need for research that supports (and fails to support) the theories and intervention methods we use in occupational therapy. I also observed in her someone who has always valued the use of purposeful activity as a therapeutic mechanism.

Still later, after completing my doctorate, I began teaching with Gary Kielhofner. We worked together on a number of projects. With some resistance, I learned about, and ultimately became immersed in, the Model of Human Occupation. At the time, I was editing a textbook on sensory integration (Fisher, Murray, & Bundy, 1991). Kielhofner drew a figure of how he visualized the interrelationship between sensory integration and the Model of Human Occupation (see Figure 46.1). The figure was like an hourglass constructed of two overlapping triangles. The top triangle was inverted to show that the Model of Human Occupation stressed occupation and barely acknowledged the role of the brain in occupational behavior (Kielhofner, 1985). The lower triangle was upright to show that sensory integration theory stressed brain functioning, with minimal discussion of the occupational nature of humans (Ayres, 1972). About this figure, Kielhofner said that if we can bridge the gap and fill in the void so as to construct a rectangle, we will have a richer view of occupational therapy.

I believed strongly in the value of occupation as a therapeutic agent. I had not forgotten the man with the spinal cord injury who wanted to build a radio. And I had not forgotten Spelbring's view that we should return physical restoration to the physical therapists. No doubt, she would also have us return remediation of psychiatric impairments to the psychiatrists, the psychologists, and the social workers. Trombly helped me to recognize the importance of implementing research to validate occupational therapy theory and practice. But, even with all that, I still lacked a vocabulary to explain to others what I did, how what I did was unique, and how my role could be clearly differentiated from that of the physical therapist, the nurse, the social worker, and so on. My work with Kielhofner on the Model of Human Occupation paved the way for me to finally conceptualize the unique contribution of occupational therapy within the health care arena and to articulate the important role of occupation as a therapeutic agent (Fisher, 1994, 1995, 1997d).

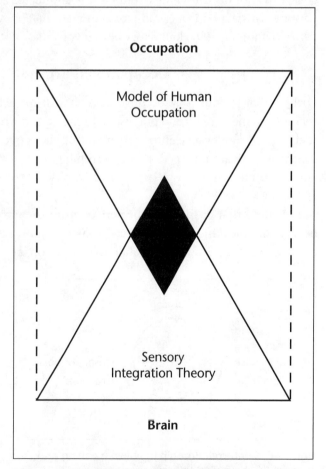

Figure 46.1. Schematic relationship between the Model of Human Occupation and sensory integration theory.

Occupation:
A Noun of Action

I came to realize the incredible power of the term *occupation*. The term occupation is a noun of action. Occupation is defined as *the* action of seizing, taking possession of, or occupying space or time. It is also defined as *the* holding of an office or position, such as one's role. Finally, in the sense of action, occupation refers to *the* being engaged in something (*The Oxford English Dictionary*, 1989).

As I have argued elsewhere, occupational therapy practitioners enable their clients to seize, take possession of, or occupy the spaces, time, and roles of their lives (Fisher, 1994). When we speak of the action of seizing, taking possession of, or occupying space, we can think of the actions our clients must perform to occupy their homes, their schools, their workplaces, and the places where they engage in recreation or leisure. Similarly, when we speak of the action of seizing, taking possession of, or occupying time—and being engaged in something—we can think that as our clients engage in task performances, they engage in a course of action that unfolds over time. We can also think about our client's need to occupy time, not just in the sense of "being busy," but also in a sense that connotes the action of doing a mental, physical, or social task that is meaningful to the person. Lastly, when we speak of the action of seizing, taking possession of, or occupying roles, we can think about the performances our clients must enact in order to assume their life roles.

Occupation is a wonderful word. Think of it—a noun of action—it is about "doing!" It conveys the powerful essence of our profession—enabling people to perform the actions they need and want to perform so that they can engage in and "do" the familiar, ordinary, goal-directed activities of every day in a manner that brings meaning and personal satisfaction (American Occupational Therapy Association [AOTA], 1993, 1995; Clark et al., 1991; Evans, 1987; Kielhofner, 1997; Rudman, Cook, & Polatajko, 1997).

Occupation: Purposeful and Meaningful Activity

I believe that we must view occupation as not just any activity, not even just any purposeful activity, but as activity that is both meaningful and purposeful to the person who engages in it. As I use the term here, *meaning* pertains to the personal significance of the activity to the client (see Figure 46.2). Meaningfulness is important as it provides a source of motivation for performance (Trombly, 1995a). As I use the term *purpose,* it pertains to the client's personal aim, reason for doing, or intended goal. Purposefulness is important as it helps organize the client's performance (Trombly, 1995a).

I believe that purpose can be derived from the meaning one makes of a situation (Nelson, 1988), but I also believe that meaning can be derived from one's purpose for engaging in the activity (Fisher, 1994). Meaning and purpose, when considered in relation to occupation, are inextricably interrelated.

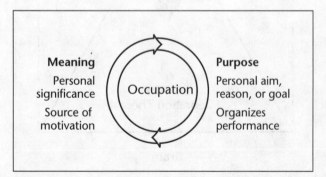

Figure 46.2. Interrelationship between meaning and purpose when applied to occupation.
Note. Copyright © 1998 by Anne G. Fisher. Reprinted with permission.

Consider the following example. Ken is a minister. Each Sunday, he puts on slacks and dress shoes instead of his usual jeans and tennis shoes. Over that he dons his vestments and a cross. He does this for "appearance"—to be socially appropriate and to wear the "correct" attire. But he also wears them to make a statement about who he is and what he believes. For Ken, they are tied to tradition, and they are symbolic of his Christian faith. Ken's purpose and Ken's meanings are virtually inseparable.

But why does Ken wear the particular cross he does? Ken wears the cross he does because of the symbolism embedded within its design. The design is that of a desert rose. Imagine a rose blooming in the desert—a rose growing out of nothing. For Ken, this is a symbol of the Resurrection—in the darkest part of our lives we can bloom; we can heal and grow. This is a belief tied to his Christian faith, but the significance of Ken's wearing of this cross is also very personal.

Ken was very ill. He had to give up his position as senior pastor and discontinue all physical activity. He went on disability. He had excruciating pain and was heavily medicated. He says, "I was like a zombie." He could not talk, and he could only eat through a straw. He became even more ill and had to be hospitalized. There was concern that Ken might not live. But then he was given a new medication. He went into remission. With guidance from others, he developed strategies to deal with his residual disability. Six months ago, Ken resumed his ministry. Last week he went skiing. He has plans to begin rollerblading once again this spring.

Ken wears the cross he does as a symbol of his own life transition:

> I went from being a responsible professional, working 70 hours a week, to basically nothing. I went from 7 days a week being busy to having no purpose or meaning in life. I went from that to getting it all back.

The point is: Purposefulness is important, but it is not enough. Occupation is both purposeful and meaningful. If we can identify activities that have potential to be meaningful to the person, we can use them to increase motivation and a sense of purpose. In this process, we cannot confuse our purposes or meanings with those of our clients.

Defining Occupation Within a Practice Context

As I have traveled internationally, I have continued to be confronted with an apparent paradox—occupational therapy practitioners who know, implicitly, that they possess unique and important expertise but who have difficulty, just as I have had, articulating their uniqueness. Moreover, they often use evaluation and intervention methods that are so similar to those of their colleagues in physical therapy, neuropsychology, social work, and nursing that any distinctions between occupational therapy and these professions become blurred and even abolished.

Since the beginning of our profession, occupation has been viewed as both a means and an end (Clark, 1917; Dunton, 1928; Gritzer & Arluke, 1985; "Occupational Therapy in the General Hospital," 1917; Quiroga, 1995; Upham, 1917). Our uniqueness has been in the use of occupation as a curative or restorative force as well as in the view that enhanced occupational performance is the desired goal of therapy. These beliefs continue to be reflected in current official statements from within our profession. According to the AOTA (1997), occupational therapy practitioners use purposeful and meaningful activities in two ways: to restore underlying capacities and to develop meaningful occupations.

As I have talked with occupational therapy practitioners both here in North America and abroad, I have found that we indeed share an understanding of occupation, but that understanding often seems to be detached from what I observe in their daily practice. Our unique focus on occupation is not always obvious in practice.

Common Intervention Methods

To clarify what I mean, I will describe the intervention methods occupational therapy practitioners currently use in their everyday practice. The focal point here will be the characteristics of the activities in which clients are engaged. As I introduce the general activity types, the astute reader will no doubt think of activities that do not fall neatly within one of these groups. It may help, therefore, to begin by thinking of four continua (see Figure 46.3).

The first continuum indicates that an activity may be more contrived or offered as exercise, or the activity may be more naturalistic and offered as occupation. The second and third continua indicate that the purpose and the meaning of the activity, respectively, may be generated more by the practitioner or generated more from within the client. Finally, the focus of the intervention may be more on remediation of impairments or more on enhanced occupational performance. These four continua can be used to evaluate the characteristics of any activity we might use as intervention. As I proceed to describe each of the major activity groups, certain key characteristics of the activities will move from left to right along one or more of the continua.

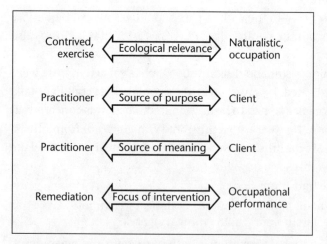

Figure 46.3. Four continua that can be used to evaluate the characteristics of any activity used as occupational therapy intervention.
Note. Copyright © 1998 by Anne G. Fisher. Reprinted with permission.

Exercise. The first group of activities I have termed *exercise.* The most salient feature of this type of activity is that the client is engaged in rote exercise or practice. The activity may have a purpose or goal, but more often than not, the purpose originated with the practitioner and not the client. In all probability, therefore, the exercise has little or no meaning to the client. Finally, the focus of the exercise is on the remediation of impairments. Examples of exercise include having the client draw a series of straight vertical lines on lined paper to develop eye-hand coordination, stretch Thera-Band®[1] or lift weights to develop strength, or stack cones to develop reach.

Contrived occupation. The second group of activities I have termed *contrived occupation.* Contrived occupation includes exercise with "added purpose" and occupation with a "contrived" component. Again, there may be a purpose or a goal, but if there is, the purpose most likely originated with the practitioner and not the client. Because the purpose originates with the practitioner, the meaningfulness of the activity to the client remains minimal. Finally, as with exercise, the focus is on the remediation of impairments.

Exercise with added purpose is exercise embedded in an activity in which both task objects and any potential meanings or purposes are contrived. One example would be to have a woman practice picking up golf balls from the floor with a reacher and placing them in a nearby bucket. Another example would be to have a man place cones on a shelf, telling him that he should pretend that they are glasses and that he is putting the dishes away. The key element is that golf balls and cones have little relevance to the actual tasks that are being simulated.

In *occupation with a contrived component,* the objects are real and not simulated. Having a boy pound nails into a board, encouraging him to pretend that he is going to build a birdhouse, is one example. The objects are real and relevant to the *practitioner-specified* purpose, but there is to be no real birdhouse. Asking a girl to throw bean bags at a target without her engagement in a game is another example. In both of these examples, the purpose and the meaning have been contrived; they are more those of the practitioner than they are those of the children.

Therapeutic occupation. The third group of activities I have termed *therapeutic occupation.* A critical characteristic of therapeutic occupation is that the client actively participates in occupation. They are activities the *client identifies* as purposeful and meaningful. And, to the greatest extent possible, the occupational performance is naturalistic and contextual. The client performs the activities using real objects in natural environments. The focus of therapeutic occupation remains on the remediation of impairments.

An example of therapeutic occupation would be to use *graded occupation* to treat impairments of balance or reach. For example, Lillian loves to read. She has expressed concern that she is experiencing difficulty maintaining her balance while reaching for objects, including books, from shelves. Together, we decide to go to her library and work on her problem areas. By progressively grading the task in terms of the challenges to her balance or the extent of reach required, engagement in an activity that has purpose and meaning to the client can be used to remediate her underlying impairments that are limiting her occupational performance. As her underlying abilities improve, she can begin to retrieve from or return to higher shelves books that are heavier.

---

[1] Thera-Band Products, The Hygenic Corporation, 1245 Home Avenue, Akron, OH 44310.

Another example of therapeutic occupation involves *direct intervention* of impairments in the context of occupation. Here, the occupational therapy practitioner might work on social abilities while a group of adolescents make a cake for one of their mothers. Or the practitioner might attempt to remediate attentional deficits as the person engages in a favored card game.

Adaptive or compensatory occupation. The final group of activities I have termed *adaptive or compensatory occupation.* As with therapeutic occupation, a critical characteristic is the client's active participation in occupations that are chosen by the client. Again, the activities are purposeful and meaningful to the client, and the occupational performance is naturalistic and contextual. In fact, the major distinction between adaptive occupation and therapeutic occupation is that adaptive occupation is focused on improved occupational performance and not on the remediation of impairments. When we use adaptive occupation, we provide assistive devices, teach alternative or compensatory strategies, or modify physical or social environments. No attempt is made to remediate the underlying impairments.

An example of adaptive occupation might involve engaging Roy, who has lung cancer and resultant low endurance, in a desired grocery shopping task. While he is shopping for his needed groceries, the occupational therapy practitioner would use education to teach him alternative ways to manage his shopping. One strategy might be to teach him to put only a limited number of items into a bag. Another might be to teach him to use a cart to transport his groceries. The key characteristic of adaptive occupation is the use of adaptation to alter or change the activity so that the client can perform it successfully (Mosey, 1986). The goal is not to improve Roy's endurance.

Legitimate Activities for Occupational Therapy

What then are the legitimate activities for occupational therapy? Kielhofner (1997) has argued that the emerging paradigm of occupational therapy requires that we recognize occupation as the level of intervention. I believe that this should be true whether the intervention involves engaging the person in therapeutic occupation for purposes of remediation or engaging the person in adaptive occupation to directly enhance occupational performance. Certainly, if we tie current practice to our philosophical base, then the clear *emphasis* must be therapeutic occupation and adaptive occupation. At the same time, we must heed Spelbring's advice and return exercise and most of our use of contrived occupation to their legitimate "owners."[2]

We do not like to think that what we are doing is not legitimate occupational therapy. But, whether we want to admit it to ourselves or not, there are still many occupational therapy practitioners here in the United States and internationally who continue to *emphasize* the use of exercise or contrived occupation to remediate impairments, justifying their programs to themselves and others by stating that their *ultimate* goal is improved occupational performance. We are challenged to ask ourselves, how are these programs any different from those of physical therapy, neuropsychology, and others?

Conceptualizing an Occupational Therapy Intervention Process Model

How can we make the philosophical foundations of our profession a reality of everyday practice? I believe that we do that by uniting practice and theory in an occupational framework. That is, we must conceptualize and implement practice in a manner that explicitly ties what we do to our unique focus on occupation as a therapeutic tool.

---

[2] I believe that there is some justification for the *occasional* use of contrived occupation, especially with clients who lack motivation or who are too fearful to engage in activities that we might believe are more relevant to their daily life needs. In this case, group, craft, or play and leisure activities may be used early in the intervention in an attempt to facilitate the client's active participation and to increase motivation. The client may initially "go through the motions" of implementing the task performance, but his or her sense of purpose and meaning in relation to the activity likely is minimal. The hope is that purpose and meaning will emerge. If, however, the use of such activities has no apparent therapeutic benefit, and the client remains unwilling to engage in occupation, then perhaps we should turn the intervention over to other professionals whose methods and focus may be more appropriate.

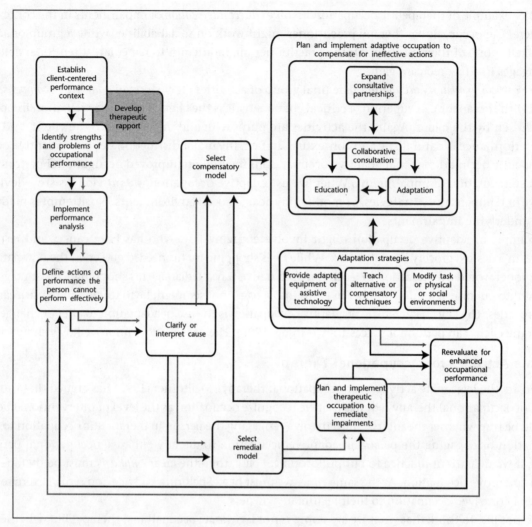

Figure 46.4. Schematic representation of the Occupational Therapy Intervention Process Model.
Note. Copyright © 1998 by Anne G. Fisher. Reprinted with permission.

If we are to remain a viable profession and avoid the risk of being viewed as redundant, we must continue the move away from the mechanistic paradigm and reconnect to our philosophical foundations.

In the remainder of this lecture, I will propose the Occupational Therapy Intervention Process Model as a structure for realizing this objective (see Figure 46.4). This model stresses the use of a top-down approach to evaluation. It also provides a framework to guide professional reasoning that leads to implementation of adaptive occupation for purposes of compensation as well as therapeutic occupation for purposes of remediation.

Establish the Client-Centered Performance Context

The first step of the Occupational Therapy Intervention Process Model is to establish the client-centered performance context. The client-centered performance context provides the framework for understanding, evaluating, and interpreting the person's occupational performance. Occupational performance unfolds as a transaction between the person and the environment as he or she enacts a task (see Figure 46.5). Therefore, the person's motivational characteristics, roles, and capacities are just as critical as are the task and the features of the environment for providing the framework that is needed to understand why, and how, a person performs the tasks he or she does and why certain aspects of the task performance may result in the person experiencing difficulty or dissatisfaction. This view is in contrast to the view that defines the context as being limited to the environment or all that is external to the person (Christiansen & Baum, 1997; Dunn, Brown, & McGuigan, 1994; Haugen & Mathiowetz, 1995).

Dimensions of the client-centered performance context. The following interrelated dimensions define the client-centered performance context:[3]

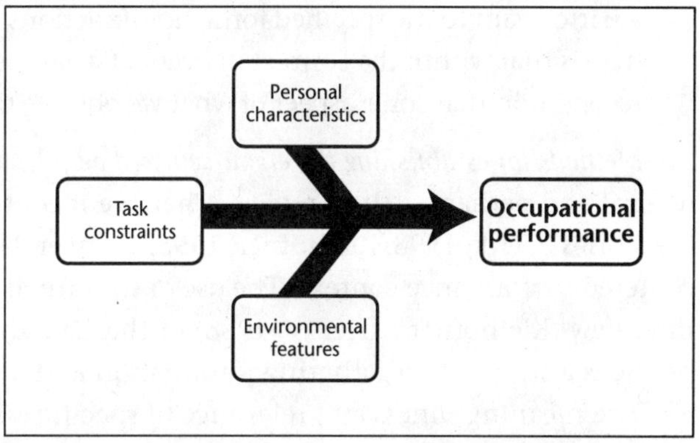

1. The *temporal dimension* places the client's occupational performance within context of his or her past; present; and possibilities, priorities, and hopes for the future.

2. The *environmental dimension* includes the persons who are present, the objects that are present, and the physical spaces where the task performances occur.

3. The *cultural dimension* pertains to the shared beliefs, values, and customs of one's cultural group that influence where one performs tasks, what tasks one performs, how one performs them, and what tools and materials are used.

Figure 46.5. Schematic representation of occupational performance unfolding as a transaction between the person and the environment as he or she enacts a task. *Note.* Copyright © 1998 by Anne G. Fisher. Reprinted with permission.

4. The *societal (institutional) dimension* includes one's available community resources, relevant economic factors, and implicit or explicit rules and regulations, including medical precautions.

5. The *social dimension* includes one's connections and relationships with others as well as the extent of collaboration that occurs between the client and others during occupational performance.

6. The *role dimension* pertains to the relationship between one's roles and the related collection of task performances that must unfold in a logical, timely, and socially appropriate manner. We must understand the person's perceived roles and any incongruities between his or her role behavior and the role behavior that is expected by society or desired by the person.

7. The *motivational dimension* pertains to one's values, interests, and goals that give meaning to activity and provide a source of motivation.

8. The *capacity dimension* pertains to the clients's diagnosed condition and the broad clinical picture of his or her neurologic, musculoskeletal, cognitive, and psychosocial capacities and impairments we gain through our initial observations and interview with the client. These are the *initial* impressions we have of a client that *begin* to inform us about the client's potentials for change, delimiters to progress, and precautions we might need to consider during intervention.

9. The *task dimension* includes both the task to be performed and the constraints that define that task. The task constraints are a set of culturally defined task characteristics that result in shared recognition that "this" person is performing "this" task (Fisher, 1997c). These culturally defined task characteristics specify the appropriate context, the tools and materials to be used, the norms or rules for the performance, and the necessary temporal order of the task actions. They are a component of what Nelson (1988) has called *occupational form*. When a person does not enact the specified occupational form, we recognize such deviations as errors. Such errors may reflect inefficiencies in organizing time or space, inappropriate or unsafe object use, inappropriate actions that

---

[3] The dimensions included within the client-centered performance context may be likened to what Christiansen and Baum (1997) termed *performance enablers.* In fact, their term, *performance enablers,* is preferred to the term *performance components* (AOTA, 1994b). The use of the term *performance components* tends to imply small (component) units of the enactment of a task performance rather than the intended underlying supporting framework. The small, goal-directed units of a task performance are *actions,* not the person's underlying capacities. For that reason, I have deliberately avoided referring to performance components during this lecture, substituting instead terms such as *capacities, abilities, limitations,* and *impairments.*

are irrelevant to the specified form, unsafe actions that place the person at risk, and so on. The important point here is that within the context of occupational therapy, we recognize "problems of performance" through the recognition that some aspect of what we observe the client doing is "out of form."

Methods for establishing the client-centered performance context. Establishing the context begins with an initial referral and perhaps a chart review. Then we meet the client. Through interview, observation, and the use of life stories (Clark, 1993; Kielhofner, 1995; Spencer, Davidson, & White, 1996), we begin to construct the client-centered performance context. The use of structured interviews, such as the Occupational Performance History Interview (Kielhofner & Henry, 1988) or the Canadian Occupational Performance Measure (Law et al., 1994), provides a structure to gathering information and identifying the client's goals.

The meaningfulness and relevance of specific task performances to the client are of critical importance in the evaluation and intervention process. Learning about the tasks that are most important to the person, the meaning of those tasks, and the nature of the contexts within which those task performances are likely to be enacted requires taking the time and effort to establish the client-centered performance context. This step is critical, and it must occur, even under the pressures of cost containment, reduced duration of care, staff cuts, and increased accountability. In fact, there is some evidence that taking more time, initially, to establish the client-centered performance context will result in overall outcomes being enhanced and overall costs reduced (Bowen, 1996; Neistadt, 1995).

Consistent with a top-down approach, it is important to point out that we do not begin to formally assess the person's underlying capacities and abilities until later (Fisher & Short-DeGraff, 1993; Trombly, 1993). Rather, at this stage in the evaluation process, we consider only the person's diagnosed condition and what we learn through informal observation and interview.

For example, before I actually met Jim, I was aware that he had sustained a brain injury several years ago and that he was experiencing difficulty finding satisfying employment. This information led me to suspect that he might have either physical or cognitive limitations, but if he did, they were unlikely to change. My first contact with him was by telephone. During our conversation, I became aware that he has expressive aphasia but that he is able to communicate most of his ideas in a manner that I could understand.

Later, when I met Jim, I noticed that he does not use his right arm. He allows it to hang at this side. As Jim and I began to talk, I quickly learned that he is bilingual—he knows both American Sign Language and English. Jim cues himself visually, using sign language, when he has difficulty verbalizing what he wants to say. During our conversation, I sensed that Jim has good comprehension and no major memory deficits. He is outgoing and appears to have good social skills. Things he said also led me to infer that he likely has good self-awareness and problem-solving abilities. But a critical feature here is that I did not formally test any of Jim's capacities. I did not ask him to move his right arm. I did not ask him to tell me the meaning of a saying like "a rolling stone gathers no moss." I did not ask him to remember and repeat number sequences or count backward from 100 by 7s.

Instead, I learned about his history, his interests, his values, and his goals. Jim is 28 years of age. He sustained a brain injury in an automobile accident 12 years ago as he was driving to diving practice. He had been a champion diver in state competition. He has had occupational therapy and speech therapy. He learned how to use a variety of assistive devices. He loves music and has taught himself to play both acoustic and electric guitar one-handed. When I asked him how he did it, he said, "Practice, practice, practice." He writes music, paints, and composes poetry. He is currently working on an album where his poetry will be set against his music. He speaks poignantly through his poetry:

I am angry . . .
  Where is the blame.
I am alive . . .
  If I find the treasure of life.
I am alone . . .
  Communications breakdown. (Cacciatore, 1994)

Jim is highly motivated to work and earn an income so that he can live on his own, but all of his past jobs have been low paying. He has worked as a companion for another young man with a brain injury. He tried working as a cashier, but found the work too stressful. He currently has a job gathering carts from the parking lot of a large warehouse department store. He has good work skills; he is friendly, on time, and able to carry out routine sequences. He has a small T-shirt company. He uses a computer to design the graphics and adds his own words. Jim wants to be a graphic designer, but he lacks the needed skills. He went to a local community college to study graphic design but did not complete the final course in English as it was too difficult. He did not earn the degree.

He says about himself, "I've adapted—I take a 'don't worry, be happy' attitude." He has maintained hope, but still he is concerned about work and wants very much to move out of his parents' home and live independently in his own apartment.

Develop Therapeutic Rapport

As I talk with Jim, I not only establish the client-centered performance context, but also begin the critical step of developing therapeutic rapport (Tickle-Degnen, 1995). "Rapport is the process of establishing and maintaining a comfortable, unconstrained relationship of mutual confidence and respect between a practitioner and client" (Mosey, 1981, p. 96). This is the beginnings of a collaborative (consultative) partnership between Jim and myself that will continue to develop throughout the time we work together (depicted by the lighter gray line in Figure 46.4). Collaboration with the client *throughout the intervention process* is required by the AOTA's (1994a) *Code of Ethics*. Effective goal setting and treatment planning demand the development of a collaborative partnership between the practitioner and the client. The practitioner brings to this partnership expertise related to available intervention strategies and knowledge related to potential outcomes. The client brings his or her values, interests, goals, and priorities. If the collaborative partnership is to be effective, there must be open sharing of each other's motivations and rationales (Bowen, 1996).

Identify Strengths and Problems of Occupational Performance

As I progress downward and narrow the focus of the evaluation, I identify tasks that are currently supporting or hindering Jim's role behavior. Task performances that support Jim's role behavior are Jim's strengths. Those that he experiences as problematic or that hinder his role behavior are his problems of occupational performance. In the process of narrowing the focus of the evaluation, I remain alert to potential discrepancies between my estimation of Jim's potential problem areas and those actually identified by him. I will include those tasks among those I will observe Jim performing. For example, Jim indicated that playing guitar is a strength; I wanted to verify his ability. I suspected that preparing meals that are not ready made may pose a problem, even though Jim did not identify cooking as a problem area. I also wanted to know more about his computer and graphic design skills.

Implement Performance Analysis

As I proceed downward to the next step of the evaluation process, I implement a performance analysis (Fisher, 1997a, 1997d). Performance analysis is defined as the observational evaluation of a person's task performance to identify discrepancies between the demands of a task and the skill of the person. The person's problems and strengths are described in terms of the quality of the goal-directed actions that comprise the occupational performance, not the client's underlying capacities and impairments. Performance analyses should not be confused with task or activity analyses, which are intended for purposes of identifying the underlying impairments that limit occupational performance or the inherent therapeutic value of a task for remediating those impairments (AOTA, 1993; Hagedorn, 1995, 1997; Llorens, 1993; Trombly, 1995b; Watson, 1997).

Implementing a performance analysis requires that we observe the quality of the transaction between the client and the environment as the client performs a task that is familiar, meaningful, purposeful, and relevant.

The Assessment of Motor and Process Skills (AMPS) (Fisher, 1997b) is a standardized performance analysis. The performance analysis also can be accomplished through informal observation of a person's occupational performance.

Because I used the AMPS to evaluate Jim, I will describe a few of its key features. The AMPS skill actions are small units of the enactment of a daily life task. An important feature of the skill actions is that they are goal directed. Most frequently, the goal of the AMPS skill action pertains to an action or step embedded within the overall task performance—*reaching* for and *lifting* the jar from the shelf or *gathering* the lettuce to the table. For other AMPS skill actions, the goal pertains more to the overall task performance—*heeding* the client-specified goal (i.e., the client's doing what the client said he or she would do) or *sequencing* the steps of the task in a logical manner such that the person–environment transaction unfolds as a coherent and recognizable routine.

An important feature of scoring an AMPS observation is that no judgment is made regarding the person's underlying capacities. That is, a person may be assigned a low score on the AMPS skill action *Sequences* for reasons other than decreased sequencing capacity. Similarly, a high score on the AMPS skill action *Lifts* would not necessarily mean that the person has good lifting capacity. Because the AMPS is a test of the quality and effectiveness of a person's occupational performance (and not underlying capacities), the person is scored on the basis of what was observed—the transaction of the person with the environment as he or she performs a familiar and chosen task. More specifically, the quality of the performance is what is graded, not the "quality" of the person's underlying capacities nor the "quality" of the environment or task objects with which the person interacts. Those judgments are deferred to the interpretation stage (i.e., Clarify or Interpret Cause), where the practitioner uses professional reasoning and perhaps further assessment to determine person, environmental, task, or sociocultural factors that may be limiting performance.

Define Actions of Performance That the Person Cannot Perform Effectively

Having observed Jim perform tasks, I proceed to define the actions that he can and cannot perform effectively. When I implemented an informal performance analysis and observed Jim set up and play his guitars, I learned that he is able to do so and, indeed, he is able to play very well using a hammer and "draw" method. When I used the AMPS and observed him prepare toast and coffee, I learned that he is able to lift, transport, and grip task objects effectively. He chose and used appropriate tools and materials, and he heeded the goal of the client-specified task. He had moderate difficulty, however, with effectively stabilizing the toast while buttering it, organizing his workspace, and adapting to problems he encountered during his task performance. Plans are under way to evaluate Jim's computer and graphic skills.

Clarify or Interpret Cause

Having identified the actions that Jim cannot perform effectively, I proceed to clarify or interpret the underlying cause of his ineffective performance. In Jim's case, the underlying cause was obvious. He has hemiplegia, and, during his task performance, he did not use any of the many assistive devices he had received earlier in his rehabilitation. Part of clarifying the cause of Jim's ineffective performance, however, will be to inquire as to why he did not use any assistive devices.

In other cases, as we seek to understand the underlying cause of a person's ineffective occupational performance, we can think in terms of impairments (e.g., John cannot put his arm into the sleeve of his shirt because of limitations in range of motion at the shoulder). We can think in terms of physical environments (e.g., Mary cannot reach the glasses from the cupboard shelf because they are too high). We can think in terms of social environments (e.g., Steven does not finish his school work tasks because the classroom environment is noisy and chaotic). We can consider societal constraints (e.g., Lillian must not bend her hip beyond 90° and reach to put on her shoes because of total hip precautions). And finally, we can consider societal expectations (e.g., Bill's work performance is not acceptable because his low productivity affects company profits).

When the underlying cause is not clear, the occupational therapy practitioner may choose to implement further assessment. Selected practice models, such as the Model of Human Occupation (Kielhofner, 1995) or the Ecology of Human Performance framework (Dunn et al., 1994), provide conceptual structures for assessing characteristics of the person or the environment that limit and support occupational performance. Occupational therapy practitioners are never at a loss for tests of the person's underlying neurologic, musculoskeletal, cognitive, or psychosocial capacities. Finally, a wide range of environmental assessments also are available (Letts et al., 1994).

Select Compensatory Model

Now that I have clarified Jim's problems and the reasons for his limitations, I am ready to select one or more intervention models. I select remedial models when I believe that restoration of underlying capacities will result in improved occupational performance. I select the compensatory model when I believe that remediation is unlikely to affect occupational performance significantly; when remediation will be "too costly in terms of time, energy, or money" (Trombly, 1993, p. 255); or when I am directed by legislation to focus on occupational performance and role behavior. I also can implement both model types simultaneously. Because I suspect that remediation will not benefit Jim, I select the compensatory model.

Plan and Implement Adaptive Occupation to Compensate for Ineffective Actions

Once the compensatory model is chosen, the next step is to plan and implement adaptive occupation. The desired outcome is the design of adaptive occupation to compensate for the client's ineffective actions. Specific details have been published elsewhere (Duran & Fisher, in press; Fisher, 1997a; Trombly, 1995c), but I will present an overview here so as to demonstrate the process of implementing the compensatory model.[4]

Expand consultative partnerships. When we first meet a client and begin to develop therapeutic rapport, we develop a collaborative (consultative) partnership with the client. Once we know that we will be implementing adaptative occupation, we also must enter into shared *consultative partnerships* with those persons who have access to needed information or who will be affected by the proposed changes. For example, members of the client's family who are living with him or her, or persons who will be providing the client with assistance, are important members of the consultative partnership.

Collaborative consultation, education, and adaptation. Once the members of the consultative partnership are identified, the practitioner implements methods of collaborative consultation (Fisher, 1997a), education (teaching–learning) (Mosey, 1986; Trombly, 1995c), and adaptation (Fisher, 1997a; Trombly 1995c). Through collaborating with the client and his or her family, client-centered goals are established. Then, building on the development of collaborative relationships, the members of the consultative partnership work together to propose and develop strategies for intervention that are based on the principles of adaptation. Finally, the members of the consultative partnership responsible for implementing the interventions are trained in how to do so on the basis of the principles of education. These persons may include the client, caregiver, service extender, or another professional.

Adaptation strategies. As I noted earlier, adaptation includes providing adapted equipment or assistive technology, teaching the client alternative strategies or compensatory techniques, and modifying the task or the physical or social environment. Marla uses a special keyboard and mouse to lessen the effects of repetitive motion. Jim has

---

[4] The compensatory model has been called the *rehabilitation* (compensatory) model by Trombly (1995c) and the *expanded rehabilitation* model by Fisher (1997a). In this lecture, I have chosen to call it the *compensatory model* as the term *rehabilitation* implies physical restoration and remediation of impairments. When the compensatory model is used in isolation of the Occupational Therapy Intervention Process Model, it includes all steps included in Figure 46.4, except Select Remedial Model and Plan and Implement Therapeutic Occupation to Remediate Impairments (Duran & Fisher, in press; Fisher, 1997a).

learned to tie his shoes one-handed. He has also taught himself how to play his guitar, using a one-handed hammer and "draw" method. Ken was taught to use lists to remember which of his many medications to take when. He uses a stool to sit and preach because one of his medications has caused peripheral neuropathy in his feet. Because of continued safety risk, Lillian requires standby assistance when standing and transferring to and from her wheelchair. For occupational therapists, who are experts in adaptation, the list of possibilities is endless.

Reevaluate for Enhanced Occupational Performance

Once the adaptations have been implemented, the client's occupational performance is reevaluated. We again use performance analyses to verify whether the client has met his or her goals. Finally, documentation of the effectiveness of our occupational therapy interventions is a critical step toward communicating the unique role of occupational therapy as well as justifying payment of occupational therapy services by health care payers.

Redefine Actions of Performance That the Person Cannot Perform Effectively

If the performance analysis implemented during the reevaluation results in the identification of additional problems, the actions the person cannot perform effectively must be redefined, and the cycle of clarifying the cause, selecting a model, and so on, is repeated.

Select Remedial Model—Plan and Implement Therapeutic Occupation to Remediate Impairments

In the event that the occupational therapy practitioner judges the client to be a good candidate for remediation, the practitioner can select one of many remedial models (e.g., biomechanical, sensory integration). Activity analysis and synthesis (Mosey, 1986) are then used to design therapeutic occupations to remediate the person's impairments that are limiting occupational performance. Ideally, the practitioner reevaluates for enhanced occupational performance, documents changes in performance, and reenters the cycle if further intervention is indicated. If the remediation is not effective, or if recovery plateaus, the practitioner can abandon the use of therapeutic occupation and select the compensatory model.

Conclusions

I realize that we all face the ongoing challenges of changing health care. Many of you, especially those of you affected by managed care and prospective payment, will view what I say as idealistic. I disagree. I believe that my view is the more realistic one. As Karen Selley DeLorenzo (personal communication, March 15, 1998) has so clearly articulated, there will be reduced monies available for rehabilitation services. We will no longer have the luxury of providing intervention for as long as functional gains can be documented. Therefore, we must make every effort to enable our clients to achieve maximum gains within the limited time available. The only way to do this is to introduce adaptive occupation and consultation from day one. Remediation is time consuming, and there is growing evidence that remediation may have limited effects on functional outcomes.[5]

---

[5] I base this assertion on research that has not demonstrated a strong enough relationship between underlying impairments and occupational performance to support the basic assumption that if the underlying cause (i.e., neuromuscular, biomechanical, cognitive, or psychosocial impairments) of limitations in occupational performance can be identified and treated, then the effects will generalize to improved occupational performance (Bernspång, Asplund, Eriksson, & Fugl-Meyer, 1987; Jongbloed, Brighton, & Stacey, 1988; Lichtenberg & Nanna, 1994; Pincus et al., 1989; Reed, Jagust, & Seab, 1989; Skurla, Rogers, & Sunderland, 1988; Teri, Borson, Kiyak, & Yamagishi, 1989). I also make this assertion despite the fact that some researchers (Judge, Schechtman, Cress, & the FICSIT Group, 1996) continue to claim strong relationships between discrete physical performance measures and instrumental activities of daily living performance even though 75% of their observed relationships were $r < .50$ (<25% explained variance) and 100% of their observed relationships were $r < .60$ (<36% explained variance). Additional evidence to support my assertion lies in studies that indicate that the effectiveness of remedial approaches may be limited (Benedict et al., 1994; Fetters & Kluzik, 1996; Hutzler, Chacham, Bergman, & Szeinberg, 1998; Kaplan, Polatajko, Wilson, & Faris, 1993; Law et al., 1997; Nakayama, Jørgensen, Raaschou, & Olsen, 1994; Neistadt, 1992).

These challenges also provide us with opportunities. In an environment where we are expected to provide quality service in less time, we face a critical need to communicate who we are, why we are important, and that what we do is unique. Case managers and teachers should be the primary targets of these educational efforts. We need to make a philosophical shift. We may need to let go of the type of thinking that is *driven* by a focus on remediation of impairments. Instead, we need to focus on what the person wants and needs to do and work with the person to enable him or her to perform tasks that are meaningful to the person and in a manner that brings satisfaction. This means that we need to rethink what is really important from the perspective of the person—occupational performance or his or her impairments. We need to rethink the evaluation process, using a top-down approach that focuses on occupation. We need to revise our intervention strategies and focus more on adaptation, education, and collaborative consultation and less on remediation. Focusing on occupational performance instead of remediation does not mean that remediation will not occur. The man who built the radio developed better strength and coordination even though that was neither his goal nor mine. Restoration of self-esteem, interests, and values also can, and should, occur through participation in adaptive occupation. When we do focus on remediation, we need to tie our interventions to our philosophical base through the application of therapeutic occupation. And, although I have said little about it during this lecture, I will add that we need to recognize the need to set goals and document efficacy in terms of occupational performance and not impairments or performance components.

Are you prepared to heed Jim's final words?

I will accept and go on.
It is my problem, not you.
What are you going to do about it? (Cacciatore, 1994)

Acknowledgments

I thank my many colleagues and students, here and abroad, who have contributed so much to the development of this lecture through their support and assistance. Many of them have also provided constructive feedback either in the context of the classroom or through ongoing dialogues that, in some cases, have gone on for years. This feedback has played a critical role in the evolution of my thinking about occupation and occupational therapy. I also thank Carol Wassell, Coordinator, Instructional Services, Colorado State University, for her preparation of the figures included in this lecture.

References

American Occupational Therapy Association. (1993). Position paper: Purposeful activity. *American Journal of Occupational Therapy, 47,* 1081–1082.

American Occupational Therapy Association. (1994a). Occupational therapy code of ethics. *American Journal of Occupational Therapy, 48,* 1037–1038.

American Occupational Therapy Association. (1994b). Uniform terminology for occupational therapy—Third edition. *American Journal of Occupational Therapy, 48,* 1047–1054.

American Occupational Therapy Association. (1995). Position paper: Occupation. *American Journal of Occupational Therapy, 49,* 1015–1018.

American Occupational Therapy Association. (1997). Statement—Fundamental concepts of occupational therapy: Occupation, purposeful activity, and function. *American Journal of Occupational Therapy, 51,* 864–866.

Ayres, A. J. (1972). *Sensory integration and learning disorders.* Los Angeles: Western Psychological Services.

Benedict, R.H.B., Harris, A. E., Markow, T., McCormick, J. A., Nuechterlein, K. H., & Asarnow, R. F. (1994). Effects of attention training on information processing in schizophrenia. *Schizophrenia Bulletin, 20,* 537–546.

Bernspång, B., Asplund, K., Eriksson, S., & Fugl-Meyer, A. R. (1987). Motor and perceptual impairments in acute stroke patients: Effects on self-care ability. *Stroke, 18,* 1081–1087.

Bowen, R. E. (1996). The issue is—Should occupational therapy adopt a consumer-based model of service delivery? *American Journal of Occupational Therapy, 50,* 899–902.

Brunnstrom, S. (1970). *Movement therapy in hemiplegia: A neurophysiological approach.* New York: Harper & Row.

Cacciatore, J. (1994). *Head injury aggression.* Unpublished poem.

Christiansen, C., & Baum, C. (1997). Person–environment occupational performance: A conceptual model for practice. In C. H. Christiansen & C. M. Baum (Eds.), *Occupational therapy: Enabling function and well-being* (2nd ed., pp. 47–70). Thorofare, NJ: Slack.

Clark, F. (1993). Occupation embedded in a real life: Interweaving occupational science and occupational therapy. 1993 Eleanor Clarke Slagle Lecture. *American Journal of Occupational Therapy, 47,* 1067–1078.

Clark, F. A., Parham, D., Carlson, M. E., Frank, G., Jackson, J., Pierce, D., Wolfe, R. J., & Zemke, R. (1991). Occupational science: Academic innovation in the service of occupational therapy's future. *American Journal of Occupational Therapy, 45,* 300–310.

Clark, F. P. (1917). The beneficial effects of work therapy for the insane. *Modern Hospital, 8,* 392–393.

Dunn, W., Brown, C., & McGuigan, A. (1994). The ecology of human performance: A framework for considering the effect of context. *American Journal of Occupational Therapy, 48,* 595–607.

Dunton, W. R. (1928). *Prescribing occupational therapy.* Springfield, IL: Charles C Thomas.

Duran, L., & Fisher, A. G. (in press). Occupational therapy assessment and treatment of a client with disorder of executive abilities. In C. Unsworth (Ed.), *Cognitive and perceptual dysfunction: A clinical reasoning approach to assessment and treatment.* Philadelphia: F. A. Davis.

Evans, K. A. (1987). Nationally speaking—Definition of occupation as the core concept of occupational therapy. *American Journal of Occupational Therapy, 41,* 627–628.

Fetters, L., & Kluzik, J. (1996). The effects of neurodevelopmental treatment versus practice on the reaching of children with spastic cerebral palsy. *Physical Therapy, 76,* 346–358.

Fisher, A. G. (1994). Functional assessment and occupation: Critical issues for occupational therapy. *New Zealand Journal of Occupational Therapy, 45*(2), 13–19.

Fisher, A. G. (1995). *Assessment of Motor and Process Skills.* Fort Collins, CO: Three Star Press.

Fisher, A. G. (1997a). An expanded rehabilitative model of practice. In A. G. Fisher, *Assessment of Motor and Process Skills* (2nd ed., pp. 73–86). Fort Collins, CO: Three Star Press.

Fisher, A. G. (1997b). *Assessment of Motor and Process Skills* (2nd ed.). Fort Collins, CO: Three Star Press.

Fisher, A. G. (1997c). Background information. In A. G. Fisher, *Assessment of Motor and Process Skills* (2nd ed., pp. 11–34). Fort Collins, CO: Three Star Press.

Fisher, A. G. (1997d). Introduction. In A. G. Fisher, *Assessment of Motor and Process Skills* (2nd ed., pp. 1–9). Fort Collins, CO: Three Star Press.

Fisher, A. G., Murray, E. A., & Bundy, A. C. (1991). *Sensory integration: Theory and practice.* Philadelphia: F. A. Davis.

Fisher, A. G., & Short-DeGraff, M. (1993). Nationally speaking—Improving functional assessment in occupational therapy: Recommendations and philosophy for change. *American Journal of Occupational Therapy, 47,* 199–202.

Gritzer, G., & Arluke, A. (1985). *The making of rehabilitation.* Berkeley University of California Press.

Hagedorn, R. (1995). *Occupational therapy: Perspectives and processes.* Edinburgh, Scotland: Churchill Livingstone.

Hagedorn, R. (1997). *Foundations for practice in occupational therapy* (2nd ed.). New York: Churchill Livingstone.

Haugen, J. B., & Mathiowetz, V. (1995). Contemporary task-oriented approach. In C. A. Trombly (Ed.), *Occupational therapy for physical dysfunction* (4th ed., pp. 510–527). Baltimore: Williams & Wilkins.

Hutzler, Y., Chacham, A., Bergman, U., & Szeinberg, A. (1998). Effects of a movement and swimming program on vital capacity and water orientation skills of children with cerebral palsy. *Developmental Medicine and Child Neurology, 40,* 176–181.

Jongbloed, L., Brighton, C., & Stacey, S. (1988). Factors associated with independent meal preparation, self-care and mobility in CVA clients. *Canadian Journal of Occupational Therapy, 55,* 259–263.

Judge, J. O., Schechtman, K., Cress, E., & the FICSIT Group. (1996). The relationship between physical performance measures and independence in instrumental activities of daily living. *Journal of the American Geriatrics Society, 44,* 1332–1341.

Kaplan, B. J., Polatajko, H. J., Wilson, B. N., & Faris, P. D. (1993). Reexamination of sensory integration treatment: A combination of two efficacy studies. *Journal of Learning Disabilities, 26,* 342–347.

Kielhofner, G. (1985). *A model of human occupation: Theory and application.* Baltimore: Williams & Wilkins.

Kielhofner, G. (1995). *A model of human occupation: Theory and application* (2nd ed.). Baltimore: Williams & Wilkins.

Kielhofner, G. (1997). *Conceptual foundations of occupational therapy* (2nd ed.). Philadelphia: F. A. Davis.

Kielhofner, G., & Henry, A. D. (1988). Development and investigation of the Occupational Performance History Interview. *American Journal of Occupational Therapy, 42,* 489–498.

Law, M., Baptiste, S., Carswell, A., McColl, M. A., Polatajko, H., & Pollock, N. (1994). *Canadian Occupational Performance Measure* (2nd ed.). Toronto, Ontario: CAOT Publications.

Law, M., Russell, D., Pollock, N., Rosenbaum, P., Walter, S., & King, G. (1997). A comparison of intensive neurodevelopmental therapy plus casting and a regular occupational therapy program for children with cerebral palsy. *Developmental Medicine and Child Neurology, 39,* 664–670.

Letts, S., Law, M., Rigby, P., Cooper, B., Stewart, S., & Strong, S. (1994). Person–environment assessments in occupational therapy. *American Journal of Occupational Therapy, 48,* 608–618.

Lichtenberg, P. A., & Nanna, M. (1994). The role of cognition in predicting activities of daily living and ambulation functioning in the oldest-old rehabilitation patients. *Rehabilitation Psychology, 39,* 251–262.

Llorens, L. A. (1993). Activity analysis: Agreement between participants and observers on perceived factors in occupation components. *Occupational Therapy Journal of Research, 13,* 198–211.

Mosey, A. C. (1981). *Occupational therapy: Configuration of a profession.* New York: Raven.

Mosey, A. C. (1986). *Psychosocial components of occupational therapy.* New York: Raven.

Nakayama, H., Jørgensen, H. S., Raaschou, H. O., & Olsen, T. S. (1994). Compensation in recovery of upper extremity function after stroke: The Copenhagen Stroke Study. *Archives of Physical Medicine and Rehabilitation, 75,* 852–857.

Neistadt, M. E. (1992). Occupational therapy treatments for constructional deficits. *American Journal of Occupational Therapy, 46,* 141–148.

Neistadt, M. E. (1995). Methods of assessing clients' priorities: A survey of adult physical dysfunction settings. *American Journal of Occupational Therapy, 49,* 428–436.

Nelson, D. L. (1988). Occupation: Form and performance. *American Journal of Occupational Therapy, 42,* 633–641.

Occupational therapy in the general hospital. (1917). *Modern Hospital, 8,* 425–427.

Pincus, T., Callahan, L. F., Brooks, R. H., Fuchs, H. A., Olsen, N. J., & Kaye, J. J. (1989). Self-report questionnaire scores in rheumatoid arthritis compared with traditional physical, radiographic, and laboratory measures. *Annals of Internal Medicine, 110,* 259–266.

Quiroga, V.A.M. (1995). *Occupational therapy: The first 30 years, 1900 to 1930.* Bethesda, MD: American Occupational Therapy Association.

Reed, B. R., Jagust, W. J., & Seab, J. P. (1989). Mental status as a predictor of daily function in progressive dementia. *Gerontologist, 29,* 804–807.

Rudman, D. L., Cook, J. V., & Polatajko, H. (1997). Understanding the potential of occupation: A qualitative exploration of seniors' perspectives on activity. *American Journal of Occupational Therapy, 51,* 640–650.

Semans, S. (1967). The Bobath concept in treatment of neurological disorders. *American Journal of Physical Medicine, 46,* 732–785.

Skurla, E., Rogers, J. C., & Sunderland, T. (1988). Direct assessment of activities of daily living in Alzheimer's disease: A controlled study. *Journal of the American Geriatrics Society, 36,* 97–103.

Spencer, J. C., Davidson, H. A., & White, V. K. (1996). Continuity and change: Past experiences as adaptive repertoire in occupational adaptation. *American Journal of Occupational Therapy, 50,* 526–534.

Stockmeyer, S. A. (1967). An interpretation of the approach of Rood to the treatment of neuromuscular dysfunction. *American Journal of Physical Medicine, 46,* 900–956.

Teri, L., Borson, S., Kiyak, H. A., & Yamagishi, M. (1989). Behavioral disturbance, cognitive dysfunction, and functional skill: Prevalence and relationship in Alzheimer's disease. *Journal of the American Geriatrics Society, 37,* 109–116.

The Oxford English dictionary (2nd ed.). (1989). Oxford, UK: Clarendon.

Tickle-Degnen, L. (1995). Therapeutic rapport. In C. A. Trombly (Ed.), *Occupational therapy for physical dysfunction* (4th ed., pp. 277–285). Baltimore: Williams & Wilkins.

Trombly, C. (1993). The Issue Is—Anticipating the future: Assessment of occupational function. *American Journal of Occupational Therapy, 47,* 253–257.

Trombly, C. A. (1995a). Occupation: Purposefulness and meaningfulness as therapeutic mechanisms. 1995 Eleanor Clarke Slagle Lecture. *American Journal of Occupational Therapy, 49*, 960–972.

Trombly, C. A. (1995b). Purposeful activity. In C. A. Trombly (Ed.), *Occupational therapy for physical dysfunction* (4th ed., pp. 237–253). Baltimore: Williams & Wilkins.

Trombly, C. A. (1995c). Retraining basic and instrumental activities of daily living. In C. A. Trombly (Ed.), *Occupational therapy for physical dysfunction* (4th ed., pp. 289–318). Baltimore: Williams & Wilkins.

Upham, E. G. (1917). Some principles of occupational therapy. *Modern Hospital, 8*, 409–413.

Watson, D. E. (1997). *Task analysis. An occupational performance approach.* Bethesda, MD: American Occupational Therapy Association.

47

1999 Eleanor Clarke Slagle Lecture

Defining Lives: Occupation as Identity:
An Essay on Competence, Coherence, and the Creation of Meaning

Charles H. Christiansen, EdD, OTR, OT(C), FAOTA

The anthropologist Bateson (1996) has written that

> The capacity to do something useful for yourself or others is key to personhood, whether it involves the ability to earn a living, cook a meal, put on shoes in the morning, or whatever other skill needs to be mastered at the moment. (1986, p. 11)

In this article, I assert that occupations are key not just to being a person, but to being a *particular* person, and thus creating and maintaining an identity. Occupations come together within the contexts of our relationships with others to provide us with a sense of purpose and structure in our day-to-day activities, as well as over time. When we build our identities through occupations, we provide ourselves with the contexts necessary for creating meaningful lives, and life meaning helps us to be well.

In this article, an important distinction is made between being well and being healthy. The ultimate goal of occupational therapy services is well-being, not health. Health enables people to pursue the tasks of everyday living that provide them with the life meaning necessary for their well-being. As Englehardt said in describing the virtues of occupational therapy, *"people are healthy or diseased in terms of the activities open to them or denied them."* (1977, p. 672)

Overview

In addressing the complex topic of personal identity, I begin by reviewing key concepts from the literature, noting particularly how our use of language gives us important insights into how we think about ourselves. I then discuss how identity is thought to be formed during the crucial developmental stages of our lives, and how it seems to be of immense importance to us as we make our way through the stages of life. After this, I consider how daily occupations serve the important purpose of enabling us to experience or realize our personal identities. I then address the implications of incomplete or blemished identities on personal well-being, and conclude with observations on the implications of identity-making for the practice of occupational therapy in the new millennium.

Propositions

My presentation is based on four propositions, all centered on the assertion that one of the most compelling needs that every human being has is to be able to express his or her unique identity in a manner that gives meaning to life. This assertion was influenced greatly by an ethnographic study of adaptive strategies reported in *The American Journal of Occupational Therapy* (McCuaig & Frank, 1991). That study described a middle-aged woman [Meghan]

Originally published 1999 in *American Journal of Occupational Therapy, 53,* 547–558.

with severe athetoid cerebral palsy who had great difficulty with voluntary movement that profoundly affected her mobility and speech. Somehow, without much professional assistance, the woman was able to devise adaptive strategies so that she could use her limited voluntary movement and assistive technology to get along in daily life. Despite rather considerable postural deformities and difficulty with hearing, she was able to live in an apartment, requiring only modest assistance of friends and neighbors to live independently.

In considering the study, I found Meghan's motivations for choosing strategies, rather than the nature of her adaptations, of greatest interest. It seemed that one very important consideration underlying her choices—especially when they were to be viewed by others—was whether or not they would show her to be an intelligent, competent woman. In short, they were issues of identity.

I remember being surprised by this observation, thinking that someone as disabled as she was would be driven by the functional necessities of life, with little reserve time or energy to be consumed by thoughts of how she might be viewed in the eyes of others. But as I thought about it more deeply, I realized that life around me was teeming with indications[1] that people (with disabilities or without) are universally concerned about their social identity and acceptance by others. The ethnographic study also pointed squarely to the reality that daily occupation was the primary means through which the woman was able to communicate her identity as a competent person.

My further thinking and study about the relationships between daily occupations and selfhood led to four premises that may be useful to the process of considering identity issues in occupational therapy. Because there is yet much work to be done in establishing the validity of theories of how identity is constructed and maintained, each proposition must be viewed as tentative.

Proposition 1: Identity is an overarching concept that shapes and is shaped by our relationships with others.

Personal identity can be defined as the person we think we are. It is the self we know. Note that this is not the same as self-concept nor is it the same as self-esteem, although these important concepts are related to identity. Baumeister (1986, 1997), an often-cited authority on the study of identity, has noted that the most obvious things in daily life are sometimes the most difficult to define. We use the word *self* in our everyday language several times a day. When we say *self,* we include the direct feeling we have about our thoughts and feelings and sensations. This begins with the awareness of our body and is augmented by our sense of being able to make choices and initiate action. It also encompasses the abstract and complex ideas that embellish the self.

The term *self-concept* refers to the *inferences* we make about ourselves. It encompasses our understanding of personality traits and characteristics, our social roles, and our relationships. We are motivated as adults to achieve some consistency in terms of how we view ourselves, and we want this view to be favorable. In general, we strive to maintain favorable views and to dispute or avoid feedback that is discrepant from our view of self (Swann, 1987; Swann & Hill, 1982). To the extent that we perceive discrepancies between our perceived and ideal selves, we are motivated to change.

A third concept is self-esteem. This refers to the evaluative aspect of the self-concept. Self-esteem is related to identity in the sense that our esteem is related to our ability to demonstrate efficacious action, which gains social approval and thus influences our overall concept of self (Baumeister, 1982; Franks & Marolla, 1976).

Finally, *identity* refers to the definitions that are created for and superimposed on the self. Identity is a composite definition of the self, and includes an interpersonal aspect (e.g., our roles and relationships, such as mothers, wives, occupational therapists), an aspect of possibility or potential (that is, who we *might* become), and a values aspect (that suggests importance and provides a stable basis for choices and decisions). Self-concept is entirely created in one's mind, whereas identity is often created by the larger society, even though it is often negotiated with others and refined

---

[1] Consider the prevalence (and popularity) of monograms, tattoos, vanity license plates, titles, degrees, pierced body parts, autobiographies, and unique names (changed or not).

by the individual as a result of those social negotiations (see Figure 47.1).

In summary, identity can be viewed as the superordinate view of ourselves that includes both self-esteem and the self-concept, but also importantly reflects, and is influenced by, the larger social world in which we find ourselves. This definition of identity leads logically to a second proposition:

Proposition 2: Identities are closely tied to what we do and our interpretations of those actions in the context of our relationships with others.

It is interesting to note that in North America, after an exchange of names between strangers, the next part of a conversation often turns on the expression, "What do you do?" The resulting dialogue provides for shared meaning by situating each person in a context the other understands or attempts to understand through further dialogue.

This everyday exchange illustrates the close connection between doing and identity, and also points out the important role that language has in creating understanding and meaning. Were it not for our social existence, there would be no need for language and communication, and it is generally believed that thought itself is a product of language. That is, when we think, we carry on an internal dialogue with ourselves. Vygotsky (1981) maintained that language provides children with the tools to gain self-awareness and, consequently, voluntary control of their actions. Thus, our understanding of the world around us is shaped as much by language, a system of spoken and written symbols, as it is by direct experience.

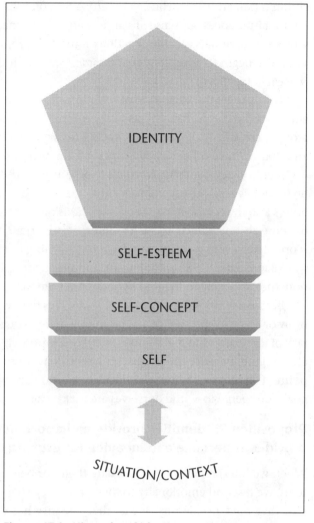

Figure 47.1. Hierarchy of identity concepts.

For example, when we learn the word *stove* as toddlers, we are also apt to learn the words *hot* and *danger*. We may also discover that if we ignore our parents' admonitions and touch a hot stove, we may burn our fingers. At the same time, we may experience disapproval for not having behaved as our parents expected.

Piaget (1954) and others (Kagan, 1981) have shown that as infants and as toddlers, the experience of coming to know the world very much involves *doing*. As children, we learn that we can intentionally act on our environment and change it. It is this acting on the environment with observable consequence that gives us our sense of selfhood, that teaches us that we are active agents, separate from our environment.

As children explore cause-and-effect events, they learn that they can have an effect on inanimate objects, such as toys, and that they can also elicit reactions from animate objects, such as pets and other people. Mostly, a child's early experiences in this regard are positive because doting parents and grandparents tend to regard any behavior as cute and, as a consequence, are very forgiving of transgressions. Later, this tolerance becomes more selective, and parents can then also communicate disapproval when a child disobeys. Yet, already, children have become active agents in the world, exerting an effect on objects and on people. Using dolls or toy figures, they can even pretend that objects *are* people.

Thus, children learn that they can get the attention of others through their actions and that their actions can be approved or not. Studies have shown that *good* and *bad* are among the words most frequently spoken to young children (Kagan, 1981). Thus, very early on, a connection is made between behavior and social approval in a manner that influences our sense of self. The point to be made here is that already, at an early age, children know themselves as individuals capable of acting on the world, and they understand that their actions have a social meaning. They also begin to appreciate that their approval as individuals is often contingent on what they do (Keller, Ford, & Meacham, 1978).

This is to be the beginning of a lifetime of understanding the interdependence of self and the social groups to which we are connected. It is also the beginning of understanding ourselves as having an identity that is related to group membership. For example, as children we learn that we are members of a family, that we are male or female, and that we have other characteristics in common or in contrast with others.

Identity development continues to be influenced by social relationships as children mature. Beginning at preschool age, self-concept and identity are shaped by a person's competencies and capabilities in comparison to others and in relationship to social standards or expectations (Ruble, 1983). During adolescence, identity is shaped by more abstract concepts, such as interpersonal traits, values, and preferences (Erikson, 1968). For adults, identity is oriented toward goals; often related to becoming a certain kind of person and not becoming another kind of person (Baumeister, 1986). Adolescent and adult identity development, although based more on abstractions, is nonetheless largely influenced by social phenomena.

Because symbolic communication involves behaviors as well as language, children learn also that a raised eyebrow or an awkward silence can be among many forms of communicating disapproval. As maturity develops, the task of understanding what constitutes social approval takes on even greater importance, and becomes even more challenging, because the feedback adults receive in social settings is much more ambiguous and indirect. At this point, it should be obvious that identity has no existence outside of interpersonal relationships. Our views of our goals, our behaviors, and ourselves are inextricably tied to our relationships with others.

Proposition 3: Identities provide an important central figure in a self-narrative or life story that provides coherence and meaning for everyday events and life itself.

When we interpret events, we evaluate them for personal meaning. If they are meaningful, they have significance to us, we respond emotionally to them, and they shape our behavior and perceptions of life. When people believe that they have no identity or that their identity has been spoiled, life becomes less meaningful and can become meaningless (Debats, Drost, & Hansen, 1995; Moore, 1997; van Selm & Dittmann-Kohli, 1998).

Our interpretation of life events and situations takes place within the framework of life stories or narratives. Other people are part of our life stories, and we are part of the life stories of others. Our lives are interwoven within the lives of others and, therefore, if our identities change, this influences our life as well as the lives of others. In this sense, identities are socially interconnected and distributed, yet understood in the context of ongoing life stories.

Proposition 4: Because life meaning is derived in the context of identity, it is an essential element in promoting well-being and life-satisfaction.

Each of us hopes for a satisfactory outcome for the particular goals we are pursuing at the moment as well as for the life we are leading, which we are aware will end at some point. To the extent that we can successfully weave together the various and multiple short stories that comprise our lives into a meaningful whole, we can derive a sense of coherence and meaning and purpose from our lives. I am proposing that our identities provide us with the context through which we interpret and derive meaning from the events we experience. Our identities also provide us with a view for future possibilities.

Theoretical Contexts

Having elaborated four propositions regarding identity, it is useful to create a context from which to view them and evaluate their implications for occupational therapy practice. There are three roots of selfhood that will serve as a framework for understanding. The first is the experience of reflexive consciousness, derived from the traditions of symbolic interactionism. This allows us to think about ourselves and the influence of our actions on others. The second is the interpersonal aspect of selfhood, the reality that identities are shaped within a social setting, where we receive acceptance, approval, and validation as worthwhile persons. The third is the agential aspect of identity, that aspect of demonstrating influence on the world around us that allows us to make meaning in our lives. When we create, when we control, when we exercise choice, we are expressing our selfhood and unique identities.

Reflexive Consciousness

The ability to think about ourselves and to have these thoughts modify our behavior is a distinctly human characteristic, and it depends on symbolic communication. Using symbols or language, we not only are able to categorize, think about, and act in socially influenced ways, but we also are able to reflect on ourselves from the perspective of others.

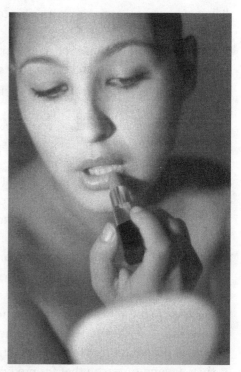

Figure 47.2. Reflexive self-consciousness—The dialogue between the *I* and the *me*.
Note. Image © 1999 PhotoDisc, Inc. Used with permission.

When we think about ourselves, we carry on the equivalent of an internal dialogue between two aspects of self, the experiencing self and the thought of self. These two aspects of the self can be labeled the *I* and the *me*. The I is the active creative agent doing the experiencing, thinking, and acting, and the me is the perspective or attitude toward oneself that one assumes when taking the roles of specific others or the generalized community. In this approach, the me's, or perspectives of the self, are the social selves—who we are in our own and others' eyes. Thought of in another way, when we consider the image of ourselves reflected in a mirror, the I is looking at and thinking about the me, all the while making grooming adjustments to improve it (see Figure 47.2).

The reflexive nature of the self is exemplified by everyday language that illustrates its duality. When we speak of self-discipline, we are talking about one aspect of the self keeping the other under control. Similarly, when we observe that Sue has "let herself go," we imply that she no longer has self-control or that she no longer cares about her public identity.

The Interpersonal Nature of Selfhood

The ideas of symbolic communication and the reflexive nature of the self are derived from a tradition of social psychology known as symbolic interactionism. This tradition goes back to the turn of the century and several prominent behavioral scientists of the time, beginning with William James (1892). Later, the famous sociologist Charles Horton Cooley (1902) made the observation that our views of ourselves are very much influenced by the reactions of others to what we do. He formulated what is known as the "looking glass theory," which maintained that the reactions of others reflect their approval and disapproval and thus constitute a primary means of developing an awareness of ourselves.

The psychologist George Herbert Mead extended this thinking in the 1930s, advancing the theory even further. In *Mind, Self and Society,* Mead (1934) held that society is created, sustained, and changed through the process of symbolic communication. In other words, social reality is constructed and negotiated through interactions with others. In these interactions, people seek to present images of the self for others to see and evaluate. The primary purposes of these social selves are to gain approval from others and to be able to gain influence, which occurs through social status and power. Mead believed that by using the reflexive processes of communication, the dialogue between I and me, we are able to imagine how we appear to others or what reactions others will have to our behaviors.[2]

Because of the dependence on others for feedback about the self, Mead (1934) believed that there is a mutual interdependence of self and society. By seeking the approval of others, a person's behavior may be moderated, but this occurs only to the extent that people are capable of exercising the self-control necessary for them to gain social approval.

Many people are reluctant to accept a view of self that suggests that every action they take is calculated to gain the approval of others because it sounds manipulative or deceptive. However, in reality, people are not able to exercise conscious control over their behaviors in a manner that permits them to plan calculated actions at every moment in every social relationship. To a certain extent, however, the rules and conventions of social interaction are such that we preserve and enhance our identity through conformity and careful reflection about the anticipated results of our behaviors on others.

As expressions of identity, people often exhibit spontaneity and creativity that test the boundaries of conformity or risk social disapproval. Unconventional behavior is often risky. This is one of the things that makes the world such an interesting place. Occasionally, acts of spontaneity and creativity are embraced and adopted by the larger group with the result that such innovations create change or progress in the culture. In this way, the reciprocal influence between self and society described by Mead (1934) is completed. That is, social expectations influence the individual, and the individual, through acts of creativity, sometimes influences the larger society. A proposal of symbolic interactionism views that the individual and society are interdependent. That is, they depend on each other for predictability and stability as well as for progress.

To summarize, the basic ideas underlying symbolic interactionism are that (a) we communicate symbolically much of the time and that the language of social life consists of both spoken and unspoken messages; (b) through our conversations with ourselves, we are able to modify our behaviors to gain social approval; and (c) the need for social approval encourages conformity, which promotes stability and predictability, but occasionally also yields individual creativity that, when adopted, serves to advance the social group.

Social Constructionism and Distributed Selves

In recent years, views of the social nature of self-identity have been extended with a school of thought called social constructionism. Theorists in this tradition propose that selves are distributed. That is, the person and their social context cannot be easily separated. Social constructionists argue that although we perceive a private and self-contained world inside our heads, it would be more accurate to describe this image as a snapshot from a constantly changing public panorama (Bruner, 1990; Gergen, 1991; Polkinghorne, 1988).

When we think of our multiple expressions of self, our children, our friendships, our marriages, our journals, and our daily interactions, we realize that our identities are indeed distributed throughout our social environments. These "pieces of self" are part of us. They define who we are, and yet they exist in other mediums, distributing identities well beyond the boundaries of a physical body. This distribution of the self only occurs through social interaction.

The social constructionist view suggests that people's identities not only are social, they also are multifaceted, yet they are perceived not so much as fragments, but as part of a comprehensive and understandable self (cf. Kondo,

---

[2] It is worth noting that Mead's assertion that our identity is totally dependent on the feedback of others has been shown to be incomplete (Schrauger & Schoeneman, 1979), mainly because research has shown that people deceive themselves by perceiving that others evaluate them more favorably than is actually the case (Greenwald, 1980).

1990). Ordinarily, we do not think of ourselves as fragmented, but as complex people with many dimensions of self. In short, we piece together our experiences to fashion an intelligible self, an identity that is comprehensible to both ourselves and others.

Life Stories

How is it that our identities can be complex and distributed while at the same time seem to be stable and predictable? The answer to this question lies in our understanding of our lives as evolving narratives or life stories. Through stories, we understand life events as systematically related. As Gergen and Gergen wrote: "One's present identity is thus not a sudden and mysterious event, but a sensible result of a life story" (1988, p. 55).

In a sense, our stories are unfolding and being rewritten as we live them. All narrative shares the similar characteristic of having a temporal order. That is, our life stories consist of events in progressive sequences. In order for our stories to have meaning, the events in our lives must be interpreted in ways that give them a relationship to each other. In this manner, they have coherence and unity. It helps that our everyday routines, our personality traits, and other factors, such as our genetic make-up, influence us in ways that provide a degree of consistency to our behavior. This makes it easier to interpret our life stories in an understandable way.

Making Sense of Experiences

The problem of how people make sense of their life experiences has been central to the work of McAdams (1997). He has analyzed life stories to derive insights into the processes people use to construct their identities within a coherent structure. His work suggests that one of the central purposes of the life story is to create unity and purpose in daily life. In constructing and interpreting life stories, people seek to fashion identities that make sense to themselves and others. Importantly, because people are not passive participants in their life stories, they can enact or create the events that express their identities in the manner they would like others to view them. This brings us to the third requirement of identity, that of human agency, or expressing the self through acting on the world around us.

Selfing: Shaping Identity Through Experience

It is the reflexive dialogue between the I and me that McAdams (1996, 1997) suggests ties human agency to identity. The I, he argues, is not a noun, but a process, which McAdams and others refer to as *selfing*. That is, by experiencing our actions and our lives as our own, we adopt them as part of ourselves, as belonging to the me. Selfing is responsible for human feelings of agency.

McAdams (1996) suggests that selfing is inherently a unifying, integrative, synthesizing process. Ego psychologists (e.g., Loevenger, 1976), building on Freud (as cited in Stachey, 1990), viewed the ego as the organizational medium of the mind that promotes healthy adaptation to life through learning, memory, perception, and synthesis (Kris, 1952). It permits the gaining of competence that White (1959) viewed as so important to successful adaptation. To quote McAdams: "The I puts experience together—synthesizes it, unifies it, makes it mine. The fact that it is mine—even when I see the sunset, I am seeing it; that when you hurt my feelings those were my feelings, not yours that were hurt—provides a unity to selfhood without which human life in society as we know it would simply not exist" (1997, p. 57). To *self* is to maintain the stance of the self in the world, It is the being and becoming that Fidler (Fidler & Fidler, 1978) has written about. In other words, selfing is the shaping of identity through daily occupations.

Occupations are more than movements strung together, more than simply doing something. They are opportunities to express the self, to create an identity.

Creating Life Meaning Through Selfing

When we create our life stories through doing, or selfing, as McAdams would say, we are living for a purpose, and deriving a sense of meaning in our lives in the process. Sommer and Baumeister (1998) have observed that people seek meaning in ordinary events along the same lines that they seek meaning in life generally. That is, they try to fulfill four basic needs. These needs are *purpose, efficacy, value,* and *self-worth.* By definition, our daily occupations, whether they pertain to work, leisure, or maintenance of self, are goal directed and, therefore, provide purpose in the moment. When we achieve success in reaching our goals, we derive a sense of efficacy and believe that we have some measure of control over our environments (Langer & Rodin, 1976).

Meaning is also derived from believing that we have done the right thing, that our actions are justifiable under the circumstances. Finally, and not least importantly, we derive meaning from our feelings of self-worth. We meet this need through the approval of others and by viewing our own traits and abilities favorably. We want to feel good about ourselves, and we want to believe that we are worthy of other people's attention and affection.[3]

This discussion should emphasize the important relationships between identity, occupations, competence, and meaning. There is clearly an important interplay between these concepts. We cannot gain the recognition of others without competent action, nor can we meet our needs for meaning without engaging in occupation in a way that receives social validation. Moreover, the things we do, even when validated by others as competent, must be understandable to ourselves within a meaningful life context.

Identity—Goals and Occupational Performance

It may be helpful here to elaborate on the important relationship between occupations and identity. To speak of occupation is to describe goal-directed activity in the context of living. Goals work as motivators precisely because we imagine how we will be affected directly or indirectly when the goal is met. Thus, goals serve as motivators because we view them in the context of self, whether we are dressing for the day or seeking a promotion. We put on the blue blazer because we imagine what we will look like and anticipate that it will be satisfactory or appropriate for the day's activities.

Similarly, when we work late, or when we willingly take on an added responsibility in volunteer activities, we imagine ourselves as being viewed as virtuous, hardworking, and worthwhile people. We may imagine getting praised, getting a promotion, or receiving a raise or recognition as a result of those efforts. These views of our identity in the future are imagined selves, and they are powerful motivators of goal-directed action. Markus and colleagues (Markus, 1977; Markus & Nurius, 1986) have called these motivating images *possible selves.* They have suggested that a goal can have an influence on behavior to the extent that an individual can personalize it by building a bridge of self-representations between the current state and the hoped-for state.

Possible selves can consist of both positive as well as negative images. They not only may represent what we would like to become, they also may represent what we are afraid of becoming. Either type of possible self can be a motivator. Thus, we may strive to become the wealthy self, the shapely self, or the well-respected and loved self; while we dread, and thus, try to avoid becoming the lonely, depressed, or incompetent self (Ogilvie, 1987).

---

[3] The British psychologist and philosopher Rom Harré (1983) has used the term *identity projects* to refer to self-directed development and expression of self. Identity projects may take the form of pursuit of fame or status or recognition of some kind. Or they may be concerned with the more personal aspects of ourselves and the way we think about ourselves. This may involve developing our potentials to create and to relate to others, or enriching our experience and understanding. Harré (1998) has also written extensively about the importance of discourse in shaping agency. A complete treatment of his propositions is beyond the scope of this article, but highly recommended for readers interested in a more in-depth analysis of the psychology of selfhood.

Possible Selves as Images of Action

Markus and her colleagues have contended that possible selves give personal meaning and structure to a person's thoughts about the future. That is, when we think about actions we might take, we project images of ourselves into those thoughts, and we view ourselves taking the actions. In other words, possible selves provide a very useful and direct mechanism for translating thoughts into actions. Goals that individuals view as important, and to which they are committed, are effective because these goals are self-relevant and self-defining.

Goals differ between people because the nature of possible selves depends on the nature of one's core self or complex identity system. Goal-directed and motivated behavior and personal identity are thus reciprocally related. Studies (Pavot, Fujita, & Diener, 1997) have shown that as we perceive ourselves becoming more like the person we want to be, our life satisfaction increases. When we do not perceive ourselves as progressing toward our desired identities, we tend to exhibit signs of unhealthy adaptation (Heatherton & Baumeister, 1991).

Social Approval and Competent Performance

Social approval and competent performance are instrumental to our thoughts of actions that will help us avoid or realize possible selves. Research shows that people will go to great lengths to alter their behavior (and indeed, even their appearance) in order to gain social approval and avoid rejection (Crowne & Marlowe, 1964).

To a large extent, our ability to gain this approval depends on our ability to portray ourselves as competent people. Through implicit expectations associated with social standing and the performance of roles, social groups help define the levels of competence necessary for acceptance, approval, and recognition.

In other words, self-appraisal is highly dependent on the extent to which we believe that we will be accepted by others. Research has also shown that it is related to efficacious action or competent performance, meaning that we must demonstrate to others that we are competent people as part of the acceptance process (Franks & Marolla, 1976).

Competent Performance

To be competent suggests that we are effective in dealing with the challenges that come our way (White, 1971). If we experience success in the challenges we undertake, we enhance our view of ourselves as competent beings (Bandura, 1977; Gage & Polatajko, 1994). This encourages us to explore and to engage the world in ways that give us our sense of autonomy and selfhood.

As we experience successes, our views of ourselves as efficacious or competent become strengthened. Thus, completing a task successfully adds to our sense of being competent human beings and, in a sense, prepares us for new challenges by bolstering our self-confidence. The term *self-confidence* is an interesting expression because it establishes a clear link between our identity and our belief in the things that we can do. Rogers (1982) asserted that developing a sense of the self as a competent agent in the world requires the expression of choice and control. Through choice, we express autonomy and, through control, we express efficacy. Brewster Smith summed it up nicely in: "The crucial attitude toward the self is self-respect as a significant and efficacious person" (1974, p. 14).

Performance Deficits

If our identities are crafted by what we do and how we do it, then it follows that any threat to our ability to engage in occupations and present ourselves as competent people becomes a threat to our identity. On a daily basis, occupational therapists come into contact with persons whose identities are threatened by virtue of performance limitations. These identity crises may occur as the result of normal aging, which often deprives us of the sense of competence we once had, or result from congenital disorders, injuries, and diseases that leave lasting or progressive disability.

To the extent that disabilities interfere with the competent execution of tasks and roles, they threaten the establishment of an identity based on competence. In some cases, injury, disease and disability also result in bodily disfigurement, which further assaults the person's identity and increases the challenges associated with establishing an identity that receives social approval (Goffman, 1963). Facial scars or anomalies, involuntary movements related to motor planning deficits, balance disorders, and unwanted tics are among the many observable signs of disorders that gain unwanted public attention and increase the challenge of fashioning a social identity that is acceptable to self and others.

Stigma

Goffman (1959) suggested that a socially competent performance involves more than simply getting the job done. There are certain stylistic and procedural expectations that must be fulfilled in order for the person to be considered by others to have performed competently and credibly. When we convince others that we have performed credibly, we are engaging in what Goffman called *impression management.*[4]

It is widely acknowledged within the cultures of people with activity limitations that impression management is an important strategy to undertake. It is a practiced skill to develop such social proficiency that one's impairment is hardly noticed. Indeed, there is a word for this, *passing,* which means that one has hidden one's devalued characteristics from others successfully, so that one has been able to pass as "normal" or able-bodied.

The ability to manage the impressions of others is often so compelling that actual performance may be secondary to preserving identity by leaving a good impression. Studies of prosthetic and assistive technology devices show that their acceptance and use may be as dependent on appearance and perceived social acceptability as their functional benefits (Batavia & Hammer, 1990; Pippin & Fernie, 1997; Stein & Walley, 1983).

Of course, the easiest way to avoid rejection is to increase control and the possibility of rejection by avoiding social interaction altogether. In confronting the risk of social rejection, it is not unusual to find people with observable disability to retreat to the safety and emotional security of interactions limited to close friends and associates. These people, it is reasoned, know the person beyond the disfigurement. Avoidance strategies are more understandable when one considers that social disapproval is not simply an uncomfortable situation that evokes feelings of embarrassment or shame. It is, quite directly, an assault on one's identity.

Researchers have shown that while passing is a useful strategy for avoiding stigma, it can result in an unhealthy adaptation to disability if it results in denial. Successful adaptation to one's individual differences requires the ability to acknowledge one's differences and to integrate them into an identity that permits a confident expression of self (Weinberg & Sterritt, 1986). One of the challenges of acquired disability is reintegration into social patterns that promote acceptance of self and a more comfortable relationship with able-bodied persons. This comfort leads to more positive acceptance by those persons.

Disability and Identity Adaptations

A surprising number of studies have directly or indirectly studied the identity consequences of children and adults with chronic illnesses and disabling conditions. These have often shown that preserving and developing one's identity are often at the heart of adaptational strategies (Charmaz, 1994; Estroff, 1989; Monks, 1995; Ville, Ravaud, Marchal, Paicheler, & Fardeau, 1992; Weinberg & Sterrit, 1986).

---

[4] It is worth mentioning that stigma affects those with whom one shares identity. Consistent with the idea of distributed selves, spouses and family members may also endure the social cost of disfigurement, poor role performance, or deviance. For example, stigma accrues to families whose members have HIV or mental illness, or who have committed suicide.

For example, a study by Charmaz (1994) of men with chronic illnesses is relevant here. She found that when men did awaken to the changes in their bodies and accept the uncertainties of their futures, they engaged in reflection and reappraisals that often improved their awareness of self and personal priorities. It is noteworthy that reappraisals of productivity, achievement, and relationships were central to this process. As a result of these reappraisals, some men changed jobs, others retired or renegotiated their work assignments, and many followed health regimens, such as exercising, more devotedly.

One recurring theme in these and other studies of adaptation to illness and disability is the role of identity in creating a sense of coherence or continuity over time. When people experience loss and change, the continuity of their lives is disrupted. Identity is the great integrator of life experience. We interpret events that happen to us in terms of their meaning for our life stories. This gives life a sense of coherence.

Identity, Sense of Coherence, and Well-Being

People with a sense of coherence view their lives as understandable, meaningful, and manageable. The concept emanates from Aaron Antonovsky (1979), who proposed a model that would explain how some people are able to cope with stressors without experiencing the negative consequences to health experienced by others. Antonovsky proposed that a sense of coherence was central to this ability to cope with stress, suggesting that people who interpret their experiences within a meaningful and understandable framework, and who perceive that their challenges are manageable, are better equipped to deal with life's unexpected turns.

Research on the sense of coherence during the past 20 years has shown that people with this attribute, or way of viewing the world, are healthier and better adjusted than people without a strong sense of coherence. For example, significant relationships have been found between sense of coherence and blood pressure, emotional stability, global health, subjective well-being, and coping skills (Antonovsky, 1993). Sense of coherence is different from, but related to, another factor found in coping studies called hardiness (Kobasa, 1979).

Of importance to this discussion is the finding that sense of coherence seems to measure a human dimension that intersects with identity. Because it reflects one's efficacy or sense of agency, because it reflects meaning, and because it reflects a person's sense of how the events in their lives fit together, sense of coherence is related in important ways to the issue of identity (Baumeister & Tice, 1990; Korotkov, 1998). In fact, this relationship is borne out in studies of personal projects done by Little and others (Little, 1989; Christiansen, Backman, Little, & Nguyen, 1999). This research, using personal projects analysis (cf. Christiansen, Little, & Backman, 1998), seeks to connect occupations of everyday life with personality traits. Findings have shown a relationship between identity dimensions of personal projects and sense of coherence. This provides a small but important piece of evidence supporting the hypothesis that identity and sense of coherence are related, and possibly overlapping, concepts (see Figure 47.3).

Issues of coherence, personal identity, meaning, and well-being have been nicely tied together in research reported by Wong (1998). He has used an implicit theories

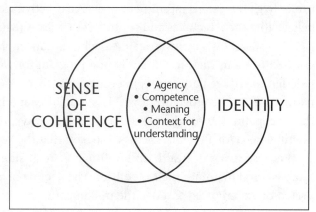

Figure 47.3. Concepts that link sense of coherence to identity.

---

[5] The nine factors are achievement striving, religion, relationship, fulfillment, fairness–respect, self-confidence, self-integration, self-transcendence, and self-acceptance.

approach to study how people define their lives as personally meaningful. Through analysis of the responses of subjects in different age groups, he has identified nine factors that collectively provide a profile of an ideal meaningful life.[5] Four of these factors focus directly on the self. In these studies, Wong has found that when people have higher profiles on these factors, their subjective well-being increases.

We can summarize by noting that research has shown that people shape their identities through their daily occupations, which are performed in a social context that gives them symbolic meaning. Over time, our evolving identities and our actions are woven together to provide a coherent life story. The central place of occupations in shaping identity and creating life meaning is so powerful that one cannot help but marvel at their implications for occupational therapy practice.

Implications for Occupational Therapy Practice

Nearly 20 years ago, Bing (1981) provided a historical review of the people and ideas that have influenced occupational therapy since its inception. In his identification of themes that have provided particular relevance for the field, he included this principle: "The patient is the product of his or her own efforts, not the article made nor the activity accomplished" (p. 501). This principle suggests that the work of therapy involves identity building.

Therapy becomes identity building when therapists provide environments that help persons explore possible selves and achieve success in tasks that are instrumental to identities they strive to achieve, and when it enables them to validate the identities that they have worked hard to achieve in the past.

Occupational Therapy as Identity Building

There is much opportunity for occupational therapy as a special and unique service that provides opportunities for people to establish, maintain, or reclaim their identities. Particularly in North America, the demographics of aging will bring the declines in function that are a threat to identity (Kunkel & Applebaum, 1992; Statistics Canada, 1993). It is no accident that late life depression is one of the most common mental health problems in adults 60 years of age and older. Although there are many causes of depression, late life depression can arise from a loss of self-esteem, a loss of meaningful roles, declining social contacts, and reduced functional status (Karp, 1994; Reker, 1997). Research on psychosocial theories of depression has shown that depression can be averted when people are given an opportunity to gain personal meaning from everyday activities, when their sense of optimism is renewed, and where they believe that there is choice and control in their lives (Baumeister, 1990; Brewer, 1993; Kapci, 1998; Rodin, 1986).

This was shown by investigators (Jackson, Carlson, Mandel, Zemke, & Clark, 1998) at the University of Southern California in their recent study of a program for well elderly persons. That successful program used lifestyle redesign to engage participants in occupations that provided both structure and meaning to the participants. The participants in the program showed less morbidity and higher morale than a control group, demonstrating clearly that occupations, through the mechanism of identity, provide the purpose, structure, and global meaning that is an essential need for all human beings. I suggest that the key link here is identity building.

Because issues of health and well-being are at stake, society needs services concerned with helping people establish and maintain their identities. The decline of abilities that comes with normal aging need not be interpreted or experienced as a decline in competence. The key to successful aging may very well be related to the acceptance of a changed body along with opportunities for demonstrating competence and control in mastering late life challenges that create the beginnings so necessary for satisfactory endings. Coming to terms with the end of life may be facilitated through occupations that lead to an enduring presence of self and the sense that one can derive meaning from all that has happened during one's life.

Beyond the demographics of aging, there are other developments that call out for a profession that can help people find meaning in their lives. The recently released global burden of disease study contains some astonishing statistics. This study, completed at Harvard University but sponsored by the World Health Organization and the World Bank, is a careful epidemiological projection of the kinds of health-related problems the world will be dealing with in the year 2020 (Murray & Lopez, 1996).

The most interesting finding from the study is that unipolar major depression will become the second leading threat to life quality in the world. It is projected to increase significantly from 1990 levels in the developed countries. Besides dementia and osteoarthritis, other conditions showing major increases will be alcohol use and self-inflicted injuries. Although the projected pattern for the world in the year 2020 will show a general increase in overall health owing to the control of infectious diseases in the developing countries, many other health challenges will be of a nature that traditional medicine is currently unequipped to handle. Depression, self-inflicted injuries, and alcohol abuse have one thing in common—they are diseases of meaning; therefore, they can be linked to social conditions that permit people to lose their identity and sense of purpose and meaning in life.

Summary

In this article, I have made the claim that occupations constitute the mechanism that enables persons to develop and express their identities. I have asserted that identities are central features of understanding the world in an evolving self-narrative, and that the continuity provided by identity enables life to be comprehended in a manner that helps minimize the uncertainties and stresses of daily life. I have maintained that it is the imagined self that provides the context for motivation and purpose and that competence is interpreted as the capable expression of identity within a social world. And finally, and most importantly, I have argued that that identity is the pathway by which people, through daily occupations and relationships with others, are able to derive meaning from their lives.

As a profession concerned with enabling people to engage in meaningful daily occupations, occupational therapy is positioned uniquely to meet the challenges confronting people whose identity is threatened by impairments, limitations to activity, and restrictions on their participation as social beings. We have seen that, in the years ahead, our friends and colleagues will be challenged with assaults on their identities brought by age, health problems, and social conditions.

Englehardt (1986) once described occupational therapists as technologists and *custodians of meaning*. As an outsider, he saw the same opportunity and unfulfilled promise that Adolph Meyer (1922) described in the founding years of occupational therapy. Yet, a full and genuine appreciation of the power of occupation to enable health and well-being has not yet made its way across the landscape of the profession.

Just as individual persons create their unique identities and life meaning through occupations, so too do professions, which represent groups of people with shared purposes, values, and interests, realize their identities through collective action. Biomedicine will experience many great advances in the years ahead. But no genetic code, no chemical intervention, and no microsurgical technology will be invented to repair broken identities and the assault on meaning that accompanies them. Because of this, the new millennium will realize the health-enabling, restorative potential of occupation, and the promise of occupational therapy will be fulfilled.

Acknowledgments

This lecture is dedicated to my friend and mentor, Robert K. Bing, EdD, OTR, FAOTA; to my special colleague and friend, Carolyn Baum, PhD, OTR/L, FAOTA; to my parents; and especially to my wife, Pamela, a pediatric occupational therapist; and, not least of all, to my children, Carrie, Erik, and Kalle.

I thank Cindy Hammecker, Charles Hayden, and Natalie Sims for their invaluable assistance in the preparation of this paper. I am indebted to my colleagues Kenneth Ottenbacher, PhD, OTR, FAOTA, and Beatriz Abreu, PhD, OTR, FAOTA, for their expressions of confidence and support.

References

Antonovsky, A. (1979). *Health, stress and coping: New perspectives on mental health and physical well-being.* San Francisco: Jossey-Bass.

Antonovsky, A. (1993). The structure and properties of the Sense of Coherence Scale. *Social Science and Medicine, 36,* 725–733.

Bandura, A. (1977). Self-efficacy: Toward a unifying theory of behavioral change. *Psychological Review, 84,* 191–215.

Batavia, A. I., & Hammer, G. S. (1990). Toward the development of consumer based criteria for the evaluation of assistive devices. *Journal of Rehabilitation Research, 27,* 425–436.

Bateson, M. C. (1996). Enfolded activity and the concept of occupation. In R. Zemke & F. Clark (Eds.), *Occupational science: The evolving discipline* (pp. 5–12). Philadelphia: F. A. Davis.

Baumeister, R. F. (1982). Self-esteem, self-presentation and future interaction. A dilemma of reputation. *Journal of Personality, 50,* 29–45.

Baumeister, R. F. (1986). *Identity: Cultural change and the struggle for self.* New York: Oxford University Press.

Baumeister, R. F. (1990). Suicide as escape from self. *Psychological Review, 97*(1), 90–113.

Baumeister, R. F. (1997). Identity, self-concept and self-esteem. In R. Hogan, J. Johnson, & S. Briggs (Eds.), *Handbook of personality psychology* (pp. 681–711). San Diego, CA: Academic Press.

Baumeister, R. F., & Tice, D. M. (1990). Self-esteem and responses to success and failure. Subsequent performance and intrinsic motivation. *Journal of Personality, 53,* 450–467.

Bing, R. K. (1981). Occupational therapy revisited: A paraphrastic journey. 1981 Eleanor Clarke Slagle Lectures. *American Journal of Occupational Therapy, 35,* 499–518.

Brewer, B. W. (1993). Self identity and specific vulnerability to depressed mood. *Journal of Personality, 61*(3), 343–364.

Bruner, J. S. (1990). *Acts of meaning.* Cambridge: Harvard University Press.

Charmaz, K. (1994). Identity dilemmas of chronically ill men. *Sociological Quarterly, 35*(2), 269–288.

Christiansen, C. H., Little, B. R., & Backman, C. (1998). Personal projects: A useful approach to the study of occupation. *American Journal of Occupational Therapy, 52,* 439–446.

Christiansen, C. H., Backman, C., Little, B. R., & Nguyen, A. (1999). Occupations and well being: A study of personal projects. *American Journal of Occupational Therapy, 53,* 91–100.

Cooley, C. H. (1902). *Human nature and the social order.* New York: Scribner.

Crowne, D. P., & Marlowe, D. (1964). *The approval motive.* New York: Wiley.

Debats, D. L., Drost, J., & Hansen P. (1995). Experiences of meaning in life: A combined qualitative and quantitative approach. *British Journal of Psychology, 86*(3), 359–375.

Englehardt, T. (1977). Defining occupational therapy: The meaning of therapy and the virtues of occupation. *American Journal of Occupational Therapy, 31,* 666–672.

Englehardt, T. (1986). Occupational therapists as technologists and custodians of meaning. In G. Kielhofner (Ed.), *Health through occupation* (pp. 139–144). Philadelphia: F. A. Davis.

Erikson, E. H. (1968). *Identity, youth and crisis.* New York: W. W. Norton.

Estroff, S. E. (1989). Self, identity and subjective experiences of schizophrenia: In search of the subject. *Schizophrenia Bulletin, 15*(2), 189–196.

Fidler, G. S., & Fidler, J. W. (1978). Doing and becoming: Purposeful action and self actualization. *American Journal of Occupational Therapy, 32,* 305–310.

Franks, D. D., & Marolla, J. (1976). Efficacious action and social approval as interacting dimensions of self-esteem: A tentative formulation through construct validation. *Sociometry, 39*(4), 324–341.

Gage, M., & Polatajko, H. (1994). Enhancing occupational performance through an understanding of perceived self-efficacy. *American Journal of Occupational Therapy, 48,* 452–461.

Gergen, K. J. (1991). *The saturated self: Dilemmas of identity in modern life.* New York: Basic.

Gergen, K. J., & Gergen, M. M. (1988). Narrative and the self as relationship. In L. Berkowitz (Ed.), *Advances in experimental and social psychology* (pp. 17–55). San Diego, CA: Academic Press.

Goffman, E. (1959). *The presentation of self in everyday life.* Garden City, NY: Doubleday.

Goffman, E. (1963). *Stigma: Notes on the management of a spoiled identity.* Englewood Cliffs, NJ: Prentice-Hall.

Greenwald, A. G. (1980). The totalitarian ego: Fabrication and revision of personal history. *American Psychologist, 35,* 603–613.

Harré, R. (1983). *Personal being.* Oxford, U.K.: Blackwell.

Harré, R. (1998). *The singular self.* London: Sage.

Heatherton, T. F., & Baumeister, R. F. (1991). Binge eating as escape from self-awareness. *Psychological Bulletin, 110,* 86–108.

Jackson, J., Carlson, M., Mandel, D., Zemke, R., & Clark, F. (1998). Occupation in lifestyle redesign: The well elderly study occupational therapy program. *American Journal of Occupational Therapy, 52,* 326–336.

James, W. (1892). *Psychology: The briefer course.* New York: Henry Holt & Co.

Kagan, J. (1981). *The second year: The emergence of self-awareness.* Cambridge, MA: Harvard University Press.

Kapci, E. G. (1998). Test of the hopelessness theory of depression: Drawing negative inference from negative life events. *Psychological Reports, 82*(2), 355–363.

Karp, D. A. (1994). Living with depression: Illness and identity turning points. *Qualitative Health Research, 4*(1), 6–30.

Keller, A., Ford, L. H., & Meacham, J. A. (1978). Dimensions of self-concept in preschool children. *Developmental Psychology, 14,* 483–489.

Kobasa, S. C. (1979). Stressful life events, personality and health: An inquiry into hardiness. *Journal of Personality and Social Psychology, 37,* 1–11.

Kondo, D. (1990). *Crafting selves: Power, gender and discourses of identity in a Japanese workplace.* Chicago: University of Chicago Press.

Korotkov, D. L. (1998). The sense of coherence: Making sense out of chaos. In P.T.P. Wong & P. S. Fry (Eds.), *The human quest for meaning: A handbook of psychological research and clinical applications* (pp. 51–70). Mahwah, NJ: Erlbaum.

Kris, E. (1952). *Psychoanalytic explorations in art.* New York: International Universities Press.

Kunkel, S. R., & Applebaum, R. A. (1992). Estimating the prevalence of long-term disability for an aging society. *Journal of Gerontology: Social Sciences, 475,* S253–S260.

Langer, E. J., & Rodin, J. (1976). The effects of choice and enhanced personal responsibility for the aged: A field experiment in an institutional setting. *Journal of Personality and Social Psychology, 34*(2), 192–198.

Little, B. R. (1989). Personal projects analysis: Trivial pursuits, magnificent obsessions, and the search for coherence. In D. M. Buss & N. Cantor (Eds.), *Personality psychology: Recent trends and emerging directions* (pp. 15–31). New York: Springer-Verlag.

Loevenger, J. (1976). *Ego development.* San Francisco: Jossey-Bass.

Markus, H. (1977). Self-schemata and processing information about the self. *Journal of Personality and Social Psychology, 35,* 63–78.

Markus, H., & Nurius, P. S. (1986). Possible selves. *American Psychologist, 41,* 954–969.

McAdams, D. P. (1996). Personality, modernity, and the storied self: A contemporary framework for studying persons. *Psychological Inquiry, 7,* 295–321.

McAdams, D. P. (1997). Multiplicity of self versus unity of identity. In R. D. Ashmore & L. Jussim (Eds.), *Self and identity: Fundamental issues* (pp. 46–78). New York: Oxford University Press.

McCuaig, M., & Frank, G. (1991). The able self: Adaptive patterns and choices in independent living for a person with cerebral palsy. *American Journal of Occupational Therapy, 45,* 224–234.

Mead, G. H. (1934). *Mind, self and society.* Chicago: University of Chicago Press.

Meyer, A. (1922). The philosophy of occupation therapy. *Archives of Occupational Therapy, 1,* 1–10.

Monks, J. (1995). Life stories and sickness experience: A performance perspective. *Culture, Medicine and Psychiatry, 19*(4), 453–478.

Moore, S. L. (1997). A phenomenological study of meaning in life in suicidal older adults. *Archives of Psychiatric Nursing, 11*(1), 29–36.

Murray, C.J.L., & Lopez, A. D. (1996). Alternative visions of the future: Projecting mortality and disability 1990–2020. In C.J.L. Murray & A. D. Lopez (Eds.), *The global burden of disease* (pp. 325–396). Geneva, Switzerland: World Health Organization.

Ogilvie, D. M. (1987). The undesired self: A neglected variable in personality research. *Journal of Personality and Social Psychology, 52,* 379–385.

Pavot, W., Fujita, F., & Diener, E. (1997). The relation between self-aspect congruence, personality and subjective well-being. *Personality and Individual Differences, 22*(2), 183–191.

Piaget, J. (1954). *The construction of reality in the child.* New York: Basic.

Pippin, K., & Fernie, G. R. (1997). Designing devices that are acceptable to the frail elderly: A new understanding based upon how older people perceive a walker. *Technology and Disability, 7*(1/2), 93–102.

Polkinghorne, D. (1988). *Narrative knowing and the human sciences.* Albany, NY: State University of New York Press.

Reker, G. T. (1997). Personal meaning, optimism, and choice. Existential predictors of depression in community and institutional elderly. *Gerontologist, 37*(6), 709–716.

Rodin, J. C. (1986). Aging and health: Effects of the sense of control. *Science, 233*(4770), 1271–1276.

Rogers, J. (1982). Order and disorder in medicine and occupational therapy. *American Journal of Occupational Therapy, 31,* 29–35.

Ruble, D. (1983). The development of social comparison processes and their role in achievement-related self-socialization. In E. T. Higgins, D. Ruble, & W. Hartup (Eds.), *Social cognition and social behavior: Developmental perspectives* (pp. 134–157). New York: Cambridge University Press.

Schrauger, J. S., & Schoeneman, T. J. (1979). Symbolic interactionist view of self-concept: Through the looking glass darkly. *Psychological Bulletin, 86,* 549–573.

Smith, M. B. (1974). Competence and adaptation: A perspective on therapeutic ends and means. *American Journal of Occupational Therapy, 28,* 11–15.

Sommer, K. L., & Baumeister, R. F. (1998). The construction of meaning from life events: Empirical studies of personal narratives. In P.T.P. Wong & P. S. Fry (Eds.), *The human quest for meaning: A handbook of psychological research and clinical applications* (pp. 143–161). Mahwah, NJ: Erlbaum.

Stachey, J. (Ed.). (1990). *The standard edition of the complete psychological works of Sigmund Freud.* New York: W. W. Norton.

Statistics Canada. (1993). *Population ageing and the elderly: Current demographic analysis.* Cat. No. 9I-533E. Ottawa, Canada: Government of Canada.

Stein, R. B., & Walley, M. (1983). Functional comparison of upper extremity amputees using myoelectric and conventional prostheses. *Archives of Physical Medicine and Rehabilitation, 73,* 1169–1173.

Swann, W. B. (1987). Identity negotiation: Where two roads meet. *Journal of Personality and Social Psychology, 53,* 1038–1051.

Swann, W. B., & Hill, C. A. (1982). When our identities are mistaken: Reaffirming self-conceptions through social interaction. *Journal of Personality and Social Psychology, 43,* 59–66.

van selm, M., & Dittmann-Kohli, F. (1998). Meaninglessness in the second half of life: The development of a construct. *International Journal of Aging and Human Development, 47*(2), 81–104.

Ville, I., Ravaud, J. F., Marchal, F., Paicheler, H., & Fardeau, M. (1992). Social identity and the international classification of handicaps: An evaluation of the consequences of facioscapulohumeral muscular dystrophy. *Disability and Rehabilitation, 14*(4), 168–175.

Vygotsky, L. S. (1981). The instrumental method in psychology. In J. V. Wertsch (Ed.), *The concept of activity in Soviet psychology* (pp. 134–143). Armonk, NY: M. E. Sharp.

Weinberg, N., & Sterritt, M. (1986). Disability and identity: A study of identity patterns in adolescents with hearing impairments. *Rehabilitation Psychology, 31*(2), 95–103.

White, R. W. (1959). Motivation reconsidered: The concept of competence. *Psychological Review, 66,* 297–333.

White, R. W. (1971). The urge toward competence. *American Journal of Occupational Therapy, 25,* 271–274.

Wong, P.T.P. (1998). Implicit theories of meaningful life and the development of the personal meaning profile. In P.T.P. Wong & P. S. Fry (Eds.), *The human quest for meaning: A handbook of psychological research and clinical applications* (pp. 111–140). Mahwah, NJ: Erlbaum.

48

The 1990s: Discussion Questions and Learning Activities

The Lectures

Fine, S. B. (1991). Resilience and human adaptability: Who rises above adversity? (1990 Eleanor Clarke Slagle Lecture). *American Journal of Occupational Therapy, 45,* 493–503.

Clark, F. (1993). Occupation embedded in a real life: Interweaving occupational science and occupational therapy (1993 Eleanor Clarke Slagle Lecture). *American Journal of Occupational Therapy, 47,* 1067–1078.

Grady, A. P. (1995). Building inclusive community: A challenge for occupational therapy (1994 Eleanor Clarke Slagle Lecture). *American Journal of Occupational Therapy, 49,* 300–310.

Trombly, C. A. (1995). Occupation: Purposefulness and meaningfulness as therapeutic mechanisms (1995 Eleanor Clarke Slagle Lecture). *American Journal of Occupational Therapy, 49,* 960–972.

Nelson, D. L. (1997). Why the profession of occupational therapy will flourish in the 21st century (1996 Eleanor Clarke Slagle Lecture). *American Journal of Occupational Therapy, 51,* 11–24.

Fisher, A. G. (1998). Uniting practice and theory in an occupational framework (1998 Eleanor Clarke Slagle Lecture). *American Journal of Occupational Therapy, 52,* 509–521.

Christiansen, C. H. (1999). Defining lives: Occupation as identity: An essay on competence, coherence, and the creation of meaning (1999 Eleanor Clarke Slagle Lecture). *American Journal of Occupational Therapy, 53,* 547–558.

Learning Activities

1. Investigate the occupational profile of most Americans in the 1990s. Some useful bibliographical references to explore appear in Appendix B.
   - What was the average family size?
   - What was the average salary? What were some typical jobs?
   - What did homes cost?
   - What were the clothing styles of the decade?
   - What was significant about the popular culture of the decade (e.g., music, film, books)?
2. If you have access to a complete collection of the *American Journal of Occupational Therapy,* scan the table of contents for each issue. What were some common topics? Can you identify any patterns in these topics? How do these relate to the messages of each Eleanor Clarke Slagle Lecture?
3. Try to summarize each Eleanor Clarke Slagle Lecture in a sentence that captures the main theme. Complete the sentence "This lecture was about. . . ."
4. Consider each lecture. Are there common threads among them that you identify? Are there any common themes that emerge when you consider these lectures together?

5. Review the biography of each lecturer of this decade (see Appendix A). Read some of the other work by the lecturer to gain an insight to the reasons why each one received this honor.

6. Consider what was happening in the history of the occupational therapy profession at the time of each Eleanor Clarke Slagle Lecture. Appendix C provides some useful bibliographical references for the history of the profession in the United States, and Appendix D has references for the global history of the profession.

7. Review what each president of the American Occupational Therapy Association presented as his or her vision for the profession at the time of each Eleanor Clarke Slagle Lecture. (A list of these presidents appears in Appendix E.) How do the lectures relate to these visions? The presidents addressed the profession through several forums, including columns in the *American Journal of Occupational Therapy,* such as "President's Address," "Nationally Speaking," and "The Issue Is."

8. Review each lecture in light of the *Centennial Vision*. What themes of the *Vision* stand out the most? What additional insights into the *Vision* do the lecturers offer?

Discussion Questions

1. Sharon Farber recognized that occupational therapy was developing in many new and exciting areas but needed something that would weave these different areas together. She argued that this common denominator or integrating force could be neuroscience. Summarize her rationale for this, and contrast it with the notion that "occupation" should be the integrating force as other Slagle lecturers argued.

2. Explain ways in which the notion of "psychoneuroimmunomodulation" can be appropriately incorporated into occupational therapy practice.

3. Susan B. Fine stated that trauma is processed through "inner structures." What are these structures? Explain each, and give examples from your practice that illustrate these structures in real situations.

4. How did Fine define "resilience"? Explain why she thought resilience was important for occupational therapists to discuss. What is the role of the occupational therapist in fostering resilience of clients?

5. Florence Clark stated that "acute care [is] consuming more and more resources, leaving less available for occupational therapists to improve the life opportunities of people with chronic disease and disability." Do you agree with this? How has this taken place in your practice? To what degree has this been a result of blaming external factors rather than taking responsibility for practice outcomes?

6. Clark quoted Penny reflecting on her rehabilitation as saying, "The individuals [occupational therapists] made an impression on me, but not the therapy that much." What caused such an impression? Do you think this is a common opinion among patients? What can occupational therapists do to change this perception?

7. How did Ann Grady define the occupational therapy values of "choice," "relevance," and "active participation in meaningful occupations"?

8. According to Grady, why should occupational therapists re-examine the meaning of the words *community* and *unity*? How would this re-examination change the practice of occupational therapy?

9. According to Catherine Trombly, from where do occupational therapists derive the belief that activities are therapeutic? Why would it be advantageous to discover *how* occupation brings about therapeutic change?

10. According to Trombly, what are the different ways in which occupation has been defined over the years, and which of these definitions does she consider problematic? Why?

11. Explain the difference(s) between *occupation-as-end* and *occupation-as-means* as proposed by Trombly. What implications do these two concepts have for occupational therapy as a profession?

12. David Nelson posited that the profession's understanding of occupation could support future roles for occupational therapists in the health care system in the independent living movement, technology, wellness, public health, and hospital-based practice. Choose 2 of these, and explain how you have seen opportunities open up in these areas, giving examples.

13. How would you explain occupational therapy assertively to the world using Nelson's Conceptual Framework for Occupational Therapy?

14. How did Anne Fisher contrast *purposeful* and *meaningful* occupation? What are the results of using either of these in intervention? How have you seen each of these characteristics support or negate the value of occupational therapy to others?

15. Fisher argued that occupational therapists must replace the traditional "remediation" approach for other approaches of intervention. What are those, and how do you think they should be implemented? How do you think future practitioners should be prepared to be competent in the implementation of these new approaches?

16. How does Charles Christiansen link the concepts of identity and occupation? Do you agree with his assertion that "identity is the pathway by which people, through daily occupations and relationships with others, are able to derive meaning from their lives"? How is this connected to the practice settings?

17. Christiansen stated that "occupations are key not to just being a person, but to being a particular person, and thus creating and maintaining an identity." Would you agree? Do occupations create and maintain the identity, or does the identity create and maintain occupations?

18. How is identity affected by disability? How can occupational therapy help an individual build identity?

19. Christiansen stated that "occupations are key not just to being a person, but to being a particular person, and thus creating and maintaining an identity." Give an example of a time in your life when one of your occupations changed (either by choice or not), and describe the effect you believe this had on your identity.

20. What are Christiansen's 3 roots of selfhood, and how do they (or do they not) relate to occupational therapy?

21. Christiansen stated that "one of the most compelling needs that every human being has is to be able to express his or her unique identity in a manner that gives meaning to life." What does he mean by this, and what does this statement mean to occupational therapy?

22. In your opinion, which of Christiansen's 4 propositions of human identity is most applicable to occupational therapy? Why?

23. Applying Christiansen's words regarding how "therapy becomes identity building," explain how this "virtual environment" has helped you to "explore your possible self and achieve success in tasks that are instrumental to the identity you strive to achieve" as a competent scholar and student. Further, explain how this course has enabled you to "validate your identity [as an occupational therapist] that you have worked hard to achieve in the past," as you integrate previous learning with the new knowledge acquired through this course.

24. Applying Christiansen's 4 propositions regarding identity development, how has your personal growth process throughout this course enabled you to further develop your identity as an occupational therapist? Which of the Slagle lectures has contributed most toward your quest for knowledge and why?

25. Christiansen cited 4 propositions centered on the assertion of the compelling need of each individual to have a unique identity to give meaning to his life. Describe these 4 ideas.

26. Christiansen explored the difference between the *I* and the *me*. Using his definitions of *I* and *me*, discuss the role of occupational therapy in facilitating the client establishing his or her self-identity. Use clinical examples if possible.

27. How does Christiansen's statement that "our identities can be complex and distributed while at the same time seem to be stable and predictable" affect occupational therapy intervention?

28. Christiansen quotes anthropologist Bateson (1996) as stating that "the capacity to do something useful for yourself or others is key to personhood." Describe ways in which your doing something useful for yourself has affected your "personhood." Describe a way you have affected another's sense of personhood through your practice of occupational therapy.

29. Christiansen stated that "The ultimate goal of occupational therapy services is well-being, not health." Does his vision support or differ from those espoused by Wilma West, Geraldine Finn, and Carolyn Baum?

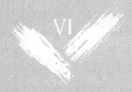

THE 2000s
The New Millennium

Historical Context of the 2000s

Around the World[1]

With the end of the Cold War and the collapse of the Soviet Union, conflict between the United States and Russia appeared much less likely by the turn of the new millennium. Both reduced stockpiles of nuclear warheads. The concerns of political strategists shifted to other areas of the world on what has been called "the dawn of a second nuclear age." Leftover cold war arsenals are still governed by the policy that prevailed during the Cold War, the doctrine of nuclear deterrence, which holds that rival great powers are safest when each has the power to annihilate each other.

Fear of nuclear proliferation turned first to Asia. Analysts worried that the U.S. conflict with the People's Republic of China over the independence of Taiwan would spin out of control in a military buildup that eventually would end in a nuclear conflict. Further, India and Pakistan have waged several wars over possession of the area of Kashmir. Conflicts in Afghanistan and the Middle East considerably influence Pakistani policy, and many see the enduring Pakistani–Indian conflict as the most likely to escalate into nuclear war (Emmott, 2008; Russett, Starr, & Kinsella, 2009; Sridaran, 2007). Various factors—including the opportunity for a useful long-term alliance against China and also Pakistan's economic collapse amid fears of Islamic fundamentalism—fueled the closest-ever India–U.S. relationship. The United States, India, and Pakistan are locked in an asymmetrical, delicate triangle. Analysts (Ganguly & Sapur, 2010; Russett et al., 2009) now argue that by tilting toward India, the United States may have inadvertently strengthened Pakistan's Islamicist right, legitimized India's Hindu supremacists, and encouraged the pursuit of nuclear weapons in both countries. In southeast Asia, North Korea has well-developed nuclear and missile programs and has steadfastly refused to enter negotiations for their reduction despite sanctions by the United Nations as well as significant political and economic isolation. Given the heat in the region, there is a growing push in Japan to alter its Constitution, which still forbids the development of offensive military forces, including nuclear weapons.

A second potential nuclear danger lies in the Middle East. As the first decade of the new millennium closes, concern over the nuclear capabilities of countries in this region have all but dominated international attention. Israel alleges it has produced nuclear weapons to confront powers hostile to it in the region—Arab countries and Iran—and that the presence of such strategic deterrence ensures its continued existence and averts attempts for a collective attack. Iran, on the other hand, has repeatedly claimed its nuclear program is peaceful amid controversy over its failure to declare sensitive enrichment and reprocessing activities to the International Atomic Energy Agency. Iran has continually insisted that acceptance of the Islamic republic as a nuclear power is the "first step" toward normalizing relations with the West. In 2007, the U.N, Security Council imposed sanctions in an effort to pressure Iran into declaring its current nuclear capabilities and deter further development of its uranium enrichment technology. These sanctions seemed only to increase Iran's resolve, escalating tensions with the West, particularly with the

---

[1]*The information contained in this introduction is accurate as of November 2010.*

United States. In July 2009, the United States explicitly ruled out the possibility that it would allow Iran to produce its own nuclear fuel, even under intense international inspection.

Some historians (Osterhammel & Petersson, 2009; Perkins, 2005; Robertson, 2003; Russett et al., 2009) have called the 2000s the "Era of Globalization," during which the benefits of free trade agreements initiated in earlier decades were expected to be reaped. In the literal sense, *globalization* refers to the increased connectivity among societies around the world due to the explosive revolution in transportation and communication technologies. The great hope of globalization was that it would raise living standards throughout the world by giving poor countries access to oversees markets; by allowing foreign investments in order to lower prices of new products; and by opening borders so people can travel to be educated, work, and send home earnings to help their families and fund new businesses. The greatest exchange has been economical, and many national borders have become eroded through international agreements leading to regional or global financial systems such as the World Trade Organization, the International Monetary Fund, and the European Union, among others. Barriers for international trade have been considerably lowered through international free trade agreements such as the General Agreement on Tariffs and Trade and the North American Free Trade Agreement.

Leading economists now claim the evidence is overwhelming that globalization has failed to live up to its potential. Globalization has permitted closer contact between different parts of the world and increased possibilities of personal exchange, mutual understanding, and friendship between "world citizens." However, it also has had the negative effect of allowing for-profit multinational corporations to circumvent the bounds of local laws and standards to take advantage of cheaper labor and services in less-developed regions. Population growth has continued to outpace economic growth, and now some 40 percent of the world's 6.5 billion people live in poverty. Many developing countries face huge burdens of foreign debt accrued in an attempt to attract foreign investors. In many cases, loans were obtained to industrialize, which did not necessarily lead to opening markets or higher levels of employment, education, and health. The problem was accentuated when investors lost confidence in the value of securitized mortgages in the United States, which resulted in a global liquidity crisis, and prompted some industrialized governments to inject capital into the financial markets. At the time of this writing, the industrialized world is experiencing the end of a recession or marked deceleration of economic activity, a sharp drop in international trade, rising unemployment, and slumping commodity prices. Only China, with its vast natural resources, appears to have been able to maintain economic growth. Its massive population represents not only a large domestic market but also a cheap labor source of some 800 million people. In August 2010, China overtook Japan to become the world's second-largest economy behind the United States.

The resulting *transculturation*, or the merging and converging of cultures, has become a concern. Fears that globalization really means Westernization or Americanization have fueled resistance around the world. Because of the complexity of the financial and political interests involved, many groups who resist this Westernization have been driven underground, becoming increasingly radicalized and unleashing terrorism around the globe.

Old terrorist groups grew and new ones emerged around the world, each with its own motivations and targets. Substantial coordination between these groups is doubtful because, although their campaigns may be global, their interests seem to be geographically localized. Thus, terrorist attacks in Russia, Ireland, Spain, the Philippines, Indonesia, Pakistan, and Israel have become nearly a daily experience. International terrorism reached U.S. soil on September 11, 2001, when members of the extremist group al-Qaeda hijacked several airplanes and flew them into the World Trade Center in New York City and the Pentagon near Washington, DC, killing 2,752 people. By October of that year, forces from the United States, Great Britain, and Australia invaded Afghanistan as part of the "War on Terror." The main purpose of the invasion was to capture al-Qaeda leader Osama bin Laden, who was suspected of masterminding the September 11 attacks, as well as the Taliban government that was providing him with a safe haven. By summer 2002, Taliban forces were subdued, and the remaining al-Qaeda rebels, presumably including bin Laden, melted away into the mountains and into neighboring Pakistan. Nevertheless, coalition forces linger in Afghanistan, the government remains unstable, continued violence threatens to re-emerge, the Taliban is regaining strength, and bin Laden remains at large. To date the reported coalition force casualties in Afghanistan exceed 5,000 while available conservative estimates place the death toll of civilians at 11,000 (CNN International, 2010).

After Iraq was forced out of Kuwait in the early 1990s, it was reported that Iraq began producing weapons of mass destruction (WMD). There was growing frustration in the United Nations over Iraq's failure to comply with inspections and interference with weapons inspectors. Fearing that it was only a matter of time before Saddam Hussein used these weapons or provided them to terrorists, in 1998 the U.S. Congress passed the Iraq Liberation Act, which stated the United States intended to remove Saddam Hussein from power. U.N. General Secretary Kofi Annan brokered an agreement between Hussein and the United Nations stating that Iraq would allow weapons inspectors greater access to suspected Iraqi manufacturing plants.

After the 2001 terrorist attacks in the United States, Iraq was perceived by many as a potential provider of weapons to terrorist groups. The United Nations passed several resolutions requiring Iraq to account for and dismantle all of its WMD. Iraq did not allow weapons inspectors into the country until December 2002. In February 2003, the United States argued that Iraq had failed to account for all weapons and, after an intense debate in the United Nations, the United States led a coalition force in the invasion of Iraq in March of that year. Several countries strongly objected to the invasion, arguing that diplomatic measures had not yet been exhausted. Approximately 3 weeks after the beginning of the invasion, these forces captured the Iraqi capital, Baghdad, and Hussein's regime was declared ended. However, Hussein and many key members of his cabinet had disappeared. Coalition troops searched for them, and Hussein was captured in December 2003. A court found him and two others guilty of crimes against humanity and sentenced him to death by hanging, which was carried out in 2006. Transition to a civil government has been slow, but coalition forces began their withdrawal from Iraq in the summer of 2010, with many troops re-deploying into Afghanistan. Continued civil unrest and partisan killings have raised fears that Iraq will burst into violence again after coalition combat troops depart. At this writing now the estimates of casualties continue to mount, varying widely between 100,000 and 300,000 Iraqis and nearly 6,000 coalition soldiers (CNN International, 2010).

As costly as the War on Terror has been in human lives, the loss through internal wars and ethnic hatreds around the world has been far more devastating. The animosities between ethic groups in Rwanda and Bosnia that escalated into genocide in the mid-1990s are well on their way to be overshadowed by the ethnic cleansing taking place in Darfur, the western region of Sudan. The United Nations puts the death toll at roughly 400,000, with up to 2.5 million Darfuris living as refugees around the world. In addition, the threat of devastation wrought by AIDS looms even larger. In Africa as a whole the infection rate has not lessened in the past decade. More than 25 million people are estimated to be HIV positive, and in the worst affected countries, one-third of the adults carry HIV. Wars and migrant labor have spread disease, and poverty and lack of health care have led to early death of the young, productive population. Unless the rest of the world takes action, the outlook for Africa looks catastrophic.

In the United States

Florida became the center of national attention in 2000 during the hotly contested U.S. presidential election. Texas Governor George W. Bush and Vice President Al Gore contested results of the election because, although Gore had obtained a majority of the popular vote, Bush had obtained a majority of electoral votes. Confusion over how votes were counted and problems in the polls supported Gore's motion that Florida's votes be re-counted, and a series of appeals went through the national court system. It took over a month for the recount, and eventually Gore conceded the election, although the controversy was never completely cleared.

The decade began with evidence that globalization would be a national issue in the United States as well. By far the event that has most significantly marked the new millennium is the September 11, 2001, terrorist attack on the World Trade Center, the Pentagon, and rural Pennsylvania. Through a series of coordinated suicide missions, members of the al-Qaeda terrorist group used hijacked commercial airplanes as missiles to attack U.S. targets. The U.S. government used these attacks, together with intelligence that bin Laden was hiding in Afghanistan and that Hussein might have a link with bin Laden, as justification to initiate the War on Terror, which included the invasions of Afghanistan and Iraq.

The 9/11 attacks had immediate and overwhelming effects on the U.S. population, prompting a patriotic tidal wave across the country in support of U.S. retaliation against the countries suspected of sponsoring the attacks. The

United States and other countries around the world were placed on a high state of alert against potential subsequent attacks, and the sense that such an attack is imminent remains part of the collective consciousness. As the months progressed, the effectiveness of the government's actions to protect its citizens became one of the most important issues debated in the 2004 and 2008 presidential elections.

The number of U.S. forces in Iraq grew as insurgents resisted their presence after the capture of Hussein. News that the number of U.S. casualties in Afghanistan and Iraq were being underreported and that there was no real target date for U.S. military withdrawal from those countries prompted massive anti-war protests across the country. After a public relations scandal exposed that combat veterans wounded in Iraq were left waiting weeks and even months for proper medical attention at military bases and inadequate hospital facilities, the Pentagon admitted that there was no adequate mechanism to accurately track the number of wounded troops. To date, of the estimated 31,000 wounded soldiers, about 630 have received amputations and needed extensive rehabilitation to return to duty or be retrained for civilian life (GlobalSecurity.org, 2010).

The decade began with evidence that globalization would be a dominant national issue in the United States. More than 200,000 refugees from Somalia and other countries have been resettled to the United States since 2000. Legal immigration increased about 15%, and a net of at least 700,000 illegal immigrants, mostly of Hispanic origin, arrived each year to join the 12,000,000 to 20,000,000 already in the country. While the majority of illegal aliens continue to concentrate in places with existing large communities of Hispanics, illegal immigrants are increasingly settling throughout the rest of the country. They can be found working mostly in service industries and in construction, with a small percentage working in agriculture. Further, an estimated 13.9 million people live in families in which the head of household or the spouse is an unauthorized immigrant. Illegal workers are estimated to pay about $7 billion per year into Social Security, and experts disagree as to whether illegal immigrants contribute more in taxes than they cost in social services.

All levels of government were criticized for the delayed and inadequate response to natural disasters, particularly Hurricane Katrina, which in 2005 wreaked catastrophic damage on Mississippi and Louisiana, left 80% of New Orleans flooded, and killed more than 1,600 people. After the storm, New Orleans had close to no population for several months. Volunteers from across the nation have worked for 5 years and, although about 80% of the population has returned, the rebuilding of the city may take decades to complete. Three years later, another hurricane made landfall in Galveston, Texas, flooding much of that city. The combined damage caused by both hurricanes is estimated to be greater than $100 billion, stretching regional and national disaster budgets to their limits. A sense of vulnerability remained through much of the decade as oil prices rose sharply after these hurricanes.

Health care ethics were challenged on several fronts in the first decade of the millennium. The case of a Florida woman Terri Schiavo, who had severe brain damage but had survived for 15 years, drew national attention when her husband's request to discontinue life support was challenged by her parents. The case was heard more than 20 times in Florida courts. Every time, the court ruled that the decision was her husband's to make, upholding the sanctity of marriage long respected by legal precedent. Politicians inserted themselves into the fray. The case was the catalyst for Florida's controversial "Terri's Law," which gave Governor Jeb Bush the authority to have Schiavo's feeding tube re-inserted when a court ruled that her husband could have it removed. The case was elevated to the Supreme Court, which refused to intervene, stating the Governor and Ms. Schiavo's parents had failed to demonstrate the merits of their claims. Some disability activists repudiated the decision, stating that it sent the message that people with disabilities were not worth the cost of the technology needed to keep them alive.

Through much of the first decade of the 21st century, human cloning has been the subject of considerable public attention and sharp moral debate. Since the announcement in 1997 of the first successful cloning of a mammal (Dolly the sheep), several species of mammals had been cloned, suggesting that the eventual cloning of humans must be considered a serious possibility. The U.S. Congress twice took up the matter and in 2001 passed a strict ban on all human cloning, including the production of cloned human embryos. However, the debate over human cloning has become further complicated by researchers' ability to isolate human embryonic stem cells. Many scientists believe that these cells are capable of becoming any type of cell in the body and therefore hold great promise for understanding and treating many chronic diseases and conditions. Some scientists also believe that stem cells derived from cloned human embryos, produced explicitly for research, might prove uniquely useful for studying many genetic diseases and devising novel therapies. In March of 2009 President Barack Obama signed an executive order clearing the way for a significant increase in federal dollars for embryonic stem cell research. An injunction on this funding was filed the following year in a Washington, DC, district court halting the implementation of President Obama's order, but an appeals court later made permanent a stay of that injunction in August 2010. As of this writing, however, several cloning-related bills remain under consideration in the Congress and Senate.

In 2007 a student with a mental illness killed 32 people at Virginia Tech University before shooting himself. This tragedy brought many issues back to the American consciousness, including gun control and mental health care. In a victory for gun control opponents, the U.S. Supreme Court ruled in 2008 that the Constitution prohibits the kind of outright ban that was being proposed in the U.S. Congress. Nevertheless, that same year Congress passed mental health parity legislation that broadly outlawed health insurance discrimination against Americans with mental health and substance use conditions in employer-sponsored health plans.

The drive to promote women and minorities in decision-making positions gained momentum at the turn of the new century, making it a decade of many "firsts." In 2007, Nancy Pelosi (D–CA) became the first woman to lead the U.S. House of Representatives. In 2008, after an eventful election campaign, Barak Obama was elected the first African-American President. During the same race, Alaska Governor Sarah Palin won the Republican nomination for Vice President, and Hillary Rodham Clinton, wife of former President Bill Clinton, became the first woman to nearly win the Democratic presidential nomination. The following year, Sonya Sotomayor became the first Hispanic woman to become a U.S. Supreme Court Justice.

Within the first few months of President Obama's presidency, he faced the consequences of a stock market crash, addressed a significant economic depression, and met the demands of U.S. military actions around the world. Further, an estimated 45 million Americans do not have health insurance, and at the time of this writing, the merits of a significant attempt at health care reform, the Patient Protection and Affordable Care Act of 2010 (P.L. 111-148), portions of which are scheduled to go into effect beginning in 2012, are still being debated, giving momentum to an unofficial third party in U.S. politics, the TEA (Taxed Enough Already) Party, which opposes the potential costs of this new law as well as other government spending, including the various financial measures used to stabilize the U.S. economy during the longest recession in post–World War II history. However, within the first year of his term, President Obama received the Nobel Peace Prize in recognition of the "extraordinary efforts to strengthen international diplomacy and cooperation between peoples." President Obama and the country undoubtedly will face many other issues of great concern for the profession of occupational therapy during his presidency.

References

CNN International (2010). *U.S. and Coalition casualties.* Available online at http://www.cnn.com/SPECIALS/2004/oef. casualties/index.html

Emmott, B. (2008). *Rivals: How the power struggle between China, India and Japan will shape our next decade.* New York: Houghton MifflinHarcourt

Ganguly, S., & Kapur, P. (2010). *India, Pakistan, and the bomb: Debating nuclear stability in south Asia.* New York: Columbia University Press.

GlobalSecurity.org (2010). *Military reports.* Available online at http://www.globalsecurity.org/military/library/report/ index.html

Osterhammel, J., & Petersson, N. (2009). *Globalization: A short history.* Princeton, NJ: Princeton University Press.

Perkins, J. (2005). *Confessions of an economic hit-man.* New York: Plume.

Robertson, R. (2003). *The three waves of globalization: A history of a developing global consciousness.* London: Zed Books.

Russett, B., Starr, H., & Kinsella, D. (2009). *World politics: The menu for choice.* Belmont, CA: Wadsworth.

Sridaran, E. (2007). *The India–Pakistan nuclear relationship: Theories of deterrence and international relations.* New York: Routledge.

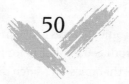

50

2000 Eleanor Clarke Slagle Lecture

Our Mandate for the New Millennium:
Evidence-Based Practice
Margo B. Holm, PhD, OTR/L, FAOTA, ABDA

If the next several patients you were to see asked you, "How do you know that what you do and how you do it really works?" would you be able to provide them with research evidence similar to that found in the pamphlets that come with your prescription medications? The evidence would include a summary of research on each occupational therapy intervention option you are considering. It would delineate the percentage of patients who benefited from each option and the percentage of those who did not. It would also clearly describe *what* each intervention consists of and *how* each is to be implemented for yielding the best outcomes for particular patient populations. Additionally, the data that support the recommended frequency and duration for each intervention would be included. It is unlikely that you could provide such evidence today. Will you be able to provide the evidence by 2010? As professionals, we have gone on record committing ourselves to evidence-based practice in Principle 2.B. of our *Occupational Therapy Code of Ethics,* which states, "Occupational therapy personnel shall fully inform the service recipients of the nature, risks, and potential outcomes of any interventions" (American Occupational Therapy Association [AOTA], 1994, p. 1037). *Can we meet this commitment?*

In this year's Slagle Lecture, I will use a common definition of *evidence-based practice* and discuss why it has meaning for the context in which our profession finds itself today. First, I will use a five-level measuring stick (see Table 50.1) to examine the strength of the evidence or the lack of evidence associated with occupational therapy interventions—*what* we do and *how* we do it—the same measuring stick that is also being used by referring physicians, educational services administrators, and health maintenance organization purchasers of services as they appraise our evidence. Second, I will raise throughout the lecture dilemmas that face us when we try to reconcile some of the principles in our Code of Ethics with the practice of occupational therapy based on limited evidence. Third, I will use the framework of continued competency to discuss what is needed to practice occupational therapy, based on research evidence, in the new millennium.

Evidence-Based Practice

As we are all aware, the health care environment of the past quarter century underwent numerous evolutionary processes that greatly affected *how* occupational therapy services were provided! For example, in many practice settings, we were confronted with prospective payment reimbursement, capitation models, reduced staffing ratios, and job losses. Additionally, we are now being judged by the functional outcomes our patients achieve. The fact that patient outcomes are improved with occupational therapy services is no longer sufficient to justify our services, unless we can also explain *what* we do and *how* we do it so that others can replicate our interventions and achieve similar outcomes with comparable patients with like needs, wants, and expectations. The emphasis on

Originally published 2000 in *American Journal of Occupational Therapy, 54,* 575–585.

Table 50.1. Hierarchy of Levels of Evidence for Evidence-Based Practice

Level	Description
I	Strong evidence from at least one systematic review of multiple well-designed randomized controlled trials
II	Strong evidence from at least one properly designed randomized controlled trial of appropriate size
III	Evidence from well-designed trials without randomization, single group pre–post, cohort, time series, or matched case-controlled studies
IV	Evidence from well-designed nonexperimental studies from more than one center or research group
V	Opinions of respected authorities, based on clinical evidence, descriptive studies, or reports of expert committees

Note. From "Evidence-Based Everything," by A. Moore, H. McQuay, & J.A.M. Gray (Eds.), 1995, *Bandolier, 1*(12), 1. Copyright © 1995 by Bandolier. Reprinted with permission.

justifying our practice patterns has been reflected in the increasing numbers of requests for the research-based evidence that supports what we are doing.

So, what is evidence-based practice? It has been defined as "integrating individual clinical expertise" with the "conscientious, explicit and judicious use of current best evidence in making decisions about the care of individual patients" (Sackett, Rosenberg, Gray, Haynes, & Richardson, 1996, p. 71). Thus, in our Code of Ethics we have also affirmed our commitment to evidence-based practice in Principle 3.D., "Occupational therapy personnel shall perform their duties on the basis of accurate and current information" (AOTA, 1994, p. 1037). *Can we meet this commitment?*

Gray (1997) described the evolution of evidence-based practice as progressing from providing services as efficiently and cheaply as possible, to "doing things better," then to *"doing things right,"* and finally to "doing the right things" (p. 17). He has also proposed that evidence-based practice for the new millennium must focus on "doing the right things right" (p. 17). In other words, the necessary shift to the evidence-based practice of occupational therapy will require us to justify *why* we do *what* we do in addition to *how* we do it. Of course, Gray's proposal implies that for any given patient population, we *know* what is "right" and, furthermore, that we *know* the "right" way to do what we do. Silverman (1998) put it another way: "How do we go about drawing a line between 'knowing' and 'doing' . . . and when do we know enough about the . . . consequences of our interventions to proceed with confidence" (p. 5)?

As occupational therapy practitioners, we have always used multiple sources of evidence, or "ways of knowing," to guide our "doing," including evidence derived from the oral tradition, our own beliefs and values, patient preferences, assessment data, the opinions of experts, and research evidence (Brown, 1999; Bury & Mead, 1998). Historically, our evidence resided within individual practitioners and was handed down from practitioner to practitioner; thus, it was not accessible to all. With the advent of occupational therapy textbooks and journals, opinions of experts and research evidence have been published and are now accessible to all. Although each source of evidence has inherent value for some aspect of our practice, no single source of evidence, or even all of them together, enables us to know enough to proceed to our "doing" with *absolute* confidence.

Information Overload and Hierarchies of Evidence

Our level of confidence in our clinical decisions should be based, in part, on the strength of the evidence we use. Fortunately, the evidence that is available has been expanding at an exponential rate; however, this expansion has created two problems: (a) There is too much evidence to sift through, and (b) the quantity of evidence does not equal quality of evidence. Shenk (1997) addressed the problem of expansion when he noted, "Just as fat has replaced starvation as [the] number one dietary concern, information overload has replaced information scarcity" (p. 29). An editorial in the *Journal of the American Medical Association (JAMA)* expressed concerns about the second problem: the quality of the evidence in which we may place our confidence. Rennie (1986) lamented that publication alone does not mean quality. The author noted wryly that there is no study too fragmented, no hypothesis too trivial, no literature citation too biased or too egotistical, no design too warped, no methodology too bungled, no presentation of results too inaccurate and too contradictory, no analysis too self-serving, no argument too circular, no conclusion too trifling or too unjustified, and no grammar and syntax too offensive for a paper to end up in print. (p. 2391)

It is because of the glut of evidence and concerns about quality control that ranking systems, or hierarchies, were developed to rate the strength of the research designs being used to generate the evidence (Moore, McQuay, & Gray, 1995; Sackett, Haynes, & Tugwell, 1985; Sackett, Richardson, Rosenberg, & Haynes, 1997). These *hierarchies of evidence* were designed to help practitioners sort through the options and select the "current best evidence" available to guide decisions about *what* to do and *how* to do it for a particular patient or patient population.

Examples of Occupational Therapy Evidence

Although evidence hierarchies vary somewhat in their rigor, the rank order of the levels of evidence is similar, with the best evidence ranked at Level I and less convincing evidence ranked at lower levels (see Table 50.1). Each level represents the research strategies that were used to structure the investigations. At the top of the hierarchy are those designs deemed (a) least vulnerable to bias, (b) more generalizable, and (c) more likely to yield patient outcomes that can confidently be attributed to the intervention being studied (see Table 50.1). Therefore, if it is current, and available, you want the "best" evidence, which is a Level I research design. The evidence hierarchy, or measuring stick, that I will use has five levels (Moore et al., 1995). At the top of the hierarchy, or Level I, are studies in which we, and those we must convince about the efficacy and effectiveness of occupational therapy, should have the most confidence. They are also the studies that we must strive to plan, implement, and publish.

Level I evidence. Level I studies are defined as "strong evidence from at least one systematic review of multiple well-designed randomized controlled trials" (Moore et al., 1995, p. 1). Level I systematic reviews usually take one of two forms: (a) meta-analytic studies or (b) systematic reviews. Both methods (a) require adherence to rigorous procedures, with well-defined study criteria for inclusion, and (b) are usually restricted to studies that use randomized controlled clinical trials. Additionally, both methods use statistical analyses to evaluate the data from each study and the studies in total.

So, what does this mean for everyday practice? Picture yourself in this scenario: You work on a neurorehabilitation unit and a new medical resident asks you, "Why does my patient need both a physical therapy exercise program and occupational therapy? What evidence do you have that cooking tasks, adapted checkers games, and those other things you do make any difference in upper-extremity motor performance?" An appropriate response would be the provision of *current best evidence* in the form of a Level I study. Occupational therapy researchers Lin, Wu, Tickle-Degnen, and Coster (1997) carried out a meta-analytic study of 17 articles, including 4 articles on studies of patients with neurological impairments. They found that in studies designed to improve the motor performance of patients with neurological impairments, the outcomes were significantly better when the patients' exercises were embedded into everyday tasks than when the patients only performed rote exercises. This study is just one example of evidence that you can use to support *what* we do and *how* we can do it to yield improvements in patients with neurological impairments and upper-extremity motor deficits.

What about Level I current best evidence for other areas of practice? A meta-analytic study of the efficacy of sensory integration treatment was recently conducted by an occupational therapy researcher (Vargas & Camilli, 1999). This rigorous meta-analysis of 22 studies considered every possible influence on the outcomes of sensory integration treatment, including (a) adherence to sensory integration treatment criteria, (b) total treatment hours, (c) diagnosis and age, (d) design and sampling, (e) number of outcomes and measurement categories, (f) professional affiliation of the researchers, (g) geographic location of the studies, and (h) publication years. The results of the study, however, provide us with a stark reminder of the difference between preferred practice and evidence-based practice.

Many therapists prefer to use a sensory integration approach to intervention with both children and adults. But *current* best evidence, namely those studies published since 1983, indicated "an absence of sensory integration effects in recent studies and the equivalence of sensory integration and alternative treatments," neither of which yielded improvement in the sensory–perceptual area (Vargas & Camilli, 1999, p. 197). In other words, the experimental groups' outcomes following sensory integration interventions were no better than those of the control groups that received no treatment, regardless of the outcome being measured. When compared with alternative types of treatment, outcomes of the sensory integration groups were equivalent but not very effective. Although we may *prefer* to ignore the findings of this study, our actions would be in conflict with Principle 2.B. of our Code of Ethics in which we commit to "fully inform the service recipients of the nature, risks, and potential outcomes of any interventions" (AOTA, 1994, p. 1037), especially if their effectiveness is in question. Tickle-Degnen (1998) developed excellent sample dialogues for communicating mixed or nonsupportive evidence about proposed interventions to patients.

The failure of these studies to demonstrate the superiority of sensory integration techniques over no treatment does not negate the possibility that (a) the outcome measures were insensitive to the changes produced, (b) the wrong outcomes were measured, or (c) the effects were obscured by the application of sensory integration techniques to inappropriate populations. Another possibility is that the statistical power, or sample size, may have been inadequate. Ottenbacher and Maas (1999) pointed out that often the effect sizes in our studies, or the magnitude of the difference between the experimental and control groups, indicate that our interventions do yield clinically worthwhile differences. However, we often do not have large enough samples to reject the null hypotheses, and therefore we conclude wrongly that our interventions are not effective (Mulligan, 1998; Ottenbacher & Maas, 1999; Vargas & Camilli, 1999).

Just as our practices change over time, so too should the evidence base of our practice. It will be important to revisit the evidence to see whether new sensory integration interventions being used in clinics and promoted in workshops, new measures such as those related to the family's perspective suggested by Cohn and Cermak (1998), or larger sample sizes can provide better support for *what* we do and *how* we do it when using sensory integration interventions.

Now, put yourself into this second scenario: The budget administrator in your hospital is questioning the use of life skills groups with a chronic mental health population. You do a computer search, and using the Cochrane Database of Systematic Reviews (www.update-software.com/cochrane/cochrane-frame.html), you find a review entitled, "Life Skills Programmes for People With Chronic Mental Illness" (Nicol, Robertson, & Connaughton, 1999). The review examined life skills programs that focused on interpersonal skills, self-care, time management, financial management, nutrition, and household skills as well as use of community resources. Unfortunately, only two randomized clinical trials were found that met the criteria, and both were conducted more than 15 years ago. Even though evidence was sparse and not what one would call current, it was the best evidence available, and the reviewers proceeded to conclude that

> there is next to no evidence that life skills training programmes are of value to those with serious mental illnesses . . . [and] until such time as any evidence of benefit is available it is questionable whether recipients of care should be put under pressure to attend such programmes. (Nicol et al., p. 10/21)

The reviewers went on to state, "If life skills training is to continue as a part of rehabilitation programmes a large, well designed, conducted and reported pragmatic randomized trial is an urgent necessity" (p. 2/21), but then they added, "There may even be an argument for stating that maintenance of current practice, outside of a randomized trial, is unethical" (p. 2/21).

Providing this current best evidence for life skills training with a chronic mental health population to any budget administrator could pose a threat or an opportunity. The threat comes if only the reviewers' conclusions are noted, namely that occupational therapy life skills groups are ineffective for chronic mental health populations at best and unethical at worst. If we provide no new evidence that counteracts the findings of the Cochrane reviewers, then it could be implied that we are in tacit agreement with the recommendation. If we take this stance, however, the threat could be generalized to other settings or populations in which life skills programs are used.

We then would have to ask ourselves the next logical question: "If there is no evidence that life skills programs make any difference with chronic mental health populations (with whom they have been used since time immemorial), what evidence is there that life skills programs are effective with developmental disability or traumatic brain injury populations?" Our opportunity lies in responding to the reviewers' *recommendation* to design, carry out, and report the findings from a large, randomized controlled trial, a design that is also known as a Level II study in our evidence hierarchy. This is the next level of evidence.

Level II evidence. The evidence needed to confirm or reject the Cochrane database findings about life skills programs is not found in the ivory towers of universities but, rather, in occupational therapy clinics and community-based practices. The study suggested by the Cochrane reviewers was a Level II research design, which consists of "strong evidence from at least one properly designed randomized controlled trial of appropriate size" (Moore et al., 1995, p. 1). For example, to conduct a randomized controlled trial in a clinic, this would mean that after a practitioner has collected baseline performance data on a patient, any patient who meets the criteria already established for participation in a life skills program would be randomly assigned to one of three groups: (a) a control group or attention group (no occupational therapy), (b) an alternative therapy group (e.g., a social work group that talks about life skills), or (c) an occupational therapy life skills group. Typically, randomized clinical trials include large numbers of participants. These participants can be accrued either slowly over time at one site or more quickly through collaboration among multiple clinical sites. The latter, multisite studies can dampen the spirits of even the most enthusiastic of researchers because of scheduling problems, budgeting issues, and philosophical differences. The problems with randomized control trials at single or multiple sites can be overcome by planning carefully, educating therapists in systematic data collection methods, ensuring that research intervention protocols are delivered in a standardized manner, and monitoring adherence to research procedures.

The common argument against doing randomized trials is the belief that patients who are randomized to the control or placebo conditions will not benefit or progress if they do not participate in occupational therapy treatment, for example, the sensory integration interventions or life skills groups. However, Portney and Watkins (1993) noted that

> in situations where the efficacy of a treatment is being questioned because current knowledge is inadequate, it may actually be more ethical to take the time to make appropriate controlled comparisons than to continue clinical practice using potentially ineffective techniques. (p. 29)

Three examples of Level II randomized controlled occupational therapy clinical trials, which accurately followed intent-to-treat principles—in other words, carried out their statistical analyses on the basis of the number of participants that entered the study, not only those who completed it—were published in *JAMA* (Ray et al., 1997), *Lancet* (Close et al., 1999), and the *Journal of the American Geriatrics Society (JAGS)* (Cummings et al., 1999). These studies examined the impact of occupational therapy interventions on falls reduction among nursing home residents and community-based frail older adults. In the large multicenter nursing home study published in *JAMA*, the proportion of recurrent fallers in the experimental facilities was significantly less ($p = .03$) than in the control facilities (Ray et al., 1997). In addition to the physician and nursing components, the occupational therapy interventions consisted of wheelchair positioning and maintenance and resident and staff instruction on safe transfers.

In the study of community-based older adults with a history of falls published in *Lancet,* the experimental group had significantly fewer falls ($p = .05$) at the 12-month follow-up than the control group. The experimental group had received a home visit and a follow-up phone call by an occupational therapist that focused on home safety and modification of the home environment (Close et al., 1999).

In the study published in the *JAGS,* community-based older adults who presented to hospital emergency rooms after falls were randomly assigned to either a post-acute-event occupational therapy intervention group or a control group. The occupational therapy intervention consisted of home safety recommendations, education, and minor home modifications. At the 12-month follow-up, the risk of falling, the risk of recurrent falls, and the odds of being admitted to a hospital were significantly lower in the occupational therapy group than in the control group (Cummings et al., 1999).

These three studies provide strong Level II evidence of the efficacy of occupational therapy for falls reduction among nursing home residents and community-based frail older adults. These are but three examples of Level II studies that you can provide to nursing home administrators, outpatient rehabilitation coordinators, or emergency room physicians as supporting evidence that *what* we do and *how* we do it can make a significant positive difference to older adults at risk for falling.

Level III evidence. However, what happens when Level I and Level II studies are not available? According to Gray (1997), "The absence of excellent evidence does not make evidence-based decision making impossible; in this situation, what is required is the best *evidence available,* not the best evidence possible" (p. 61). For example, picture yourself in this third scenario: The new physiatrist at your rehabilitation facility came from a setting where the occupational therapists used Bobath axial rolls for patients with stroke who had hemiplegia and shoulder subluxation, and she writes specific orders for their use. You are not convinced that the axial rolls work very well, and you prefer the type of sling that you have been using for the past 10 years—the same one that your physical disabilities professor preferred. In addition, the axial rolls seem to increase your patients' shoulder pain. Even though you found no Level I or Level II studies in your literature search, you located four studies that meet Level III criteria (Brooke, Lateur, Diana-Rigby, & Questad, 1991; Hurd, Farrell, & Waylonis, 1974; Williams, Taffs, & Minuk, 1988; Zorowitz, Idank, Ikai, Hughes, & Johnston, 1995).

Level III studies derive their "evidence from well-designed trials without randomization, single group pre–post, cohort, time series, or matched case-controlled studies" (Moore et al., 1995, p. 1). Although you are pleased to find that the best evidence available indicated that the Bobath axial roll made no difference, or even increased shoulder displacement (Zorowitz et al., 1995), you also find that the sling that you prefer fared no better. In fact, you find that the evidence for use of an axial roll, a sling, or a wheelchair trough for reducing shoulder displacement is mixed at best, and some of the most recent evidence indicates that the sling you prefer actually increases vertical asymmetry (Brooke et al., 1991). At that moment, Principle 1.C. of our Code of Ethics comes to mind—"occupational therapy personnel shall take all reasonable precautions to avoid harm to the recipient of services" (AOTA, 1994, p. 1037)—only now its relevance has new meaning. You have learned two lessons from your search: (a) You are appalled to learn that your preferred intervention may have done harm, and (b) you have learned that although you are not from a state that requires continuing education for licensure, the relevance of one aspect of our Code of Ethics (Principle 3.C.) is now clearer: "Occupational therapy personnel shall take responsibility for maintaining competence by participating in professional development and educational activities" (AOTA, 1994, p. 1037).

Next, imagine that you are an occupational therapy practitioner employed by a skilled nursing facility. You frequently encounter new residents who qualify for rehabilitation services because of a 3-day hospital stay. However, because they have a primary diagnosis of dementia of the Alzheimer type and severe memory impairments, their ability to benefit from any rehabilitation is frequently challenged. A Level III study combining occupational therapy compensatory strategies and behavioral techniques featured in *JAGS* (Rogers et al., 1999) may have the type of evidence you are looking for. The study found that during a 1-week occupational therapy skill intervention condition using compensatory strategies and a structured environment, the residents with dementia significantly increased the proportion of time they engaged in self-dressing and significantly decreased their disruptive behaviors compared with the usual care. During the 3-week occupational therapy habit training condition that followed, residents were able to maintain their gains. Additionally, during both occupational therapy intervention conditions, the use of labor-intensive physical assists decreased significantly. A Level III study such as this can be used to provide fiscal intermediaries with supporting evidence that *what* we do and *how* we do it can benefit even nursing home residents who are severely disabled and cognitively impaired.

The next Level III study could be helpful if you find yourself in the following scenario: You work for a private therapy company that provides services to several group homes for adults with developmental disabilities. The owner of the homes tells you that he had been "surfing the Net" and had found the Cochrane Database Systematic Review on the ineffectiveness of life skills groups. Given the conclusions of the reviewers, he wants to know what evidence you have that indicates that the life skills groups you are implementing are effective. You tell him that you also read the review and point out that applying the findings from the Cochrane review to his clients might not be in their best interest because the participants in the studies described in the review had chronic mental illness and were in hospital-based programs—a population very different from his community-based clients with developmental disabilities. You explain that since reading the review, you have been using the methods and outcomes described in a Level III study by Neistadt and Marques (1984), whose participants also had developmental disabilities. You then show him the data you have collected over the past 3 months, documenting the specific life skills groups each client in his facilities has participated in as well as their outcomes. You note that all clients have made gains.

A fourth example of a Level III study pertains to school-based practice and pediatrics wherein occupational therapy practitioners are frequently associated with *fine motor* skills training. This association with fine motor skills is not surprising, though, because when you use the key words fine motor to search through the 10 million journal articles indexed in MEDLINE, 1 of the 10 subject headings you are presented with, and the only profession, is *occupational therapy*. A Level III intervention study by Case-Smith et al. (1998) found that preschoolers with fine motor delays who received direct occupational therapy services improved their fine motor skills and related functional performance significantly, and the rate of gain was greater than that of their peers who had no fine motor delays (p. 788). The next time you need to convince your educational services administrator about the benefits that occupational therapy can offer to preschool populations with fine motor delays, bring this supporting evidence, along with a Level IV study by McHale and Cermak (1992).

Level IV evidence. According to Moore et al. (1995), Level IV studies consist of "evidence from well-designed nonexperimental studies from more than one center or research group" (p. 1). Sometimes our inquiry into the need for, or effectiveness of, an intervention begins with a multisite descriptive study. The Level IV study by McHale and Cermak (1992) described the time allocated to fine motor activities and tasks in six elementary classrooms. Minute-by-minute data collection indicated that 30% to 60% of the day was dedicated to fine motor tasks, with writing tasks predominating. This study provides the context and relevance of occupational therapy interventions for preschoolers with fine motor delays—preschoolers who will soon become elementary school students.

Level V evidence. The lowest level of the hierarchy of evidence is Level V, which is defined as "opinions of respected authorities, based on clinical evidence, descriptive studies, or reports of expert committees" (Moore et al., 1995, p. 1). Unlike Level IV descriptive studies, Level V studies do not need to be from multiple centers or research groups. Studies that use qualitative designs are also identified as Level V studies. One such study published recently in the *Occupational Therapy Journal of Research (OTJR)* (Bye, 1998) involved in-depth interviews of therapists who worked with terminally ill patients. For a profession that is used to facilitating functional gains in patients rather than in preparing them for death, this Level V study provides a framework for guiding the practice of occupational therapy in end-of-life care. The study had as its core aim "Affirming Life: Preparing for Death" (Bye, 1998, p. 8). Interventions focused on "building against loss," achieving "normality within a changed reality," regaining "client control" over daily routines and activities, providing "supported and safe" environments, and finding "closure in some aspects of their lives" (p. 8). It is Level V studies like this one that enable researchers to describe and probe aspects of our practice that cannot be accomplished with Level I and Level II studies and simultaneously pave the way for future research. Level V evidence also can help us define new programs that have the potential to benefit populations not typically associated with rehabilitation or occupational therapy and point the way to new areas of inquiry and program development.

Also included in Level V evidence are the opinions of respected authorities. Although all the other examples of evidence I have cited were based on research, or from external sources, Level V evidence allows for the evidence *residing within the practitioner*. When we use opinion-based evidence, we are grounding our clinical reasoning and therapeutic decisions and actions in the advice of experts, established practices, continuing education information, or reference texts by known leaders in the field (Brown, 1999; Bury & Mead, 1998). It is not unusual for fieldwork students, entry-level practitioners, and practitioners changing practice areas to rely primarily on the opinions of master practitioners, supervisors, or therapists with specialty certification. It is also not unusual for us to continue to provide interventions that are based on the wisdom of the "form in the file drawer," which represents established practices that have "always been done that way."

When we use Level V evidence based on clinical experience and expertise to guide decision-making with our patients, we must be aware of how our own values, beliefs, and biases influence our decisions. In a study of physicians' perceptions of their patients' preferences, patients were asked to rate four preferred courses of action for a life-threatening illness, and their physicians were asked to predict their patients' preferences as well as to state their preferences for themselves. Unfortunately the physicians' predictions of their patients' preferences more closely matched their own preferences than those of their patients (Schneiderman, Kaplan, Pearlman, & Teetzel, 1993). It is because of the potential power associated with clinical expertise that ethicists Lidz and Meisel (1983) remind us that we must take care that we do not view the decision-making process with patients as one of merely persuading the patient to accept what we believe to be the proper course.

However, it is precisely our clinical experience, clinical expertise, and clinical reasoning that Sackett et al. (1996) referred to in their definition of evidence-based practice when they speak of "*integrating individual clinical expertise*" [italics added] with the "use of current best evidence in making decisions about the care of individual patients" (p. 71). I would like to emphasize that if we are to practice evidence-based occupational therapy, evidence can only be used to inform clinical expertise, not replace it, and clinical expertise must be used in conjunction with the best available evidence, not substituted for it (Bury & Mead, 1998; Sackett et al., 1996).

We have made a commitment in our Code of Ethics to "collaborate with service recipients or their surrogate(s) in determining goals and priorities throughout the intervention process" (AOTA, 1994, p. 1037). It is in the fulfillment of this commitment that patient and practitioner together must consider the evidence before them and make informed decisions about the occupational therapy interventions that will best meet the patient's needs, wants, and expectations. *Can we meet this commitment?*

Collective evidence. I have applied a five-level measuring stick to some of our evidence and cited examples of evidence associated with each level. But what about the strength of our collective evidence as a scholarly profession? To get a snapshot of the bigger picture, I applied the same hierarchy to all articles published in *OTJR* for the past 5 years (1995–1999). I chose the *OTJR* because it is "devoted to the advancement of knowledge through scientific methods" (Abreu, Peloquin, & Ottenbacher, 1998, p. 757). As you can see in Table 50.2, over the past 5 years, the preponderance of the evidence in our research journal was at Level V, which is defined as "opinions of respected authorities, based on clinical evidence, descriptive studies, or reports of expert committees" (Moore et al., 1995, p. 1). Obviously, a journal must receive manuscripts before they can be published. As our collective research competence improves, so will the levels of evidence that we are able to generate and submit for publication.

Table 50.2. Hierarchy of Evidence Applied to Articles Published in the *Occupational Therapy Journal of Research*, 1995–1999

Level	Design	Number of Articles
I	Systematic reviews, meta-analytic studies	1
II	Randomized controlled trials	6
III	Trials without randomization	21
IV	Nonexperimental studies from more than one center	11
V	Opinions of respected authorities, descriptive studies	41

Note. Based on hierarchy by Moore, McQuay, and Gray (1995).

Evidence-Based Practice and Continued Competency

At graduation, more than one class has heard the speaker say something similar to, "Half of what we taught you will not be true in 5 years. Unfortunately, we do not know which half" (Sackett et al., 1997, p. 38). Therefore, a commitment we have made to ourselves and to our service recipients in our Code of Ethics is to "take responsibility for maintaining competence by participating in professional development and educational activities" (AOTA, 1994, p. 1037). The importance of continued competency to occupational therapy practitioners was confirmed in a recent report entitled "Continued Competency in Occupational Therapy: Recommendations to the Profession and Key Stakeholders" by the National Commission on Continued Competency in Occupational Therapy (NCCCOT) (Mayhan, Holm, & Fawcett, 1999). From a survey of a stratified random sample of 550 of the 88,885 occupational therapists and 550 of the 33,512 occupational therapy assistants in the database of the National Board for Certification in Occupational Therapy (response rate = 33%), the NCCCOT found that more than 85% of the respondents endorsed the importance of continued competency for occupational therapy practitioners. Members of the NCCCOT also conducted in-depth interviews with representatives of other stakeholders in the future of our profession. These stakeholders included employers, payers, institutional and individual private accreditation program representatives, consumer advocates, and health policy analysts. These stakeholders shared the common perception that our continued competency is important to consumer protection and that individual occupational therapy practitioners have "the primary and ultimate responsibility for assuring their own continued competency" (Mayhan et al., 1999, p. 54).

Although we must be able to demonstrate competency in the core functions delineated in our *Standards of Practice* (AOTA, 1998) and the functions associated with the professional roles we fulfill (AOTA, 1993), we must also develop competence in research skills. Because of the changes in clinical practice as well as the changes in the evolving evidence base of occupational therapy, if we do not develop the research skills necessary to make use of the current best evidence for our patients, the result will be a progressive *decline* in our clinical competency.

In a special issue of *The American Journal of Occupational Therapy (AJOT)* devoted to professional competence, Abreu et al. (1998) led off their article with a prediction that in a practice environment that is continually changing, the survival of the profession depends, in part, on the "capacity of therapists to achieve competence in scientific inquiry and research" (p. 751). Then, using the levels of research competence identified by the American Occupational Therapy Foundation (1983) and Mitcham (1985), they explicated descriptors of the associated knowledge, skills, and attitudinal research competencies for practitioners at the beginning, intermediate, and advanced levels of occupational therapy research. What is necessary for continued competence in research and for our professional survival is for all of us to increase the number and level of our research competencies—not just to "maintain competence" as is the wording in our Code of Ethics but, rather, to improve our competence. *Can we meet this challenge?*

How Do I Become an Evidence-Based Practitioner?

At the *individual* level, each of us could fulfill all the research competencies identified by Abreu et al. (1998) and still not be an evidence-based practitioner, unless we also use the evidence and use it appropriately. This means that even if the evidence is clear and we decide that we can easily fit it into our preferred practice patterns, if it is not appropriate or acceptable to the patient, it is not evidence-based practice for that patient. As individuals, we must examine our practices to determine whether we are "integrating individual clinical expertise" with the "conscientious, explicit and judicious use of current best evidence" (Sackett et al., 1996, p. 71) by asking ourselves five questions. If we can answer affirmatively to any of the questions, we are making the right moves toward evidence-based practice.

Question 1: Do I Examine What I Do by Asking Clinical Questions?

The process of evidence-based practice begins by identifying the interventions that we use frequently in our practices with particular populations of patients, or for particular problems in performance, and then posing questions.

Richardson, Wilson, Nishikawa, and Hayward (1995) identified the anatomy of a clinical question as having four parts: (a) the patient, population, or problem; (b) the intervention, which may include frequency and duration; (c) the outcome of interest; and (d) the comparison intervention. An example of a clinical question using this format might be: (a) In patients who have sustained a cerebrovascular accident, (b) does the use of a resting splint on the affected hand for 3 hours each day (c) reduce tone and increase function (d) compared with no splinting?

Question 2: Do I Take Time to Track Down the Best Evidence to Guide What I Do?

To answer your clinical question, you must track down the evidence. This involves computer searches with key words and syntax that will efficiently locate the best evidence as well as hand searches (Booth & Madge, 1998). Typical databases you might search are MEDLINE, CINAHL, the Cochrane Database of Systematic Reviews, the ACP Journal Club, Evidence-Based Medicine, DARE, ERIC, PsycLit, and OT SEARCH. In addition to published articles, OT SEARCH includes manuscripts that have not been published but provide evidence that should be considered. You will also need to conduct hand searches of appropriate journals because not all articles on a specific topic will automatically show up in a database search and because not all journals are indexed. In addition to electronic and journal resources, there are human resources who can help you, and reference librarians should be at the top of the list. Additionally, researchers in related disciplines can be helpful because they may have access to important unpublished data, or they may be able to put you in touch with their colleagues who have been conducting studies relevant to the evidence you are trying to track down.

Question 3: Do I Appraise the Evidence or Take It at Face Value?

To appraise the evidence, of course, includes everything you hated about any research course you took, or why you may have avoided taking any. Appraising the evidence requires that you analyze each section of an article and apply the evidence hierarchy to determine at which level the study meets the established criteria. Article analysis is central to evidence-based practice, but it can also be very difficult. One of the structured article review instruments, such as those found on the Web sites of The Cochrane Collaboration, the University of Alberta, McMaster University, and York University, can help you get started, or you can develop a review tool based on the 1993–1994 *JAMA* article series entitled, "User's Guide to the Medical Literature." When you get to the section of the article that includes the statistics, get out the snacks and bring up Trochim's data analysis Web site at Cornell University to reduce your anxiety and start you on your way to understanding the numbers before you (Trochim, February 20, 2000).

Question 4: Do I Use the Evidence to Do the "Right Things Right"?

One way to use the evidence before you is to develop a clinical guideline for your practice and format it according to the six "rights" identified by Graham (1996): Is "the right person, doing the right thing, the right way, in the right place, at the right time, with the right result" (p. 11)? The clinical guideline for "doing the right things right" is developed by using the evidence you locate to delineate the six "rights":

1. Who is the *right* person to implement the intervention? What level of competence is required? Is special certification required? Can an occupational therapy assistant implement the intervention?
2. What is the *right* thing to do? What does the evidence tell you? Does the patient agree?
3. What is the *right* way to implement the intervention? Does the evidence suggest a protocol or specifications that must be met? Can the patient's dignity and privacy be maintained equally in all contexts in which the intervention could be implemented? Does the frequency or duration of the intervention make a difference?
4. What is the *right* place in which to implement the intervention? Is the home better than the clinic? Is the clinic better than the classroom? Is equipment required that dictates where the intervention must take place?
5. What is the *right* time to provide the intervention? Does time since onset of disability or admission to rehabilitation services make a difference? Does delaying the intervention make a difference? Does the time of day make a difference? Does time until, or since, discharge make a difference?

6. What is the *right* result? Did the intervention do what it was intended to do? Is the patient satisfied with the result? Are you satisfied with the result?

After you have implemented the evidence-based guideline, ask yourself Question 5.

Question 5: Do I Evaluate the Impact of Evidence-Based Practice?

To assess the impact of the evidence-based clinical guideline you developed in response to Question 4, you would begin with a chart audit to determine whether the guideline was actually used and, then, whether it was used as intended. Finally, patient outcomes, cost-effectiveness, patient satisfaction, and therapist satisfaction must also be considered. The impact of the latter, therapist satisfaction with evidence-based practice, is pivotal, especially given the barriers to evidence-based practice.

Barriers and Motivation for Evidence-Based Practice

As Law and Baum (1998) noted in an issue of the *Canadian Journal of Occupational Therapy* dedicated to evidence-based practice, there are many barriers to its practice at both the system level and the individual level. The barriers cited include lack of administrative support, lack of access to research evidence, lack of skill in finding the evidence, lack of skill in interpreting the evidence, and lack of time. These barriers were reiterated in a Level V study of Canadian therapists' perceptions of evidence-based practice (Dubouloz, Egan, Vallerand, & von Zweck, 1999). The authors found that although therapists perceived evidence-based practice as a way of looking for understanding of the interventions they used, it also generated feelings of inadequacy related to research skills. Additionally, there were attitudinal barriers in that the therapists perceived that the evidence they would find might threaten the ways they preferred to practice.

Gray (1997) suggested a formula that we might find helpful as we seek to identify factors that will influence our performance of evidence-based practice (see Figure 50.1). He perceived that the performance of evidence-based practice is directly influenced by motivation multiplied by competence divided by the barriers we need to overcome. Many factors in the context in which we practice today can be barriers to us; however, I am choosing to reframe them under motivation. Therefore, legislation, regulation, prospective payment system for skilled nursing facilities, capitations on reimbursement, new patient populations, new practice environments, new collaborations, and a new episodic reimbursement system for rehabilitation hospitals and exempt rehabilitation units can all be entered into the formula as motivation. I perceive them as motivators because they provide for us the impetus to describe, examine, and publish the evidence derived from what we do and how we do it. Also under motivation add the principles in our Code of Ethics that require us, for ethical practice, to "collaborate with service recipients," "fully inform . . . [them] of the nature, risks, and potential outcomes of any intervention," and "avoid harm" to them as well as to "perform . . . duties on the basis of accurate and current information" and "take responsibility for maintaining competence" (AOTA, 1994, p. 1037).

At a minimum, competence in this formula refers to competence in searching for, appraising, and applying existing evidence in everyday practice. For professional survival, however, we must be able to generate, publish, and make accessible to all the evidence that we now have to search for. This requires that we learn to gather evidence systematically in our practices as well as learn the knowledge, skills, and attitudes associated with occupational therapy research at the beginning, intermediate, or advanced levels of competence (Abreu et al., 1998).

$$Performance = \frac{Motivation \times Competence}{Barriers}$$

Figure 50.1. Factors affecting the performance of evidence-based practice (Gray, 1997, p. 7).

Although one could dwell on barriers in the work environment and in the laws, regulations, and reimbursement systems, the barrier over which we have most influence is our own attitudes. On the basis of the findings of the Canadian study (Dubouloz et al., 1999), we have been alerted ahead of time that it may not be the external barriers but, rather, our own attitudinal barriers that may hinder the practice of evidence-based occupational therapy in the United States in the new millennium.

However, there are four encouraging examples of our movement toward evidence-based practice in the United States. Perhaps in response to the evidence-based practice initiatives of our Canadian and British colleagues, the new *Standards for an Accredited Educational Program for the Occupational Therapist* developed by the Accreditation Council for Occupational Therapy Education (ACOTE) requires that occupational therapist graduates be able to "provide evidence-based effective therapeutic intervention related to performance areas" (ACOTE, 1999, p. 579). Furthermore, the AOTA Executive Board passed a motion that an evidence-based panel be formed to review and evaluate research that relates to *The Guide to Occupational Therapy Practice* (Moyers, 1999, 2000) in order to make the document evidence based. Additionally, the *AJOT* Associate Editor for Evidence-Based Practice, Linda Tickle-Degnen, instituted the Evidence-Based Practice Forum in which she guides practitioners through some aspect of evidence-based practice.

The best practice example, however, is from the notice in the *Coverage Policy Bulletin* of Aetna US Healthcare in which coverage of cognitive rehabilitation was recently announced. Although the studies were not Level I or Level II studies, the evidence was convincing. It states in the bulletin:

> The efficacy of cognitive therapy so far has been measured by its objective influence on function and the subjective value of these changes to the individual. Although current evidence supports cognitive therapy as a promising approach, definitive conclusions regarding its efficacy must await large-scale, well-conducted, controlled trials. (Aetna US Healthcare, 2000)

We can provide that evidence!

Conclusion

Eleanor Clarke Slagle was a proponent of habit development. Therefore, I will suggest two new habit patterns that we need to develop if we are to address proactively the realities of our professional exigencies. Each suggested habit pattern is followed by a question.

Habit 1: Evidence-Based Practice Now

Although the evidence for *what* we do and *how* we do it may be difficult to find, we have an obligation to become competent in, and make a habit of, searching for the evidence, appraising its value, and presenting it to those we serve in an understandable manner.

Question 1. After reading this lecture, could you provide your next several patients with a summary of the research evidence on the occupational therapy intervention options you are considering for them so that together you could make the best decisions?

Habit 2: The Evidence Base of Occupational Therapy in the New Millennium

We also have an obligation to improve our research competencies, to develop the habit of using those competencies in everyday practice, and to advance the evidence base of occupational therapy in the new millennium. Only then can we be sure that as we seek to do the "right things right," that we are fulfilling our ethical responsibility to perform our "duties on the basis of accurate and current information" (AOTA, 1994, p. 1037). I will close by asking you to think ahead one decade.

Question 2. If in the year 2010 you stand accused of practicing occupational therapy based on research, will there be enough evidence to convict you?

Acknowledgments

I thank the following colleagues for their hearty critiques of my thinking and of the Slagle manuscript: Lynette S. Chandler, PhD, PT; Denise Chisholm, MS, OTR/L; Louise Fawcett, PhD, OTR/L, FAOTA; Sharon Gwinn, MS, OTR/L; Tamara Mills, OTR/L; Sharon Novalis, MSOT, OTR/L; Varick Olson, PhD, PT; Beth Skidmore, OTR/L; Ronald G. Stone, MS, OTR/L; George Tomlin, PhD, OTR/L; and especially to my mentor, Joan C. Rogers, PhD, OTR/L, FAOTA, ABDA.

References

Abreu, B., Peloquin, S. M., & Ottenbacher, K. (1998). Competence in scientific inquiry and research. *American Journal of Occupational Therapy, 52,* 751–759.

Accreditation Council for Occupational Therapy Education. (1999). Standards for an accredited educational program for the occupational therapist. *American Journal of Occupational Therapy, 53,* 575–582.

Aetna US Healthcare. Cognitive rehabilitation. *Coverage Policy Bulletin.* Retrieved March 6, 2000 from the World Wide Web: http://www.aetnaushc.com/cpb/data/CPBA0214.htm

American Occupational Therapy Association. (1993). Occupational therapy roles. *American Journal of Occupational Therapy, 47,* 1087–1099.

American Occupational Therapy Association. (1994). Occupational therapy code of ethics. *American Journal of Occupational Therapy, 48,* 1037–1038.

American Occupational Therapy Association. (1998). Standards of practice for occupational therapy. *American Journal of Occupational Therapy, 52,* 866–869.

American Occupational Therapy Foundation. (1983). The Foundation—Research competencies for clinicians and educators. *American Journal of Occupational Therapy, 37,* 44–46.

Booth, A., & Madge, B. (1998). Finding the evidence. In T. Bury & J. Mead (Eds.), *Evidence-based healthcare: A practical guide for therapists* (pp. 107–135). Woburn, MA: Butterworth-Heinemann.

Brooke, M., Lateur, B., Diana-Rigby, G., & Questad, K. (1991). Shoulder subluxation in hemiplegia: Effects of three different supports. *Archives of Physical Medicine and Rehabilitation, 72,* 582–586.

Brown, S. J. (1999). *Knowledge for health care practice: A guide for using research evidence.* Philadelphia: Saunders.

Bury, T., & Mead, J. (1998). *Evidence-based healthcare: A practical guide for therapists.* Woburn, MA: Butterworth-Heinemann.

Bye, R. A. (1998). When clients are dying: Occupational therapists' perspectives. *Occupational Therapy Journal of Research, 18,* 3–24.

Case-Smith, J., Heaphy, T., Marr, D., Galvin, B., Koch, V., Ellis, M. G., & Perez, I. (1998). Fine motor and functional performance outcomes in preschool children. *American Journal of Occupational Therapy, 52,* 788–800.

Close, J., Ellis, M., Hooper, R., Glucksman, E., Jackson, S., & Swift, C. (1999). Prevention of falls in the elderly trial (PROFET): A randomised controlled trial. *Lancet, 353,* 93–97.

Cohn, E. S., & Cermak, S. A. (1998). Including the family perspective in sensory integration outcomes research. *American Journal of Occupational Therapy, 52,* 540–546.

Cummings, R. G., Thomas, M., Szonyi, G., Salkeld, G., O'Neill, E., Westbury, C., & Frampton, G. (1999). Home visits by an occupational therapist for assessment and modification of environmental hazards: A randomized trial of falls prevention. *Journal of the American Geriatrics Society, 47,* 1397–1402.

Dubouloz, C.-J., Egan, M., Vallerand, J., & von Zweck, C. (1999). Occupational therapists' perceptions of evidence-based practice. *American Journal of Occupational Therapy, 53,* 445–458.

Graham, G. (1996, June). Clinically effective medicine in a rational health service. *Health Director,* 11–12.

Gray, J.A.M. (1997). *Evidence-based healthcare: How to make health policy and management decisions.* New York: Churchill Livingstone.

Hurd, M. M., Farrell, K. H., & Waylonis, G. W. (1974). Shoulder sling for hemiplegia: Friend or foe? *Archives of Physical Medicine and Rehabilitation, 55,* 519–522.

Law, M., & Baum, C. (1998). Evidence-based occupational therapy. *Canadian Journal of Occupational Therapy, 65,* 131–135.

Lidz, C. W., & Meisel, A. (1983). Informed consent and the structure of medical care. In *Making health care decisions: The ethical and legal implications of informed consent in the patient–practitioner relationship* (Vol. 2). Washington, DC: U.S. Government Printing Office.

Lin, K., Wu, C., Tickle-Degnen, L., & Coster, W. (1997). Enhancing occupational performance through occupationally embedded exercise: A meta-analytic review. *Occupational Therapy Journal of Research, 17,* 25–47.

Mayhan, Y. D., Holm, M. B., Fawcett, L. C. (Eds.) & National Commission on Continued Competency in Occupational Therapy. (1999). *Continued competency in occupational therapy: Recommendations to the profession and key stakeholders.* Gaithersburg, MD: National Board for Certification in Occupational Therapy.

McHale, K., & Cermak, S. A. (1992). Fine motor activities in elementary school: Preliminary findings and provisional implications for children with fine motor problems. *American Journal of Occupational Therapy, 46,* 898–903.

Mitcham, M. D. (1985). *Integrating research competencies into occupational therapy: A teaching guide for academic and clinical educators.* Rockville, MD: American Occupational Therapy Foundation.

Moore, A., McQuay, H., & Gray, J.A.M. (Eds.). (1995). Evidence-based everything. *Bandolier, 1*(12), 1.

Moyers, P. A. (1999). The guide to occupational therapy practice. *American Journal of Occupational Therapy, 53,* 247–322.

Moyers, P. A. (2000). Letters to the editor—Author's response. *American Journal of Occupational Therapy, 54,* 113–114.

Mulligan, S. (1998). Patterns of sensory integration dysfunction: A confirmatory factor analysis. *American Journal of Occupational Therapy, 52,* 819–828.

Neistadt, M. E., & Marques, K. (1984). An independent living skills training program. *American Journal of Occupational Therapy, 38,* 671–676.

Nicol, M. M., Robertson, L., & Connaughton, J. A. (1999). Life skills programmes for people with chronic mental illness. *Cochrane Database of Systematic Reviews, 3: The Schizophrenia Group.* Retrieved January 26, 2000 from the World Wide Web: http://www.update-software.com/cochrane.htm

Ottenbacher, K. J., & Maas, F. (1999). Quantitative Research Series—How to detect effects: Statistical power and evidence-based practice in occupational therapy research. *American Journal of Occupational Therapy, 53,* 181–188.

Portney, L. G., & Watkins, M. P. (1993). *Foundations of clinical research: Applications to practice.* Norwalk, CT: Appleton & Lange.

Ray, W. A., Taylor, J. A., Meador, K. G., Thapa, P. B., Brown, A. K., Kajihara, H. K., Davis, C., Gideon, P., & Griffin, M. R. (1997). A randomized trial of a consultation service to reduce falls in nursing homes. *Journal of the American Medical Association, 278,* 557–562.

Rennie, D. (1986). Guarding the guardians: A conference on editorial peer review. *Journal of the American Medical Association, 256,* 2391–2392.

Richardson, W. S., Wilson, M. C., Nishikawa, J., & Hayward, R. S. (1995). The well-built clinical question: A key to evidence-based decisions. *ACP Journal Club, 123,* A-12.

Rogers, J. C., Holm, M. B., Burgio, L. D., Granieri, E., Hsu, C., Hardin, J. M., & McDowell, B. J. (1999). Improving morning care routines of nursing home residents with dementia. *Journal of the American Geriatrics Society, 47,* 1049–1057.

Sackett, D. L., Haynes, R. B., & Tugwell, P. (1985). How to read a clinical journal. In D. L. Sackett, R. B. Haynes, & P. Tugwell (Eds.). *Clinical epidemiology: A basic science for clinical medicine* (pp. 285–322). Boston: Little, Brown.

Sackett, D. L., Richardson, W. S., Rosenberg, W., & Haynes, R. B. (1997). Critically praising the evidence. In D. L. Sackett, W. S. Richardson, W. Rosenberg, & R. B. Haynes (Eds.), *Evidence-based medicine: How to practice and teach EBM* (pp. 38–156). New York: Churchill Livingstone.

Sackett, D. L., Rosenberg, W. M., Gray, J.A.M., Haynes, R. B., & Richardson, W. S. (1996). Evidence-based medicine: What it is and what it isn't. *British Medical Journal, 312,* 71–72.

Schneiderman, L. J., Kaplan, R. M., Pearlman, R. A., & Teetzel, H. (1993). Do physicians' own preferences for life-sustaining treatment influence their perceptions of patients' preferences? *Journal of Clinical Ethics, 4,* 28–32.

Shenk, D. (1997). *Data smog.* San Francisco: Harper Edge.

Silverman, W. A. (1998). *Where's the evidence?: Debates in modern medicine.* New York: Oxford University Press.

Tickle-Degnen, L. (1998). Quantitative Research Series—Communicating with clients about treatment outcomes: The use of meta-analytic evidence in collaborative treatment planning. *American Journal of Occupational Therapy, 52,* 526–530.

Trochim, W. (February 20, 2000). *What is the research methods knowledge base?* Retrieved from the World Wide Web: http://trochim.human.cornell.edu/kb/index.htm

Vargas, S., & Camilli, G. (1999). A meta-analysis of research on sensory integration treatment. *American Journal of Occupational Therapy, 53,* 189–198.

Williams, R., Taffs, L., & Minuk, T. (1988). Evaluation of two support methods for the subluxated shoulder in hemiplegic patients. *Physical Therapy, 68,* 1209–1213.

Zorowitz, R. D., Idank, D., Ikai, T., Hughes, M. B., & Johnston, M. V. (1995). Shoulder subluxation after a stroke: A comparison of four supports. *Archives of Physical Medicine and Rehabilitation, 76,* 763–771.

51

2001 Eleanor Clarke Slagle Lecture

The Sensations of Everyday Life:
Empirical, Theoretical, and Pragmatic Considerations

Winnie Dunn, PhD, OTR, FAOTA

The experience of being human is imbedded in the sensory events of everyday life. When we observe how people live their lives, we discover that they characterize their experiences from a sensory point of view. People talk about the intensity or dullness of an image. When they explain a dream or an event of the prior day, they use sensory words to characterize the dream's elements. Sensation is the common language by which we share the experience of being human; it provides a common ground for understanding.

Yet sensation also is so intimate and personal that we use it to define our individuality. We describe the difference between one person and another in relation to those persons' interest in, tolerance for, and pleasure with sensations. Because of our personal experiences with sensation, it is sometimes hard or even inconceivable to imagine another person's experience with an object or event or context. We want to frame the sensory experiences within our own parameters; we think of another person's description as "same," "somewhat similar," or "very different" from our own. All art is an expression of the artists' personal experiences with the universe and might be described as their personal sensory history shared in the form of the art; everyone responds differently to particular art.

The discipline of occupational therapy has had a collective interest in sensory processing across the entire evolution of our profession. We have generated and continue to generate a wealth of information about how persons process sensory information and how those methods guide choices. These choices ultimately affect a person's ability to live a satisfying life. Everyone is personally interested in the experiences of sensation, and occupational therapists can advance thinking about the contribution of sensory processing to our understanding of the human experience both in the typical course of the day and as it might interfere with living a satisfying life.

The unique contribution of occupational therapy knowledge is in attaching understanding and meaning to sensory experiences. We make the applications to daily life to which other disciplines only allude. We might characterize our role as translator: We stand in the space between abstract constructs and application to practice, looking back and forth, translating for each group what the other has to say. Therefore, we can inform colleagues about the meaning of their research and families about their situations, enabling each group to advance their own thinking and ultimately advance knowledge overall.

Background Knowledge Related to Sensory Processing

Scholars from many disciplines have studied aspects of sensory processing. Their work provides evidence about how the sensory systems contribute to the experience of being human. Neuroscientists have identified the unique qualities of each sensory system that make it possible for humans to take in information for the brain's use (Kandel, Schwartz, & Jessell, 2000). The brain initially becomes a repository for this sensory input, creating maps of the

Originally published 2001 in *American Journal of Occupational Therapy, 55,* 608–620.

body and the environment from each sensory system's point of view (Dunn, 1998). As these maps form, the brain begins to integrate information from multiple sensory systems, forming higher order schemas of performance in contexts. Throughout life, these maps are modified in relation to the person's activities, forming the background for learning and understanding.

In addition to considering the basic sensory input and processing occurring in the nervous system, scientists have reported on the nervous system's methods for mediating its own input (Kandel et al., 2000). Neural regulation occurs through mechanisms that balance excitation and inhibition, creating thresholds for responding at the point that the proper amount of input has accumulated (Dunn, 1998). Genetic and environmental factors contribute to each person's ways of responding to excitation and inhibition. Therefore, people have different thresholds for noticing, responding to, and becoming irritated with sensations; these thresholds, in turn, affect their daily choices and are reflected in their mood, temperament, and ways of organizing their lives (Baranek, 1999; Dunn, 1997, 2000; Rothbart & Jones, 1999; Zuckerman, 1994).

Cognitive mechanisms, such as attention, organization, memory, and problem solving, operate with information from the sensory systems and, therefore, illustrate balancing threshold demands. A natural tension exists in the brain's processing between internal information (sensations of the body, i.e., touch, visceral) and external information (sensations of the environment, i.e., auditory, visual). Cognitive processing is optimal when internal and external information processing afford task performance together (Gijsbers van Wijk & Kolk, 1997b). For example, Shumway-Cook and Woollacott (2000) tested cognitive processing in relation to internal and external information processing in young and older adults. They created several conditions of imbalance in internal and external information processing demands and found that older adults need to have both external (visual) and internal (somatosensory, vestibular, proprioceptive) cues available for postural control in order to perform a demanding cognitive task.

The mechanisms of sensory processing are intertwined with many other brain functions. By studying these phenomena in various combinations, the actual contributions and relationships can be revealed and then applied to other scholarly inquiries, such as the role of sensory processing in individual differences and various human conditions.

Data Indicating Individual Differences in Sensory Processing

Studies employing psychophysiological methods provide evidence about the nature of individual differences when processing sensory events in the nervous system. Researchers have produced a body of literature about sensation seeking as a biosocial phenomenon in humans (Carton, Morand, Bungenera, & Jouvent, 1995; Glicksohn & Abulafia, 1998; Sarmany-Schuller, 1999; Zuckerman, 1994; Zuckerman, Ulrich, & McLaughlin, 1993). Zuckerman (1994) reported on physiological differences in persons with high and low sensation-seeking traits. Persons who are high sensation seekers experience a reduction in heart rate with the introduction of a new stimulus, which is interpreted to be an orienting response that makes the person available to receive the stimuli. Conversely, low sensation seekers experience an acceleration of heart rate, presumably triggering fear or threat, leading to inhibition and avoidance of new stimuli.

Interdisciplinary teams, including occupational therapy researchers, have taken advantage of psychophysiology methods to investigate the relationships among the nervous system's responses and patterns of sensory processing in daily life. In studies with preschoolers (McIntosh, Miller, Shyu, & Dunn, 1999) and adults (Brown, Tollefson, Dunn, Cromwell, & Filion, 2001), researchers found distinct patterns of noticing and habituation that coincided with the four categories of sensory processing proposed in Dunn's Model of Sensory Processing (Dunn, 1997). These findings suggest that we can characterize the ways that humans take in sensation and that individual differences exist in how we use those sensations to construct our daily lives.

Data Indicating Differences in Sensory Processing Related to Human Conditions

In addition to identifying patterns of individual difference in sensory processing, researchers have studied the unique features of sensory processing that occur for persons with various conditions. These data reveal the broad influence that sensory processing has on every aspect of daily life. The studies suggest that attention to the person's sensory processing patterns may provide insight for understanding these conditions and for deriving meaning from the person's performance repertoire. Knowledge about a person's patterns of sensory processing may contribute to the design of more effective interventions and the advancement of knowledge.

Accumulating evidence identifies distinct sensory processing patterns in children and adults with various conditions (Ayres, 1989; Baranek, 1999; Baranek, Foster, & Berkson, 1997a; Brown & Dunn, in press; Brown et al., 2001; Case-Smith, Butcher, & Reed, 1998; Cermak & Daunhaur, 1997; Cooper, Majnemer, Rosenblatt, & Birnbaum, 1993; DeGangi & Greenspan, 1989; Dunn, 1999, 2000; Dunn & Daniels, 2001; Johnson-Ecker & Parham, 2000; Larson, 1982; Provost & Oetter, 1993; Royeen & Fortune, 1990; Wiener, Long, DeGangi, & Battaile, 1996). Researchers use a variety of data collection methods, including criterion measures, direct evaluation of performance, interviews, questionnaires, and observations, to characterize sensory processing. In spite of the variety of methods, researchers have reported distinct sensory processing characteristics in persons with various human conditions.

Genetic and developmental disorders. Some researchers have studied sensory processing patterns in children with genetic disorders. Belser and Sudhalter (1995) measured skin conductance and found that boys with Fragile X syndrome are more physiologically aroused by eye contact than boys with Down syndrome. They also found that boys with Fragile X syndrome who also had autism demonstrated more avoidant reactions than boys with autism only. Belser and Sudhalter concluded that difficulty with modulating arousal may be a distinguishing characteristic of Fragile X syndrome. Other researchers also have verified that both children with Fragile X syndrome and children with sensory modulation disorder responded to sensory stimuli at higher levels, at higher rates, and with lack of habituation (McIntosh, Miller, Shyu, & Hagerman, 1999; Miller et al., 1998) than peers without disabilities. Therefore, conditions that affect the nervous system, like Fragile X syndrome and Down syndrome, also change the ways that persons respond to sensory input.

Baranek et al. (1997a) studied sensory defensiveness and its relationship to stereotypic behaviors in children and adults with developmental disabilities. They reported on two factors emerging from the data: auditory and other hypersensitivities and tactile defensiveness. In another report, Baranek et al. (1997b) identified a relationship between tactile defensiveness and rigid, inflexible behavior patterns. Hotz and Royeen (1998) found that children rated their own tactile defensiveness as more intense than did their mothers, although a high correlation existed between the mothers and their own children. Kinnealey (1998) reported on a preschooler with sensory defensiveness who also had difficulty with age-appropriate learning at preschool; the child also demonstrated anxiety and need for control, which affected her school and family relationships. Kinnealey and Fuiek (1999) tested adults with sensory defensiveness and found them to be more anxious and depressed, but they did not experience more pain than their peers without defensiveness. Perhaps rigidity and inflexibility are behaviors reflective of coping with very low thresholds that quickly overwhelm some persons' nervous systems.

In another set of studies, Baranek (1999) found that children with autism and developmental disabilities displayed different ways of responding to visual, auditory, touch, and body position stimuli in relation to each other and cohorts without disabilities. DeGangi and Greenspan (1989) found tactile defensiveness, vestibular dysfunction, and poor ocular motor control in children with developmental delays and children with regulatory disorders. Lai, Parham, and Johnson-Ecker (1999) reported a strong relationship between sensory defensiveness (i.e., overresponsiveness to stimuli) and sensory dormancy (i.e., underresponsiveness to stimuli) in children with disabilities, suggesting interrelatedness between these two ways of responding. The children with disabilities in their study had a higher rate of both dormancy and defensiveness than the comparison group of children without disabilities, suggesting that modulation of input was in question.

Brain disorders. Sensory processing also affects cognitive performance for persons with brain dysfunction; auditory factors seem particularly relevant (Arciniegas et al., 1999; Denney, 1997; Madigan, DeLuca, Diamond, Tramontano, & Averill, 2000; Ragneskog & Kihlgren, 1997). Ragneskog and Kihlgren (1997) found that auditory environments affected level of cognitive awareness in patients with dementia; background music engendered calming, whereas more uncontrolled sounds increased agitation. Denney (1997) also found that persons in a rehabilitation unit demonstrated 57% less agitation after 1 week of quiet music in the dining room. The negative behaviors rebounded when the music was stopped and returned to lower levels when the music was reintroduced, providing stronger evidence that the music affects the cognitive state.

Although cognitive processing speed is slower for most persons who have had traumatic brain injury, auditory input slows these persons' processing even more (Madigan et al., 2000). For example, in a study of persons with traumatic brain injury, researchers found that attentional mechanisms failed in persons who were unable to filter stimuli and took a longer time to respond to auditory cues (Arciniegas et al., 1999). Therefore, it is possible to understand the relationship between cognition and sensory processing by looking at performance when the balance in attention to internal (body) and external (environment) sensory cues is disrupted.

Schizophrenia. Sensory processing challenges are also prominent for persons who have schizophrenia, and these challenges are linked to the cognitive impairments characteristic of the disorder (e.g., Bunney et al., 1999; Cromwell, 1993; Frith, Blakemore, & Wolpert, 2000; Hemsley, 1993; Jin et al., 1998; Light & Braff, 2000; McGhie & Chapman, 1961; Venables, 1969). In a classic article, McGhie and Chapman (1961) identified disturbances of attention, perception, and changes in motility and body awareness as key features of the onset of schizophrenia. They categorized persons' descriptions of their early experiences with schizophrenia and described them having to face an unstable and newly fluctuating relationship between perception of self (body sensations) and the environment. During this early period, persons seem to have increasing awareness of all stimuli and cannot organize the myriad of sensations, making it more and more difficult to function. Authors have proposed that delusions emerge from attempts to make meaning out of this increasingly undifferentiated sensory input (Frith et al., 2000; Light & Braff, 2000).

Fatigue. Not only chronic brain disorders provide information about sensory processing. Scholars studying fatigue also have reported relationships to sensory processing primarily related to balancing internal and external information processing. Authors have reported evidence of fatigue when persons are experiencing low internal and external information processing demands (Finkelman, 1994; Gijsbers van Wijk & Kolk, 1997a) and when persons have both too high and too low external demands (Bensing, Hulsman, & Schreurs, 1999; Rijk, Schreurs, & Bensing, 1999). For example, Rijk et al. (1999) studied fatigue in general medicine practices and found that fatigue was high when persons experienced overload of external stimuli and decreased when persons found their external stimulation attractive. Because fatigue reports are generally related to internal cues (e.g., tiredness, dullness, body complaints), Gijsbers van Wijk and Kolk (1997b) concluded that both too few (leading to boredom) and too many (leading to being overwhelmed) external cues can lead to increased attention to internal cues and, therefore, higher rates of fatigue. They recommended changes in daily life to reestablish the balance between internal and external information processing demands to reduce fatigue and therefore improve performance and satisfaction.

This review provides a sample of the extensive interdisciplinary interest in phenomena related to sensory processing and its impact on performance. Data from children and adults, persons with and without disorders, and out-of-laboratory and natural environment settings indicate that sensory processing has a pervasive influence on the human experience. Furthermore, the apparently far-reaching effect of sensory processing on peoples' ability to experience a satisfying life underscores the importance of studying sensory processing from many perspectives, including the unique perspectives offered from the discipline of occupational therapy.

Explanation of Dunn's Model of Sensory Processing

In 1997, I proposed a model for sensory processing that accounted for the nervous system's thresholds for acting and the person's propensity for responding to those thresholds (Dunn, 1997). The original model evolved from the literature, such as that described previously, and analysis of data gathered with the Sensory Profile measure from a national sample of children without disabilities (Dunn, 1999; Dunn & Brown, 1997; Dunn & Westman, 1997). This model of sensory processing has proven useful in guiding subsequent research and providing a structure for gaining insights into the nature of sensory processing across the life span.

The primary features of this model are (a) consideration of one's neurological thresholds (i.e., reactivity), (b) consideration of one's responding or self-regulation strategies, and (c) consideration of the interaction among thresholds and responding strategies. Figure 51.1 illustrates the model, with thresholds on the vertical axis and responding strategies on the horizontal axis.

In this model, thresholds and responding strategies represent a con-

Thresholds/Reactivity	Responding/Self-Regulation Strategies	
	Passive	Active
High	Low Registration	Sensory Seeking
Low	Sensory Sensitivity	Sensory Avoiding

Figure 51.1. Dunn's Model of Sensory Processing.
Note. From "The Impact of Sensory Processing Abilities on the Daily Lives of Young Children and Families: A Conceptual Model" by W. Dunn, 1997, *Infants and Young Children, 9*(4), 23–25. Copyright © 1997 by Aspen Publishers, Inc. Adapted with permission.

tinuum of possible conditions, such that a person's ways of responding to sensory events in daily life can be characterized as reflecting both a particular threshold *and* a responding strategy. Although a person's responses to sensory events could fall anywhere on this model, the four outermost interaction points are named for the purpose of dialogue. High thresholds with passive responding strategies are called *low registration;* high thresholds with active responding strategies are called *sensory seeking;* low thresholds with passive responding strategies are called *sensory sensitivity;* and low thresholds with active responding strategies are called *sensory avoiding* (see Figure 51.1). These concepts are explained in greater detail in other sources (Brown et al., 2001; Dunn, 1997, 1998, 2000; Dunn & Brown, 1997; Dunn & Daniels, 2001; Huebner & Dunn, 2000).

Description of Anchor Points in the Model

Persons who have high neurological thresholds require a lot of sensory input for responding. When persons have low registration, they do not notice sensory events in daily life that others notice readily (i.e., passive responding strategy). They may not notice when other people come into the room or food or dirt on their face and hands. Others may have to call the person's name several times or use additional cues such as touching to get the person's attention. Persons who are sensation seekers enjoy sensory experiences and find ways to enhance and extend sensory events in daily life (i.e., active responding strategy). They like physical movements such as climbing, twirling, swinging, and bouncing. They search for additional sensory experiences for themselves, such as humming and other mouth noises, touching objects, feeling vibrations in stereo speakers and appliances, wearing perfume, and smelling flowers (Brown et al., 2001; Dunn, 1997; Dunn & Brown, 1997; Dunn & Daniels, 2001).

Persons who have low neurological thresholds, or sensory sensitivity, notice sensory stimuli quite readily and more sensory events in daily life than do others. They are easily distracted by movements, sounds, or smells while in groups of people, such as in class or at the movie theatre. They notice food textures, temperatures, and spices more rapidly than others. They may be uncomfortable with clothing tags, elastic, or certain fabric textures. Their high rate of noticing while continuing to experience all of these is a more passive responding strategy (i.e., letting things happen) than is seen in sensation avoiders. Sensory avoiders find ways to limit sensory input throughout the day. They stay away from distracting settings; for example, they leave the room if others are moving, talking, or bumping into them. They create rituals for daily routines, which may be an active strategy to generate only familiar, predictable sensory patterns for themselves. They also become unhappy when these rituals are disrupted perhaps because of increasing unpredictability (Brown et al., 2001; Dunn, 1997; Dunn & Brown, 1997; Dunn & Daniels, 2001).

Sensory processing is a complex endeavor. People do not experience sensory events of daily life in a unitary manner. As the literature has shown, internal and external conditions affect the way people process sensory information. They may be more sensitive (have lower thresholds) for some types of sensory input, while being less attentive (have higher thresholds) for other types of sensory input. A model must symbolize complex processes without being complex itself so that it affords further conceptualization and synthesis. This model of sensory processing is meant to provide a framework for studying, interpreting, and gaining insights into the nature of sensory processing, including all of its complexities, and the impact of sensory processing on daily life.

Evidence Emerging From Studies Using Dunn's Model of Sensory Processing

Dunn's Model of Sensory Processing reflects concepts for consideration toward understanding the impact of sensory processing in daily life. My colleagues and I have used the various forms of the Sensory Profile—the Infant/Toddler Sensory Profile for children birth to 3 years of age, the Sensory Profile for children 3 years to 10 years of age, and the Adult Sensory Profile for adolescents and adults—to conduct studies about the nature of sensory processing as a core feature of the human experience. These measures contain descriptions of sensory events in daily life; the informant (self or parent) uses a 5-point Likert scale (almost always to almost never) to record the frequency they engage in the behaviors described in each item. We have reported good internal consistency estimates for each measure. Findings from specific studies have been and are being reported elsewhere; when considering the findings across ages and human conditions, some consistent patterns emerge that provide insights and furnish information for future interpretations and discoveries.

Sensory seeking is a prominent feature for everyone. To date, we have conducted factor analyses on infants and toddlers (Dunn, in press; Dunn & Daniels, 2001), children (Dunn, 1999; Dunn & Brown, 1997), and adults (Brown et al., 2001) without disabilities. In each case, sensory seeking has emerged as a prominent factor accounting for a large amount of the variance in the groups (infants and toddlers, 8%–11%; children, 22%; adults, 7.8%) (see Table 51.1).

Perhaps the sensory seeking factor illustrates the predominant method that people use for gathering information and keeping track of themselves and what is going on around them. As Coren, Porac, and Ward (1984) stated:

> The brain, the organ that is responsible for your conscious experience, is an eternal prisoner in the solitary confinement of the skull . . . and must rely on information smuggled into it from the senses . . . the world is what your brain tells you it is, and the limitations of your senses sets the boundaries of your conscious experience. (p. 2)

In implementing responsibility for the conscious experience, the brain exercises vigilance in monitoring the moment-to-moment changes in body integrity, environmental conditions, and the continuous and changing relationship of the body with the environment (Damasio, 1999). In all the factor structures, the sensory seeking factor contained items from multiple sensory systems. Not one sensory modality but, rather, one theme characterized sensory seeking: searching for and enjoying sensory experiences. Perhaps the sensory seeking factors provide evidence of the brain's multisensory vigilance and the universality of seeking sensation as part of the experience of being human.

The factor structures reflect thresholds and reactivity rather than sensory system organization. Evidence suggests that some children who have learning and behavioral disabilities exhibit difficulties processing input from particular sensory systems (Ayres, 1979, 1989; Ayres & Tickle, 1980; Fisher, Murray, & Bundy, 1991; Kimball, 1986). Additionally, researchers and practitioners in occupational therapy have traditionally constructed sensory histories using sensory system groupings (i.e., auditory, visual, touch, vestibular, proprioceptive, taste, smell) (Ayres, 1979;

Table 51.1. Selected Items From the Sensory Seeking Factor of Each Factor Analysis

Sensory Profile Form	Item
Infant/Toddler	My child finds ways to make noise with toys. My child enjoys physical activity (bouncing, being held up high in the air).
Child	My child twirls/spins self frequently throughout the day. My child loves to be barefoot.
Adult	I enjoy being close to people who wear perfume or cologne. I hum, whistle, sing, or make other noises.

Brown & Dunn, in press; Case-Smith et al., 1998; Cooper et al., 1993; DeGangi & Greenspan, 1989; Dunn, 1999, in press; Dunn & Daniels, 2001; Johnson-Ecker & Parham, 2000; Larson, 1982; Provost & Oetter, 1993; Royeen & Fortune, 1990). Consequently, one might hypothesize that these sensory system groupings would emerge as factors in factor analyses.

However, the findings from the factor analysis studies of the Sensory Profile indicate that the items cluster on the basis of the person's level of reactivity (i.e., thresholds for responding) rather than by sensory system (Brown et al., 2001; Dunn, in press; Dunn & Brown, 1997; Dunn & Daniels, 2001). When persons tend to seek or avoid sensory input, they are likely to seek or avoid input from more than one sensory system.

Perhaps the questions on the Sensory Profile enable persons to characterize the excitation and inhibition needs of their own nervous systems. Preliminary evidence shows that persons with distinct sensory processing patterns consistent with the quadrants in Dunn's model also have distinct patterns of amplitude and habituation responses in skin conductance measures (Brown et al., 2001; McIntosh, Miller, Shyu, & Dunn, 1999; McIntosh, Miller, Shyu, & Hagerman, 1999; Miller et al., 1998). For example, Brown et al. (2001) found that amplitude measurements were higher for persons with low threshold patterns (sensory sensitivity, sensory avoiding) than persons with high threshold patterns (low registration, sensory seeking). However, persons with sensory avoiding and low registration habituated quickly, whereas persons with sensory sensitivity and sensory seeking habituated more slowly. McIntosh, Miller, Shyu, and Hagerman (1999) also reported a similar pattern when testing children. These psychophysiology measures are considered involuntary nervous system responses. The fact that persons with distinct sensory processing matching each quadrant on Dunn's Model of Sensory Processing also displayed a unique pattern of skin conductance (i.e., the pattern of amplitude plus habituation) lends psychophysiological support to the model. Possibly the Sensory Profile measures tap persons' awareness of their own (or their child's) nervous system's responding patterns, providing valuable information about nervous system operations in an accessible format.

Patterns emerge across ages to reveal both stability and developmental factors. Most of the data from the Sensory Profile studies indicate that responsiveness and reactivity patterns remain the same across the life span. Despite the wide range of ages we have tested, generally the levels of responding remain the same across both the sensory systems and the patterns of sensory processing (i.e., the categories) from Dunn's model. These findings suggest that there is something inherent about sensory processing that is separate from specific learning or experiences. Certainly, persons learn from every experience, and sensory processing provides the information for that learning. Preliminary cross-sectional data suggest that people use consistent sensory processing patterns across time. A person who has low registration, even with variability due to biobehavioral state, environmental variables, and motivation, will likely have a range of registration that reflects lower registration than others in similar situations. Thus far, we only have cross-sectional data and will need to collect longitudinal data to verify these hypotheses.

Two notable exceptions to these stability patterns seem to reflect active changes in particular developmental periods. Our data on *infants and toddlers* indicate the existence of developmental trends for some of the sensory systems (Dunn, in press; Dunn & Daniels, 2001). In the *tactile system,* the youngest infants (birth to 6 months of age) are very responsive to their parents and rarely resist being held or cuddled. Children between 1 and 3 years of age have a wider range of responses to tactile input, with the average scores between seldom and occasionally. Perhaps as children grow older, they begin to differentiate the wider range of tactile inputs and learn about becoming part of the world outside the mother's womb. They also develop more skills for negotiating their responses during this period (Gormly, 1997). For the *visual and oral sensory systems,* scores steadily progress across the ages of birth to 3 years, with the youngest infants responding frequently to stimuli and the older toddlers responding seldom to occasionally. Again, as the children experience sensations of living in the world, they accumulate information and then habituate to some sensory events as those events become familiar patterns to the nervous system.

For older adults, low threshold factors (sensitivity, sensory avoiding) continue to function at the same level as younger adults, but high threshold factors (registration, seeking) change (Pohl, Dunn, & Brown, 2001). Specifically, after 70 years of age, registration gets worse (i.e., it gets progressively harder to notice stimuli), and persons seek stimuli less (i.e., they engage in fewer and fewer behaviors to add sensation to their experiences). One explanation for this phenomenon is that older adults have poorer sensory acuity, such as hearing and vision, thus reducing their actual input. Another explanation is related to the wider experiences of older adults; perhaps as persons grow older, more experiences are familiar, thus not triggering thresholds for responding as often as younger adults. The low threshold patterns continue throughout the adult period; consistency in low threshold patterns may reflect the nervous system's continuing vigilance for protective responses to potentially harmful stimuli, whereas familiarity with a broader range of information produces less responding in day-to-day familiar situations. Nonetheless, this finding offers information about strategies we might employ for supporting older adults to remain actively engaged and participatory as they age.

Evidence differentiates patterns of sensory processing across human conditions. Studies that include persons with various disabilities, such as attention deficit hyperactivity disorder (ADHD), autism, Asperger syndrome, schizophrenia, Fragile X syndrome, and sensory modulation disorder, indicate that sensory processing is significantly different for persons with these disorders compared with peers without disabilities (Brown et al., 2001; Dunn & Bennett, in press; Kientz & Dunn, 1997; McIntosh, Miller, Shyu, & Dunn, 1999). Additionally, some evidence suggests that disability groups are significantly different from each other in their patterns of sensory processing. For example, Ermer and Dunn (1998) conducted a discriminant analysis on data from children with autism, children with ADHD, and children without disabilities and were able to categorize the children with 89% accuracy on the basis of factor analysis scores alone. (Remember the factor scores are groupings of items that reflect Dunn's Model of Sensory Processing.) Low threshold items related to inattention and distractibility differentiated children with ADHD, whereas poor oral sensory processing differentiated children with autism.

When combined with the data presented in the earlier section about sensory processing differences across a number of human conditions, strong evidence appears to indicate that sensory processing information can enhance our understanding of human disorders specifically and the human experience in general. The normative data on the Sensory Profile suggests a continuum of responding, with persons who have disabilities occupying the ends of the ranges. Significant differences in sensory processing from the patterns most people experience may be a considerable factor contributing to the overall behavioral, cognitive, and psychosocial manifestations of particular disorders.

Integrating Data Across Disciplines Provides Insights

If we are to understand the role of sensory processing in our humanity, including how it affects people's lives, we must consider how knowledge generated across disciplines informs our conception of being human. Researchers have studied personality, temperament, self-regulation, and traits related to responsiveness to understand the nature of being human (Bagnato & Neisworth, 1999; Costa & McCrae, 1987; Rothbart, Ahadi, & Evans, 2000; Rothbart & Jones, 1999; Zuckerman, 1994). These bodies of work offer important constructs that characterize people's ways of being. When combined with sensory processing constructs, we begin to see the possible impact of sensory processing on behavioral and personality traits.

Studying temperament and personality. Just as in the sensory processing literature, temperament and personality researchers have conducted factor analytic studies to uncover the constructs underlying self-regulation, personality, temperament, and behavioral response traits (Bagnato & Neisworth, 1999; Costa & McCrae, 1987; Rothbart et al., 2000; Rothbart & Jones, 1999; Zuckerman, 1994). These scholars have found factor structures that seem to reflect levels of reactivity.

For example, Rothbart and colleagues have studied the temperament characteristics of infants and young children and identified factors they called "surgency" (i.e., positive affect, activity level), fear, irritability/anger, and persistence. These same characteristics emerge in studies of children through school age (Rothbart et al., 2000; Rothbart, Derryberry, & Hershey, 2000; Rothbart & Jones, 1999). Rothbart and Derryberry (1981) believed that these temperament characteristics of development precede and underlie the development of self-regulatory processes.

Table 51.2. Comparison of the Factor Structures of Infant/Child Temperament and Adult Temperament and Personality Scales and Sensory Processing Scales

Infant/Child Temperament	Adult Temperament and Personality	Sensory Processing
Fear	Negative affect Neuroticism	Sensory avoiding
Irritability/anger	Orienting sensitivity	Sensitivity
Surgency		
Positive affect	Intellect/openness Agreeableness Extraversion	Sensory seeking
Persistence	Effortful attention Conscientiousness	Low registration

Researchers studying adults have reported similar constructs of temperament and have linked these constructs to personality traits (Caspi, 2000; Rothbart et al., 2000; Starratt & Peterson,1997). Rothbart, Ahadi, and Evans (2000) reported a four-factor temperament structure that is consistent with the child temperament factors. They also studied the relationship between this temperament structure and the Big Five personality factor structure defined by Costa and McCrae (1987) and found considerable convergence in the two structures. Table 51.2 illustrates the convergence of constructs from the child and adult factor structures.

Hypothesizing about relationships among temperament, personality, and sensory processing. Four distinct constructs continue to emerge from the temperament and personality literature (see Table 51.2). The characteristics of these constructs appear to be consistent with the four constructs that have emerged from the sensory processing factor analyses as well. Table 51.2 also contains a column that illustrates hypothesized relationships between the constructs from Dunn's Model of Sensory Processing and the temperament and personality constructs. In this proposed set of relationships, sensory seeking is associated with agreeableness and extraversion of adulthood and surgency of childhood. Sensory avoiding is associated with fear, negative affect, and neuroticism. Sensitivity is associated with irritability and anger and orienting sensitivity. Finally, I hypothesize that the temperament characteristics of persistence and effortful attention and the personality trait of conscientiousness explain a different facet of task persistence than low registration. That is, the sensory processing pattern of low registration (high thresholds and passive responding patterns) seems to enable task performance because of lack of noticing other stimuli. Table 51.3 lists some sample items from the adult temperament and adult sensory processing measures discussed here.

Does this mean that we do not need to study sensory processing because the substantial temperament and personality literature could tell us all there is to know? I do not think so. What I believe to be true about these hypothesized relationships is that these different areas of inquiry are getting at some universal truths about being human, but from different points of view. When we have multiple viewpoints, we can inform knowledge development because one way of looking at something can only reveal a portion of the overall truth.

Illustrating relationships among temperament, personality, and sensory processing. Following the tradition of Keogh's (1982, 1994) work, Rothbart and Jones (1999), prominent researchers on children's temperament, wrote about how to apply temperament knowledge to classroom situations. They discuss the fact that positive affect and negative affect are not anchor points on the same scale—an important point because it means that children are not "doomed" to experiencing distress and fear if they have a high degree of negative affect. Rather, studies reveal that children can have various degrees of each temperament trait; thus, they can be prone to distress or fear and still possibly experience a positive affect. This complexity in the relationships among temperament traits precludes parents and teachers from labeling children according to only one feature. Rothbart and Jones concluded that this insight enables caregivers "to accentuate the child's positive tendencies, while at the same time diminishing negative reactions that could lead to discouragement or conflict" (p. 39).

Table 51.3. Sample Items From the Temperament and Sensory Processing Questionnaires

	Temperament		Sensory Processing
Fear Negative affect	• Loud noises sometimes scare me. • Sometimes I feel a sense of panic or terror for no apparent reason.	Sensory avoiding	• I wear gloves or avoid activities that will make my hands messy. • When others get too close, I move away.
Irritability/anger Orienting sensitivity	• I often notice mild odors and fragrances. • I am often aware how the color and lighting of a room affects my mood.	Sensitivity	• I become dizzy easily (e.g., after bending over, getting up too fast). • I startle easily to unexpected or loud noises (e.g., vacuum cleaner, dog barking, telephone ring).
Surgency Positive affect	• When listening to music, I usually like to turn up the volume more than other people. • I would enjoy watching a laser show with lots of bright, colorful flashing lights.	Sensory seeking	• I enjoy being close to people who wear perfume or cologne. • I enjoy how it feels to move about (e.g., dancing, running).
Persistence Effortful attention	• I can easily resist talking out of turn, even when I'm excited and want to express an idea. • When interrupted or distracted, I usually can easily shift my attention back to whatever I was doing before.	Low registration	• I don't notice when people come into the room. • I get scrapes or bruises but don't remember how I got them.

Note. Temperament questions from the Adult Temperament Questionnaire, version 1.3, Mary Rothbart. Sensory processing questions from Adult Sensory Profile, Tana Brown and Winnie Dunn.

If we add knowledge about children's sensory processing patterns to this story, we provide caregivers information about how to make adjustments to "accentuate the child's positive tendencies" and "diminish negative reactions" and supply data about why these changes might be effective in supporting the child's performance. Sensory processing knowledge adds a level of awareness about the conditions necessary for the child to negotiate the demands of the day successfully. Rothbart and Jones (1999) gave the example of creating a clear routine for a child who is highly anxious, describing a cognitive method for helping the child to develop expectations. Sensory processing knowledge would indicate which sensory systems are likely to trigger anxious reactions (e.g., low threshold responses) and which sensory input mechanisms might be easier for the child to manage. Armed with this information, the teacher could refine instructions, routines, and guidance to minimize low threshold inputs and take advantage of less sensitive forms of sensory information. Without sensory information, the teacher might create a routine that continues to employ a sensitive sensory system and conclude that the overall approach to the problem was not effective.

Speculating about sensory processing using insights from the personality and temperament literature. Many examples just like this one illustrate the importance of interdisciplinary perspectives if we are to understand universal truths about the experience of being human. However, knowledge will not advance unless each discipline considers how other perspectives might inform its work and provide a host of questions that could not be generated from a single discipline's perspective. The fact that consistent patterns about temperament, personality, and sensory processing emerge across studies of children and adults suggests that there is insight to be had in understanding how these constructs interact with each other.

For instance, we might infer some characteristics about sensory processing (a newer line of research) from the relationships we hypothesize to exist between the more established temperament and personality literature and sensory processing. Earlier in the temperament line of research, some controversy existed about whether temperament characteristics were stable throughout life and whether early temperament characteristics predicted personality traits in adulthood (Starratt & Peterson, 1997). The now substantial body of evidence seems to illuminate two important factors. First, longitudinal studies indicate fairly high stability in personality (McCrae, Costa, & Arenberg, 1980); even studies that showed some changes reported that the fluctuations were small overall (e.g., Eysenck, 1987). Cross-sectional data on sensory processing traits provide preliminary evidence that sensory processing patterns are stable across the life span. We might hypothesize that sensory processing patterns manifest as do temperament and personality (i.e., that they also are stable across ages), although our hypothesis needs to be tested explicitly.

Second, personality and temperament researchers indicate that context can affect the manifestation of one's personality traits. Starratt and Peterson (1997) suggested that people may not express their personality traits as strongly in contexts that have variable relevance for them. Perhaps this same tendency to express traits differently across contexts also occurs with one's pattern of sensory processing. A person might construct a home environment so that it minimizes sensory experiences that are more sensitive, whereas at work the person would have to confront these sensory challenges. Starratt and Peterson also hypothesized that the expression of one's personality traits may change across the context of time. Extraverts may express themselves differently in their 20s than in their 60s. We see this same phenomenon of changes across time with the infants, toddlers, and older adults in the sensory processing data (Dunn & Daniels, 2001; Pohl et al., 2001). Perhaps a person's underlying sensory processing traits remain the same, and the demands of life at different ages expose different aspects of his or her sensory processing strategies.

Speculating about personality and temperament using insights from the sensory processing literature. We are not limited to speculating from the more established personality and temperament literature to the newer sensory processing literature. We can also speculate about developed lines of research from newer work.

Some studies have linked sensory processing to cognitive, behavioral, and psychosocial performance, suggesting that linking to temperament and personality also would be fruitful. Baranek et al. (1997a) studied sensory defensiveness and its relationship to stereotypic behaviors in children and adults with developmental disabilities. They reported a relationship between tactile defensiveness and rigid, inflexible behavior patterns. Kinnealey and Fuiek (1999) tested adults with sensory defensiveness and found that they were more anxious and depressed but did not experience more pain than their peers without defensiveness. Stephens and Royeen (1998) found an inverse relationship between self-esteem and school-aged children's responses on the Touch Inventory for Elementary Children, with increasing levels of tactile defensiveness correlated with poorer self-esteem. Parham (1998) reported changing relationships between cognitive performance at school and sensory processing; reading scores were more highly related in younger grades, whereas math performance was more highly related in later elementary grades. Kinnealey (1998) reported on a preschooler with sensory defensiveness who also had difficulty with age-appropriate learning at preschool, anxiety, and need for control, which affected her school and family relationships.

With some association between sensory processing and psychosocial and cognitive performance, we can consider how sensory processing knowledge might inform the temperament work. First, sensory processing evidence informs about how to support persons to be successful in their daily lives. Although the personality and temperament literature makes clear that certain traits are more (or less) conducive to certain situations, discussions about what to do about poorly matched situations are more general. Cohn, Miller, and Tickle-Degnen (2000) found that children want to participate in social interactions, engage in self-regulation, and perceive competence in performance. Parents in the same study reported the desire to learn strategies to support their children and to obtain personal validation for their role as parents. The authors concluded that the therapeutic process needs to center on supporting children and parents in their daily lives and natural contexts; parents need specific information to do this successfully.

Jarus and Gol (1995) found that adding kinesthetic input to skills acquisition routines improved performance in both children with and children without sensory integrative dysfunction. They hypothesized that proprioceptive information gained through kinesthesia provides body scheme information for postural control to support task performance. Stratton and Gailfus (1998) used sensory integrative approaches to address overreactivity in adolescents and adults with ADHD who were abusing substances and could not persist through the substance abuse treatment sessions. They found that the sensory integrative approach enabled the clients to take advantage of the substance abuse program. Woodbury (1997) used an auditory and visual desensitization technique with children with autism. Fewer than half could complete the intervention, but those who did could participate more adaptively. This finding suggests that we must take care in applying desensitization and that it can be effective with selected persons.

Kinnealey, Oliver, and Wilbarger (1995) found that adults with sensory defensiveness had strategies for coping with their daily lives, including avoiding aversive stimuli, imbedding predictability, preparing mentally for situations, talking themselves through situations, counteracting uncomfortable sensations, and confronting discomfort. This array of strategies suggests that intervention methods must include methods not only to resolve the sensory defensiveness, but also to manage it within daily life. These persons had insight about their sensory defensiveness, yet it was still part of their identity, suggesting that low thresholds persist across an extended period of life and, therefore, may be underlying factors to one's temperament.

Second, all the temperament and personality constructs represent types of engagement. One of the sensory processing constructs, low registration, represents lack of engagement. Perhaps lack of noticing is another facet underlying the personality–temperament traits of persistence, effortful control, and conscientiousness because without being distracted by external stimuli, persons can persist at task performance. This area may be one in which sensory processing literature can inform personality and temperament research by expanding the notion of the underlying features that enable persistence.

This construct of low engagement also has been useful in studies involving disability groups. For example, persons with schizophrenia simultaneously have low registration and sensory avoiding (Brown et al., 2001). We hypothesize that this pattern of poor noticing (low registration) and hyperresponsiveness leading to withdrawal (sensory avoiding) may reflect the small range within which these persons can receive sensory input and use it to participate successfully. These possible sensory processing relationships may provide information about applying temperament constructs to disability groups because our work has been fruitful in this area.

Third, one's sensory processing patterns seem to reflect the way a person's nervous system functions (Brown et al., 2001; McIntosh, Miller, Shyu, & Dunn, 1999; McIntosh, Miller, Shyu, & Hagerman, 1999; Miller et al., 1998); one's temperament and personality may be the behavioral manifestation of one's sensory processing patterns and nervous system functions. Thus, by knowing a person's sensory processing patterns, one can construct explicit environmental conditions and activities that support both the nervous system's functions and its temperament (e.g., enhance positive affect while minimizing negative affect).

We need to conduct studies using both sensory processing and temperament–personality measures to investigate the nature of these relationships and gain further insights. Thus far, adequate evidence suggests that these lines of investigation would be fruitful.

Application to Practice

So what does this knowledge mean for practice? The idea that one's sensory processing patterns are relatively stable across one's life creates a slippery slope for possible application to practice. One could deduce that with the view that "we are what we are," there is no reason to provide intervention because it would be futile; but this would be incorrect. Human beings have many relatively stable traits, ones that characterize both our collective humanity and our individuality, such as the way the circulatory system works or our need to be connected with other human beings. Although we might characterize our need to be connected to other human beings as a limitation, we also might consider the advantages of that need for supporting the overall human experience. I think that in knowing one's "features" we might be set free to learn, evolve, and live a satisfying life.

502

I believe that the essential gift of our sensory processing knowledge is in providing opportunities for insight. Occupational therapists have crafted an entire focus in our discipline out of coming to understand sensory processing; we have information that will inform others about the nature of their humanity. *Sensory processing patterns are reflections of who we are: These patterns are not a pathology that needs fixing.* Intervention addresses the interference between our desired life and our current performance; sensory processing knowledge can narrow this gap and reduce interference, thereby affording a satisfying life.

We must take care in sharing this gift. Sensory processing is a deeply personal experience. Because our discipline has studied sensory processing, we can offer people, families, and colleagues information about the impact of sensory processing in daily life. We must not fall into the trap of thinking that in knowing something about a person, we as therapists must set out to change it. The way a person processes sensory information is just that—the way the person processes sensory information. No way of processing sensory information is inherently good or bad—it just is. People with every pattern of sensory processing are living successfully and unsuccessfully; you are not doomed to failure if you have low registration or guaranteed success if you are a sensation seeker. A sensation seeker in an impoverished environment will flounder, whereas a sensation avoider may flourish there.

So ask yourself: What would take so much effort for me to do that I would lose myself in the process? Let us consider an example. If I find the place where you can barely hear my voice, do you see it as an opportunity to work on your listening, or do you want me to just speak up? If I just speak up, this is an adaptation to support your current auditory skills so that you can participate in the ideas being shared. People who wear glasses say that they hear better with their glasses on. Glasses do not affect hearing per se; they provide support for the load on the nervous system, making attentional resources available for hearing. Conversely, if I find the place where my voice is quite irritating, do you want me to keep it up so you can adjust your frequency range, or do you want me to tone down the screeching so you can pay attention? Your nervous system is unavailable for learning when it is in a fight-or-flight mode. Knowing about your own sensory processing patterns provides you with a method for managing daily life; knowing about your needs and limits on sensory input enables you to increase or decrease input to support your needs and yield more successful outcomes.

The primary and essential intervention using sensory processing knowledge is information. Knowledge about one's own; a family member's; or a friend's, student's, or coworker's sensory processing patterns is the most powerful tool we have to give. When people have insight about why the movie theater is so challenging, the food is so difficult to eat, the concert is too boring, or the stark bedroom is so comforting, they can generalize to other life situations and make better decisions for themselves in collaboration with your ideas. Kinnealey et al. (1995) suggested that insight and designing a sensory diet are primary ways to address sensory defensiveness in adults; Cohn and Cermak (1998) concurred, stating that educating caregivers so that they can provide a nurturing sensory environment is critical for children's outcomes.

Beyond sharing information so people can know themselves better, therapeutic intervention is only appropriate when there is something the person wants or needs to do and their way of sensory processing interferes with that aspect of living a satisfying life. Intervention must focus on living; to that end, we construct intervention options based on what is respectful and compatible with the person's life. For example, persons with low registration notice much fewer cues than others. Although we have the knowledge to construct an intensive sensory program, and persons with low registration will respond to sensory intensity and might come to notice more aspects of engagement during intense sensory stimulation, it is likely that at the end of this intensity, these persons will still have low registration. Low registration is not a problem to resolve; living a satisfying life is the challenge to address. We must use our information so that the person comes to know how to construct work and living environments and establish rituals to provide intensity routinely as a support for daily life so that he or she can be successful. Many persons have low registration; only some are struggling in their daily lives. Those who are struggling may lack insight about the nature of their sensory processing and, therefore, do not make choices that support both their sensory processing needs and the activities of interest in their lives. We have the knowledge and skills to bridge this gap.

Summary

Sensory processing is a core feature of our humanity. Understanding the nature of one's sensory processing needs provides background knowledge for constructing daily life routines and contexts that are respectful of the nervous system's need for some balance of excitation and inhibition. It is possible that sensory processing mechanisms underlie the manifestations of one's temperament and personality, and these relationships need to be tested.

References

Arciniegas, D., Adler, L., Topkoff, J., Cawthra, E., Filley, C. M., & Reite, M. (1999). Attention and memory dysfunction after traumatic brain injury: Cholinergic mechanisms, sensory gating, and a hypothesis for further investigation. *Brain Injury, 13*, 1–13.

Ayres, A. J. (1979). *Sensory integration and the child.* Los Angeles: Western Psychological Services.

Ayres, A. J. (1989). *Sensory Integration and Praxis Tests.* Los Angeles: Western Psychological Services.

Ayres, A. J., & Tickle, L. S. (1980). Hyper-responsivity to touch and vestibular stimuli as a predictor of positive response to sensory integration procedures by autistic children. *American Journal of Occupational Therapy, 34*, 375–381.

Bagnato, S. J., & Neisworth, J. T. (1999). Collaboration and teamwork in assessment for early intervention. *Child and Adolescent Psychiatric Clinics of North America, 8*, 347–363.

Baranek, G. T. (1999). Autism during infancy: A retrospective video analysis of sensory-motor and social behaviors at 9–12 months of age. *Journal of Autism and Developmental Disorders, 29*, 213–224.

Baranek, G. T., Foster, L. G., & Berkson, G. (1997a). Sensory defensiveness in persons with developmental disabilities. *Occupational Therapy Journal of Research, 17*, 173–185.

Baranek, G. T., Foster, L. G., & Berkson, G. (1997b). Tactile defensiveness and stereotyped behaviors. *American Journal of Occupational Therapy, 51*, 91–95.

Belser, R. C., & Sudhalter, V. (1995). Arousal difficulties in males with fragile X syndrome: A preliminary report. *Developmental Brain Dysfunction, 8*(4–6), 270–279.

Bensing, J., Hulsman, R., & Schreurs, K. (1999). Gender differences in fatigue: An empirical study into the biopsychosocial factors of fatigue in men and women. *Medical Care, 37*, 1078–1083.

Brown, C., & Dunn, W. (in press). *The Adult Sensory Profile.* San Antonio, TX: Psychological Corporation.

Brown, C., Tollefson, N., Dunn, W., Cromwell, R., & Filion, D. (2001). The Adult Sensory Profile: Measuring patterns of sensory processing. *American Journal of Occupational Therapy, 55*, 75–82.

Bunney, W. E. J., Hetrick, W. P., Bunney, B. G., Patterson, J. V., Jin, Y., Potkin, S. G., & Sandman, C. A. (1999). Structured Interview for Assessing Perceptual Anomalies (SIAPA). *Schizophrenia Bulletin, 25*, 577–592.

Carton, S., Morand, P., Bungenera, C., & Jouvent, R. (1995). Sensation-seeking and emotional disturbances in depression: Relationships and evolution. *Journal of Affective Disorders, 34*, 219–225.

Case-Smith, J., Butcher, L., & Reed, D. (1998). Parents' report of sensory responsiveness and temperament in preterm infants. *American Journal of Occupational Therapy, 52*, 547–555.

Caspi, A. (2000). The child is father of the man: Personality continuities from childhood to adulthood. *Journal of Personality and Social Psychology, 78*(1), 158–172.

Cermak, S. A., & Daunhaur, L. A. (1997). Sensory processing in the postinstitutionalized child. *American Journal of Occupational Therapy, 51*, 500–507.

Cohn, E. S., & Cermak, S. A. (1998). Including the family perspective in sensory integration outcomes research. *American Journal of Occupational Therapy, 52*, 540–546.

Cohn, E., Miller, L. J., & Tickle-Degnen, L. (2000). Parental hopes for therapy outcomes: Children with sensory modulation disorders. *American Journal of Occupational Therapy, 54*, 36–43.

Cooper, J., Majnemer, A., Rosenblatt, B., & Birnbaum, R. (1993). A standardized sensory assessment for children of school-age. *Physical and Occupational Therapy in Pediatrics, 13*(1), 61–80.

Coren, S., Porac, C., & Ward, L. M. (1984). *Sensation and perception* (2nd ed.). Orlando, FL: Academic Press.

Costa, P. T., & McCrae, R. R. (1987). Personality assessment in psychosomatic medicine: Value of a trait taxonomy. *Advances in Psychosomatic Medicine, 17*, 71–82.

Cromwell, R. L. (1993). A summary view of schizophrenia. In R. Cromwell & C. R. Snyder (Eds.), *Schizophrenia: Origins, processes, treatment and outcomes* (pp. 335–349). New York: Oxford University Press.

Damasio, A. (1999). *The feeling of what happens: Body and emotion in the making of consciousness.* New York: Harcourt Brace Jovanovich.

DeGangi, G. A., & Greenspan, S. I. (1989). *Test of sensory functions in infants manual.* Los Angeles: Western Psychological Services.

Denney, A. (1997). Quiet music: An intervention for mealtime agitation? *Journal of Gerontological Nursing, 23*(7), 16–23.

Dunn, W. (1997). The impact of sensory processing abilities on the daily lives of young children and families: A conceptual model. *Infants and Young Children, 9*(4), 23–25.

Dunn, W. (1998). Implementing neuroscience principles to support habilitation and recovery. In C. Christiansen & C. Baum (Eds.), *Occupational therapy: Achieving human performance needs in daily living* (pp. 182–233). Thorofare, NJ: Slack.

Dunn, W. (1999). *The Sensory Profile.* San Antonio, TX: Psychological Corporation.

Dunn, W. (2000). *The Infant Toddler Clinical Edition Sensory Profile.* San Antonio, TX: Psychological Corporation.

Dunn, W. (in press). *The Infant Toddler Sensory Profile.* San Antonio, TX: Psychological Corporation.

Dunn, W., & Bennett, D. (in press). The performance of children with ADHD on the Sensory Profile. *Occupational Therapy Journal of Research.*

Dunn, W., & Brown, C. (1997). Factor analysis on the Sensory Profile from a national sample of children without disabilities. *American Journal of Occupational Therapy, 51,* 490–495.

Dunn, W., & Daniels, D. (2001). Initial development of the Infant Toddler Sensory Profile. Manuscript submitted for publication.

Dunn, W., & Westman, K. (1997). The Sensory Profile: The performance of a national sample of children without disabilities. *American Journal of Occupational Therapy, 51,* 25–34.

Ermer, J., & Dunn, W. (1998). The Sensory Profile: A discriminant analysis of children with and without disabilities. *American Journal of Occupational Therapy, 52,* 283–290.

Eysenck, H. J. (1987). The definition of personality disorders and the criteria appropriate for their description. *Journal of Personality Disorders, 1*(3), 211–219.

Finkelman, J. M. (1994). A large database study of the factors associated with work-induced fatigue. *Human Factors, 36,* 232–243.

Fisher, A. G., Murray, E. A., & Bundy, A. C. (1991). *Sensory integration theory and practice.* Philadelphia: F. A. Davis.

Frith, C. D., Blakemore, S., & Wolpert, D. M. (2000). Explaining the symptoms of schizophrenia: Abnormalities in the awareness of action. *Brain Research Reviews, 31*(2–3), 357–363.

Gijsbers van Wijk, C. M. T., & Kolk, A. M. M. (1997a). Seksevers-chillen in gezondheidsbeleving [Sex differences in perceived health]. *Nederlands Tijdschrift Voor Geneeskunde, 141*(6), 283–287.

Gijsbers van Wijk, C. M. T., & Kolk, A. M. M. (1997b). Sex differences in physical symptoms: The contribution of symptom perception theory. *Social Science and Medicine, 45*(2), 231–246.

Glicksohn, J., & Abulafia, J. (1998). Embedding sensation seeking within the big three. *Personality and Individual Differences, 25,* 1085–1099.

Gormly, A. V. (1997). *Lifespan human development* (6th ed.). Orlando, FL: Harcourt Brace Jovanovich.

Hemsley, D. R. (1993). A simple (or simplistic?) cognitive model for schizophrenia. *Behavior Research and Therapy, 31,* 633–645.

Hotz, S. D., & Royeen, C. B. (1998). Perception of behaviours associated with tactile defensiveness: An exploration of the differences between mothers and their children. *Occupational Therapy International, 5*(4), 281–292.

Huebner, R., & Dunn, W. (2000). Introduction and basic concepts of sensorimotor approaches to autism and related disorders. In R. Huebner (Ed.), *Autism and related disorders: A sensorimotor approach to management* (pp. 3–40). Gaithersburg, MD: Aspen.

Jarus, T., & Gol, D. (1995). The effect of kinesthetic stimulation on the acquisition and retention of gross motor skill by children with and without sensory integration disorders. *Physical and Occupational Therapy in Pediatrics, 14*(3/4), 59–73.

Jin, Y., Bunney, W. E., Jr., Sandman, C. A., Patterson, J. V., Fleming, K., Moenter, J. R., Kalali, A. H., Hetrick, W. P., & Potkin, S. G. (1998). Is P50 suppression a measure of sensory gating in schizophrenia? *Biological Psychiatry, 43,* 873–878.

Johnson-Ecker, C. L., & Parham, L. D. (2000). The evaluation of sensory processing: A validity study using contrasting groups. *American Journal of Occupational Therapy, 54,* 494–503.

Kandel, E., Schwartz, J., & Jessell, T. (2000). *Principles of neural science.* New York: McGraw-Hill.

Keogh, B. (1982). Children's temperament and teacher's decision. In R. Porter & G. Collins (Eds.), *Temperamental differences in infants and young children* (pp. 269–278). London: Pitman.

Keogh, B. (1994). Temperament and teachers' views of teachability. In W. Carey & S. McDevitt (Eds.), *Prevention and early intervention: Individual differences as risk factors for the mental health of children* (pp. 246–256). New York: Brunner/Mazel.

Kientz, M. A., & Dunn, W. (1997). Comparison of the performance of children with and without autism on the Sensory Profile. *American Journal of Occupational Therapy, 51,* 530–537.

Kimball, J. G. (1986). Prediction of methylphenidate (Ritalin) responsiveness through sensory integrative testing. *American Journal of Occupational Therapy, 40,* 241–248.

Kinnealey, M. (1998). Princess or tyrant: A case report of a child with sensory defensiveness. *Occupational Therapy International, 5*(4), 293–303.

Kinnealey, M., & Fuiek, M. (1999). The relationship between sensory defensiveness, anxiety, depression, and perception of pain in adults. *Occupational Therapy International, 6*(3), 195–206.

Kinnealey, M., Oliver, B., & Wilbarger, P. (1995). A phenomenological study of sensory defensiveness in adults. *American Journal of Occupational Therapy, 49,* 444–451.

Lai, J., Parham, D., & Johnson-Ecker, C. (1999, December). Sensory dormancy and sensory defensiveness: Two sides of the same coin? *Sensory Integration Special Interest Section Quarterly, 22,* 1–4.

Larson, K. A. (1982). The sensory history of developmentally delayed children with and without tactile defensiveness. *American Journal of Occupational Therapy, 36,* 590–596.

Light, G. A., & Braff, D. L. (2000). Do self-reports of perceptual anomalies reflect gating deficits in schizophrenia patients? *Biological Psychiatry, 47,* 463–467.

Madigan, N. K., DeLuca, J., Diamond, B. J., Tramontano, G., & Averill, A. (2000). Speed of information processing in traumatic brain injury: Modality-specific factors. *Journal of Head Trauma Rehabilitation, 15,* 943–956.

McCrae, R. R., Costa, P. T., Jr., & Arenberg, D. (1980). Constancy of adult personality structure in males: Longitudinal, cross-sectional and times-of-measurement analyses. *Journal of Gerontology, 35,* 877–883.

McGhie, A., & Chapman, J. (1961). Disorders of attention and perception in early schizophrenia. *British Journal of Medical Psychology, 34,* 103–116.

McIntosh, D. N., Miller, L. J., Shyu, V., & Dunn, W. (1999). Overview of the Short Sensory Profile (SSP). In W. Dunn (Ed.), *The Sensory Profile* (pp. 59–74). San Antonio, TX: Psychological Corporation.

McIntosh, D., Miller, L., Shyu, V., & Hagerman, R. (1999). Sensory modulation disruption, electrodermal responses and functional behaviors. *Developmental Medicine and Child Neurology, 41,* 608–615.

Miller, L., McIntosh, D., McGrath, J., Shyu, V., Lampe, M., Taylor, A., Tassone, F., Neitzel, K., Stackhouse, T., & Hagerman, R. (1998). Electrodermal responses to sensory stimuli in individuals with fragile X syndrome: A preliminary report. *American Journal of Medical Genetics, 83*(4), 268–279.

Parham, L. D. (1998). The relationship of sensory integrative development to achievement in elementary students: Four-year longitudinal patterns. *Occupational Therapy Journal of Research, 18,* 105–127.

Pohl, P., Dunn, W., & Brown, C. (2001). *Interacting with sensory information from daily life: The Sensory Profile of Older Adults.* Manuscript submitted for publication.

Provost, B., & Oetter, P. (1993). The sensory rating scale for infants and young children: Development and reliability. *Physical and Occupational Therapy in Pediatrics, 13*(4), 15–35.

Ragneskog, H., & Kihlgren, M. (1997). Music and other strategies to improve the care of agitated patients with dementia: Interviews with experienced staff. *Scandinavian Journal of Caring Sciences, 11*(3), 176–182.

Rijk, A. E., Schreurs, K. M. G., & Bensing, J. M. (1999). Complaints of fatigue: Related to too much as well as too little external stimulation? *Journal of Behavioral Medicine, 22,* 549–573.

Rothbart, M. K., Ahadi, S. A., & Evans, D. E. (2000). Temperament and personality: Origins and outcomes. *Journal of Personality and Social Psychology, 78*(1), 122–135.

Rothbart, M., & Derryberry, D. (1981). Development of individual differences in temperament. In M. Lamb & A. Brown (Eds.), *Advances in developmental psychology* (Vol. 1, pp. 37–86). Hillsdale, NJ: Erlbaum.

Rothbart, M., Derryberry, D., & Hershey, K. (2000). Stability of temperament in childhood: Laboratory infant assessment to parent report at seven years. In V. Molfese & D. Molfese (Eds.), *Temperament and personality development across the life span* (pp. 85–140). London: Erlbaum.

Rothbart, M. K., & Jones, L. B. (1999). Temperament: Developmental perspectives. In R. Gallimore, L. Bernheimer, & T. Weisner (Eds.), *Developmental perspectives on children with high-incidence disabilities. The LEA series on special education and disability* (pp. 33–53). Mahwah, NJ: Erlbaum.

Royeen, C. B., & Fortune, J. C. (1990). Touch Inventory for Elementary-School-Aged Children. *American Journal of Occupational Therapy, 44,* 155–159.

Sarmany-Schuller, I. (1999). Procrastination, need for cognition and sensation seeking. *Studia Psychologica, 41*(1), 73–85.

Shumway-Cook, A., & Woollacott, M. (2000). Attentional demands and postural control: The effect of sensory context. *Journal of Gerontology: Medical Sciences, 55A*(1), M10–M16.

Starratt, C., & Peterson, L. (1997). Personality and normal aging. In P. D. Nussbaum (Ed.), *Handbook of neuropsychology and aging: Critical issues in neuropsychology* (pp. 15–31). New York: Plenum.

Stephens, C. L., & Royeen, C. B. (1998). Investigation of tactile defensiveness and self-esteem in typically developing children. *Occupational Therapy International, 5*(4), 273–280.

Stratton, J., & Gailfus, D. (1998). A new approach to substance abuse treatment: Adolescents and adults with ADHD. *Journal of Substance Abuse Treatment, 15*(2), 89–94.

Venables, P. H. (1969). Sensory aspects of psychopathology. *Proceedings of the Annual Meeting of the American Psychopathological Association, 58,* 132–143.

Wiener, A. S., Long, T., DeGangi, G., & Battaile, B. (1996). Sensory processing of infants born prematurely or with regulatory disorders. *Physical and Occupational Therapy in Pediatrics, 16*(4), 1–17.

Woodbury, P. P. (1997). Students with autism: A light/sound technology intervention. *Dissertation Abstracts International Section A: Humanities and Social Sciences, 57*(11-A), 4651.

Zuckerman, M. (1994). *Behavioral expressions and biosocial bases of sensation seeking.* New York: Cambridge University Press.

Zuckerman, M., Ulrich, R. S., & McLaughlin, J. (1993). Sensation seeking and reactions to nature paintings. *Personality and Individual Differences, 15,* 563–576.

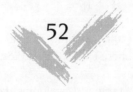

52

2003 Eleanor Clarke Slagle Lecture

Chaotic Occupational Therapy:
Collective Wisdom for a Complex Profession

Charlotte Brasic Royeen, PhD, OTR, FAOTA

The Telling of a Trip[1]

Let's go on a trip with nary a dip, until we reach the tip of 2003.
  The year of the she.
Don't let yourself flip and be a good pip, while I let myself quip. All of it free.
The year of the three. Habits of the mind, habits of the heart, and habits of the art.
The habit of three. Freedom within art, using daily actions of mind and heart.
  Just do your part.
Engage in thee.

In her Eleanor Clarke Slagle lecture, Brunyate (1957) quotes from Ms. Slagle's 1920 Presidential Address, stating, "this happens to be my turn" (p. 195). And so it is. I thank you for the honor. Sincere appreciation is extended to those among you, especially the American Occupational Therapy Foundation (AOTF), who have helped to raise this scholar, as well as to my dear friends and beloved family. As Cokie Roberts (2003) suggested in her opening ceremony address and in her book (1998), we are our mothers' daughters. In recognition of her supposition, please acknowledge my mother Harriet Schmudde Brasic Bound Pewitt. This telling is dedicated to the memories of Paula Flanders Amphlett and Robert Bing.

In order to get real, you have to be surreal.[2] Time is relative and wrinkled (Hawking, 1993). Nearly 100 years ago our foremothers formed the National Society for the Promotion of Occupational Therapy, the precursor of the American Occupational Therapy Association (AOTA). Ten years ago Florence Clark (1993) presented her Eleanor Clarke Slagle lecture (henceforth referred to as a Slagle), using "the genre of interpretative occupational science" that had implications for occupational therapy (p. 1067). It is only fitting that I take from something nearly 100 years ago, and from something 10 years ago, and using a space-time singularity—better known as a wormhole or a wrinkle in time (L'Engle, 1962)—wrinkle or fold them into equivalent and corresponding forms as a profession, occupational therapy, and as a discipline, occupational science.[3] Yet, within the telling of 10 and 100, I have a wrinkle of my own.

Chaucer referred to "lyfe so short, the craft so long to lerne." Besides life being too short, occupational therapy is that craft that I have labored to love and learn for 31 years. Just now I am beginning to discern its true self; the authentic occupational therapy of Yerxa's (1966) Slagle—a craft so long to learn.

Per Ursula K. LeGuin (2000), I shall do a telling—to perform, to act, to tell—hoping to dispel the surreal separation of intellect and passion presumed by Western civilization since the time of Descartes (1596–1650) based upon Plato (428–347 B.C.) and Socrates (469–399 B.C.). As the communications theorist Marshall McLuhan

Originally published 2003 in *American Journal of Occupational Therapy, 57,* 609–624.
Please note that there was no Eleanor Clarke Slagle Lecture in 2002.

(1911–1980) wrote, "the medium is the message" (McLuhan & Fiore, 2001) and as occupational therapy plays forth,[4] the medium is the message. Such is true for many levels of meanings in this Slagle lecture as well as most everything in daily life. Chaos theory provides the challenge of finding order, or levels of meanings, within apparent disorder. Since King (1978) in her Slagle stated that doing with meaning promotes individual adaptation, I leave that for you to do, as part of art.

I shall endeavor to practice the craft of occupational therapy today, with a blend of science, heart, and art: having two foci. One is on *herstory* or the pattern that connects. The other focus is on theory, a missing link, the invisible theoretical model, which we have implicitly known, embraced, and envisioned without explicitly knowing, namely, chaotic occupational therapy. I request that you review the emotional experiences you undergo during this telling. Thus, in the end I will challenge you to enact meta-emotion of occupation, an evolving concept based upon occupation, related—in part—to Fine's (1991) import regarding response of feelings about a situation in her Slagle.

Herstory and Professional Identity Founded Upon Occupation

Occupational therapy emerged as a health profession in the 1910s, incorporating the mind, body, and spirit in a holistic approach to health. Unlike other professions, however, we have had a challenge explaining what constituted occupational therapy since its inception (Quiroga, 1995), being what Primeau, Clark, and Pierce (1989) called the "invisible profession." Let us temper occupation with a simple technical analysis, a tangible treatment of occupation having tassels of terms for the populace. The Tetralogy of Occupation is such a tempering. The Tetralogy of Occupation,[5] which may help ameliorate our tautology[6] concerning occupation, consists of four simple concepts:[7] (a) purposeful activity, (b) activity plus meaning, (c) doing with meaning, with (d) participation in context.

Note that fundamental to the Tetralogy of Occupation is the decision to most appropriately consider occupation as a process, and not a product. Such an action takes exception to our profession's long-standing tainting tautology when talking about occupation in a dual manner—as a means and as an end. Trombly (1995) discussed occupation in this manner in her Slagle: occupation-as-end or goal and occupation-as-means or change agent. The issue was evident at an occupational therapy research consensus conference (Hasselkus, 2000). Dual use of the term is confusing to external audiences. Metaphorically speaking, one simply cannot have one's cake and eat it too! Thus, let us give up the cake by eating it, and focus upon occupation as a process, or occupation as means (Rebeiro & Cook, 1999), thereby minimizing the confusion that ambiguous use of the word purveys.

Additionally, being a bit of a wit, rather than reinventing the wheel, I looked to the past or *herstory* to find wheels or word forces of others that well-illustrate, in this manner, occupation as process or occupation for the populace. In presenting a framework for activity as an intervention in her Slagle, Allen (1987) stated that, "Activity actualizes a person's strengths" (p. 573). In her Slagle, Johnson (1973) specifically referred to occupational therapy as a process wherein ". . . man learns to make decisions about the quality and style of life he seeks to achieve and to influence his health" (p. 3).

In the same manner that Christiansen (1999) linked personal self-esteem to the development of personal identity in his Slagle, armed with professional identities created by (a) the Tetralogy of Occupation, (b) knowledge of occupation as process, and (c) the sage words of our foremothers, we have the tools necessary to further enhance our professional self-esteem and related professional identity. Armed accordingly, we shall lift off from the tarmac of timidity and go boldly forth where no occupational therapists, and no occupational scientists, have gone before. Our target is not to take down the axis of evil, but rather, using what Huss (1977) referred to in her Slagle as "a caring touch," to build the axis of good in service to society, consistent with our professional origins in a fourth professional identity of values (i.e., moral roots). Our moral roots are what Reed (1986) called humanism in her Slagle; Bing (1981) called moral treatment[8] in his Slagle; Grady (1995) called active participation in her Slagle; and Wilcock (2000) called occupational justice.

The fundamental worth of these sentiments was well-articulated by Stattel (1956) in her Slagle, ". . . [W]e have been given a wonderful professional heritage of courage and wisdom and as we continue to extend our hand to the benefit of mankind, may we continue to believe and search for further knowledge" (p. 194).

The timeless values of our past provide a solid foundation for the professional identity of occupational therapy in the present and henceforth. In order to move forward, thus, we shall go back for the future.

Back for the Future

In her Slagle, Jantzen (1974) stated that receipt of the Eleanor Clarke Slagle lecture award was established by AOTA in 1954 to honor Ms. Slagle (1876–1942). According to Wegg (1960) in her Slagle, "Ms. Slagle is recognized as a pioneer occupational therapist who established principles of occupational therapy for the advancement of the field" (p. 65). Ms. Slagle did innovative work in habit training, program implementation (Serrett, 1985), and served in leadership roles in AOTA (Meyer, 1937).

In her Slagle, Sokolov (1957) was "awed by the honor of being an Eleanor Clarke Slagle lecturer" (p. 13). In 2002, when I was daunted by this honor, I reverted to my habit training in order to cope. A scholar's habit training includes historical review and immersion in original literature, so I found myself, for the latter part of 2002, sitting in the archives of the AOTF under the tutelage of Ms. Mary Binderman, librarian extraordinaire![9] And, as Eleanor Clarke Slagle wrote to William R. Dutton, "You may know that I did not fool away many minutes" (correspondence 1929–1937 of Dutton & Slagle). Sitting in the archives with my white, cotton gloves and sharpened, number-two pencils (graciously provided by Ms. Binderman),[10] I spent many an afternoon reading through the original correspondence of Ms. Slagle.[11]

- First, the lyricism of writings of that era has been lost.
- Second, politics are politics—meaning how you do and do not get along with people to accomplish a goal—whether it is the early 1900s or now, remain constant.
- Third, Eleanor Clarke Slagle, as did many others, believed in occupation as a process and occupational therapy as a service to society.
- Fourth, Eleanor Clarke Slagle believed that a college degree is a desirable prerequisite for occupational therapists (correspondence of Eleanor Clarke Slagle, 1925–1929; The National Society for the Promotion of Occupational Therapy, Annual Meetings, 1917–1924). So, in our current move to postbaccalaureate level entry we have finally caught up to the standards Eleanor Clarke Slagle expected in 1920 and 1934.

Personally, I have no doubts that were Ms. Slagle still with us, she would advocate for education at the doctoral level of entry for occupational therapists. Action toward this goal might be a step towards, what Fiorentino (1975) in her Slagle talked about as "the need to change in order to establish the profession of occupational therapy" (p. 19). I think the clinical doctorate is another step in the development of our profession.[12] I believe that we must move to a doctoral level of entry if we are to remain a viable profession delivering health and human services. Remember Chaucer's line: "lyfe so short, the craft so long to lerne."

The fifth and single most profound discovery, for me, was the Standards of the National Society for the Promotion of Occupational Therapy set forth in 1925. These standards, I believe, reflect the craft it has taken me over a quarter of a century to really learn—the art, heart, and science of occupational therapy. Paraphrasing a handwritten note from Dr. Robert Bing in the AOTA archives, these 15 standards or principles were developed by an AOTA committee of physicians, chaired by William R. Dutton, finally presented in 1925 but never officially adopted by AOTA (The National Society for the Promotion of Occupational Therapy. Annual Meetings, 1917–1924). The principles were published in *Occupational Therapy and Rehabilitation,* a precursor of *The American Journal of Occupational Therapy (AJOT),* in August 1925 as part of a lecture outline on occupational therapy for medical students and physicians (Bing, 1981). I have taken poetic license and adapted these timeless principles of occupational therapy as a focus forward for 2025. They have been translated to language of our current time and culture, and are presented in Figure 52.1.

1. Occupation is a process of participation in meaningful activity to promote quality of life and health.
2. Goals of engagement in occupation include social participation, self-esteem, self-efficacy, health and wellness, mitigation of the effects of disease or injury or both, flow, and capacity for engagement in fulfilling life roles as well as societal responsibility and membership.
3. In applying occupational therapy, three main areas are of concern:
   a. *Habits of the Mind:* Use of scientific methods including evidence-based care, theoretical foundations, and clinical reasoning.
   b. *Habits of the Heart:* The virtues of doing good, including care, compassion, as well as kindness, and a humanistic approach.
   c. *Habits of the Art:* The art of practice including therapeutic use of self, refinement of intuition, and noncognitive actions.
4. Occupational therapy service must be administered under the supervision of a licensed or fully certified occupational therapist, and must be delivered in a manner consistent with the highest standards for and reflective of best practices regarding interprofessional collaboration and communication.
5. Occupational therapy is founded upon an individual's or population's needs, interests, culture, and idiosyncratic characteristics.
6. Occupational therapy practice may extend from individuals to populations. And occupational therapy practice should occur in natural environments with either individuals or groups. The advantage of group work is value added in terms of interpersonal and psychosocial interactions and feedback in situ for generalizability.
7. Any activity in which a client chooses to engage should be within the zone of the just right challenge: within their skills, interests, and abilities.
8. All activities in which a client chooses to engage should be regularly graded and adapted to assure flow, challenge, and change.
9. The most valid outcome measure of occupational therapy intervention is the effect it has on the client—the value it has for the client—and his or her familial or social systems or both.
10. Regardless of the unique characteristics a client may present, ranging from disablement or despair to disease or societal conditions, from the occupational therapist, usual and customary standards of care, standards of performance, as well as moral behavior, should be expected in the therapeutic encounter.
11. During meta-emotion of occupation, or thinking or feeling about thinking or feeling while doing with meaning, various perceptions may be desired—depending upon circumstances—including flow, joy, and happiness.
12. Novelty, variety, individual or group meaning or both, social, and cultural value all influence the occupational process in which one engages, with observable activity as the outcome.
13. Financial gain or conflict of interest or conflict of commitment should never interfere with virtues of occupational therapy practice or any partner (client, therapist, family member) involved.
14. All occupational therapists must be proficient in patient education. They should further be expert in therapeutic use of self and matching their psychosocial style to the client or family member needs.
15. All forms of the process of doing with meaning constitute engagement in the process of occupation. Thus, the scope of occupational therapy is holistic, widespread, and integrated into most all human functions as reflected in the Occupational Therapy Practice Framework, and is an entitlement of all humans in the form of occupational justice.

Figure 52.1. 1925–2025 occupational therapy's legacy of humanistic ways, occupational justice, and timeless truths.

In her Slagle, Hollis (1979) stated that "none of us has any idea what the world, and specifically occupational therapy, will be like in 2020 A.D." (p. 499). Her statement holds true for 2025 as well: We cannot presume to know what the world will be like then. But, as Bing (1981) suggested, we can and should consider old values "such as these principles" as "we chart new directions" (p. 514), and I suggest we continue to explore these values through what Mosey (1985) in her Slagle termed "philosophical inquiry" (p. 505).

This fractal piece of *herstory* presents us with principles and patterns that provide a framework for the future, built on the past. Thus, we have gone back to the past to encapsulate a vision or focus forward for the future. The care and enactment of the principles so presented relates to three areas of habits in occupational therapy, corresponding to the scientific, ethical, and artistic dimensions of clinical reasoning suggested by Rogers (1983, p. 616) in her Slagle. I propose that three habit areas for occupational therapy are habits of the mind, habits of the heart, and habits of the art.

Habits of the Mind (the Scientist)[13]

These are based upon use of scientific evidence, theory, and clinical reasoning, what Rogers (1983) referred to as systematic and the scientist's way of thinking. Included herein would also be what Grady referred to as the science of occupation (1992, p. 584). Further included herein would be the call for scientific evidence about the effects of practice, what Holm (2000) discussed as the mandate for evidence-based practice in her Slagle.

Habits of the Heart[14] (the Ethicist)

These habits pertain to the morality of doing good, caring, compassion, and humanism, what Rogers (1983) referred to as responsive and the ethicist's way of thinking. This is a particular form of ethical theory called virtue ethics.

Habits of the Art (the Artist)

These habits relate to use of creativity and intuition, surrealism, and the therapeutic use of self, which further relates to what Rogers (1983) identified as convincing as well as the artist's way of thinking. She summarized it well, stating, "Artistry involves the orchestration of broad strategies for grappling effectively with the uncertainties inherent in clinical practice" (p. 614). And, it also pertains to what Grady (1992) identified as "the purposefulness of occupation will always remain as our art" (p. 584). Much of the work of Peloquin (Abreu, Peloquin, & Ottenbacher, 1998; Peloquin, 1989, 1996, 1997, 2001, 2002) speaks to this neglected area of appreciation.

In a seminal Slagle, Finn (1972) identified that imagination has been dulled in the technological society of today. And, that "it is this process of creative thinking which is required of us, as occupational therapists, in order to interpret our knowledge about human potential, growth and development . . . so that it becomes functional materials for developing . . . the health of a community" (p. 63).

According to Manthey (1997), mutual respect or respect between people is built upon individual respect, or respect for oneself. Let us respect our profession and revel in our cherished and honorable past principles that wrinkle in time across 1925 to 2025. By honoring our profession's timeless truths, we have potential for individual self-respect so important for mutual respect; required for interprofessional practice; essential to build an axis of good in service to society. In her Slagle, Dunn (2001) argued for "the importance of interdisciplinary perspectives if we are to understand . . . truths about the experience of being human (p. 615). Only with individualized and mutual respect can this be accomplished. Remember that a single bangle does not jangle.[15]

Now that we have looked to the past, let us look to what else may be a key for our future. In her Slagle, West (1968) stated, "Let us turn, then, from any comfortable reflection on our past to the infinitely more exciting exercise of projecting our future" (p. 10). I shall share with you a piece of my own. For Grady (1992) states, "above all, vision means seeing possibilities" (p. 1062).

A Piece of My Own for Occupational Science and Occupational Therapy

Possibilities. . . . I propose chaos theory as a missing link to help integrate our science and our profession. It can assist in integrating the tenuous tangle of tangents of occupation into a whole, tolerant of Mosey's (1985) pluralistic approach to the profession using many theories, frames of reference, and technologies. Chaos theory has research implications for the discipline and allows for a technical analysis of occupation, which, heretofore, we have been slow to address. It is high time to move from the lens of linearity to the kaleidoscope of chaos in occupational science and occupational therapy. As charged by Henderson (1988) in her Slagle, "We must recognize the importance of theory in the growth of professional knowledge. We must see theory building as something we *can* do, and each of us must accept responsibility for our part in theory development" (p. 574). I suspect that we shall be the Dadaists of linearity.

Occupation as a concept is undergoing a scholarly renaissance for which occupational science has served as a catalyst (Wilcock, 2002; Yerxa, 2000). I shall add to the scholarly discourse on occupational science by elaborating on occupation using chaos theory, extending Yerxa's authentic occupational therapy into chaotic occupational therapy and responding to Henderson's charge. According to Whewell (1847/1967), in the early phases of a discipline, struggle with definitions, conceptualizations, and key constructs pertaining to that discipline are part of the method of science. Kuhn[16] (1962/1970) reiterated this, as well as many other concepts in 1962 and 1970 in his book, *The Structure of Scientific Revolutions*. So, in our struggle to define and refine, we as a profession and as a discipline are perfectly normal. Thank goodness!

Chaos Theory

Chaos theory, as used here, refers to dynamical systems or the interwoven forces and motions of nonlinear systems. The science of chaos, or chaos theory, purports that chaos is a form of order disguised as disorder (Coffey, 1998). That is, chaos theory suggests that even in cases of extreme disorder, what appears as chaos actually has an underlying pattern or order. Just as I hope this complex telling does. Thus, what might appear as chaos, indeed, typically has an underlying order—if only we could discern, understand, or "see" it.

Why is chaos theory important? First, according to Pediani (1996) as based upon Coppa (1993), chaos theory is important because scientific models may be limited in their use for understanding and predicting complex relationships thereby identifying the limits of the ability of humans to predict. Second, in a sense, chaos theory is postmodernism coming to science and to occupational therapy (Royeen & Luebben, 2002). In medicine, the limits of prediction and knowing, closely linked to chaos theory as a metaphor for the limits of knowing, have been the source of hot debate (Goodwin, 1997; Theodooropoulous, 1998). And the debate occurs within one of "the last bastions of the modernist belief that all things are potentially knowable" (Goodwin, p. 1399), which relates to human beings and their sins of arrogance: How can we presume to know all things? Might chaos theory assist us in our challenge to describe human occupation in context over time?

Third, the reductionistic approach of breaking a system into component parts is being replaced with a dynamical approach of looking at how systems function (Shepperd, 1996) *in situ* or *in toto* or both. Simply put, using a gestalt view that the working whole is greater than the sum of the parts calls for a chaotic approach to analysis. This is a holistic approach to which occupational therapy has long laid claim. By understanding and using chaos theory, we may begin to address, among many things, how and why we occupational therapists do holistic practice. We may do so in a manner similar to how Buell and Cassidy (2001) use chaos theory to understand the nature of quality of care in early childhood education, or how Collins (2001) used chaos and complexity theories to explore self awareness in human adaptation.

Chaos theory is based on the work of many individuals from diverse fields. Related to dynamical system theories or nonlinear dynamics and complexity science (Plexus Institute, 2003), however, chaos theory is based—in part—on the work of Prigogone and Stengers (1984), in which they noted that changing patterns of organization were apparent from liquids at boiling point.[17] Much of the interest in more recent developments regarding chaos theory can be traced to the work of the meteorologist Lorenz, who first postulated something termed sensitivity to initial conditions as characteristic of chaos theory. Sensitivity to initial conditions refers to a unique configuration of the interactions of multiple variables in multiple systems, such that the initial conditions are so complex and variable that the eventual outcome of their interactions cannot be predicted. This explains why long-range weather forecasting, more than 4 to 5 days, is not possible—the sensitivity of initial conditions is simply too complex to reliably predict specific outcomes. Is human engagement in occupation in context across time any less complex than the weather?

Related to the concept of sensitivity to initial conditions is the concept of the butterfly effect as postulated by Lorenz in 1960s, delineating sensitivity to initial conditions such that a butterfly flapping its wings in the Amazon can change the path of a tornado in Texas (Warren, Franklin, & Streeter, 1998). Certainly, we can predict generalities such as in the northern hemisphere, it is hotter in the summer and cooler in the winter. We cannot, however, reliably predict specific complexities about a specific individual. So much for evidence-based practice as a mantra![18] At some point in application, our science must give way to the heart and art for the practice of occupational therapy.

Since World War II, chaos theory has developed out of dynamical systems theory, which has replaced general systems theory as a dominant scientific paradigm (Abraham, 1994; Remer, 1996; Warren et al., 1998). Chaos theory transcends disciplinary boundaries and has been extended from basic sciences into the social sciences including ecology, sociology, sociometry, and psychology (Abraham & Gilgen, 1995; Remer, 1996; Thelen & Smith, 1994). Now is the time for chaos to also permeate occupational science and occupational therapy.

A Fractal View of Chaos Theory

Five key assumptions underlie chaotic systems. I summarize each of these assumptions briefly in turn.

Interactions Between and Among Variables Are Nonlinear

Western culture is based upon underlying assumptions about linear relationships between variables. Assuming linearity, for every increment in variable "x," there is a proportionate increase in variable "y." The fundamental assumption of linearity permeates Western society, ranging from increases in class time and schooling in order to improve student achievement, to the predominate use of parametric statistics in research, to diets based upon decreased caloric intake to decrease weight. Chaos theory rejects such notions of linearity and, instead, is predicated upon complex, nonlinear relationships among variables. Has the intervention outcome trajectory of a client with whom you have worked ever been linear?

Variables Co-Effect One Another and Are Interdependent

In chaos theory, there is no such thing as independence. Instead, just as in real life, all things are related to all other things in some manner, but not in a linear relationship. Take, for example, the concept of wind and rock. Wind will wear down a rock through the centuries, and the rock will redirect the wind patterns. The variables, the wind and the rock, co-effect each other. Neither is isolated from the other, but is interdependent in terms of existence. Does not an occupational therapist and her client exist in an interdependent, co-effecting manner creating a *herstory*?

Chaotic Systems Exist in Far-From Equilibrium States of Flux or Turbulence

Chaotic systems, or those systems not in evident order or regularity, do not exist in equilibrium (where forces are equal and cancel each other out). Rather, they exist in states where forces are not equal—the edge of chaos. Consequently, flux or turbulence (disturbance) is created within the system. The classic example of this chaotic state is weather, which is forever changing. Is this not also true of the healthy human condition?

Chaotic Systems Are Self-Guided, Self-Organizing, Nonhierarchically Based, and Demonstrate Emergent Behavior

Chaotic systems are thought to organize or, in some manner, order themselves as they emerge and evolve. And they are not based upon a single authority or power controlling the rest of the system. Rather, a collection of forces come together and intrinsically guide the overall organization of the system. One may consider the interplay of genetic predisposition, environmental experiences, occupational participation, and emotional tone as—in part—the collection of forces that organize in an individual human to create a unique person.

Chaotic Systems Possess an Underlying Order

In spite of apparent disorder or randomness, associated chaotic systems are thought to possess an underlying order. Consider the desk of someone writing a paper. Piles are generally everywhere, notes scattered about, and a view of disorder usually reigns. But the author typically knows the underlying order of what information is in which pile, and how to access a particular nugget. The order is there, if one knows or understands the system behind it. Chaotic systems are like that. Life is like that. Occupational therapy is like that.

I shall now present a telling about occupation in six parts, evolving out of my own understanding of chaos and occupation. Many of these ideas are not new, rather the "newness lies in formulation of the idea" (Stattel, 1956, p. 194).

Charlotte's Web of Chaos

I shall put forth provisional constructs about occupation using chaos theory. Indulge me while I pay homage to E. B. White and call it Charlotte's Web of Chaos presented in Figure 52.2.

These constructs are related and interacting layers of occupational (a) complexity, (b) patterns and metapatterns, (c) process, (a) shaping, (e) variance, and (f) transience. I put these forth as an invitation to scrutinize that which could evolve to be our mainstay: an analysis of the web of occupation.

Occupational Complexity[19]

Occupational complexity refers to the many variables or processes that influence or co-effect one another within the many contexts in which occupation occurs (Dunn, Brown, & McGuigan, 1994), including adaptation (Frank, 1996), flow (Csikszentmihalyi, 1990), meaning (Christiansen, 1994), motivation and volition (Kielhofner, 1995), occupational identity (Christiansen, 1999), occupational appeal and intactness (Pierce, 1998), and intentionality

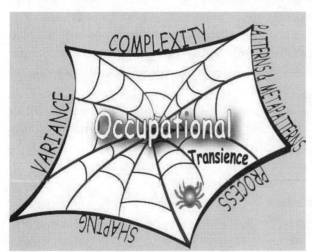

Figure 52.2. Charlotte's Web of Chaos.

and meaning of occupational engagement (Crabtree, 1998; Jackson, 1996; Magnus, 2001; Pierce, 1998; Zemke & Clark, 1996). Using the 1995 AOTA position paper, Golledge (1998) suggests that an emphasis on the dimensions (performance, contextual, temporal, psychological, social, symbolic, and spiritual) of occupation reflects occupational complexity. Wilcock's theory of the need for human occupation (Wilcock, 2002) including theological need and sociocultural factors might be an analogous way to view occupational complexity.

In linking such complexity to chaos theory, occupational complexity transcends a parallel distributed processing system, wherein dimensions of occupation consist of systems or networks, or webs, which are heterarchially (Spitzer, 1999) arranged into an overall system. As used here, occupational complexity refers to the interaction of variables (dimensions) within one of these systems, as well as to the dynamical interaction of multiple systems undergirding occupation within a given person. Thus, I hypothesize that three networks of systems, that is, internal occupational processes (the brain), occupational performance (the body), and occupational contexts (the environment) comprise or encompass the dynamical systems of occupation for which any or all of these networks, or webs, or subcomponents of networks may be control parameters thereby illustrating the dynamics of neuro-occupation. Any of the individual dimensions of occupation may be control parameters. Control parameters refer to key variables that, if changed or varied, influence (not control) the entire operation of the occupational system(s), or webs.

To illustrate, we know that if we vary a control parameter such as volition (psychological) through use of a reinforcement system, occupational performance can be changed. Further, if we vary context, the occupational performance is affected and consequently changed. Thus, variation of key control variables manipulates or changes the operation of the systems or of the entire system, or the occupational complexity (neuro-occupation), of that individual. Neuro-occupation, a term coined by Padilla and Peyton (1997) and used by others (Gutman & Biel, 2001; Howell, 1999; Lohman & Royeen, 2002; Walloch, 1998; Way, 1999) refers to the interactive, interdependent development or symbiosis between the human nervous system and engagement in occupation. Many Slagle lecturers such as Ayres (1963) and Farber (1989) foreshadowed the concept of neuro-occupation in discussing the effect of atypical nervous system activity upon human performance whereas others, such as Reilly (1962), emphasized the reverse, or the effect of purposeful human activity upon health. The concept of neuro-occupation integrates the two approaches into a single, emerging interfield theory as defined by Bechtel (1998).[20]

Occupational Patterns and Metapatterns

The patterns of occupation—occupational forms (Nelson, 1997) or designs—shape and form our lives. Occupational patterns refer to the design or configuration of occupations or proto-occupations in a human or primate (Fortune, 1996; Wood, Towers, & Malchow, 2000). I hypothesize that occupational patterns are, in and of themselves, chaotic systems that are self-organizing, self-guided and, in states of health, far from equilibrium. And, the personal meaning of our occupational patterns constitutes occupational identity as suggested by Christiansen (1999).

Patterns overall "tend to repeat themselves not exactly, not perfectly, but still enough to be recognized" (Remer, 1996). Clark (1997) has hypothesized that patterns of occupation should be identifiable and discernible regarding which patterns will promote health. I further hypothesize that additional occupational patterns can also be identifiable such as (1) those not conducive to health, (2) those promoting disease, or (3) those putting one at risk for injury, (4) those promoting joy, and (5) those promoting happiness or contentment.

If chaos is, indeed, order disguised as disorder, the challenge to occupational science and occupational therapy is to discern the pattern of occupations giving rise to varying conditions or states such as health, disease, injury, or happiness. In theory, occupational patterns apply to individuals across the lifespan. Our myopia, however, may prevent our ability to discern patterns while we are in the midst of them. Only by larger picture "gestalts" can occupational patterns be discerned. One needs either a view over time (longitudinal) or across dimensions (fractal geometry) to see how pieces or fractals or bits contribute to the larger "whole" or intact pattern.

To illustrate, just as one may need a psychologist or psychotherapist to discern psychological patterns behind behaviors of an individual, an occupational therapist may be needed to discern occupational patterns characterizing the person's unique manifestation of activities of daily living, leisure, work, parenting, and stress-release activities. To illustrate, Clark (1997) referenced understanding of an occupation to past, present, and future events.

As used by Clark (1997), the temporality of occupational patterns refers to the ability to see the design of occupations over a given time, what Bateson (1996) refers to as composition. Occupational patterns, however, may also be metapatterns (e.g., groups of bits in routines or configurations of occupations by groups of individuals, or by societies). In chaos theory, metapattern refers to the world as comprised of patterns (Goertzel, 1995). As applied to occupation, metapattern refers to the patterns of a single individual during a temporal "slice of life," or when repeated occupational patterns last across the lifespan. According to another Bateson (1979), metapatterns are "The pattern which connects." In the case of morning routines, pilot research suggests that the result of one's morning routine is *carpe diem,* or seize the day.

Occupational Process

Fisher (1998), in her Slagle, stressed the importance of process to occupational therapy. Similarly, a chaotic construction of occupation should emphasize that occupation is a process, and not a product that can be simplistically observed as a performance, action, or activity. Occupation is so much more than just activity!

Dynamical systems theory presupposes the evolving nature of a process over time. Similarly, a single occupational process evolves or unfolds over time. And, a single occupational process is interrelated with other occupational processes of a given individual in a specific situation, unfolding at the same time, at overlapping times, or at different times. Any given occupational process rarely, if ever, unfolds in isolation.

I hypothesize that more typically, multiple occupational processes are ongoing, and related to one another simultaneously, sequentially, or both (e.g., they co-effect one another with a web). For example, I regularly exercise on a treadmill and watch a favorite television show while dinner is cooking. This illustrates a web of at least three ongoing, co-effecting occupational processes: (a) exercising on the treadmill for health and wellness; (b) watching television for humor, stress release, and passage of time; and (c) cooking dinner, an occupation that is part of my caregiver role. Segal (2000) uses the term enfolding to refer to performance of "more than one occupation at a time." I use the phrases "web of occupational processes," or "webbing." Related to this, Cokie Roberts (2003) talked about "multitasking" by women in her opening ceremony presentation.

Occupational processes imply that occupation is not just a product (like "meal" or a "garden"), but is a process— a force that fosters order (occupation) out of chaos (nonuniformity). Conceptualization in this manner allows for a larger view of occupation not just as an event, but as a continually self-generating system, where the doing provides the meaning for generating more doing, and so on.

Occupational processes, perhaps, are the web of life![21]

Narrowly defining occupation as "activities of daily living" or "work" or "leisure" lacks the larger richness and diversity, and—indeed—the sequencing and emergent aspects, of occupation in all of our lives. How occupations enfold into one another and how occupations are multiplied while enacting them is discussed by Bateson (1996). Thus, multiple occupational processes enfolding over the lifespan, and enfolding across cultures over generations is the essence of what is meant by occupational process, a chaotic process so much more complex than a single event or activity.[22] Finally, the human drive to engage in occupational processes as a self-organizing function (Kielhofner & Forsyth, 1997) is that which gives life richness and meaning. Instead of Descartes' phrase, *"Cogito ergo sum"* (I think, therefore I am), I propose that occupational science and occupational therapy use *"Ago, ergo sum"* (I do [with purpose], therefore I am).

Occupational Shaping

In a chaotic process, wind is a force that shapes rock (Abraham, 1994). Similarly, occupation can be considered a chaotic process that shapes a human (e.g., occupational shaping). The total of our beliefs and sense of self comes from the occupational shaping of the web of a lifetime—be it a few days or over 80 years.

Just as a rock has a physical structure transformed by wind, the human species has a genetic blueprint shaped by occupational engagement. The interdependence presupposed in chaos theory renders nature versus nurture moot (Abraham & Gilgen, 1995). So too, nature versus nurture is irrelevant in a chaotic conceptualization of occupation. Rather, this chaotic elaboration of occupation, including occupational shaping, places our attention where it needs to be: upon the multiple webs of occupation.[23] It places our attention upon the nature of occupational engagement and the changes that take place within an organism, the environment, and society overall due to the engagement in the occupational process, also referred to by Law (2002) as participation. Well before the International Classification of Functioning, Disability, and Health (World Health Organization [WHO], 2001), participation has been a component of many foremothers' Eleanor Clarke Slagle lectures including Zimmerman (1960), Ackley (1962), and King (1978).

One may surmise that occupational shaping is developmentally based. It may be. A developmental framework, however, would have to be flexible and incorporate the wide range of variation that is normal and typical. It is theorized that occupational shaping occurs within development networks or webs of typically occurring occupations in which those of a given age and culture most typically engage.

Research in the *Proceedings of the National Academy of Sciences* (Maguire et al., 2000), and widely reported in popular media provides strong data supporting the construct of occupational shaping in very concrete terms. The investigators reported evidence of significantly larger posterior hippocampi of a group of London taxi drivers as compared to control subjects. This is clear evidence of occupational shaping of the brain, in a literal sense!

Occupational Variance

Occupational variance refers to the degree to which occupational processes are free to vary related to the control parameters of the individual's dynamical systems. In this case, degree of freedom refers to the variables that influence the process (i.e., the number and kinds of things that compose the system) (Freeman, 1995). Thus, occupational complexity is determined, in part, by the variance allowed for by the degrees of freedom. Occupational science may be the identification and delineation of the webs (networks and networks of systems, internal occupational processes, occupational dimensions, and occupational contexts) and the key control variables or control parameters. Accordingly, occupational therapy would be the-planned-for perturbation (or force-creating adaptations) of control parameters impinging upon the web designed to promote health and well-being. This may be what Nelson (1997) called occupational synthesis, which is based upon the creative process (Hasselkus, 2002; Pierce, 2001, 2003).

Occupational Transience

Occupational perseverance is the continued or prolonged engagement in an occupation directly related to previous or former engagement in that occupation (Carlson, 1996). I propose an antithetical concept: occupational transience. I define transience as the new temporariness in everyday life and propose that occupation is a transient structure or temporal state that exists interspersed between chaotic modes and that chaotic modes are the rich milieu of nonuniformity that is life, which exist when occupation is absent or in flux. Consequently, occupational process orders chaos in our lives as human performance that is organized (Carlson, 1996). Occupational transience, therefore, is a chaotic state in which we exist in between occupations. I hypothesize that based upon Toffler's (1970) notion of transience, individuals will have varying metapatterns of high or low transience of occupations.

Occupational transience may be the negative space within a web. Metaphorically speaking, occupational transience may be the equivalent of "living in the state of stuck."[24] Admittedly, this is an oversimplification since, indeed, there are only degrees of chaos and order resulting from occupation, not absolute states or quantities. And, as based in chaos theory, Warren et al. (1998) further hypothesized that the time of greatest change is related to the degree of chaos in a given state (e.g., the greater the degree of chaos),[25] the greater the susceptibility to perturbation. Such a concept has potentially profound implications for the practice of occupational therapy. We should practice near the edge of chaos! No protocols need apply.

Occupation is the organization of nonuniformity into a new form through participation. Thus, chaos theory allows the use of occupation as a normalizing process, regardless of the presence or absence of a disability or impairment. In this case, occupation, as a normalization process, allows for participation and activity as consistent with the ICF (WHO, 2001).

Cautions About Chaos

Having given enthusiastic support and endorsement of chaos as a foundational concept for occupation as a telling herein, I provide a note of caution. Chaos is not to be construed as a grand theory, but rather as a pragmatist's (Hooper & Wood, 2002) working tool for integration of occupational science and occupational therapy concepts, knowledge, and science by providing a broader perspective (Remer, 1996), although allowing for the unique case of an individual's experience. For, much like complexity theory in nonlinear dynamical systems, chaos is not a comprehensive theory but a collection of ideas, concepts, observations, and models (Waliszewski, Molski, & Konarski, 1998).[26] Further, use of chaos in occupation will be beneficial only as it facilitates continued development of a body of knowledge about occupation and therapy. As Baum (1980) stated, "We must do more than speak of our theories. We must develop a rage for knowledge and document our principles as a scientific discipline" (p. 508). We must always remember, however, that per our timeless principles and values, being a good occupational therapist may not be possible without being a good human being—and no theoretical reference is going to make us good human beings.[27] Only our morals will do that.

Conclusions About Chaos

In this telling of occupation, I have presented chaos theory, which transcends our culturally normed reference of linearity. Use of chaos to reconstruct occupation will allow incorporation of most all theoretical and research work done to date in occupational science and occupational therapy, as well as allow for a practical distinction between the two. The potential value of such a meta theory to provide a cohesive core for the science of occupation is great.

According to Arndt and Bigelow (2000), order and chaos are in a delicate balance. I would argue that chaos will predominate, and that those who embrace, understand, and use chaos theory will succeed. At the beginning of this telling I shared a quote from Chaucer. Nearing the end of this telling, another quote attributed to Chaucer seems apt: "Ful wys is he that can himselfven knowe!" With liberal revising for our current time, I suggest—full wise is she who can know herself, her profession of occupational therapy, and her discipline of occupational science.

The Ending of a Telling

Pay Your Professional Tax

First, we have the arsenal to move occupational therapy forward in service to society. Professional identity means responsibility. We must take off from the tarmac of timidity and enter the tableau of occupation. We shall take the concept of occupation, the theories of occupation, and instead of the lens of linearity, use the collide and scope of chaos. In her Slagle, Fidler (1966) referred to professional tax as the privileges and obligations "that come with a profession" (p. 1). Brunyate (1957) believed that privilege is bound in duty. So it is. You are charged to pay for your privilege of being an occupational therapist. You are charged to pay your professional tax and take up the scholarship of occupation—as an art, science, and therapy! Llorens (1970) said it best in her Slagle: "I would like to share a rather startling discovery I made some time ago. It was that 'they,' whoever 'they' were that I should be doing something to objectify our knowledge and raise the level of our practice included 'me.' I, herewith, challenge each of you to join me in that task so that we can move toward facilitating growth and development and fulfilling the promise of occupational therapy" (p. 101).

Engage in and Encourage Meta-emotion of Occupation

In her Slagle, Moore (1976) foreshadowed the proposed concept of meta-emotion of occupation stating that, ". . . humans need to understand emotional self before they can fully participate in intellectual life" (p. 19). So too Reilly (1962) valued the inexorable import and integration of thinking and feeling, stating that "man, through the use of his hands, can creatively deploy his thinking, feelings, and purposes to make himself at home in the world and to make the world his home" (p. 2). Ask yourself the following questions: "What do I feel about this telling?" "What did I feel when it started?" "How do I feel that it has ended?" Development of such an awareness of feeling or thinking about feeling or thinking while doing with meaning is the meta-emotion of occupation (Royeen & Duncan, 2001; Royeen, Duncan, & McCormack, 2001).[28] Reflection on thinking or feeling and thinking or feeling while doing over time builds our knowledge and understanding of ourselves, of practice, and of those whom we serve—a dimension of meaning we have not fully addressed in our profession and our discipline. The concept of meta-emotion of occupation is based upon the commonly accepted term metacognition, which means thinking about how one thinks to achieve a cognitive task such as addition or subtraction. Meta-emotion further incorporates aspects of the concept of somatic marker as discussed by Damasio (1994).

Honor the Pattern That Connects

Bing (1981) stated, "We are influenced by those who come before us more than we can truly know. . . . The past assists us in fashioning our future" (p. 516). As homage to our former Eleanor Clarke Slagle lecturers, and as homage to the metaphor "I am my motherdaughter," I have included a meaningful reference to each previous Eleanor Clarke Slagle lecturer as a part of this telling.[29]

Rood (1958) stated, "We benefit by the drive and vision of those who have gone before and we in turn have a responsibility to add our particulate share whatever it might be" (p. 326). West (1968) called this professional responsibility and consciousness (p. 13). The pattern that connects is, indeed, part of what has shaped us in the present and will continue to do so in the future. The medium is the message—look for and honor the pattern that connects.

Surrealism as Our Art

Occupational therapists see the surreal in order to help people get real. We can see what is not possible, and through occupation can create and adapt the world to make things doable with meaning. Creativity is the key to our art, and according to Rogers (1983), perplexity spurs on our artistry (p. 616). As Nietzche (1961/1969) expressed in *Thus Spoke Zarathustra* through the character Zarathustra, "I tell you: one must have chaos in one, to give birth to a dancing star. I tell you: you still have chaos in you" (p. 46).

Summary

In her Slagle, Gilfoyle (1984) suggested that we must question the three areas in occupational therapy. I use her three areas as a guide to summarize, in a very small nutshell, this complex telling. First, Gilfoyle suggested we must question our value system. Herein I have presented a timeless value system for elaboration and delineation to practice based upon appreciation and review of our *herstory*. Second, she suggested we must question the demands of practice. Herein I have provided a provisional exploration of Charlotte's Web of Chaos to liberate us from a linear view of reality, which does not match practice. Third, Gilfoyle suggested that we question educational requirements. Herein I have suggested that the entry-level clinical doctorate should become our norm.

Closing Blessing

In his Eleanor Clarke Slagle lecture, Dr. Robert Bing (1981) quoted the grand dame herself. I shall do the same as a blessing to end this telling: "The integrity of your profession is in your hands. I bid you Godspeed in your work" (Eleanor Clarke Slagle as cited in Bing, 1981, p. 516).

Acknowledgments

If it takes a village to raise a child, then it takes a vast network to raise a scholar to write and present a Slagle. To acknowledge just a few of my vast network, I give my heartfelt thanks to Marlene Aitken, PhD (occupational therapy), for general proofreading; Cindy Coirritore, PhD (management information systems and technology), for technology advisement and the veeper; John Fleming, OT (occupational therapy), for theoretical advising; Julie Gasper, PhD (business), for the veeper voice of Eleanor Clarke Slagle; Gail Jensen, PhD (physical therapy), for repeatedly instructing me to "just move the field forward"; Beverly Kracher, PhD (business ethics), for assistance in the history of philosophy; Ivelisse Lazzarini, OTD (occupational therapy), for assistance in technology; Aimee Luebben, EdD (occupational therapy), for Latin translation and editing; Carol Peters and Sue McGahan, for expert secretarial support and assistance; Doris Pierce, OT (occupational therapy), for helping me practice occupation; Barbara Rider, PhD (occupational therapy), for support, feedback, and inspiration; Laura Strickland, EdD, OT (occupational therapy), for theoretical assistance; Sidney Stohs, PhD (toxicology), who modeled great scholarship and closed his eyes while I took an unofficial sabbatical; and Patricia Wilbarger, MEd, OT (occupational therapy), for support, inspiration, and clinical understanding of chaos in action.

References

Abraham, F. D., & Gilgen, A. R. (Eds.). (1995). *Chaos theory in psychology.* Westport, CT: Praeger.

Abraham, R. (1994). *Chaos, gaia, eros: A chaos pioneer uncovers the three great streams of history.* New York: Harper Row.

Abreu, B. C., Peloquin, S. M., & Ottenbacher, K. (1998). Competence in scientific inquiry and research. *American Journal of Occupational Therapy, 52,* 751–759.

Ackley, N. (1962). The challenge of the sixties. *American Journal of Occupational Therapy, 16,* 273–281.

Allen, C. K. (1987). Activity: Occupational therapy's treatment method. 1987 Eleanor Clarke Slagle Lecture. *American Journal of Occupational Therapy, 41,* 563–575.

Allport, G. W. (1960). Personality and social encounter. Boston: Beacon Press.

Arndt, M., & Bigelow, B. (2000). Commentary: The potential of chaos theory and complexity science. *Health Care Management Review, 25*(1), 35–38.

Ayres, A. J. (1963). The development of perceptual-motor abilities: A theoretical basis for treatment of dysfunction. Eleanor Clarke Slagle Lecture. *American Journal of Occupational Therapy, 17,* 221–225.

Bateson, G. (1979). *Mind and nature: A necessary unity.* New York: Bantam Press.

Bateson, M. C. (1996). *Enfolded activity and the concept of occupation.* In R. Zemke & F. Clark (Eds.), *Occupational science: The evolving discipline* (pp. 5–12). Philadelphia: F. A. Davis.

Baum, C. M. (1980). Occupational therapists put care in the health system. 1980 Eleanor Clarke Slagle Lecture. *American Journal of Occupational Therapy, 34,* 505–516.

Bechtel, W. (1998). *Philosophy of science: An overview for cognitive science.* Hillsdale, NJ: Erlbaum.

Bellah, R. N., Masden, R., Sullivan, W. M., Swindler, A., & Tipton, S. M. (1985). *Habits of the heart; individualism and commitment in American life.* Berkeley, CA: University of California Press.

Bing, R. K. (1981). Occupational therapy revisited: A paraphrastic journey. 1981 Eleanor Clarke Slagle lecture. *American Journal of Occupational Therapy, 35,* 499–518.

Brunyate, R. (1957). Powerful levers in little common things. 1957 Eleanor Clarke Slagle Lecture. *American Journal of Occupational Therapy, 12,* 193–202.

Buell, M. J., & Cassidy, D. J. (2001). The complex and dynamic nature of quality in early care and educational programs: A case for chaos. *Journal of Research in Childhood Education, 15*(2), 209–219.

Cahnmann, M. (2003). The craft, practice, and possibility of poetry in educational research. *Educational Researcher, 32*(3), 29–36.

Capra, F. (1996). *The web of life: A new scientific understanding of living systems.* New York: Random House.

Carlson, M. (1996). The self-perpetuation of occupation. In R. Zemke & F. Clark (Eds.), *Occupational science: The evolving discipline* (pp. 143–180). Philadelphia: F. A. Davis.

Chavez, V. (2002, November). *A single bracelet does not jingle: Teaching community building at SFSU*. Paper presented at the Building Community to Improve Health: The Power, the Proof, the Promise, Sacramento, CA.

Christiansen, C. (1994). Classification and study in occupation. A review and discussion of taxonomies. *Journal of Occupational Science (Australia), 1*(3), 3–21.

Christiansen, C. (1999). Defining lives: Occupation as identity: An essay on competence, coherence, and the creation of meaning. 1999 Eleanor Clarke Slagle Lecture. *American Journal of Occupational Therapy, 53*, 547–558.

Clark, F. (1993). Occupation embedded in real life: Interweaving occupational science and occupational therapy. 1993 Eleanor Clarke Slagle Lecture. *American Journal of Occupational Therapy, 47*, 1067–1078.

Clark, F. (1997). Reflections on the human as an occupational being: Biological need, tempo and temporality. *Journal of Occupational Science (Australia), 4*(3), 86–92.

Coffey, D. S. (1998). Self-organization, complexity and chaos: The new biology for medicine. *Nature Medicine, 4*(8), 882–885.

Collins, M. (2001). Who is occupied? Consciousness, self awareness, and the process of human adaptation. *Journal of Occupational Science, 8*(1), 25–32.

Coppa, D. F. (1993). Chaos theory suggests a new paradigm for nursing science. *Journal of Advanced Nursing, 18*(6), 985–991.

Correspondence of W. R. Dutton and Eleanor Clarke Slagle. (1929–1937). Archives of the American Occupational Therapy Association. *Box 3, Folder 27*.

Correspondence of Eleanor Clarke Slagle. (1925–1929). Archives of the American Occupational Therapy Association. *Box 24, Series 5, Folder 160*.

Crabtree, J. (1998). The end of occupational therapy. *American Journal of Occupational Therapy, 52*, 205–214.

Csikszentmihalyi, M. (1990). *Flow: The psychology of optimal experience*. New York: Harper and Row.

Damasio, A. R. (1994). *Emotion, reason, and the human brain*. New York: Avon Books.

Duncan, M., & Royeen, C. B. (2000, November). *Grounded learning in context: Neuro-occupation*. Paper presented at Society for Neuroscience Annual Meeting, New Orleans, LA.

Dunn, W. (2001). The sensations of everyday life: Empirical, theoretical, and pragmatic considerations. 2001 Eleanor Clarke Slagle Lecture. *American Journal of Occupational Therapy, 55*, 608–620.

Dunn, W., Brown, C., & McGuigan, A. (1994). The ecology of human performance: A framework for considering the effect of context. *American Journal of Occupational Therapy, 48*, 595.

Farber, S. D. (1989). Neuroscience and occupational therapy: Vital connections. 1989 Eleanor Clarke Slagle Lecture. *American Journal of Occupational Therapy, 43*, 637–646.

Fidler, G. S. (1966). Learning as a growth process: A conceptual framework for professional education. 1965 Eleanor Clarke Slagle Lecture. *American Journal of Occupational Therapy, 20*, 1–8.

Fine, S. B. (1991). Resilience and human adaptability: Who rises above adversity? 1990 Eleanor Clarke Slagle Lecture. *American Journal of Occupational Therapy, 45*, 493–503.

Finn, G. L. (1972). The occupational therapist in prevention programs. 1971 Eleanor Clarke Slagle Lecture. *American Journal of Occupational Therapy, 26*, 59–66.

Fiorentino, M. R. (1975). Occupational therapy: Realization to activation. 1974 Eleanor Clarke Slagle Lecture. *American Journal of Occupational Therapy, 29*, 15–21.

Fisher, A. G. (1998). Uniting practice and theory in an occupational framework. 1998 Eleanor Clarke Slagle Lecture. *American Journal of Occupational Therapy, 52*, 509–521.

Fortune, T. (1996). The proto–occupation/occupation interface: An explanation of human occupation and its symbolic origins. *Journal of Occupational Science (Australia), 3*(3), 91.

Frank, G. (1996). The concept of adaptation as a foundation for occupational science research. In R. Zemke & F. Clark (Eds.), *Occupational science: The evolving discipline* (pp. 47–55). Philadelphia: F. A. Davis.

Freeman, W. J. (1995). The kiss of chaos and the sleeping beauty of psychology. In F. D. Abraham & A. R. Gilgen (Eds.), *Chaos theory in psychology* (pp. 19–31). Westport, CT: Praeger.

Gilfoyle, E. M. (1984). Transformation of a profession. 1984 Eleanor Clarke Slagle Lecture. *American Journal of Occupational Therapy, 38*, 575–584.

Goertzel, B. (1995). Evolutionary dynamics in minds and immune systems. In F. D. Abraham & A. R. Gilgen (Eds.), *Chaos theory in psychology* (pp. 169–180). Westport, CT: Praeger.

Golledge, J. (1998). Distinguishing between occupation, purposeful activity and activity. Part 1: Review and explanation. *British Journal of Occupational Therapy, 61*(3), 100–105.

Goodwin, J. S. (1997). Chaos, and the limits of modern medicine. *JAMA, 278,* 1399–1400.

Grady, A. (1992). Occupation as vision. *American Journal of Occupational Therapy, 46,* 1062–1065.

Grady, A. P. (1995). Building inclusive community: A challenge for occupational therapy. 1994 Eleanor Clarke Slagle Lecture. *American Journal of Occupational Therapy, 49,* 300–310.

Gutman, S. A., & Biel, L. B. (2001). Promoting the neurological substrates of well being through occupation. *Occupational Therapy in Mental Health, 17*(1), 1–22.

Hasselkus, B. R. (2000). From the desk of the editor: Habits of the heart. *American Journal of Occupational Therapy, 54,* 247–248.

Hasselkus, B. R. (2000). From the desk of the editor: Reaching consensus. *American Journal of Occupational Therapy, 54,* 127–128.

Hasselkus, B. R. (2002). *The meaning of everyday occupation.* Thorofare, NJ: Slack.

Hawking, S. W. (1993). *Hawking on the big bang and black holes.* Singapore: World Scientific.

Henderson, A. (1988). Occupational therapy knowledge: From practice to theory. *American Journal of Occupational Therapy, 42,* 567–576.

Hollis, L. I. (1979). Remember? 1979 Eleanor Clarke Slagle lecture. *American Journal of Occupational Therapy, 33,* 493–499.

Holm, M. B. (2000). Our mandate for the new millennium: Evidence-based practice. 2000 Eleanor Clarke Slagle Lecture. *American Journal of Occupational Therapy, 54,* 575–585.

Hooper, B., & Wood, W. (2002). Pragmatism and structuralism in occupational therapy: The long conversation. *American Journal of Occupational Therapy, 56,* 40–50.

Howell, D. (1999). Neuro-occupation: Linking sensory deprivation and self-care in the ICU patient. *Occupational Therapy in Health Care, 11*(4), 75–85.

Huss, A. J. (1977). Touch with care or a caring touch? 1976 Eleanor Clarke Slagle Lecture. *American Journal of Occupational Therapy, 31,* 295–310.

Jackson, J. (1996). Living a meaningful existence in old age. In R. Zemke & F. Clark (Eds.), *Occupational science: The evolving discipline.* (pp. 339–361). Philadelphia: F. A. Davis.

Jantzen, A. C. (1974). Academic occupational therapy. A career specialty. 1973 Eleanor Clarke Slagle Lecture. *American Journal of Occupational Therapy, 28,* 73–81.

Johnson, J. A. (1973). Occupational therapy: A model for the future. 1972 Eleanor Clarke Slagle Lecture. *American Journal of Occupational Therapy, 27,* 1–7.

Kielhofner, G. (1995). Introduction to the Model of Human Occupation. In J. P. Butler (Ed.), *A Model of Human Occupation: Theory and application* (2nd ed., pp. 1–25). Baltimore: Williams & Wilkins.

Kielhofner, G., & Burke, J. P. (1977). Occupational therapy after 60 years: An account of changing identity and knowledge. *American Journal of Occupational Therapy, 31,* 675–689.

Kielhofner, G., & Forsyth, K. (1997). The Model of Human Occupation: An overview of current concepts. *British Journal of Occupational Therapy, 60*(3), 103–110.

King, L. J. (1978). Toward a science of responses. 1978 Eleanor Clarke Slagle Lecture. *American Journal of Occupational Therapy, 32,* 429–437.

Kuhn, T. S. (1962/1970). *The structure of scientific revolutions* (2nd ed.). Chicago: University of Chicago Press.

Law, M. (2002). Distinguished scholar lecture: Participation in everyday life. *American Journal of Occupational Therapy, 56,* 640–649.

LeGuin, U. K. (2000). *The telling.* New York: Harcourt.

L'Engle, M. (1962). *A wrinkle in time.* New York: Farrar, Straus, & Giroux.

Llorens, L. A. (1970). Facilitating growth and development: The promise of occupational therapy. 1969 Eleanor Clarke Slagle Lecture. *American Journal of Occupational Therapy. 24,* 93–101.

Lohman, H., & Royeen, C. B. (2002). Posttraumatic stress disorder and traumatic hand injuries: A neuro-occupational view. *American Journal of Occupational Therapy, 56,* 527–537.

Lyons, B. G. (1983). Purposeful versus human activity. *American Journal of Occupational Therapy, 37,* 493–495.

Magnus, E. (2001). Everyday occupations and the process of redefinition: A study of how meaning in occupation influences redefinition of identity in women with a disability. *Scandinavian Journal of Occupational Therapy, 8,* 115–124.

Maguire, E. A., Gadian, D. G., Johnsrude, I. S., Good, C. D., Ashburner, J., Frackowlak, R., & Frith, C. D. (2000). Navigation-related structural change in the hippocampi of taxi drivers. *Proceedings of the National Academy of Sciences, USA, 97,* 4398–4403.

Manian, F. A. (1997). Letter to the editor: Chaos, and the limits of modern medicine. *JAMA, 278,* 1399–1400.

Manthey, M. (1997). Chaos theory and the partnership concept. *Creative Nursing Management, 3*(1), 3.

McLuhan, M., & Fiore, Q. (2001). *The medium is the message.* New York: Ginko Press. (Original work published in 1967)

Meyer, A. (1937). Address in honor of Eleanor Clarke Slagle. *Occupational Therapy in Mental Health, 5*(3), 109–113.

Moore, J. C. (1976). Behavior, bias and the limbic system. 1975 Eleanor Clarke Slagle Lecture. *American Journal of Occupational Therapy, 30,* 11–19.

Mosey, A. C. (1985). A monistic or a pluralistic approach to professional identity? 1985 Eleanor Clarke Slagle lecture, *American Journal of Occupational Therapy, 39,* 504–509.

National Society for the Promotion of Occupational Therapy. Correspondence of W. R. Dutton and Eleanor Clarke Slagle. (1929–1937). Archives of American Occupational Therapy Association. *Box 3, Folder 27.*

National Society for the Promotion of Occupational Therapy. Correspondence of Eleanor Clarke Slagle. (1925–1929). Archives of American Occupational Therapy Association. *Box 24, Series 5, Folder 160.*

National Society for the Promotion of Occupational Therapy. (Annual Meetings 1917–1924). Archives of the American Occupational Therapy Association. *Box 1, Series 1, Folder 1.*

National Society for the Promotion of Occupational Therapy. (Annual Meetings, 1917–1924). Archives of the American Occupational Therapy Association. *Box 3, Series 1, Folder 27.*

Nelson, D. L. (1997). Why the profession of occupational therapy will flourish in the 21st century. 1996 Eleanor Clarke Slagle Lecture. *American Journal of Occupational Therapy, 51,* 11–24.

Nietzche, F. (1961/1969). *Thus spoke Zarathrustra.* New York and London: Penguin Group.

Padilla, R., & Peyton, C. G. (1997). Neuro–occupation: Historical review and examples. In C. B. Royeen (Ed.), *Neuroscience occupation: Links to practice* (pp. 1–31). Bethesda, MD: American Occupational Therapy Association.

Pediani, R. (1996). Chaos and evaluation in nursing research. *Journal of Advanced Nursing, 23,* 645–646.

Peloquin, S. M. (1989). Sustaining the art of practice in occupational therapy. *American Journal of Occupational Therapy, 43,* 219–226.

Peloquin, S. M. (1996). Art: An occupation with promise for developing empathy. *American Journal of Occupational Therapy, 50,* 655–661.

Peloquin, S. M. (1997). The spiritual depth of occupation: Making meaning and making lives. *American Journal of Occupational Therapy, 51,* 167–168.

Peloquin, S. M. (2001). Confluence: Moving forward with affective strength. *American Journal of Occupational Therapy, 55,* 69–77.

Peloquin, S. M. (2002). Reclaiming the vision of "reaching for heart as well as hands." *American Journal of Occupational Therapy, 56,* 517–526.

Peshkin, A. (2000). The nature of interpretation in qualitative research. *Educational Researcher, 29*(9), 5–9.

Pierce, D. (1998). What is the source of occupation's treatment power? *American Journal of Occupational Therapy, 52,* 490–491.

Pierce, D. (2001). Occupation by design: Dimensions, therapeutic power, and creative process. *American Journal of Occupational Therapy, 55,* 249–259.

Pierce, D. (2003). *Occupation by design: Building therapeutic power.* Philadelphia: F. A. Davis.

Pierce, D., & Peyton, C. (1999). A historical cross-disciplinary perspective on the professional doctorate in occupational therapy. *American Journal of Occupational Therapy, 53,* 64–71.

Plexus Institute. (2003, March). Complexity in practice: Understanding and acting to improve health and health care. *An International Plexus Institute Summit Conference.* Jointly sponsored with Mayo Clinic and the Center for the Study of Healthcare Management. University of Minnesota. Preconference workshop in Introduction to Complexity Science. (March 20). Rochester, MN.

Prigogone, I., & Stengers, I. (1984). *Order out of chaos: Man's dialogue with nature.* Toronto, Ontario, Canada: Bantam.

Primeau, L. A., Clark, F., & Pierce, D. (1989). Occupational therapy alone has looked upon occupation: Future applications of occupational science to pediatric occupational therapy. *Occupational Therapy in Health Care, 6*(4), 19–32.

Quiroga, V.A.M. (1995). *Occupational therapy: The first 30 years: 1900–1930.* Bethesda, MD: American Occupational Therapy Association.

Rebeiro, K. L., & Cook, J. V. (1999). Opportunity, not prescription: An exploratory study of the experience of occupational engagement. *Canadian Journal of Occupational Therapy, 66*(4), 176–187.

Reed, K. L. (1986). Tools of practice: Heritage or baggage? 1986 Eleanor Clarke Slagle Lecture. *American Journal of Occupational Therapy, 40,* 597–605.

Reilly, M. (1962). Occupational therapy can be one of the great ideas of 20th century medicine. 1961 Eleanor Clarke Slagle Lecture. *American Journal of Occupational Therapy, 16,* 1–9.

Remer, R. (1996, Winter). Chaos theory and the canon of creativity. *Journal of Group Psychotherapy, Psychodrama, and Sociometry,* 145–154.

Roberts, C. (1998). *We are our mothers' daughters.* New York: William Morrow.

Roberts, C. (2003, June). *Keynote address.* Session presented during the opening ceremony of the American Occupational Therapy Association's 83rd Annual Conference & Expo, Washington, DC.

Rogers, J. C. (1983). Clinical reasoning: The ethics, science, and art. 1983 Eleanor Clarke Slagle Lecture. *American Journal of Occupational Therapy, 37,* 601–616.

Rood, M. S. (1958). Every one counts. Eleanor Clarke Slagle Lecture. *American Journal of Occupational Therapy, 12,* 326–329.

Royeen, C. B. (2002). Occupation reconsidered. *Occupational Therapy International, 9*(2), 112–121.

Royeen, C. B., & Duncan, M. (2001). *Meta-emotion of occupation: A new twist for mental health.* Paper presented at the American Occupational Therapy Association Annual Conference & Expo, Philadelphia, PA.

Royeen, C. B., Duncan, M., & McCormack, G. (2001). Reconstruction of the Rood approach for occupation based treatment. In S. Pedretti (Ed.), *Occupational therapy: Practice skills for physical dysfunction* (5th ed., pp. 576–587). St. Louis: Mosby.

Royeen, C. B., & Luebben, A. J. (2002). Annotated bibliography of chaos for occupational therapy. *Occupational Therapy in Health Care, 16*(1), 63–80.

Scherer, M. J. (2000). *Living in the state of stuck: How assistive technology impacts the lives of people with disabilities* (3rd ed.). Newton Upper Falls, MA: Brookline Books.

Segal, R. (2000). Adaptive strategies of mothers with attention deficit hyperactivity disorder: Enfolding and unfolding occupations. *American Journal of Occupational Therapy, 54,* 300–306.

Serrett, K. D. (1985). Eleanor Clarke Slagle: Founder and leader in occupational therapy. *Occupational Therapy in Health Care, 5*(3), 101–108.

Shepperd, J. (1996). Chaos theory: Implications for homeopathy. *European Journal of Classical Homeopathy, 2*(5–6), 36–41.

Sokolov, J. (1957). Therapist into administrator. Eleanor Clarke Slagle Lecture. *American Journal of Occupational Therapy, 11,* 13–19, 34.

Spitzer, S. L. (1999). Dynamic Systems Theory: Relevance to the theory of sensory integration and the study of occupation. *Sensory Integration Special Interest Section Quarterly, 22*(2), 1–4.

Stattel, F. (1956). Equipment designed for occupational therapy. 1955 Eleanor Clarke Slagle Lecture. *American Journal of Occupational Therapy, 10,* 194–198.

Thelen, E., & Smith, L. B. (Eds.). (1994). *A dynamical systems approach to the development of cognition and action.* Cambridge, MA: MIT Press.

Theodooropoulous, D. S. (1998). Chaos and the limits of modern medicine [Letter to the editor]. *JAMA, 279,* 11.

Toffler, A. (1970). *Future shock.* New York: Random House.

Trombly, C. A. (1995). Occupation: Purposefulness and meaningfulness as therapeutic mechanisms. 1995 Eleanor Clarke Slagle Lecture. *American Journal of Occupational Therapy, 49,* 960–972.

Waliszewski, P., Molski, M., & Konarski, J. (1998). On the holistic approach in cellular and cancer biology: Nonlinearity, complexity, and quasi-determinism of the dynamic cellular network. *Journal of Surgical Oncology, 68,* 70–78.

Walloch, C. L. (1998). Neuro-occupation and the management of chronic pain through mindfulness meditation. *Occupational Therapy International, 5*(3), 238–248.

Warren, K., Franklin, D., & Streeter, C. L. (1998). New directions in systems theory: Chaos and complexity. *Nursing Administration Quarterly, 22*(2), 40–47.

Way, M. (1999). Parasympathetic and sympathetic influences in neuro-occupation pertaining to play. *Occupational Therapy in Health Care, 12*(1), 71–86.

Wegg, L. S. (1960). The essentials of work evaluation. Eleanor Clarke Slagle Lecture. *American Journal of Occupational Therapy, 14,* 65–79.

West, W. L. (1968). Professional responsibility in times of change. 1967 Eleanor Clarke Slagle Lecture. *American Journal of Occupational Therapy, 22,* 9–15.

Whewell, W. (1847/1966). *The philosophy of the inductive sciences founded upon their history.* London: Frank Cass Publications.

Wilcock, A. A. (2000). Development of a personal, professional and educational philosophy: An Australian perspective. *Occupational Therapy International, 7*(2), 79–86.

Wilcock, A. A. (2002). A theory of the human need for occupation. *Journal of Occupational Science, 9*(1), 17–24.

Wood, W., Towers, L., & Malchow, J. (2000). Environment, time-use, and adaptedness in: Implications for discerning behavior that is occupational in nature. *Journal of Occupational Science, 7*(1), 5–18.

World Health Organization. (2001). *ICF: International Classification of Functioning, Disability and Health.* Geneva: Author.

Yerxa, E. J. (1966). Authentic occupational therapy. 1966 Eleanor Clarke Slagle Lecture. *American Journal of Occupational Therapy, 21,* 1–9.

Yerxa, E. J. (2000). Occupational science: A renaissance of service to humankind through knowledge. *Occupational Therapy International, 7*(2), 87–98.

Zardetto-Smith, A. M., Mu, K., Phelps, C. L., Houtz, L. E., & Royeen, C. B. (2002). Brains rule! Fun = learning = neuroscience literacy. *The Neuroscientist, 8*(5), 396–404.

Zemke, R., & Clark, F. (Eds.). (1996). *Occupational science: The evolving discipline.* Philadelphia: F. A. Davis.

Zimmerman, M. E. (1960). *Devices: Development and direction.* Paper presented at the 1960 American Occupational Therapy Association Conference.

Endnotes

1. A multidimensional exploration using poetry as scholarly inquiry (Cahnmann, 2003) with full recognition of the role of self in this paper (Peshkin, 2000).
2. The literary and artistic genre of surrealism grew out of Dadaism, an art movement prior to WWI founded upon defying rationality through artistic expression. Surrealism's goal was to blend the unconscious and conscious into an authentic, or surreal, reality.
3. Development of a discipline includes responsibility as a steward of the discipline.
4. The concept related to play, specifically fun, has been shown to be highly correlated with learning (Zardetto-Smith, Mu, Phelps, Houtz, & Royeen, 2002).
5. See Royeen (2002).
6. Please see p. 564 of Allen (1987) for a parallel discussion of Soviet psychology's use of the word "activity" as a principle and focus of study as a tautology.
7. For a thorough review of purposeful activity, please see Lyons (1983).
8. For a historical review of humanistic moral treatment in occupational therapy, see Kielhofner and Burke (1977).
9. It is interesting to note that Bing (1981) suggested that "The history of occupational therapy is the most neglected part of our professional endeavors" (p. 514).
10. These are environmental conditions required to maintain the integrity of historical documents.
11. My fact-finding and constant comparative methodology, using historical review, resulted in five themes.
12. See Pierce and Peyton (1999) for an historical overview of clinical doctorates in the health fields.
13. The phrase used by Hooper and Wood (2002).
14. Bellah, Madcsen, Sullivan, Swindler, and Tipton (1985) as cited in Hasselkus (2000) in an *AJOT* "From the Editor" section titled "Habits of the Heart."
15. Adapted from "A single bracelet does not jingle" (Chavez, 2002, p. 24).
16. What Kuhn referred to as paradigm and paradigm shift is similar to consilience and consilience of induction as discussed by Whewell (1847/1967).

17. Dr. Prigogone died in June 2003.
18. It is beyond the scope of the current paper to delineate how and why chaos theory renders much of evidence-based practice moot; suffice to say that humans are complex systems and though we can reliably predict the course of a disease across populations, we cannot presume to predict how any given individual will react in a particular set of circumstances given a particular disease condition! Rogers (1983) well-articulated this on p. 607 of her Slagle.
19. Occupational, as used here, is based upon Gilfoyle's 1984 Eleanor Clarke Slagle definition, "Occupational is defined as a process of action in which a person is the action agent or doer" (p. 578).
20. Ayres referred to the profession and field of study called neurophysiologists. Early founders talked of occupationologists. (The National Society for the Promotion of Occupational Therapy, Annual Meetings 1917–1924.) I hope we see an analogous profession and discipline evolve: neuro-occupationologists.
21. A phrase borrowed from Capra (1996).
22. Activity is but a teaser for occupation!
23. Allen (1987) identified that the only social science to address activity as a central focus is Soviet psychology.
24. This phrase is borrowed from Scherer (2000) but may be used somewhat differently from her intent.
25. Just short, that is, of going beyond the edge of chaos into madness.
26. According to Allport (1960), General Systems Theory was seen as the hoped for unifier for a monistic approach. I see chaos theory allowing for Mosey's (1985) pluralistic approach.
27. Adapted from Manian's (1997) statement about physicians in reference to chaos theory.
28. Actually defined as appreciation (including conscious, subconscious, and unconscious processing of information) of the feelings that occur during engagement in the process of *occupation* (Royeen, 2002, p. 620).
29. *AJOT* could not accommodate the listing of all Eleanor Clarke Slagle lecturers that was developed. I have recommended to AOTA that it be posted on the AOTA Web site, and be maintained henceforth.

2004 Eleanor Clarke Slagle Lecture

Time, Space, and the Kaleidoscopes of Occupation

Ruth Zemke, PhD, OTR, FAOTA

Time and space have been studied at many levels from cosmic, evolutionary, to human. Cosmic time and space is the story of the origins of the universe. Evolutionary time and space is that of living creatures on earth. Human time and space are understood in the course and activity of a human life (Tuan, 1977, pp. 132–134). Each uses a different set of kaleidoscopic mirrors through which we can view our occupations. Each results in a different picture, but all depend upon the basic elements of occupation for their design.

Cosmic Time and Space

The cosmic level of time and space has engaged philosophers and theologians in every culture as it is intertwined with basic issues of humanity, represented by Paul Gauguin's 1897 painting, "Where do we come from? What are we? Where are we going?" The painting shows (from right to left) the life cycle—birth, life, death representing respectively our origin, our identity, and our destiny, human concepts that are linked to cosmic ones. Humans can trace our lives back through time and space, through generations, through animal ancestry, early forms of living matter, through the elements of matter in the universe, through the energy that is interconvertible to matter, that is both particles and waves.

Einstein's cosmology suggested that in the beginning was Oneness of time, space, matter, and energy; a Singularity, where everything was an infinitesimal point in space, an infinitesimal instant of time; everything was zero size. About 15 billion years ago, the universe, space, time, matter, and energy burst forth in a searing hot fireball of the "big bang" in which space, naturally dynamic, expanded with time, "carrying matter like driftwood on the tide" (Veneziano, 2004, p. 56). As the fireball expanded and cooled, tiny subatomic particles coalesced into atoms. Einstein's theory of general relativity equations were based on a four dimensional geometry including both time and space. Gravity was a curve or bend in the time–space continuum near matter. Atoms thus merged under the action of gravity to form galaxies and stars. Some stars developed planetary systems, and some of these planets—at least one that we know about—developed life.

Evolutionary Time and Space

In adapting to the environment across evolutionary time, animal species have relied upon adaptation through natural selection from variations in populations of a species *over time and space*. Edelman's theory (1987, 1989, 1992) of the development of the mind suggested that *adaptation of the individual brain* also occurs through a *selection process,*

Originally published 2004 in *American Journal of Occupational Therapy, 58,* 608–620.

in this case, selecting from the *variety of the population* of neurons in the brain. He pointed out that from the moment of conception of the individual, time and place determine the formation of groups of cells as they divide and migrate and organize. Our individuality is determined by the temporal and spatial history of the developing cells, embryo, fetus. A primary repertoire or basic group of brain cells is shaped through our individual interactions with the environment time and space. This shaping occurs through neural synapses forming and strengthening. Successive stimuli are organized sequentially and in locations producing different patterns of neuronal discharge producing perceptions of change that become our initial perspective of time and space. These neural connections form what Edelman calls "local maps" of our experience with the world around us. These local maps are groups of neurons that linked together because the sensations of occupational engagement of the person with their environment was one in which the stimuli from the environment were also linked together closely in time and space. These groups of local maps, neural maps of instants of our experience, gradually organize, forming global maps. Living creatures' brain maps of the reality within and outside themselves allow them to begin to acknowledge self versus nonself. They also begin to recognize patterns in their actions in the environment and patterns in the environment itself, patterns in time and space.

Paul MacLean (Former Director of Brain & Behavior Lab at NIMH) developed a model of the human brain as triune or three-part (Jacobs, 2003; MacLean, 1978). The triune brain is an evolutionary model that describes the ancient reptilian brain (brainstem), the early mammalian, emotional brain (limbic system), and the higher mammalian, cerebral neocortical brain developing "on top of" each other. To assist in understanding its anatomical structure, Ornstein and Thompson (1984) ask us to picture a rambling house, added on to over the years. In contrast, Caine & Caine (1991) suggest that, to understand the complex functions of the triune human brain, we think of it as three family members living together, working together. I like to think of the Brain family of three sisters.

The oldest sister Brainstem Betty is in charge of maintenance: providing food and waste disposal, attending to general security and comfort of their home place. She functions in an automatic way, loves order and security, and resists change and novelty. When she attends to sex, it's for reproduction. She never truly thinks of herself as separate from the others, nor from the home in which they live. In her concrete world, time is now and place is here. Since she doesn't use language, she's the strong silent one.

Betty (and early humans) were so directly immersed in the world that objectivity was not likely because there was little distinction between one's self and the outside (Jacobs, 2003, p. 13). These differentiations are made possible by Edelman's global maps, which are the beginning of conscious awareness—distinguishing self from nonself, developing boundaries between self and nonself, inside and outside, developing concepts, abstractions, and categories of knowledge of time and space of the world inside and outside of the self.

The second sister in the Brain family is a "Sensitive, New Age" kind of woman. Limbic Louise is deeply emotional and shares her feelings with a variety of facial expressions and body language unknown to Betty. Lou treasures affiliation, ritual, and celebration. She has emotions related to time and space, bringing the feelings from past experience into her present location. Lou vacillates between competition and cooperation. Her sexual focus is on romantic feelings or occasionally the pain of rejection. She is afraid of being alienated from the group or cut off from the emotional satisfaction of membership in the group or with important "others." To Lou, time means past feelings and future anxiety, space means being near or far from people and things she cares about.

The youngest and largest of the sisters is Neocortical Nell. She's the Brain family's pride and joy. She has creative skill in language and art, and yet is capable of complex scientific analysis and high level abstract thought. Nell wants meaningful occupation, challenge, novelty, stimulation. She deplores boredom, occupational deprivation, stagnation. Her sisters occasionally wish she were not quite so self-aware and introspective, or at least that she didn't talk about herself and to herself so much. It's as though Neocortical Nell concocts her own version of internal and external reality, of time and space, in contrast to their sensory or emotional perceptions of the external world. She keeps track of the family history, the past, and places they have been, but most keenly focuses on the future and the potential to turn the family homestead into a model place. She can anticipate, plan for the future, and carry out plans for the entire Brain family, although she shares the decision making with the others. Whereas the sisters are proud of what Nell can do, there are times when they "downshift" to Lou's emotional control of situations or even let Betty loose, with her less smooth, more aggressive behaviors. Those are times such as when Nell is bored with routine or habitual occupations or deprived of meaningful occupations, when Lou makes them feel anxious or stressed, or Betty's alarm goes off warning the others that their safety is threatened!

The abstractions that are so natural for Neocortical Nell produce filters, substitutions of concepts for sensory perceptions, thus a loss of immediate experience putting her somewhat out of touch with the real world. Humans in Western culture, like Nell, came to see themselves, not as part of natural selection, but as dominating nature. As we separated self from all else we began to observe the natural world rather than participate in it. We began to see things—nature, others—in terms of their utility and purpose relative to us. We can shut out actual experiences of engagement with the outside world—we may miss seeing the sunset because we're driving and fretting over our day at work; we can disengage from what we are doing and from fully "being" in and experiencing the moment, the place, and the occupation (Jacobs, 2003, p. 14; Langer, 1989).

Occupation is defined and described in many ways: those that emphasize the external, observable nature of occupation, the ordinary and familiar things that people do everyday (American Occupational Therapy Association [AOTA], 1995) and those that emphasize the experience of engagement in an activity (Pierce, 2001, 2003). Human time and space also have two aspects: an external or locational one, such as clock time or a geographical position, and an experiential aspect that is "lived space" (Parkes & Thrift, 1980) and time. This experiential aspect is subjective, one in which "the experiencer lives and moves and searches for meaning" (Buttimer, 1976, p. 282). When we include this experiential definition of occupation, it reminds us to also consider the experiential aspects of time and space.

Time/Temporality

Traditionally we have thought of time in its cosmic sense: the indefinite or unlimited extent in which events have happened, are happening, or are going to happen; every moment that has ever been or ever will be. We have studied the external locational dimension of time: clock time, the moment at which something has happened, is happening, or will happen, the duration of an event or between events.

Christiansen (1996) reviewed traditional concepts of occupational balance in our field and their relationship to time, including time use. Time use studies have reported international results, occupational patterns of how people spend their time in many countries (e.g., Robinson & Godbey, 1997; Szalai et al., 1977; Szalai & Andrews, 1980) and discussed appropriate research methods for data collection and analysis (Pentland, Harvey, Lawton, & McColl, 1999). All of these have used locational views of time as the measure of occupation. In this tradition, Minato & Zemke (2004) studied the time use of persons with schizophrenia living in the community in Japan to explore the stresses of their daily occupational patterns and their strategies of occupational choice related to stress. We found that although the participants chose to spend time in stress reducing occupations as a short-term strategy, they also chose to use their time in stressful participation in worklike activities within the day care program, a co-op sheltered workshop, or a part-time job because of the long-range skill development and practice in controlling their reactions to stress. Erlandsson, Rognvaldsson, & Eklund (2004) offer a more recent method to study occupational patterns in time as they transformed "yesterday diaries" into time-and-occupation graphs and analyzed the complexity of the patterns described by the graphs. They cited the need for further development of a process describing patterns of occupation in terms of other occupational characteristics, such as the value and meaning of the occupations and their relationship to health and well-being (Erlandsson, Rognvaldsson, & Eklund, p. 12).

Perhaps a better match for the concept of occupation that I wish to explore today, that of the experience of engagement, might be the concept of temporality; the experience of time, the perception of time, the meaning of time. We are familiar with the temporal aspects of occupations—"the rhythm (patterns of tasks within the occupation), tempo (rate or speed [of the process] of the occupation), synchronization (with other coparticipants), duration . . . and sequence (ordering of tasks)," which contribute to the patterns of our daily occupations (Larson & Zemke, 2004, p. 82). We experience time in occupations, not in identical clock or calendar units. I believe that our focus in occupational therapy and occupational science should be on occupational temporality, the experience of time as shaped by engagement in occupations (Larson & Zemke, 2004; Zemke & Clark, 1996, p. 92). For example, some occupations must be continued to completion and thus determine the pace and amount of time that will be required, such as childcare occupations, in which the child's tempo may be more important than the adult's schedule (Krieger, 1996; Larson, 2000; Larson & Zemke, 2004).

Human perception of time shows the blend of characteristics of the Brain family. We must "perceive succession, simultaneity, and duration within each sensory system; integrate these perceptual patterns; organize this information to give a clear sense of present in relation to past and future; and organize these aspects of time within the sociocultural milieu" (Blanche & Parham, 2001, p. 188). Beginning with infancy's awareness, similar to that of Brainstem Betty's, of discomfort—hunger, thirst, fatigue, cold—and of duration as the time satisfaction and comfort are obtained. The accompanying internal and external reactions to discomfort and comfort are formed into the basic emotional repertoire of Limbic Louise, who shows increasing complexity, but reacts strongly to time's meaning as conditioned by those around her. Neocortical Nell is the clock reader of the family, cognitively perceiving the rational concepts of a temporal world of supposedly equal units of seconds, minutes, hours, and years, using her PalmPilot™ calendar and schedules. Together they shape our experience of time within engagement in occupation throughout our lifespan. Cottle and Klineberg (1974) discussed the lifespan development of our experience of time, our temporality.

People experience a variety of temporalities shaped by occupational engagement. How is our view of time affected by our occupations? We perceive time to move at different rates within different occupations. Sometimes we lose track of time completely because we are so involved in a challenging activity that we focus on the occupational experience itself, not on external time.

Flaherty's studies (1999) have discussed the underlying qualities that might produce three temporalities: Temporal Compression, Temporal Protraction, and Synchronicity. Temporal Compression occurs when we experience less time is passing (has passed) than clock time indicates. Sometimes, as we say, "time flies when you're having fun"—as though the clock has speeded up its movement. In contrast, Temporal Protraction occurs when we experience more time passing than the clock time indicates. At times, when we are bored, for example, we feel that time drags—as though the clock has slowed down. Flaherty also identified Synchronicity, a match of perceived, experiential time and clock time. Much of our day probably entails engagement in occupations that produce this experience, especially in this society where we have clocks everywhere and watches on most every arm.

Other occupational temporalities have been described. Csikszentmihalyi (1990) and Csikszenmihalyi and Csikszentmihalyi (1988) described specific qualities of occupations that might lead us to experience Flow, an intense focus upon our engagement in occupation that includes a feeling of timelessness. Other experiences of disrupted temporality include Temporal Rupture, the distortion of time in a life changing event such as acute or chronic illness and onset of disability. It is as though the "fabric" of time were torn by the incident and its repair was a very gradual and slow process of return to familiar temporalities as one's gradual involvement in satisfying occupations returns. A temporary but intense emotional and cognitive disruption can occur under extreme circumstances of intense impact. An example of this extreme temporal experience is seen in the following video clip. At a Memorial Day program last May, the WWII U.S. Army Air Force fighter pilot, Lt. Colonel Victor Bast, who is my father, was invited to speak about the meaning of his experiences in that distant time and place. Within his reminiscences, he recalled the moment before an air battle, when for him, time stopped.

Few of us experience such a dramatic disruption of our temporality as that; however, most of us have frequently experienced temporal compression, protraction, synchronicity, and occasionally, flow. Larson studied what I have referred to as occupational temporality, the experience of time during engagement in occupation, using Experience

Sampling Methods (ESM) with 35 occupational therapy students in the Midwestern and Western United States who responded via an e-mail paging system to questions about their occupational experience (Larson, in press). They named the occupation, place, and social circumstances at the time of being paged, and they answered questions about such occupational characteristics as the novelty, complexity, and skill used in the occupation; about participatory experience including their emotional and intellectual engagement and their focus on self and on the occupation, as well as their perception of the temporality of the occupational experience. She found, using Structural Modeling analysis, that the occupational features of novelty and complexity and individual's skill use were good predictors of engagement, which in turn predicted temporality. Her model of Dynamic Occupations in Time (DOiT) (Larson, in press) illustrated the complex relationships predicted from literature and the results of her data.

Larson's further examination of the data with Configural Frequency Analysis (Bergman, 1998; Von Eye, Spiel, & Wood, 1996) was an attempt to find patterns of the factors (novelty, complexity, emotional and intellectual engagement, attention to self, and attention to occupation) at high or low level and the temporalities that might be associated with them. Her findings supported the existence of patterns of characteristics that occurred more often than would be expected statistically, but also that the six composite "types" or patterns that she described were associated with the range of perceived temporalities. Based on analysis of open-ended questions to the participants, she suggests that additional occupational and individual characteristics should be included to better predict temporality including such elements as enjoyment of the occupation, satisfaction with performance of the occupation, performance stress, and how closely we approach goal attainment.

In response to the feelings of time pressure in American society we are encouraged to prioritize our goals (Covey, 1989), to attempt to cut down on the things we have to do. Economically well-to-do, this country's people suffer from a perception of time poverty; we have too many things (occupations) to do in the time available. Compared to others in the world, do Americans seem money rich and time poor? With a limit of the same 24 hours a day the rest of the world has, can we get time rich? Our attempts at solving this dilemma include time deepening (Robinson & Godbey, 1997). In a polychronic culture (Hall, 1983), several occupations can be performed within the same time frame. This multitasking is what we have referred to as enfolded occupations (Bateson, 1996; Larson & Zemke, 2004; Zemke & Clark, 1996, p. 91). Primeau described "trip-chaining" for the combination of more than one purpose in an automobile trip (1996, p. 120). For the realtor who is driving, involved in a cell phone conversation with a customer, searching the computerized Web site for real estate listings for yet another customer from his laptop, while commuting to a third customer's "for sale" site, we may have "space deepening" as well. It may not have been possible to be in more than one place at a time, but with technology, we are trying.

Space/Place

While the 18th and 19th centuries, philosophically, were an era of temporocentrism (Casey, 1997, p. x), where space was usually studied in terms of time, 20th century philosophy emphasized the foundational quality of space and place in human life and the equally intertwined quality of space and time. If we think of cosmic time as the infinite extent in which things can happen, every moment that has and will exist, then a similar cosmic view defines space as the expanse extending in all directions in which all material things exist. If a locational view of time is a moment at which something happens, the duration of or between things, then a similar dimension of space is a location of things, the area of or between things. Our occupational interest in space is related to our human position within it and movement through it through engagement in occupations.

We are embodied, spatially dimensional as well as temporally. We are moved through space—our expanding universe, our planet's rotation around the sun, and in my home in California, the earthquake movement of the earth beneath our feet. We also act, we move in space, as does matter within our bodies, blood, air, and chemicals that are our food and waste. Our internal and external movements change the relationship within our body, between our own and other bodies, between our planet and other astronomical bodies, between all the elements of matter of our universe. These changing relationships produce the perception of time and the experience of temporality. Similarly, the experiential nature of space may be in our recognition of place, the perception of, and meaning of place as shaped by our occupations, our "occupatio-spaciality."

Because we are (embodied) "beings," we are "doers" (act and move), we are "becoming," we are spatiotemporal creatures, located in and experiencing both space and time. If our life is a tapestry, then its design is formed of our location and experience of space and time, the warp and the weft, woven together through the patterns of our occupations. A pattern is a design; an arrangement or disposition of elements. In this case, occupational patterns are the designs of our occupations in time and space, the arrangement of temporal and spatial locations and experiences.

The gradually developing awareness of space, as of time, begins with our own body. Merleau-Ponty noted, "Far from my body's being for me no more than a fragment of space, there would be no space at all for me if I had no body" (1962/2002, p. 112). Henderson directed occupational therapists' and scientists' attention to our interaction with the spatial environments of body space (our body and body surface perceptions, known through proprioception or kinesthesis), grasping space (the area within our reach, known by functional movement of our upper extremities), and distal space (that area beyond reach through which we move our bodies) (Blanche & Parham, 2001; Henderson, 1996). Perceiving space requires the brain to process multiple sources of sensory information from the level of Brainstem Betty's differentiation of predator or prey, through Limbic Lou's feelings stimulated by a whiff of familiar aftershave lotion, to Neocortical Nell's cognitive construction of the map of a trip to work, or image of cyberspace. But just as the experience of temporality is different from the physical cosmic time, physical space too has its experiential partner.

How does "space," a physical entity, become "place," a meaning entity? What makes a house or an apartment, a castle or a hovel, "home"? Place is made both physically and symbolically. In Relph's (1976) classic presentation of the phenomenology of place, he identifies the essence of the subjective experience of place which makes it so different from space. Although a place is commonly but not necessarily an identifiable location, there must be some recognizable qualities, natural or constructed appearance, or something reflecting human activities and values. The stadiums of our cities are easily recognizable places. Its essence is that "Place is a centre of action and intention, it is 'a focus' where we experience the meaningful events of our existence" (Norberg-Schulz, cited by Relph, 1976, p. 42). "Space is transformed into place as it acquires definition and meaning" (Tuan, 1977, p. 136). Place develops from the patterns of occupational interaction that occur there and their meaning to us, indeed "some events and actions are significant only in the context of certain places" (Relph, 1976, p. 42). What occupations are enacted in what kinds of places or spaces? What is a "sacred" place (church, temple, shrine, "green cathedral")? What is a public place versus a private place?

Place attachment is a bonding of person to place. We feel connected to a place based on our occupational past there and our perception of occupational potential within it (Altman & Low, 1992). "[A] place has personal significance, a significance established through time spent in or with the space . . . personal experiences, either direct or vicarious, lead the person to attach meaning . . . linking significant life events, key developmental themes, or identity processes with a particular environment. . . . Place attachment is not a state but a process that continues throughout life" (Rubenstein & Parmalee, 1992, pp. 142–143). "While it takes time to form an attachment to place, the quality and intensity of experience matters more than simple duration" (Tuan, 1998, p. 198).

Rowles's (1991) findings illustrate the importance of quality, intensity, and duration of experience with place in his study of elders in their small home town: that place became a component of self. Over many years of living in the same community, the spatial environment had developed an historical time-depth of meaning, with layer upon layer of meaningful life experience accumulating. It became linked to their personal history and became a part of their self-identity. It was a place, not a space, and their self-identity had place identity. When I describe myself as "an American; a Californian transplanted at midlife from Wisconsin," I believe I am not just reciting my temporal history, my spatial geography, but saying something about myself.

Placemaking is the act of creating and maintaining places (for example, homemaking)—a human occupation often in collaboration with others. Hasselkus (1999) defined occupational therapists' unique act of placemaking, making a therapeutic occupational place, in terms of the experience of intimacy and connection between therapist and client defined by the doing of occupation. The act of making and maintaining that therapeutic place takes time, first developing rapport and understanding of the situation; then, engagement in the therapeutic occupation; and finally reaching the state of relative well-being brought about by therapy.

Time and Space, Temporality and Place

"We have a sense of space because we can move and of time because, as biological beings, we undergo recurrent phases of tension and ease. . . .When we stretch our limbs we experience space and time simultaneously—space as the sphere of freedom from physical constraint and time as duration in which tension is followed with ease. . . .A pace is not only something we can see—the span between one foot and another—but it is also felt in the muscles. How is the pace (step) . . . related to time? A pace is a unit of time because it is felt as a biological arc of effort and ease, strain and relaxation. One hundred paces means one hundred units of a biological rhythm that we know intimately" (Tuan, 1977, pp. 118, 129–130).

Hall (1983) noted that the study of time and space "has led the human species out into the universe, down into the heart of the atom, and is the basis of much of the theory concerning the nature of the physical world" (p. 203). Space and time constitute important elements of the set of patterns we call culture. Time talks and space speaks, as part of our silent cultural body language (Hall, 1959/1981). Space and time have held the attention of others (Bachelder, 1964) who have defined the nature of time and space through the experience of time and space by individuals within their culture.

Rowles (2003) reminded us that the "experience" of time and space also can be vicarious participation in spatially or temporally displaced environments. For example, we may experience temporal and spatial displacement with reflective involvement while paging through an old photo album or watching family slides, home movies, or videos from our past. (I certainly felt momentary displacement when I saw some of those slides of me that Dr. Royeen showed us!) We experience vicarious projection into places that are geographically displaced from our current location while reading literature, watching movies, playing video games, or surfing the Internet.

Time and space can constrain or enable occupations. In the real world, a time–space prism (Dear, 1996) determines where, when, and, in some ways, what occupations we can do. The time it takes to move through space limits the distance we can travel between occupations. Certain activities are constrained or enabled in certain times and places. We have a certain degree of occupational time and place dependence. That is, we depend upon times and places to allow us to "be" and "do" our selfhood through our occupations. They provide temporal and spatial occupational affordances for our activity, like the physical affordances of surfaces and objects. Places are "behavior settings" (Barker, 1968), where individuals and their surroundings together create systems from which emerge a certain behavioral status quo, the stability of place. Place influences the type, frequency, duration, and style of behavior, and through occupational behavior, influences lifestyle and well-being (Hamilton, 2004). Location in developmental time can enable but also constrain our occupations, often for the benefit of others rather than our own health and well-being, as when any age group is limited by the phrase "act your age!"

Life is continuous development of occupational horizons, or boundaries of our perceptions of the spatial and temporal world, and Blanche and Parham (2001) offer tentative examples of some of them. For example, the infant's beginning organization of occupation is within the horizon of its own Body Space in the Present (p. 191). For the infant, co-occupations within this horizon are breastfeeding and cuddling with their caregiver. An adult may find occupations such as meditation or receiving a massage within that same horizon. Another spatiotemporal horizon of occupation is that of Reach Space in Proximal Time (p. 192), or interactions within what Hall (1966/1982) called personal space, occurring within a time frame of minutes to hours in infant occupations such as manipulation or mouthing of toys (Pierce, 1997) and for adult occupations such as computer keyboarding. A spatiotemporal horizon called Moving Through Proximal Space and Time is exemplified by occupations such as dancing, playing football, or maneuvering through a crowded public space. Expanding horizons even further, Moving Through Cognitive Space in Extended Time, the individual is able to organize time and space to "orchestrate a stream of occupations into a daily round of activities" (Blanche & Parham, 2001, p. 193). The furthest horizon of time and spatial organization of occupations they suggested was Imagining Action in Distant Time (p. 193). They posit that praxis is the "organizational process that manifests itself in motor control as well as in general organization of behavior" (p. 183) and that a "dysfunction in this basic spatiotemporal organizational mechanism [such as developmental dyspraxia or adult apraxia] manifests itself throughout the lifespan" (p. 183). It is the role of the occupational therapist not only to address organization of simple motor behavior in proximal space and time, but to consider treatment approaches that will help our clients organize space and time in occupations across "increasingly more abstract and complex spatiotemporal horizons" (p. 198).

Rowles's (1991, 2003) research reflects these occupational temporal-spatial horizons in our everyday activities as we move through our daily life along our familiar pathways. His research found a rhythm, in time and space, of routine taken-for-granted occupations. One pattern was development of body awareness of one's home and objects in it. Repetition of occupations in a familiar setting with familiar objects over the years allowed elderly participants to handle space on an unconscious level and helped them adapt for changing sensory abilities. Body awareness in the larger environment beyond the home was part of an occupational pattern of their routine community participation, like a familiar dance, with people and places in temporal, spatial, and social synchrony.

We mix time and space; in our thinking time is described in "length," or even volume (having a big time out!). And space is measured in time. Modern life means we wonder how long (spatial term for time) we will have to look for a parking space and whether we should have allotted a bigger block (spatial term for time) for our next appointment. Tuan (1998) explains, "An explanation for the wide use of time to measure distance is the fact that units of time convey a clear sense of effort. The useful answer to questions of distance tells us how much effort is needed—what resources of energy are required—to achieve a goal" (p. 128).

Occupational engagement requires attention as well as muscular energy, and our choices of occupation are constrained by limited attentional resources. Because of limited energy for attention, optimal choices of occupations throughout the lifespan are important to support development. (Csikszentmihalyi, 1974, 1990; Csikszentmihalyi & Csikszentmihalyi, 1988; Csikszentmihalyi & Larson, 1984). Csikszentmihalyi recommends a purposeful, agentic occupational life resulting in feelings of temporospatial harmony in which one's varied activities fit together into a unified flow experience, producing a meaningful life experience. It's hard to attain this level of meaning in our life, and adolescents are an age group that seems to have particular difficulty finding ideal occupations for its development. Adolescents frequently do not experience the state of flow where their skills and the challenges of their occupations are above average, but well-matched. Instead, they engage in occupations in which they experience a state of apathy or boredom, with low skills and challenges (Farnworth, 2000). An example of this is seen in research from my recent grant project (Zemke, 2000), the work of Qu (2003), reported at this Minneapolis AOTA Conference (Qu, Zemke, Chu, & Sun, 2004), studying the quality of occupational experience of young adolescents during smoking.

We carried out an ESM study of over 100 children in the Los Angeles area. These middle school 12-year-olds reported their experience of occupations in over 3,000 "beeped" responses on their Palm III PDAs. Forty-three percent of the students were categorized as smokers or experimenters, somewhat lower than the over 50%–60% of teens usually categorized as such. The time of day of smoking incidents reflected school breaks, after school, late-afternoon, and early-evening peaks, and over 10% of the places where they smoked were that back corner of the school grounds that we all probably remember from our school days, out on the urban street, and alone in their bedrooms. In addition to smoking, secondary occupations they were sometimes engaged in were passive, "just thinking," TV, or listening to music. Their experiential state during smoking was one of apathy, what Csikszentmihalyi and Larson (1984) called an entropic or disordered cognitive state, with below average affect, low levels of activation, low cognitive efficiency, low motivation, and low self-concept. Even more interesting was their experiential pattern previous to, during, and after smoking. When beeped prior to smoking, their responses commonly indicated below average responses to most of the measures of their experience. The trend that was seen in 22 of 28 measures was that those low feelings dropped even lower during smoking, but then were higher when beeped after the smoking incident. It would appear that smoking may be an adaptive strategy used by the young people to improve their experience of life, although making it worse before it gets better. Nonsmoking students showed similar patterns of occasional apathy with improvement following engagement in a variety of occupations. These results suggest directions for development of a program of Lifestyle Redesign for the young people, assisting them to find and choose healthier occupational strategies for improving their daily experience.

Time, Space, and Occupation: Home and Work

"Time and space are directed when one is actively planning. Plans have goals. Goal is a temporal as well as spatial term. . . . In purposeful activity, space and time become oriented with to the active self" (Tuan, 1977, p. 128).

Let's look briefly at some examples of such purposeful activity, the occupations carried out at home and work, in terms of their temporal and spatial dimensions. For adult Americans, work is a descriptor of the self. This holds true even for some Americans who have little to no job opportunity and thus feel lower self-worth because of unemployment (Wilson, 1998). Ehrenreich (2001), in her "undercover" role as minimum wage worker, noted that few of her coworkers felt deceived. But then she realized that people knew her as the waitress, cleaning person, nursing home aide, or retail clerk not because she was acting like one, but because that is who she was, at least at that time and place. In the closing of a furniture manufacturing plant in the South, Bamberger and Davidson (1998) noted the impact on the workers of the loss of their temporospatial activity, work, at White Furniture Company. The blue-collar workers who stayed at the plant for years before and then during its closing chose to stay because, to them, it was a career, their life, not just a job. These people constantly used metaphors of death to describe the loss of their workplace and work time because they felt that something of themselves died when White Furniture closed.

Let's consider the routine of going to work in the morning and returning home at night. This is such a habit for us as we move in time and space that we give it little thought. Yet ritual surrounds these to-and-fros. Each day is a new day. In the morning, work lies ahead, in one's future. Movement to it is forward movement. Although work may be routine much of the time, novelty is always a possibility if only because one may meet strangers whose behavior cannot be predicted, or external events may be unpredictable. Uncertainty and the potential for surprise are characteristics of the future and contribute to a sense of the future. At the end of the day the worker prepares to return home. "We return—tracing our steps back in space—and going back in time—to the familiar haven of the home" (Tuan, 1977, p. 127). Home is where one starts from and where one returns in this daily journey (Casey, 1993). Home is a place full of familiar objects that we have chosen and know well through frequent daily use. "Home is an intimate place . . . 'where every day is multiplied by all the days before it'" (Stark, cited by Tuan, 1977, p. 145). "Home place and quotidian life feel real. . . .The real is a familiar daily round, unobtrusive like breathing" (Tuan, 1977, pp. 145–146).

Larson and Zemke's (2004) discussion of occupatio-temporality is nested within a review and synthesis of factors in the orchestration and synchronization of daily activities for dyads and groups in both work and home place contexts. For most of us, occupational boundaries, our lines between home and work, are drawn through the dimensions of time and space. We put physical, mental, and behavioral edges or borders or bridges between these two occupational settings. Nippert-Eng (1995) speaks of the "territory" of the self, presenting the self not just as a mental construct, but as located in space and time, manifest as the behavior of our embodied self. We embed this self in and associate it with particular environments, such as home and work, which evoke associated activity. Not only unique "doings," but unique "ways of being" may accompany our engagement within the temporal and spatial boundaries of work or home or the transitions between them. A comparison of workplace and home reflects the way aspects of the self are situated within or shared through these occupational settings' spatiotemporality. As we change times and places, commuting between work and home, our occupations may be self-integrating, supporting our common self, or self-segregating, separating different aspects of our self. For example, in "public" time and spaces we are normally accessible and accountable to others, while in "private" time and space we are relatively inaccessible and unaccountable (Zerubavel, 1985). Work is associated culturally and historically with more public temporalities and places, in contrast to home. Although we traditionally think of physical separation or segmentation of these realms of activity as occurring in time and space, Nippert-Eng (1995) reminds us that an even more definitive mental segmentation and transition accompanies our physical ones. Time and space and the physical journeys within them are not the essence of the boundaries and transitions between occupations, but, rather, the "grease that helps our mental gears shift" between the ways of thinking, being, and doing. Zerubavel (1991) suggested that the worlds of work and home required a mental leap to transition, whereas Nippert-Eng suggests that if they are more integrated, they may require only a mental stroll. Dickie (1996) reported on the fluid spatiotemporal boundaries between the "productive" work and "reproductive" family obligations of people who produce craft work in their home. However, in our segmented contemporary American society, frequent transitions are required of most of us.

Liminality (Turner, 1967, 1974; Van Gennep, 1960) refers to cultural transformations in which people leave one social status and enter another. Although it has not usually been applied to a daily repeated dis- and relocation of status and selfhood, the concept fits the daily commute well:

> Relative to home and work, the journey between them is a spatially, temporally, and socially "interstructural" location. For this reason, it offers the perfect opportunity for mental transitions between realms. As the journey physically dislocates and relocates us, it simultaneously encourages us to mentally detach from and reattach to the realms and selves on either side. (Nippert-Eng, 1995, p. 119)

As a commuter in Los Angeles for the last 25 years, I had never thought of my time in the long, narrow parking lot called the freeway as a liminal experience, daily changing my status and self from homemaker to employee and back. Would greater segregation or greater integration of my time, space, and self have eased that burden?

Occupation, Time, and Space Within the Kaleidoscopes of Culture

As an occupational scientist, I find culture interesting mainly as a group's view of what occupations are important to engage in and why, when, where, and how we do them. Bonder, Martin, and Miracle (2004) promote a dynamically focused view of culture as a "system that emerges through the everyday interaction of individuals" (Bonder et al., 2004, p. 162). Thus time and place both affect the expression of culture. Culture is learned and its values are local (developed through interactions at particular times in particular locations). The "ability of cultures to incorporate new ideas, to borrow from other cultures, to assimilate new information, is a strength that enables cultures to persist" (p. 164). As a cultural group, we Western occupational therapists need to carefully assess how our ideas of time, space, and occupation should be shared globally.

Blanche and Henny-Kohler (2000) suggest three ways of sharing knowledge between geographic regions, reflecting potential styles for occupational therapy in the United States and other countries. The first style is one of dependence or colonialism, perhaps many people's view of globalism today. It means importing ideas and techniques into one geographic area from another without evaluation of their fit to regional ideology and practices. The second way, independence or nationalism, protects tradition in an area by rejecting imported ideas and techniques, but results in a lack of information from outside our own familiar ideas and practices. The third, interdependent style favors regional or local research and education along with international exchange. American occupational therapy and occupational science have developed research and practices that are being shared globally. However, for most effectiveness, they must be evaluated for their relationship to local culture and ideology.

"Each culture believes that every other space & time is an approximation to or perversion of the real space and time in which *it* lives" (Mumford, 1963, p. 18). "Temporal patterns are at the crossroads of a vast web of cultural characteristics; they permeate the personality of a place" (Levine, 1997, p. 188). "We become conscious of this thing named culture when we leave our world and come up against differences—substantive and stylish differences in the way the ordinary practices of life are carried out, differences in what matters and what doesn't" (Dickie, 2004, p. 170).

Between 1998 and 2002, I spent from several months to half of the year in Japan, consulting and teaching in a developing graduate program. I was faced by much that was familiar in my home and work settings, but much that was different. The temporal and place qualities of the occupational category of "work" in Japan and the United States may be considered cultural forms (Trice, 1993), forms that contrast the cultures on the surface and also reflect underlying cultural ideologies. This overlay is exemplified in Dickie's discussion of family reunions (2004, p. 172) in which the forms may change as immigrant families acculturate, but the underlying ideology valuing family is retained.

As Hall (1966/1982) and Levine (1997) explored other cultures, they noted that the Japanese view of time and of place, or *BA,* includes another important basic cultural concept of *MA.* To Westerners, this is the space between two things, the time interval between two events, an emptiness. To the Japanese, one aspect of *MA* is that of *HASHI,* or bridging in both time and space. It recognizes not only the edges, boundaries, and the spaces between these occupational settings, but bridges between them (Hall, 1983, p. 210). As *MA,* the space between a table and a chair is not empty, but "full of nothing," acting as a bridge between them. *MA* is reflected in many aspects of daily life. The temporal give and take of conversation and dialogue is different. In Japan, as in most Asian countries, it is important to wait before speaking, to indicate time spent in thinking over what the other has said before thoughtfully entering one's own comments. The meaning of the silence is culturally recognized by the Japanese. In fact, one way to say no without saying it may be in a significant pause before saying yes. That pause if full of meaning to others in the culture, although not to a Western listener. "To most Westerners, a lack of overt activity signals that nothing is happening." But in Japan, "periods of nonactivity are understood to be necessary to any meaningful action" (Levine, 1997, p. 197). As Iwama (2003, 2004) notes, "*becoming, being,* and then *doing* may be a more understandable progression to the Japanese experience" than Wilcock's (1998) "doing, being, and becoming" (p. 249).

Because of the American focus on the individual, children learn to express their unique self, to attend to their own needs, request that these be met, to use their ability to do what is necessary to meet them. In contrast, Japanese children learn instead to harmonize with the group, that belonging is more important than doing in defining self (Iwama, 2003, 2004). They expect that in exchange people will be kind and considerate, that it is not appropriate to ask for things because what you need will be given to you by the group.

The temporality and place of the Japanese workplace has its roots in the group-oriented principle of *GIMU* (Benedict, 1946/1989; Kondo, 2004), obligation to others. "Virtually every social relationship is structured around clearly delineated duties" (Levine, 1997, p. 179). Core obligations are to one's home (family) and work (company). A major source of happiness and well-being is the "pride that the Japanese feel when successfully repaying their ON (Levine, 1997, p. 179) or debt (Benedict, 1946/1989) to these groups. The sense of obligation and responsibility to the group is strongly linked to a sense of *shoga-nai,* accepting conditions, being situated, knowing one's place in the group at any time (Kondo, 2004). This place includes *Gaman-suru,* enduring the hardship of a junior or beginning place and time in the group.

According to Levine (1997), the Japanese, being so group-oriented, seem to demand less private time (home time, leisure time) than do people in the United States, tending instead to stay around the group in the more public workplace, spend worktime developing and strengthening their relationships, go out to eat and drink together. The resulting *WA* (harmony) drives the motivation of the Japanese workforce. The relatively fuzzy boundary between work and social life reflects fundamental attitudes toward the nature of work and nonwork time (Levine, 1997, p. 179). Social relationships similar to friendships are expected to develop in the workplace and time. Sharing social "'down time' . . . is necessary for the *WA* (harmony) that . . . colleagues and Japanese society in general . . . value so highly" (p. 180). What Americans might view as "wasting time" in the workplace is a very important part of the job. Long hours at work are their obligation to their workplace, but with time, seniority will bring rewards. "SENYU KORAKU," struggle now, enjoy later, is a proverb. This belief—that what they are doing is part of the group effort—may be their principal buffer against stress.

"The impact of globalization on localized cultures must . . . be addressed. The development of occupational therapy theories that are sensitive to particular cultures is apt to lead to more culturally sensitive practice. . . .It would seem that best practice in any localized culture must take the universal as well as culture specific aspects of occupation into account" (Kondo, 2004, p. 182). Universal as well as local theories of occupation and occupational therapy theories need to be developed (Clark, Sato, & Iwama, 2000; Hocking & Whiteford, 1997; Kondo, 2004).

Time and Place: NowHere

The mirrors and lenses of the kaleidoscopes of time and place illustrate multiple facets of the complexity of occupation. If we look through the lenses of Here and Now, we can see the image that Friedland and Boden (1994) called "NowHere." What do we see for our role as occupational therapists, given our focus on occupation? Our new AOTA president, Carolyn Baum, has encouraged us to "create a process to identify topics for, and develop position papers on, key issues important to society" (LaGrossa, 2004, p. 15). We can begin to identify appropriate topics for such engagement by looking at our beliefs, assumptions, and current evidence regarding occupation. First, we can ask, "How is occupation related to health?" Based on Yerxa (2000) and our current Framework, we can think of health as existing when people's resources enable them to achieve valued goals through meaningful occupational patterns of participation in their communities. The occupational health of individuals and of societies are linked together—the problems of an economic recession resulting in widespread unemployment is a societal health problem and to the individuals affected a personal occupational one as well, resulting in occupational insufficiency or deprivation. Accepting that link, then when we look for key issues important to society and ask "What is a healthy society?" One answer is that a healthy society is one that enables meaningful occupation for all (Westhorp, 1995; Wilcock, 2003). A society that enables occupation for all will require not only health care change, but political, economic, and other social change. The suggestions for how to get that change are not new ones. The World Health Organization's Ottawa Charter for Health Promotion (1986) proposed that action was needed in five major directions: (1) building healthy public policy; (2) creating supportive environments; (3) strengthening community action; (4) developing personal skills; and (5) reorienting health services beyond the provision of clinical and curative services toward the pursuit of health. These are ideals we can accept and use to identify topics and our positions to respond to this key issue of developing a healthy society enabling occupations for the health of all the people!

"Subtlety and modesty are appropriate for nuns and therapists, but if you're in business, you'd better learn to speak up and announce your significant accomplishments to the world–nobody else will" (Trump, 2004, p. 2). Well, Mr. Trump, these therapists are ready, in this place and time, Here and Now, to stand up and announce our accomplishments to the world. The Fund To Promote Awareness of Occupational Therapy speaks with the voice of each one of us! We speak for our field—occupational therapy, for our discipline—occupational science, and for those whom we teach and serve. We work for the full participation through a healthy round of occupations of all people in their communities (their meaningful places) around the globe (today and tomorrow), each day of their lives! We work for participation in healthy occupation for EVERYBODY, EVERYWHERE, EVERY DAY!

References

Altman, I., & Low, S. (Eds.). (1992). *Place attachment*. New York: Plenum Press.

American Occupational Therapy Association. (1995). Position paper: Occupation. *American Journal of Occupational Therapy, 49,* 1015–1018.

Bamberger, B., & Davidson, C. (1998). *Closing. The life and death of an American factory*. New York: Norton.

Barker, R. (1968). *Ecological psychology*. Stanford, CA: Stanford University Press.

Bergman, L. (1998). A pattern-oriented approach to studying individual development: Snapshots and processes. In R. Cairns, L. Bergman, & J. Kagan (Eds.), *Methods and models for studying the individual* (pp. 83–122). Thousand Oaks, CA: Sage.

Blanche, E., & Henny-Kohler, E. (2000). Philosophy, science and ideology: A proposed relationship for occupational science and occupational therapy. *Occupational Therapy International, 7*(2), 99–110.

Blanche, E., & Parham, D. (2001). Praxis and organization of behavior in time and space. In S. Smith-Roley, E. Blanche, & R. Schaaf (Eds.), *Sensory integration with diverse populations* (pp. 183–200). San Antonio, TX: Psychological Corporation.

Bonder, B., Martin, L., & Miracle, A. (2002). *Culture in clinical care*. Thorofare, NJ: Slack.

Bonder, B., Martin, L., & Miracle, A. (2004). Culture emergent in occupation. *American Journal of Occupational Therapy, 58,* 159–168.

Carlson, M., & Clark, M. (1991). The search for useful methodologies in occupational science. *American Journal of Occupational Therapy, 45,* 235–241.

Casey, E. (1993). *Getting back into place. Toward a renewed understanding of the place-world*. Bloomington: Indiana University Press.

Casey, E. (1997). *The fate of place. A philosophical history*. Berkeley: University of California Press.

Clark, F., Sato, T., & Iwama, M. (2000). Bankoku kyotu no sagyo teigi no kochiku ni mukete: Sagyo kagaku no shiten [Toward the construction of a universally acceptable definition of occupation: Occupational science perspective]. *Sagyo Ryoho Janaru, 34,* 9–14.

Cottle, T., & Klineberg, S. (1974). *The present of things future. Explorations of time in human experience*. New York: Macmillan.

Covey, S. R. (1989). *The 7 habits of highly effective people. Restoring the character ethic*. New York: Simon & Schuster.

Csikszentmihalyi, M. (1990). *Flow. The psychology of optimal experience*. New York: Harper & Row.

Csikszentmihalyi, M., & Csikszentmihalyi, I. (Eds.). (1988). *Optimal experience. Psychological studies of flow in consciousness*. Cambridge, England: Cambridge University Press.

Csikszentmihalyi, M., & Larson, R. (1984). *Being adolescent. Conflict and growth in the teenage years*. New York: Basic Books.

Dear, M. (1996). Time, space and the geography of everyday life of people who are homeless. In R. Zemke & F. Clark (Eds.), *Occupational science: The evolving discipline* (pp. 107–114). Philadelphia: F. A. Davis.

Dickie, V. (2004). Culture is tricky: A commentary on culture emergent in occupation. *American Journal of Occupational Therapy, 58,* 169–173.

Edelman, G. (1987). *Neural Darwinism: The theory of neuronal group selection*. New York: Basic Books.

Edelman, G. (1989). *The remembered present: A biological theory of consciousness*. New York: Basic Books.

Edelman, G. (1992). *Bright air, brilliant fire: On the matter of the mind*. New York: Basic Books.

Ehrenreich, B. (2001). *Nickle and dimed. On (not) getting by in America*. New York: Henry Holt.

Farnworth, L. (2000). Time use and leisure occupations of young offenders. *American Journal of Occupational Therapy, 54,* 315–325.

Friedland, R., & Boden, D. (1994). *NowHere. Space, time and modernity*. Berkeley: University of California Press.

Gallagher, W. (1993). *The power of place. How our surroundings shape our thoughts, emotions, and actions*. New York: HarperCollins.

Hall, E. (1959/1981). *The silent language*. New York: Doubleday.

Hall, E. (1966/1983). *The hidden dimension*. New York: Doubleday.

Hall, E. (1983). *The dance of life. The other dimension of time*. New York: Doubleday.

Hamilton, T. (2004). Occupations and places. In C. Christiansen & E. Townsend (Eds.), *Introduction to occupation: The art and science of living*. Upper Saddle River, NJ: Prentice Hall.

Hasselkus, B. (1999). Occupational space and occupational place. *Journal of Occupational Science, 6,* 75–79.

Henderson, A. (1996). The scope of occupational science. In R. Zemke & F. Clark (Eds.), *Occupational science: The evolving discipline* (pp. 419–424). Philadelphia: F. A. Davis.

Hocking, C., & Whiteford, G. (1997). What are the criteria for development of occupational therapy theory? A response to Fidler's lifestyle performance model. *American Journal of Occupational Therapy, 51,* 154–157.

Iwama, M. (2003). The issue is—Toward culturally relevant epistemologies in occupational therapy. *American Journal of Occupational Therapy, 57,* 582–588.

Iwama, M. (2003). Revisiting culture in occupational therapy: A meaningful endeavor [Editorial]. *OTJR: Occupation, Participation and Health, 24,* 2–3.

Jacobs, G. D. (2003). *The ancestral mind.* New York: Viking Penguin.

Kondo, T. (2004). Cultural tensions in occupational therapy practice. Considerations from a Japanese vantage point. *American Journal of Occupational Therapy, 58,* 174–184.

Krieger, M. (1996). A phenomenology of motherhood. In R. Zemke & F. Clark (Eds.), *Occupational science: The evolving discipline* (pp. 243–246). Philadelphia: F. A. Davis.

LaGrossa, J. (2004). 2004 RA: Revamping OT credibility. *Advance for Occupational Therapy Practitioners, 20*(8), 14–16.

Langer, E. (1989). *Mindfulness.* New York: Addison-Wesley.

Larson, E. (2000). The orchestration of occupation: The dance of mothers. *American Journal of Occupational Therapy, 54,* 269–280.

Larson, E. (in press). The time of our lives: The experience of temporality in occupation. *Canadian Journal of Occupational Therapy.*

Larson, E., & Zemke, R. (2004). Shaping the temporal patterns of our lives: The social coordination of occupation. *Journal of Occupational Science, 10,* 80–89.

Levine. (1997). *A geography of time.* New York: Basic Books.

MacLean, P. (1978). A mind of three minds: Educating the triune brain. In J. Chall & A. Mirsky (Eds.), *Education and the brain* (pp. 388–342). Chicago: University of Chicago Press.

Merleau-Ponty, M. (1965/2002). *Phenomenology of perception* (C. Smith, Trans.). New York: Routledge. (Original work published 1945 in French)

Mumford, L. (1963). *Technics and civilization.* New York: Harcourt, Brace & World.

Nippert-Eng, C. (1995). *Home and work. Negotiating boundaries through everyday life.* Chicago: University of Chicago Press.

Ornstein, R., & Thompson, R. (1984). *The amazing brain.* Boston: Houghton Mifflin.

Parkes, D., & Thrift, N. (1980). *Times, spaces, and places: A chronogeographic perspective.* Chichester, U.K.: Wiley.

Pentland, W., Harvey, A., Lawton, M. P., & McColl, M. (1999). *Time use research in the social sciences.* New York: Kluwer Academic.

Pierce, D. (2001). Untangling occupation and activity. *American Journal of Occupational Therapy, 55,* 138–146.

Primeau, L. (1996). Human daily travel: Personal choices and external constraints. In R. Zemke & F. Clark (Eds.), *Occupational science: The evolving discipline* (pp. 115–124). Philadelphia: F. A. Davis.

Qu, W. (2003). *Quality of daily occupational experience and its relationship with adolescent tobacco smoking.* Ann Arbor, MI: UMI Dissertations Services.

Qu, W., Zemke, R., Chu, Y., & Sun, P. (2004). Quality of daily occupational experience and its relationship with adolescent tobacco smoking. Paper presented at the 84th Annual American Occupational Therapy Association Conference, Minneapolis.

Rechtschaffen, S. (1996). *Timeshifting.* New York: Doubleday.

Relph, E. C. (1976). *Place and placelessness.* London: Pion.

Relph, E. (2001). The critical description of confused geographies. In P. Adams, S. Hoelscher, & K. Till (Eds.), *Textures of place: Exploring humanist geographies* (pp. 150–166). Minneapolis: University of Minnesota Press.

Robinson, J., & Godbey, G. (1997). *Time for life. The surprising ways Americans use their time.* University Park: Pennsylvania State University Press.

Rowles, G. (1991). Beyond performance: Being in place as a component of occupational therapy. *American Journal of Occupational Therapy, 45,* 265–271.

Rowles, G. (2003). The meaning of place as a component of self. In E. Crepeau, E. Cohn, & B. Schell (Eds.), *Willard & Spackman's occupational therapy* (10th ed., pp. 111–119). Philadelphia: Lippincott Williams & Wilkins.

Rubenstein, R., & Parmalee, P. (1992). Attachment to place and the representation of the life course of the elderly. In I. Altman & S. Low (Eds.), *Place attachment* (pp. 139–163). New York: Plenum.

Szalai, A. S., et al. (Eds.). (1972). *The use of time: Daily activities of urban & suburban populations in 12 countries.* New York: Moulton.

Szalai, A. S., & Andrews, F. M. (Eds.). (1980). *The quality of life: Comparative studies.* Beverly Hills, CA: Sage.

Terkel, S. (1972). *Working.* New York: Avon Books.

Trice, H. (1993). *Occupational subcultures in the workplace.* Ithaca, NY: ILR Press.

Trump, D. (2004, April 15). Quote of the day. *Orange County Register,* Business, p. 2.

Tuan, Y.-F. (1977). *Space and place: The perspective of experience.* Minneapolis: University of Minnesota Press.

Tuan, Y.-F. (1982). *Segmented worlds and self.* Minneapolis: University of Minnesota Press.

Turner, V. (1974). *The ritual process.* New York: Pelican Books.

Van Gennep, A. (1960). *The rites of passage.* Chicago: University of Chicago Press.

Veneziano, G. (2004). The myth of the beginning of time. *Scientific American, 290*(5), 54–65.

Von Eye, A., Spiel, C., & Wood, P. (1996). Configural frequency analysis in applied psychological research. *Applied Psychology—An International Review, 45,* 301–352.

Wilson, W. (1998). *When work disappears. The world of the new urban poor.* New York: Random House.

Wilcock, A. (1998). *An occupational perspective of health.* Thorofare, NJ: Slack.

Wilcock, A. (2003). Population interventions focused on health for all. In E. Crepeau, E. Cohn, & B. Schell (Eds.), *Willard & Spackman's occupational therapy* (pp. 30–45). Philadelphia: Lippincott Williams & Wilkins.

World Health Organization. (1986). *Ottowa charter for health promotion.* Ottowa, Canada: Author.

Zemke, R. (2000). *Quality of time use and adolescent smoking.* Los Angeles: Transdisciplinary Tobacco Use Research Center, University of Southern California.

Zemke, R., & Clark, F. (1996). The dimensions of occupation. In R. Zemke & F. Clark (Eds.), *Occupational science: The evolving discipline* (pp. 89–93). Philadelphia: F. A. Davis.

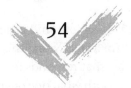

54

2005 Eleanor Clarke Slagle Lecture

Embracing Our Ethos, Reclaiming Our Heart

Suzanne M. Peloquin, PhD, OTR, FAOTA

This lecture holds familiar themes drawn from sentiments, values, and thoughts found in occupational therapy literature and elucidated through images, fables, and stories with human interest. In essence, this work is a historical and philosophical attempt to cast light on the ethos of occupational therapy. It is my hope to illuminate our ethos—the beliefs that guide us—and to do so in such a way that a fresh perspective on current challenges is possible. In the end, I will set before you this idea that asks affect and will to join with thought: To advance into the future embracing the ethos that has characterized occupational therapy since its inception is to reclaim the profession's heart.

I prepared for this day with a synthesis of my prior work, gathering new ideas to lift those thoughts to higher ground. In the process, an insight emerged. Over the years, many of you have told me that my work strikes a resonating chord, some of you naming that chord soulful, others philosophical, and still others poetic or lyrical. I believe that you discerned in my writing glints of an ethos that always has resonance, and your discernment sealed my choice of topic.

Any hope to cast light on an ethos is large enough to give one pause. This effort is but a start. I've read widely, thought deeply, and sifted many works for the beliefs that guide us. From dauntingly many iterations, I've culled themes wellworn and ethological. I've chosen words with care, seeking fidelity to our forebears and a quintessence that endures. The guiding beliefs that I propose are but my take on many other takes, here now for your taking, remaking, or leaving altogether.

The Meaning of a Professional Ethos

Dictionary definitions of the term *ethos* include these: a person's character or disposition; an individual's moral nature; the characteristic spirit or prevailing sentiment of a group; the genius—that extraordinary and distinctive capacity or aptitude—of a people or institution; the guiding beliefs, standards, or ideals that pervade and characterize a group; the spirit that motivates the ideas or practices of a community; the complex of fundamental values that permeate or actuate major patterns of thought and behavior (Simpson & Weiner, 1989).

A profession's ethos is thus an interlacing of sentiment, value, and thought that captures its character, conveys its genius, and manifests its spirit. An ethos carries beliefs so fundamental and sound that they endure, both transcending and supporting the particularities of shifting paradigms. The idea of a professional ethos kindles hope that one can apprehend and articulate a profession's character. Physician Larry Churchill (1975) said that

Originally published 2005 in *American Journal of Occupational Therapy, 59,* 611–625.

ethological beliefs are "often loosely identified, seldom find articulate form, and generally operate inconspicuously in the routines of a given community" (p. 31). Physical therapist Christine Stiller (2000) understood a professional ethos as core beliefs held in a dynamic that responds to change. Nurse Anthony Tuckett (1998) said that an ideal ethos has moral integrity in addressing both what one ought to do and how one ought to be. Each thought a profession's ethos discoverable.

Metaphors reveal its functions. An ethos serves as touchstone against which individuals strike their actions to know their worth. As inner voice, an ethos inspires individuals and calls them back when they stray too far. An ethos sets a profession's course in ever-changing times. It is bare-bones plot in a heroic tale. Bold standard raised in a milling crowd, an ethos leads those with diverse roles and views to say, "That's right!" The pull of an ethos is unbroken, sometimes undertow in currents less ideal. Its confluence of sentiment, value, and thought yields *guiding* beliefs, both vital and lasting.

It is important at the outset to distinguish our profession's ethos from other more familiar of its characterizations. Intimations of the profession's character, genius, and spirit nest in key documents of the American Occupational Therapy Association. The official definition, for example, describes occupational therapy's unique purpose, focus, and populations (American Occupational Therapy Association [AOTA], 2004). The philosophical statement reveals our grasp of the nature of persons and of occupation (AOTA, 1979). The *Code of Ethics* sets guidelines for moral practice and relationships, linking them to cherished principles (AOTA, 1994). The core values and attitudes paper culls values from our documents and uses nursing's language to cast them as commitments (AOTA, 1993). *The Guide to Occupational Therapy Practice* describes to a broad audience the scope and actions of our therapy (Moyers, 1999). The *Occupational Therapy Practice Framework* lays out the domain and process of our work (AOTA, 2002). Singly and collectively these documents draw from, organize, standardize, or recognize aspects of our ethos. They reflect its contours and honor its substance. Even together, however, they neither constitute nor state our ethos.

Also drawing from and leading back to our ethos is discourse about the profession's paradigms, models, and legitimate tools—hallmarks of our knowledge and interventions. Especially close to the ethos are discussions of the art, science, and ethics of the profession and thoughts about our culture and integrative values (Hansen, 2003; Hasselkus, 2002, Hubbard, 1991; Kielhofner 1997; Mosey, 1981; Reed & Sanderson, 1999; Rogers, 1983; Shannon, 1977; West, 1984; Wilcock, 1998; Wood, 1995, 2004; Yerxa, 1967). Not yet within our literature, however, is there an exposé of the guiding beliefs that serve as ethos.

Absent from easy access, therefore, is the ground on which Robert K. Bing (1986) suggested we stand when he said this: "Where we will find comfort, safety, and stability is in those decades-old fundamentals and principles developed by our founders and practiced by our pioneers . . . our beliefs, our values—they form the rock upon which we must stand" (p. 670). The rock is there; we need only cast light on it.

The Ethos of Occupational Therapy

The early decades of the 20th century shaped the context from which our ethos emerged. Physician Sidney Licht (1967) shared a glimpse of those times from his lived experience. A loaf of bread cost a nickel, then. Eggs were 40 cents a dozen. A man who bought a 5 cent beer could eat all the hard-boiled eggs he wanted. There was neither radio nor television. Milk was brought to homes 7 days a week by horse-drawn wagons. Toast was made atop a gas range. Houses were heated with wood or coal, and neither electric refrigeration nor supermarkets existed. It cost a penny to send a postcard, a penny more to mail a letter. All telephones were black. Street lights were turned on by men called lamplighters; there were no traffic lights or parking meters. Ford's touring car sold for $360.00.

A recently industrialized society rued the effects of machines that maimed bodies at an alarming rate. Arts and crafts societies emerged against the monotony and lost autonomy of factory work. Sanitation was poor. Social workers such as Jane Addams saw the ill effects of city life among poor immigrants and offered community activities in neighborhood settlement houses. Engineers such as the Gilbreths advanced techniques to make people and machines more efficient. War was in the news. The ways through which neighboring countries supported their soldiers prompted readiness to do the same here.

In 1917, our profession's founding year, Binet proposed the IQ test; Dewey endorsed learning by doing. Many condemned the failure of hospitals to ready patients for return to society. Inhumane conditions for mental illness earned public exposure, and the National Committee for Mental Hygiene, launched by former patient Clifford Beers, sought better treatment. Human behavior was examined in the lights of inner purpose and environmental cause. Philosophers spoke of holism, common sense, and practical consequences (Peters, 1953; Roback, 1952). I've but skimmed the wellspring from which our ethos emerged.

Early supporters of the use of occupation, the founders of the Society for the Promotion of Occupational Therapy, and early occupational workers drew from this context and their experiences a common understanding: Occupation could help. In discussing the power of occupation and a therapy built around it, they reiterated central themes with visionary zeal. From their discussions, five beliefs emerged with guiding potential, each a confluence of sentiment, value, and thought. Each had the capacity to shape character, establish reputation, and carry the profession's spirit across changing times. Each became part of our ethos.

Because each ethological belief captures a distinct and equally important dimension of occupation or occupational therapy, each relates to the others existentially rather than sequentially or hierarchically. The end result is a complex of guiding beliefs, an ethos. It is this: (1) time, place, and circumstance open paths to occupation; (2) occupation fosters dignity, competence, and health; (3) occupational therapy is a personal engagement; (4) caring and helping are vital to the work; and (5) effective practice is artistry and science. Taken together, these beliefs capture that which we profess—declare and affirm—in the world.

I offer a sampling of each of these early beliefs and, on this golden anniversary of the first Eleanor Clarke Slagle Lecture in 1955, follow each sampling with thoughts from Slagle lecturers who extended them across time. These thoughts complement kindred ideas taken from all such lectures and showcased during today's prelecture time. If they evoke others from your memory, I am pleased.

Time, Place, and Circumstance Open Paths to Occupation

One guiding belief is that time, place, and circumstance open paths to occupation, challenges notwithstanding. Situated in life circumstances of all kinds, persons *occupy* time and place (Reed & Sanderson, 1999). Adolf Meyer (1922), a neuropathologist and champion of the profession, saw time's path to occupation. Sharing his philosophy of occupational therapy when professor of psychiatry at Johns Hopkins University, he said: "Man learns to organize time and he does it in terms of *doing* things . . . and one of the things he does we call work and occupation—we might call it the ingestion and proper use . . . of time with its successions of opportunities" (pp. 9–10).

Meyer (1922) cited philosopher Pierre Janet, noting that proper use of time is "the realization of reality, bringing the very soul of man out of dreams of eternity to the full sense and appreciation of actuality." Our role as occupation workers, Meyer said, consists of "giving opportunities rather than prescriptions" (p. 7). If a person's use of time was a doing, it was also and more essentially a becoming, a realization of the soul (Peloquin, 1990, 1997a; Wilcock, 1998). Meyer continued, "The awakening to a full meaning of time as the biggest wonder and asset of our lives and the valuation of opportunity and performance as the greatest measure of time; those are the beacon lights of the philosophy of the occupation worker" (p. 9).

Watching groups of mentally ill patients engaged in handwork, Meyer (1922) saw "a pleasure in achievement, a real pleasure in the use and activity of [one's] hands and muscles and a happy appreciation of time" (pp. 3–4). He said that valuing time led to a "conception of mental illness as *problems of living*" rather than as only problems with thinking, or diseases, or disorders of constitution (p. 4).

Taking a complementary if pragmatic view, Allan Cullimore (1921), chief of Educational Service in Letterman Hospital in San Francisco, spoke of time's worth. He applauded occupational therapy's *real* work as therapeutic agent, cautioning against busy work. "Occupational therapy planned to kill time," he said, "stands in the same relation to the real occupational therapy as that of first aid to medical treatment based on examination and careful diagnosis" (p. 537). "Occupations must lead somewhere," Cullimore said, "and the patient must want to follow" (p. 538). Time and circumstance, we note, open paths to occupation. Place and circumstance do so as well.

Many places of the time called for occupations: hospitals for the insane; wards in general hospitals, from pediatric to psychopathic to orthopedic; hospital workshops; sanitaria for the treatment of tuberculosis; tents and army barracks; schools for defectives; institutions for the blind; convalescent homes; and private dwellings. Meyer's (1922) philosophy included harmonic engagement with place: "Our conception of man is that of an organism that maintains and balances itself in the world of reality and actuality by being in active life and active use . . . and acting its time in harmony with its own nature and the nature about it" (p. 5). He supported an "orderly rhythm in the atmosphere" of mental hospitals, using among disturbed patients the habit training approach to life tasks—dressing, eating, working, playing—developed by Eleanor Clarke Slagle (Meyer).

Other early practitioners saw occupation at the interface of place and circumstance. Susan Tracy (1913), nurse and early practitioner, wrote, "The occupation room provides a new environment. It takes the patient away from his individual apartment and from the living rooms of the institution which may be filled with the suggestion of invalidism. It presents a cheerful atmosphere of quiet activity and a satisfying sense of something worthwhile being accomplished" (p. 4).

Discussions of helpful atmospheres led to the making of places that grew them. Thomas Kidner (1923), Canadian architect and founder, published designs for recreation halls, workshops, and theaters to accommodate occupations. A few years later, Louis Haas (1927), director of Men's Therapeutic Occupations at Bloomingdale Hospital in White Plains, New York, published more designs, noting reciprocal ties between occupation and place: "In occupational therapy," he said, "any corner that would hold a couple of chairs was at first considered a place in which this treatment could be given. . . . The treatment itself was used as a means of transforming, not only the patient, but the very inadequate floor spaces and unsightly walls, into more inspiring surroundings" (p. 285). Many instances of environmental transformations appear in our literature (Carlova & Ruggles, 1946; Slagle, 1938).

Thoughts about occupation's emergence from time, place, and circumstance have endured. In her Slagle lecture, Anne Fisher (1998) made the connection succinctly and well. She said: "The term occupation conveys the powerful essence of our profession—enabling people to seize, take possession of, or occupy the spaces, time, and roles of their lives" (p. 511). Some 30 years earlier, Gail Fidler (1966) had said in her lecture, "Man's innate drive to fulfill his needs for self-identity and realization through productive transactions with his object and interpersonal world is and has been the cornerstone of occupational therapy" (p. 8). Our ethos, in part, is this: Time, place, and circumstance open paths to occupation. Guided by this belief, occupational therapy practitioners are pathfinders.

Occupation Fosters Dignity, Competence, and Health

Another guiding belief is that occupation fosters dignity, competence, and health. Founder William Rush Dunton, Jr. (1919) conveyed his belief in the healing role of occupation in a creed that prefaced a book on wartime work, known as reconstruction therapy. He wrote:

> That occupation is as necessary to life as food and drink. That every human being should have both physical and mental occupation. That all should have occupations which they enjoy. . . . That sick minds, sick bodies, sick souls, may be healed through occupation. (p. 17)

Almost 10 years earlier, Robert Carroll (1910), a physician in Asheville, North Carolina, had noted the worth of occupation in terms of dignity and competence, confidently proposing a "Law of Work" and asserting that "work truly is life." He said:

The greatest influence, the true and lasting benefit in work as a therapeutic agent, rests in the moral uplift, the great mastering of self which comes when one is taught to work right, when one knows the joy and forgets the burden of doing, when self-mastery displaces indulgence, when doubt of one's strength is replaced by faith. (p. 2034)

Whether endorsed as moral creed or scientific law, the belief was this: Occupation fosters dignity, competence, and health. Meta Anderson (1920) thus said that occupational therapy "should inspire the feeling of pleasure and self-respect which comes from being useful, and the feeling of power which comes from progressive daily achievement" (p. 326). Most poignant is her story, told in the language of the day:

> An official was visiting the work of the feebleminded in a certain school. The teacher reported the good work done by the various schoolchildren. When she had finished, a low grade girl member of the class tugged at her sleeve and said, "Tell him that I cleaned the garbage can." She had cleaned the garbage can and had done it very well. She beamed over the praise given to her after she had called attention to her accomplishment. She had been useful and her joy was unbounded. (p. 326)

One soldier gave this testimonial to occupation: "I got a new vision of life. . . . [I] saw the dignity of labor made new and interesting, and even more powerful because of the handicap" (Cooper, 1918, pp. 24–25).

Belief in the healing power of occupation—in its capacity to help individuals become hale and whole—has endured. What bolder affirmation than that in the Slagle lecture of Mary Reilly (1962): "The hypothesis that I presented for evidence of proof was that man, through the use of his hands, as they are energized by mind and will, can influence the state of his own health. I asked if this were a kind of idea that America could subscribe to and to that I replied with a resounding yes" (p. 8). Our ethos, in part, is this: Occupation fosters dignity, competence, and health. Guided by this belief, occupational therapy practitioners enable occupations that heal.

Occupational Therapy Is a Personal Engagement

A third guiding belief holds that occupational therapy is a personal engagement. Engagement—the commitment to involve and occupy oneself and be bound by mutual promise—was thought necessary for patient and therapist alike. George Barton (1920), an architect and founder informed by nursing courses and his own disability, clarified the aim of occupational work:

> Not in the making of a product, but in the making of a MAN, of a man stronger physically, mentally, and spiritually than he was before, for just as his body can be strengthened by carefully graded exercise from week to week, as his mind can be strengthened and be improved in the same way, so also may his spirit be reborn in greater strength and purity by the effort for, and the realization of his triumph over disability and despair. (p. 308)

Such engagement and cocreation were essentially and deeply personal.

Also personal were responses among patients such as those ill from tuberculosis. These touched Bayard Crane (1919), a physician in Rutland, Massachusetts. He said, "In them pain will create outcry or fright. Monotony will produce depression, discouragement, or desperation. Uselessness will break down initiative and ambition" (p. 63). Crane sought occupational workers who could "help meet the individual patient more on his own terms. . . . I am pleading" he said, "for a method which aims to further individualize with the temperament of each patient. . . . It is an attempt to instill in the treatment enspiring [*sic*] influences created by diversion, by occupation of mind, by stimulation of flagging interests, and by reeducation of faith and self-confidence" (p. 64). The need for occupational workers to engage as and with persons was clear.

Charlotte Moodie (1919), nurse and director of Social Service at Grace Hospital in Detroit, described patients who were engaged:

> Here, in his wheelchair we find Joe, recovering from a fractured thigh, busily engaged in carving a breadboard or bookrack. Close by, lying flat on his back is Max, a bright cheery young chap . . . tuberculosis of the spine . . . ties him to his bed. He is now making a wool sweater by means of which Miss Tracy calls "rake knitting." In the women's ward is Mrs. Schuster making a basket, something she has always wanted to do. (p. 314)

This scene of patients much engaged evokes the image of a practitioner who had explored capacity, interest, and meaning, inspired confidence and courage, and personally engaged.

Years earlier, Tracy (1913) had described the requisite engagement, noting that occupational nurses "are constantly being impressed with the fact that the technical and mechanical part of their work is but one aspect of their professional duty, that a broader conception must be attained—a sense of obligation to minister to the individual as well as to the disease" (p. 9) and to be "thoughtful of the deeper needs of her patient" (p. 11). Therapeutic obligation included deep consideration.

Meyer (1922) spoke of the integrity implicit in such engagement: "It takes rare gifts and talents and rare personalities to be real pathfinders in this work. There are no royal roads; it is all a problem of being true to one's nature and opportunities and of teaching others to do the same with themselves" (p. 7). Being true and real were important. Equally vital to the engagement were other ways of being endorsed by Kidner (1929) in an address to graduating students:

> May you realize in increasing measure the value of certain spiritual things which are the real making of life, but which we call by many common names. Kindness, humanity, decency, honor, and good faith—to give these up under any circumstances whatever, would be a loss greater than any defeat, or even death itself. (p. 385)

Perceptions of occupational therapy as a personal engagement have endured. Elizabeth Yerxa (1967) spoke eloquently of this view in her Slagle lecture:

> We cannot really help clients unless *we are there*; that is we feel, we encounter, we take time, we listen and we *are* ourselves. . . . Personal authenticity as an occupational therapist means that the therapist allows himself to feel real emotion as he enters into mutual relation with the client. . . . Philosophically, we do not see man as a "thing" but as a being whose choices allow him to discover and determine his own Being. Our media, our emphasis upon the client's potentials, the necessity for him to act and the mutuality of our relationship with him provide a milieu in which his suffering can be translated into the resolve to become his true self. (p. 8)

Our ethos, in part, is this: Occupational therapy is a personal engagement—a mutual commitment to involve and occupy the self and be bound by promise. Guided by this belief, occupational therapy practitioners cocreate daily lives.

Caring and Helping Are Vital to the Work

A fourth guiding belief within our ethos is that caring and helping are vital to the work. Herbert Hall (Hall & Buck, 1915), physician and early practitioner, spoke with deep feeling of any individual left idle or bereft. He said, "Put yourself in that man's place—imagine the despair and the final degeneration that must sap at last all that is brave and good in life" (p. viii).

Ora Ruggles (Carlova & Ruggles, 1946), reconstruction aide during World War I, enacted the empathy endorsed by Hall. She explained the caring effects of such empathy: "I don't see what's missing. I see what's there. I see real manhood. I see great courage. I see tremendous strength. I see true spirit. That's what gives me courage, strength, and spirit. I gain as much or more as the men I try to help" (p. 76). She said that she had made a great discovery, simple, yet so effective: "It is not enough to give a patient something to do with his hands," she said. "You must reach for the heart as well as the hands. It's the heart that really does the healing" (p. 69). Early practitioners sought to develop traits that shaped such caring. Moodie (1919) valued, "above all, infinite patience, the ability to teach and to criticize without causing offense or discouragement, the power of inspiring confidence in others, and last but not least an optimistic temperament and a sense of humor" (p. 314).

Hall (1922a) described the nature of our helping: "Occupational therapy . . . attempts to restore the general effectiveness of people who have become incapacitated through illness and who are not able to make satisfactory progress by their own unguided efforts" (p. 163). Respect for personal dignity was central to such helping. Susan Wilson (1929), chief occupational therapist at Brooklyn State Hospital, said that "the patient's every moment is carefully supervised," but "the treatment must not become too paternal, killing the patient's sense of responsibility for his own person" (p. 191). Similarly, Crane (1919) characterized our therapy as one which "makes the patient a creator, a doer" (p. 64).

Affirmations of our caring have endured. In her 1980 Slagle lecture, Carolyn Baum called us back to this belief at a time when health delivery systems had turned less caring. She said:

> Occupational therapy harnesses will and gives the individual control through activity. That is human, that is care. We are respected by physicians and the health care system for that caring . . . through our professional relationships we reach out and with empathy to show that we care, hoping that from this caring the person will find his own strength. (p. 515)

And exhortations to help have endured, as June Sokolov (1957) reminded us in her lecture:

> In this role of helping people to achieve commonly held objectives, nothing is more rewarding than our deepening awareness of human strength and frailty. One learns to hold aloft the ideal, to expect from people the most and the best of which they are capable yet to respect human frailty and hence to treasure the least of the offerings. (pp. 18–19)

Affirming respect for dignity in our helping, Jerry Johnson (1973) said in her Slagle, "The client and the therapist participate in a collaborative process . . . whereby the therapist provides an experiential learning environment in which the client can initiate or participate in occupational performance meaningful to him" (p. 3). Our ethos, in part, is this: Caring and helping are vital to our work. Guided by this belief, occupational therapy practitioners reach for hearts as well as hands (Peloquin, 2002a).

Effective Practice Is Artistry and Science

A fifth guiding belief is that effective occupational therapy is at once artistry and science. The interpersonal art is part of our ethos. A patient told Ruggles (Carlova & Ruggles, 1946), "You're an artist in the greatest medium of all. You're an artist in people" (p. 92). Slagle (1927), in her management roles, saw art's necessity among occupational workers. She said:

> For, if lacking in this—in understanding, in give and take, in spiritual vision of the "end problem" of all too many cases, the craftsman may make some initial showing, but the work will eventually flag and be largely a failure. (p. 126)

Supporting such artistry and vision, physician Addison Thayer (1908) of Portland, Maine, told a colleague using occupation, "It is not so much the work as the way you inspire the person to take it up" (p. 1486).

Artistry of the apt intervention is also part of the ethos. As an example, an anonymous piece in *The Modern Hospital* read in 1922, "Every OT worker of experience has seen hard, rebellious men and women soften and become teachable under the influence of quiet work . . . which may carry over into the machine life a new sense of humanity, a growing love of creative accomplishment" (p. 374). When Tracy (1921) personified occupational therapy as a wise woman walking swiftly through hallways to her patients, she included artful interventions:

> A young house painter who has fallen hurt from a staging and is pretty badly hurt. . . . Next, a psychopathic patient in a bed held in a restraining jacket. . . . Third, a man who repairs furniture. Only one of his hands are [sic] available at present. Then a three-year-old baby with a new arm in place of one crushed by an automobile. Occupational Therapy sets down her basket—There is something interesting for each person. (Tracy, 1921, p. 398)

Belief in the value of our art, in its interpersonal and interventional aspects, has endured. Geraldine Finn (1972) argued for both in her Slagle lecture, saying,

> It is this process of creative thinking which is required of us, as occupational therapists, in order to interpret our knowledge about human performance . . . and human relations . . . in the service of maintaining the health of a community. It is necessary for us to begin to think creatively about our particular understanding of man's needs and to start to build new images around this knowledge. (p. 63)

Science has been of equal value. Hall (1922b) called occupational therapy "the science of prescribed work" (p. 245). Elizabeth Upham (1918), director of the art department at Milwaukee Downer College, framed it more deeply as "the science of healing by occupation" (p. 13). Calling for records and statistics in occupational therapy, Horatio Pollock (1929), director of the Statistical Bureau of the New York Department of Mental Hygiene, regarded occupational therapy "as a scientific effort for the restoration to health of the mentally and physically ill" (p. 416).

Barton's (1915) scientific hypotheses, thought extreme, included one that any medicine of the day listed in *materia medica* books had an occupational equivalent. If doctors prescribed benzol as a leucotoxin, he said, occupational therapists could engage the same patient in canning work so that benzine fumes could yield the same effect (Barton, 1915). Signs of scientific pursuit were everywhere. Harry Mock (1919), a lieutenant colonel, supported the Walter Reed way of noting motion gained. He included a photograph of a soldier flexing to view his measurements. The caption read, "Visualizing results encourages the patient" (p. 13).

Belief in science as part of our ethos has endured. In the first Slagle lecture, Florence Stattel (1956) said this: "We have been given a wonderful professional heritage of courage and wisdom and as we continue to extend our hand to benefit mankind, may we continue to believe and search for further knowledge" (p. 194). Our long-standing belief in science has grown to recognize a discipline of occupational science well-represented by the Slagle lectures of Florence Clark (1993) and Ruth Zemke (2004).

The idea of an integrated practice based on art and science permeates cases published in our early years. One is representative:

> Private J. was studying law when he was drafted. . . . He was wounded by shrapnel in his left arm and a stiff, flexed elbow had resulted. Reading law books would hardly benefit his condition but J. was interested also in making mission furniture out of old boxes and lumber. . . . Using his left hand chiefly, he soon became adept at hammering, sawing, planing, and other movements which necessitated a certain amount of flexion and extension of the elbow joint. Every week the amount of motion in the joint was measured and a careful record made. When J. saw by actual measurement that his range of motion in this joint was increasing, he was indeed happy and redoubled his efforts. Practically full joint movement had been restored when he was finally discharged. (Mock, 1919, p. 14)

Beliefs about practice as artistry *and* science have endured. Joan Rogers' (1983) Slagle lecture discussed our reasoning as a confluence of science, art, and ethics. In the very next lecture, Elnora Gilfoyle (1984) noted kinship in art and science: "Imagination," she said, "is the common quality in both science and art" (p. 578). She elaborated:

> In science, imagination organizes experiences into concepts, and in art imagination allows us to enter into the human experiences. Science offers explanations and rational knowledge, whereas art carries an awareness of intuitive knowledge. Science of therapy is a creation to explain, and the art of therapy is a creation to relate. (p. 578)

Our ethos, in part, is this: Effective practice is artistry and science. Guided by this belief, occupational therapy practitioners are distinctly artists and distinctly scientists, both at the same time, all the time (Collins & Porras, 1994).

The Guiding Power of Our Ethos

Consider the guiding potential of our ethos: (1) time, place, and circumstance open paths to occupation; (2) occupation fosters dignity, competence, and health; (3) occupational therapy is a personal engagement; (4) caring and helping are vital to the work; and (5) effective practice is artistry and science. Each belief is expressive, persuasive, and thoughtful. Each evokes the best of who we are; each plumbs the depth of what we do. Together they afford us this view: We are pathfinders. We enable occupations that heal. We cocreate daily lives. We reach for hearts as well as hands. We are artists and scientists at once. This is our character; this is our genius; this is our spirit.

Ours is an ethos of engagement—a commitment to involve and occupy ourselves and be bound by mutual promise. Were we to distill the complex of our guiding beliefs into one brief account, our ethos might be this: Engagement for the sake of persons and their occupational natures. We engage so that others may also engage (Moyers, 1999).

Formed in the youth of our profession, our ethos calls to mind a clear-sighted youth from *The Little Prince*. Antoine de Saint-Exupéry (1943) there argued that as many individuals mature, they lose their capacity to imagine, discern deeply, and thus understand. Remembering a childhood drawing, he said:

> I showed my masterpiece to the grown-ups, and asked them whether the drawing frightened them. But they answered "Frighten? Why should anyone be frightened by a hat?" My drawing was not a picture of a hat. It was a boa constrictor digesting an elephant. But since the grown-ups were not able to understand it, I made another drawing: I drew the inside of the boa constrictor, so that the grown-ups could see it clearly. . . . The grown-ups' response, this time, was to advise me to lay aside my drawings of boa constrictors from the inside or the outside, and devote myself instead to geography, history, arithmetic and grammar. That is why, at the age of six, I gave up what might have been a magnificent career as a painter. (p. 4)

Similar experiences pull many from their imaginative capacities. Devoting themselves to routine matters, they weaken their powers of discernment. But when the 6-yearold in this story matured, he used his childhood drawing to predict the quality of understanding that he might expect from others. He explained:

> I have lived a great deal among grown-ups. I have seen them intimately, close at hand. . . . Whenever I met one of them who seemed to me at all clear-sighted, I tried the experiment of showing him my Drawing Number One, which I have always kept. I would try to find out, so, if this was a person of true understanding. But whoever it was, he, or she, would always say: "That is a hat." Then I would never talk to that person about boa constrictors, or primeval forests, or stars. . . . I would talk to him about bridge, and golf, and politics, and neckties. And the grown-up would be pleased to have met such a sensible man. (de Saint Exupéry, 1943, p. 5)

De Saint Exupéry clung to the clear-sightedness of his youth. He preserved his imaginative capacities while considering grown-up matters. Similarly, we might hold close the clarity, imagination, and perspective of our ethos as we consider matters grown up in our profession.

Challenges to the Integrative Ethos

We mostly agree that in spite of rich contributions to our development, views from medical and business models can wither our health care, educational, and scholarly aims. Among those views are an emphasis on rational fixing, a reliance on method and protocol, a drive for efficiency and profit (Peloquin, 1993a). Embrace of such views could lead to these beliefs, each true in its way but stark in its omission: Time, place, and circumstance produce profit margins. Performance fixes dysfunction. Therapy is a detached transaction. Problem solving is essentially the work. Effective practice is best-researched protocol.

Complaints from many sectors of our profession discern in such beliefs a disregard (Peloquin, 1993a). Consider this: If time, place, and circumstance produce profit margins, paths to occupation can get blocked. If performance fixes dysfunction, quests for dignity, competence, and health can be thwarted. If occupational therapy is a transaction, personal engagement can get lost. If problem solving is key, caring can matter less. If effective practice is best-researched protocol, artistry can seem esoteric. In this way, one might mistakenly think organizational profit opposed to professed aims, therapeutic purpose at odds with personal meaning, technical efficiency preempting human presence, competent solutions more prized than caring actions, and scientific reasoning sounder than artful intuition. Such polarized thought is not surprising in view of Churchill's (1975) argument that ethological norms, typically integrative and complex, are vulnerable to dualisms. Polarized thought can temporarily disintegrate an ethos.

A practitioner's felt-experience of a disintegrating trend is a sense of juggling, a struggle to stand in place with some views held but briefly, a stretch to keep tossed items safe but still within reach. Pressed to disregard functions that they deem valuable, practitioners feel deep consequences in every realm of practice. We've named one *depersonalization*.

Depersonalization evokes a radical image in its removal of persons. When personal care is hollowed from health delivery, practitioners feel the assault, and those seeking care are devastated (Peloquin, 1993b). René Magritte rendered the angst well in a work called *The Therapist*. A seated and caped figure sits squarely under a slivered moon and flattened hat. Face and chest are gone, replaced by emptiness. Doubtful that this therapist could find paths to occupation. The promise of engagement is slim. Caring expressions seem improbable, helping unlikely. Depersonalization mutes our call to engage for the sake of persons and their occupational natures. It spawns disheartening times, places, and circumstances. The realities and dangers of depersonalization permeate cultural images. As forms of art, they help us discern de Saint-Exupéry's boa consuming the elephant. And we *should* be frightened by this hat.

We must ask: Is our ethos the problem? Is its interlacing of sentiment, value, and thought outdated fancy to be put aside? I think not. I propose instead a reframing of disheartening contexts in the clear light of our ethos. Listen to the Parable of Two Frogs (author unknown, 1999):

> A group of frogs were hopping contentedly through the woods, going about their froggy business, when two of them fell into a deep pit. All of the other frogs gathered around the pit to see what could be done to help their companions. When they saw how deep the pit was, they agreed that it was hopeless and told the two frogs that they should prepare themselves for their fate, because they were as good as dead. . . .

> The two frogs continued jumping with all their might, and after several hours of this, were quite weary. Finally, one of the frogs took heed to the calls of his fellow frogs. Exhausted, he quietly resolved himself to his fate, lay down at the bottom of the pit, and died. The other frog continued to jump as hard as he could, although his body was wracked with pain and he was quite exhausted.

> Once again, his companions began yelling for him to accept his fate, stop the pain and just die. The weary frog jumped harder and harder and, wonder of wonders, finally leaped so high that he sprang from the pit.

> Amazed, the other frogs celebrated his freedom and then, gathering around him asked, "Why did you continue jumping when we told you it was impossible?" The astonished frog explained to them that he was deaf, and as he saw their gestures and shouting, he thought they were cheering him on. What he had perceived as encouragement inspired him to try harder and to succeed against all odds.

We too can reframe disheartening contexts. Our ability to do so rises from the capacity for resilience that Susan Fine (1990) described in her Slagle lecture. She asked, "Who rises above adversity?" (p. 493) I say that *we* do. We acknowledge an enormous cleft of land in Arizona, a dangerously deep pit and obstacle to circumvent, but reframe it positively as the Grand Canyon. Likewise, we can reframe challenges to our ethos as calls for its reclamation. The challenges can cheer us on.

A Fresh Perspective on Current Challenges

Five reflections follow, each framing a current challenge in light of a guiding belief. Together they suggest actions so grounded in our ethos that they promise reclamation of our heart. Let me explain. Dictionary definitions of the term *heart* yield a more fulsome meaning than we sometimes suppose. Heart is the seat of feeling but is also the seat of understanding and thought. It is the depths of soul or spirit. Heart is the source of life and its vital principle; heart is one's disposition, temperament, and character; heart is courage; it is the source of human ardor, enthusiasm, or energy; heart is the innermost part of anything (Simpson & Weiner, 1989). Because the full-bodied meaning of *heart* is so like that of ethos connotationally and metaphorically, an embrace of the profession's ethos seems an embrace of our heart.

We Are Artists *and* Scientists

Guided by the belief that effective practice is artistry *and* science, we are artists and scientists at once (Collins & Porras, 1994). Honoring our ethos, we strive toward integrative practices (Peloquin, 1994, 2002a). Gestalt visions grounded our ethos in it origins, images of whole persons possessed of mind, body, *and* spirit; hands *and* hearts; physical *and* mental health. How can we reclaim those? For one, we can prompt the imagination that drives our science and art. Consider a beach scene. Sand and water come together at seaside, quite distinct but dynamically related. Seaside *is* because of land and ocean. Grains of sand and waves of sea together make seaside. Seaside would not *be* if one were gone.

More images may fire our gestalt capacities. A nesting doll holds others within itself. A dance evokes rhythmic moves, some made in tandem. Woodland streams send many-sourced waters in shared directions. A butterfly draws one form from another. A symphony makes harmony from differing sounds. A tapestry brings warp and weft to pleasing patterns (Baum, 1980; Wood, 1995). A cyclist pedals two wheels smoothly and at once. Yin-yang magatamas show goodness of fit in neatly opposed designs. Each image disrupts our dichotomies. Each prompts integrative thought.

Add to such imagery the question asked by William James (1947) about whether we walk more essentially with the right or the left leg. Clearly we need both. And if we drift to polar thinking, we might consider ski poles, together lending support and balance. Can we not imagine cosupportive synergies drawn from science *and* art (Peloquin, 1994)? If so, we can see intervention, education, and inquiry as venues for the integration of competence *and* caring, professional purpose *and* personal choice, productivity *and* self-actualization, problem solving *and* collaboration, evidence *and* meaning. That perspective captures our ethos.

Even in the business world, James Collins and Jerry Porras (1994) endorsed the "genius of the and" noting that "a highly visionary group will aim to be distinctly yin and distinctly yang, both at the same time, all the time" (p. 45). When, in light of our ethos, we envision and enact our belief that effective practice is artistry *and* science, we realize a vital principle of our profession. And in doing so we reclaim our heart.

We Are Pathfinders

Guided by the belief that time, place, and circumstance open paths to occupation, we are pathfinders. But how can we find paths to occupation in managed care and other disintegrating environments? We must first see overly managed systems as polarized. Management—skillful handling and control—is a distinct part of good care, but even in the realm of horse training, where the term *management* originated, experts suggest this broader view:

> We shall have to give up our inclination to control our horse by force. Instead we shall have to try to learn to respect the way that he wants to do things. . . . And, instead of trying to impose on our particular animal the idea of what he should be able to achieve, we must first seek to learn what his capabilities really are . . . we shall have to add to our analytical capability an equal capacity for intuitive thought. . . . Without this, our relationship with our horse will be one of spiritual warfare instead of harmony and beauty. (Hassler, 1994, p. 16)

Strife occurs in health systems when control preempts care. Without harmonious relationships and respect for choice, management fails (Curtin, 2003). If we had galloping costs, unbridled excesses, and runaway procedures, these called for taming. But they did not warrant the split vision that has made an oxymoron of managed care (Peloquin, 1996). To see the split is to discern the missing care. And that discernment opens paths for its return.

In his reflections about educational systems, Gordon Davies (1991) asked a hard question of those on governing boards with control: "Are we helping to create an environment" he asked, "in which teaching and learning are honored and can flourish?" (p. 58). He saw in governance a pathfinding role. He heard a call to engender restlessness throughout the system, disturb complacency, and insist that rules be broken for the sake of learning (Davies). Likewise we might ask, "Are we making environments in which occupation can flourish?" Our activists, theorists, and innovators have asked. They have seen their pathfinding roles. They cause restlessness and disturb complacency as they challenge oppressive policy, affirm occupation as central, and make new practice sites—in clubhouses, workplaces, and community centers—for the sake of occupation.

Others make paths in quiet ways. Practitioners nest kindness, choice, and respect in approved interventions, working within payment rules to enhance performance. They foster dignity. Practitioners working in cramped spaces share big and courageous ideas that help clients remake their lives. They foster competence. Practitioners with huge caseloads in rushed circumstances craft cogent letters that extend occupational therapy. They foster health. Blocked as some may be from real occupation, they feel its steady pull. They heed its innermost call for dignity, competence, and health. They shape circumstances that hasten its return. Their efforts call to mind the words of Nkosi Johnson (Wooten, 2004), an African child and activist who died of AIDS at the age of 12: "Do all you can with what you have in the time you have in the place you are" (Norris, 2004).

If health care environments seem disintegrative, they are not unique. Educators face a press for what Kerry Walters (1991) called a vulcanization of students, a Spocklike penchant for rational problem solving that stunts affective growth. Technologies proliferate, some putting interpersonal ken and harmony at risk. Through confluent models that foster learning with, about, and for whole persons, occupational therapy educators grow human potential and blaze trails to occupation (Peloquin, 2002b). Scholars face cut-throat trends to earn grant funds for institutional gain. Some are pushed toward discontinuous projects that neither flow from preferred inquiry nor grow the profession's work (Mosey & Abreu, 1998). Through mindfulness, integrative methods, and a compass set on occupation, scholars make pathways back to our ethos (Abreu, Peloquin, & Ottenbacher, 1998).

Practitioners who honor occupation in disintegrating environments are pathfinders. When, challenges of all kinds notwithstanding, we affirm the belief that time, place, and circumstance open paths to occupation, we enact the courage of our profession. And we reclaim our heart.

We Reach for Hearts as Well as Hands

Guided by the belief that caring and helping are vital to our work, we reach for hearts as well as hands. Nine decades after he first said them, Hall and Buck's (1915) words still ring clear: "Put yourself in that man's place—imagine the despair" (p. viii). Depersonalized contexts in our times can fire such imagination and stoke our wills. Listen to Alfie Kohn (1990):

> No imported solution will dissolve our problems of dehumanization and coldness. No magical redemption from outside of human life will let us break through. The work that has to be done is work, but we are better equipped for it than we have been led to believe. To move ourselves beyond ourselves, we already have what is required. We are human and we have each other. (pp. 267–268)

How are we equipped to move ourselves beyond ourselves? Stories from the autobiography of Ora Ruggles point to our capacity for empathy (Peloquin, 1995). At its core a disposition toward fellowship, empathy is a turning toward another not just to solve a problem but to care and to help. Ora's turning enabled her reaching, made clear in her work with a girl named Edith (Peloquin, 1995).

Ora launched a program at Olive View sanatorium, knowing that a board of directors would inspect her work before granting space or funds. She first intervened with Edith, a teen with spinal tuberculosis so severe that she lay arched and prone in a Bradford Frame. Ora found a mirror that let Edith see her hands; she built her a worktable. Noting Edith's flair for style and skill at sewing, she nurtured her potential as a dress designer and suggested doll clothes as a start. Edith produced fine work.

When county board members visited Edith, Ora heard a woman nicknamed "Hawkeye" regret time spent on such a "hopeless case." Ora said, "No one is hopeless who wants to be helped, and there's nobody in this place who wants to be helped more than Edith does. That's why I'm working with her and that's why I'm going to continue working with her." She smiled at Edith. "And that's why she's going to get well" (Carlova & Ruggles, 1946, p. 168). Hawkeye said that such sentiment was fine, but the board sought clear results.

Edith was to have shin bone segments grafted to her unstable spine. She yearned to pay for her surgery but doubted such income from doll clothes. Ora considered the situation. She made stylized figures from pipe cleaner and suggested that Edith clothe and group these to show rhythm and life. Edith caught on, creating ballets, skaters on a pond. Other patients joined in, making backgrounds and bases. The doll clothes sold readily in Los Angeles, and Edith's share of the profits funded her surgery.

At the next visit of the board, a physician reviewed Ora's work, and even Hawkeye was impressed. They approved a workshop that Ora helped design. Edith was discharged. She attended a fashion design school, became a well-known dress designer, supported her family, and funded patients at Olive View. The story is a tribute to Edith's spirit. It tells of Ora's empathy *and* good management sense.

John Gums (1994) would applaud the work of Ruggles, whose reaching for hearts and hands spread fellowship broadly. Gums said:

> Every human being is born with the capacity to empathize. Most medical professionals, through their training, are taught to squeeze out that natural ability. Rediscovering it later in our professional life is a goal we should all have. Evidence suggests that to do so, emphasis must be placed on consideration of human life. (p. 251)

The rediscovery of empathy is not an add-on task to juggle alongside others, but more like the act of a cyclist turning the wheels of competence and caring at once. Elsewhere I've suggested that empathy is a considered way of being brought to our doing, no matter what that doing is (Peloquin, 1995). Being present to another in time is not the same as having lots of time. Consider interactions during checkout at a grocery store. In a few minutes, some cashiers forge real connections. We have much more time than most cashiers, and we connect well through our doing. And if being present admittedly *takes* energy, it paradoxically restores it, unlike the drain toward emptiness of depersonalization.

When, in light of our ethos, we affirm to ourselves and to others that caring and helping are vital to our work, when we empathically dispose ourselves toward that end, we share the ardor of the profession. In doing so, we reclaim the profession's heart.

We Cocreate Daily Lives

Guided by the belief that occupational therapy is a personal engagement, we cocreate daily lives. But how can we engage in cocreation when so much pulls us elsewhere? Media messages say that a clock has filled our souls. We wear time-machines strapped to our bodies. We're out of sorts without them. We tick with the many things that we must do. We stay wound up and out of touch with ourselves and others; we buzz within. We race with time, hoping to beat it. While seeking a control that eludes us, we turn from healthy rhythms of occupation and relationship. We loathe the idea of getting behind, or worse, of getting worn, ugly, and old. We have nearly forgotten what it means to engage with the world and connect with others (Peloquin, 1990).

If we hope to engage—to involve and occupy ourselves and others and be bound by mutual promise—we must expand our views of time. Consider the book *Cheaper by the Dozen*, about Frank Gilbreth, honorary member of the Society for the Promotion of Occupational Therapy. Gilbreth's son described his father's passion for efficiency. Fully clothed and sitting on the carpet, Gilbreth taught his 12 children the most expedient way to bathe while extending the life of the soap. If we see time only as a commodity, we have split his larger vision. Gilbreth's son, Frank Jr. (1948) shared what we have missed:

> Someone once asked Dad: "But what do you want to save time *for*? What are you going to do with it?
>
> "For work, if you love that best," said Dad. "For education, for beauty, for art, for pleasure."
>
> He looked over the top of his pince-nez. "For mumbletypeg if that's where your heart lies." (p. 237)

We mark time; we count units of productivity because we must. But only if we engage with the world will we find where our hearts lie. And only if we engage with others can we help them find what they love best.

Most media messages that commodify time differ from a sense of time's wonder, like that of our forebears, found in the story of *The Velveteen Rabbit* (Williams, 1978). The Rabbit, new to a young boy's nursery, asked the Skin Horse, a kindly older toy, a question that we too ask:

"What is REAL?" asked the Rabbit one day. . . . "Does it mean having things that buzz inside you and a stick-out handle?"

"Real is not how you are made," said the Skin Horse. "It's a thing that happens to you. When a child loves you, then you become Real."

"Does it hurt?" asked the Rabbit.

"Sometimes," said the Skin Horse, for he was always truthful. "When you are Real you don't mind being hurt."

"Does it happen all at once, like being wound up," he asked, "or bit by bit?

"It doesn't happen all at once," said the Skin Horse. "You become. It takes a long time. That's why it doesn't often happen to people who break easily, or have sharp edges, or who have to be carefully kept. Generally, by the time you are Real, most of your hair has been loved off, and your eyes drop out and you get loose joints and are very shabby. But these things don't matter at all, because once you are Real you can't be ugly, except to people who don't understand. (pp. 16–17)

When engaged and real, Yerxa (1967) said that "we feel, we encounter, we take time, we listen and we *are* ourselves" (p. 8). A modern-day story reveals such engagement.

I sustained a severe, complicated injury to my right dominant hand. . . . I was prescribed occupational therapy treatment. . . . As at many previous sessions, I was seated across from Karen (the occupational therapist), prepared to begin my treatment. However, this time was different. I gazed down at my right hand resting on the tabletop and suddenly regarded it in a totally different light than ever before—I became aware that I was permanently disfigured. . . . Overwhelmed by this realization, tears welled in my eyes, and I whispered, "It's so ugly."

Without missing a beat, Karen . . . explained that my emotions were a normal reaction to my injury . . . reassured me that this was a normal response and that we could discuss the process during therapy sessions . . . she assured me that I wasn't alone; we would work through it together. When Karen finished, I was utterly speechless. Karen had given voice to my despair. . . . For the first time since the accident, I felt as if someone could truly empathize with my plight. (Ponsolle-Mays, 2003, pp. 246–247)

The storyteller, Michelle Ponsolle-Mays (2003), later became an occupational therapist. She wrote, "And when I now use my right hand to help someone with an activity, what I see is no longer ugly—it is my personal swan" (p. 247). To the extent that we engage with others so that they can create their daily lives, we become real.

As part of our mutual promise, we can also engage as professional citizens, speaking for persons and their occupational natures. That voice—raised to secure meaningful pursuits for all—can be the defining character of our organizations (Sullivan, 1999). Professional citizenship will balance market forces if we hold what Harold Perkin (1989) called "the professional social ideal," a commitment to society as a fellowship rather than only as a marketplace in which persons become consumers and profit matters most (Peloquin, 1997b). Only then will we integrate social justice and economic solvency to shape real reform (Perkin, 1989). Only then will profit support real profession.

When, in light of our ethos, we commit to the personal engagement of occupational therapy, when we engage with others so that they might seize their daily lives, we practice real occupational therapy. We share the innermost core of the profession, and we reclaim our heart.

We Enable Occupations That Heal

Guided by the belief that occupation fosters dignity, competence, and health, we enable occupations that heal. When asked to see what we do as performance that fixes dysfunction, we might recall Meyer's (1922) vision of our dual beacon lights of performance *and* opportunity. Ours is a unique perspective. We see everyday activities as a making of lives and worlds, a broader and deeper view than that of mere performance or function, and one steeped in opportunity. Philosopher Elaine Scarry (1985) noted the world-making function of persons:

As one maneuvers each day through the realm of tablecloths, dishes, potted plants, ideological structures, automobiles, newspapers, ideas about families, streetlights, languages, city parks, one does not at each moment actively perceive the objects as humanly made; but if one for any reason stops and thinks about their origins, one can with varying degrees of ease recognize that they have human makers. (p. 312)

The image of someone in the act of making is one in which human being—its character, heart, and spirit—flows into personal doing. The difference between doing and making is one of substance and not semantic. Human making is a creation, our humane engagement a cocreation (Peloquin, 1997a).

Consider activities of daily living. We name hair care grooming, but we can see it as an act of making oneself presentable, attractive, or even likeable. What we call cooking we could easily call the making of a meal nested within larger makings—of hearth, home, or tradition. What we call work is more deeply the making of a living, a family, a reputation, a community, a society. Wherever it falls in Abraham Maslow's (1970) scheme of need, health, and hope, we see human making in daily tasks (Peloquin, 1997a). We see occupations as vital links to dignity, competence, and health. That perspective can lift our clever line, *Occupational therapy, skills for the job of living,* to higher and more healing ground where living is more than a job. And from there we might say, *Occupational therapy, making daily lives* (Peloquin, 2002a). That perspective captures our ethos.

In her poem, Janet Petersen (1976) casts even simple occupations as expressions of the human spirit:

There is a shouting SPIRIT deep inside me:

TAKE CLAY. It cries,

TAKE PEN AND INK,

TAKE FLOUR AND WATER,

TAKE A SCRUB BRUSH,

TAKE A YELLOW CRAYON

TAKE ANOTHER'S HAND

AND WITH ALL THESE SAY YOU,

SAY LOVING. (p. 61)

Through occupations such as these, the human spirit emerges, manifesting itself in small and large ways. Its emergence graces photographs of individuals seized by occupation (Menashe, 1980).

Practice stories revere this spirit. Therapist Betty Baer (2003) introduced us to a Vietnam veteran with a high-level spinal cord injury and from a remote part of Texas; he called himself a "Mountain Man." Betty wrote:

J. was self-conscious about the hole left in his throat from the tracheotomy. He thought that an Indian choker necklace would be a good way to cover up the hole. Unfortunately, he was unable to make this himself, even with the best of OT compensatory techniques and gadgets. Since I had a little experience with beadwork, we decided that he would create the design and I would be his "hands"—following his directions to produce the choker necklace. We thought this would be a good experience. It was important for J. to direct his care—why not direct his creativity as well?

This was a big challenge for both of us. It was difficult for him to put into words the steps of the activity his hands knew how to do so well. It was challenging for me to follow his instructions, and not just improvise on the knowledge of beadwork that I already possessed.

To our mutual amazement, the choker . . . looked great.

J. wore it with pride and received many compliments. This activity not only transformed a handful of beads into a necklace, but it also transformed J.'s role from a passive patient to active teacher. It was a truly wonderful OT/patient experience . . . one I will never forget. (p. 5)

When, in spite of constraints, practitioners make their interventions meaningful, lively, and even fun, they infuse therapy's purposive aims with its capacity to encourage and inspire. Acting on the belief that occupation fosters dignity, competence, and health, we embrace the spirit of the profession. As we enable healing occupations, we reclaim our heart.

Conclusion

We can stand on the rock that is our ethos and from there proclaim our view: Time, place, and circumstance open paths to occupation. Occupation fosters dignity, competence, and health. Occupational therapy is a personal engagement. Caring and helping are vital to the work. Effective practice is artistry and science. Our profession takes this stand for the sake of persons and their occupational natures. We engage—we involve and occupy ourselves and commit to mutual promise—so that others may also engage. This is our character; this is our genius; this is our spirit.

Mihaly Csikszentmihalyi (1993), a modern-day friend of occupational therapy, offered thoughts to guide a profession through this millennium. His thoughts reverberate with our ethos. "You are a part of everything around you," he said. "You shall not deny your uniqueness. You are responsible for your actions. You shall be more than what you are" (pp. 289–290).

The reflective part of this lecture began with de Saint-Exupéry's story, to which I now return. Here, a wise fox shares goodbyes with the little prince:

"Goodbye," [the little prince] said.

"Goodbye," said the fox. "And now here is my secret, a very simple secret; it is only with the heart that one can see rightly; what is essential is invisible to the eye."

"What is essential is invisible to the eye," the little prince repeated, so that he would be sure to remember. (1947, p. 87)

The ethos of occupational therapy restores our clear-sightedness so that we see what is essential: We are pathfinders. We enable occupations that heal. We cocreate daily lives. We reach for hearts as well as hands. We are artists and scientists at once. If we discern this in ourselves, if we act on this understanding every day, we will advance into the future embracing our ethos of engagement. And we will have reclaimed a magnificent heart.

Acknowledgments

My thanks go to those who preceded me in the Slagle tradition; those who nominated and introduced me; those who shared stories, images, or songs; those who helped find resources; those who warmed seeds of this work in Texas, California, Pennsylvania, and Oklahoma; those who gave me PowerPoint hints; those who gentled my prelecture mix into being; those who helped me today. I also thank those who have taught me, read me, challenged me, and worked beside me. You have all encouraged me. I especially thank each of you for being here—family, friends, teachers, students, and colleagues—because without an audience, a lecture hardly exists. Unlike interactive lectures that fill my days, this is a reading. I hope that you still feel included.

References

Abreu, B., Peloquin, S. M., & Ottenbacher, K. (1998). Competence in scientific inquiry and research. *American Journal of Occupational Therapy, 52,* 751–759.

American Occupational Therapy Association. (1979). Resolution C, 531-79. The philosophical base of occupational therapy. *American Journal of Occupational Therapy, 33,* 785.

American Occupational Therapy Association. (1993). Core values and attitudes of occupational therapy practice. *American Journal of Occupational Therapy, 47,* 1085–1086.

American Occupational Therapy Association. (1994). Occupational therapy code of ethics. *American Journal of Occupational Therapy, 48,* 1037–1038.

American Occupational Therapy Association. (2002). Occupational therapy practice framework: Domain and process. *American Journal of Occupational Therapy, 56,* 609–639.

American Occupational Therapy Association. (2004). Definition of occupational therapy practice for the AOTA Model Practice Act. (Available from the State Affairs Group, AOTA, Bethesda, MD.)

Anderson, M. L. (1920). Mental reconstruction through occupational therapy. *Modern Hospital, 14,* 326–327.

Anonymous. (1999). Parable of two frogs. *The Lord's grace. General stories of God's grace.* Retrieved February 23, 2004, from http://lordsgrace.com/stories

Anonymous. (1922). What David Belasco said. *Modern Hospital, 18,* 373–374.

Baer, B. (2003). The mountain man and the bead lady. *Revista OT,* April, 5.

Barton, G. E. (1915). Occupational therapy. *Trained Nurse and Hospital Review, 54,* 138–140.

Barton, G. E. (1920). What occupational therapy may mean to nursing. *Trained Nurse and Hospital Review, 64,* 304–310.

Baum, C. M. (1980). The 1980 Eleanor Clarke Slagle Lecture—Occupational therapists put care in the health system. *American Journal of Occupational Therapy, 34*, 505–516.

Bing, R. K. (1986). The subject is health: Not of facts but of values. *American Journal of Occupational Therapy, 40*, 667–671.

Carlova, J., & Ruggles, O. (1946). *The healing heart.* New York: Messner.

Carroll, R. S. (1910). The therapy of work. *JAMA, 54*, 2032–2035.

Churchill, L. R. (1975). Ethos and ethics in medical education. *North Carolina Medical Journal, 36*, 31–33.

Clark, F. (1993). The 1993 Eleanor Clarke Slagle Lecture—Occupation embedded in a real life: Interweaving occupational science and occupational therapy. *American Journal of Occupational Therapy, 47*, 1067–1078.

Collins, J. C., & Porras, J. (1994). *Built to last. Successful habits of visionary companies.* New York: Harper Collins.

Cooper, G. (1918). Re-weaving the web: A soldier tells what it means to begin all over again. *Carry On, 1*, 23–26.

Crane, B. T. (1919). Occupational therapy. *Boston Medical and Surgical Journal, 181*, 63–65.

Csikszentmihalyi, M. (1993). *The evolving self: A psychology for the third millennium.* New York: Harper Collins.

Cullimore, A. R. (1921). Objectives and motivation in occupational therapy. *Modern Hospital, 17*, 537–538.

Curtin, L. (2003). Ethics in management. A relationship ethos might help. *Journal of Clinical Systems Management, 5*, 8–9.

Davies, G. K. (1991). Teaching and learning: What are the questions? *Teaching Education, 4*, 57–61.

de Saint-Exupéry, A. (1943). *The little prince.* New York: Harcourt Brace Jovanovich.

Dunton, W. R., Jr. (1919). *Reconstruction therapy.* Philadelphia: Saunders.

E. E. (1921). Occupational therapy. *Hospital Progress, 2*, 265.

Fidler, G. S. (1966). Learning as a growth process: A conceptual framework for professional education. *American Journal of Occupational Therapy, 20*, 1–8.

Finn, G. (1972). The occupational therapist in prevention programs. *American Journal of Occupational Therapy, 26*, 59–66.

Fine, S. B. (1990). The 1990 Eleanor Clarke Slagle Lecture. Resilience and human adaptability: Who rises above adversity? *American Journal of Occupational Therapy, 45*, 493–503.

Fisher, A. G. (1998). The 1998 Eleanor Clarke Slagle Lecture—*American Journal of Occupational Therapy, 51*, 509–521.

Gilbreth, F. B. (1948). *Cheaper by the dozen.* New York: Thomas Y. Cromwell.

Gilfoyle, E. (1984). The 1984 Eleanor Clarke Slagle Lecture—Transformation of the profession. *American Journal of Occupational Therapy, 38*, 575–584.

Gums, J. (1994). Empathy to apathy: A consequence of higher education? *Pharmacotherapy, 14*, 250–251.

Haas, L. J. (1927). The next step in occupational therapy development. *Occupational Therapy and Rehabilitation 6*, 283–302.

Hall, H. J. (1922a). American Occupational Therapy Association. *Archives of Occupational Therapy 1*, 163–165.

Hall, H. J. (1922b). "Science so-called." *Modern Hospital, 18*, 558–559.

Hall, H. J., & Buck, M. M. (1915). *The work of our hands.* New York: Moffat, Yard.

Hansen, R. A. (2003). Ethics in occupational therapy. In E. B Crepeau, E. C. Cohn, & B. A. Boyt Schell (Eds.), *Willard and Spackman's occupational therapy* (pp. 953–961). Philadelphia: Lippincott Williams & Wilkins.

Hasselkus, B. R. (2002). *The meaning of everyday occupation.* Thorofare, NJ: Slack.

Hassler, J. K. (1994). *Beyond the mirror—The study of the mental and spiritual aspects of horsemanship.* Quarryville, PA: Goals Unlimited.

Hubbard, S. (1991). Towards a truly holistic approach to occupational therapy. *British Journal of Occupational Therapy, 54*, 415–418.

James, W. (1947). *A new name for some old ways of thinking.* New York: Longmans, Green.

Johnson, J. (1973). The 1972 Eleanor Clarke Slagle Lecture—Occupational therapy: A model for the future. *American Journal of Occupational Therapy, 27*, 1–7.

Kidner, T. B. (1923). Planning for occupational therapy. *Modern Hospital, 21*, 414–428.

Kidner, T. B. (1929). Address to graduates. *Occupational Therapy and Rehabilitation, 8*, 379–385.

Kielhofner, G. (1997). *Conceptual foundations of occupational therapy.* Philadelphia: Davis.

Kohn, A. (1990). *The brighter side of human nature.* New York: Basic.

Licht, S. (1967). The founding and the founders of the American Occupational Therapy Association. *American Journal of Occupational Therapy, 21*, 269–277.

Maslow, A. H. (1970). *Religions, values and peak experiences.* New York: Viking.

Menashe, A. (1980). *Inner grace. Photographs by Abraham Menashe.* New York: Alfred A. Knopf.

Meyer, A. (1922). The philosophy of occupational therapy. *Archives of Occupational Therapy, 1*, 1–10.

Mock, H. E. (1919). Curative work. *Carry On, 1*, 12–17.

Moodie, C. S. (1919). The value of occupational therapy to the nursing profession. *Hospital Social Service Quarterly, 1*, 313–315.

Mosey, A. C. (1981). *Occupational therapy: Configuration of a profession*. New York: Raven.

Mosey, A., & Abreu, B. A. (1998, April). *Research as a tool rather than an end of inquiry*. Short course presented at the American Occupational Therapy Association Annual Conference & Expo, Baltimore.

Moyers, P. (1999). The guide to occupational therapy practice. *American Journal of Occupational Therapy, 53*, 247–322.

Norris, M. (Interviewer). (2004, December 1). *All Things Considered* [Radio broadcast]. Washington, DC: National Public Radio.

Peloquin, S. M. (1990). Time as a commodity: Reflections and implications. *American Journal of Occupational Therapy, 45*, 147–154.

Peloquin, S. M. (1993a). The patient–therapist relationship: Beliefs that shape care. *American Journal of Occupational therapy, 47*, 935–942.

Peloquin, S. M. (1993b). The depersonalization of patients: A profile gleaned from narratives. *American Journal of Occupational Therapy, 47*, 830–837.

Peloquin, S. M. (1994). Occupational therapy as art and science: Should the older definition be reclaimed? *American Journal of Occupational Therapy, 48*, 1093–1096.

Peloquin, S. M. (1995). The fullness of empathy: Reflections and illustrations. *American Journal of Occupational Therapy, 49*, 24–31.

Peloquin, S. M. (1996). The issue is—Now that we have managed care, shall we inspire it? *American Journal of Occupational Therapy, 50*, 455–459.

Peloquin, S. M. (1997a). The spiritual depth of occupation: Making worlds and making lives. *American Journal of Occupational Therapy, 51*, 167–168.

Peloquin, S. M. (1997b). Should we trade person-centered service for a consumer-based model? *American Journal of Occupational Therapy, 51*, 612–615.

Peloquin, S. M. (2002a). Reclaiming the vision of *Reaching for Heart as Well as Hands*. *American Journal of Occupational Therapy, 56*, 517–526.

Peloquin, S. M. (2002b). Confluence: Moving forward with affective strength. *American Journal of Occupational Therapy, 56*, 69–77.

Perkin, H. (1989) *The third revolution: Professional elites in the modern world*. London and New York: Routledge.

Peters, R. S. (Ed.). (1953). *Brett's history of psychology*. New York: Macmillan.

Petersen, J. (1976). *A book of yes*. Niles, IL: Argus.

Pollock, H. M. (1929). The need, value, and general principles of occupational therapy statistics. *Occupational Therapy and Rehabilitation, 8*, 415–420.

Ponsolle-Mays, M. (2003). My ugly duckling. In D. R. Labowitz (Ed.), *Ordinary miracles. True stories about overcoming obstacles and surviving catastrophes* (pp. 246–247). Thorofare, NJ: Slack.

Reed, K. L., & Sanderson, S. N. (1999). *Concepts of occupational therapy*. Philadelphia: Lippincott Williams & Wilkins.

Reilly, M. (1962). Occupational therapy can be one of the great ideas of 20th century medicine. *American Journal of Occupational Therapy, 16*, 1–9.

Roback, A. A. (1952) *History of American psychology*. New York: Library Publishers.

Rogers, J. C. (1983). The 1983 Eleanor Clarke Slagle Lecture—Clinical reasoning: The ethics, science, and art. *American Journal of Occupational Therapy, 37*, 606–616.

Scarry, E. (1985). *The body in pain: The making and unmaking of the world*. New York: Oxford University Press.

Shannon, P. (1997).The derailment of occupational therapy. *American Journal of Occupational Therapy, 31*, 229–234.

Simpson, J. A., & Weiner, E. S. C. (Eds.). (1989). *The Oxford English dictionary*. Oxford: Clarendon Press.

Slagle, E. C. (1927). To organize an "OT" department. *Occupational Therapy and Rehabilitation, 6*, 125–130.

Slagle, E. C. (1938). From the heart. *Occupational Therapy and Rehabilitation, 16*, 343–345.

Sokolov, J. (1957). Therapist into administrator. Ten inspiring years. *American Journal of Occupational Therapy, 11*, 13–19.

Stattel, F. M. (1956). Equipment designed for occupational therapy. *American Journal of Occupational Therapy, 10*, 194–198.

Stiller, C. (2000). Exploring the ethos of the physical therapy profession in the United States: Social, cultural, and historical influences and their relationship to education. *Journal of Physical Therapy Education, 14,* 7–15.

Sullivan, W. M. (1999). What is left of professionalism after managed care? *Hastings Center Report, 29,* 7–13.

Thayer, A. (1908). Work cure. *JAMA, 51,* 1485–1486.

Tracy, S. E. (1913). *Studies in invalid occupation.* Boston: Whitcomb and Barrows.

Tracy, S. E. (1921). Getting started in occupational therapy. *Trained Nurse and Hospital Review, 67,* 397–399.

Tuckett, A. G. (1998). An ethic of the fitting: A conceptual framework for nursing practice. *Nursing Inquiry, 5,* 220–225.

Upham, E. (1918). Rehabilitation of disabled soldiers and sailors—Teacher training for occupational therapy. *Training of teachers for occupational therapy for the rehabilitation of disabled soldiers and sailors.* Washington, DC: Federal Board for Vocational Education: Government Printing Office.

Walters, K. S. (1991). Critical thinking, rationality, and the vulcanization of students. *Journal of Higher Education, 61,* 448–467.

West, W. (1984). A reaffirmed philosophy and practice of occupational therapy for the 1980s. *American Journal of Occupational Therapy, 38,* 15–23.

Wilcock, A. A. (1998). Reflections on doing, being, and becoming. *Canadian Journal of Occupational Therapy, 65,* 248–256.

Williams, M. (1978). *The velveteen rabbit or how toys become real.* New York: Avon.

Wilson, S. C. (1929). Habit training for mental cases. *Occupational Therapy and Rehabilitation, 8,* 189–197.

Wood, W. (1995). Weaving the warp and weft of occupational therapy: An art and science for all times. *American Journal of Occupational Therapy, 49,* 44–52.

Wood, W. (2004). The heart, mind, and soul of professionalism in occupational therapy. *American Journal of Occupational Therapy, 58,* 249–257.

Wooten, J. (2004). *We are all the same.* New York: Penguin.

Yerxa, E. J. (1967). The 1966 Eleanor Clarke Slagle Lecture—Every one counts. *American Journal of Occupational Therapy, 12,* 1–9.

Zemke, R. (2004). The 2004 Eleanor Clarke Slagle Lecture—Time, space, and the kaleidoscopes of occupation. *American Journal of Occupational Therapy, 58,* 608–620.

55

2006 Eleanor Clarke Slagle Lecture

The World of Everyday Occupation:
Real People, Real Lives[1]

Betty Risteen Hasselkus, PhD, OTR, FAOTA

Many roots are in the heartland of the United States. I was born in Wisconsin and have lived there all my life. Wisconsin is home to me. But "home" to me throughout my career in occupational therapy has always been the concept of **everyday occupation.** By *everyday occupation* I mean the phenomenology or lived experiences of day-to-day life (Pollio, Henley, & Thompson, 1997).

Everyday occupation is not necessarily occupation that occurs every day; it may, but it also may not. But even when it is less frequent, what I call everyday occupation is embedded in or drawn directly from those regular, daily occupations of our lives. An example of such a regular, daily everyday occupation might be preparation of a meal. A variation of this everyday occupation is preparation of a holiday meal. By my definition, even though the holiday meal is something special and does not occur daily, it still represents a form of everyday occupation because of its embeddedness in the context of daily life. Everyday occupations are all part of the rhythms of daily life; they are the occupational fabric of our everyday experiential worlds.

Everyday occupation is a primary means by which we organize the worlds in which we live; the intermeshed patterns of ordinary occupations are what give shape to our daily lives. I propose that it is around these features of everyday living that we build meaning and community in our lives (Hasselkus, 2002). And yet, the everyday occupation of people is often "seen but unnoticed" (Garfinkel, 1964, p. 226).

The purpose of this Slagle lecture is to highlight this seen but often unnoticed aspect of our occupational lives. By raising our awareness of the beauty, complexity, and "delicate layerings" (de Certeau, 1998, p. xvi) of everyday occupation, by sharing the theoretical and conceptual literature on everyday occupation, by describing some of the intriguing and compelling research on everyday occupation that is being carried out inside and outside our profession, and by recognizing the soul-wrenching state of humans for whom little meaningful daily occupation exists, I aim to demonstrate the essential relevance of everyday occupation to our quality of life and to our world of occupational therapy and occupational science. To that end, I hope to promote understandings of everyday occupation as a therapeutic entity, as a focus for teaching and training, and as an area of research inquiry with vast potential.

When our son was 8 years old, he had a school assignment to write a paragraph describing his "home." John's short paragraph included the following sentence about home: "At night I lie in bed and listen to my mother sewing, and my dad brushing his teeth." What a lovely tribute to the centrality and meaning of everyday occupation in our lives. Even to an 8-year-old little boy, the meaning of life at home is embodied in the everyday occupations of the house-hold—his mother sewing and his dad brushing his teeth.

Originally published 2006 in *American Journal of Occupational Therapy, 60,* 627–640.

[1]*The idea for this title came from a phrase written down in my notes—"real people living real lives"— and attributed to Elliot G. Mishler; neither he nor I, however, can remember its origin.*

Everyday Occupation: "Seen But Unnoticed"

Kathleen Norris (1998) says, "It is in ordinary life that our stories unfold . . ." (p. 77). In other words, the familiar world of everyday life is what we know as the *real* world; familiar scenes of everyday life are what we perceive as normal, what we hold in common with others, and what we take for granted (Garfinkel, 1964). Everyday life provides the "points of departure and return" (Garfinkel, 1964, p. 225) for every kind of variation in daily life we impose on ourselves; we say things like, "Oh, it's so good to get back to normal" after having house guests, or after a period of remodeling, or after a time of travel—all temporary departures from our usual routines. Everyday life is like an anchor in our lives. A fourth century scientist, philosopher, and theologian, Gregory of Nyssa, is quoted as saying, "Let us remember that the life in which we ought to be interested is 'daily' life. We can, each of us, only call the present time our own" (cited in Norris, 1998).

Everyday life is also a paradox in our lives. The small behaviors that make up the realm of daily life for each one of us are more than what we have in common with others; they also represent our own exquisite individuality and distinction. We may all brush our teeth every day, perhaps more than once a day, but it's probably fair to assume that we each have our own particular way of doing this tooth brushing. So on one level, we are all doing the same thing, but on another level we are *not* doing the same thing. I believe that the vast majority of occupational therapy that addresses daily life issues and skills has been based on the assumption that we are doing basically the same things, all of us, and therapy personnel have often not delved deeper to get at the singularities embedded in individual daily life. And yet, as Michel de Certeau (1998) has said, understanding of these ordinary activities "comes to light only in the details" (p. ix).

Anonymity of the Everyday

Herein lies one of the reasons that everyday occupations tend to be "seen but unnoticed." They are *seen* as commonalities across people, countries, and even cultures—something we all do. And commonality leads to lack of distinction, loss of individuality and personality. Kort (1996) says the culture is obsessed with commonalities and unities, and will produce them in order to "simplify and manipulate the world" (pp. 98–99). Rather strong words—that the overall cultural tendency in our world is to seek unity and social cohesion in order that we may render the world manageable and within our control. Kort further states that this tendency leads to the "anonymity of the everyday" (p. 105).

I see some truth in Kort's declarations, and I see tendencies toward this search for unity and commonalities within our profession of occupational therapy and our discipline of occupational science. In our efforts to define our world of practice, we create and re-create unities in the form of categories, definitions, and modalities. We strive for ways that we can reduce what we do to simple, understandable terms—terms that are accessible not only to physicians, nurses, social workers, and other health professionals but also to all the lay people, insurance people, sales people, government employees, etc., with whom we work and interact. In other words, we strive for concepts and terms that are common denominators.

Creating occupational categories. Early efforts to define our professional domain divided the concept of occupation into three dimensions—work, leisure, and self-maintenance. These three dimensions were often depicted as three large intersecting circles. Sometimes the intersections of the circles were elaborated to portray types of occupation that overlapped categories, such as the occupation of an artist, which might constitute an overlap between work and leisure. Primeau (1996a, 1998) has argued that schema such as these reflect simplistic notions of everyday occupation; she used household tasks to demonstrate the many meanings of occupation that are ignored by such models. Similarly, Lobo (1998) examined the meaning of leisure, especially its interrelationship to what we call work, revealing complexities well beyond the leisure concept in the model of three basic dimensions. Primeau and Lobo were ahead of me in their expanded thinking. For years in my university teaching, I clung tenaciously to what I now call the "big three"; I used these three categories of *work, self-maintenance,* and *leisure* to organize my teaching and writing about occupation. This model offered me a way to manage classroom content and helped me articulate the ideas I was trying to present.

In 2002, the American Occupational Therapy Association published the *Occupational Therapy Practice Framework: Domain and Process* (American Occupational Therapy Association [AOTA], 2002). By this time, my own thinking had changed, and I found myself wishing that this important document had gone further outside the box in terms of our conceptualization of occupation. Yet, at least the new breakdown of occupational categories in the framework did begin to offer nuances and a hint of the complexities inherent in the performance areas. The *Framework* elaborates the categories of occupation beyond the "big three" to include *activities of daily living, instrumental activities of daily living, education, work, play, leisure,* and *social participation; performance skills and patterns; contextual components* such as *temporality;* and *cultural* and *social* demands are sub-listed.

The danger in categories. If we look across these two models, we can see some progression toward increasing complexity. Yet models, by their very nature, reach for the inclusive, the common denominator, unity. Is this bad? No, of course not. We are searching for ways to define our territory and ourselves and to understand the essence of our profession, and we are looking for ways to communicate with colleagues and clients. Our culture demands this of us. But the models are paradoxically both helpful and dangerous; they can mold and shape us in ways that are defining but also limiting. Once we internalize the categories of occupation, we begin to fit people and their needs and our own skills into those categories. "What are you seeing that patient for?" "ADL." Our worlds of therapy seem much more manageable when we can describe and explain things in clear, simple terms. In our use of the big categories, we risk losing sight of the unique contexts and individual small behaviors of everyday life and everyday occupation that make up those sweeping categories.

So one reason that everyday occupation is often *seen but unnoticed* is because we have a penchant for pulling things together into entities that give us a sense of unity, into categories. What is *seen* is the common denominator, the anonymity of the everyday; what are often *unnoticed* are the complexities and singularities of the everyday.

Powerlessness of Words

A second reason that everyday occupation is often seen but unnoticed is the matter of social power. *Words* have a lot of power—or not. The words that are used to describe everyday occupation in the English language are words without power. I'm not sure if this applies to other languages as well. But think of the words we use in English to describe what we do in our daily lives: *routine, mundane, ordinary, commonplace, run-of-the-mill, usual, fundamental, elementary, familiar, basic, taken for granted.* These are not words with power in our lexicon. These are words that are humdrum, boring, unexciting. These are words to skip over so we can get on with the stimulating and stirring parts of language and life.

Devaluing the ordinary. Serious and wide-ranging consequences can result from the powerlessness in the words we use to describe everyday-ness in our lives. As an example, for years in our society, women's work in the home was referred to as routine, day-to-day, ordinary. Daniels (1987) describes the cultural separation that emerged between "the public world where men went out to work and the private world where women remained at home to raise a family" (p. 404). Work in the private world became largely invisible, fell outside the boundaries of what was considered valuable production, and seemed only to be noticed when absent (Daniels, 1987; de Certeau, Giard, & Mayol, 1998; DeVault, 1991; Wadel, 1979). Giard (1998) quotes the words of a song sung by women in Quebec: "Mom don't work 'cause she got too much to do" (p. 156). What women have "to do" has not been considered work. As a corollary, work in the private home domain has also been regarded as less important than that in the public domain. And as Daniels suggests, the lesser importance ascribed to work in the private domain led to women themselves devaluing their work even more generally: "The lack of validation attendant upon women's work in the family, in volunteer worlds, and in women's occupations affects the definitions women make of their own efforts" (p. 408).

My mother brought this realization to me when she was dying; we were talking about the funeral arrangements she wanted to have, and she made a comment that had a poignancy I still feel as a daughter and a woman. She told me that she had already written her obituary and shared with me some of what she had included about her life, a not unimpressive list of volunteer activities in the community and church, as well as teaching mathematics part-time in the junior high school. Yet, near the end of our discussion, she summed up her life by saying, and I quote verbatim, "Of course, it isn't as interesting as a man's." Women have, perhaps, been particularly affected by the invisibility of the everyday in our society; women, like my mother, internalized this invisibility and translated it to mean that what they did with their lives was not worth noticing very much, could be skipped over in deference to other more exciting and important aspects of life.

The everyday as an "immense remainder." Michel de Certeau (1998) refers to the *language* of everyday practices as a "murmuring" and a "chiaroscuro" in life (pp. 199–200). He says ordinary practices do not "speak"; they are part of what he calls an "immense remainder," meaning they are part of our experience that is not symbolized in our language and is, thus, relegated to obscurity and the background. He gives as an example the shopper in the supermarket who must synthesize what is in the refrigerator at home; the tastes, appetites, and moods of family or upcoming guests; the best buys and their possible combinations with what is already on hand at home, etc. The synthesis of these various elements takes the form not of discourse, however, but of the decision itself, the act and manner in which the opportunity is seized. The shopper does not talk through this everyday shopping practice, but rather the shopper pretty much silently decides and acts. Because of the paucity of language available to describe the everyday, the practices of daily life end up marginalized, belonging to no one, being without singularity or individual owners—an immense remainder.

The Problem Framework in Therapy

The cultural tendency to seek unity and commonality in our everyday worlds, plus the powerlessness and the paucity of language used to describe everyday-ness in our lives, are, thus, reasons why we may see but not notice the essential nature of everyday occupation in our therapeutic work. We don't want to focus on what we perceive to be the ordinary, already familiar, routine aspects of life. We don't want to be identified with the "immense remainder" of life. We want to be respected; we want to have a voice that will be listened to, not skipped over, in the social, educational, and medical hierarchies that exist in our worlds of therapy; we want to be considered highly skilled, not do-ers of the ordinary and mundane, or that which cannot be well articulated. Our core values and very essence may be embodied in everyday occupation, but these values and this focus are not likely to generate attention or respect from the powers of influence in our society.

One of the approaches we have taken historically in our development as a profession has been to conceptualize the everyday within a *problem* framework. We have linked our focus on occupation to a context of disability—making everyday occupations part of a problem. In the everyday world as a problem, the commonplace became not only seen, but also noticed (Garfinkel, 1964). With the link to disability, what was basically familiar and routine became unfamiliar and challenging; with this emphasis, occupational therapists found themselves able to develop and demonstrate high-level skills and to gain a sense of self-respect as well as respect from colleagues and clients. But we must recognize that with this link came, also, the medical perspective and the illness model as determinants of many aspects of the profession. In such a situation, the everyday world may become an abstraction—a world described by categories and unities instead of "the actualities of the everyday experience" (Smith, 1987, p. 89).

The premise of this Slagle lecture is that the small experiences of everyday life and everyday occupation have complexity, beauty, meaningfulness, and relevance to health and well-being that belie their aura of ordinariness and routine. For in the unique and small experiences that comprise each individual's daily life, we, as occupational therapy personnel, can derive deep understandings about the nature of the lived occupational experiences of human beings and about human occupation more broadly. And these understandings can help dissolve the anonymity of the everyday and give voice to the "immense remainder" of human experience that, at present, does not speak. Such understandings can embrace and have relevance to people with and without disabilities.

The Small Experiences of Daily Life

The 20th-century sociologist Erving Goffman (1967) used the phrase *small behaviors* to describe little external signs of social engagement—glances, facial movement, gestures, body positioning, and verbal utterances (p. 1). His attention to these small behaviors of social interaction "that most of us seldom notice" has been referred to as brilliant (Cahill, 1992, p. 194). Goffman's writings (1959, 1961, 1963, 1967) address themes such as behavior in public places, stigma, forms of talk, the presentation of self in everyday life, interaction rituals, and impression management. Goffman's analytical descriptions of even the most fleeting of social interactions help one realize just how "immense" the remainder of human experience really is. I'm using the parallel phrase *small experiences* to refer to the many seen-butseldom-noticed commonplace small experiences of our daily occupational lives— our everyday occupation.

The small behaviors and experiences of everyday occupation can be hugely important in therapeutic practice (Hasselkus, 1998). They can be the very essence of practice in some settings and with some clients. Think of children with autism, people with dementia or deep depression, and patients in semiconscious states. And these small behaviors can be the backbone of evidence for therapeutic effectiveness in our reporting—*if* they are not only seen but noticed, and *if* they are given voice. For, in reality, these nuances of everyday occupation offer, in these contexts, powerful evidence that our practice *does* make a difference.

Small Experiences and Family Research

A scholarly focus on the small behaviors and experiences of everyday life is found at the Center on Everyday Lives of Families (CELF), housed at the University of California–Los Angeles, Department of Anthropology, with branch centers in Sweden and Italy [retrieved July 20, 2005, from http:// www.celf.ucla.edu]. The list of papers coming out of the UCLA center is provocative and very relevant to us as occupational therapists; a primary focus on the small experiences of everyday occupation is apparent. A few titles of research papers in progress, part of a much longer list, include

- Habits of the Hearth: Children's Bedtime Routines as Relational Work
- Children in the Home, Toys in the Tub: Middle-Class Contexts of Work and Play
- Learning About Work at Dinnertime: Language Socialization in Dual-Earner American Families
- Doing Things With Play: The Play of Everyday Life
- Space, Time, and Activities in the Everyday Lives of Working Families
- Establishing Ties to the Community: Gay Fathers and the Work of Alliance Building in Everyday Family Life.

The UCLA center integrates scholars across four subfields of anthropology, along with scholars from the fields of applied linguistics, education, and psychology. One of its four primary goals is to generate "public dialogue on how working families accomplish routine family and household activities and the centrality of these activities for building family and community relationships and world views." I can't help but think that an occupational science researcher would be a perfect addition to the team.

Small Experiences and Occupational Therapy

In occupational therapy, we, too, have begun to create new knowledge about everyday occupation through our practice and research. My own research has been on the everyday experiences of caregiving—both of family members caring for elderly family members (Hasselkus 1989, 1992, 1998) and, with Virginia Dickie, of occupational therapy personnel caring for patients and clients of all ages (Hasselkus & Dickie, 1994). Also in our literature is research on the everyday experiences of mothering for children at different stages of childhood (Francis-Connolly, 2000) and for children with disabilities (Larson, 2000; McGuire, Crowe, Law, & VanLeit, 2004). The daily occupations and routines of persons with schizophrenia (Suto & Frank, 1994), spinal cord injuries (Thibodaux, 2005), and Alzheimer's disease (Josephsson, 1994; Nygård & Borell, 1998; Öhman & Nygård, 2005) have been studied, as have the lifestyle patterns of well elderly (Carlson, Clark, & Young, 1998; Jackson, Carlson, Mandel, Zemke, & Clark, 1998). The nature and meaning of play in childhood has been studied cross-culturally (Bazyk, Stalnaker, Llerena, Ekelman, & Bazyk, 2003). Others have studied the construction of self-care routines in mothers with disabled children and in older non-disabled women (Kellegrew, 2000; Ludwig, 1998). In the past decade, the American Occupational Therapy Foundation has offered two conferences on "habits" (see special supplement issues of *The Occupational Therapy Journal of Research*, Vol. 20, Fall 2000, and *OTJR: Occupation, Participation and Health*, Vol. 22, Winter 2002). This sampling of research in our own profession provides ample testimony to the potential breadth of topics on everyday occupation that have relevance for occupational therapy.

Everyday Occupation Related to Food

Because the concept of "everyday occupation" is so broad, I will narrow my focus at this point to one aspect of our daily lives, that is, to everyday occupation *related to food*. I will use this food-specific focus to illustrate the singularities and many-faceted nature of all everyday occupation. Food, after all, plays a central role in the everyday lives of most, if not all, people (de Certeau et al., 1998; Silva & Nelson, 2005).

My sister Eleanor was a poet. One of her poems is entitled "Oranges, Really," and it is a poem that describes an amazing array of distinguishing characteristics of this common household food. I think the "Really" part of the title is intended to help us give more than the usual attention to this ordinary food of our daily life, to not only see but to notice, to begin to appreciate all the sensations and visual stimulants present in this common fruit that we can find any day at the grocery store as we go about our everyday occupations.

ORANGES, REALLY
ELEANOR RISTEEN GORDON

the fruit the color
the color the fruit   ORANGE

I touch the assembled heads of oranges,
the thickened stippled skin.
How beautiful the names of oranges:
Sunkist, Sun Treat
Seald Sweet
Pure Gold
Bob White, Blue Goose, Indian River.
I bask in their fragrance,
lift from red tissue nest
pressed breast-round
juice gone solid in my hand,
navel-tucked.
With muffled white sound,
thumbnail in orange hide
splits
soft-lined peel from fruit;
tiny membrane pockets burst and squirt—
jets of dimestore orangedrink machines.
The orange in halves:
sweet vulvas of orange sections
force their shapes upon each other.
I bite—
orange smacks my tongue,
orange floods the gates of my throat.

So, what are some of the powerful attributes of the humble orange? Color. Shape. Taste. Outside and inside. Solid and liquid. The whole and the parts. Soft and not so soft. Scent and fragrance. Beauty. Sensuousness. All that in the common ORANGE . . . Really! So, the poem awakens us to the complexity and beauty of one very small part of our everyday world experience—a piece of fruit, an orange. Therapeutically, the orange is a virtual treasure trove of sensory stimulation. Selecting and picking up an orange, holding an orange, peeling an orange, breaking it into sections, bringing the sections to the mouth, biting off pieces and chewing and swallowing—all accompanied by the sights, sounds, tastes, and fragrances of the orange—is perhaps therapy at its finest.

Now that we have given it our attention, the orange no longer seems ordinary and mundane; it seems almost elegant, full of sensations to be experienced and appreciated, offering opportunities for a myriad of small behaviors and experiences. My sister has given the orange "voice," enabled the everyday to "speak."

Contextual layers of eating. I have just recently worked with a colleague from the University of Ulster, Northern Ireland, to analyze data from a study of family caregivers caring for family members with dementia (Hasselkus & Murray, in press). The data are from telephone interviews conducted with family caregivers in Wisconsin, and one question we asked each participant was "Can you think back and describe a very satisfying experience in your caregiving?" The data were narratives of caring for family members with dementia, and one of the stories related to food was the following:

> Last year for Thanksgiving, my father hadn't been eating, and we went to pick him up [at the nursing home] and brought him to my house for Thanksgiving dinner. My father had always loved prime rib, so I had fixed prime rib for Thanksgiving dinner. I had turkey and everything, but I also had prime rib. When I fixed my father's plate, I said, "Dad, this is prime rib," and I put a piece in his mouth. My father tasted it, and for some reason, he just started grabbing, reaching for the plate. I could not get it in him fast enough. He started chewing, and he hadn't chewed in almost a month. That was the most [pause], it was the most uplifting . . . it was just a miracle, that's about all I can say. That made Thanksgiving beautiful.

Many people with cognitive impairments, as the father in this caregiver's story, lose both the pleasure previously found in eating and the ability to carry out the eating process (Volicer et al., 1989). Occupational therapy personnel who work in geriatrics may have experienced firsthand the agonizing ethical struggles that result in such situations— questions related to feeding tubes, force-feeding, autonomy (Åkerlund & Norberg, 1985; Corcoran & Gitlin, 1996; Gubrium, 1975; Kane & Caplan, 1990; Moody, 1992). In such situations, eating is reduced to a purely consumptive activity—without joy or pleasure for anyone. The breakthrough witnessed by the daughter in the prime rib story represents the very satisfying experience for her of finding a way to restore her father's occupation of eating to one that offered both consumption of food and apparent pleasure. The writer Wendell Berry (2002) said in his agrarian essays, "The pleasure of eating . . . may be the best available standard of our health" (p. 326). To this daughter, her father's small behaviors during that Thanksgiving meal—chewing and swallowing, grabbing for the food—reflected a rare moment of relative well-being and health in his life. And as she said, "That made Thanksgiving beautiful." So there, too, is the "beauty" in everyday occupation—everyday occupation deeply embedded in the family's unique history, individual preferences, memories, and familiar routines; everyday occupation far beyond the simple act of getting food into the body.

In another study of occupation and dementia, I focused on satisfying and dissatisfying experiences of day-care staff members, using a sample of day-care centers in Wisconsin (Hasselkus, 1998). Here is a story from a day care staff person about a participant with dementia, and this story, too, is related to food:

> This particular client would become very agitated being with the group, especially at mealtime. And he was not eating well. What we had suggested doing was to bring him back into the office area where it's somewhat more quiet . . . And when he would be in a quiet, more controlled situation, he just did very well . . . He would actually sit down with his meal and bless himself and his food . . . he ate much better and he was even concerned, you know, if he would spill something, and just seemed to be much more in touch with reality . . . This was very satisfying, you know. . . he was very much in contact with his past and the real situation of sitting down to eat a meal.

In the previous story, the father's moment of relative well-being was likely *facilitated* by the familiar routines of the family around the dinner table at Thanksgiving. Alternatively, being with others at mealtime increased this client's agitation and led to him "not eating well." His was a different history, a history of being accustomed to eating alone, or at least in a very quiet environment. He had a routine that he was used to following, including a blessing for himself and the food—a routine that was totally lost in the group meal situation of the center. In the quiet of the office, this man was able to connect with his meal, carry out his usual familiar routines, take care of himself, and eat better. In Warde and Hetherington's (1994) study of routine food practices, they make the statement that "For some people, what and where they eat is a very conscious expression of their personal identities and style of life" (p. 769). The day-care participant, upon moving to the office to eat in a space of relative quiet, was able to live, once again, the rituals, habits, and routines still held in his memory from days gone by.

Kathleen Norris (1998), a writer on the everyday, speaks of the humble, daily occupations such as washing the body, drinking enough water, and, I would add, eating nutritious food, as "acts of self-respect" (p. 40). And it is around such small acts of self-respect during the day that we build quality in our daily lives. For the man at the day care center, sitting by himself in the office transformed the everyday occupation of eating a meal into, once again, an act of self-respect—an occasion that allowed him to reconnect with his past and to reenact the meaningful small experiences of the past in his present life with dementia.

The making of a meal. Another kind of everyday activity related to food is the making of a meal—meal preparation. In occupational therapy, a study of meal preparation is being carried out by researchers from three countries—New Zealand, Thailand, and the United States (Hocking, Wright-St. Clair, & Bunrayong, 2002; Wright-St.Clair, Bunrayong, Vittayakorn, Rattakorn, & Hocking, 2004; Wright-St. Clair, Hocking, Bunrayong, Vittayakorn, & Rattakorn, 2005). The study examines the experiences of older women as they carry out food preparations for a holiday. The researchers used focus groups to interview the women and to elicit narratives of their experiences in preparing and sharing foods—at Christmastime in New Zealand and the United States, and for the Songkran water festival in Thailand.

The New Zealand component of the study included a sample of 16 women (Wright-St. Clair et al., 2005). The four gold standards for the food preparation, derived from the data, were preparing home-cooked foods; following traditions of making foods from scratch; being thrifty and practical in shopping for food; and preparing and serving food in abundance (having leftovers was definitely required). Long-used family recipes held special place in the planning. Ordinary everyday cooking objects sometimes held special significance, such as great-grandmother's wooden spoon or mixing bowl. The food preparation, in a way, enabled the women to relive their memories of working together with several generations of women kinfolk in the kitchen and provided opportunities to come together and share once again in the work of making the meals.

In the New Zealand study, holiday food preparation and sharing were also ways to make and remake the family identity. Who they were as a family unit and what they ate when they came together at Christmas in New Zealand connected families to their cultures and histories. Adaptations occurred over the years as the women cleverly mixed the old with new and different foods, sometimes starting new traditions. As families expanded and grew more complex with marriages, divorces, remarriages, extended families, etc., the women struggled to meet the needs of all; "gathering together over home-cooked food" remained the focal point for the family Christmas.

Giard (1998) states, "*doing-cooking* is the medium for a basic, humble, and persistent practice that is repeated in time and space, rooted in the fabric of relationships to others and to one's self, marked by the 'family saga' and the history of each, bound to childhood memory just like rhythms and seasons" (p. 157). The international study of food occupations by our colleagues is an imaginative in depth study of the meaning of food and holiday traditions as relates to the women's identities, family identities, blending of old and new rituals, and food preparation as a source of self-validation. We are way beyond food as mere sustenance here.

We can probably *all* think of our own holiday traditions, our own adaptations across the years to what we knew as children, how we continue certain traditions and incorporate new ones, which traditions are most valued and which are not. Togetherness around the family table is the subject of a book by Doris Christopher (1999). In the chapter on holiday meals, Christopher quotes one friend as saying, "New recipes are fine for any other day . . . but on Thanksgiving, I want those yams with marshmallows, and the Jell-O salad" (p. 102). For me, I want the turkey stuffing made from my mother's recipe—no way would I substitute a package of stuffing mix, nor would I substitute an exotic stuffing of apricots or sausage. Our own feelings about the concept of "made from scratch" and "home-made" foods, or, what in my case constitutes "real" stuffing, can be powerful.

And what does this all mean for the older woman who becomes disabled? As occupational therapists, we might be advising her to no longer do much cooking, to take shortcuts, to use more prepared foods, to let some other member of the family do most of the work now, to give up some of the usual family traditions, etc. Do we appreciate the emotional depths of these changes we are recommending? What can we do, with our expertise in homemaking skills, to better help such a client weather this huge wrench in her life patterns and identity within a family?

The presentation of food. Other aspects of food-related occupations to consider are the small experiences associated with the *presentation* of food. By "presentation" I am referring to everything from the way the food is arranged and garnished on the plate, to the way the table is decorated; the use of paper plates versus china plates; eating outside on a picnic table or inside at the dining room table; eating at home or in a restaurant, at a table or at a counter, by a window or in a corner against a far wall. The food items on the menu and their presentation constitute a system of messages and codes for food-related occupations: formal or informal; special or ordinary; fancy or plain; home-cooked or carryout; a lot of work or easily put together (Delamont, 1983; Douglas, 1972). Presentation made all the difference in the world to the participant at the day care center who was offered the opportunity to eat alone in the office instead of in the common area with all the other participants.

In the introduction to Wendell Berry's book on agrarian living, we are reminded that "Food, rather than simply being fuel, is the most concrete and intimate connection between ourselves and the earth that exists" (Wirzba, 2002, p. xviii). Maybe. In Gubrium's (1975) early ethnography of nursing home life, he describes the presentation of food in the dining room at Murray Manor:

> At the Manor, clientele are not aware of the menu for any meal before they actually see their food on the table . . . When food trays are about to be distributed, a relative hush comes over the dining room . . . entrees are placed on heated plates that have covers. Clientele don't know what the main course is until they either remove the cover themselves or hear the comments of others in the room who already have done so. (pp. 172–173)

To have one's meal arrive under cover, so to speak, and to have no idea what one is going to be eating until the cover is removed, seems a practice that eliminates all personal associations to the food. Probably little or no "intimate connection" exists between the residents and Mother Earth in settings such as Murray Manor.

A practice that distances the "eater" from the food even more is that found in a different institutional setting—namely, a prison. About a year ago, a group of prisoners in one of Wisconsin's maximum-security prisons produced a videotaped program with the title "You Don't Want to Live in My House" (NEWIST/CESA 7, 2005) (Available from NEWIST/CESA 7, 2420 Nicolet Drive, Green Bay, Wisconsin 54311; e-mail newist@uwgb.edu; telephone 1-800-633-7445). This video is one in which men in the prison provide firsthand accounts of the experience of everyday life in a maximum-security prison. Their hope is that the video will act as a strong deterrent for young people on the outside who are leading lives that put themselves at risk for imprisonment. One section of the videotape focuses on the "Chow Hall." The prisoner–narrator describes how the food trays are handed to the prisoners *through a hole in the wall:* "You don't see who serves it, you don't see who prepares it, you don't get to say what you want." Surely such a procedure maximizes the sense of *dis*connection between the person eating the food and the world from whence the food comes. Additionally, the routines and rules of the prison, including those of the Chow Hall, exemplify a quintessential level of commonality and anonymity in the everyday. As the security director states on the videotape, the routine is the "same thing, day in, day out, 24 hours a day." And, as the prisoner in the video states, they get the same institutional food "day after day, week after week, year after year"—and for some, "it's for the rest of their lives." The food routines of the prison reflect the beliefs that keeping everything the same for everybody, day after day and year after year, will help create social stability among the prisoners and staff, and that such stability will keep the prison and its inmates manageable and under control.

In sharp contrast to prison life, a different situation of severe constraints in everyday occupation exists for people who are homeless. To survive as a homeless person *requires* individual ingenuity to get through every hour of every day. In a book I discovered, titled "Hidden Kitchens" (Silva & Nelson, 2005), a homeless man named Jeffry describes his daily life on the streets of Chicago: "When you're homeless and living on the streets, you've got to look around . . . It's called trailblazing. You've got to blaze the trail, you know" (p. 22).

Trailblazing has taught Jeffry where he can get a free cup of coffee. He knows who will give him a doughnut and who won't and when they're giving free haircuts in the parks. On Sundays he knows which churches are serving and what the Salvation Army is offering for supper. Some nights Jeffry would slip into Cook County Hospital. He describes his routine at the hospital as follows:

> You go in coughing, you know, and they give you one of those little plastic bracelets. And when they call your name, you don't answer. And you got a band around your wrist, so now you can sit there half the night and go to sleep or look for a hospital microwave to cook your cup o' noodles in . . . They'd say, "Have a cup of coffee," and I'd see there was a microwave in the lunchroom . . . Mostly I just wanted a place to pop my popcorn. Sometimes I survived for days on popcorn. (pp. 22–23)

There's no keeping everything "the same for everybody" here, as there was in the prison. Instead of having to bow to the demands and needs of an institutional system, Jeffry has *no* system in place around which to build his everyday occupation; he must create some kind of system for himself, make bits and pieces of the existing infrastructure work for him, satisfy his wants and needs to the best of his ability—for food, warmth, a place to sleep, and a microwave in which to make popcorn. The human geography of Jeffry's everyday world is complex and laden with risk at the level of his very survival. His network of informal supports is the result of his own entrepreneurial actions. He has, in fact, devised patterns of everyday occupation unique to his life circumstances, and food-related occupations are at the heart of his daily existence.

Social Forces and Occupational Deprivation

After giving special attention to everyday occupations related to food, I want to broaden our thinking again back to everyday occupation more generally, expanding on situations in which severe occupational constraints are present. For example, in another part of the prison video, the men were asked to share what they "miss most" from their previous lives outside the prison. The emphasis on missing the everyday-ness of life is unmistakable and moving. Their words describing what they "miss most" offer compelling testimonies about the importance of everyday occupations to the quality of our lives—"making breakfast for my kids," "going to the park," "just looking at the sky," "going to the store," "taking a shower when I want to," "making a phone call or writing a letter." As one of the prisoners said, "The simple things that didn't matter to me out there *matter* to me now."

Beyond individuals to communities. In situations such as prisons, where everyday occupation is severely constrained, the term *occupational deprivation* applies. Occupational deprivation is an outcome of societal conditions in which individuals are prevented from engaging in personally gratifying activities—conditions such as poverty, lack of employment opportunities, illiteracy, stigma, homelessness, disability, violence, or other social circumstances such as incarceration or institutionalization (Duncan, 2004; Wilcock, 1998). We have new and thought-provoking literature in our profession that examines the meaning of occupation and occupational deprivation in social situations such as these (Kronenberg, Algado, & Pollard, 2005; Watson & Swartz, 2004). The writers in these texts are challenging us as therapists as well as the occupational therapy profession more broadly to expand beyond the Western ideologies of individualism and independence; beyond the medical model; and beyond the traditional occupational categories of work, leisure, and self-maintenance. The aim is to reorient occupational therapy away from its overwhelming focus at only the individual level and toward the social forces that affect whole communities and populations, so that we may act as "catalysts for social transformation" (Hasselkus, 2004, p. xiv). The focus of these texts is on people's rights, specifically the *right* of people everywhere to engage in meaningful occupation in their daily lives.

The Occupational Enablement Group. The recent text edited by Ruth Watson and Leslie Swartz (2004)—*Transformation Through Occupation*—presents the philosophy and practice of occupational therapy as viewed through the lens of South Africa. The chapters contain descriptions of occupational therapy-initiated programs and research in communities near Cape Town, such as program development for families living in poverty and violence, women and youth in the criminal justice system, youth at risk in the community, and families living with HIV/AIDS. The philosophical emphasis is on the socio-cultural infrastructure of the region and the need for structural changes, even as the aim is also for improved quality of life for individuals.

As just one example from the book, the Occupational Enablement Group is described—a program offered by occupational therapy students for men at a homeless shelter in the metropolitan area of Cape Town (Duncan, 2004). In setting the context for this project, the author of this chapter states,

> Marginalized men abound in every major city in South Africa. You pass them waiting for casual jobs on the side of the road or begging at traffic lights . . . Most are semi-skilled and semi-literate; some are graduates and highly skilled . . .

> Most have families they never see; some have squandered their wealth on gambling and drugs while others have been in prison or hospital so long they don't know how to live in society any more. Many are refugees or exiles from war-ravaged or politically volatile countries bordering South Africa. They all suffer from lost dignity, apathy, mental and emotional distress, and occupational alienation." (pp. 210–211)

As Duncan states further, homelessness is not simply lack of a home; homelessness is also lack of privacy, security, safety, and sense of belonging. Using Townsend's (2000) concept of enabling occupation, the students in this project strived to facilitate the ability of the men living at the shelters to "choose, organize, and perform" occupations they found useful and meaningful by rediscovering forgotten occupational interests and abilities, and by increased awareness of the capacity for renewal through occupation (Duncan, 2004, p. 210, 211).

Smith (1987), in her book on the everyday world as problematic, makes the strong point that the everyday world is not only the world as directly experienced by each of us, within which our consciousness begins. The everyday world is also constituted of unseen social and cultural forces. These unseen forces arise out of social systems and organizations that are not necessarily part of the local setting, yet they create changes and intrude on people's lives. Such are the economic forces that lead to poverty, the social forces that lead to violence, the environmental forces that lead to disease and ill health, and the political forces that lead to powerlessness and absence of autonomy.

Invisible social forces in Western societies. The South African text edited by Watson and Swartz (2004) and the global text edited by Kronenberg et al. (2005) offer potent testimony to the occupational needs of populations in developing countries around the world. Yet these social forces exist in all societies. Our literature is beginning to contain examples of inquiry that address these culturally and socially organized forces of influence on everyday occupation (homelessness, incarceration, community health, health service utilization, street kids, hospitalization, disability, unemployment) both at home and abroad (Benedict & Farel, 2003; Crepeau, 1994; Cutchin, 2000; Denshire, 1996; Farnworth, 2000; Finlayson, Baker, Rodman, & Herzberg, 2002; Henry & Lucca, 2002; McColl, 2005; Molineux & Whiteford, 1999; Snyder, Clark, Masunaka-Noriega, & Young, 1998; Suarez-Balcazar, 2005).

The UCLA Center on Everyday Lives of Families, referred to earlier, made my hometown newspaper one day in March 2005 with an article about their study of how working families in America manage the demands of their day-to-day lives (Verrengia, 2005). In the article, a linguistic anthropologist with the center summarized findings from 32 Los Angeles working families by saying, "There isn't much room for the flow of life, those little moments when things happen spontaneously." In America, families are experiencing what these researchers call a "seismic shift" in response to both economic and sociocultural pressures of daily life. Four trends in family dynamics seem to be evolving in the increasingly scheduled lives of working families: growing indifference in the way people treat each other, less and less unstructured time, accumulation of clutter/stuff, and decreasing time together as an entire family. Who of us cannot see hints of these dynamics in our own lives, if not outright full-blown realities?

At times, these largely invisible social forces that severely constrain meaningful everyday occupation become visible to us in our therapeutic work with individuals, as can be found in the words of a young South African man with quadriplegia who described his day-to-day at-home existence as a "life sentence" (cited in Fourie, Galvaan, & Beeton, 2004, p. 78), or, in the United States, a caregiver for her husband with dementia who told me her life was "plain hell, in two words—it was just practically like being in a prison." Apparently, a sense of being imprisoned can be experienced locally, even in one's own home, as it can be experienced in a large maximum-security facility in Green Bay, Wisconsin.

The disruptions of everyday occupation imposed by illness or disability are the usual targets of our occupational therapy. But as the young man with quadriplegia and the caregiver for her husband with dementia clearly illustrate, the illness or disability is one thing, but larger forces contribute to their occupational deprivation. Both that which is experienced directly as well as that which exists at the level of an unseen social and institutional force in our lives are important to address. Both are part of our everyday world; both affect our personal and community lives; and both are important to our work in occupational therapy as we seek equity for people in their day-to-day occupations (Townsend & Whiteford, 2005).

Letting Go

The Clothes We Wear

In preparing this Slagle lecture, I had to let go of several types of everyday occupation that I originally wanted to include. I had looked forward to developing part of the lecture on everyday occupation related to *the clothes we wear*—the meaning of how we dress ourselves, concepts about fashion, the relationship of what we wear to concepts of impression management and the presentation of self in everyday life (Goffman, 1959, 1963). I wanted us to think together about the relationship of our apparel to our identities and to our sense of well-being. What statements do people believe they are making to society by what they wear?

Being able to dress oneself independently and appropriately has great prominence as a therapeutic goal in a number of areas of practice. Do we include in our therapy sensitivities to the meaning of clothing to the person with whom we are working? Clothing is sort of a protective coating that we put on the body to protect it from the elements, but it is also a form of expression. What is expressed by the positioning splint that we are asking a client to wear, the orthopedic shoes, the prosthesis, or the bib in the dining room of the nursing home? Ann NevilleJan—colleague in occupational therapy, scholar, and wearer of orthopedic shoes—has said that "discourse about shoes and clothing for people with disabilities is grounded in the medical model to the exclusion of contemporary fashion and style . . . While styles and designs of shoes have dramatically changed over time, the 'orthopedic' shoe has remained style-less and androgynous" (presentation at the 15th Annual Occupational Science Symposium, University of Southern California, Department of Occupational Science & Occupational Therapy, "Managing Appearance: The Oppression of Shoes," Jan. 17, 2003). With our focus on independence and the need for adapted clothing to simplify the dressing process for clients, do we ignore the other important aspects of fashion and wearing apparel—thereby inadvertently contributing to what our colleague has referred to, using what I assume was purposely chosen strong language, as "oppression"?

Where We Put Things

I had looked forward to developing a section of the lecture on *where we put things*—front room, back room, closet, shelf, pantry, top drawer, bottom drawer, attic, basement, kitchen. What does where we put things say about our occupational lives and our identities and our sense of wellbeing? Virginia Dickie (2003), in her study of the identity of home crafters as workers, found that those craft people who had a designated place to store supplies and to work on craft products seemed to have stronger identities as crafters and workers. The way they organized their space, including where they put things, made a statement about their sense of value of themselves as workers.

One of my graduate students did a qualitative study on the experience of older women who had recently been prescribed the use of a cane (Euhardy, 1998). One of the primary themes of meaning derived from the data was related to where the women *put* their canes: "The cane is hanging on the bedroom door . . . That's where I keep it. If I need it, I know where it is" (p. 34). Outside the home environment, where to put the cane was described as a significant problem for some of the women; situations in restaurants and churches were especially troublesome: "It's an awful nuisance, you don't know where to put it . . . it's always in other people's way . . . you just don't know where to put it. Or what to do with it" (pp. 40–41).

I don't think, in our literature on assistive devices, the problem of where to put the devices has been identified as a possible reason for lack of use—yet, such a reason may very well exist. In our published research, study participants give other reasons for non-use, such as the device is not needed, does not work well, is too cumbersome, or is too difficult to use (Gitlin, Levine, & Geiger, 1993; Mann et al., 2005). Problems with *where to put the thing* may very well be embedded in some of these statements.

When we ask a client to keep cooking utensils out on the counter for ease of use, or on the lowest shelf to be more reachable, or to install a grab bar on the side of the tub, to move a bed from the bedroom upstairs to the dining room downstairs, to get rid of the throw rugs, or to put a telephone on the bedside table, these seemingly reasonable suggestions—from our point of view—may or may not fit with the person's own sense of where things belong and what should be present in what place. Like preparation of a meal, where we put things likely draws strongly on our family history, and memories of where our mother or father put things, and how things were stored in our growing-up years. I still think, to this day that I should keep a little dish of butterscotch candy in the dining room cupboard and that the second drawer down in my dresser should contain my underwear.

Travels in Daily Life

I wanted to talk about our *travels in daily life* and expand on how those travels are related to our everyday occupation. The occupational purposes of adult daily travel, the nature of the travel itself, and the constraints on travel are all of interest (Primeau, 1996b).

But of equal interest is the travel of children in their everyday occupations—to and from school, of course, but also in their paths of travel in their neighborhood play. In Roger Hart's creative study on Children's Experience of Place, conducted in the mid-1970s, he mapped out the territories of the children in his research—the farthest distances of free range, the farthest distances of "with permission," the farthest distances of "with permission and with other children." He described their paths and shortcuts, where they went on foot or on bicycles; he described their scary places, secret places, magic places.

What would be the free range of children today in urban settings? What social forces have come to bear on the freedom of children to roam their neighborhoods or to walk to school? My sister and I walked eight blocks to our elementary school, a route that included a path through an orchard next to a woods and then crossed a main street as well as a number of side streets. There were no crossing guards and no traffic lights; we looked both ways and ran across when there was a break in the flow of traffic. If my parents worried about our safety, I was unaware of it. I remember no worries about safety on my part. The times were different, and some of the dark forces that seem to be present today were either ignored, extremely rare, unknown, or nonexistent in those years. What are the effects of this more fearsome world today on children's senses of adventure, self-confidence, independence, freedom, and play? What are the effects, in other words, on the developmental trajectory of a child in this day and age?

Awakening to the Everyday

We can, each of us, only know the world as we experience it (Dietz, Prus, & Shaffir, 1994). I have presented a viewpoint in this lecture that, in order to understand people, "it is necessary to become intimately familiar with their lifeworlds: to see how people make sense of the situations they encounter in their daily routines and how they deal with these situations on an ongoing basis" (Dietz et al., 1994, p. 2). Our everyday living is governed by certain unassailable givens such as our families of origin, birth cultures, our genetic physical and mental capabilities, and the institutional forces of our society, but our human selves can transform these nascent beginnings into lives that possess countless and prolific variations on our common humanity.

I believe that the ordinary rhythm of daily living is the deep primordial nourishment of our existence. It is the "truth"—the primary reality for each one of us. After all, everyday occupation is present in our lives at *all* times and in *all* places.

As Michel de Certeau (1998) has stated, the legitimacy of our everyday ways of operating and doing things will be achieved if these practices "no longer appear as merely the obscure background of social activity, and if a body of theoretical questions, methods, categories, and perspectives, by penetrating this obscurity, make it possible to articulate them" (p. xi). As occupational therapists—in this profession that we love—we have the potential to be an exception to the generalized *in*visibility of everyday occupation in people's lives. We can do this by awakening to its already existing presence in our philosophy, in our education, in our research, and in our therapeutic practices. *With our clients,* such a heightened awareness will enable us to enter the rich and singular spaces of their everyday lives, maximizing our abilities to work together effectively toward the maintenance and renewal of meaningful day-to-day living. *With the public,* an awareness such as this will contribute toward broader and deeper insights into the importance and meaning of everyday occupation in the social fabric of our lives, thereby helping people find value in their everyday practices (Wadel, 1979).

May it be so.

Acknowledgments

I extend my heartfelt gratitude to Wendy Wood for nominating me for the Eleanor Clarke Slagle Lectureship Award; to quote Thomas Jefferson, "Friendship is precious, not only in the shade, but in the sunshine of life." Thank you, Wendy, for your friendship in this moment of sunshine. I also give special thanks to good friend and colleague Ruth Benedict for her very able (and patient) assistance with the technological aspects of the lecture.

References

Åkerlund, B. M., & Norberg, A. (1985). An ethical analysis of double bind conflicts as experienced by care workers feeding severely demented patients. *International Journal of Nursing Studies, 22,* 207–216.

American Occupational Therapy Association. (2002). Occupational therapy practice framework: Domain and process. *American Journal of Occupational Therapy, 56,* 609–639.

Bazyk, S., Stalnaker, D., Llerena, M., Ekelman, B., & Bazyk, J. (2003). Play in Mayan children. *American Journal of Occupational Therapy, 57,* 273–283.

Benedict, R. E., & Farel, A. M. (2003). Identifying children in need of ancillary and enabling services: A population approach. *Social Science & Medicine, 57,* 2035–2047.

Berry, W. (2002). *The art of the commonplace: The agrarian essays of Wendell Berry* (N. Wirzba, Ed.). Washington, DC: Shoemaker & Hoard.

Cahill, S. (1992). Erving Goffman. In J. M. Charon (Ed.), *Symbolic interactionism: An introduction, an interpretation, an integration* (pp. 185–200). Englewood Cliffs, NJ: Prentice Hall.

Carlson, M., Clark, F., & Young, B. (1998). Practical contributions of occupational science to the art of successful ageing: How to sculpt a meaningful life in older adulthood. *Journal of Occupational Science, 5,* 107–118.

Christopher, D. K. (1999). *Come to the table: A celebration of family life.* New York: Warner Books.

Corcoran, M., & Gitlin, L. N. (1996). Managing eating difficulties related to dementia: A case comparison. *Topics in Geriatric Rehabilitation, 12*(2), 63–69.

Crepeau, E. B. (1994). Three images of interdisciplinary team meetings. *American Journal of Occupational Therapy, 48,* 717–722.

Cutchin, M. P. (2000). Retention of rural physicians: Place integration and the triumph of habit. *Occupational Therapy Journal of Research Supplement, 20,* 106S–111S.

Daniels, A. K. (1987). Invisible work. *Social Problems, 34,* 403–415.

de Certeau, M. (1998). *The practice of everyday life, Vol. 1* (S. Rendall, Trans.). Berkeley, CA: University of California Press. (Original work published 1984)

de Certeau, M., Giard, L., & Mayol, P. (1998). *The practice of everyday life, Vol. 2* (T. J. Tomasik, Trans.). Minneapolis: University of Minnesota Press. (Original work published 1998)

Delamont, S. (1983). Lobster, chicken, cake and tears: Deciphering wedding meals. In A. Murcott (Ed.), *The sociology of food and eating* (pp. 141–151). Aldershot, England: Gower Publishing Co. Ltd.

Denshire, S. (1996). A decade of creative occupation: The production of a youth arts archive in a hospital site. *Journal of Occupational Science: Australia, 3,* 93–98.

DeVault, M. L. (1991). *Feeding the family: The social organization of caring as gendered work.* Chicago: University of Chicago Press.

Dickie, V. (2003). Establishing worker identity: A study of people in craft work. *American Journal of Occupational Therapy, 57,* 250–261.

Dietz, M. L., Prus, R., & Shaffir, W. (1994). *Doing everyday life: Ethnography as human lived experience.* Mississauga, Ontario, Canada: Copp Clark Longman Ltd.

Douglas, M. (1972). Deciphering a meal. *Daedalus, 101 (Winter),* 61–81.

Duncan, M. (2004). Promoting mental health through occupation. In R. Watson & L. Swartz (Eds.), *Transformation through occupation* (pp. 198–218). London: Whurr Publishers.

Euhardy, R. (1998). *Canes as cultural objects in the lives of elderly women.* Unpublished master's thesis, University of Wisconsin–Madison.

Farnworth, L. (2000). Time use and leisure occupations of young offenders. *American Journal of Occupational Therapy, 54,* 315–325.

Finlayson, M., Baker, M., Rodman, L., & Herzberg, G. (2002). The process and outcomes of a multi-method needs assessment at a homeless shelter. *American Journal of Occupational Therapy, 56,* 313–321.

Fourie, M., Galvaan, R., & Beeton, H. (2004). The impact of poverty: Potential lost. In R. Watson & L. Swartz (Eds.), *Transformation through occupation* (pp. 69–84). London: Whurr Publishers.

Francis-Connolly, E. (2000). Toward an understanding of mothering: A comparison of two motherhood stages. *American Journal of Occupational Therapy, 54,* 281–289.

Garfinkel, H. (1964). Studies of the routine grounds of everyday activities. *Social Problems XI,* 225–250.

Giard, L. (1998). The nourishing arts. In M. de Certeau, L. Giard, & P. Mayol (Eds.), *The practice of everyday life, Vol. 2* (pp. 151–169), (T. J. Tomasik trans.). Minneapolis: University of Minnesota Press.

Gitlin, L., Levine, R., & Geiger, C. (1993). Adaptive device use by older adults with mixed disabilities. *Archives of Physical Medicine & Rehabilitation, 74,* 149–152.

Goffman, E. (1959). *The presentation of self in everyday life.* Garden City, NY: Doubleday.

Goffman, E. (1961). *Asylums: Essays on the social situation of mental patients and other inmates.* Garden City, NY: Doubleday & Co., Anchor Books.

Goffman, E. (1963). *Behavior in public places.* New York: Free Press.

Goffman, E. (1967). *Interaction ritual: Essays in face-to-face behavior.* Chicago: Aldine.

Gubrium, J. F. (1975). *Living and dying at Murray Manor.* New York: St. Martin's Press.

Hart, R. (1979). *Children's experience of place.* New York: Irvington Publishers.

Hasselkus, B. R. (1989). The meaning of daily activity in family caregiving for the elderly. *American Journal of Occupational Therapy, 43,* 649–656.

Hasselkus, B. R. (1992). The meaning of activity: Day care for persons with Alzheimer disease. *American Journal of Occupational Therapy, 46,* 199–206.

Hasselkus, B. R. (1998). Occupation and well-being in dementia: The experience of day care staff. *American Journal of Occupational Therapy, 52,* 423–434.

Hasselkus, B. R. (2002). *The meaning of everyday occupation.* Thorofare, NJ: Slack.

Hasselkus, B. R. (2004). Foreword. In R. Watson & L. Swartz, Eds., *Transformation through occupation* (pp. xiii–xv). London: Whurr Publishers.

Hasselkus, B. R., & Dickie, V. A. (1994). Doing occupational therapy: Dimensions of satisfaction and dissatisfaction. *American Journal of Occupational Therapy, 48,* 145–154.

Hasselkus, B. R., & Murray, B. J. (in press). Everyday occupation, well-being and identity: The experience of caregivers in families with dementia. *American Journal of Occupational Therapy.*

Henry, A. D., & Lucca, A. M. (2002). Contextual factors and participation in employment for people with serious mental illness. *Occupational Therapy Journal of Research Supplement, 22,* 83S–84S.

Hocking, C., Wright-St. Clair, V., & Bunrayong, W. (2002). The meaning of cooking and recipe work for older Thai and New Zealand women. *Journal of Occupational Science, 9,* 117–127.

Jackson, J., Carlson, M., Mandel, D., Zemke, R., & Clark, F. (1998). Occupation in lifestyle redesign: The well elderly study occupational therapy program. *American Journal of Occupational Therapy, 52,* 326–336.

Josephsson, S. (1994). *Everyday activities as meeting-places in dementia.* Doctoral dissertation, Department of Clinical Neuroscience and Family Medicine, Section of Geriatric Medicine, Karolinska Institute, Stockholm.

Kane, R. A., & Caplan, A. L. (Eds.). (1990). *Everyday ethics: Resolving dilemmas in nursing home life.* New York: Springer.

Kellegrew, D. H. (2000). Constructing daily routines: A qualitative examination of mothers with young children with disabilities. *American Journal of Occupational Therapy, 54,* 252–259.

Kort, W. A. (1996). *"Take, read": Scripture, textuality, and cultural practice.* University Park, PA: Pennsylvania State University Press.

Kronenberg, F., Algado, S. S., & Pollard, N. (Eds.). (2005). *Occupational therapy without borders: Learning from the spirit of survivors.* London: Elsevier Limited.

Larson, E. A. (2000). The orchestration of occupation: The dance of mothers. *American Journal of Occupational Therapy, 54,* 269–280.

Lobo, F. (1998). Social transformation and the changing work-leisure relationship in the late 1990s. *Journal of Occupational Science, 5,* 147–154.

Ludwig, F. M. (1998). The unpackaging of routine in older women. *American Journal of Occupational Therapy, 52,* 168–175.

Mann, W. C., Kimble, C., Justiss, M. D., Casson, E., Tomita, M., & Wu, S. S. (2005). Problems with dressing in the frail elderly. *American Journal of Occupational Therapy, 59,* 398–408.

McColl, M. A. (2005). Disability studies at the population level: Issues of health service utilization. *American Journal of Occupational Therapy, 59,* 516–526.

McGuire, B. K., Crowe, T. K., Law, M., & VanLeit, B. (2004). Mothers of children with disabilities: Occupational concerns and solutions. *OTJR: Occupation, Participation and Health, 24,* 54–63.

Molineux, M., & Whiteford, G. E. (1999). Prisons: From occupational deprivation to occupational enrichment. *Journal of Occupational Science, 6,* 124–130.

Moody, H. R. (1992). *Ethics in an aging society.* Baltimore, MD: John Hopkins University Press.

Neville-Jan, A. (2003, January 17). *Managing appearance: The oppression of shoes.* Paper presented at the 15th Annual Occupational Science Symposium, University of Southern California, Department of Occupational Science & Occupational Therapy.

NEWIST/CESA 7. (Producer). (2005). You don't want to live in my house [Videotape]. (Available from NEWIST/CESA 7, 2420 Nicolet Drive, Green Bay, Wisconsin 54311, e-mail newist@uwgb.edu)

Norris, K. (1998). *The quotidian mysteries: Laundry, liturgy and "women's work."* New York: Paulist Press.

Nygård, L., & Borell, L. (1998). A life-world of altering meaning: Expressions of the illness experience of dementia in everyday life over three years. *Occupational Therapy Journal of Research, 18,* 109–136.

Öhman, A., & Nygård, L. (2005). Meanings and motives for engagement in self-chosen daily life occupations among individuals with Alzheimer's Disease. *OTJR: Occupation, Participation and Health, 25,* 89–97.

Pollio, H. R., Henley, T. B., & Thompson, C. J. (1997). *The phenomenology of everyday life.* New York: Cambridge University Press.

Primeau, L. A. (1996a). Work and leisure: Transcending the dichotomy. *American Journal of Occupational Therapy, 50,* 569–577.

Primeau, L. A. (1996b). Human daily travel: Personal choices and external constraints. In R. Zemke & F. Clark (Eds.), *Occupational science: The evolving discipline* (pp. 115–124). Philadelphia: F. A. Davis.

Primeau, L. A. (1998). Orchestration of work and play within families. *American Journal of Occupational Therapy, 52,* 188–195.

Silva, N., & Nelson, D. (2005). *Hidden kitchens: Stories, recipes, and more from NPR's The Kitchen Sisters.* New York: Holtzbrinck Publishers.

Smith, D. E. (1987). *The everyday world as problematic: A feminist sociology.* Boston: Northeastern University Press.

Snyder, C., Clark, F., Masunaka-Noriega, M., & Young, B. (1998). Los Angeles street kids: New occupations for life programs. *Journal of Occupational Science, 5,* 133–139.

Suarez-Balcazar, Y. (2005). Empowerment and participatory evaluation of a community health intervention: Implications for occupational therapy. *OTJR: Occupation, Participation and Health, 25,* 133–142.

Suto, M., & Frank, G. (1994). Future time perspective and daily occupations of persons with chronic schizophrenia in a board and care home. *American Journal of Occupational Therapy, 48,* 7–18.

Thibodaux, L. R. (2005). Habitus and the embodiment of disability through lifestyle. *American Journal of Occupational Therapy, 59,* 507–515.

Townsend, A. (2000). Enabling occupation. *Journal of Occupational Science, 7,* 42–43.

Townsend, E., & Whiteford, G. (2005). A participatory occupational justice framework: Population-based processes of practice. In F. Kronenberg, S. S. Algado, & N. Pollard (Eds.), *Occupational therapy without borders: Learning from the spirit of survivors* (pp. 110–126). London: Elsevier Limited.

Verrengia, J. B. (2005, March 21). Families cut intimacy, spontaneity out of lives. Associated Press/*Wisconsin State Journal,* p. A1.

Volicer, L., Seltzer, B., Rheaume, Y., Karner, J., Glennon, M., Riley, M. E., et al. (1989). Eating difficulties in patients with probable dementia of the Alzheimer type. *Journal of Geriatric Psychiatry and Neurology, 2,* 188–195.

Wadel, C. (1979). The hidden work of everyday life. In S. Wallman (Ed.), *Social anthropology of work* (pp. 365–384). New York: Academic Press.

Warde, A., & Hetherington, K. (1994). English households and routine food practices: A research note. *Sociological Review, 42,* 758–778.

Watson, R., & Swartz, L. (Eds.) (2004). *Transformation through occupation.* London: Whurr Publishers.

Wilcock, A. A. (1998). *An occupational perspective of health.* Thorofare, NJ: Slack.

Wirzba, N. (2002). Introduction. In W. Berry, *The art of the commonplace* (pp. vii–xx), Washington, DC: Shoemaker & Hoard.

Wright-St. Clair, V., Bunrayong, W., Vittayakorn, S., Rattakorn, P., & Hocking, C. (2004). Offerings: Older Thai women taking food to the temple for Songkran. *Journal of Occupational Science, 11,* 115–124.

Wright-St. Clair, V., Hocking, C., Bunrayong, W., Vittayakorn, S., & Rattakorn, P. (2005). Older New Zealand women doing the work of Christmas: A recipe for identity formation. *Sociological Review, 53,* 332–350.

56

2007 Eleanor Clarke Slagle Lecture

Becoming Innovators in an Era of Hyperchange

Jim Hinojosa, PhD, OT, FAOTA

We are living in a time of rapid and unpredictable change. Advances in knowledge and technology have made our lives more interconnected and complex. New expectations are changing the dynamics of our personal and professional lives. We're speeding up and struggling to hold onto control of all our responsibilities, both personally and professionally. We are living in a time of *hyperchange*.

I've become extremely aware of how it is affecting my life and the people around me. My personal to-do list seems endless, and deadlines are getting shorter and shorter. Everyone around me seems too busy. I'm not sure exactly what they're doing, but they're busy doing it. I have to make professional decisions quicker than ever before. The very pace of my work world seems faster. Sometimes I feel overwhelmed with the amount of new knowledge and emerging technologies I'm expected to master.

How is hyperchange altering our personal and professional roles and responsibilities? How is it affecting occupational therapy education, practice, and research? In preparing this lecture, I came across a tale from India about three fish.[1] I think the fable's moral is particularly fitting with this topic:

> Three fish lived in a pond. One was named "Plan Ahead," another was "Think Fast," and the third was called "Wait and See." One day, they heard a fisherman say that he was going to cast his net in their pond the next day.
>
> "Plan Ahead" said, "I'm swimming down the river tonight!"
>
> "Think Fast" said, "I'm sure I'll come up with a plan!"
>
> "Wait and See" said, "I just can't think about it now!"
>
> When the fisherman cast his nets, "Plan Ahead" was long gone. But "Think Fast" and "Wait and See" were caught! "Think Fast" quickly rolled his belly up and pretended to be dead.
>
> "Oh, this fish is no good!" said the fisherman, and threw him safely back into the water. But "Wait and See" ended up in the fish market.
>
> And so the saying goes: "In times of danger, when the net is cast, plan ahead or think fast!" (Forest, 2006)

As occupational therapists, we cannot afford to "wait and see." I propose that we must both plan ahead *and* think fast. We must plan with an understanding of hyperchange and its influences on our lives. We must plan to ensure that we maintain our professional competence. We must plan for an unsure future with a vision of the world we want to live and work in.

In these rapidly and unpredictably changing times, uncertainty about the future is natural. Hyperchange is abrupt, erratic, and random. It makes long-term forecasting and planning increasingly difficult and risky. Decisions

Originally published 2007 in *American Journal of Occupational Therapy, 61*, 629–637.

must be made faster, particularly at the professional level. If we do not participate timely and effectively in the decision-making process, we risk being swept aside.

In 2001, for instance, the U.S. Surgeon General challenged health professionals to assess their roles and take action in preventing and decreasing obesity (U.S. Department of Health and Human Services, 2001). The report notes that people are spending too much time in inactive behaviors and watching television. But the report does not mention occupational therapy. There is no reference to occupation or changes in family routines or activities.

Why? Because occupational therapy is not recognized as a viable profession to prevent disability. Occupational therapy is not understood as a profession that has the potential for increasing people's participation in life activities. And, thus, by extension we've not been seen as a profession that can assist in the fight against obesity. Yet, every day we help people change their routines and actions so they can willingly engage in meaningful, healthy activities. Occupational therapy was not part of the national plan to address obesity because we did not respond immediately to the U.S. Surgeon General's call.

In occupational therapy, we are acutely experiencing the effects of hyperchange. Consider the expansion of knowledge and related skills needed to provide competent therapy services today. Think of all the information that practitioners need today to be effective and ensure qualification compared to only 5 years ago. Today, beyond reading scholarly articles and attending continuing education workshops, practitioners need to be aware of what is on the Internet and what colleagues are writing on practice-related e-mail groups as well as what evidence is available supporting their interventions. We also have to be aware of changing policies and advancing technologies.

Society's knowledge as a whole is expanding rapidly. It's obvious in our development of new information. As knowledge expands, some becomes outdated. Pat Lynch ("ERC 2000 Spring Conference Review," 2000), president of the consulting firm Potential, believes that 90% of what we know today will be irrelevant in 5 years. Professional competence is not easy to maintain within this context. The amount of new information we need to process each day can be overwhelming. With so much new input and so many changes, it is very easy to begin to feel that we cannot keep up with all the demands of proficiency and packed schedules.

Four conditions that characterize hyperchange are increasing uncertainty, rapid pace of change, growing ambiguity, and increased complexity in the workplace. We experience growing ambiguity in the workplace when everyday problems seem to become resistant to routine solutions. We have more complex responsibilities and live with ever-increasing performance expectations. For many of us (personal life stresses aside), these work expectations are the most stressful. The systems and institutions we work in are changing and evolving every day. Many are changing their missions, policies, and goals, even their basic organizational structures. For those of us in private practice, competition is greater than ever, and outside payers are engaging in aggressive cost containment practices.

In these years of instant information and high value cost-effectiveness, clients and employers expect affordable, high-quality interventions. For therapists, a clear focus on practice is absolutely necessary today to provide interventions that result in immediate outcomes. Therapists are under incredible pressure to increase productivity with fewer resources.

When expectations of employers and clients can't be met, it is easy to feel ambiguous about our work and professional lives. We struggle to merge our fantasized view of occupational therapy with the reality of practice in today's world. Our values often come in conflict with workplace demands and employer and business models. These issues are just a few we deal with as a profession.

---

[1]*Note:* From "Stories in a Nutshell," by H. Frost, 2000, Story Arts Online, retrieved October 18, 2007, from www.storyarts.org/library/nutshell/index.html. Copyright © 2000 by Heather Frost. Reprinted with permission.

I began preparing for this lecture by reading literature on times of change, planned change, and effective management both past and present. I was amazed at how this issue seems to be on so many people's minds today. But these concerns really aren't new. Charles Darwin captured the notion best when he said, "It is not the strongest of the species that survives, nor the most intelligent, but the one most responsive to change." As for resistance to change, Earle (n.d.) summarizes it with "the only person who truly welcomes lots of changes is a baby with a full diaper."

As occupational therapy practitioners, are we aware of the implications of hyperchange? Or are we just living within it, coping each day without any awareness of what is happening? I think we all realize the world is changing rapidly, and I think many of us recognize the negative consequences. But for the sake of our profession and for the benefit of our professional lives, we *must* alter our views and behaviors to meet the challenges of life in hyperchange. We cannot wait and see.

In 1962, Thomas Kuhn described the concept of a *paradigm shift* in science. He saw change coming from breaking old ways of thinking and proposed that thought is strongly determined by a person's assumptions and theories about the world. Paradigms are our individual worldviews that influence our thinking and, therefore, our actions. Some scholars have objected to the term *paradigm* because they feel it's overused. I've chosen to use it because it captures the importance of examining beliefs, perceptions, and actions in the context of our worldviews. To adapt to this rapidly changing world, we must alter our ways of thinking. *We must create paradigm shifts*.

In 2006, Weiner and Brown echoed Kuhn. Instead of talking about a paradigm shift, they emphasized *thinking clearly*. They asserted that our assumptions, prejudices, prejudgments, and even yearnings influence our thinking and that to deal effectively with change, we must become *innovators*.

So then, how do we do this? How do we shift our paradigms? We must determine where to focus our energies and how to acknowledge our potentials and learn when to use reasoning skills to advance practices and interactions. We must recognize and draw on personal and professional relationships for the advancement of the profession and ourselves.

In the past, occupational therapy leaders have challenged us to shift or change our paradigms. But usually the challenge was to get us to accept a single one. This will not work today. Our responsibilities and roles are too varied to fit within one way of thinking. This won't lead to innovation but rather to stagnation in our abilities to think "outside of the box."

Take, for instance, the American Occupational Therapy Association's (AOTA; 2002) mandate for absolute professional acceptance of the *Occupational Therapy Practice Framework: Domain and Practice*. This document restrains practitioners. It limits how we look at occupational therapy, and it blinds us to new conceptualizations about our domain of practice. No one document, single theory, or intervention paradigm should be considered more important than any other.

In the December 2006 issue of *Popular Science*, I was startled that the Grand Award for Best Innovation of 2006 was given to the Bostitch Harriquake nail. A redesign of the simple nail was selected because of its far-reaching effect on many people's lives (Clynes, 2006). The judges selected it in a year when innovations included the growth of new body organs, the cloning of a lamb, and a 253-mph car. Why a nail? It had existed for more than two centuries without any major modifications. But researchers found that during the recent hurricanes more damage was done to homes and buildings when they were ripped apart because of a limitation in the nail's design. The function and purpose of the nail determined its redesign (Clynes, 2006).

This innovation and change in thinking closely parallels an important aspect of occupational therapy. Like therapists' interventions, the nail redesign emerged from a functional need and its relevance to people's daily lives. And like many interventions, the development was not particularly exciting. The nail designers observed its function and design. They noted its positive aspects and also where there were problems. They adapted and modified its overall structure to meet newly identified realities. It blended into people's lives and was not considered important enough to make the nightly news. Most people who benefit from the intervention will never even be aware of the amount of work and reasoning that led to the innovation.

If we are to become innovators, we must accept our individualities and operate from three basic principles. First, we must anticipate hyperchange and accept that the world is erratic but still full of opportunities. Second, we must look for what changes are really taking place. We must observe, reflect, and confirm our conclusions with others. Third (and most difficult), we must stop ignoring ideas or events because they do not fit in our current thinking.

Today, occupational therapy practitioners may share core values, knowledge, and skills, but there can be no one right theoretical approach or perspective on practice. Innovation requires that we not accept just one set of rules. Innovators are willing to challenge past attitudes and ways of thinking. Innovators recognize that some limits to what we can do are within ourselves. Innovators reflect and create new realities, dream, and are not afraid to take chances (Rumball, 1998).

But even though we may share values, knowledge, and skills, what we do and how we do it varies in many ways. We must consider what influences our thinking and reasoning. Barnitt and Partridge (1997) studied occupational and physical therapists' reasonings. They determined that physical therapists adopted a diagnostic or procedural style, whereas occupational therapists used a narrative style. When trying to understand a client, occupational therapists are more likely to consider the social context and the client's point of view. But while these are important, we must not let our reliance on narrative reasoning blind us from considering other options.

In fact, in some practice situations, diagnostic or procedural reasoning may be the most appropriate style to use. If a young client, for example, has a wrist fracture, the goal is to return functional use to the hand. The occupational therapist would be most effective by focusing on the diagnostic aspects and realizing that resolving those issues will lead to the client's return to function and participation in daily life activities.

In this situation, an occupational profile is of little use in treatment planning. The critical factors are the client's specific deficits and limitations. Of course, as treatment progresses, ongoing evaluation of the client by the therapist will provide information to develop a profile of the person as an occupational being in his or her life context. But initially, the therapist should use procedural reasoning to obtain the information needed to develop realistic, functional, and achievable goals based on clear, baseline data.

If we see the world as static, believing that occupational therapy is limited by what we currently can do, then we will act and respond consistently with those beliefs and views. But if we stretch our viewpoints and welcome change, realizing interventions must be based on a client's problems or needs, we will act accordingly. We can shift our paradigms.

Becoming innovators in adapting practices to meet the new realities of the world is essential to our profession's continuing development. Innovation begins by examining a situation and reflecting on it from different perspectives. This reflection is critically important. We have to examine our own beliefs, values, and biases. We must look for patterns and common themes. We should confer with others more and try to understand their perceptions.

Occupational therapists tend to engage in narrative reasoning in attempting to understand a client's story. We can be more innovative, though, if we also try to learn what others around us think and see. Understanding a physical therapist's diagnostic concerns can add to our options as we reflect on a client's case. Repeated reflections of our own ideas will not lead to new treatment options. But reflecting on our thoughts while also taking into consideration the ideas of others will facilitate new alternatives. And talking with others who may not share our philosophical views and perceptions of the world will expand our ideas and thus lead to even more potential alternatives.

In 1998, Barrett proposed a paradox process that he called the "recipe for life in an era of hyperchange" (p. 1). He suggested thinking opposite to what is conventional. In fact, he encouraged trying to think of two opposites simultaneously. These combined opposites will result in the synthesis of new and creative ideas. Let's consider how we usually think about discharging a client. Our usual options are discharge or continue therapy. In other words, one or the other.

If, however, we try to consider both at the same time—discharge and continuing therapy—it opens a whole new range of options. The possibilities for discharge and continuing therapy may become transitioning to a new setting, providing short-term outpatient therapy or home-based intervention, or continuing therapy with new priorities. Innovative thinkers consider opposites in order to synthesize new ideas.

Today, I'm going to discuss the need for innovative interventions in three important areas of our profession: organization, education, and practice.

Professional Organization

Three organizational structures support our profession. Most notably, AOTA has wide-ranging activities at the national level. State associations (which often are less structured) have state-specific goals. And local groups offer membership support and continuing education opportunities. But are these organizational structures effective? Do they really support the needs of our profession and colleagues?

Looking for innovative change here begs two simple questions: If we were to create our professional association today, what would its purpose and function be? How would it be structured?

In this time of hyperchange, professional organizations must evolve and change. Activities that may have been effective and important 10 years ago may not be so today. I served for 12 years on AOTA's Commission on Practice. I chaired the commission from 1989 to 1995. It was an incredible learning experience, and I value the personal and professional relationships I made during those years. I strongly believed in the importance of our activities.

But today I question the need for some of AOTA's commissions. Does a professional association need governance commissions to develop papers and perform administrative functions? Do these papers and activities meet the needs of the profession and practitioners? I think our national association needs to focus its limited resources on other areas. We must recognize the difference between the profession and the professional association.

Occupational therapy, as a profession, has established a sound philosophical and theoretical base for its existence. The professional associations exist to support this profession. In a young profession, the association devotes resources to defining language, articulating a philosophical base, and educating society about the profession. As a profession matures, as occupational therapy has, the professional association's purpose changes to address more external issues affecting the profession.

Our associations must develop mechanisms for dealing with rapid change and shifting priorities. I believe that the professional associations need to reorganize their structures to directly support their purposes. The associations should explore smaller administrative structures that can make timely decisions. They also must support activities that promote the long-term viability of the profession. They must monitor legislative and reimbursement policies. They must advocate with other organizations to support the profession's present and future goals.

Unlike in the past, our associations do not need to direct the philosophical or theoretical development of the profession. This is happening among our scholars and will continue to do so. The professional association's responsibility today is to provide outlets for dialogue and the sharing of ideas from multiple perspectives.

Education

To survive into the future, occupational therapy educational programs must develop clearly defined research agendas and develop timely and relevant curricula. Colleges and universities across the country are increasing expectations for faculty to engage in research and scholarship. Faculty must conduct research, publish, and provide university service. Programs are expected to be integrated consistently into the institution as a whole. If a program is isolated, then it would be better doing training outside of the expensive environment of a university.

In 2002, our department at New York University (NYU) was examined as part of a systematic review of all programs in the Steinhardt School of Education. The university president clearly stated that programs can continue to exist in the research university only if they had clear research agendas and faculty who were actively contributing to the development of knowledge. He made it very clear that it was not enough for professional programs to graduate competent professionals.

For decades, our faculty have prided themselves in graduating outstanding, competent, and ethical occupational therapists. As the university review process began, though, we realized we needed to realign our priorities. We needed to revise immediately our research agenda and shift to focusing on hiring highly qualified, tenure-track faculty. And we needed to develop working relationships with faculty in other departments across the university.

In less than a year, the department faculty responded to the challenges, and we reorganized to become a better, more integrated department within NYU. While we continue to graduate competent therapists, our priorities now are consistent with the goals and guidelines of the university. In the future, I believe the survival of occupational therapy programs in research universities will depend on our willingness today to move beyond education and include the continued development of our profession's body of knowledge and increased collaboration with others in the institution.

I know we're not alone in having to respond to such challenges. Dr. Paula Kramer (personal communication, February 9, 2007) from the University of the Sciences in Philadelphia reports that faculty in her institution are expected to engage in research or activities that inform teaching. Faculty have responded by developing and implementing community-based, grant-funded service learning projects and exploring the scholarship of teaching. This response has been viewed positively by the university.

In the future, I believe all occupational therapy programs will have to have clearly defined research or community agendas consistent with their college or university's mission and goals. In all institutions, faculty will have to become integrated members of the larger institutional communities.

Another concern for all occupational therapy educators is to make sure that the curriculum remains relevant. Many curricula will need to be revised consistent with the educational goals of the university or college. They also will need to be revised to meet students' learning needs and styles. Ninety percent of what students learn today will be irrelevant in 5 years. Educators need to adjust curriculums to teach students *how* to learn rather than focusing only on skills, procedures, and techniques. There also will be increased pressures for interdisciplinary, interactive curriculums.

Prensky (2006) observed that most educators have not prepared themselves for the 21st century. Kids entering college today are the first generation to have spent their entire lives using computers, videogames, digital music players, video cams, and cell phones. A college student today has spent 10,000 hours playing video games, answered 200,000 e-mails, watched 20,000 hours of television, seen 500,000 commercials, and spent nearly 5,000 hours reading books (Prensky, 2001a).

Innovators in occupational therapy education must develop effective teaching styles compatible with the students that enter our programs. The next generation of occupational therapy students may think and reason differently because of their life experiences and because they live in a highly technological world (Prensky, 2001b). They may have different learning styles that require different or new instructional methods. Occupational therapy educators need to build new, innovative curriculums based on sound teaching and learning theories. Some occupational therapy educators have begun to explore new instructional methods, such as problem-based learning (McNulty, Crowe, & VanLeit, 2004). But revised curriculums will need to go beyond philosophical beliefs and content concerns to include new teaching and learning theories.

In revising and developing curriculums, occupational therapy educators need to realize that there is no one correct teaching or learning theory appropriate for all students. To respond to today's practice demands, occupational therapy graduates need to be able to reason and solve problems in a timely, efficient, and cost-effective manner. Educators should explore alternative teaching and learning theories beyond the domain of occupational therapy to develop new curriculums that give students the knowledge and skills to succeed in a rapidly changing world. Curriculums need to focus more on reasoning and problem solving and less on specific knowledge and intervention techniques. For example, a curriculum does not need to focus on learning conditions; instead, students need to learn to use resources to find relevant information in an efficient manner.

Practice

Graduates of occupational therapy programs are entering an exciting but very demanding work world. Reimbursers, payers, and consumers all are demanding increased accountability and documentation. Payers expect services that are cost effective and result in immediate functional outcomes. Therapists are under incredible pressure to increase productivity with fewer resources.

In response, occupational therapy practice has become less individualized and more routine, based on accepted treatment protocols. Therapists spend less time with clients and focus more on specific treatment techniques. From my perspective, innovation in practice requires a new focus on theory-based intervention and attention paid to our personal and professional relationships.

It's only natural that when a practitioner is expected to treat more patients, he or she will focus on productivity and efficiency. Some therapists will develop treatment protocols that standardize interventions based on clients' diagnoses or conditions. Others will select a preferred treatment approach for all clients.

Take "Jane": Jane works at a large metropolitan hospital in a rehabilitation unit. She is expected to treat six or more patients with a wide range of diagnoses each day. Patients spend an average of 2 weeks on the unit. She doesn't have time to develop individualized treatments for each client because she feels overwhelmed with evaluations and discharge summaries. She has to document everything she does.

Or "Sally": Sally is an itinerant therapist working at three different schools. She is frustrated at not having opportunities to talk and work with her colleagues. She feels that the administrations do not support collaboration because it could take away from treatment times. She believes their only concern is the child's IEP (individualized education program) completion. She feels like her treatment services are being defined by curricula and are resulting in her having to treat too many children who need help with handwriting. She thinks principals are not concerned about the quality of interventions.

In these examples, therapists reported spending less actual therapy time with clients. Their concerns were centered on efficiency over effectiveness. They have mixed feelings about this because they value client-centered priorities but feel forced to focus primarily on productivity. To cope, they focus on establishing routine treatment protocols specific to their client's problems. They deliver what they consider to be the most efficient treatments. But this shift is away from attending to the individual to focusing only on efficiency. Therapy becomes about protocols, techniques, and procedures rather than driven by the theory of practice.

Like medicine, occupational therapy is a science-based profession. Guidelines for interventions or frames of reference are based on theories that have been developed by the scientific disciplines. As professionals, we have an ethical responsibility to provide interventions based on these established theories. A theoretical base for a frame of reference is an integrated whole. It's not the whole theory, and it's usually developed using several theories. That theoretical base is the foundation for the guidelines for intervention.

Occupational therapy scholars and researchers must engage in applied research to establish the efficacy of occupational therapy frames of reference. Researchers should focus on applied research designs concerned with the practical question of whether a frame of reference does what it is designed to do. Does the frame of reference lead to successful remediation of the problem? Applied research focuses on the validity, reliability, and efficacy of a theoretically-based guideline for intervention (Mosey, 1996). The challenge for occupational therapy scholars and researchers will be to develop research protocols acceptable to the scientific community. We must look beyond the criteria set by basic research to obtain evidence supporting the efficacy of our interventions.

Theory-based interventions are critical. Society grants occupational therapy practitioners the right to practice because of our expertise and unique skills. We must, then, be able to provide society with evidence supporting our expertise. We must be able to provide theory-based interventions built on valid theories. Would you go to a doctor who gave you medication but could not tell you what to expect? Of course not. Likewise, occupational therapy practitioners should be able to inform clients about possible outcomes of an intervention. We can do this only when our interventions are based on solid theories, which give us the knowledge we need to make educated predictions.

Theory-based frames of reference direct how we then use our therapeutic modalities and techniques. For innovation, practitioners must apply treatment techniques or modalities as they are directed through theory-based frame of reference. A theoretically based frame of reference describes how a specific modality will be applied and under what conditions based on a client's needs. Practitioners should look beyond modalities to ensure that they are consistent with valid theories.

A therapist's conscious use of self, a basic modality in almost all treatments, varies depending on how the theory guides the therapist to interact with a client and the environment. A therapist applying a frame of reference based on Bandura's (1977) social learning theory, for instance, would apply the conscious use of self by modeling and reinforcement. But a therapist applying the neurodevelopmental frame of reference would use physical handling and social interactions.

Providing competent and effective interventions is a challenge for any occupational therapy practitioners given today's rapidly changing service delivery models and treatment environments. Society, payers, and consumers are demanding that practitioners describe the specific outcomes of interventions. Innovation in treatment means that all practitioners must now be able to explain a theory that underlies a frame of reference. Just as we expect doctors to tell us what the effects of a medication may be, consumers and payers expect occupational therapists to be able to explain rationales for intervention and what outcomes might result. Innovation also demands that therapists look for new theories and develop new frames of reference or guidelines for intervention. Some may need to be modified based on revised theories and still others with questionable validity may no longer be appropriate to use. New or revised frames of reference or guidelines for interventions must address the needs of clients in today's world.

Athena Tsai, an NYU occupational therapy student, developed a frame of reference in 1996 called "Patient's Acceptability of Using Humor for Pain Relief." In exploring the literature, she discovered McCaffery's (1979) theory of reducing pain with humor. After developing this frame of reference, she studied its viability in a nursing home with clients who were experiencing upper-limb pain. All five of her participants found that humor—in this case, telling a *Reader's Digest* joke—created a joyful atmosphere and reduced their pains. This new frame of reference has great potential for older clients with chronic pains. It innovatively addresses both the physical and psychological needs of its target population.

Being innovative in occupational therapy does not mean always turning to the latest techniques or strategies. It means addressing the basic concerns that underlie practice. We must provide interventions that will address the wide range of activities people participate to give their lives meaning. Take self-care and personal hygiene, for example. Yes, they are routine and not very glamorous, but they are important for human dignity. Innovators will realize the value of these important human activities and ensure that they remain a treatment priority. Innovators will ensure that these interventions are treated as relevant and meaningful to clients. A person's ability to complete self-care determines his or her ability to participate in society. We should rethink how we address self-care. Occupational therapists often spend time working with a client on his or her ability to complete specific self-care tasks out of context. Shifting goals from a client's ability to do self-care to a focus on a client's participation in society may change interventions. The innovation is in addressing a client's needs in the context of society today.

The need for innovation in our professional organizations, educational models, and practice strategies is obvious. But what about our basic interactions, like sitting with a client, meeting a coworker in the hall? Anne Cronin

Mosey (1981, 1986) argued that therapists can only create environments for change; they can't change a client directly. A skilled occupational therapy practitioner uses himself or herself with other tools to create situations that encourage positive change. Fundamentally, this therapeutic use of self is core to occupational therapy practice. Occupational therapy occurs in our interactions with clients and colleagues. It's the nature and scope of our modern relationships that makes becoming innovators so difficult. Today, practice innovations have to be constructed to take place within our rushed workplace interactions. As a profession that values the person and personal choice, our innovations must address our relationships with others.

Transformational thinking in innovation highlights the importance of human behaviors and interactions with others. To be effective, relationships should be fostered on understanding and respect as professionals. A relationship-oriented approach to living allows us to come up with new and different solutions in our rapidly changing world.

To become person-centered, reflect on the following questions: What would your colleagues, patients, and people you care about say about you? What characteristics would you like to have? What contributions do you make to your family, friends, clients, people you work with, and all those you cherish in your life? What difference would you like to make in the lives of others? We cannot truly separate our work lives from our personal lives. And we can't let our work dominate our free time.

In this time of hyperchange, it is so important that we recognize the value of personal and professional relationships. In our daily efforts to get everything done, we may not be giving enough attention to developing and maintaining relationships. It is too easy to lose contact with others or to communicate in impersonal methods such as e-mail, text messages, or voice mail. And yet, relationships are essential to being innovative and to having a satisfying personal and professional life. Without such connections, we will not have the support systems we need to respond to the stresses of hyperchange. No innovation can be realized if others don't recognize and accept it as well.

Occupational therapists need to re-examine practice. Interventions are changing. Service delivery models are changing. Expectations for outcomes are changing. And, at the very heart of it all, the relationships we have with others are changing and often at the expense of productive collaboration. We must find efficient ways of establishing rapport with other therapists and work for the benefit of clients. Our goal should be to have interactions that enhance interventions and effectiveness. "We" are the only part of the relationship that we can be responsible for. We need a paradigm shift in how we view our modern interactions.

We can redefine collaboration in this time of hyperchange. We must make a personal commitment to work in partnership with others. We also must welcome change as a challenge, not a burden. We should embrace innovations, practice flexibility, and take time to reflect on practice.

Recognizing change as a challenge means we need to recognize that we often feel overwhelmed with new knowledge, technologies, and busy schedules. Think about and remember the strategies and skills that you have. Acknowledge your strengths. Learn to enjoy the challenges of change. And finally, manage change; don't let it manage you.

Innovation is, of course, essential for positive change. It includes advancing knowledge, modernizing techniques, and developing new technologies. A major responsibility for a professional is to translate these innovations to practice. Each of us must make sure that occupational therapy innovations are used to improve the lives of the clients we serve. Embracing innovation will ensure competence and improve practices. Embracing innovation ensures that we use innovation for good rather than becoming a victim of it.

There is a tendency today to increase regulations and develop policies to try to control our world. We create rules and rigid procedures. We start looking for efficiency over effectiveness. But when we become rigid and structured, we lose the ability to respond to an individual as a person. Developing flexibility in thinking and action will help us respond to these tendencies.

When you take time to reflect on your practices and actions, you can learn from what you've done and improve on who you are. Thomas Paine wrote that "The real man smiles in trouble, gathers strength from distress, and grows brave by reflection." Reflection is the one tool we have to improve our relationships with others. We are a part of a profession that cares about people. We care about the individual. We work to put people back in control of their lives. We must make the time to reflect on all of this.

The scope of occupational therapy practice has expanded over the years in response to changes in society and the needs of consumers. It also has changed in response to the demands and expectations of payers. Managed care, hospital-based programs, and home-based and education-based services each have their own cultures of interactions and communications. Systems delineate a person's professional responsibilities and the kinds of relationships that are appropriate.

Nevertheless, we still can find effective ways to establish relationships with colleagues and ways to work together for the benefit of our clients and ourselves. Our goal must be to foster interactions that enhance interventions and treatment effectiveness. While working together, we must act consistently with our professional responsibilities, supporting our profession's values and scope of practice. Use self-reflection to promote your competence. Become comfortable with inter-professional conflict. There is no single "right" way to resolve a conflict. Consider the disadvantages and advantages to each action. Remember the principles of a fair argument. Stick to the issues; don't attack the person. And always remember that your position may not be the best or only option.

As occupational therapy practitioners today, we often pride ourselves in our ability to adapt. But, at this time in our history, we are uniquely challenged. Today many people still do not understand what occupational therapy is. As all professions, we are evolving and changing with society. We must clearly explain to society what we contribute, and we must provide evidence that supports that our interventions are effective.

But many occupational therapy scholars and researchers continue to focus primarily on the philosophical underpinnings of the value of occupation rather than on establishing specific, effective interventions. When we have evidence that interventions are not effective—such as sensory integration (Mulligan, 2002; Pollock, 2006; Shaw, 2003; Vargas & Camilli, 1999)—we argue that the studies are invalid rather than working to change our interventions. I'm not saying that we should abandon sensory integration, for instance, but I think we may need to modify the frame of reference to assure its efficacy.

Conclusion

We live in exciting and challenging times. Occupational therapy practitioners must respond to rapid and unpredictable change. We must become innovators to meet our responsibilities as therapists and as individuals. Our profession's future depends not on what AOTA develops but on how each of us creates lives as modern professionals. The future of occupational therapy is in our control. I challenge you all to become innovative, reflective practitioners who embrace life in an era of hyperchange. It is time to plan ahead and think fast.

Acknowledgment

I thank Catherine Hensly for her editorial assistance.

References

American Occupational Therapy Association. (2002). Occupational therapy practice framework: Domain and process. *American Journal of Occupational Therapy, 56,* 609–639.

Bandura, A. (1977). *Social learning theory.* Englewood Cliffs, NJ: Prentice Hall.

Barnitt, R., & Partridge, C. (1997). Ethical reasoning in physical therapy and occupational therapy. *Physiotherapy Research International, 2,* 178–194.

Barrett, D. (1998). *The paradox process: Creative business solutions, where you least expect to find them.* New York: AMACOM.

Clynes, T. (2006, June). Dr. Nail versus monster. *Popular Science,* 106–109.

Earle, R. (n.d.) Thriving in hyperchange: A case study in personal stress control. *The Sources HotLink.* Retrieved March 14, 2007, from www. hotlink.ca/HL1110-Hyperchange.htm

Forest, H. (2006). *Three fish: A tale from India.* Retrieved December 29, 2006, from www.storyarts.org/library/nutshell/stories/threefish.html

Kuhn, T. S. (1962). *The structure of scientific revolutions.* Chicago: University of Chicago Press.

McCaffery, M. (1979). *Nursing management of the patient with pain* (2nd ed.). Philadelphia: Lippincott.

McNulty, T. M., Crow, T., & VanLeit, B. (2004). Promoting professional reflection through problem-based learning evaluation activities. *Occupational Therapy in Health Care—Special Topic: Best Practices in Occupational Therapy Education, 18,* 71–82.

Mosey, A. C. (1981). *Occupational therapy: Configurations of a profession.* New York: Raven Press.

Mosey, A. C. (1986). *Psychosocial components of occupational therapy.* New York: Raven Press.

Mosey, A. C. (1996). *Applied scientific inquiry in the health professions : An epistemological orientation* (2nd ed.). Bethesda, MD: American Occupational Therapy Association.

Mulligan, S. (2002). Advances in sensory integration research. In A. C. Bund, S. Lane, E. A. Murray, & A. G. Fisher (Eds.), *Sensory integration: theory and practice* (2nd ed., pp. 397–411). Philadelphia: F. A. Davis.

Pollock, N. (2006). *Keeping current: Sensory integration.* (Issue Brief No. 3). Hamilton, ON: CanChild Centre for Childhood Disability Research. Retrieved October 18, 2007, from http://www.canchild.ca/ Default.aspx?tabid=1237

Prensky, M. (2001a). Digital natives, digital immigrants. *On the Horizon, 9*(5). Retrieved February 19, 2007, from www.marcprensky.com/writing/Prensky%20-%20Digital%20Natives,%20Digital%20Immigrants%20-%20Part1.pdf

Prensky, M. (2001b). Digital natives, digital immigrants, part II: Do they really *think* differently? *On the Horizon, 9*(6). Retrieved February 19, 2007, from www.marcprensky.com/writing/Prensky%20%20Digital %20Natives,%20Digital% 20Immigrants%20-%20Part2.pdf

Prensky, M. (2006, December 2005/January 2006). Listen to the natives. *Educational Leadership, 63,* 8–13.

Rumball, D. (1998). *The innovation report.* Toronto: Ministry of Small Business and Entrepreneurship. Retrieved January 28, 2007, from www.sbe.gov.on.ca/ontcan/sbe/downloads/wisdom_exchange/we_ report_innovationreport.pdf

ERC 2000 Spring Conference review. (2000, June). *Runzheimer Reports on Relocation, 19,* 1–6.

Shaw, S. R. (2002). A school psychologist investigates sensory integration therapies: Promise, possibility, and the art of placebo. *NASP Communique, 31,* 5–6.

Tsai, A. (1996). *Patient's acceptability of using humor for pain relief.* Unpublished master's thesis, New York University, New York.

U.S. Department of Health and Human Services. (2001). *The Surgeon General's call to action to prevent and decrease overweight and obesity.* Rockville, MD: Author. Retrieved October 18, 2007, from www.surgeongeneral.gov/topics/obesity/calltoaction/CalltoAction.pdf

Vargas S., & Camilli G. (1999). A meta-analysis of research on sensory integration treatment. *American Journal of Occupational Therapy, 53,* 189–198.

Weiner, E., & Brown, A. (2006). *Future think: How to think clearly in a time of change.* Upper Saddle River, NJ: Pearson/Prentice Hall.

Embracing Ambiguity:
Facing the Challenge of Measurement

Wendy J. Coster, PhD, OTR/L, FAOTA

I will introduce the topic of this paper with a story:

The summer that I turned 10 was very full. After living in Naples, Italy, for 3 years, my family and I were moving north to Milan. I was leaving the American school I had attended and would start attending a new Italian school in the fall. In between, we returned to the United States for the summer. We traveled by ship each way, each trip lasting over a week with stops along the way in exotic places such as Gibralter, Morocco, Majorca, and Cannes.

In the United States, we traveled around in a big, old, used Cadillac my father had bought to visit family and friends across New York and around Washington, DC. We celebrated several birthdays and the christening of my baby sister, went for a long hike with my uncle and dad and got lost, and watched hours of Saturday morning cartoons—a novel experience for us because Italy didn't really have television at that time.

Upon arrival in Milan my brothers and I had a few weeks of tutoring in Italian and then started at our new school. The first day my teacher gave the class what must be the universal first-week-of-school assignment: to write about "what I did over the summer." I picked up the unfamiliar dip pen, dipped it in the inkwell, and scratched out (not very neatly): "Io sono andato a America." "I went to America. I went on a boat. I came to Milan." At that point I had exhausted my knowledge of Italian grammar and vocabulary and stopped. I knew that what I had written looked like a first-grader's essay, including the blotches that came from my unruly, unfamiliar pen. For a previously competent student it was embarrassing and demoralizing not to be able to do better. However, getting a bad grade was not my worst fear. What was more important to me was that my teacher might think that those few simple sentences I had managed to produce told the whole story of my adventurous summer—that she would think that essay was ME.

Facing the Challenge of Measurement

My teacher was actually very kind and understanding on that day long ago, but the experience became like a grain of sand in my consciousness, an irritant that never quite went away. I had realized the discrepancy between what we can tell or show and what the experience really is, between the *measure* of a person's ideas or abilities and reality. Eventually that insight led to the question that has fascinated and challenged me for many years: How can we reconcile the need to design and use measures in our research and practice with the knowledge that the information they give us is inadequate, often ambiguous, and sometimes misleading?

In our society today there are very strong forces pressing us to treat the data from standardized measures as the person's "full story." From reimbursement decisions based on scores on the Functional Independence Measure™

Originally published 2008 in *American Journal of Occupational Therapy, 62,* 743–752.

(FIM; Uniform Data System for Medical Rehabilitation 1997) to high-stakes achievement tests in schools, there is pressure to simplify very complex decisions through the application of numbers. Occupational therapy's concern for the whole person is being challenged daily by this pressure in our practice and in our research.

An effective response to this challenge will need to go beyond selecting instruments with the best reliability or predictive accuracy, or the application of modern methods such as Rasch analysis. We also must examine and challenge some of the assumptions underlying the current use of measures and the conclusions being drawn from this use. The phenomena at the core of occupational therapy's concern are complex and, as our attention moves from the domain of body structures and functions to activity and participation, they also are increasingly abstract. Our concerns encompass both directly observable events—the doing—and experiences that can be conveyed only through some intermediary mechanisms—the phenomena we call *meaning, feeling, being,* and *quality of life.*

To try to capture a picture of these phenomena for use in our practice or research, occupational therapy often has turned to the methods and instruments developed in other disciplines whose concerns, priorities, and knowledge may not be the same as ours. One source has been medicine, a discipline whose primary concern is observable phenomena such as the integrity of body functions and performance of physical tasks. Another has been psychology, which focuses more on abstract unobservable processes such as the cognitive, social, and emotional dimensions of experience. Although each of these bodies of knowledge has contributed in valuable ways to the tools we use, each has also brought influences and assumptions that have often gone unexamined for their compatibility with occupational therapy. This paper examines several of these important issues:

- How we define what we are measuring;
- How we derive and interpret quantitative data from our instruments; and
- How the social nature of the assessment process influences the results we obtain.

I will end with some thoughts about how a better understanding of these issues can help us to achieve the ideals of occupational therapy practice and to advance our research.

Power of Words

Words connote reality. When we have extracted a pattern from the array of stimuli we experience, we mark the pattern with a name—a word. Almost immediately the word takes on the power to influence our thoughts and feelings. We know from cognitive science, for example, that speaking or seeing the word first makes it more likely that we will perceive a particular stimulus (Bueno & Frenck-Mestre, 2002). Words reduce ambiguity to enable us to live socially in a world of objects. I can show you the object I give the name to, and we can agree to use that name whenever we speak about that object. Cultures vary in the extent to which they differentiate within particular categories, but they all have ways of marking or pointing out with words the features that differentiate the categories that are meaningful within their culture.

The sciences vary in the degree of precision in their naming processes. For example, in physics the phenomenon given a particular name may have a very precise mathematical reference such as an equation (Lightman, 2005). In biology some terms have very precise referents (e.g., fern, poodle) that can be readily identified from their observable features. However, when we begin to study human experience scientifically, terms begin to appear that have varying degrees of uncertainty or ambiguity in their referents. We cannot demonstrate pain with a microscope or point out health as clearly as we can identify a cell.

Metaphor often comes into play to express aspects of phenomena that are less easily pointed out or defined (Brown, 2003). These metaphors are shaped by a culture's values and orientation to human affairs (Lakoff & Johnson, 1980). For example, the metaphors related to disease in U.S. culture evoke images of disease as an enemy: Viruses *attack* our cells, we *fight off* a cold, and we *beat* or *succumb* to an illness. Our metaphor of disease describes it as a foreign invader, something with distinct boundaries that is separate from ourselves.

However, other cultures may hold different metaphors about disease. For example, disease may be understood as a storm within us, caused by disturbance of natural harmony between body and soul, or as a disturbance in the balance between opposing forces (Karasz, 2005; Storck, Csordas, & Strauss, 2000). In these metaphors, disease is on a continuum with health and is not exclusively caused by outside influences.

The important point is that different approaches to diagnosing and treating illness will appear correct or "right" to cultures that hold these different metaphors. If the cause of disease is believed to be external to ourselves, then it makes sense to search for a primary cause using measures that focus on external observable factors. However, if illness and disorder reflect a disturbance of balance among internal and external forces, we are more likely to consider multiple causal forces as relevant and to use a combination of objective and subjective measures to examine these possibilities.

Implicit meaning associated with words is not limited to metaphors. Consider the word *recovery*, a term used frequently in medical rehabilitation outcome studies. In common usage *recovered* means "restored fully to health," such as recovered from the flu. However, the same term is currently applied in research with a very different meaning. Duncan and her colleagues illustrated this problem in an analysis of results from stroke outcome studies (Duncan, Jorgensen, & Wade, 2000). Twenty-seven of these studies used the Barthel Index as their outcome measure, which examines the person's need for assistance to perform basic activities of daily living, including eating, dressing, grooming, and walking. All studies used a cut-off score to identify patient groups whom they labeled as either recovered or not recovered. However, Duncan et al. (2000) found that, across the 27 studies, 7 different cut-off scores had been used to define *recovered* and *not recovered* groups and the choice of cut-off point was not explained in several of the studies. This variability in the definition of "recovered" affected the conclusions drawn about the proportion of patients likely to improve over a particular period of time or as a result of intervention. Conclusions about the effectiveness of intervention would have been different in several studies if cut-off score had been used.

Whose Definition Is This?

The impact of variability in the operational definition of *recovery* is not the only concern raised by Duncan et al.'s (2000) findings. Regardless of which cut-off score they used, by choosing "recovery" to describe the focus of their research, these investigations all accepted the implicit meaning of the term as defined by the measure, which is "not needing physical assistance with most basic ADLs." Whose definition is this? Most likely it is that of the payers, who are concerned with how many days the person must be treated in an expensive facility and when the person can go home without need for specialized or extra support. Is that a meaningful focus of concern? Of course it is. Health care is an expensive resource, and it is reasonable for the companies and agencies involved in financing it to be concerned about efficient allocation of this resource.

However, using "recovery" to describe the results of this research also pulls in the usual meaning of the term to most people reading it. The implicit message being communicated to the reader is that the participants are now "well," back to the way they were before, and their major health issues are resolved. Perhaps, according to a very narrow physical health standard, they are. But occupational therapy practitioners, family members, and the clients themselves know that this isn't the case. As Radomski expressed so well in the title of her article, "There is more to life than putting on your pants" (Radomski, 1995).

The use of a cut-off score on a measure to define recovery rests on the assumption that recovery of function can be marked distinctly in the same way that we can define whether someone does or does not have a fever. This approach has roots in medicine's focus on success as measured by cure rate. However, in this context it denies the ambiguity inherent in processes, such as functional recovery, that are slow and continuous and that often vary depending on contextual factors present at a given moment. The medical researchers reporting these studies are applying the same framework to a very different type of experience and treating it as if it is the same.

This research evidence may then be used to determine whether treatment is authorized, or a service is deemed medically necessary.

In the field of mental health, introduction of the term *recovery* in the 1990s represented a radical reframing of assumptions about services for people with serious mental illness. In this case the leaders in the field argued forcefully for a dynamic conceptualization of recovery as a *process* focused on meaningful participation in life even though the illness may not be cured (Anthony, 1993). Recovery as defined here clearly requires consideration of more than whether the person is able to complete basic ADLs, and it cannot be evaluated using cut-off scores on a single measure.

Meaning Depends on the Measure

Duncan et al.'s (2000) review of stroke research is a rare example of a scientist looking carefully at the impact of decisions about measures on the results of research and the conclusions drawn from these results. The paucity of such critical reviews stands in striking contrast to the level of scrutiny and amount of discussion one can find in the literature on sample selection methods, controls for bias in the *administration* of measures, or selection of appropriate data analysis methods. Although considerable attention is paid to evaluating the *psychometric* properties of the instruments used, little is paid to the *appropriateness* of the measures selected for the question being investigated. In many research reports it seems sufficient to report that the measures selected are "reliable and valid" before moving on to other weightier issues. Yet the validity of even the best-designed randomized clinical trial ultimately depends on whether the outcome measure used is appropriate for the question and responsive to the expected amount of change (e.g., Matson, 2007).

This word *recovery*, as well as other terms we frequently use, such as *function, disability, activity,* and *participation,* share the common feature that their definition (their meanings) depend heavily on the measure used in the particular context. Our habits of thought and communication lead us to expect that a word like *function* always refers to approximately the same construct or has the same meaning. However, depending on the measures chosen, the reality at present is that there may be very little overlap in content and often quite variable degrees of association between clinical instruments that purport to measure the same thing (e.g., Coster et al., 2004). As a consequence, when a study reports that a treatment is or is not effective, it is impossible to draw any conclusions about the implications of these results until we know how the outcomes were measured and the criteria used to define effectiveness.

Borrowed Ideas

Medicine meets the behavioral sciences in the arena of disability and rehabilitation. Here the medical orientation to objective phenomena and preference for clear-cut distinctions meets the complexity, unpredictability, and ambiguity of people's daily behavior. We can see the influences of both of these disciplines played out in the design of various measures used in the field (Streiner & Norman, 1995). Medicine has a pragmatic focus on "what works" in terms of differentiating groups with different diagnoses or predicting outcomes of professional interest. It has not concerned itself particularly with identifying or defining underlying constructs. Not surprisingly, the discipline tends to emphasize physical performance in measures of function and to emphasize signs, symptoms, and diagnosis during the assessment process.

In contrast, psychology has consistently concerned itself with abstract constructs presumed to reflect processes underlying observed behavior. As a science, it also views itself as seeking facts or truths about persons, but the primary objects of its theory and research—constructs such as memory, self-efficacy, and attention—are not fully present in nature. Instead, their existence and influence is inferred based on what can be observed. Definitions of abstract concepts such as these are particularly likely to reflect cultural orientation and values. They represent what a given group considers distinctive, worth knowing about, or real.

For example, Westerners believe that we can identify and measure a set of personality traits that influence the behavior of a person across situations (Ozer Benet-Martínez, 2006). This view is consistent with a cultural value and philosophy that view the person as an active, autonomous agent and historically has had difficulty acknowledging how much the environment (both social and physical) influences our behavior (Danzinger, 1997). Considerable research in social psychology has been done to identify and name these traits and to investigate the relations between measures of these traits and other phenomena of interest.

However, in many Eastern systems of thought individuals are considered to be an inextricable part of a larger whole and their characteristics can only be understood in relation to the social context of which they are a part (e.g., Iwama, 2003; Nisbett, Peng, Choi, & Norenzayan, 2001). This alternative view challenges the Western approach, asserting that it does not reflect all reality and cannot be assumed to capture universal truths. Although Western measures might be translated and administered to Asian people, this does not guarantee that their data can validly be interpreted using the same Western framework.

From Numbers to Measures

In its early days, in order for psychology to be considered a science rather than remain a branch of philosophy, it had to find a way to assign numbers to the abstract qualities of interest or find things to count that were accepted as representative of these qualities. Numbers were the language of science and the means of measurement.

Another story will serve well to introduce some important features of measurement. There is a bridge in Boston crossing the Charles River named the Harvard Bridge, although it crosses from Boston over to MIT. If you walk across the bridge you will notice that the pavement is marked at regular intervals with lines indicating that this distance is equal to so many "smoots." The bridge is 364.4 smoots—"plus or minus an ear"—long. This fact was discovered when the Lambda Chi Alpha fraternity used the body of their shortest freshman pledge, Oliver Smoot, to measure the bridge back in 1958. The fraternity, with the support of the city, has maintained this unique measuring system every since (reported in Tavenor, 2007).

This story is a humorous reminder of the original relation between measures and the form of the human body, which is still preserved in our "foot" ruler, and the need for measures to solve practical problems such as determining the length of a field or the correct height for a doorway. Systematic application of measures was necessary for order and harmony in early societies (e.g., to ensure that a square house was built with equal corners and parallel walls of the same height). From the beginning measures also had important social value as they were needed (e.g., to mark boundaries of land ownership or to determine appropriate charges for the weight of goods being sold; Tavenor, 2007).

Since ancient times secret qualities and powers have also been associated with numbers and mathematics (Livio, 2002). For the Greeks, numbers and the proportions described in geometry reflected the structure and harmony of the universe. They could be used to represent the systematic relations of musical notes and the patterns seen in nature. Thus the study of mathematics revealed important truths about the universe.

As subsequently discovered by Newton, Galileo, and other scientists, mathematics also could be used to express precisely the laws governing many physical phenomena. Descartes subsequently summarized the view of the scientific age, arguing that because *qualities* are the product of our unreliable senses, *quantity* is a more reliable measure of reality than quality (Tavenor, 2007). From that point on in Western history, it was not a large leap to begin to view quantity as a measure of ultimate value. This view was also consistent with the industrial era's valuing of productivity and standardization of units of industrial products (Danzinger, 1997).

We don't have to look far to see the expression of this thinking in psychology. In many of the instruments designed to measure human abilities, the capacity to do more (e.g., complete more puzzles, solve more arithmetic problems) is the means used to rank persons. The numbers obtained from these measures are believed to provide a more objective way to determine individuals' standing on a culturally important dimension such as intelligence. A subtle but important conclusion that has followed from this reasoning is that if these numbers were obtained through rigorous and standardized procedures, then they must reflect reality (Gould, 1981).

Some constructs of interest to the behavioral and social sciences are not as readily measured by observation of performance. An alternative approach to generating the numbers needed for scientific analysis is needed. Here another leap of reasoning is made. If qualities of experience, like self-efficacy, or confidence, goal-orientation, or disability, are assumed to exist on a continuum, then we can use ordered response scales to locate each person on that continuum. So we ask the person whether each of several of statements about his or her confidence is true or not on a scale from 1 to 7, from "not at all true" to "definitely true," or we ask the person who is recovering from a stroke how much difficulty, on a scale from 1 to 4, from "cannot do" to "no difficulty," she has performing a set of daily activities. If we add or average the resulting item scores, we now have a number we can use to rank people on their confidence or their function or to correlate with scores from other measures.

There are several of problems with this approach to developing measures. For one, it rests on the assumption that the items and ratings on the instrument divide the dimension of confidence, disability, or self-efficacy into equivalent units like the inch markings on a ruler (Wright & Linacre, 1989). Therefore, a score of 20 is interpreted as indicating that the person has twice the confidence, function, or self-efficacy as the person whose score was 10, and half the confidence, function or self-efficacy as the person who scored 40. Or, as another example, we assume that achieving a positive change in one's confidence from a score of 1 to a score of 2 is equally significant as achieving an improvement from a score of 3 to a score of 4.

We know from clinical practice that not all tasks or levels of performance are equally challenging or meaningful, and yet this is what we assume when we add these kinds of scores together. In reality when we subject our measures to modern analytic approaches, such as item response theory or Rasch analysis (Bond & Fox, 2001), the picture often looks quite different: Sometimes it is a short step to improve from one rating level to the next, and sometimes it is a very big step. In other words, our untested measures of these complex constructs may well give a distorted picture of reality. They may give equal weight to easy and difficult achievements or underestimate the degree of progress a person has made toward important goals.

The Social Context of Measurement

The construction of a measure is a human process. Therefore, by definition, the process is embedded in a social system of values and ideas about people (Danzinger, 1990). This social influence often is quite hard to see when we are part of the same system, but it becomes apparent if we ask, Who is not well-described by this measure? For example, practitioners know that many standardized tests do not provide a differentiated profile of their clients with significant disabilities. As a psychology intern I saw this clearly when I tested several community-living adults with developmental disabilities. It was apparent from observing and interacting with these clients that their profiles of cognitive strengths and limitations were very different, but they all achieved identical (low) scores on the IQ test I administered.

This odd situation results from the fact that the primary objective for the developers of these instruments was to maximize the differentiation among the majority of people in the population: those who score between ±2 standard deviations from the mean in the distribution of the ability or trait (Anastasi & Urbina, 1997). Therefore, most of the items provide useful information only about individuals within that range. Unfortunately, that is not the part of the population we typically serve. The choices the developers made when selecting the items and creating the scoring system may have made it impossible for the person with a motor or communication impairment to obtain a score above 0. The implication of such a score is that this person's performance reveals *nothing of significant interest,* a value judgment that is embedded in the design of the instrument.

The practitioners who were involved in pilot testing of the School Function Assessment (SFA; Coster, Deeney, Haley, & Haltiwanger, 1998) recognized—and resisted—the negative social implication of 0 scores.

When an earlier version of the SFA used performance ratings that were on a scale of 0 to 3, they almost never gave a student a score of 0, even though it was obvious from other data in the form that a score of 0 would have been the appropriate rating. When we asked why, they explained that they hated the connotations of giving a child a 0 score because it seemed so pessimistic and because others often interpreted these scores to mean that the student *couldn't do anything*.

Impact of Our Choice of Measurement Lens

Our instruments provide a way to extract a pattern from the performance of an individual for some purpose. However, the complexity of a person's behavior can be viewed through many lenses, each of which may detect a different pattern. In turn, the choice of lens has a profound influence on the picture that the user forms of the person who is being assessed. It can emphasize deficit, as measured by standard deviations below the mean, or it can call attention to achievements, as measured by a score that reflects the current repertoire of daily life skills.

More importantly, the type of picture constructed by an instrument often leads to very different kinds of dialogues about the person's needs, potentially useful interventions, and likely outcomes. To illustrate, a study by Linehan, Brady, and Hwang (1991) presented teachers with two different assessment reports on the same 12-year-old student with severe disabilities. One report summarized the student's performance on standardized test items, such as standing on one foot for 5 seconds, cutting out a circle, or drawing a cross. The other report provided descriptions of how the student accomplished various tasks during the school day, indicating that he could dress himself independently except for tying shoes and could travel independently from his classroom to the lunch-room. When asked to project the student's likely level of achievement of goals on his individualized educational plan for the year, those who read the second description expected significantly higher achievement than those who read the first one.

Since Rosenthal and Jacobson (1968) published their classic book *Pygmalion in the Classroom,* there have been ample other demonstrations of the power of evaluative information to influence expectations and, in turn, to influence outcomes in situations that include classrooms, research labs, physicians' offices, and social encounters (Rosenthal, 1976). Our measures are a major source of information in our practice and our research.

In the past decade the United States has increasingly moved toward decision making on the basis of instrument numbers. In national surveys to guide policy decisions, a person is counted as having a disability based on whether he or she has difficulty performing two or more specific daily activities (e.g., Walsh & Khatutsky, 2007). In some settings one must qualify for services by scoring sufficiently low on a particular test (e.g., at least 1.5 standard deviations below the mean). The argument often made in support of these approaches is that an objective method is being applied because numbers from standardized measures are being used and that objective methods are more trustworthy, reasonable, and fair. But is this true? Behind these numbers is a human decision to select a particular instrument that emphasizes certain tasks or abilities and minimizes the importance of others. It is a human decision to set or accept a particular criterion. That decision often is based on pragmatic or economic reasons and not on science or on an understanding of the strengths and limitations of measures. Nevertheless, these decisions affect our practice and the services our clients can obtain.

The situations I have been describing fall in the domain of what Messick (1980, 1989) has termed the *consequential aspects of validity:* Are the *social* consequences that follow from administration of the test appropriate, given the nature of the test? Messick and others (e.g., Cronbach, 1988) have argued that both meaning and values are *always* involved in the validation of measures and therefore validators must examine whether an application of a measure has *appropriate consequences* for individuals and institutions. It is hard to resist the apparent legitimacy of numbers, but we need to examine existing practices by asking questions, such as

- Is this an appropriate measure to use for identifying clients whose functional limitations are of a type and degree that require intervention and support services?
- Is requiring that a student must score minus 1.5 *SD* deviations on a specific standardized test in order to obtain occupational therapy services consistent with the legal definition of students to whom those services should be provided?
- Does this measure sample the appropriate content using appropriate methods to identify whether occupational therapy services have helped the client progress toward important goals?

If the answer to any of these questions is no, then I believe we have a professional and ethical obligation to challenge these misapplications of measurement and to advocate strongly for more appropriate alternatives.

Sources of Bias in Measurement

Assessment is always a social process. For one, assessment is most often conducted in some kind of face-to-face exchange between practitioner and client. In addition, the majority of clinical assessment tools require that a person (the practitioner or the client) determine the appropriate quantitative measure (a score or rating) to assign for a given item. These social features of the assessment context may exert more influence over the data obtained from measurement than we realize. Most efforts to ensure the quality of assessment data focus on reducing random sources of inconsistency across occasions or raters. These random influences are the sources of potential error that traditional reliability studies examine. But there is a substantial literature demonstrating that consistent biases also may influence the outcomes of measurement (Gilovich, Griffin, & Kahneman, 2002).

One source of bias is our susceptibility to influence by elements of a situation of which we are not even aware, or which we believe (wrongly, as it turns out) we are able to resist. For example, two studies done with the FIM (UDS, 1997) showed that raters were systematically influenced in their own ratings by seeing the ratings of other items that had already been completed by other team members (Doctor, Wolfson, McKnight & Burns, 2003; Wolfson, Doctor, & Burns, 2000). Studies with other instruments have shown that respondents are systematically influenced by the anchor or range of the scale. When asked to rate an experience such as the frequency of feeling irritated or sad, respondents gave different answers depending on whether the scale extended over a short or longer period (e.g., "in the past week" vs. "in the past month"; Chapman & Johnson, 2002). Nevertheless, raters consistently claim that they *were not influenced* by variations such as these when making their judgments.

Respondents also appear to use the structure of items and scales (and features of the assessment context) to make inferences about what the examiner is really most interested in (Redelmeier, Schull, Hux, Tu, & Ferris, 2001; Redelmeier, Tu, Schull, Ferris, & Hux, 2001; Schwartz, 1999). Then they respond according to this inferred purpose, perhaps by emphasizing certain types of experiences and minimizing others. Thus, cues suggesting that the examiner is most interested in physical function may lead respondents to under-report experiences reflecting their emotional well-being, or vice versa. These cues may be as subtle as the pictures on the wall of the rooms where the assessment is conducted.

Instruments developed without input from people with disabilities frequently present quandaries of interpretation. For example, the well-known SF-36 (Ware & Sherbourne, 1992) and other health-related, quality-of-life measures introduce questions about a person's positive or negative daily experiences with the phrase, "Does your health limit you. . . ?" The person with a recent stroke may include stroke-related impairments as part of his or her definition of current health state when answering these items. However, the teenager with cerebral palsy or an athlete with a decade-old spinal cord injury may not consider his or her disability to be a health problem and may wonder how to answer a question such as, "During the past 4 weeks were you limited in the kind of work or other regular daily activities you could do as a result of you physical health?" If a study compares the quality-of-life of these groups using the SF-36, can we be sure that the responses from each group are capturing the same experiences? (Hays, Hahn, & Marshall, 2002) The SF-36 is considered the gold standard among measures of health-related-quality-of-life and is applied widely in clinical research. But is an item that asks whether or not the person is "limited in walking more than 1 mile" a valid indicator of quality of life (Meyers & Andresen, 2000)?

Clinical assessment also is a judgment process that requires a complex integration of information from multiple sources. Studies in cognitive psychology have documented that in situations with complex processing demands people often reason by applying heuristics, which are thinking short-cuts that help reduce the complexity of information processing by applying a general guideline to arrive at a judgment (Tversky & Kahneman, 1974). These shortcuts actually work quite well in many problem-solving situations of daily life. However, they also make us susceptible to systematic errors, particularly when we try to synthesize results from multiple sources of assessment information (Croskerry, 2003; Garb, 1998). For example, we are susceptible to confirmatory bias, which is the tendency to notice only information that supports our working hypothesis about the source or nature of a person's problem, so we fail to seek out or account for contradictory information. Another well-known cognitive bias is *search satisfying,* the tendency to call off a search (e.g., for an explanation of assessment results) once a plausible answer has been found. This tendency may lead us to conclude our consideration of the data prematurely, before we have completed a full examination of all the findings.

These cognitive biases are an outcome of how our human brain functions, and they operate outside of our awareness. They have been studied extensively in psychology as well as in medicine, and their impact on diagnostic reasoning is described in the recently popular book *How Doctors Think* (Groopman, 2007). The reality of their influence is yet another reason we should draw conclusions from our measures with caution.

Where Should We Go From Here?

The discovery that the tools and processes we have thought of as objective, scientific, or sound are, in fact, fraught with uncertainty can be disconcerting. Confronted with this evidence of pervasive ambiguity we may want to throw up our hands and say "Oh, well, it is what it is" and continue with our usual habits. Alternatively we may consider abandoning the whole enterprise as hopeless. However I would like to urge another alternative, which is to use the power that a deeper understanding of measures gives us to work toward more positive outcomes.

Becoming a Positive Subversive

The story at the beginning of this paper introduced the idea that measures have the power to shape the story that others hear about a person. I have presented several examples where that power has resulted in a narrow, truncated, impoverished, or misleading view of the person. However, that power also can be used to positive ends to challenge these limitations and bring the larger story to life. We can all play a part in this important enterprise.

For years I had a title ready for a talk I hoped to give someday: "Test Development as a Subversive Activity." In this talk I would tell about how I discovered, from working on the Pediatric Evaluation of Disability Inventory (PEDI; Haley, Coster, Ludlow, Haltiwanger, & Andrellos, 1992) and School Function Assessment (Coster et al., 1998), that the design of an instrument could actually cause the people using it to think differently about the children they were assessing. After using one of these assessments it was common to hear comments from parents, teachers, and therapists like the one from a mother who said, "This was the first team meeting where we talked about Jeremy's strengths, not just his deficits."

Thinking differently also leads to different decisions being made in the context of intervention or research. For example, when the PEDI was first used in early studies of dorsal rhizotomy surgery for children with cerebral palsy, it revealed that meaningful functional changes could occur even without significant changes in impairment-level measures (Dudgeon et al., 1994; Nordmark, Jamlo, & Hagglud, 2000). This was a significant challenge to existing approaches to evaluating interventions, which had assumed that changes in impairment must precede changes in function. Now, use of functional outcome measures is routine in clinical trials of surgical and pharmacological interventions for children with cerebral palsy.

Here is an incredible power for positive change if one can design an instrument that simultaneously fits well enough within the existing system to be adopted but incorporates enough differences to change thinking in a positive way—in other words, making test development a subversive activity. To be an effective subversive one must first thoroughly know the existing system—its rules, policies, priorities, resources, and ways of thinking—so that the new instrument is designed to meet the system's essential criteria well enough to be given serious consideration. The instrument developer also must have a vision of a new way to bring the client's story forward and must be able to persuade the powers-that-be that this new alternative is *just what they need*. Who knew that instrument development also might require political strategy and skills? But it does. And it must so that we can persuade powerful entities, like the Centers for Medicare and Medicaid Services and other policy-making bodies, to adopt or accept the new measures we develop.

An effective, positive subversive must be willing to try a different way to capture the client's story. Occupational therapy's holistic and client-centered philosophy, values, and practice provide excellent preparation for this creative role. We have seen many wonderful examples of this creativity in the development of instruments such as the Activity Card Sort (Baum & Edwards, 2008), the Children's Assessment of Participation and Enjoyment (King et al., 2004), and the Occupational Self-Assessment (Baron, Kielhofner, Jenger, Goldhammer, & Wolenski, 2002), which have influenced practice and research both within and beyond occupational therapy by enabling a richer portrait of the client's life and concerns to emerge.

Routinely using instruments such as these in occupational therapy practice is one way that we can change the dialogue with clients, family members, and other professionals. But we also need to acquire and use sophisticated knowledge about measures to challenge current assessment practices that are overly narrow in focus or require use of instruments in inappropriate ways, such as when qualifying students for services. These practices not only limit the client's ability to tell his or her full story, but they also restrict our profession.

We need to challenge interpretations of research evidence that draw inappropriate conclusions from the measures that were used, particularly when those interpretations are used to restrict occupational therapy practice or to establish overly narrow service guidelines. If a study or a systematic review concludes that a therapy program "does not improve function," then we must examine whether the outcome measures examined more than basic physical function and challenge the conclusions if they do not. If a study concludes that little further recovery is seen after the first six months following a traumatic brain injury, then we must examine how recovery was defined and whether the measure used to do so is sensitive to smaller amounts of functional change. And if a study purports to examine participation, then we should make sure that the content of the outcome measure examines more than basic ADLs or whether the person can walk a mile and asks about social relationships and engagement in family and community life, work, play and leisure. A life of quality is about *so* much more than buttoning a shirt or tying shoes. We must make sure that our measures capture its richness and complexity.

Acknowledgment

There are many, many people whose support, encouragement, and belief in me helped to bring this work to fruition. I would especially like to thank my students at Boston University for the energy and intelligence that makes teaching them such a joy; Ellen Cohn and Sue Berger for nominating me and the rest of the creative and generous faculty at Boston University for being the best colleagues one could ever hope to have; and my family, whose love and good humor keep me going.

References

Anastasi, A., & Urbina, S. (1997). *Psychological testing* (7th ed.). Upper Saddle River, NJ: Prentice Hall.

Anthony, W. A. (1993). Recovery from mental illness: The guiding vision of the mental health service system in the 1990s. *Psychosocial Rehabilitation Journal, 16*(4), 11–23.

Baron, K., Kielhofner, G., Jenger, A., Goldhammer, V., & Wolenski, J. (2002). *Occupational Self-Assessment Version 2.1.* Chicago: Model of Human Occupation Clearinghouse.

Baum, C. M., & Edwards, D. (2008). *Activity Card Sort* (2nd ed.). Bethesda, MD: AOTA Press.

Bond, T. G., & Fox, C. M. (2001). *Applying the Rausch model: Fundamental measurement in the human sciences.* Mahwah, NJ: Erlbaum.

Brown, T. L. (2003). *Making truth: Metaphor in science.* Urbana: University of Illinois Press.

Bueno, S., & Frenck-Mestre, C. (2002). Rapid activation of the lexicon: A further investigation with behavioral and computational results. *Brain and Language, 81,* 120–130.

Chapman, G. B., & Johnson, E. J. (2002). Incorporating the irrelevant: Anchors in judgments of belief and value. In T. Gilovich, D. Griffin, & D. Kahneman (Eds.), *Heuristics and biases: Then and now* (pp. 120–132). New York: Cambridge University Press.

Coster, W. J., Deeney, T., Haley, S. M., & Haltiwanger, J. (1998). *School Function Assessment.* San Antonio, TX: Psychological Corporation.

Coster, W. J., Haley, S. M., Andres, P., Ludlow, L., Bond, T., & Ni, P. (2004). Refining the conceptual basis for rehabilitation outcome measurement: Personal care and instrumental activities domain. *Medical Care, 42*(Supp. 1), I62–I72.

Cronbach, L. J. (1988). Five perspectives on validation argument. In H. Wainer & H. Braun (Eds.), *Test validity* (pp. 3–17). Hillsdale, NJ: Erlbaum.

Croskerry, P. (2003). The importance of cognitive errors in diagnosis and strategies to minimize them. *Academic Medicine, 78,* 775–782.

Danzinger, K. (1997). *Naming the mind: How psychology found its language.* Thousand Oaks, CA: Sage.

Danzinger, K. (1990). *Constructing the subject: Historical origins of psychological research.* Cambridge: Cambridge University Press.

Doctor, J. W., Wolfson, A. M., McKnight, P., & Burns, S. P. (2003). The effect of inaccurate FIM instrument ratings on prospective payments: A study of clinician expertise and FIM rating difficulty as contributing to inaccuracy. *Archives of Physical Medicine and Rehabilitation, 84,* 46–50.

Dudgeon, B. J., Libby, A. K., McLaughlin, J. F., Hays, R. M., Bjornson, K. F., & Roberts, T. S. (1994). Prospective measurement of functional changes after selective dorsal rhizotomy. *Archives of Physical Medicine and Rehabilitation, 75,* 45–53.

Duncan, P. W., Jorgensen, H. S., & Wade, D. T. (2000). Outcome measures in acute stroke trials: A systematic review and some recommendations to improve practice. *Stroke, 31,* 1429–1438.

Garb, H. N. (1998). *Studying the clinician: Judgment research and psychological assessment.* Washington, DC: American Psychological Association.

Gilovich, T., Griffin, D., & Kahneman, D. (Eds.). (2002). *Heuristics and biases: Then and now.* New York: Cambridge University Press.

Gould, S. J. (1981). *The mismeasure of man.* New York: Norton.

Groopman, J. (2007). *How doctors think.* New York: Houghton-Mifflin.

Haley, S. M., Coster, W. J., Ludlow, L., Haltiwanger, J., & Andrellos, P. (1992). *Pediatric Evaluation of Disability Inventory (PEDI).* Boston: Trustees of Boston University.

Hays, R. D., Hahn, H., & Marshall, G. (2002). Use of the SF-36 and other health-related qualify of life measures to assess persons with disabilities. *Archives of Physical Medicine and Rehabilitation, 82*(Suppl. 2), S4–S9.

Iwama, M. (2003). The Issue Is: Toward culturally relevant epistemologies in occupational therapy. *American Journal of Occupational Therapy, 57,* 582–588.

Karasz, A. (2005). Cultural differences in conceptual models of depression. *Social Science and Medicine, 60,* 1625–1635.

King, G., Law, M., King, S., Rosenbaum, P., Kertoy, M., & Young, N. L. (2004). *Children's Assessment of Participation and Enjoyment (CAPE).* San Antonio, TX: Psychological Corporation.

Lakoff, G., & Johnson, M. (1980). *Metaphors we live by.* Chicago: University of Chicago Press.

Lightman, A. (2005). *A sense of the mysterious*. New York: Vintage Books.

Linehan, S. A., Brady, M. P., & Hwang, C. (1991). Ecological versus developmental assessment: Influences on instructional expectations. *Journal of the Association of Persons With Severe Handicaps, 16,* 146–153.

Livio, M. (2002). *The golden ratio*. New York: Broadway Books.

Matson, J. L. (2007). Determining treatment outcome in early intervention programs for autism spectrum disorders: A critical analysis of measurement issues in learning-based interventions. *Research in Developmental Disabilities, 28,* 207–218.

Messick, S. (1980). Test validity and the ethics of assessment. *American Psychologist, 35,* 1012–1027.

Messick, S. (1989). Meaning and values in test validation: The science and ethics of assessment. *Educational Researcher, 18,* 5–11.

Meyers, A. R., & Andresen, E. M. (2000). Enabling our instruments: Accommodation, universal design, and access to participation in research. *Archives of Physical Medicine and Rehabilitation, 81*(Supp. 2), S5–S9.

Nisbett, R. E., Peng, K., Choi, I., & Norenzayan, A. (2001). Culture and systems of thought: Holistic versus analytic cognition. *Psychological Review, 108,* 291–310.

Nordmark, E., Jamlo, G. G., & Hagglund, G. (2000). Comparison of the Gross Motor Function Measure and Paediatric Evaluation of Disability Inventory in assessing motor function in children undergoing selective dorsal rhizotomy. *Developmental Medicine and Child Neurology, 42,* 245–252.

Ozer, D. J., & Benet-Martínez, V (2006). Personality and the prediction of consequential outcomes. *Annual Review of Psychology, 57,* 401–421.

Radomski, M. V. (1995). Nationally Speaking: There's more to life than putting on your pants. *American Journal of Occupational Therapy, 49,* 487–490.

Redelmeier, D. A., Schull, M. J., Hux, J. E., Tu, J. V., & Ferris, L. E. (2001). Problems for clinical judgment: I. Eliciting an insightful history of present illness. *Canadian Medical Association Journal, 164,* 647–651.

Redelmeier, D. A., Tu, J. V., Schull, M. J., Ferris, L. E., & Hux, J. E. (2001). Problems for clinical judgment: 2. Obtaining a reliable past medical history. *Canadian Medical Association Journal, 164,* 809–813.

Rosenthal, R. (1976). *Experimenter effects in behavioral research*. New York: Irvington.

Rosenthal, R., & Jacobson, L. (1968). *Pygmalion in the classroom*. New York: Holt, Rinehart, & Winston.

Schwartz, N. (1999). Self-reports: How the questions shape the answers. *American Psychologist, 54,* 93–105.

Storck, M., Csordas, T. J., & Strauss, MM. (2000). Depressive illness and Navajo healing. *Medical Anthropology Quarterly, 14,* 571–597.

Streiner, D. L., & Norman, G. R. (1995). *Health measurement scales: A practical guide to their development and use* (2nd ed.). Oxford: Oxford University Press.

Tavenor, R. (2007). *Smoot's ear: The measure of humanity*. New Haven: Yale University Press

Tversky, A., & Kahneman, D. (1974). Judgment under uncertainty: Heuristics and biases. *Science, 185,* 1124–1131.

Uniform Data System for Medical Rehabilitation. (1997). *Guide to the Functional Independence Measure*. Buffalo: State University of New York.

Walsh, E. G., & Khatutsky, G. (2007). Mode of administration effects on disability measures in a sample of frail beneficiaries. *Gerontologist, 47,* 838–844.

Ware, J. E., & Sherbourne, C. D. (1992). The MOS 36-item short-form health survey (SF-36). I. Conceptual framework and item selection. *Medical Care, 30,* 473–483.

Wolfson, A. M., Doctor, J. N., & Burns, S. P. (2000). Clinician judgments of functional outcomes: How bias and perceived accuracy affect rating. *Archives of Physical Medicine and Rehabilitation, 81,* 1567–1574.

Wright, B. & Linacre, J. (1989). Observations are always ordinal. Measurements however must be interval. *Archives of Physical Medicine and Rehabilitation, 70,* 857–860.

58

2009 Eleanor Clarke Slagle Lecture

Reclaiming Our Heritage:
Connecting *the* Founding Vision *to the* Centennial Vision

Kathleen Barker Schwartz, EdD, OTR, FAOTA

I am delighted to have the pleasure of exploring with you the *Founding Vision* of occupational therapy. As the *Centennial Vision* is poised to lead the profession in the beginning of the 21st century, I would like to take us back in time to the early years of the 20th century, when the profession of occupational therapy was founded. There are many parallels between that founding period and now. In this lecture, I will examine the ideas and values that underlie the vision articulated by the founding generation of occupational therapists and describe the similarities and differences between the *Founding Vision* and the *Centennial Vision*. I propose that the commonalities within the two visions create continuity between our past and present—that the *Centennial Vision* does not represent a new set of values but rather builds on values that the profession has held since its inception in 1917.

It is the purpose of history to elucidate connections in the hope that we can learn from our rich past and feel more related to it. Understanding the connection between the values articulated in the *Founding Vision* and those expressed in the *Centennial Vision* can give practitioners of today a sense of continuity and community with earlier generations of occupational therapists and an understanding that many of the contemporary values we currently hold were first articulated by occupational therapy's founding generation almost 100 years ago.

Let us first compare the two visions. The *Founding Vision* states, "The particular objects for which the corporation is formed are as follows: The advancement of occupation as a therapeutic measure; for the study of the effect of occupation upon the human being; and for the scientific dispensation of this knowledge" (National Society for the Promotion of Occupational Therapy [NSPOT], 1917).

The *Centennial Vision* states, "We envision that occupational therapy is a powerful, widely recognized, science-driven, and evidence-based profession with a globally connected and diverse workforce meeting society's occupational needs" (American Occupational Therapy Association [AOTA], 2007, p. 613). These visions share a focus on (1) successful promotion of occupation as a vital force to meet society's needs and (2) engagement in and dissemination of scientific research that supports the effectiveness of occupational therapy.

In short, within both visions there is a concern with *occupation* and *science*. Let us examine the similarities and differences with which the founding generation and today's generation view these concepts.

Originally published 2009 in *American Journal of Occupational Therapy, 63,* 681–690.

Progressive Era: 1890–1920 and Hull House

Before we discuss the *Founding Vision* of occupational therapy, it is helpful to understand the ideas and events that shaped the early years of the 20th century, frequently referred to as the *Progressive Era* (Hofstadter, 1969). Similar to today, the United States faced many problems at the beginning of the 20th century, including war, immigration, industrialization, exploitation of workers, poor schools, and inadequate medical care. However, despite the daunting list of problems, the Progressive Era represented a time of great optimism and confidence in the idea that societal problems could be successfully addressed through progressive reforms.

The *reformers* were people with strong views about democracy and social justice, and they held a firm belief in the power of science to influence proposed social, educational, and meddical reforms. In particular, the reform movements involving arts and crafts, moral treatment, scientific management, and women's suffrage would have a significant and direct influence on the founders of the profession of occupational therapy.

A perfect example of the reformers is Jane Addams of Hull House. In 1889, Jane Addams and Ellen Gates Starr established Hull House in the neighborhood that was the point of entry for immigrants who came to Chicago (Addams, 1911). The purpose of Hull House was to create social and economic reform by providing educational programs and social services.

By the 1920s, the programs at Hull House served more than 9,000 people and included courses for children and adults taught by volunteer professionals from all walks of life, including doctors, lawyers, college professors, craftspeople, artists, and musicians. Addams used her celebrated connections to persuade renowned professionals such as John Dewey and Adolf Meyer to present lectures. It was at Hull House that Eleanor Clarke Slagle took her "invalid occupations" course, and thus became educated in the concept of occupational therapy.

Founders

On March 15, 1917, in Clifton Springs, New York, NSPOT—later to become AOTA—was legally incorporated. It was a modest beginning: Five founders gathered together in a small village in upstate New York. And it was a bold act: These individuals were committed to creating an organization that would spread a vision throughout the United States—a vision of something in which they deeply believed and one they hoped would change society.

Those at the founding meeting included Eleanor Clarke Slagle, a social welfare reformer; George Edward Barton, an architect; William Rush Dunton, Jr., a psychiatrist; Susan Cox Johnson, a teacher; and Thomas B. Kidner, an architect (Figure 58.1). Susan Tracy, a nurse who valued "invalid occupations," was invited but was unable to

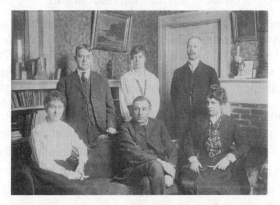

Figure 58.1. Front row, from left to right: Susan Cox Johnson, George Edward Barton, Eleanor Clarke Slagle. Back row, from left to right: William Rush Dunton, Jr.; Isabelle Newton Barton; Thomas B. Kidner.

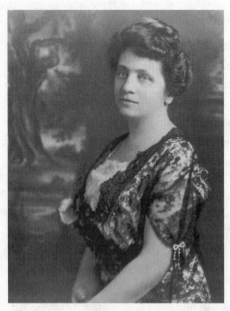

Figure 58.2. Eleanor Clarke Slagle.

attend. Herbert Hall, a physician, is also considered to be a founder, although he did not attend this meeting. As one of my graduate students characterized the founders, they were two doctors, two architects, two Susans, and one Eleanor!

Time does not permit me to discuss all of the founders, so I have chosen Eleanor Clarke Slagle, George Edward Barton, and William Rush Dunton as those who best exemplify the themes I will explore.

Eleanor Clarke Slagle

Eleanor Clarke Slagle (Figure 58.2) strongly believed in the promise of therapeutic occupations and spent her long professional career "spreading the gospel of occupational therapy," as she described her mission in a letter to Dunton (Slagle, 1918). At the retirement banquet held in her honor in 1937, Slagle's compatriot, Harriet Robeson, described her as a "pioneer by nature, with a searching mind and a keen interest in social problems and their psychological aspects" (Robeson, 1937, p. 3). To give you an idea of Slagle's influence, speakers at her retirement banquet included Eleanor Roosevelt, Adolf Meyer, and the Commissioner of Mental Hygiene for the State of New York.

Robeson (1937) described Slagle's contribution in this way: "Mrs. Slagle has directed and laid the solid foundation stones on which our profession and our natural organization rest today" (p. 4). During her years with AOTA, Slagle held many jobs within the association. Robeson invites us to "[i]magine the duties of a President, Treasurer, Executive Secretary, Specialist, Traveling Salesman, Promoter, Advocate, and Ghost Writer, combined into one job and that would be but a part picture of the office Mrs. Slagle has filled these past 20 years in the AOTA" (Robeson, 1937, p. 3).

Much of Slagle's work for AOTA was done on a volunteer basis because she also held a full-time job. Slagle provided steady leadership for the association from 1917 to 1937. Robeson (1937) said of Slagle's tenure, "Officers have come and gone. Boards have changed; but Mrs. Slagle has remained, steadfastly to guide our craft through often foggy seas" (p. 3). The Eleanor Clarke Slagle Lectureship was created in recognition of her significant contribution to the profession.

To provide a little history about the Slagle Lectureship, it was here in Houston 56 years ago that the AOTA House of Delegates and the Board approved its creation. The motion reads in part,

O.T. Honorary Guest Lectureship: As is done in medicine and other professional scientific fields, we [the AOTA membership at large] extend the single honor each year at our Annual Conference of having an Honorary Occupational Therapy Guest Lectureship, to be called out of deference to one of our most outstanding O.T. pioneers—the "Eleanor Clarke Slagle Lectureship." . . . The lecturer each year would be some outstanding occupational therapist who has made significant contributions to the field. (AOTA, 1953)

The minutes of the discussion show that the delegates raised issues such as geographical representation, payment of travel expenses, educational background, whether a non–occupational therapist could be considered to be a Slagle lecturer, and whether 10 years of experience was a good minimum for such consideration. One of the delegates wanted to know what would happen if you had a "red-hot OT" with just 8 years experience? The response was, "If they are so good at 8 years, think how wonderful they will be a 10 years" (AOTA, 1953). The debate ended in unanimous approval of the creation of the Slagle Lectureship.

Slagle was an exception for the times: She sought out educational experiences at a time when many women did not, she lived alone and financially supported herself (she had been married and later separated from her husband), and she had professional ambitions. The most "acceptable" professions at that time for women were nurturing jobs such as nursing, teaching, or social welfare. That three women—one from each of the "acceptable" professions—were involved in the founding of our profession is noteworthy and had a significant influence on the development of occupational therapy.

We will let Slagle describe in her own words her early education in occupational therapy. She wrote,

Covering a period of years of interest in the unfair social attitude toward the dependency of mentally and physically handicapped, followed by lectures on Social Economics by Professor Henderson, Chicago University, Jane Adams, Hull House, Julia Lathrop, now of the Children's Bureau . . . I took up [in] 1910 special courses in occupations and educational methods, Chicago School of Civics and Philanthropy, now a part of the University of Chicago, followed by a 6-month study of hospitals, charitable institutions and dependency of mental and physical cases. (Slagle, n.d., p. 1)

For this course of study, Slagle earned a certificate. In April 1912, Slagle was hired as director of occupational therapy by Adolf Meyer of Phipps Psychiatric Clinic, Johns Hopkins Hospital in Baltimore, Maryland. Meyer was instrumental in helping to conceptualize occupational therapy. Indeed, Slagle names Meyer, along with Addams and Lathrop of Hull House, as responsible for sowing the "seed of occupational therapy for mental patients" (Slagle, 1922, p. 11). Because of her background in social welfare, Slagle was interested in the environmental influences on mental illness and joined with Meyer to create and administer a habit-training program at Phipps Clinic. The program was designed for individuals with severe schizophrenia, known at that time as *dementia praecox*. The habit-training program was based on the assumption that "occupation used remedially serves to overcome some habits, to modify others, and construct new ones to the end that habit reactions will be favorable to the restoration and maintenance of health" (Slagle, 1922, p. 14).

After Slagle left Phipps Clinic, she returned to Chicago where, among other activities, she headed a school of occupational therapy named for Chicago physician Henry P. Favill. Slagle then moved to New York and became the director of occupational therapy for New York Mental Hygiene Department. One of her first acts was to create a habit-training program similar to the one at Phipps Clinic. Although Slagle also supervised the development of other occupational therapy services such as ward activities and occupation centers that ultimately served nearly 70,000 patients in New York's state hospitals, it was the habit-training programs that held a particular attraction for her. She told training aides, "It takes consecration and genuine love of the human family to understand the direction and participation in habit training classes among patients who have been in hospitals anywhere from 5 to 20 years" (Slagle, 1922, p. 13).

Slagle (1924) defined the primary goal of occupational therapy as "help[ing] patients to readjust themselves, both socially and industrially, through organized occupations" (p. 98), and she spent her professional life creating and supervising programs that achieved that goal. She also was mindful of the value of validating the effectiveness of occupational therapy and reminded therapists of the "value of accurate notes" (Slagle, 1922, p. 17). She admonished those in change of conducting research in New York's Mental Hygiene Department to include study of the effects of occupational therapy in addition to psychiatry. She said, "Surely it is not too much to expect that equally valuable contributions in the field of occupational therapy would result if the institute undertook research into its underlying principles and its mode of application" (Slagle, 1924, p. 104).

Slagle was heavily influenced by social justice concerns for those who had landed in the "discard of life" to attain a modicum, at least, of self-respect and dignity (Slagle, 1922, p. 13), and she saw occupation as the means to achieve it. She saw scientific research as the means to help establish the value of the occupational therapy profession and ensure its longevity. She dedicated her life to shaping, directing, and promoting the profession, thereby advocating for those not held in high regard by society.

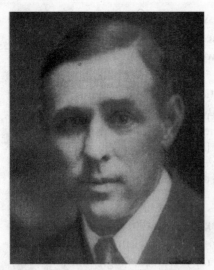

Figure 58.3. George Edward Barton.

George Edward Barton

George Barton (Figure 58.3) came to believe in the healing power of occupation through his own personal experience. In 1901, Barton learned he had tuberculosis. In 1912, he developed gangrene on his left foot while doing an environmental survey, and following surgery he developed hysterical paralysis on the left side of his body. Barton was desolate when he sought the spiritual counsel of Rev. Elwood Worcester, rector of the Emmanuel Church in Boston. The good reverend convinced Barton that although he might feel that life might not be worth living for himself alone, "It would be worthwhile to prove for the sake of others that a man in his condition could overcome his disabilities and teach others to do the same" (Licht, 1967, p. 270). Thus Barton's new vocation in occupational therapy was born.

Barton was an architect by training and interested in the effect that the environment can have on individuals. For a time he worked in London with William Morris, the leader of the Arts and Crafts Movement, who inspired in him a concern for the relationship between the environment and social problems. On his return to the states, Barton served as the first secretary of the Boston Society of Arts and Crafts. As a man sensitive to the enviroment, he found hospital conditions deplorable. Paramount in Barton's mind was the need to create an environment that would promote healing.

He purchased a house in Clifton Springs, New York, which he named Consolation House, and remade it to reflect the tenets of William Morris: Your home should contain only what you know to be useful and believe to be beautiful (Boris, 1986). Barton created the opposite of the hospital experience that he had found so debilitating. His wife, Isabelle Newton Barton, describes Consolation House: "Consolation House is merely a little colonial dwelling, with its shop and garden, in a sleepy upstate village, wherein a sick person, who, convalescing, hates the very thought of the hospital, can be far away from all 'sick' atmosphere, and at the same time learn something to be of value to him" (Newton, 1917). In other words, it "represented the efforts of a man to get away from institutional life toward one through which he could be happy, get well, and become self-supporting" (Newton, 1917).

George Barton (1922) chose the Phoenix, "which burns itself up with its own fire and is reborn from its own ashes," as the emblem of Consolation House to represent the "triumph over disability and despair" (p. 308). That engagement in occupation might ultimately result in patients becoming self-supporting was a critical factor for Barton. In part, Barton was operating under a strong social norm at that time. As he wrote, "A man is not a *normal* man just because his temprature is 98.6°. A man is not a normal man until he is able to provide for himself" (Barton, 1922, p. 305).

Consolation House provided a healing environment where Barton and others would recover was his solution to the debilitating effects of institutional life. He devised his own self-treatment, primarily using the occupations of carpentry and gardening. As Mrs. Barton described him, "Starting alone, with no prospect of help, paralyzed on his left side so that he could scarcely do more than stand, and with no motion possible in his left hand and arm, he used his own body as a clinic to work out the problems of re-educating himself. He made a beginning by reclaiming a weed patch" (Newton, 1917).

After he gradually recovered, Barton focused on providing occupational treatment for others. He wrote, "I am going to try to prove that the patient can spend the long enforced hours of convalescence . . . in preparing himself for the life which he has got to lead when that convalescence is ended" (Barton, 1914b, p. 330).

Barton did not have a medical background, and he initially expressed his interest in occupation in terms of a social and educational perspective. He asserted, "I am not a doctor and have no particular interest in medicine, but I may perhaps lay some slight claim to being a socialist however insignificant, and my great aim is to use the hospital as a re-educational institution" (Barton, 1914a). However, Barton's view changed over time, and by 1917 he was insisting that the word occupational *therapy* be used instead of *re-education* because he wanted to have the "health-giving side emphasized" (Barton, 1917b). This change probably reflected Barton's realization that the profession of occupational therapy would be better accepted and promoted as a therapeutic service that was part of the scientific medical community.

Barton had a close affinity for the engineering sciences, probably because of his technical education as an architect. He was specifically taken with the ideas about measurement and efficiency underlying the popular movement of the time known as *scientific management.* Barton was particularly interested in the time and motion studies of Frank and Lillian Gilbreth. Indeed, he wrote a letter to Frank Gilbreth, offering the services of the NSPOT to contribute to the "Plan to Re-educate Our Men Maimed in the War" (Barton, 1917c). In addition, in a piece he wrote about measuring efficiency, Barton asked, "What is an efficiency expert? An 'efficiency expert' . . . is simply an engineer who substitutes accurate measurement for personal opinion . . . and unscientifically derived conclusions" (Barton, n.d., pp. 77–78). Barten then took the idea of devising methods of measurement to address practical problems in scientific management and applied the principles of measurement to occupational therapy. You can understand the appeal to George Barton of a science that could help occupational therapists to measure patients' movements and match the correct occupation with the corresponding motion. Barton incorporated time and motion studies into his work and developed a form of activity analysis: "Mr. Barton first considers what motions are possible or impossible, desirable and undesirable; then he finds some occupation which involves those possible and desired motions" (Newton, 1917).

Barton died in 1923 and therefore did not live long enough to see many of his ideas implemented. In a letter from Mrs. Barton to Dunton, dated July 12, 1923, she states,

> His enthusiasm and vision were too energetic for his frail body, and, after a really heroic winter working under great difficulties . . . he collapsed thirteen days before he died on April 27, with a return of his tuberculosis. It, of course, seems very hard to me, but I am happy in possessing the finest sturdiest little 2½ year-old son, who bids fair to possess such a body that he can perhaps accomplish things his father failed in becuase of his own physical drawbaks. (Newton, 1923)

Through his own journey of self-healing Barton learned the value of occupation. This experience led him to dedicate the rest of his life to helping others achieve the physical, emotional, and financial recovery that he had achieved. Barton was a man of action and ideas. Influenced by the Arts and Crafts and Scientific Management movements, Consolation House represents Barton's attempts to create an aesthetic, healing environment that also incorporated a scientific approach to treatment.

Barton had a prickly personality; he was easily offended and held strong views. However, I believe that on balance the passion he possessed for occupational therapy compensates for his eccentricities. Consolation House was an extraordinary undertaking in which he tried to put into practice his ideas about occupation and science. In fact, years later, in a keynote address given at the 50th Annual Occupational Therapy Conference, the following question was posed: "Does it sound too visionary to suggest that there be a Consolation House within walking distance of every urban dweller?" (Bockoven, 1971, p. 224).

William Rush Dunton, Jr.

William Rush Dunton, Jr. (Figure 58.4) is frequently referred to as the "father of occupational therapy" because of his many contributions to the development and promotion of the profession (Quiroga, 1995). He was a strong believer in the value of therapeutic occupation and a tireless promoter of research in occupational therapy. He wrote in his "Credo for Occupational Therapists":

> That occupation is as necessary to life as food and drink
>
> That every human being should have both physical and mental occupation
>
> That all should have occupations which they enjoy.

(Dunton, 1919, p. 10)

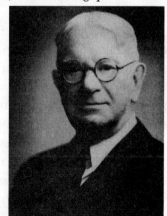

Figure 58.4. William Rush Dunton, Jr.

Dunton was a man of principle and independent thought. He was a member of a prominent Philadelphia family and a descendent of Benjamin Rush, one of the signers of the Declaration of Independence. After he graduated from medical school at the University of Pennsylvania, it was assumed he would follow in his uncle's footsteps—his uncle being a prominent physician. However, Dunton broke with his family's wishes that he marry a woman from an equally privileged background and instead chose Edna Hogan, a nursing superintendent at Children's Hospital in Philadelphia. This ended his professional relationship with his uncle, forcing Dunton to strike out on his own. He ultimately became a psychiatrist and was appointed supervisor of occupation classes at the Sheppard Asylum (now Sheppard Pratt Hospital) in Maryland.

It was Dunton's life-long interest in crafts that helped him understand that occupation was a valuable form of therapy for himself and others (1943). He first became interested in crafts as a child. In a tongue-in-cheek autobiographical sketch titled *How I Got that Way,* he wrote,

> Perhaps my parents were to blame. Father was mechanically minded and by precept and example fostered an instinct or craving in me to know how things are put together or why wheels go round [and] we must blame some gene in me which came from my great grandfather, William Rush, who made his living as a wood carver and sculptor [and] Mother was a most accomplished needlewoman, and, being the baby of the family, I was naturally with her a great deal and grew familiar with crocheting . . . and almost all forms of needlework. (Dunton, 1943, p. 244)

Evidence that Dunton retained a lifelong interest in arts and crafts is provided in his extensive list of publications (Dunton, 1946). It shows several articles on quilts and quilting, gardening, toy making, chintz work, and a study of craftts.

Of course, most of Dunton's publications are related to promoting occupational therapy. He wrote books and articles to help medical students, physicians, nurses, and occupational therapists understand the use of therapeutic occupation. His perspective was a humanistic one. At the founding meeting, Dunton proposed that the philosophy underlying the moral treatment movement of the mid-1800s was one to which occupational therapy should adhere through its valuing of a humanistic, occupation-based approach to care for the mentally ill (Dunton, 1917). He also was holistic in his view of treatment, arguing in a 1928 article that it was impossible to separate the mental and the physical. He used a quote from Thomas Salmon to highlight the importance of this psychobiological view: "The old, unproductive controversy over what is 'mental' and what is 'physical' is ending . . . only an approach broad enough to permit . . . the psychobiological point of view throws light upon their nature" (Salmon, as cited in Dunton, 1928b, pp. 9-10).

Although Dunton advocated this enlightened view, he also understood that for many of his fellow physicians, the holistic versus reductionistic and the mind versus body debates were not decided. Thus his 1928 and 1945 editions of the textbook *Prescribing Occupational Therapy* explained the use of occupations within the context of medical diagnoses.

Dunton's most important contribution to the promotion of occupational therapy was in his role as publisher, editor, and author. In large part, he was responsible for creating and preserving the written legacy of the profession (McDaniel, 1971). When the NSPOT was formed in 1917, Dunton was editor of the *Maryland Psychiatric Quarterly*. Dunton made the *Quarterly* the official journal of the association until 1921, when he inaugurated the profession's first official journal, the *Archives of Occupational Therapy*. It was renamed *Occupational Therapy and Rehabilitation* in 1924. Dunton remained its owner and editor until AOTA took over responsibility for the profession's journal, and the first issue of the *American Journal of Occupational Therapy* was published in 1947. Dunton's editorial contributions totaled more than 25 years, all of which were without remuneration.

One of Dunton's greatest challenges was obtaining sufficient work of high-enough quality to publish. He worked tirelessly to ensure that sufficient material was available, often prevailing upon his friends, such as Adolf Meyer, Eleanor Clarke Slagle, Susan Tracy, and Herbert Hall, to write. He also wrote many articles himself. Out of desperation he developed one strategy that he described in a letter to a member of the editorial board for an upcoming conference: "By the way, will you arrange with Slagle about the papers which are read? The best plan is to snatch them out of the reader's hand" (Dunton, 1928a).

Dunton's challenge was particularly difficult because occupational therapy had not yet established itself as a research-based profession. As a physician, Dunton understood that it was necessary for the profession to conduct scientific research in order to demonstrate its effectiveness within the medical community, and he tried to convince occupational therapists of this necessity. He wrote, "It should be remembered that without a record of the data, the value of the work accomplished may be questioned since it is not available for the use of others unless put in proper written form" (Dunton, 1934, p. 328).

Dunton understood that research and publication were the best ways to promote and justify the profession. He also saw cultivation of a scientific approach as something that would invigorate occupational therapists themselves as well as the profession. He observed, "Unless one has the desire to develop one's work, to analyze it, to improve it, then it becomes irksome and we are little more than robots. It is this spirit that has advanced occupational therapy so far in the past two decades" (Dunton, 1928c, p. 347).

Part of the challenge for the profession was to articulate the occupation process in a way that would be scientifically persuasive. Dunton understood that it was difficult to convince those who held a scientific view that what appeared to be a seemingly simple process of engagement in occupation was actually quite complex and of considerable scientific merit. He said,

> Probably we enthusiasts for occupational therapy are to blame because we have not presented the subject to these doubters in a form in which they could understand it. . . . We have talked too simply of the virtues of occupational therapy and have praised it in one-syllabled [sic] words, whereas we should have used highly technical terms and shown by fractions, tangents, and co-sines the mental effect of making a basket. (Dunton, 1934, p. 325)

Part of the problem of articulating occupational therapy lay in the dearth of research instruments that could measure the full complexity of the individual and his or her successful engagement in occupation. Dunton wrote,

> [W]e are unable to present the results of research because the psychologists have not given us formulae for judging the emotional effect of pounding a copper disk into a nut dish or other occupations . . . Nor have the physiological chemists given us a test whereby if we lay a bit of paper on a patient's tongue we may judge that by its turning a pale pink he is enjoying his weaving to a mild degree, whereas his neighbor shows a crimson when tested because he is having a wonderful time putting a jig saw puzzle together. In other words we lack a quick and snappy means of measuring the emotions. (Dunton, 1934, pp. 325-326)

Thus, Dunton describes in his own inimitable fashion what we continue to struggle with today in terms of providing evidence-based outcomes research.

Dunton believed in both occupation and science. He was humanistic and holistic in his view of the ability of therapeutic occupation to heal both mind and body. He also valued science and understood that scientific research was required in order for the profession to prove its effectiveness to the medical community. Like his fellow founders, Dunton was a man of thought and action. Throughout his long career, he tirelessly promoted the profession through advocacy, publishing, and editing. He almost single-handedly helped to preserve the written legacy of the profession, and he inspired others to write and publish and cultivate an inquiring mind.

To summarize, the founders deeply believed in the benefits of therapeutic occupation and created a profession whose mission was to spread their vision throughout the country. They expressed a vision of occupational therapy that was holistic, humanistic, and scientific. Their goals were as follows:

- To promote occupational therapy as a way to help individuals reclaim dignity and self-respect; to heal the body, mind, and spirit; and to become productive members of society
- To develop a systematic approach to the use of occupation
- To encourage engagement in scientific research in order to demonstrate the effectiveness of occupational therapy and establish its legitimacy within the medical community.

Centennial Vision: The Profession's Contemporary View of Occupation and Science

In 2003, the AOTA Board of Directors initiated a strategic planning process that culminated in the *Centennial Vision*. The process involved close to 2,000 practitioners, educators, and researchers united in developing a "roadmap for the future of the profession" (AOTA, 2007, p. 613). The *Vision* unites all of us in developing and promoting a profession dedicated to meeting society's occupational needs. The profession is envisioned as "powerful, widely recognized, and science-driven . . . with a globally connected and diverse workforce (p. 613)." In other words, the *Centennial Vision* puts occupation at the heart of what we do, recognizes that scientific research is critical to our survival, and emphasizes our interconnectedness with occupational therapy practice throughout the world.

A major thread that connects the *Founding Vision* with the *Centennial Vision* is a profound belief in the healing nature of occupation. However, the *Centennial Vision* broadens the definition of occupation envisioned by the founders to include "preventing and overcoming obstacles to participation" in valued occupations (AOTA, 2007, p. 613), thus incorporating a social perspective into the view of engagement in occupations.

This incorporation of a social perspective within the *Centennial Vision* reflects the movement within society from a medical illness model to a prevention wellness model exemplified by the World Health Organization's (WHO's) introduction of their 2001 classification system. The *International Classification of Functioning, Disability and Health* promotes a view of health as something that is achieved through the individual working in collaboration with medical and social support systems to break down any environmental barriers in order to achieve a full, productive life (WHO, 2001). Within the occupational therapy profession, a blending of the medical and social perspectives is represented in the *Occupational Therapy Practice Framework, 2nd Edition* (AOTA, 2008), which was introduced in 2002 and revised in 2008 to provide a structure for articulating practice that centers on active participation of the client in a context that promotes engagement in chosen occupations.

The emphasis on science remains strong in both the *Founding* and *Centennial* visions. One difference is that the profession has gone from aspiration to accomplishment; that is, we no longer simply aspire to do research but are actively engaged in it. The profession's success in demonstrating effectiveness of therapeutic interventions has improved as more occupational therapists earn PhDs and conduct scientific inquiry. Yet Dunton's concern—ensuring that the research models and measurements reflect the complexities of engagement in occupation—still remains a challenge today. Although the importance of evidence-based practice is well understood, the need for more research and better instruments is still pressing (Holm, 2000; Coster, 2008).

Finally, the *Centennial Vision* takes the practice of occupational therapy beyond the United States, linking it to the global community. This represents a realization that to meet society's occupational needs, the profession of occupational therapy has to serve the world (Kronenberg, Algado, & Pollard, 2005). Each country's practice and research can—and must—inform and support one another's practice and research. In comparison, the *Founding Vision* does not explicitly reflect an international perspective. The founders' awareness of the importance of international events and community was surely there, however, because the United States was deeply involved in fighting World War I—an event that certainly created an understanding of the interconnectedness of countries and the impact that their actions can have on the rest of the world. With today's advanced technology and economic interdependency, productive and collaborative international relationships are of paramount importance.

Achieving the Centennial Vision by Embracing Our History

We can achieve our *Centennial Vision* through reclaiming our historical legacy. We can do this if we take the steps outlined below.

1. Retain the founders' vision of a humanistic–scientific practice and dedicate ourselves to bridging that divide between the two paradigms.

The founders believed in a vision of occupational therapy that was holistic and humanistic as well as scientific. But the world has changed since 1917. In 2009, we are living in a world where the scientific medical model has achieved dominance in much of U.S. health care. This creates a conflict of competing values between the holistic, socially oriented humanistic paradigm and the reductionistic, medical model, scientific paradigm (Kielhofner & Burke, 1977). The challenge that the profession faces is to be scientific in its interventions, documentation, and measurement of outcomes and still hold true to its original humanistic values. Thus it is imperative that today's occupational therapists bridge the humanistic and scientific paradigms.

In the current practice arena, this is not easy to do if the predominant perspective of the setting is the medical model. Even in school-based and community practices, the medical model is the basis of referral for therapy, and reimbursement agencies expect that practitioners will provide scientific evidence of effectiveness. Thus occupational therapists must blend the scientific and humanistic perspectives in order to achieve occupational therapy's vision: A vision where occupation is at the heart of our intervention, *not a diagnosis.*

Leaders within the profession have developed theoretical and research models and frameworks that place client-centered occupation at the core of intervention (Christiansen & Townsend, 2010; Kielhofner, 2008; Law, 1998). Therapists not familiar with these models should become so in order to be able to introduce occupation-centered approaches to evaluation and intervention in their settings. Students and new graduates who have been educated to view occupational therapy practice as occupation and client centered should carry that vision into their various practice arenas and be prepared to fight for this vision when it does not fit with the prevailing treatment approach of the agency.

Adolf Meyer (1922) wrote that there are no "royal roads" to being an occupational therapist (p. 7). By that he meant that no one was going to roll out a red carpet for those promoting this new profession. Occupational therapists would have to face many challenges to help ensure the profession's success. Like our founders, we must be pioneers and risk-takers to promote our *Vision.*

2. We can achieve our Centennial Vision *if we emulate the founders as role models of leadership.*

There has been considerable focus on history during the recent U.S. presidential transition and discussion of how the lessons from history could be applied to our troubled times. In particular, Franklin Delano Roosevelt and Abraham Lincoln have been held up as leaders President Barack Obama could emulate. Similar to what is happening on the political level, I am suggesting that we in the profession of occupational therapy look to our history and our founders for lessons in leadership.

In this lecture I have tried to provide the biographical essence of three of the founders and discuss the qualities that made them leaders. One quality that stands out in my mind is their personal and professional courage. For example, George Barton developed his own self-cure when the medical community offered him little in the way of treatment. Eleanor Clarke Slagle separated from her husband and established herself as financially self-sufficient and professionally successful at a time when this was relatively rare for a woman to do. William Rush Dunton married a woman outside his accepted social circles, even when it meant being ostracized by his family and having to professionally establish himself without their support.

In addition to courage, creating a profession takes optimism and innovative thinking, and it takes a leap of faith. The founders saw a need and a way to fill it. They were pioneers committed to a vision, and they committed themselves to the hard work that it takes to implement a vision. If it meant working long hours and sometimes doing mundane tasks to be an advocate for the profession, Slagle did it. If it meant snatching the conference papers out of the hands of presenters so the work of occupational therapy could be preserved in written publications, Dunton did it. If it meant overcoming the exhaustion that is part of having a chronic illness to make the dream of Consolation House a reality, George Barton did it.

The founders also had confidence and an unyielding belief in occupational therapy. As Susan Tracy (1921) reminds us, "The real success of the movement often depends upon the faith of the launchers. If occupational therapy be 'tried' with a feeling of possible failure, the odds will be against it. There is no success in doubt, there is no success in fear, there is no success in division of purpose. Convince yourself of the value of occupational therapy, and then establish its use" (p. 399).

The founders displayed confidence, courage, hard work, creativity, and a willingness to take risks. These characteristics are what we need to cultivate if we are going to lead our profession in implementing the *Centennial Vision*. As President Moyers Cleveland reminded us, "Without champions for our *Vision*, there will not be a *Vision*" (Moyers, 2007, p. 625).

Call to Action: Now It Is Our Turn to Lead

In conclusion, I would like to issue a call to action to all in this audience. Today I have described the contributions of three of the founders of occupational therapy: Eleanor Clarke Slagle, George Edward Barton, and William Rush Dunton. They were creative risk takers, visionary leaders, and tireless advocates for their patients and the profession. You could say that their presence was historical karma—they were the right people at the right time in the right place. Their act of founding the profession—creating a profession that had hitherto not existed—gave them the opportunity to put their many talents and skills to work. It enabled them to live up to their potential and exert an influential role on a fledgling profession.

I would argue that, almost a century later, we are at another pivotal point in our profession. We are at the beginning of the 21st century and we have a vital mission: implementing the *Centennial Vision,* a *Vision* that will help us to flourish in this new century. In the United States and around the world, increasing attention is being paid to the rights of all people to participate in society. Like the founders, we are confronted with inequities and disparities in society that affect people's health, quality of life, and participation. Like the founders, we have a powerful tool—the use of engagement in occupation—as both a means and end to health. What we have that the founders did not is a growing body of evidence to support the efficacy of what we do, and we have the power of numbers. Each of you, through your innovative, evidence-based practice and commitment to participation for all, can enact the social justice values of our founders while creating the powerful, science-driven profession that we envision today.

I would further argue that you are the right people at the right time in the right place. The United States has elected a new president who has pledged to provide health care for all. President Obama's health policy team is asking everyone for their views on what our health care system should become. Now is the perfect opportunity for occupational therapists to voice our vision.

This lecture should serve to remind you that, like our forefathers and foremothers, we all have the potential to be political activists, risk takers, and confident leaders. Indeed, are you so different from the founders? Are you not tireless promoters of occupational therapy like Slagle? Are you not innovators in your work as was Barton? And are you not all promoters of evidence-based practice like Dunton? If you are not, now is your opportunity to be.

Our founders remind us of what can be done with talent and commitment. And history can strengthen our resolve by helping us to understand that as occupational therapists of today we have a heritage of strong leaders, from the initial founders through succeeding generations of occupational therapists whose innovations in clinical practice, theory, measurement, and research reflect the values that the *Founding Vision* and the *Centennial Vision* share. Now it is our turn to take up the challenge as we enter a new century of occupational therapy.

References

Addams, J. (1911). *Twenty years at Hull House.* New York: MacMillan.

American Occupational Therapy Association. (1953). *House of Delegates minutes.* Houston, TX: Author.

American Occupational Therapy Association. (2007). AOTA's *Centennial Vision* and executive summary. *American Journal of Occupational Therapy, 61,* 613–614.

American Occupational Therapy Association. (2008). Occupational therapy practice framework: Domain and process (2nd ed.). *American Journal of Occupational Therapy, 62,* 625–683.

Barton, G. E. (1914a). Personal correspondence to Dunton on November 30, 1914 [Letter]. Bethesda, MD: Wilma West Library Archives.

Barton, G. E. (1914b). A view of invalid occupation. *Trained Nurse and Hospital Review, 52,* 327–330.

Barton, G. E. (1917a). Personal correspondence to William Rush Dunton on February 6, 1917 [Letter]. Bethesda, MD: Wilma West Library Archives.

Barton, G. E. (1917b). Personal correspondence to Frank Gilbreth on June 26, 1917 [Letter]. Bethesda, MD: Wilma West Library Archives.

Barton, G. E. (1917c). Inoculation of the bacillus of work. *The Modern Hospital, 8*(6), 399–403.

Barton, G. E. (1922). What occupational therapy may mean to nursing. *Trained Nurse and Hospital Review, 64,* 304–310.

Barton, G. E. (n.d.). *Movies and the microscope.* Bethesda, MD: Wilma West Library Archives.

Bockoven, J. S. (1971). Legacy of moral treatment: 1800s to 1910. *American Journal of Occupational Therapy, 25,* 223–225.

Boris, E. (1986). *Art and labor: Ruskin, Morris, and the craftsman ideal in America.* Philadelphia: Temple University.

Christiansen, C., & Townsend, E. (2010). *Introduction to occupation: The art and science of living* (2nd ed.). Upper Saddle River, NJ: Pearson Education.

Coster, W. (2008). Embracing ambiguity: Facing the challenge of measurement (Eleanor Clarke Slagle lecture). *American Journal of Occupational Therapy, 62,* 743–752.

Dunton, W. R. (1917). History of occupational therapy. *Modern Hospital, 8*(6), 380–382.

Dunton, W. R. (1919). *Reconstruction therapy.* Philadelphia: W. B. Saunders.

Dunton, W. R. (1928a). Personal correspondence to Harriet Robeson on June 8, 1928 [Letter]. Bethesda, MD: Wilma West Library Archives.

Dunton, W. R. (1928b). *Prescribing occupational therapy.* Baltimore, MD: Charles C. Thomas.

Dunton, W. R. (1928c). The three "r's" of occupational therapy. *Occupational Therapy and Rehabilitation, 7,* 345–348.

Dunton, W. R. (1934). The need for and value of research in occupational therapy. *Occupational Therapy and Rehabilitation, 13,* 325–328.

Dunton, W. R. (1943). How I got that way. *Occupational Therapy and Rehabilitation, 22,* 244–246.

Dunton, W. R. (1945). *Prescribing occupational therapy* (2nd ed.). Baltimore, MD: Charles C Thomas.

Dunton, W. R. (1946). *Bibliography of W. R. Dunton, Jr.* Bethesda, MD: Wilma West Library Archives.

Hofstadter, R. (1969). *The Age of Reform: From Bryan to FDR.* New York: Alfred Knopf.

Holm, M. (2000). Our mandate for the new millennium: Evidence-based practice (Eleanor Clarke Slagle lecture). *American Journal of Occupational Therapy, 54,* 575–585.

Kielhofner, G., & Burke, J. P. (1977). Occupational therapy after 60 years: An account of changing identity and knowledge. *American Journal of Occupational Therapy, 31,* 675–689.

Kielhofner, G. (2008). *Model of human occupation* (4th ed.). Philadelphia: Lippincott Williams & Wilkins.

Kronenberg, F., Algado, S., & Pollard, N. (2005). *Occupational therapy without borders.* Philadelphia: Elsevier/Churchill Livingstone.

Law, M. (Ed.). (1998). *Client-centered occupational therapy.* Thorofare, NJ: Slack.

Licht, S. (1967). The founding and founders of the American Occupational Therapy Association. *American Journal of Occupational Therapy, 21,* 269–277.

McDaniel, M. (1971). Forerunners of the *American Journal of Occupational Therapy. American Journal of Occupational Therapy, 225,* 41–46.

Meyer, A. (1922). The philosophy of occupation therapy. *Archives of Occupational Therapy, 1*(1) 1–10.

Moyers, P. A. (2007). A legacy of leadership: Achieving our *Centennial Vision* (Presidential Address). *American Journal of Occupational Therapy, 61,* 622–628.

National Society for the Promotion of Occupational Therapy. (1917). *Certificate of incorporation.* Clifton Springs, NY: Author.

Newton, I. (1917) Consolation House. *Reprint from Trained Nurse and Hospital Review.* Bethesda, MD: Wilma West Library Archives.

Newton, I. (1923). Personal correspondence to William Rush Dunton on July 12, 1923 [Letter]. Bethesda, MD: Wilma West Library Archives.

Quiroga, V. (1995). *Occupational therapy: The first 30 years.* Bethesda, MD: American Occupational Therapy Association.

Robeson, H. A. (1937). *Eleanor Clarke Slagle: Testimonial to Mrs. Eleanor Clarke Slagle, annual banquet, 21st annual meeting of the American Occupational Therapy Association.* Bethesda, MD: Wilma West Library Archives.

Slagle, E. C. (1918). Personal correspondence to William Rush Dunton on November 23, 1918. Bethesda, MD: Wilma West Library Archives.

Slagle, E. C. (1922). Training aides for mental patients. *Archives of Occupational Therapy, 1*(1), 11-18.

Slagle, E. C. (1924). A year's development of occupational therapy in New York state hospitals. *Modern Hospital, 22*(1), 98–104.

Slagle, E. C. (n.d). *Experience of Eleanor Clarke Slagle.* Bethesda, MD: Wilma West Library Archives.

Tracy, S. E. (1921). Getting started in occupational therapy. *The Trained Nurse and Hospital Review, 67*(3), 397–399.

World Health Organization. (2001). *Introduction to the ICIDH–2: The international classification of functioning, disability and health.* Geneva, Switzerland: Author.

59

2010 Eleanor Clarke Slagle Lecture

What's Going On Here?
Deconstructing the Interactive Encounter

Janice Posatery Burke, PhD, OTR/L, FAOTA

The Slagle gave me an unprecedented opportunity to read and savor many of the great thoughts of my predecessors. They are the leaders of our field and an impressive group of thinkers. I am grateful for the opportunity I spent this past year with their work.

I have often sought to understand our leaders and their drive for success and passion for our field. They climbed a century-high mountain and obtained a towering history of creativity and clinical excellence. The excitement and enthusiasm of those wise individuals who created our profession gave us our foundation, and I am sure their passion represents the push that got many of us into occupational therapy and here this evening.

As they expressed their hopes for occupational therapy, they set a very high standard for success and challenged us to do our best for the profession. They often sought what seemed to be unachievable heights and made us all dream. They are very hard acts to follow.

I viewed the honor of working on the Slagle as an intellectual expedition. This past year, I set out on a journey to reach the base camp established by those who came before. I wanted to expand my thinking and seek a path that would enhance my sphere of knowledge about our profession. The expedition quickly became a catalyst for me to seek in-depth information about ideas that I would not normally have had the time to explore as I worked on my desire to find a new way of "knowing" the experience we call *occupational therapy*.

Like the peak of a distant mountain, the long hike often seemed too great a distance to travel, too high a step to reach, or simply too far in the future to be real. My colleagues, friends, and family helped make the journey enjoyable. They softened the bumps on the road; straightened the many hairpin turns that threatened the expedition; and comforted me with good conversation, insightful thoughts, and exceptional counsel. My work tonight reflects the culmination and synthesis of all who have helped me. Because of them, I know that what I present tonight is not just mine. I am very thankful for their support.

Scope of the Talk

As I worked on this presentation, I realized the importance of the journey. This past year, I had the chance to forge a new path to information that resides outside the commonplace of occupational therapy. I worked to clear a trail that will more fully explain the interactional space and interpersonal relations that occupational therapists create during the occupational therapy encounter.

I can trace my deep interest in the idea of interaction to my early experiences as a young clinician. During those first years, I worked in different settings: a rehabilitation center, an outpatient clinic, and schools with both adults

Originally published 2010 in the *American Journal of Occupational Therapy, 64,* 855–868.

and children. In those treatment environments, I wondered why it was that some therapy sessions felt so very different from others. I began to consider how a therapist (me) could deliberately shape the treatment session to promote its "success." Simply put, I wanted to know more about why certain human interactions in therapy worked. I wanted to discover the secret of success as a clinician and define ways to replicate that success time and time again.

I had further glimpses of this goal when I was working on my master's degree at the University of Southern California (USC), creating a model of occupational behavior that included personal causation, role, and socialization and later while defining the Model of Human Occupation. I moved further along when I taught in a clinical faculty position at USC.

Those brief moments of clarity helped inform my work as I established my first private practice, Therapy West in Los Angeles, and later, when I moved to Thomas Jefferson University in Philadelphia. My objectives matured as I worked full time with university students as well as in my small private practice with young children and their families and while I finished my dissertation and doctorate. The ephemeral emergence of interaction I observed and reflected on became more lasting and permanent as I became a seasoned therapist and educator and shaped the first independent research I did as I observed clinicians in action.

To this day, every time I observe or step inside the clinical interaction, I ask myself, What more can I see here? What are the nonverbal interactions that help or hinder this therapy? How are others reacting to my words and actions? The answers collected over the years inform my talk today.

Passion for Interaction

I have a passion for interaction. The conduct of an interaction is endlessly fascinating. It's a riddle. It is always different, yet it includes the same parts and structure each time (beginning, middle, end). It can be new but also has an old familiarity. It can happen over a long period of time (as in an hour-long team meeting) or very quickly (during a short elevator ride or a walk down a corridor). It has a physical quality (where you are in relation to another), but it does not require touch. It may have visual features (eye contact, a common point of focus) and even sound, but neither is essential. It happens in starched, formal settings as well as in relaxed, informal ones.

My initial observation of and later fascination with people-to-people interaction came about because of my family (always a good target for blame). My mother knew many people in the small city where we lived. She had four siblings and many cousins, aunts, and uncles who shared a common last name. My father had also grown up there and had a business in this same city. We lived near the city center, where everyone went out on foot to complete their customary round of daily activities. These routines included scheduled visits to families in their homes and incidental, brief exchanges on the street or in stores. I became privy to the numerous encounters that my mother would have with relatives, friends, and acquaintances when she took me around. At her side, I absorbed the rhythm of the conversations, the movement of the speakers as they moved in close to share particular intimacies or opened up the circle of conversation to be joined by others or to acknowledge a familiar passerby. I absorbed the different forms of greetings that were used, depending on familiarity, and the variances in small talk that established common ground. I cannot count how many times I would hear a conversation that started something like, "You look very familiar. Do I know you from. . . ?" and inserted was the name of a neighborhood, a school, or a community location. These interactions were the fabric and social engagement of my childhood.

My fascination with the conduct of interaction gets me into trouble with my friends and family, who sometimes bargain with me before going out to eat or to shop. They often say something like, "Are we just going to go there directly, or are you going to stop and talk to everyone on the way?" I guess they are trying to decide if they should wear comfortable shoes for standing around or, in the case of my son when he was younger, bring something to play with in anticipation of the inevitable pauses in the action. Often they extract a pledge when we enter a store that goes something like, "Promise me you will not be too friendly once we get inside." They may add a "tag" that includes a particular reason like, "We don't want to be there all day." Or they may just worry aloud, saying, "If you are too friendly, they'll know we're not from around here."

I supremely appreciate observations of person-toperson interaction and have a profound interest in how people relate with each other throughout their daily activities. It is an easy jump from this interest to a more focused look at the interactions that occur within a helping profession like occupational therapy, where we address how people navigate the occupations of their life and look for openings into those lives.

Resources in the Literature

This lecture series honors [Eleanor Clarke] Slagle and her desire for others to reflect on and learn from therapy experiences. During my journey to "base camp Slagle," I filled the time between great ideas and landscapes with reading. I'd like to give you a quick glimpse of the literature I used to focus my attention on the study of interaction.

I started by getting to know the depth of literature within occupational therapy related to therapeutic use of self. I needed to understand how we use verbal and nonverbal behaviors to facilitate communication and found that although these specific skills received acknowledgment, they were not recognized for the depth of contribution they could make.

I read much of the literature generated by Adam Kendon (1990) and his associates in *Conducting Interaction*, including his work addressing what he called responses to Erving Goffman's early focus highlighting the need for in-depth study of "the countless patterns and natural sequences of behavior occurring whenever persons come into one another's immediate presence" (p. ix). Kendon (1990) and others describe the details of what occurs between people, including "where they look, when they speak or remain silent, how they move, how they manage their faces, orient to one another, and position themselves spatially" (p. 3). Examining these materials allowed me to develop an appreciation for the contribution that nonverbal behaviors make to the overall communication and interaction event. I came to understand and appreciate the experience when two people spot one another across a room and then, while walking toward each other, look away and prepare so that by the time they are close they can remake eye contact and greet one another. These behaviors are important when I consider how the therapy event is organized, how we prepare and conduct our own behavior with our patients and our colleagues in the work setting, . . . manage miscommunication and awkward moments, and repair our own missteps.

During the many hours between the switchbacks and mountain roads moving toward base camp, I considered the use of gesture—and, in particular, Neapolitan priest Andrea deJorio's work *Gesture in Naples and Gesture in Classical Antiquity* (2000)—and came to recognize the use of one's face and facial expressions as well as one's hands in conveying an additional dimension to the communication process and how that may play out in interactions between therapists, patients, families, and staff. In addition, the conceptual and research literature addressing sequence organization in interaction, pragmatics in human communication, and quantification of kinetic behavior were helpful in constructing my understanding of movement and its role in interaction during a therapy session.

The body of work I explored also included patterns of organization in public behavior that led me to ask questions about my day-to-day movement in all of the different spaces I inhabit as I go about work and play in and around Philadelphia. How do I escape bumping into others as I negotiate the public transportation maze, crossing paths with throngs of people, jockeying for seats on the train, or finding where to stand on the subway platform? I became keenly aware of the idea of collision avoidance as well as the miraculous phenomena of interpersonal coordination and monitoring that allow us to remain in a continuous state of movement while reading one another's anticipated actions. This information is enormously useful in the negotiations of therapy spaces in the rehabilitation setting, clinic corridors, and the evercrowded hospital cafeteria.

I studied the classic, foundational work in verbal and nonverbal communication, including Edward T. Hall (1959, 1969, 1976) and Erving Goffman (1963, 1967, 1971). This influenced my understanding of the complex relations and "sequential temporal patterns of speech and gaze in dialogue" (Kendon, 1981) that we therapists manage each time we meet a new patient, attend a staffmeeting, and participate in a case conference.

We use visual information and often do not thinkmuch about it, but I spent time developing an introductory understanding of the elegance of graphic display that Edward Tufte (1990, 2001) explained as he defined ways to visually represent and explain data. This provided some ideas for considering nontraditional data displays.

And, of course, I read the deep body of work in verbal and nonverbal communication in the medical visit and other patient clinician encounters, including work on patient satisfaction and the impact on outcomes, and gained momentum in my conviction that we must attend to verbal and nonverbal behaviors if we are to create data that prove the efficacy of occupational therapy.

In looking for explanations of visual and nonverbal storytelling, I struck gold in the literature of film and the consideration of the process of directing, including *mise-en-scène* or, as I learned, the things put in the frame to tell the story. In addition, I found that screenwriters use a prescribed plot paradigm to build visual stories with words and that an actor's ability to reenact and replicate emotion and action on demand defines that profession (Bordwell & Thompson, 2010;Monaco, 2009; Osgood & Hinshaw, 2009). I realized that therapists use similar methods when they "direct," "write," and participate in the therapeutic process.

Therapy as Interaction

The physical, emotional, and social context of any interaction is framed by its purpose. The interaction of a therapy session is unique. It is not the same as the interaction that we have in our casual exchanges with others. Occupational therapists conduct the business of therapy within a distinct frame of improving performance. Occupational therapists use physical space, therapeutic objects, their bodies, their voices, and their reasoning skills to create an interaction that produces therapeutic outcomes.

Creating Meaningful Encounters

Our lives as therapists are filled with certain kinds of encounters. For our patients and their families, the evaluation, consultation, and every particular therapy session has the potential to hold lasting meaning that is profoundly important. In therapy, we set the stage and begin the next chapter of the patients' story, giving them the skills to write what comes next and propelling them forward toward whom they will be. That ability to create those stories is the foundation upon which our profession is built. This is the way that we as professionals make a lasting impact on an individual's health and well-being. Finding the way to that success requires defining the story of the therapy encounter. For lasting meaning to occur and change in the course of a life, a therapist must be committed to behaviors that create interactional relationships.

With this said, occupational therapy is interpersonal interaction. Although the space that each of us creates as an occupational therapist reflects unique experiences and training, our profession's unifying commitment to the interactional relationship drives all of us to focus on the same priorities: providing our patients and their families with glimpses of what is possible, what can be done, and what it will take to get there.

You all bring clinical stories with you today. This convention hall is filled with those stories. They are exceptional and are the experiences that belong to all of us as occupational therapists. Those stories define our profession and speak to our commonality. This is why no matter where you are, what you are doing, or what your background might be, if you meet other occupational therapists, you immediately know who they are and what they do. You know what their life is like. We relate to one another immediately. This is the culture of our profession, and that shared culture creates the common experience of being an occupational therapist.

To define the interactional story, I plan to deconstruct a group of therapeutic encounters based on interactional time and events to answer questions that include, What happens in therapy sessions? What is the shared experience of being an occupational therapist? What defines our commonality? What do we typically do or say? And how do we set the space and move ourselves in and out of the action?

From the beginning of this project, I speculated that there is a particular set of verbal and nonverbal behaviors that must be in place to create a successful therapeutic encounter. I figured that if I could hear and see therapeutic stories being created, I would find common threads. These threads would lead me to a wealth of information about the verbal and nonverbal strategies that therapists use every day. To this end, I analyzed the data from a study with occupational therapists and their patients. Although the study was completed in a pediatric setting, I believe that you will see that many of the interaction findings apply to a wide variety of occupational therapy settings and patient populations. I have myself experienced their application to a broad range of patient encounters, including when I observe occupational therapists in adult acute care and rehabilitation, hear stories about working with adults who have developmental delays, review cases from our Alzheimer's disease projects, or watch students in patient simulations with individuals who have psychosocial difficulties.

The Study

In the study I am discussing this evening, qualitative data were collected from four occupational therapists who worked in an early intervention, community-based setting. Each of them was observed and recorded in at least two clinical encounters. They performed evaluations using the Peabody Developmental Motor Scales (Folio & Fewell, 2000) and collected additional physical and historical information about other aspects of the child's performance contributing to the overall evaluation. Some of the observations were initial evaluations in which the therapists, young children, and families were new to one another and occupational therapy or new to one another but familiar with occupational therapy. Some of the sessions were reevaluations with therapists, children, and families sharing the camaraderie of interacting with one another over a period of time, creating change and celebrating improvements that reflected the investment of time and effort, worry, and concern. Evaluations were conducted in homes and in the early intervention agency. Some sessions were with just the therapist, child, and parent or grandparent. Others included members from the team or multiple family members.

Interactional Model

I recognized some basic interactive and contextual information about the therapists in the study that could be organized and analyzed by developing a simple model (Figure 59.1).

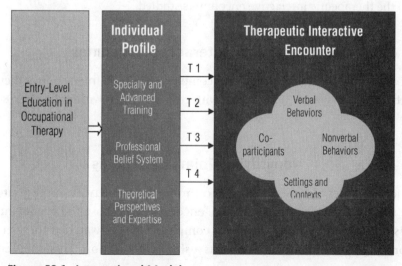

Figure 59.1. Interactional Model.

Entry Education in Occupational Therapy

The first commonality is professional education. The four therapists who participated in this project had completed their entry-level education in occupational therapy from four different educational programs via two different entry routes (bachelor's and master's).

Individual Profile

Following their graduation, the therapists developed their own unique *individual profile*. Like a fingerprint, a therapist's profile is distinctive. It represents a composite of experiences that are formed as each therapists works, reads, is mentored, observes other therapists, and matures into a professional.

Specialty and Advanced Training

The therapists accumulated specialty and advanced training based on their individual interests. They attended different conferences and workshops, continuing education programs, and in-depth specialty training and studied for advanced degrees (two specialized in early childhood).

Professional Belief Systems

Their unique profiles revealed individual *professional belief systems*. These belief systems guide, focus, and determine what a therapist will do in a given situation and are demonstrated when occupational therapists focus on different concerns during an evaluation or treatment. Professional belief systems are evident in the selection or exclusion of topics addressed during the course of the session and the amount of time devoted to each particular topic.

For example, some therapists were more concerned with a line of inquiry about movement; others focused more attention on development, play, family time, daily routines, or mealtime. Similarly, some therapists excluded some topics (disease management, sleeping or digestive issues, dietary problems), as they did not see them falling into their domain of concern.

Theoretical Perspectives and Expertise

Finally, individual profiles included preferred theoretical perspectives and expertise. These are based on an individual's education, training, and preferences as well as their professional expertise developed in different work settings.

These four therapists (depicted in this model as T1, T2, T3, and T4) brought their professional education and individual profiles to the therapeutic interactive encounters studied.

Therapeutic Interactive Encounter

Once engaged in the encounter, the therapists directed complex action and interaction as they (1) used verbal behaviors, (2) used nonverbal behaviors, and (3) interacted with co-participants within the given settings and contexts of the evaluation.

Identifying Points of Analysis

Given this interactional model, the next issue to confront was to identify appropriate places to launch an analysis within the real-time therapeutic interactive encounters. Because the events unfold in a more or less orderly fashion, it is possible to find like points for comparisons. As I watched these encounters, I identified points of analysis or a point in time where there was a shift in the action. This point could be identified as a *therapeutic juncture*.

Examples of therapeutic junctures include a point when the therapist does something that demands action. The therapist can ask a question, move to the next task, provide a new movement challenge, and so on. The juncture provides a point at which the interaction between the therapist and patient or family member can be observed, analyzed, and deconstructed. These junctures cause shifts in action that allow the encounter to exponentially expand as the encounter progresses. What better place to deconstruct an encounter than at these single junctures?

Argentine writer Jorge Luis Borges (1962), winner of the first international publisher's award, wrote a short story about this moment titled *The Garden of Forking Paths*. In the story, the antagonist discovers that the particular path taken after entering an ancient garden of forking paths defines the future. These paths sometimes reconverge and cross over a vast labyrinth in time and space. That labyrinth leads to many possible ends in differing times at different places. The short story, written over 60 years ago, is considered the birth of modern hypertext stories and remains current today as the foundation of many popular television programs, from *Lost* to *Flash Forward*.

It is interesting to think of "differing paths" as they apply to the therapeutic encounter. In this project, I chose a set of single junctures where a path begins and where I could observe, analyze, and deconstruct verbal and nonverbal behaviors. By taking these single junctures, I could discover how therapists create therapeutic interaction, manage information, and direct action during therapy sessions. This knowledge provided insight into the scope of behaviors used and decisions made throughout therapeutic encounters.

What I Learned

The data obtained exemplified the variety and complexity of roles that therapists must take as they produce and direct a successful encounter. In all, the occupational therapists were clearly highly skilled professionals who knew what they needed to do and how to make it happen. I came to see therapists in a role very much akin to that of the director of a film. Like film directors, therapists "work closely with the cast and production crew and involve others in the process of storytelling while taking responsibility and making important decisions" (Osgood & Hinshaw, 2009, p. 6). Film directors fully conceive the project well in advance of the first day of production. Therapists need to conceive and know the possibilities that a therapeutic interaction can produce and, like directors, need to "possess experience in the production process and have a strong sense of story development" (Osgood & Hinshaw, 2009, p. 6).

Reciprocal, Reflexive, and Complementary

The complex nexus of therapeutic interaction occurs in real time during face-to-face encounters. It engages coparticipants in reciprocal, reflexive, and complementary interactions. Therapeutic interaction is reciprocal and reflexive in that it occurs based on relationships of alternating, sequencing experiences across successive moments of real time. I say or do something, and in turn you respond by saying or doing something. Every action begins with a motivation and creates a reaction.

Verbal and nonverbal partners also react in retrospective actions. They take into account what the other is doing or has done and prospectively anticipate what will happen next.

Finally, interaction is complementary. It depends on relationships between simultaneous actions of interactional partners. It unfolds in a natural order like any turntaking event that requires you to take account of another and make a reasonable response. Sometimes responses can be unreasonable. Sometimes they can be fraught with missed signals and divergent streams of talk.

Social and Cultural Conventions

There are social and cultural constructs or conventions that contribute to the organization and construction of the interaction, and they vary based on the persons who are present. Likewise, therapeutic interactions are also socially and culturally constructed. You know this from your own experiences. Patients who are recent immigrants, older or younger, male or female, working class or professional, will respond quite differently to the experience of being seen in a hospital, clinic, rehabilitation center, private office, or their own home. Each brings with himself or herself his or her own understanding of what is to be done and how one must conduct oneself. The interaction occurs as a partnership between therapist and the intended coparticipant. That it occurs simultaneously and with a synchrony is testimony to each participant's ability to read and respond to one another and the therapist's ability to direct this complex set of action and words.

Fine-Grained Detail of Occupational Therapy

The fine-grained detail of occupational therapy is revealed using a technique called *microanalysis*. Looking at videotaped material at normal speed will be a realtime analysis. I wanted to slow down real time to understand the very subtle things that happen between therapists and patients in the therapeutic space at those key junctures.

Microanalysis is a technique that allows each action or movement or sound to be slowed down. Using microanalysis, each interaction is viewed in 1/30-second increments. It is a frame-by-frame analysis of action and sound. To understand this level of specificity, recognize that each 1-hour therapy session yields 108,000 frames. Each of these frames can be individually analyzed. Although I looked at all 108,000 frames for each session, I only chose a set of frames to analyze. Of those selected, I mapped each action and sound change frame by frame so that single actions could be microanalyzed. These sets of frames represent similarities and differences across the recorded therapeutic junctures. I'll turn now to the analysis.

Analysis of Verbal Behaviors

Therapist use both *direct* and *indirect* verbal requests throughout a session. In the data set, both types of requests were used to elicit information. In addition, it appears that verbal remarks are used to draw a participant's attention to specific actions. Therapists might want to indicate that they are noting a change and improvement in the child, and so they say, "I see we like to color, don't we?" They may wish the parent to say or do something to encourage the child, indicating that desire by saying, "Make a picture for Mommy" or "String a necklace for Mommy." They also use what I call "out-loud" talk to signal the importance of what they are observing: "I see you are using both hands" or "You've got very nice sitting balance." This type of interaction is a way of drawing attention to the purpose of occupational therapy.

Participants in a State of Readiness

Therapists expect the parents, or who I am calling the participants, to give their complete attention to the action at hand, to be "in the moment," and to be ready to provide information as requested. As a result, participants are in a state of attentive readiness. They must be alert, recognize requests, and supply the requisite information or action.

Participants hold up their end. They return the therapist's eye gaze, turn to face them, answer questions, and show interest and willingness to share talk and action for a common purpose. They engage in a joint construction of the interaction. As you will see, this latter behavior requires some experience on the part of the participant.

Direct and Indirect Requests

Direct requests and responses can be mapped out in a diagrammatic structure (Figure 59.2). The point of comparison is between new or *novice participants* (those for whom this is the first occupational therapy experience) and *experienced participants* (those who have been actively engaged with their child in occupational therapy for at least 6 months). The experience of therapy for each of these two groups of participants was clearly different.

The novice participants are fresh to the therapy interaction. They are essentially "feeling their way," figuring out the terrain in this new land. They are in the beginning stages of forming an understanding of what an occupational

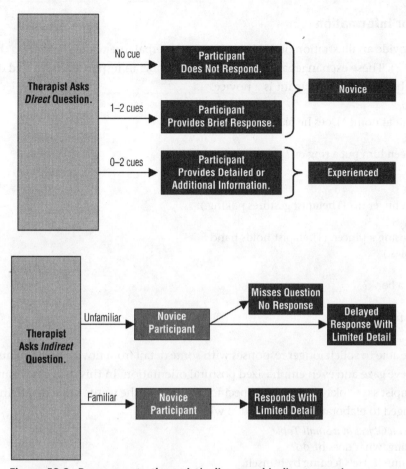

Figure 59.2. Responses to therapist's direct and indirect questions and cues.

therapist does during an occupational therapy session, the primary areas of focus, the materials used, and the types of questions asked.

When asked direct questions, novice participants tend to give short answers (1–5 words) that have little to no detail, or they may simply head nod or shake their head in response.

An interaction is initiated by the therapist in the form of making a direct verbal request. If the direct request does not have a cue (e.g., eye gaze, use of the participant's name), then it is not recognized as a request by novice participants. As a result, they do not respond.

In the second iteration, the therapist makes a verbal request to a novice participant, but this time he or she tags it with a cue, an eye gaze directed at the novice participant, or the use of the participant's name. In this instance, the new participant recognizes the request and will respond, albeit briefly.

The novice participants are compared with those who have been receiving occupational therapy or have previously received occupational therapy or a similar intervention (e.g., physical therapy, speech therapy). I refer to these individuals as *experienced participants*. Because of their ongoing interaction with the occupational therapist, they understand the kind of information that is needed, and they can apply what they have learned from previous sessions.

Experienced participants respond regardless of whether there is a cue to them. They are able to recognize the request based on their past experiences. They know therapists are constantly collecting information, and they are willing to participate in this endeavor by providing detailed or additional information. Let's look at some examples of this type of interaction.

Direct Requests for Information

These first samples provide an illustration of the back-and-forth verbal interaction between a therapist and a novice participant (Figure 59.3). These exchanges are characteristically short in response length and detail (they may consist only of a gesture) because the participant is a novice.

Child With Ring Stack
T: Does he have this at home? Does he play with it?
M: No, he doesn't.
T: Have you ever seen him put a ring on?
M: No.

Child Poking Finger
T: Will he poke his finger in? (Therapist gestures poking.)
M: (Mother nods yes.)
T: He seems to be using a pincer. (Therapist holds hand
up and demonstrates.)
M: Yes.
T: Does he look at a book?
M: Yeah.
T: Does he look at pictures?
M: Yeah.

Therapists may be able to solicit longer responses with some detail from novice participants when they are close by and using intense eye gaze and even emphasized postural orientation. In this next case example, the answers are longer when the therapist says "okay" or asks for specifics, indicating she wants more detail. In this way, the novice participant is encouraged to elaborate when provided with prompts.

Child Playing With an Object at a Small Table
T: In terms of feeding, what does he do?
M: Real good by himself. He's feeding by himself.
T: Using?
M: He tries to use the spoon.
T: Okay.
M: (no response)
T: Okay.
M: (no response)
T: Drinking?
M: He would rather drink from a cup.
T: His choice is the cup?
M: Yeah, his choice is the cup.

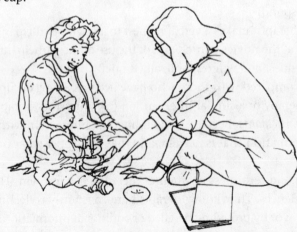

Figure 59.3. Line drawing of therapist, child, and mother.

In this sequence, we heard the continuous turn taking that is emblematic of interaction. The sequence is a beginning: It provides a first step toward interaction that is reciprocal, reflexive, and complementary with the simultaneous action of the interactional partners. The parent sustained a longer chain of information as the therapist supported each response and provided prompts to encourage even more answers.

A Word About the Line Drawings

As a point of reference, line drawings were sketched directly from the images grabbed off of the videotape recordings. The drawings are used in the same manner and for the same reason that Kendon (2004) described in his work *Gesture: Visible Action as Utterance*. He suggested that "drawings are generally preferable to camera-ready picture frames pulled directly from the videotape. Not only can one show, in the drawing, just the details that are pertinent for the exposition, but the problem of showing photographs of people who might wish to remain anonymous is completely avoided" (Kendon, 2004, p. vii). In this way, line drawings allow me to focus your attention on the action that I was attending to in the analysis without distracting you with the extraneous details that were present in the backdrop of the real-life setting. In addition, the line drawings avoid the temptation of critiquing the setting, the materials, the dress, or other similar off-the-point (irrelevant, unconnected, or secondary) details of the action.

Direct Requests With Experienced Participants

The direct-request situation is substantially different when the participant is experienced—someone who has "been here before." Experienced participants are acquainted with the rhythm and the timing of the session, they are aware of the information that is of primary concern to the occupational therapist, they recognize the openings and opportunities for providing that information, and they understand the kinds of responses that are expected of them and how they contribute to the session and to the therapeutic enterprise.

Direct requests with experienced participants are answered with more precise, detailed information. For example, the therapist asks, "What kind of stroller is he in?" The mother answers, "It has back support." The mother has shaped the information with specific detail based on what she understands the therapist cares about and needs to know. Let's look at some more examples.

On the first visit to the community-based agency, a little boy is accompanied by his mother and his cousin, who is visiting for the summer. Within the first minutes of the session it becomes apparent that the mother is an experienced participant. She knows her way around therapy—what occupational therapists are interested in— and she gives information within that framework. In response to the therapist's questions, she explains her son's behavior with thick, richly detailed descriptions. In contrast to the novice examples, her experience is evident by the length and detail as well as her use of key words.

This mother demonstrates that she knows what occupational therapy is about and what therapists focus on, as evidenced by the kinds of things she chooses to talk about (e.g., he likes being in the water and the connection to aquatherapy), the language used to describe her son's behavior (e.g., reaching and using his trunk), and other details (e.g., "I see him trying a lot harder"). Similarly, she shows her understanding of the relationship between therapy and function, commenting that she saw him sitting up by himself more after therapy. In other portions of the interview, she gives thick, detailed descriptions of how her son eats, his use of his hand, and his resistance to others feeding him. With her knowledge of occupational therapy, she is able to observe her own child in other settings and at home and bring those details of her child's strengths and needs to the therapist.

Indirect Responses

Indirect questions are more subtle in nature and more difficult to identify as a question to be answered. When an indirect question is asked about an unfamiliar topic, the novice participant may miss the question and make no response or give a delayed response with limited detail. When the topic is about something that is familiar to the participant, the novice participant responds with limited detail.

The next example represents the kinds of responses that occur with a novice participant. This is the first home visit for this family. The child being seen is one of a set of twins. The little girls are 6 months old and were born prematurely. The first 6 months of parenthood with these twins was spent addressing a host of issues secondary to their prematurity.

At the start of the visit, the mother recounts the history with doctors to date. From her stories, it is clear that she is used to being in the role of listener. She shares her experiences with experts who, in her words, "don't say much." Based on this mother's comments and her experiences in settings such as the neonatal intensive care unit, we can safely speculate that her role has primarily consisted of being a silent observer: watching the expert.

In contrast, this occupational therapy session in her home is a dramatic change and, in all likelihood, is the first time she will be asked to participate in a collaborative way. The start of this session is rocky as she gets her "sea legs" and begins to understand what occupational therapy is all about.

The mother is seated on the sofa, holding one of her twin babies. The therapist has positioned herself on the floor with the other twin, directly in front of the mother. The therapist observes the baby while making notes. She continues to look at the baby while asking what I have categorized as an *indirect question*, and it is to the baby. It goes like this:

T: "You don't mind being on your back. Are you looking at the light?"

The mother makes no response. The therapist knows the baby won't answer, but she expects that the mother will. This is not the case, because this mother is new to occupational therapy and does not quite understand how it works. The therapist, an ever-vigilant director of the interaction, recognizes that things have not gone as expected and makes the necessary corrections and modifications.

Ten seconds later, the therapist asks her next question and provides an added cue—her eye gaze to the mother. She says, "Does she always lay to one side?" In this instance, the mother sees the eye contact, recognizes the question is for her, and responds, "Yeah."

For the most part, novice participants miss requests that are indirect and unfamiliar to them. This is evident in this case. In some instances, novice participants are able to catch a therapist's request, even if it is indirect. They understand the request because it is familiar—something any mother, father, or grandparent is routinely asked, because they are a mother, father, or grandparent.

In this next example, mother and therapist are in the same position. The therapist is visually involved with the child without any eye contact or other cues for the mother, such as use of her name. But in this interaction, the talk is familiar. The therapist says, "Who is older? You or your sister?" The mother answers for her child, "I am." The response is noted in the change of her eye gaze to the therapist. She responds to this indirect request because it is about a familiar topic and one she has heard and will hear time and time again as the mother of twins.

How Do Novice Participants Gain Experience?

Therapists teach participants about the verbal and nonverbal behaviors that are common in the world of occupational therapy. They do this by working with the participant and establishing a mutual focus on the specific skills and concerns that warrant their attention. They shape questions as direct requests, such as "I wanted to ask you. . . ." and place themselves at eye level, looking right at the participant. They also talk out loud in an effort to make the participant aware of what they are doing, what they are observing, the reasons why they are doing it, and the expectations they have for the future. Therapists say things like, "I'm looking at what he does with one hand and with two" or "He's starting to transfer. He's letting go." Within a short period of time, novice participants learn from their therapists and gain experience. In this way, a novice participant becomes an experienced one.

Experienced Participants Respond to Therapists Indirect Questions

In contrast to novices, experienced participants recognize opportunities to provide information regardless of whether the question is familiar or unfamiliar. They see this as a way to give details about what is going on beyond the four walls of therapy.

This next example takes place during a reevaluation in a community-based setting with the grandmother, therapist, and child. The action occurs within the first moments of the evaluation session. The therapist is waiting for me to indicate that the recording crew is ready to begin. While they wait, the therapist and child play around. The grandmother watches and recognizes an opportunity for the child to show what she is beginning to do at home.

With impeccable timing, this grandmother, an experienced participant, recognizes what is needed and not only provides information during the play time, such as, "Say your alphabet; she's starting to say her alphabet," but also modifies it once the therapist begins rattling off the alphabet too quickly, adding, "No, slower, just one at a time." The grandmother knows that this is the kind of information this therapist focuses on and could be of use to this therapist right now. These verbalizations contribute to the interaction's success.

Experienced participants take active roles in the session. They bring up their own familiarity and understanding of the behaviors that are the focus of the occupational therapy and they initiate related topics.

Ignoring Topics

Therapists may (1) ignore topics or (2) interrupt participants over the course of an interactive encounter. These two behaviors are a direct consequence of the therapist's responsibility for keeping the focus of the interaction on topic and accomplishing what he or she set out to do within a given time period. These behaviors also seem to reflect therapists' willingness to address only topics within their defined theoretical perspectives and expertise. This type of response to off-topic material is extensively written about in the medical encounter literature. For example, when therapists define behavior problems as residing outside of their professional belief system and expertise, then in all likelihood, topics related to behavior will be ignored. This may not be an example of "best practice," especially if we believe that our role is to understand the whole person, but it does occur.

Similarly, novice participants who are not yet familiar with what is included and excluded in occupational therapy may introduce off-subject topics. These topics may be ignored or given minimal attention by the occupational therapist. For example, when a therapist was asked to speculate about a young child with cerebral palsy and his potential to be a wheelchair athlete, the therapist acknowledged the comment and redirected to a new therapy-oriented topic.

Experienced participants are also inclined to make their own requests, remind therapists of topics that need to be addressed in the session, or bring up areas of concern that may be off topic. Therapists work to redirect the focus, even if it takes some time. Here is an example from a reevaluation. The therapist has just shifted the action from playing with a toy that facilitated the child's reach, grasp, and release. The child kept putting the toy in his mouth, and now the therapist is turning her attention to his oral–motor skills. The therapist's and mother's words overlap, and the therapist repeatedly attempts to redirect the topic.

T: *How ya doing with eating?*   *Oh, well then*
M: He had a whole jar of baby food before we came here, um…

T: *you should be full. Look at you. Yor goin need a bath.*
M.   But we're giving him juices — And instead of so much milk

T: *Is that helping? With the congestion?*
M: all the time, we're giving him more juices and - and water —   *Umm,I*

T: *You looking at*
M: don't know if it's helping. I'm trying to see if it'll help his bowels to go more easily…

T: *yourself? Who's that kid?*

M: Because most of the time that Pediasure is not doing it, for me. I mean,

T: *He's getting tired.*   *Not as bad?*

M: it's like… He's straight now, not as bad as he used to. but the

T: *Let's try one more thing.*

M: pediasure milk, boy, I'm telling you, that stuff is expensive. I've got to walk three

T: *One of things I want to do.*

M: blocks away to get it.

The mother brings up a topic that is of concern to her, (her child's eating and digestion) that she knows has been of interest to this child's team, in response to the therapist who has asked about eating. The therapist is not concerned with the dietary and digestive aspects of the issue (she indicated in a follow-up interview that she believed the issue was best discussed with the team's nurse), so she works to move to a topic within her domain of concern.

Forming and Reforming Interactional Space

In the eight evaluation sessions, therapists all engaged in forming and reforming interactional space. Therapists seemed to be quite deliberate in placing themselves and the participants in ways that facilitated interaction and communication. They did this for two key reasons: (1) to elicit the child's best performance and (2) to provide signals of their intentions to others. Each therapist seemed to have "customary ways," or unique styles, to set up and use the four walls of the interactional space. They created these spatial arrangements to be sensitive to nonverbal information and have access to head movements, eye gaze, body movements, and gestures.

In an example of forming and reforming an interactional space, the therapist introduces a ring stack toy; moves away a small table; adjusts the child's feet, setting them apart; turns the ring stack upright; and holds it for him to facilitate his performance all within a dense complex of seconds.

To shed some light on this dense complexity of words and actions, I want to tell you about an analytic technique used for displaying the local geography of action. In searching for a way to visualize the complex and multiple foci of action in a video sample, I considered a number of options. One in particular was the idea of developing an adaptation of musical scoring, mapping the different movements and dialog of the participants like the orchestration for multiple instruments. This was very foreign to me because I only know how to read music at a very elementary skill level. At any rate, I later discovered a technique that I called *conversation convention*, short for *conversation and movement convention*, and my research team quickly adopted that language. When we sat down and began to deconstruct the dialog and action, it became apparent to me that we needed a more elaborate way to map the multiple parts presented by the therapist, parent participant, and child, each of whom contributed words and actions. We quickly changed over to the established vernacular of displaying local geography of action.

Based on Christian Heath's (1986) work *Body Movement and Speech in Medical Interaction*, we were able to decode the precise words and actions of all participants during an encounter and the location of the various elements and their interrelation at points in the data. Heath's "rough and ready" method proved useful in mapping focus on the action and provided "an analytic device for developing a sense and picture of its detail" (pp. 18–19). The convention used here is my own iteration of his technique. Figure 59.4 illustrates the total voice and action that occurs in 11 seconds. You see the name of the speaker and the dialogue in large, bolded print. You also see a notation for the time and a small v or caret, which is the convention used to indicate the origin point for the action. Each line above the dialogue is labeled for the person contributing the action. Coincidentally, this type of notation is extremely similar to that used in the professional editing of video and sound.

In this illustration, we can get a real sense of the complexity of action that the therapist is directing. Specifically, the therapist is talking, and the child, mother, and therapist are all moving and participating in the action. When these segments are scrolled in real time, you can get a sense of the ongoing stream of interaction that occurs throughout an encounter.

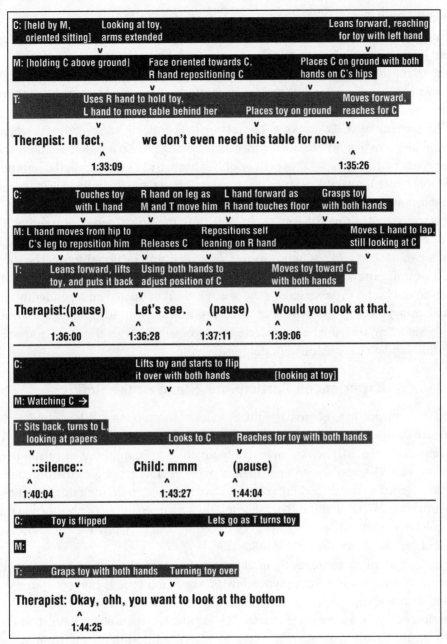

Figure 59.4. Total voice and action.
Note. C = child; M = mother; T = therapist; R = right; L = left; ^ or v = origin point for action.

Therapists seem to have exemplary interaction skills. They move themselves, others, and objects within short periods of time into positions that make sense for the task at hand. They use verbal comments to announce their intentions and underscore what they see.

In this next example, the therapist carefully plans the timing of the re-formation of the interactional space. She takes into account a number of variables and waits until the time is right for success. She re-forms the interactional space based on a number of key factors, namely (1) what she knows about children in this developmental stage and how to get them to do something you want them to do; (2) what she knows about this child in particular, since he has just developed a strong interest in using a marker; (3) what she knows from her repertoire of experience about the kinds of positions and surfaces she needs to accurately assess his skill level; and, finally, (4) what she believes will work in a situation like this.

The session begins with the child sitting on a chair at a table. He quickly tires of the confinement, and the therapist is able to set up a new center of action on the mat. Now they have come to the line-drawing challenge of the Peabody assessment (Folio & Fewell, 2000), and the therapist finds herself stranded on a mat.

When she presents the line challenge, the child is sitting. The child responds by lying on his side and beginning to draw. Once the therapist has recognized the problem (the child will not be able to do his best in this position), she allows him to "give it a go" while she formulates an alternative plan of how she will get him into a seated position for drawing based on his own initiative (i.e., making the tabletop look enticing, moving those very desirable markers to the table, and having him move as his own idea rather than placing him in a seated position) and then executes it with a remarkable precision. The therapist proves to be quite effective in using herself, the setting, and the props.

Therapists are able to use interactional space, even when it is extremely limited and they are, in a sense, constrained by the environment. This example is from the evaluation session in a very small row home in Philadelphia. The mother is seated on the sofa between two people from the early intervention center. The therapist is on the floor, supporting the child in a standing position. A fourth member of the early intervention team is beside the therapist, as are two of the child's siblings. In this very small interactional space, the therapist was able to reform it and make postural shifts that allowed her to signal others that she was giving her full attention to the child. Later, when she completes the assessment, she sets the child up to play independently with a toy; puts her assessment materials away; picks up her papers; and makes postural shifts, turning herself toward the mother on the sofa and clearly signaling that she had completed her assessment with the child and was ready to ask the mother some questions and give her some important information.

Experienced Participants Stand at the Ready

Novice participants are more likely to observe the therapist and offer support for their child during an interaction. In contrast, experienced participants appear more comfortable being involved and responding. They "stand at the ready," poised to respond if needed, and become actively involved to support the successful performance of their child. They are the backup. Therapists often offer them a position close by or give them signals to move into the action when they are needed to roll up a child's sleeves, coax the child to do something, and to remove "troublesome" objects from the child's line of vision. They develop their own repertoire of positions so they can move in or out of the action quickly, unnoticed, without words or direction, and they provide "frontline" information about an emerging skill that they know the therapist is following.

Experienced participants are able to insert themselves into the frame of action and extract themselves as needed. This is strikingly evident when we look at the synchrony of words and actions that occur in a very short period of time across a session with a young child, experienced participant, his mother, and a cousin.

Remarkable action occurs in a segment that lasts 22 seconds. The therapist has finished asking all of her initial questions, and she is beginning to move into the "handson," child-oriented portion of the assessment. She has shifted her postural orientation from the mother to the child and re-formed her interactional space and her eye gaze to the child, clearly sending the signal that this is where her focus of attention is for the time being.

The mother, an experienced participant, is seated to the left toward the back of the child. A cousin is in the foreground. The therapist reaches to her left to bring in a colorful toy, which is a set of plastic links fastened together as a chain to capture the child's attention. She places it in front of the child. The mother, an experienced participant, recognizes what is going on: The therapist wants to attend to and assess the child's sitting balance, and so she verbally moves into the action to shift her child's attention away from the what the therapist is doing (challenging his balance—something she knows her child does not like), saying, "Wow, look at all of those beautiful colors." Her son hears her and responds to her words by looking in her direction.

Then, without any prompt, she reaches into the play space to draw her son's attention to the toy, unlinks it, sets it down in front of him, and ends up handing it to him. Once the child has the toy, he brings it to his mouth while his cousin catches hold of the other end in a playful gesture. The therapist is able to continue her physical assessment of the child without protest from him.

Sometimes the parent is a catalyst for the therapist to shift her own focus, letting the mother have a hand at the action. With experience, participants are able to place themselves in the action and fully participate without verbal or physical prompts or even eye contact with the therapist.

Conclusion

In this talk, I have shared my passion for interaction and showed how it directly connects to the very core of our profession. I have established a model of interaction and defined the components that shape the therapeutic actions and space created by occupational therapists.

In doing so I have summarized what I have learned as I journeyed to the base camp that Eleanor Clarke Slagle founded so long ago. I guess that if this was one of my Slagle dreams, we'd all be dressed in climbing gear, ready to scale and conquer the mountain that still looms before us.

Tonight, I know that the journey I took beyond base camp defines a new route to the mountain peak and points a way for others to see interaction as the cornerstone of our profession. Interaction can be a powerful way to understand the efficacy of occupational therapy and share the reasons why our therapeutic approach works so well. This new understanding can change the conversation about the exceptional contributions our profession makes to health and wellness.

I hope this fresh viewpoint will situate others to look deeply at the basic interaction that defines our profession. This pioneering direction can stimulate innovative areas of research—areas that build on the strength of our founders' foresight and redefine a shared vision for our future.

Acknowledgments

My thanks go out to my colleagues and friends at Jefferson, AOTA, and beyond who believe in me and gave me wonderful support along the way; my assistant Kerri O'Rourke, who is fast, smart, and just plain fun; my sweet son and my amazing daughter-in-law, who always made time and space to ask about my progress on the Slagle; and my husband, Neil, who knows when to step in and out of the frame, isn't afraid of heavy lifting, and has a remarkable gift for argumentation and organizational detail.

References

Bordwell, D., & Thompson, K. (2010). *Film art* (9th ed.). New York: McGraw Hill.

Borges, J. (1962). The garden of forking paths. In J. Borges, *Ficcones* (pp. 89–101). New York: Grove Press.

deJorio, A. (2000). *Gesture in Naples and gesture in classical antiquity*. Bloomington: Indiana University Press.

Folio, M. K., & Fewell, R. R. (2000). *Peabody Developmental Motor Scales* (2nd ed.). Austin, TX: Pro-Ed.

Goffman, E. (1963). *Behavior in public places: Notes on the social organization of gatherings*. New York: Free Press.

Goffman, E. (1967). *Interaction ritual: Essays on face-to-face behavior*. Garden City, NY: Anchor Books.

Goffman, E. (1971). *Relations in public: Microstudies of the public order*. New York: Harper & Row.

Hall, E. T. (1959). *The silent language*. New York: Anchor Books/Doubleday.

Hall, E. T. (1969). *The hidden dimension*. Garden City, NY: Anchor Books.

Hall, E. T. (1976). *Beyond culture*. Garden City, NY: Anchor Press/Doubleday.

Heath, C. (1986). *Body movement and speech in medical interaction*. Cambridge, UK: Cambridge University Press.

Kendon, A. (Ed.). (1981). *Nonverbal communication, interaction, and gesture*. New York: Mouton.

Kendon, A. (1990). *Conducting interaction: Patterns of behavior in focused encounters*. Cambridge, UK: Cambridge University Press.

Kendon, A. (2004). *Gesture: Visible action as utterance*. Cambridge, UK: Cambridge University Press.

Monaco, J. (2009). *How to read a film: Movies, media, and beyond* (4th ed.). New York: Oxford University Press.

Osgood, R. J., & Hinshaw, J. (2009). *Visual storytelling, videography, and postproduction in the digital age*. Boston: Wadsworth/Cengage Learning.

Tufte, E. R. (1990). *Envisioning information*. Cheshire, UK: Graphic Press.

Tufte, E. R. (2001). *The visual display of quantitative information* (2nd ed.). Cheshire, UK: Graphic Press.

The 2000s: Discussion Questions and Learning Activities

The Lectures

Holm, M. B. (2000). Our mandate for the new millennium: Evidence-based practice (2000 Eleanor Clarke Slagle Lecture). *American Journal of Occupational Therapy, 54,* 575–585.

Dunn, W. (2001). The sensations of everyday life: Empirical, theoretical, and pragmatic considerations (2001 Eleanor Clarke Slagle Lecture). *American Journal of Occupational Therapy, 55,* 608–620.

Royeen, C. B. (2003). Chaotic occupational therapy: Collective wisdom for a complex profession (2003 Eleanor Clarke Slagle Lecture). *American Journal of Occupational Therapy, 57,* 609–624.

Zemke, R. (2004). Time, space, and the kaleidoscopes of occupation (2004 Eleanor Clarke Slagle Lecture). *American Journal of Occupational Therapy, 58,* 608–620.

Peloquin, S. M. (2005). Embracing our ethos, reclaiming our heart (2005 Eleanor Clarke Slagle Lecture). *American Journal of Occupational Therapy, 59,* 611–625.

Hasselkus, B. R. (2006). The world of everyday occupation: Real people, real lives (2006 Eleanor Clarke Slagle Lecture). *American Journal of Occupational Therapy, 60,* 627–640.

Hinojosa, J. (2007). Becoming innovators in an era of hyperchange (2007 Eleanor Clarke Slagle Lecture). *American Journal of Occupational Therapy, 61,* 629–637.

Coster, W. (2008). Embracing ambiguity: Facing the challenge of measurement (2008 Eleanor Clarke Slagle Lecture). *American Journal of Occupational Therapy, 62,* 743–752

Schwartz, K. B. (2009). Reclaiming our heritage: Connecting the founding vision to the *Centennial Vision* (2009 Eleanor Clarke Slagle Lecture). *American Journal of Occupational Therapy, 63,* 684–693.

Burke, J. P. (2010). What's going on here? Deconstructing the interactive encounter (Eleanor Clarke Slagle Lecture). *American Journal of Occupational Therapy, 64,* 855–868.

Learning Activities

1. Investigate the occupational profile of most Americans in the early 2000s. Some useful bibliographical references to explore appear in Appendix B.
   - What is the average family size?
   - What is the average salary? What are some typical jobs?
   - What do homes cost?
   - What are the clothing styles of the decade?
   - What is significant about the popular culture of the decade (e.g., music, film, books)?
2. If you have access to a complete collection of the *American Journal of Occupational Therapy,* scan the table of contents for each issue. What are some common topics? Can you identify any patterns in these topics? How do these relate to the messages of each Eleanor Clarke Slagle Lecture?

3. Try to summarize each Eleanor Clarke Slagle Lecture in a sentence that captures the main theme. Complete the sentence "This lecture was about. . . ."

4. Consider each lecture. Are there common threads among them that you identify? Are there any common themes that emerge when you consider these lectures together?

5. Review the biography of each lecturer of this decade (see Appendix A). Read some of the other work by the lecturer to gain an insight to the reasons why each one received this honor.

6. Consider what was happening in the history of the occupational therapy profession at the time of each Eleanor Clarke Slagle Lecture. Appendix C provides some useful bibliographical references for the history of the profession in the United States, and Appendix D has references for the global history of the profession.

7. Review what each president of the American Occupational Therapy Association presented as his or her vision for the profession at the time of each Eleanor Clarke Slagle Lecture. (A list of these presidents appears in Appendix E.) How do the lectures relate to these visions? The presidents have addressed the profession through several forums, including columns in the *American Journal of Occupational Therapy*, such as "President's Address," "Nationally Speaking," and "The Issue Is."

8. Review each lecture in light of the *Centennial Vision*. Which themes of the *Vision* stand out the most? What additional insights into the *Vision* do the lecturers offer?

Discussion Questions

1. What was Margo Holm's definition of *evidence-based practice (EBP)*, and why did she consider it important to the occupational therapy profession?

2. Summarize the 5 levels of occupational therapy evidence proposed by Holm. How could each type of evidence influence occupational therapy in a practice setting?

3. Holm suggested that occupational therapy practitioners ask themselves 5 questions to determine if they are engaging in EBP. Briefly summarize these questions. How do you answer these questions in your own practice?

4. What is the 5-level measuring stick Holm talked about? What are the implications for the profession?

5. Holm stated that we "have an obligation to improve our research competencies, to develop the habit of using those competencies in everyday practice, and to advance the evidence base of occupational therapy in the new millennium." Describe some ways in which you think occupational therapy education programs can assist with this and some ways in which practitioners can contribute to this. What are you doing to develop competencies that will further the evidence base of our professional practice?

6. How has Holm's clarification of the 5 levels of EBP inspired you to think about your own research?

7. What are the 5 steps Holm suggests to becoming an evidence-based practitioner? What other steps can you suggest to become an evidence-based practitioner?

8. Holm stated that "Our level of confidence in our clinical decisions should be based, in part, on the strength of the evidence we use." She then noted 2 problems regarding the use of evidence to make practice decisions. Identify these major problems, and discuss how they impede your ability to use evidence. Then propose a strategy to encourage current practitioners to actively participate in this process.

9. How can the typical occupational therapist who works in a home health setting become an evidence-based practitioner? How can practitioners who work in an acute psychiatric setting or in a school system became an evidence-based practitioner? How could this take place in other settings and your own practice setting?

10. Explain the 4 sensory processing patterns that Winnie Dunn claimed humans demonstrate (sensory seeking, sensory avoiding, sensory sensitivity, and low registration), and give examples of how you have personally experienced each pattern.

11. Dunn likened the 4 sensory processing patterns to personality traits that are fairly stable throughout a person's lifetime. Which of the patterns best describes your own experience?

12. Dunn suggested that a unique contribution of occupational therapy can be characterized as the role of "translator." Explain what she meant by that in the context of her lecture, and give examples of situations in which that has been your role in practice.

13. Considering the 4 sensory processing patterns Dunn described, how would you approach introducing stress management training to clients who each demonstrate one of these patterns?

14. Explain why it would be useful to help an occupational therapy client know his or her own sensory processing patterns as described by Dunn.

15. Charlotte Brasic Royeen argued that it is most appropriate to consider occupation as a "chaotic process" rather than a product and that the latter conceptualization confuses the public. Explain what she meant by occupation as a chaotic process and why the consideration of occupation as a product may create unnecessary confusion.

16. Royeen proposed chaos theory as an integrator of occupational science and occupational therapy. She suggested chaos theory permits a nonlinear understanding and a kaleidoscopic approach to analysis that supports holistic practice. Explain how a linear approach may limit practice and scientific development and how a "chaotic" approach, as proposed by Royeen, may engender a more holistic process.

17. Explain Royeen's argument that chaos theory brings to light the limitations of EBP.

18. Royeen explained 5 key assumptions that underlie chaotic systems. Summarize each assumption, and provide a corresponding illustration from your practice.

19. Royeen offered her "Charlotte's Web of Chaos" as a representation of how chaos theory constructs are evident in interacting layers of occupation. Explain how each construct in this web contributes to the understanding of occupation as a process.

20. Royeen recommended that professionals and clients alike engage in "meta-emotion of occupation." She suggested a reader answer 3 questions in relation to her lecture: "What do I feel about this telling?" "What did I feel when it started?" "How do I feel that it has ended?" After you answer these questions for yourself, explain how this consideration of meta-emotion may contribute to the therapeutic encounter.

21. Ruth Zemke began her lecture with a definition of a cosmic level of articulation and study of time and space. Summarize this definition, and discuss your own personal awareness of this level of time and space. What have you learned about it? When and how do you become aware of it?

22. When discussing the evolutionary level of articulation and study of time and space, Zemke used the metaphor of 3 "sisters": Brainstem Betty, Limbic Louise, and Neocortical Nell. Explain the function of each, and then describe how they work together as a family, particularly in relation to the experience and use of time and space.

23. Explain what Zemke meant by the concept of *occupational temporality* and why she believed it should be the focus of occupational therapy and occupational science.

24. Explain the distinction Zemke made between the notions of *space* and *place*. What are the characteristics of each? In what ways can this understanding influence the way in which we structure occupation with our clients?

25. Zemke argued that, although time and space are important, of greater interest to occupational therapy and occupational science are the interweaving of *temporality* and place. How did she articulate this argument? In what ways do you personally experience temporality and place in your own life? Give examples of the experience of clients with whom you have worked and for whom temporality and place were of particular importance.

26. Zemke recommended that occupational therapists and occupational therapy assistants consider treatment approaches that help clients organize space and time in occupations across complex spatiotemporal horizons. Give some examples of such possible treatment approaches, and explain the contexts in which they would be most appropriate.

27. Zemke called attention to the apparently "empty" time between occupations and "empty" space between objects, likening them to the stage of *liminality* often associated with rituals. Explain what she meant by this, and describe how this understanding might be used in the clinical encounter.

28. Explain why Suzanne Peloquin affirms that it is useful to articulate a profession's *ethos* (the interlacing of sentiment, value, and thought that captures the profession's character, conveys its genius, and manifests its spirit).

29. Peloquin noted that key documents of the American Occupational Therapy Association, such as the official definition of occupational therapy, the philosophical statement, the *Code of Ethics,* and so on, hold within them intimations of the profession's character, genius, and spirit. Is there a particular document you frequently refer to as a source of inspiration in occupational therapy? What about that document inspires you?

30. Peloquin listed 5 beliefs that emerged from the discussion of the founders for the Society for the Promotion of Occupational Therapy early in the 20th century: that (a) time, place, and circumstance open paths to occupation; (b) occupation fosters dignity, competence, and health; (c) occupational therapy is a personal engagement; (d) caring and helping are vital to the work; and (e) effective practice is artistry and science. Give examples of how you have observed each of these values in action or where you have seen failure of these values to be upheld.

31. How would you explain occupational therapy's "ethos of engagement" to various audiences, such as clients, caregivers, physicians, or third-party payers?

32. What models of thinking in today's society threaten occupational therapy's aims according to Peloquin? How do these models thwart the profession's ethos?

33. Peloquin proposes 5 reflections that together promise the reclamation of occupational therapy's heart. How might you integrate these reflections in your own practice of occupational therapy?

34. Betty Risteen Hasselkus dedicated her lecture to articulating a deep understanding of the importance and meaning of everyday occupation in the lives of clients and the general public. What importance did she ascribe to such understanding? What can be gained by this understanding, and what is the risk of the lack of such understanding?

35. Explain what Hasselkus means by "everyday occupation." What are its dimensions, and how does it manifest in peoples' lives?

36. Hasselkus claims that everyday occupation goes unnoticed, it is anonymous, and words are powerless to describe it. What does she believe is the consequence of these features in our professional understanding of the term *occupation?*

37. Jim Hinojosa described the present time as being one of *hyperchange,* or a time characterized by increasing uncertainty, rapid pace of change, growing ambiguity, and increased complexity in the workplace. Does that description fit your life? What examples of hyperchange do you experience in your personal and professional life?

38. Hinojosa suggests that in times of hyperchange occupational therapy practitioners must divest from a "wait-and-see" attitude and be adept at planning ahead and thinking fast. What examples of missed opportunities for occupational therapy are you aware of that resulted from slow action on the professional's part? What examples of successful planning ahead or thinking fast have you experienced?

39. According to Hinojosa, what dangers might the profession face by adopting too narrow a professional focus or definition of its domain of practice? Inversely, what benefits are there to permitting the coexistence of varied perspectives and practice paradigms?

40. Hinojosa calls occupational therapy practitioners to be "innovators *of* change" in order to control their own future. What examples of innovative change are called for in occupational therapy and practice? Where do you see the greatest opportunities for occupational therapy lie in the future? How could you take advantage of such opportunities and not let them pass us by?

41. Wendy Coster posits that there often is a discrepancy between what we can tell or show and what the experience really is, or between the measure of a person's abilities and ideas and reality. Illustrate this assertion with an example of your own experience.

42. Coster argues that the assumptions and modes of thinking about people that accompany the measurements and methods from disciplines such as psychology, medicine, and education are not always compatible with the val-

ues and practice of occupational therapy. What danger may be inherent in the over-reliance on such measurement tools? What benefits? Do you think such reality can best be represented?

43. Coster states that occupational therapy's concern for the whole person is being challenged daily by the pressure to use standardized measures to tell a client's "full story." In what ways have you faced such pressure? What methods do you think are better suited to represent the reality of a client's occupational functioning?

44. Coster named several sources of bias in measurement. In what ways can the social features of the assessment context exert influence over the data obtained from measurement?

45. How might the actual instruments used to obtain assessment measurements influence the way a therapist views the client? Consider both negative and positive influences.

46. Kathleen Barker Schwartz noted that there were similarities between the social contexts of the United States and the World at the beginning of the 20th century when occupational therapy was founded and today. What similarities do you see?

47. Schwartz identified Eleanor Clarke Slagle's definition of the primary role of occupational therapy as "help[ing] patients to readjust themselves, both socially and industrially, through organized occupations." In what ways do you think this definition remains the same today, and in which does it not?

48. Schwartz described George Edward Barton's "Consolation House." What features of this house are present in your practice environment, and which are not? What difference do you imagine the missing pieces would make?

49. Schwartz admonished the profession to strive to bridge the divide between the paradigms of humanistic and scientific practice. In what ways are you aware of such divide? What strategies can you implement to bridge this divide?

50. Schwartz also admonished the profession to emulate the founders as role models of leadership. What other role models of leadership can you identify in the profession? What characteristics do they share with the founders, and which characteristics would you like to emulate?

51. Janice Posatery Burke noted that the interaction of an occupational therapy session is influenced by the physical, emotional, and social context and framed by its purpose. Give examples from your own practice that illustrate this interplay. Describe changes in interaction affected by changes in each of the contextual elements or in the purpose of the interaction.

52. Burke stated that complex nexus of therapeutic interaction engages coparticipants in reciprocal, reflexive, and complementary interactions. Explain what she meant by each of these adjectives, and provide examples of instances when signals related to these interactions are missed.

53. Provide examples from your own practice in which direct and indirect interactions were used in order to reach a therapeutic outcome.

54. What did Burke mean with the phrase *forming and reforming interactional space* in relation to the therapeutic process.

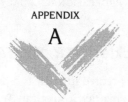

Short Biographies of the Eleanor Clarke Slagle Lecturers, 1955–2010

Compiled and written by
Yolanda Griffiths, OTD, OTR/L, FAOTA

Editor's Note

The following biographical sketches and bibliographies give an overview of the lifelong contributions made by each of the Eleanor Clarke Slagle lecturers. Certainly, a few paragraphs and a list of publications cannot do justice to these leaders' lives, spirit, energy, and commitment. Their gift to the profession is much more extensive and includes work on committees, mentoring to individuals and groups, leadership on special projects—the list is un-ending. Because of limitations of space, we have included in these bibliographies only retrievable publications. The degrees listed reflect the lecturers' current degrees, as opposed to his or her degrees at the time of the Lecture.

Most of the information that follows was graciously provided by the lecturers themselves. In circumstances in which the lecturer could not be contacted, every effort was made to summarize available published information through careful library database searches. Some of the biographies have not changed from the previous edition. We acknowledge the assistance of Ivelisse Lazzarini, OTD, OTR/L in compiling those biographies for the 2nd edition. We express appreciation to all the lecturers for sharing their time and lives with us so graciously and candidly.

Naida Ackley, OTR, FAOTA—1962

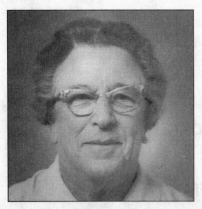

Naida Ackley retired in 1972 as director of the occupational therapy department at Trenton Psychiatric Hospital, in Trenton, New Jersey. She graduated from Sargent College (Boston University) and the Philadelphia School of Occupational Therapy (University of Pennsylvania), where she received an advanced standing certificate.

Ackley was named an AOTA Fellow in 1973 and also holds an honorary AOTA life membership and a life membership in the New Jersey Occupational Therapy Association. She was active in both state and national professional associations and held offices and committee assignments in both.

Bibliography

Anderson, M., Levine, C., Ackley, N., Cole, N., Gallagher, E., & Marr, A. (1947). OT clinic and case studies. *American Journal of Occupational Therapy, 1,* 125–127.

Flint, D. L., Anderson, M., Booth, M. D., & Ackley, N. (1947). Delegates division: Michigan; Kansas; Northern California; New Jersey. *American Journal of Occupational Therapy, 2,* 116–123.

Howard, A., Ackley, N., Pyun, E., & Black, G. A. (1949). Delegates division: Illinois; New Jersey; Hawaii; Oregon. *American Journal of Occupational Therapy, 3,* 217–220.

Collins, E., Ackley, N., & Davis, J. (1950). Meeting of the House of Delegates: American Occupational Therapy Association: Book Cadillac Hotel, Detroit, Michigan: August 21, 22, 25, 1949. *American Journal of Occupational Therapy, 4,* 128–132.

Ackley, N. (1953). People you should know: Elizabeth P. Ridgeway: A biographical sketch. *American Journal of Occupational Therapy, 7,* 138.

Ackley, N. (1957). Guide for committees: Report on the special committee on standard operating procedures for committees. *American Journal of Occupational Therapy, 11,* 116–118.

Willard, H., & Ackley, N. (1960). Nationally Speaking: From the President; From the Committee on Student Affiliation. *American Journal of Occupational Therapy, 14,* 150–156.

Ackley, N. (1961). Nationally Speaking: Accreditation of occupational therapy departments. *American Journal of Occupational Therapy, 15,* 68–72.

Ackley, N. (1962). The challenge of the sixties (1962 Eleanor Clarke Slagle Lecture). *American Journal of Occupational Therapy, 16,* 279–281.

Ackley, N. (1970). *Basic services and equipment for rehabilitation centres, occupational therapy department in a mental health hospital.* New York: United Nations Monographs.

Claudia K. Allen, MA, OTR/L, FAOTA—1987

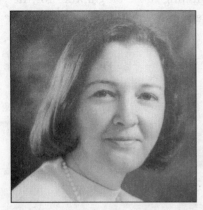

Claudia Kay Allen received her bachelor's degree from San Jose State University and her master's degree from New York University. She began her career working with children, most of whom had cerebral palsy. After two years she shifted into psychiatry and began to notice the similarities between disabled children and adults. Her commitment to people with lifelong cognitive disabilities was formed during the years of working as chief occupational therapist in at Los Angeles County/University of Southern California (USC). While serving in various positions on the faculty in the Department of Occupational Therapy at USC, she held faculty appointments in psychiatry and the behavioral sciences at the School of Medicine. Many schools throughout the United States, Canada, the United Kingdom, and Australia have invited her to be a guest lecturer and a reader for work done for graduate degrees. She never left practice because observations of people with disabilities are the database for describing the Allen Cognitive Levels.

The Allen Conceptual Model was first published in 1985, which opened additional opportunities and responsibilities. In the insurance industry, Allen worked as a consultant for Blue Cross of California and contributed to Medicare guidelines. In collaboration with S&S Worldwide, she initiated the use of craft projects as the content for standardized tests. Poor validity is a critical deficiency in functional tests for people with cognitive disabilities. The persons refuse to do the tests or say that they can do everything when they cannot. The realization that many people enjoy doing crafts and they will try their best or not get defensive about mistakes convinced Allen that crafts have a great potential as a testing vehicle. Research studies that support the validity of these tests are emerging.

Interest in the practical value of the Allen Cognitive Levels resulted in scores of continuing education workshops by Allen spanning two decades, and these workshops are being taught all over the world. A deliberate focus on universal applications has resulted in an enormous range of implementations in many cultures, within all age groups, spanning diverse diagnostic categories (psychiatry, neurology, pediatrics, gerontology, burns, tendon transplants), and applied by people in a variety of health-related professions. Throughout Allen's career, she has been known for asking a critical question, "So what?" The answer should be an improvement regarding the quality of life of people with cognitive disabilities. Allen was in the initial group of Fellows honored by the American Occupational Therapy Association (AOTA).

Linking Key Messages of the 1987 Eleanor Clarke Slagle Lecture to the AOTA *Centennial Vision:* When comparing my Slagle lecture to AOTA's *Centennial Vision*, I was struck by the number of problems and dreams that remain the same. While thinking about what can be done now, the possibility of writing definitions stimulated my curiosity. Are we at a point in our history that allows us to write definitions that are simple enough to be adopted by the general public? Adoption requires consistent and repetitive use of definitions.

Occupational therapists help disabled people do activities.

Who and what are included in this one sentence. The dictionary definition of *occupation* as employment exists. Therefore, to overcome this problem, the word *activity* must be stated. The admission criteria for therapy involve a disability. When discharged, many of patients have worrisome disabilities that require assistance. What is special about us is our ability to design activities that may enable positive performance. For most health-related professions, residual disabilities are the end of care; for us, they are the beginning of the challenge.

Occupational therapists help people with disabilities do selected activities. Individuals are evaluated to measure abilities and disabilities. Therapists consult with individuals and caregivers to select meaningful activities. Selected activities are analyzed to identify the psychical and mental abilities required to do each step in the activity. Steps in the activity can remain the same, be modified, or omitted as needed. When activity demands are matched to the person's remaining abilities, successful performance, a sense of satisfaction, and a constructive use of time and energy is experienced. Therapists teach long-term caregivers how to set up activity demands that match abilities. Mismatches produce negative experiences such as frustration, boredom, idleness, quitting, accidents, or injuries. Troublesome behaviors affect all social support systems, including families, health care systems, sanitation services, disease control, police departments, courts, and jail. Prolonged mismatches result in isolation, neglect, homelessness, and institutional warehousing. Costs are reduced or eliminated by providing alternatives, which are innocuous, pleasant, and successful.

"Why" and "how" are added to the initial definition. Without assistance, people with disabilities engage in troublesome behavior, with consequences that are scattered throughout the community. We design activities to generate alternative behaviors. In addition, the cost of facilitating constructive performance is cheaper than correcting the damage done by disturbing behaviors. What I have learned in the past 20 years is that designing for successful performance requires two scales: one for the disabled person and another for the activity. To match, ability must be equivalent to the activity demands. By matching, occupational therapists make doing possible.

—*Claudia Allen*

Bibliography

Allen, C. K., Earhart, C. A., & Blue, T. (1995). *Understanding cognitive performance modes.* Ormond Beach, FL: Allen Conferences.

Allen, C. K. (1993). Creating a need-satisfying, safe environment: Management and maintenance approaches. In C. B. Royeen (Ed.), *AOTA Self-Study Series: Cognitive rehabilitation.* Rockville, MD: American Occupational Therapy Association.

Allen, C. K., & Robertson, S. C. (1993). *A study guide for occupational therapy treatment goals for the physically and cognitively disabled.* Rockville, MD: American Occupational Therapy Association.

Allen, C. K. (1992). Cognitive disabilities. In N. Katz (Ed.), *Cognitive rehabilitation: models for intervention in occupational therapy.* Boston: Andover Medical.

Allen, C. K., Earhart, C. A., & Blue, T. (1992). *Occupational therapy treatment goals for physically and cognitively disabled.* Rockville, MD: American Occupational Therapy Association.

Allen, C. K. (1991). Cognitive disabilities and reimbursement for rehabilitation and psychiatry. *Journal of Insurance Medicine, 23*(4), 245–247.

Allen, C. K., & Foto, M. (1991). Reporting occupational therapy outcomes with the *ICIDH* codes. *Physical Disabilities Special Interest Section Newsletter, 14*(2), 2–3.

Allen, C. K. (1990). Activities: Cross-cultural similarities and difference. In *Proceedings of the 10th International Congress of the World Federation of Occupational Therapy,* Melbourne, Australia.

Allen C. K. (1990). Development of a research tradition in cognitive rehabilitation. *Mental Health Special Interest Section Newsletter, 13*(2), 1–3.

Royeen, C. B., Foto, M., Allen, C. K., Bass, C., Moon-Spelling, T., & Wilson, D. (1990). Reports that work. In C. B. Royeen (Ed.), *AOTA Self-Study Series: Assessing function*. Rockville, MD: American Occupational Therapy Association.

Allen, C. K. (1989). Treatment plans in cognitive rehabilitation. *Occupational Therapy Practice, 1*, 1–8.

Allen, C. K., Foto, M., Moon-Spelling, T., & Wilson, D. (1989). A medical review approach to Medicare outpatient documentation. *American Journal of Occupational Therapy, 43*, 793–800.

Heimann, N. E., & Allen, C. K. (1989). The routine task inventory: A tool for describing the functional behavior of the cognitively disabled. *Occupational Therapy Practice, 1*(1), 67–74.

Wilson, D. S., Allen, C. K., McCormack, G. L., & Burton, G. U. (1989). Cognitive disabilities and routine task behaviors in a community-based population with senile dementia. *Occupational Therapy Practice, 1*(1), 58–66.

Allen, C. K. (1988). Cognitive disabilities. In S. Robins (Ed.), *Mental health focus*. Rockville, MD: American Occupational Therapy Association.

Katz, N., Allen, C. K., & Burke, J .P. (1988). The development of standardized clinical evaluations in mental health. *Occupational Therapy in Mental Health, 8*(1), 1–94.

Allen, C. K. (1987). Activity: Occupational therapy's treatment method (1987 Eleanor Clarke Slagle Lecture). *American Journal of Occupational Therapy, 41*, 563–575.

Allen, C. K. (1987). Occupational therapy: Functional assessment of severity of mental disorders. *Hospital and Community Psychiatry, 39*, 140–142.

Allen, C. K., & Allen, R. E. (1987). Cognitive disabilities: Measuring the social consequences of mental disorders. *Journal of Clinical Psychiatry, 48*, 185–191.

Allen, C. K. (1985). *Occupational therapy for psychiatric diseases: Measurement and management of cognitive disabilities*. Boston: Little, Brown.

Allen, C. K. (1982). Independence through activity: The practice of occupational therapy (Psychiatry). *American Journal of Occupational Therapy, 36*, 731–739.

Lindquist, J. E., Allen, C. K., & Stocking, S. (1982). Response and commentary: A reply to Utley and Robertson. *Occupational Therapy Journal of Research, 2*, 120–124.

Copans, S., Osgood, D., Allen, C. K., Babbott, J., & Baer, E. (1971). *The home health handbook: A preliminary guide to self help and rural medicine* (3rd ed.). Brattleboro, VT: Stephen Green.

A. Jean Ayres, OTR, PhD—1963

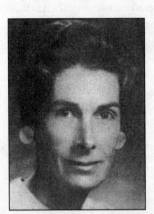

Anna Jean Ayres was professor at the University of Southern California (USC) for more than 20 years. She was born in 1923 and grew up on a farm in Visalia, California. She was married in 1969 to Franklin Baker and died in 1989 due to complications from cancer.

Ayres received bachelor's and master's degrees in occupational therapy in 1945 and 1954, respectively, and her doctorate in educational psychology in 1961, all from USC. She also undertook postdoctoral work at the Brain Research Institute, University of California, Los Angeles. The exposure provided the formal educational foundation for her work, but it was extensive reading of brain research accompanied by clinical research and practice that were most helpful in generating the ideas and theoretical concepts underlying her theory and treatment of sensory integrative dysfunction.

As a child, she struggled with learning problems similar to those she would later study. Ayres's major research focused on sensory integration and the brain and how sensory integration dysfunction affects children's learning abilities. In 1977, the Ayres Clinic was created to treat children with sensory integration dysfunction using techniques from occupational therapy. Ayres published 54 articles, two books, and numerous tests and videos related to sensory integration dysfunction and therapy. She was a frequent lecturer and was a founder of Sensory Integration International, a nonprofit organization dedicated to the promotion of sensory integration research.

Ayres is credited with pioneering the concept of sensory integration. During the latter years of her career, she conducted a private practice at her private clinic and, with the help of others, revised and expanded the Southern California Sensory Integration and Praxis Tests.

Ayres was a member of the American Psychological Association and held a California State License in psychology. She was granted a life membership from the Occupational Therapy Association of California. Her awards include the AOTA Award of Merit, 1965; Roster of Fellows, 1973; and charter membership in the Academy of Research from the American Occupational Therapy Foundation, 1983.

Bibliography

Ayres, J. (1949). An analysis of crafts in the treatment of electroshock patients. *American Journal of Occupational Therapy, 3,* 195–198.

Ayres, J. (1954). A form used to evaluate the work behavior of patients: A preliminary report. *American Journal of Occupational Therapy, 8,* 73–74.

Ayres, J. (1954). Ontogenetic principles in the development of arm and hand functions. *American Journal of Occupational Therapy, 8,* 95–99.

Ayres, J. (1955). A pilot study on the relationship between work habits and workshop production. *American Journal of Occupational Therapy, 9,* 264–276.

Ayres, J. (1955). Proprioceptive facilitation elicited through the upper extremities: Part I: Background. *American Journal of Occupational Therapy, 9,* 1–9.

Ayres, J. (1955). Proprioceptive facilitation elicited through the upper extremities: Part II: Application. *American Journal of Occupational Therapy, 9,* 57–58.

Ayres, J. (1955). Proprioceptive facilitation elicited through the upper extremities: Part III: Specific application. *American Journal of Occupational Therapy, 9,* 121–126.

Ayres, J. (1957). A study of the manual dexterity and workshop wages of thirty-nine cerebral palsied trainees. *American Journal of Physical Medicine, 36,* 6–10.

Ayres, J. (1958). Basic concepts of clinical practice in physical disabilities. *American Journal of Occupational Therapy, 12,* 300–302.

Ayres, J. (1958). The visual–motor function. *American Journal of Occupational Therapy, 12,* 130–138.

Ayres, J. (1960). *Hemiplegia: Occupational therapy reference manual for physicians.* New York: American Occupational Therapy Association.

Ayres, J. (1960). Occupational therapy for motor disorders resulting from impairment of the central nervous system. *Rehabilitation Literature, 21,* 302–310.

Ayres, J. (1960). Research for therapists. In *Proceedings of the American Occupational Therapy Association* (pp. 79–82). New York: American Occupational Therapy Association.

Ayres, J. (1961). Development of the body scheme in children. *American Journal of Occupational Therapy, 15,* 99–102.

Ayres, J. (1961). The role of gross motor activities in the training of children with visual motor retardation. *Journal of the American Optometric Association, 33,* 121–125.

Ayres, J. (1962). Integration of information. In *Approaches to the treatment of patients with neuromuscular dysfunction, Study Course IV* (Third International Congress, World Federation of Occupational Therapists). Dubuque, IA: William C Brown.

Ayres, J. (1962). Perception of space of adult hemiplegic patients. *Physical Medicine and Rehabilitation, 43,* 552–555.

Ayres, J. (1963). The development of perceptual–motor abilities: A theoretical basis for treatment of dysfunction (1963 Eleanor Clarke Slagle Lecture). *American Journal of Occupational Therapy, 17,* 221–225.

Ayres, J. (1963). Occupational therapy directed toward neuromuscular integration. In H. S. Willard & C. S. Spackman (Eds.), *Occupational therapy* (3rd ed., pp. 358–466). Philadelphia: Lippincott.

Ayres, J. (1964). *Perceptual–motor dysfunction in children.* Offset monograph from the Greater Cincinnati District, Ohio Occupational Therapy Association Conference, Cincinnati.

Ayres, J. (1964). Perceptual–motor for training for children. In *Approaches to the treatment of patients with neuromuscular dysfunction, Study Course VI* (pp. 17–22). Dubuque, IA: William C Brown.

Ayres, J. (1964). Perspectives on neurological bases of reading. In M. P. Douglas (Ed.), *Claremont Reading Conference, 28th yearbook* (pp. 113–118). Claremont Graduate School Curriculum Laboratory.

Ayres, J. (1964). Tactile functions: Their relation to hyperactivity and perceptual–motor behavior. *American Journal of Occupational Therapy, 18,* 6–11.

Ayres, J. (1965). A method of measurement of degree of sensorimotor integration. *Archives of Physical Medicine and Rehabilitation, 46,* 433–435.

Ayres, J. (1965). Patterns of perceptual–motor dysfunction in children: A factor analytic study. *Perceptual and Motor Skills, 20,* 335–368.

Ayres, J. (1966). Interrelation of perception, function, and treatment. *Journal of the American Physical Therapy Association, 46,* 641–744.

Ayres, J. (1966). Interrelations among perceptual–motor abilities in a group of normal children. *American Journal of Occupational Therapy, 20,* 288–292.

Ayres, J. (1966). Interrelationships among perceptual–motor functions in children. *American Journal of Occupational Therapy, 20,* 68–71.

Ayres, J., & Reid, W. (1966). The self-drawing as an expression of perceptual–motor dysfunction. *Cortex, 2,* 254–265.

Ayres, J. (1967). Remedial procedures based on neurobehavioral constructs. In *Proceedings, 1967 International Convocation on Children and Young Adults With Learning Disabilities,* Pittsburgh, PA.

Ayres, J. (1968). A product of sensory integrative process. In H. K. Smith (Ed.), *Perception and reading* (Proceedings of the 12th Annual Convention International Reading Association). Newark, DE: International Reading Association.

Ayres, J. (1968). Sensory integrative processes and neuropsychological learning disability. *Learning Disorders, 3*(2), 75–81.

Ayres, J. (1969). Deficits in sensory integration in educationally handicapped children. *Journal of Learning Disabilities, 2,* 160–168.

Ayres, J. (1969). Relation between Gesell development quotients and later perceptual–motor performance. *American Journal Occupational Therapy, 23,* 11–17.

Ayres, J. (1971). *The challenge of the brain.* Presented at the Perceptual Motor Conference, sponsored by the Physical Education Division of the American Association for Health, Physical Education, and Recreation, Sparks, NV.

Ayres, J. (1971). Characteristics of types of sensory integrative dysfunction. *American Journal of Occupational Therapy, 25,* 329–334.

Ayres, J. (1972). Basic concepts of occupational therapy for children with perceptual–motor dysfunction. In *Proceedings of the 12th World Congress of Rehabilitation International,* Sydney, Australia.

Ayres, J. (1972). Improving academic scores through sensory integration. *Journal of Learning Disabilities, 5,* 338–343.

Ayres, J. (1972). *Sensory integration and learning disorders.* Los Angeles: Western Psychological Services.

Ayres, J. (1972). Sensory integrative dysfunction in a young schizophrenic girl. *Journal of Autism and Childhood Schizophrenia, 2,* 174–181.

Ayres, J. (1972). Sensory integrative process: Implications for deaf-blind from learning disability children. In *Proceedings of the National Symposium for Deaf-Blind* (pp. 17–20). Garden Grove, CA: TR Publications.

Ayres, J. (1973). An interpretation of the role of the brain stem in intercessory integration. In A. Henderson & A. Coryell (Eds.), *The body senses and perceptual deficit: Proceedings of the Occupational Therapy Symposium on Somatosensory Aspects of Perceptual Deficit* (pp. 60–69). Boston: Boston University.

Ayres, J. (1975). Sensorimotor foundations of academic ability. In W. M. Cruickshank & D. Hallahan (Eds.), *Perceptual and learning disabilities in children* (pp. 35–53). Syracuse, NY: Syracuse University Press.

Ayres, J. (1977). Cluster analyses of measure of sensory integration. *American Journal of Occupational Therapy, 31,* 362–366.

Ayres, J. (1977). Dichotic listening performance in learning disabled children. *American Journal of Occupational Therapy, 31,* 441–446.

Ayres, J. (1977). A response to defensive medicine. *Academic Therapy, 13,* 149–152.

Ayres, J. (1978). Learning disabilities and the vestibular system. *Journal of Learning Disabilities, 11,* 18–29.

Ayres, J. (1979). *Sensory integration and the child.* Los Angeles, CA: Western Psychological Services.

Ayres, J. (1979). The sensory registration function in autistic and aphasic/apraxic children. In *Piagetian theory and its implications for the helping professions: Proceedings of the Ninth Interdisciplinary Conference* (pp. 35–46). Los Angeles: University of Southern California.

Ayres, J., & Tickle, L. (1980). Hyper-responsivity to touch and vestibular stimuli predict positive responses to sensory integration procedures in autistic children. *American Journal of Occupational Therapy, 34,* 375–381.

Ayres, J., & Mailloux, Z. (1981). Influence of sensory integration procedures on language development. *American Journal of Occupational Therapy, 35,* 383–390.

Ayres, J., & Mailloux, Z. (1983). Possible pubertal effects on the therapeutic gains in an autistic girl. *American Journal of Occupational Therapy, 37,* 535–540.

Ayres, J., Slavik, B. A., Kitsuwa-Lowe, J., Danner, P. T., & Green, J. (1984). Vestibular stimulation and eye contact in autistic children. *Neuropediatrics, 15,* 267–273.

Cermak, S. A., &. Ayres, J. (1984). Crossing the body midline in learning-disabled and normal children. *American Journal of Occupational Therapy, 38,* 35–39.

Ayers, A. J., & Robbins, J. (2004). *Sensory integration and the child: Understanding the hidden sensory disorders* (25th anniversary ed.). Los Angeles: Western Psychological Services.

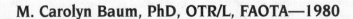

M. Carolyn Baum, PhD, OTR/L, FAOTA—1980

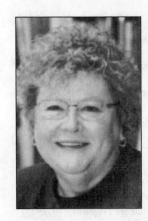

Carolyn Baum is the Elias Michael Director and Professor of Occupational Therapy and Neurology at Washington University School of Medicine in St. Louis, Missouri. She graduated from Kansas University with a bachelor's degree in occupational therapy in1966; a master's degree in health management from Webster University in St. Louis in 1979; and a doctorate in social work with a concentration in social policy and aging from the George Warren Brown School of Social Work at Washington University in St. Louis in 1993.

Baum was born in Chicago in 1943. Her father, Gibson Henry Manville, was a Pullman conductor and her mother, Nell Laverne Curry, was a teacher and later a hospital dietitian. She has a brother, a farmer, and a sister, a retired schoolteacher. She has one daughter, Kirstin Sumner, who lives in Chicago with her husband Scott and her son Graham.

Growing up in Winchester, Kansas, in a farming community, she was a member of a class of 18 students that together went from first grade through high school. Baum remembers having been involved in the 4-H Club and entering all sorts of contests and learning how to sew and cook. In fact, she relates, "Actually, I got a purple ribbon at the State for a cake, and I was awarded a Betty Crocker *Homemaker of Tomorrow* award" (C. Baum, personal communication, October 8, 2004).

Upon graduation from high school, Baum went to Kansas State to become a home economics teacher. However, she reached a turning point when visiting a cousin in Tacoma, Washington. Her cousin, an assistant director of special education for the Tacoma Public Schools, told her that although she was content with her career, if given the opportunity to do it again, she would have chosen to be an occupational therapist. Baum's cousin took her to visit occupational therapists in the local school district, which "was one of the first school districts in the country where they integrated the children with resource rooms in the mainstream school" (C. Baum, October 8, 2004), and the rest is history. Upon her return home, she transferred to the University of Kansas, changed majors, and became an occupational therapist.

Once she completed her bachelor's degree, Baum said, "I went to work at the University of Kansas Medical Center in Kansas City and started a cardiac rehabilitation program with a nurse, and within 6 months I was presenting my first paper" (C. Baum, October 8, 2004). Later she accepted a position at the Research Medical Center in Kansas City. "I went there to start the rehabilitation occupational therapy program, and I became director of rehabilitation and then director of physical medicine and rehabilitation managing occupational, physical and speech therapy. I was getting really involved in AOTA [the American Occupational Therapy Association] by that time (the 1970s) and found that Florence Cromwell, Wilma West, and others took an interest in my work and served as mentors" (C. Baum, personal communication, October 8, 2004). In 1976, Jerry Johnson recruited Baum to run the occupational therapy program at the Irene Walter Johnson Rehabilitation Institute in St. Louis.

"I came to St. Louis and joined an academic medical center, where nobody knew what occupational therapy was, and nobody saw the effectiveness. . . . There was nothing to justify our services, so I started building pilot studies and working with doctors, and I guess that is probably one of my strengths—I know how to build collaborations, because if you have got to get something done, you have got to do it with other people. "(C. Baum, personal communication, October 8, 2004)

When asked what she considers important in her career she said,

"I do what I do because I want to make a difference in the lives of the people we serve. I have always had this passion for occupational therapy, but it is because I like what we do for people. I am also passionate about our history and the fact that we are not the first generation to deal with the complexity of these problems. We just need to respect that these are difficult issues that we deal with. We are talking about social and health reform when we are talking about putting people in an environment where they can fully participate. I get frustrated when people think that we should be able to have easy answers. We are a part of a system that is always in change; we need to lead change." (C. Baum, personal communication, October 8, 2004)

When referring to what she considers major accomplishments of her career, she said,

"Building a strong academic program and a research enterprise, being able to serve the profession as president of AOTA, and building an interdisciplinary translational research program addressing issues of stroke. I also have been fortunate to be able to work with wonderful students and many colleagues around the world to improve our understanding of cognition and its impact of occupational performance." (C. Baum, personal communication, October 8, 2004)

Personally, Baum described herself as a person who has friends all over the world. She loves to travel, is an avid photographer, enjoys entertaining and cooking, and reads a lot of fiction and works that will increase her knowledge (C. Baum, personal communication, October 8, 2004). A special interest and of hers is spending time with her grandson.

Baum has been involved in two major rehabilitation policy initiatives. She served on the National Institutes of Health (NIH) committee that wrote the rehabilitation plan for Congress that implemented the National Center for Medical Rehabilitation Research. She also served on the Institute of Medicine committee that wrote the report *Enabling America for Congress,* which subsequently was published as a book. She also has been involved with the Alzheimer's Association; the County Recreation Board in St. Louis; and national, state, and local occupational therapy organizations.

Baum's research focuses on enabling older adults to live independently. Rather than focus on people's deficits, she seeks to understand what a person with chronic disease or disability can do. Her work has been recognized with funding from the NIH, the National Institute of Disability Rehabilitation Research, the James S. McDonnell Foundation, the Social Security Administration, and the Older Adults Service and Information System (OASIS). She currently is principal investigator of the McDonnell Science Foundation project "Linking Neuroscience to Everyday Life." In this initiative she has worked with colleagues to build an integrated model of cognitive rehabilitation. The project involves neuroscientists, neurologists, and occupational therapists to understand the brain and cognitive mechanisms that support everyday life.

Baum served as AOTA president from 1982 to 1983 and again from 2003 to 2007. She is also past-president of the National Board of Certification of Occupational Therapy (NBCOT). She was inducted into the Academy of Research in 2005. Her AOTA awards include the Award of Merit, the Eleanor Clark Slagle Lecture, the Roster of Fellows, the Certificate of Appreciation, and the Meritorious Service Award. Last year she received the Wilma West AOTA and AOTF President's Award.

Linking Key Messages of the 1980 Eleanor Clarke Slagle Lecture to the AOTA *Centennial Vision:*
Even as early as my Slagle Lecture, I was challenging the profession to define itself and link education and practice to build our future knowledge. I was privileged to serve as president when the AOTA Board took the challenge to create a vision that would guide the profession's actions to achieve the vision that our founders stated when they started our professional society in 1917. I was so proud that the members of the profession worked together under the leadership of Charles Christiansen, our vice president, to chart our course toward the realization of our profession's potential to serve society with knowledge and services. As a part of that vision was the need to link our resources in education, practice, and science. I have tried to lead by example. When I presented the Eleanor Clarke Slagle Lectureship Award, I was a clinician, yet I saw the importance of our collective strength. I feel even more strongly now about the importance of our collective efforts to provide a united front to serve the needs of our society's occupational needs. I occasionally re-read my lecture and think that I could have been more concise in my message; however, I think that many of the issues I proposed then are still important today, especially as we exercise our knowledge and strength as a profession that makes such a difference in people's lives.

—*Carolyn Baum*

Bibliography

Wolf, T. J., Stift, S., Connor, L. T., & Baum, C. (2010). Feasibility of using the EFPT to detect executive function deficits at the acute stage of stroke. *Work, 36*(4), 405–412.

Baum, C., & Katz, N. (2009). Occupational therapy approach to assessing the relationship between cognition and function. In T. Marcotte & I. Grant (Eds.), *Neuropsychology in everyday functioning: Translating laboratory performance to the real world.* New York: Guilford Press.

Hartman-Maeir, A., Katz, N., & Baum, C. M. (2009). Cognitive–Functional Profile (CFP) for individuals with suspected cognitive disabilities. *Occupational Therapy in Health Care, 23*(1), 1–23.

Wolf, T. J., Baum, C., & Connor, L. T. (2009). The changing face of stroke: Implications for occupational therapy practice. *American Journal of Occupational Therapy, 63,* 621–625.

Baum, C. (2008). Foreword. In C. H. Christiansen & E. A. Townsend (Eds.), *Introduction to occupation: The art and science of living* (2nd ed., pp. xv–xvi). Upper Saddle River, NJ: Pearson.

Baum, C. M., Connor, L. T., Morrison, M. T., Hahn, M., Dromerick, A. W., & Edwards, D. F. (2008). The reliability, validity, and clinical utility of the Executive Function Performance Test: A measure of executive function in a sample of people with stroke. *American Journal of Occupational Therapy, 62*(4), 446–455.

Baum, C. M. & Edwards, D. F. (2008). *The Activity Card Sort* (2nd ed.). Bethesda, MD: AOTA Press.

Foster, E., Perlmutter, M., & Baum, C. M. (2008). Evaluating occupational performance of older adults. In S. Coppola, S. Elliott, & P. Toto (Eds.), *Strategies to advance gerontology excellence: Promoting best practice in occupational therapy* (pp. 349–382). Bethesda, MD: AOTA Press.

Baum, C. (2007). Achieving our potential [Presidential Address]. *American Journal of Occupational Therapy, 61*(6), 615–621.

Edwards, D. F., Baum, C. M., Hsia, A., Kidwell, C., & Dromerick, A. W. (2007). Racial disparities in function and quality of life after first ischemic stroke. *Neurology, 68*(12), A132–A133.

Baum, C. (2006). Harnessing opportunities and taking responsibility for our future. *American Journal of Occupational Therapy, 60*(3), 249–257.

Edwards, D. F., Hahn, M. G., Baum, C. M., & Dromerick, A. W. (2006). The impact of mild stroke on meaningful activity and life. *Journal of Stroke and Cerebrovascular Diseases, 15*(4), 151–157.

Edwards, D. F., Hahn, M. G., Baum, C., Perlmutter, M. S., Sheedy, C., & Dromerick, A. W. (2006). Undetected impairment in persons with stroke: Validation of the post-stroke rehabilitation guidelines. *Neurorehabilitation and Neural Repair, 20,* 42–48.

Baum, C. (2005). Centennial challenges, millennium opportunities [Presidential Address]. *American Journal of Occupational Therapy, 60*(6), 609–616.

Baum, C., Baptiste, S., & Law, M. (2005). Using information to influence policy. In M. Law, C. Baum, & W. Dunn (Eds.), *Measuring occupational performance: Supporting best practice in occupational therapy* (2nd ed., pp. 367–374). Thorofare, NJ: Slack.

Baum, C. M., Bass Haugen, J., & Christiansen, C. (2005). A framework for decision-making occupations. In C. Christiansen & C. M. Baum (Eds.), *Occupational therapy: Performance, participation, and well-being* (3rd ed.). Thorofare, NJ: Slack.

Baum, C. M., & Christiansen, C. (2005). Outcomes of an occupation-based approach. In C. Christiansen & C. M. Baum (Eds.), *Occupational therapy: Performance, participation, and well-being* (3rd ed.). Thorofare, NJ: Slack.

Baum, C. M., & Christiansen, C. (2005). Overview of a PEOP framework to support occupation-based practice occupations. In C. Christiansen & C. M. Baum (Eds.), *Occupational therapy: Performance, participation, and well-being* (3rd ed.). Thorofare, NJ: Slack.

Baum, C., Perlmutter, M., & Dunn, W. (2005). Establishing the integrity of measurement data: Identifying impairments that can limit occupational performance and threaten the validity of assessments. In M. Law, C. Baum, & W. Dunn (Eds.), *Measuring occupational performance: Supporting best practice in occupational therapy* (2nd ed., pp. 49–64). Thorofare, NJ: Slack.

Christiansen, C., & Baum, C. M. (2005). The nature of occupations. In C. Christiansen & C. M. Baum (Eds.), *Occupational therapy: Performance, participation, and well-being* (3rd ed.) Thorofare, NJ: Slack.

Christiansen, C., & Baum, C. M. (Eds.). (2005). *Occupational therapy: Enabling function and well-being* (3rd ed.). Thorofare, NJ: Slack.

Edwards, D., & Baum, C. (2005). Occupational performance: Measuring the perspectives of others. In M. Law, C. Baum, & W. Dunn (Eds.), *Measuring occupational performance: Supporting best practice in occupational therapy* (2nd ed., pp. 93–106). Thorofare, NJ: Slack.

Edwards, D. F., Hahn, M., Dromerick, A. W., & Baum, M. C. (2005). Race differences in function and quality of life in mild stroke. *Stroke, 36*(2), 480.

Law, M., Baum, C., & Dunn, W. (2005). Challenges and strategies in applying an occupational performance measurement approach. In M. Law, C. Baum, & W. Dunn (Eds.), *Measuring occupational performance: Supporting best practice in occupational therapy* (2nd ed., pp. 375–382). Thorofare, NJ: Slack.

Law, M., Baum, C., & Dunn, W. (2005). *Measuring occupational performance: Supporting best practice in occupational therapy* (2nd ed.). Thorofare, NJ: Slack.

Law, M., Baum, C. M., & Dunn, W. (2005). Occupational performance assessment. In C. Christiansen & C. M. Baum (Eds.), *Occupational therapy: Enabling function and well-being* (3rd ed.). Thorofare, NJ: Slack.

Law, M., Dunn, W., & Baum, C. (2005). Measuring participation. In M. Law, C. Baum, & W. Dunn (Eds.), *Measuring occupational performance: Supporting best practice in occupational therapy* (2nd ed., pp. 107–128). Thorofare, NJ: Slack.

Baum, M. C. (2004). Building a professional tapestry [Presidential Address]. *American Journal of Occupational Therapy, 59*(6), 606.

Baum, C. M. (2004). Transition [Editorial]. *OTJR: Occupation, Participation and Health, 24*(2), 43.

Hahn, M. G., & Baum, M. C. (2004). Improving participation and quality of life through occupation. In G. Gillen & A. Burkhardt (Eds.), *Stroke rehabilitation: A function-based approach* (2nd ed., pp. 45–58). St. Louis, MO: Mosby.

Baum, C. M. (2003). Participation: Its relationship to occupation and health [Editorial]. *OTJR: Occupation, Participation and Health, 23*(2), 46–47.

Baum, C. M., & Edwards, D. F. (2003). What persons with Alzheimer's disease can do: A tool for communication about daily activities. *Alzheimer's Care Quarterly, 4*(2), 108–118.

Letts, L., Baum, C., & Perlmutter, M. (2003, June 2). Person–environment–occupation assessment with older adults. *OT Practice*, pp. 27–34.

Acharya, A. B., Edwards, D. F., White, D. A, Tucker, F., Sheedy, C. W., Corbetta, M., Miller, J. P., Baum, C., & Dromerick, A. W. (2002). How mild is mild stroke? Cognitive impairment in persons with mild stroke. *Neurology, 58*(7, Suppl. 3), A280–A281.

Baum, C. M. (2002). Adolph Meyer's challenge: Focus on occupation in practice and in science [Editorial]. *OTJR: Occupation, Participation and Health, 22*(4), 130–131.

Baum, C. M. (2002). Letter from the editor. *OTJR: Occupation, Participation, and Health, 22*(3), 5.

Baum, C. M. (2002). Viewpoints—Creating partnerships: Constructing our future. *Australian Occupational Therapy Journal, 49,* 58–62.

Baum, C. M. (2002). [Untitled editorial]. *OTJR: Occupation, Participation and Health, 22*(1), 3.

Baum, C. M. (2002). [Untitled editorial]. *OTJR: Occupation, Participation and Health, 22*(2).

Baum, C. M., & Baptiste, S. (2002). Reframing OT practice. In M. Law, C. M. Baum, & S. Baptiste (Eds.), *Occupation-based practice: Fostering performance and participation.* Thorofare, NJ: Slack.

Baum, C. M., Berg, C., Seaton, M., & White, L. (2002). Fostering performance. In M. Law, C. M. Baum, & S. Baptiste (Eds.), *Occupation-based practice: Fostering performance and participation* (pp. 27–40). Thorofare, NJ: Slack.

Baum, C. M., LaVesser, P., & Strong, S. (2002). Doing occupational therapy-based practice. In M. Law, C. M. Baum, & S. Baptiste (Eds.), *Occupation-based practice: Fostering performance and participation* (pp. 93–106). Thorofare, NJ: Slack.

Baum, C. M., Missiiuna, C., & Perlmutter, M. (2002). Defining occupational therapy intervention. In M. Law, C. M Baum, & S. Baptiste (Eds.), *Occupation-based practice: Fostering performance and participation* (pp. 63–78). Thorofare, NJ: Slack.

Baum, C. M., Missiiuna, C., & Perlmutter, M. (2002). Doing client-centered practice. In M. Law, C. M. Baum, & S. Baptiste (Eds.), *Occupation-based practice: Fostering performance and participation* (pp. 51–59). Thorofare, NJ: Slack.

Baum, C. M., & Wilkins, S. (2002). From diagnosis to occupational performance. In M. Law, C. M. Baum, & S. Baptiste (Eds.), *Occupation-based practice: Fostering performance and participation* (pp. 41–50). Thorofare, NJ: Slack.

Law, M., Baum, C. M., & Baptiste, S. (2002). *Occupation-based practice: Fostering performance and participation.* Thorofare, NJ: Slack.

Baum, C. M. (2001). A forum for occupation, participation and health [Editorial]. *Occupational Therapy Journal of Research, 21,* 71–72.

Baum, C. M. (2001). A married couple dealing with Alzheimer's disease. In S. E. Ryan & K. Sladyk (Eds.), *Ryan's occupational therapy assistant: Principles, practice issues, and techniques* (3rd ed., pp. 301–312). Thorofare, NJ: Slack.

Baum, C. M., & Baptiste, S. (2001). Using information to influence policy. In M. Law, C. M. Baum, & W. Dunn (Eds.), *Measuring occupational performance: Supporting best practice in occupational therapy* (pp. 269–275). Thorofare, NJ: Slack.

Baum, C. M., & Edwards, D. F. (2001). *Activity Card Sort.* St. Louis, MO: Washington University.

Baum, C., Perlmutter, M., & Dunn, W. (2001). Establishing the integrity of measurement data: Identifying impairments that can limit occupational performance and threaten the validity of assessments. In M. Law, C. M. Baum, & W Dunn (Eds.), *Measuring occupational performance: Supporting best practice in occupational therapy* (pp. 43–56). Thorofare, NJ: Slack.

Edwards, D., & Baum, C. M. (2001). Occupational performance: Measuring the perspectives of others. In M. Law, C. M. Baum, & W. Dunn (Eds.), *Measuring occupational performance: Supporting best practice in occupational therapy* (pp.77–88). Thorofare, NJ: Slack.

Law, M., & Baum C. (2001). Measurement in occupational therapy. In M. Law, C. M. Baum, & W. Dunn (Eds.), *Measuring occupational performance: Supporting best practice in occupational therapy* (pp. 3–19). Thorofare, NJ: Slack.

Law, M., Baum, C., & Dunn, W. (2001). Challenges and strategies in applying an occupational performance measurement approach. In M. Law, C. M. Baum, & W. Dunn (Eds.), *Measuring occupational performance: Supporting best practice in occupational therapy* (pp. 277–283). Thorofare, NJ: Slack.

Law, M., Baum, C., & Dunn, W. (2001). *Measuring occupational performance: Supporting best practice in occupational therapy.* Thorofare, NJ: Slack.

Archey, B., & Baum, M. C. (2000). A new language in support of enablement. *American Journal of Occupational Therapy, 54*(2), 223–225.

Baum, C. (2000). The evolution of rehabilitation science at Washington University School of Medicine. *Technology and Disability 12*(2&3), 119–122.

Baum, C. M. (2000). Occupation-based practice: Reinventing ourselves for the new millennium. *OT Practice, 5*(1), 12–15.

Baum, C. M. (2000, January 3). Reinventing ourselves for the new millennium. *OT Practice*, pp. 12–15.

Baum, C. M., & Edwards, D. F. (2000). Documenting productive behaviors: Using the Functional Behavior Profile to plan discharge following stroke. *Journal of Gerontological Nursing, 26*(4), 34–43.

Baum, C. M., Perlmutter, M., & Edwards, D. F. (2000). Measuring function in Alzheimer's disease. *Alzheimer's Care Quarterly, 1*(3), 44–61.

Everard, K. M., Lach, H. W., Fisher, E. B., & Baum, C. M. (2000). Relationship of activity and social support to the functional health of older adults. *Journal of Gerontology: Social Sciences, 55B*(4), S208–S212.

Edwards, D. F., Baum, C. M., Meisel, M., Depke, M., Williams, J., Braford, T., et al. (1999). Home-based multidisciplinary diagnosis and treatment of inner city elderly with dementia. *The Gerontologist, 39*(4), 483–488.

Baum, C. M. (1998). Achieving effectiveness with a client-centered approach: A person–environment interaction. In Gray, D.B., Quatrano, L.A., & Lieberman, M.L., (Eds.), *Designing and using assistive technology: The human perspective* (National Institute of Health Conference Proceedings, pp. 137–146). Baltimore: Paul H. Brookes.

Baum, C. M. (1998). Client-centered practice in a changing health care system. In M. Law (Ed.), *Client-centered occupational therapy* (pp. 29–44). Thorofare, NJ: Slack.

Baum, C. M., & Gray, D.B. (1998). People with disabilities, their families, and rehabilitation services: Minimizing the impact of disability on personal relationships. In McCall, M.A. & Bichenbach. J. (Eds.), *Introduction to disability*. Edinburgh, Scotland: Harcourt, Brace.

Baum, C. M., & Law, M. (1998). Community health: A responsibility, an opportunity, and a fit for occupational therapy. *American Journal of Occupational Therapy, 52*(1), 7–10.

Baum, C. (1997). The managed care system: The educator's opportunity. *Education Special Interest Section Quarterly, 7*(2), 1–3.

Baum, C. M., & Christiansen, C. (1997). The occupational therapy context: Philosophy–principles–practice. In C. Christiansen & C. Baum (Eds.), *Occupational therapy: Enabling function and well-being* (2nd ed., pp. 26–44). Thorofare, NJ: Slack.

Baum, C. M., & Law, M. (1997). Occupational therapy: Focus on occupation and occupational performance. *Israel Journal of Occupational Therapy, 6*(1), E1–E14.

Baum, C. M., & Law, M. (1997). Occupational therapy practice: Focusing on occupational performance. *American Journal of Occupational Therapy, 51*(4), 277–288.

Christiansen, C., & Baum, C. M. (Eds.). (1997). *Occupational therapy: Enabling function and well-being* (2nd ed.). Thorofare, NJ: Slack.

Christiansen, C., & Baum, C. M. (1997). The occupational therapy context: Philosophy–principles–practice. In C. Christiansen & C. Baum (Eds.), *Occupational therapy: Enabling function and well-being* (2nd ed.). Thorofare, NJ: Slack.

Christiansen, C., & Baum, C. M. (1997). Person–environment occupational performance: A conceptual model for practice. In C. Christiansen & C. Baum (Eds.), *Occupational therapy: Enabling function and well-being* (2nd ed., pp. 46–70). Thorofare, NJ: Slack.

Christiansen, C., & Baum, C. M. (1997). Understanding occupation: Definitions and concepts. In C. Christiansen & C. Baum (Eds.), *Occupational therapy: Enabling function and well-being* (2nd ed., pp. 2–24). Thorofare, NJ: Slack.

Law, M., & Baum, C. M. (1997). National Perspective—Evidence-based occupational therapy. *Canadian Journal of Occupational Therapy, 65*, 131–135.

Baum, C. M. (1996). Women as care providers and care receivers: Effective strategies. In D. M. Krotoski, M. A. Nosek, & M. A. Turk (Eds.), *Women with physical disabilities: Achieving and maintaining health and well-being* (pp. 243–257). Baltimore: Paul. H. Brookes.

Baum, C. M., McGeary, T., Pankiewicz, R., Braford, T., & Edwards, D. F. (1996). An activity program for cognitively impaired low-income inner city residents. *Topics in Geriatric Rehabilitation, 12*(2), 54–62.

Edwards, D. F., & Baum, C. M. (1996). Functional performance of inner city African American older persons with dementia. *Topics in Geriatric Rehabilitation, 12*(2), 17–27.

Baum, C. M. (1995). The contribution of occupation to function in persons with Alzheimer's disease. *Journal of Occupation Science: Australia 2*(2), 59–67.

Baum, C. M. (1995). Supporting the family: Strategies for managing neurological deficits in Alzheimer's and related disorders. In *Proceedings of the Goldie S. Cohen Memorial Conference*, Newton, PA.

Baum, C. M., & Bachelder, J. (1995). Rehabilitation of patients with progressive multiple sensory losses, including use of corrective lens and low vision aids. *Seminars in Hearing, 16*(3), 281–286.

Baum, C., & Edwards, D. (1995). AOTA's 1995 Representative Assembly Highlights—Occupational performance: Occupational therapy's definition of function. *OT Week, 9*(6), A11–A12.

Baum, C. M., Storant, M., Yonan, C., & Edwards, D. (1995). The relation of neuropsychological test performance to performance of functional tasks in dementia of the Alzheimer type. *Archives of Clinical Neuropsychology, 11*, 69–75.

Young, V. L., Seaton, M. K., Feely, C. A., Arfken, C., Edwards, D. F., Baum, C. M., et al. (1995). Detecting cumulative trauma disorders in workers performing repetitive tasks. *American Journal of Industrial Medicine, 27*, 419–431.

Baum, C. M., & Hilton, C. (1994). Occupational therapy: Moving forward to meet future needs. *Health Care Trends and Transitions, 5*(3), 25–28.

Law, M., & Baum, C. M. (1994). Creating the future: A joint effort. In *Proceedings of the CanAm Conference of the American and Canadian Occupational Therapy Associations*, Bethesda, MD.

Radomski, M. V., Dougherty, P. M., Fine, S. B., Baum, C., & Royeen, C. (1994). Case studies in cognitive rehabilitation. In *AOTA Self-Study Series—Cognitive rehabilitation*. Rockville, MD: American Occupational Therapy Association.

Baum, C. M. (1993). Cognitive rehabilitation: An adaptive approach. In C. Royeen (Ed.), *Cognitive rehabilitation*. Rockville, MD: American Occupational Therapy Association.

Baum, C. M., & Edwards, D. (1993). Cognitive performance in senile dementia of the Alzheimer's type: The Kitchen Task Assessment. *American Journal of Occupational Therapy, 47*(5), 431–436.

Baum, C. M., Edwards, D. F., & Morrow-Howell, N. (1993). Identification and measurement of productive behaviors in senile dementia of the Alzheimer type. *The Gerontologist, 33*(3), 403–408.

Baum, C. M., & LaVesser, P. (1993). Caregiver assistance: Using family members and attendants. In C. Christiansen (Ed.), *Activities of daily living activities*. Rockville, MD: American Occupational Therapy Association.

Baum, C. M. (1992). Disability in the United States: A portrait from national data [Book Review]. In S. Thompson-Hoffman & I. Storck (Eds.), *Springer Series on Rehabilitation* (Vol. 8). New York: Springer.

Baum, C. M. (1991). Addressing the needs of the cognitively impaired elderly from a family policy perspective. *American Journal of Occupational Therapy, 45*(7), 594–606.

Baum, C. M. (1991). The environment: Providing opportunities for the future. *American Journal of Occupational Therapy, 45*(6), 487–490.

Baum, C. M. (1991). Identification and use of environmental resources. In C. Christiansen & M. C. Baum (Eds.), *Occupational therapy: Overcoming human performance deficits* (pp. 788–802). Thorofare, NJ: Slack.

Baum C. M. (1991). Professional issues in a changing environment. In C. Christiansen & M. C. Baum (Eds.), *Occupational therapy: Overcoming human performance deficits* (pp. 804–817). Thorofare, NJ: Slack.

Christiansen, C., & Baum, C. M. (Eds.). (1991). *Occupational therapy: Overcoming human performance deficits*. Thorofare, NJ: Slack.

Edwards, D. F., Baum, C. M., & Deuel, R. M. (1991). Constructional apraxia in Alzheimer's disease: Contributions to functional loss. *Physical and Occupational Therapy in Geriatrics, 9*(3/4), 53–68.

Edwards, D. F., Deuel, R. K., Baum, C. M., & Morris, J. C. (1991). A quantitative analysis of apraxia in senile dementia of the Alzheimer type: Stage-related differences in prevalence and type. *Dementia, 2,* 142–149.

Dueul, R. K., Edwards, D. F., & Baum, C. M. (1990). Properties of apraxia test items that distinguish early states of dementia. *Annals of Neurology, 28*(2), 222–223.

Edwards, D. F., & Baum, C. M. (1990). Caregiver burden across stages of dementia. *Occupational Therapy Practice, 2*(1), 17–31.

Deuel, R. K., Edwards, D. F., Baum, C. M., & Mui, A. (1989). Clinical dementia stages and the occurrence of manual dyspraxia in senile dementia of the Alzheimer type. *Annals of Neurology, 26*(1), 124.

Baum, C. M. (1988). Certification: Serving the public interest. *American Journal Occupational Therapy, 42*(2), 77–79.

Baum, C. M., Edwards, D., Leavitt, K., Grant, E., & Deuel, R. (1988). Performance components in senile dementia of the Alzheimer's type: Motor planning, language, and memory. *Occupational Therapy Journal of Research, 8,* 356–368.

Baum, C. M. (1987). Research: Its relationship to public policy. *American Journal of Occupational Therapy, 41*(3), 143–145.

Baum, C. M., & Devereaux, E. (1987). General perspectives on management and planning. In *Occupational therapy* (7th ed., pp. 181–192). Philadelphia: Harper & Row.

Baum, C. M., & Devereaux, E. (1987). Managing occupational therapy. In *Occupational therapy* (7th ed.). Philadelphia: Harper & Row.

Baum, C. M. (1986). *Understanding the prospective payment system: A business perspective.* Thorofare, NJ: Slack.

Baum, C. M., & Luebben, A. J. (1986). *The clinician's guide to prospective payment.* Thorofare, NJ: Charles B. Slack.

Mann, M., Edwards, D., & Baum, C. M. (1986). OASIS: A new concept for promoting the quality of life for older adults. *American Journal of Occupational Therapy, 40*(11), 784–786.

Baum, C. M. (1985). The evolution of the United Health Care System. In *Management for occupational therapists* (pp. 3–25). Rockville, MD: American Occupational Therapy Association.

Baum, C. M. (1985). Growth, renewal, and challenge: An important era for occupational therapy. *American Journal of Occupational Therapy, 39*(12), 778–784.

Baum, C. M., & Luebben, A. J. (1985). Assessing community resources to support independent living. In M. Kirkland & S. Robertson (Eds.), *Planning and implementing vocational readiness in occupational therapy* (pp. 95–98). Rockville, MD: American Occupational Therapy Association.

Hunt-Fine, L., Baum, C. M., & Lottes, L. M. (1985). Institutional settings for geriatric occupational treatment practice. In S. Robertson & M. Kirkland (Eds.), *Role of occupational therapy and the elderly* (pp. 139–144). Rockville, MD: American Occupational Therapy Association.

Luebben, A. J., & Baum, C. M. (1985). Systems skills assessment. In M. Kirkland & S. Robertson. (Eds.), *Planning and implementing vocational readiness in occupational therapy.* Rockville, MD: American Occupational Therapy Association.

Baum, C. M., Boyle, M. A., & Edwards D. (1984). Initiating occupational therapy clinical research. *American Journal of Occupational Therapy, 38*(4), 267–269.

Baum, C. M. (1983). A look at our strength in the 80's. *American Journal of Occupational Therapy, 37*(7), 451–455.

Baum, C. M. (1983). Management of finances, communications, personnel with resources, and documentation. In H. Hopkins & H. Smith (Eds.), *Willard and Spackman's occupational therapy* (6th ed., pp. 815–825). Philadelphia: J. B. Lippincott.

Baum, C. M. (1983). Strategic integrated management system. *American Journal of Occupational Therapy, 37*(9), 595–600.

Baum, C. M., & Devereaux, E. (1983). Systems perspective: Conceptualizing and implementing occupational therapy in today's complex environment. In H. Hopkins & H. Smith (Eds.), *Willard and Spackman's occupational therapy* (6th ed., pp. 799–814). Philadelphia: J. B. Lippincott.

Baum C. M. (1982). Deregulation—Regulations of special interest to occupational therapists. *American Journal of Occupational Therapy, 36*(10), 633–635.

Baum, C. M. (1982). Opportunity for occupational therapy: The time is now. *American Journal of Occupational Therapy, 36*(6), 363–365.

Baum, C. M. (1982). A perspective of occupational therapy in the U.S. Health system. In *Proceedings of the 8th International Congress World Federation of Occupational Therapists,* Hamburg, Federal Republic of Germany.

Baum, C. M. (1981). The advocacy report: Section IV. *Occupational Therapy News, 35*(1), 23.

Baum, C. M. (1980). Independent living: A critical role for occupational therapists. *American Journal of Occupational Therapy, 34*(12), 773–774.

Baum, C. M. (1980). Occupational therapists put care in the health system (1980 Eleanor Clarke Slagle Lecture). *American Journal of Occupational Therapy, 34*(8), 505–516.

Baum, C. M. (1978). Management and documentation of occupational therapy services. In H. Smith & H. Hopkins (Eds.), *Willard and Spackman's occupational therapy* (5th ed.). Philadelphia: J. B. Lippincott.

Baum, C. M. (1978). *Third-party reimbursement manual.* Rockville, MD: American Occupational Therapy Association.

Baum, C. M. (1972). A management tool: The department audit. *American Journal of Occupational Therapy, 26,* 299–301.

Robert Kendall Bing, EdD, OTR, FAOTA—1981

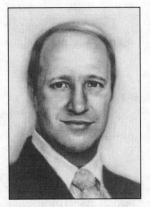

Robert Kendall Bing was professor and dean emeritus, School of Allied Health Sciences, University of Texas Medical Branch (UTMB), Galveston. He was born March 2, 1929. His parents, Kenneth L. and Ruth T. Bing, were school teachers in Cambridge, Nebraska. He grew up in North Carolina, Minnesota, Georgia, and Missouri and graduated from Central High School, Cape Girardeau, Missouri.

He began his college studies at Southeast Missouri State University and then transferred to the University of Illinois College of Medicine to complete his degree in occupational therapy under the direction of his mentor, Beatrice Wade. Following military service, Bing matriculated at the Institute for Child Study, University of Maryland, College Park, and received an MA and an EdD. He was a member of Phi Kappa Pi honorary fraternity.

Bing joined the faculty and staff of the School of Allied Health Sciences, UTMB, in 1966 and became the founding dean of the School of Allied Health Sciences in 1968. He remained in this position until late 1980, when he stepped down to return to his first loves, teaching and research. Subsequently, Bing left Galveston and taught for a brief period at Elizabethtown College in Pennsylvania, then retired to Galveston in 1987. He remained active as visiting professor, Occupational Therapy, University of South Dakota for several years and wrote chapters for various texts. He retained his extensive interests in history, particularly in medicine and health care.

During his extensive career he practiced in Virginia, Connecticut, Illinois, and Texas. He held academic appointments at Virginia Commonwealth University; Towson State University; the Universities of Nebraska, Florida, and Illinois Colleges of Medicine; and the University of Texas Medical Branch at Galveston. He was visiting professor at the University of Western Australia in 1979.

Bing was very active in professional organizations, serving as president of two state societies, as member or chair of numerous national committees and councils, and as AOTA president. Awards include AOTA's Roster of Fellows and Award of Merit. He also was named Honorary Citizen of Hidalgo for his volunteer work in the Lower Rio Grande Valley, Texas, in 1977; received the Outstanding Alum Award in 1987 from the College of Applied Health Sciences, University of Illinois at Chicago; and was named an Unsung Hero by the *Galveston County Daily News* in 1991. During his retirement, he served as an active volunteer with the AIDS Coalition of Coastal Texas.

Bing died May 15, 2003, at the age of 75, at his home in Galveston, after a lingering illness. He dedicated his lifetime of service toward advancing the profession, which he so dearly loved. Bing generously shared his wisdom, leadership, and personal integrity in promoting the highest standards of education and research as well as developing future leaders of the profession. His legacy to occupational therapy will never be forgotten. The Wilma L. West Library and the AOTA archives are the grateful recipients of most of Bing's collection of professional papers, photographs, and books. They will provide invaluable resources to affirm the history of occupational therapy and support the continuation of its scholarship.

Bibliography

Bing, R. K. (1961). *William Rush Dunton, Jr.—American psychiatrist: A study in self.* Baltimore: University of Maryland.

Bing, R. K. (1967). William Rush Dunton, Jr.: American psychiatrist and occupational therapist, 1868–1966. *American Journal of Occupational Therapy, 21,* 172–175.

Offenkrantz, W., Bing, R. K., Buckley, C., Hayes, H., Kelley, J., King, J., et al. (1967). A psychiatrically oriented case conference for occupational therapy students. *American Journal of Occupational Therapy, 21,* 70–75.

Bing, R. K. (1968). Discussion: Recapitulation of ontogenesis: A theory of practice of occupational therapy. *American Journal of Occupational Therapy, 22,* 433–435.

Bing, R. K. (1969). Requisites for relevance: Changing concepts in occupational therapy education. *Annals of the New York Academy of Science, 166,* 1020–1026.

Bing, R. K. (1981). Occupational therapy revisited: A paraphrastic journey (1981 Eleanor Clarke Slagle Lecture). *American Journal of Occupational Therapy, 35,* 499–518.

Bing, R. K. (1983). Nationally Speaking: Beliefs at a new beginning. *American Journal of Occupational Therapy, 37,* 376–379.

Bing, R. K. (1983). Nationally Speaking: The industry, the art, and the philosophy of history. *American Journal of Occupational Therapy, 37,* 800–801.

Bing, R. K. (1983). Nationally Speaking: Professional nationalism. *American Journal of Occupational Therapy, 37,* 301–304.

Bing, R. K. (1984). Living forward, understanding backward, part 1. *American Journal of Occupational Therapy, 38,* 363–366.

Bing, R. K. (1984). Living forward, understanding backward, part 2. *American Journal of Occupational Therapy, 38*, 425–439.

Bing, R. K. (1984). Nationally Speaking: To survive, to become: Our way of life. *American Journal of Occupational Therapy, 38*, 785–798.

Bing, R. K. (1985). Nationally Speaking: On getting from here to there to anywhere. *American Journal of Occupational Therapy, 39*, 771–776.

Bing, R. K. (1986). The American Occupational Therapy Association Inc. viewpoint. *Pediatrics, 78*, 184–186.

Bing, R. K. (1986). Nationally Speaking: The subject is health: Not of facts but of values. *American Journal of Occupational Therapy, 40*, 667–671.

Bing, R. K. (1986). Report to members. *Occupational Therapy News, 40*(6), 4.

Bing, R. K. (1987). Who originated the term occupational therapy? *American Journal of Occupational Therapy, 41*, 192–194.

Bing, R. K. (1992). Point of departure (A play about founding the profession). *American Journal of Occupational Therapy, 46*, 27–32.

Bing, R. K. (1997). Looking back: "And teach the agony to sing": An afternoon with Eleanor Clarke Slagle. *American Journal of Occupational Therapy, 51*, 220–227.

Ruth Brunyate Wiemer, MEd, OTR, FAOTA—1957

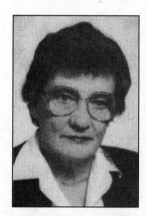

Ruth Brunyate Wiemer received a bachelor's degree in sociology from Hollins College in 1938, a certificate from the Philadelphia School of Occupational Therapy in 1940, and a master's degree in education from John Hopkins University in Baltimore in 1967. She was awarded an LHD by Towson State University in 1980.

Brunyate worked with Dr. Winthrop M. Phelps doing pioneering work in cerebral palsy at the Children's Rehabilitation Institute in Maryland from 1941 to 1961. She held various positions, including staff therapist, director of occupational therapy services, administrative assistant to the executive director, and acting executive director in 1957. Brunyate became assistant professor and acting director of the Department of Occupational Therapy at Milwaukee Downer College in 1961.

Brunyate joined the Maryland State Department of Health as a consultant in 1962 and was named chief of the Division of Occupational Therapy in 1966. She continued as chief when the agency became the Department of Health and Mental Hygiene in 1970. She retired in 1980 and lives on Maryland's Eastern Shore.

She held many appointed and elected positions in the Maryland Occupational Therapy Association, including the presidency. Brunyate was the first elected AOTA president, serving from 1961 to 1966. As chair of the Legislation Committee, she provided the impetus for establishment of the AOTA Government Affairs Division. She was an incorporator and board member of the American Occupational Therapy Foundation and served on its Research Development Committee.

Brunyate was honored numerous times throughout her career. She received the AOTA Award of Merit; the Roster of Fellows Award; a Certificate of Appreciation of the Commission on Education; the Lindy Boggs Award; the Maryland Occupational Therapy Association Roster of Merit and Presidential Commendation Award; the Community College of Baltimore's Brunyate Lectureship; the University of Texas School of Allied Health Sciences Class Dedication; Who's Who in America; Who's Who in American Women; Who's Who in Health Care; the State of Maryland Governor's Citation; and the Department of Health and Mental Hygiene Certificate of Appreciation. In 1996, Brunyate received the Wilma L. West Presidential Commendation for her 57 years of service to the profession. After Brunyate's friend West died in 1996, Brunyate said she had decided, "Never could I come to a conference without her. But how could I resist something like this [award]." She died in June 2008.

Bibliography

Editor's note: *Bibliographical information appears as indexed with alternative author names "Brunyate, R. W." or "Wiemer, R. B."*

Brunyate, R. W. (1946). Occupational therapy in cerebral palsy clinics. *Canadian Journal of Occupational Therapy, 13*, 27, 33.

Brunyate, R. W. (1947). Occupational therapy for patients with cerebral palsy. In H. Willard & C. Spackman (Eds.), *Principles of occupational therapy* (pp. 274–287). Philadelphia: Lippincott.

Brunyate, R. W. (1949). Occupational therapy means freedom for parents. *Crippled Child, 26*, 11.

Brunyate, R. W., & Phelps, W. M. (1950). Occupational therapy in the treatment of cerebral palsy. In W. Dunton & S. Licht (Eds.), *Occupational therapy principles and practice*. Springfield, IL: Charles C Thomas.

Brunyate, R. W. (1951). People you should know: Mrs. Elizabeth Martin Wagner, OTR; Beatrice D. Wade: A biographical sketch. *American Journal of Occupational Therapy, 5*, 213–214.

Brunyate, R. W. (1952). The importance of pre-skill activities in occupational therapy for the cerebral palsied. In *Proceedings of the Second Cerebral Palsy Institute*. New York: Coordinating Council for Cerebral Palsy.

Brunyate, R. W. (1952). The featured occupational therapy department. *American Journal of Occupational Therapy, 5,* 219–221.

Brunyate, R. W. (1954). Occupational therapy for patients with cerebral palsy. In H. Willard & C. Spackman (Eds.), *Principles of occupational therapy* (2nd ed., pp. 301–329). Philadelphia: Lippincott.

Brunyate, R. W. (1954). A study of the use of magnetic toys in the treatment of cerebral palsied children. *American Journal of Occupational Therapy, 8,* 151.

Brunyate, R. W., & Phelps, W. M. (1957). Occupational therapy in the treatment of cerebral palsy. In W. Dunton & S. Licht (Eds.), *Occupational therapy principles and practice* (2nd ed., pp. 173–187). Springfield, IL: Charles C Thomas.

Brunyate, R. W. (1958). Powerful levers in little common things (1957 Eleanor Clarke Slagle Lecture). *American Journal of Occupational Therapy, 12,* 193–202.

Brunyate, R. W. (1962). The clinical center: An integral part of the education program. *American Journal of Occupational Therapy, 16,* 61–65.

Brunyate, R. W. (1962). Graphs: Their value as a record form in the management of the cerebral palsied. *American Journal of Occupational Therapy, 16,* 13–21.

Brunyate, R. W. (1963). Occupational therapy for patients with cerebral palsy. In H. Willard & C. Spackman (Eds.), *Principles of occupational therapy* (3rd ed., pp. 264–307). Philadelphia: Lippincott.

Brunyate, R. W. (1963). The student in pre-clinical education: Impressions of a clinically-oriented therapists. *American Journal of Occupational Therapy, 17,* 181–186.

Brunyate, R. W. (1964). Nationally Speaking: From the president elect. *American Journal of Occupational Therapy, 18,* 69.

Brunyate, R. W. (1966). Keynote address. *American Journal of Occupational Therapy, 20,* 9–16.

Brunyate, R. W. (1967). After fifty years, what stature do we hold? *American Journal of Occupational Therapy, 21,* 262–267.

Brunyate, R. W. (1967). Nationally Speaking: From the president, Ruth W. Brunyate. *American Journal of Occupational Therapy, 21,* 54–55.

Brunyate, R. W. (1967). Nationally Speaking: From the president, Ruth W. Brunyate: A modification of role for nursing home service. *American Journal of Occupational Therapy, 21,* 126–127.

Cromwell, F., & Brunyate, R. W. (1968). Nationally Speaking: The newest of our member categories: The COTA. *American Journal of Occupational Therapy, 22,* 377–379.

Brunyate, R. W. (1969). Nationally speaking. *American Journal of Occupational Therapy, 23,* 209–212.

Cromwell, F., & Brunyate, R. W. (1970). Nationally speaking. *American Journal of Occupational Therapy, 24,* 89–90.

Wiemer, R. B., & West, W. L. (1970). Occupational therapy in community health care. *American Journal of Occupational, Therapy 24,* 323–328.

Wiemer, R. B. (1972). Nationally Speaking: What is National Health Council? Is AOTA's membership in it worthy of budget priority? *American Journal of Occupational Therapy, 26,* 3A–4A.

Wiemer, R. B. (1972). Some concepts of prevention as an aspect of community health: A foundation for development of the occupational therapist's role. *American Journal of Occupational Therapy, 26,* 1.

Clarke, D., Cromwell, F. S., Fanning, L., Fidler, G., Gillette, N., Hightower, M., Hill, M., Nathan, C., Spelbring, L., Ward, J., Wiemer, R. B., & Johnson, J. A. (1974). Association report I: Task force on target populations. *American Journal of Occupational Therapy, 28,* 158–163.

Brunyate, R. W. (1979). Traditional and nontraditional practice areas. In American Occupational Therapy Association (Ed.), *Occupational therapy: 2001 AD*. Rockville, MD: Editor.

Brunyate, R. W. (1984). Student transition from academics to fieldwork. In American Occupational Therapy Association (Ed.), *Fieldwork manual*. Rockville, MD: Editor.

West, W., & Wiemer, R. B. (1991). The Issue Is: Should the Representative Assembly have voted as it did, when it did, on occupational therapists' use of physical agent modalities? *American Journal of Occupational Therapy, 45,* 1143–1147.

Janice Posatery Burke, PhD, OTR/L, FAOTA—2010

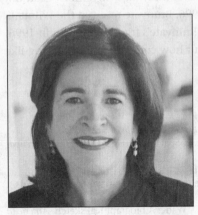

Janice Posatery Burke's rich and productive academic, research, and clinical career includes substantial service to the community, teaching, collaboration on research and theory projects, and occupational assessment and intervention with patients and their families. She is Professor and Chair in the Department of Occupational Therapy and Founding Dean of the Jefferson School of Health Professions at Thomas Jefferson University (TJU) in Philadelphia.

At TJU, Burke also serves as Executive Director of Jefferson Elder Care (JEC), a nationally recognized program offering evidenced-based occupational therapy service to older adults and their caregivers. To build the workforce to meet the health and wellness challenges of the older adult population, JEC trains occupational therapists to use evidenced-based techniques to address the needs of older adults with dementia, including providing a program of Skills2Care, home safety, and dementia services. JEC also provides interdisciplinary educational support to the families and the health professionals who serve them.

Burke has received training funds from federal, state, and local agencies, including the U.S. Department of Education, for more than 15 years. With this support she has implemented a variety of specialty practice projects housed in both community and regional health facilities. These training activities are designed to prepare occupational therapists for positions in early intervention and school-based settings.

A member of the first graduating class of occupational therapists at Utica College of Syracuse University, Burke later entered the profession at Burke Rehabilitation Center in White Plains, New York, and has maintained an active clinical practice since that time. She attended the University of Southern California (USC), where she received certification from the Andrus Gerontology Center and obtained a master's degree in occupational therapy. At USC she studied under Mary Reilly, which proved an important turning point for Burke. The critical skills learned while under the guidance of Reilly helped prepare Burke for the theoretical and analytic work that is the cornerstone of her career and her contribution to the field.

Burke's research activities began with her master's thesis that looked issues related to personal causation, locus of control, and social role. Her early theoretical work built on that of Reilly and was published in seminal papers that defined the Model of Human Occupation. Her love of the profession and interest in the history of occupational therapy, nurtured by Reilly and Florence Cromwell, manifested itself when she coauthored a paper documenting the founding of the profession.

Although imbued with a strong theoretical interest, research, and curiosity, Burke was never far from the clinical practice that centered her activities as a professional and is the bedrock of her theoretical work and research. She has developed and implemented community and school-based services, as well as has provided consultations and individualized therapy since 1975 when she was appointed Director of Training in Occupational Therapy at the University Affiliated Program (UAP) at Children's Hospital of Los Angeles (CHLA). The time spent working as a member of an interdisciplinary team at the nationally recognized regional clinical center helped solidify both her high standards for excellence and primary clinical interest in serving children with developmental, learning, and sensory integration problems and their families. After leaving CHLA in 1983, she received advanced training in sensory integration while under the supervision of A. Jean Ayres and was cofounder of Therapy West, a private practice centered in Culver City, California.

Burke moved to Pennsylvania in 1988 to join the faculty at Thomas Jefferson University (TJU). She continued both her clinical and academic activities by working with students at TJU, with individuals and their families in private practice, and in clinical settings at Children's Hospital of Philadelphia and the Children's Seashore House. She soon entered the University of Pennsylvania as a doctoral student and was awarded her PhD after researching and writing a dissertation on frames of meaning. Her research has focused on education, culture, and society and her qualitative research methodology on the interaction that occurs inside the therapy space.

Burke has continued to see patients and families during her academic career spanning nearly a quarter-century. Recently, she consulted and participated in research projects that address issues of traumatic brain injury in adults, Alzheimer's disease, and related dementia, particularly how these conditions affect older adults and their caregivers. Today she maintains a strong involvement in research related to occupational therapy. This interest is reflected in the 2010 Slagle lecture. Her current research and theory projects include the study of both verbal and nonverbal behaviors that occur during therapist, parent, and child assessment interactions. Her curiosity and drive to understand the particular therapeutic intervention and success of occupational therapy connects her divergent interests in gerontology and children. This line of research has matured since her days in Los Angeles. Her long-term and diverse experience has helped her as she works to develop a unified model of practice that brings relevancy and success to contemporary occupational therapy primed for the changing health care environment of the 21st century.

Burke has served as a Director on the American Occupational Therapy Association (AOTA) Board of Directors and is an AOTA Fellow. She has served as a board member of the American Occupational Therapy Foundation (AOTF) and is a well-known and respected national and international scholar and lecturer. She is an active member of her local community, having served on the board of her township library, as a member of the Parent–Teacher Organization, and as a therapist serving children and their families in various surrounding school districts. She is the recipient of numerous awards from local, state, and national organizations, including the A. Jean Ayres Award from AOTF, the Burlington Resources Foundation Faculty Achievement Award and the Lindback Award for Distinguished Teaching from TJU, and the Pennsylvania Occupational Therapy Association Award for Outstanding Achievement.

Linking Key Messages of the 2010 Eleanor Clarke Slagle Lecture to the AOTA *Centennial Vision:* The *Centennial Vision* for occupational therapy excites my curiosity and provides rich and fertile ground filled with opportunities to work with many entities, including (1) students in the class and in the community; (2) children and their families with individualize care; and (3) older adults with dementia in clinical evaluation, treatment, and research. In addition, I am inspired to collaborate with researchers and therapists to better understand sensory integration, develop evidenced-based interventions for individuals with Alzheimer's disease and their caregivers, and bring the uncommon perspective of occupational therapy to decipher the divergent needs of a various patient populations all seen within the therapeutic space of the working occupational therapist.

—Janice Posatery Burke

Bibliography

Black, H. K., Gitlin, L. N., & Burke, J. P. (2010). Context and culture: African American elders' experiences of depression. *Mental Health, Religion, and Culture.* DOI: 10.1080/13674676.2010.505233

Burke, J. P. (2010). What's going on here? Deconstructing the interactive encounter (2010 Eleanor Clark Slagle Lecture). *American Journal of Occupational Therapy, 64*(6), 216–227.

Collins, L., Schimmer, A., Diamond, J., & Burke, J. P. (2010). Evaluating verbal and non-verbal communication skills in an ethnogeriatric OSCE. *Patient Education and Counseling.*

Schaaf, R. C., Benevides, T., Blanche, E., Brett-Green, B. E., Burke, J. P., Cohn, E., et al. (2010). Parasympathetic function in children with sensory processing disorder. *Frontiers in Neuroscience, 4*(4), 1–11.

Gitlin, L. N., Winter, L., Vause-Earland, T., Herge, E. A., Chernett, N., Piersol, C. V., & Burke, J. P. (2009). Practice Concepts—The Tailored Activity Program (TAP) to reduce behavioral symptoms in individuals with dementia: Feasibility, acceptability, and replication potential. *The Gerontologist,* doi: 10.1093/geront/gnp087

Stineman, M., Rist, P., & Burke, J. P. (2009). Through the clinicians' lens: Objective and subjective views of disability. *Qualitative Health Research, 19*(1), 17–29.

Burke, J. P., & Schaaf, R. (2008). Family narratives and play assessment. In L. D. Parham & L. Fazio (Eds.), *Play in occupational therapy for children* (2nd ed., 195–215). St. Louis, MO: Mosby.

Gitlin, L. N., Winter, L., Burke, J. P., Chernett, N., Dennis, M. P., & Hauck, W. W. (2008). Tailored activities to manage neuropsychiatric behaviors in persons with dementia and reduce caregiver burden: A randomized pilot study. *American Journal Geriatric Psychiatry, 16,* 229–239.

Kurz, A. E., Saint-Louis, N., Stineman, M., & Burke, J. (2008). Exploring the personal reality of disability and recovery: A tool for empowering the rehabilitation process. *Qualitative Health Research, 18*(1), 90–105.

Mailloux, Z., & Burke, J. P. (2008). Play and the sensory integrative approach. In L. D. Parham & L. Fazio (Eds.), *Play in occupational therapy for children* (2nd ed., 263–278). St. Louis: Mosby.

Mailloux, Z., May-Benson, T., Summers, C., Miller, L. J., Brett-Green, B., Burke, J. P., et al. (2007). The Issue Is—Goal Attainment Scaling as a measure of meaningful outcomes for children with sensory integration dysfunction. *American Journal of Occupational Therapy, 61*(2), 254–259.

Parham, L. D., Cohn, E., Spitzer, S., Koomar, J., Miller, L. J., Burke, J. P., et al.. (2007). Fidelity in sensory integration intervention research. *American Journal of Occupational Therapy, 61*(2), 216–227.

Burke, J. P. (2006). Foreword. In S. Smith-Roley, & R. C. Schaaf (Eds.), *Workbook for understanding the nature of sensory integration with diverse populations.* Tucson, AZ: PsychCorp.

Kurz, A. E., Saint-Louis, N., Stineman, M., & Burke, J. (2006). Exploring the personal reality of disability and recovery: A tool for empowering the rehabilitation process. *Archives of Physical Medicine and Rehabilitation, 87*(10), E1–E33.

Burke, J. P., & Lomba, T. B. (2005). Measurement of occupational performance. In M. Law, C. Baum, & W. Dunn (Eds.), *Occupational therapy outcomes: Assessing occupational performance* (2nd ed.). Thorofare, NJ: Slack.

Roley, S. S., Burke, J. P., Cohn, E., Koomar, J., Miller, L. J., Schaaf, R., et al. (2005). A strategic plan for research in a clinical profession. *Sensory Integration Special Interest Section Quarterly, 28*(2), 1–3.

Schaaf, R. C., & Burke, J. P. (2004). Program of research in occupational therapy and sensory integration. *Sensory Integration Special Interest Section Quarterly, 27*(4), 3, 6.

Burke, J. P. (2003). Philosophical basis of human occupation. In P. Kramer, J. Hinojosa, & C. Brasic Royeen (Eds.), *Perspectives in human occupation* (pp. 32–44). Philadelphia: Lippincott Williams & Wilkins.

Burke, J. P. (2001). Clinical reasoning and the use of narrative in sensory integration assessment and treatment. In S. Smith-Roley, E. Blanche, & R. C. Schaaf (Eds.), *Understanding the nature of sensory integration with diverse populations* (pp. 203–214). Tucson, AZ: PsychCorp.

Burke, J. P. (2001). How therapists' conceptual perspectives influence early intervention evaluations. *Scandinavian Journal of Occupational Therapy, 8*(1), 49–61.

Burke, J. P. (2000). Measurement of occupational performance. In M. Law, C. Baum, & W. Dunn (Eds.), *Occupational therapy outcomes: Assessing occupational performance* (pp. 195–202). Thorofare, NJ: Slack.

Burke, J. P. (1999). Foreword. In S. Miller Porr & E. Berger Rainville (Eds.), *Pediatric therapy: A systems approach.* Philadelphia: F. A. Davis.

Burke, J. P. (1998). Clinical interpretation of "Health and the Human Spirit for Occupation." *American Journal of Occupational Therapy, 52*(6), 419–422.

Burke, J. P. (1998). Play—The life role of the infant and young child. In J. Case-Smith (Ed.), *Pediatric occupational therapy and early intervention* (2nd ed., pp. 189–205). Boston: Butterworth-Heinemann.

Burke, J. P., & Schaaf, R. (1997). Family narratives and play assessment. In L. D. Parham & L. Fazio (Eds.), *Play: A clinical focus in occupational therapy for children* (pp. 67–84). St. Louis, MO: Mosby.

Mailloux, Z., & Burke, J. P. (1997). Play in conjunction with sensory integrative procedures. In L. D. Parham & L. Fazio (Eds.), *Play: A clinical focus in occupational therapy for children* (pp. 112–125). St. Louis, MO: Mosby.

Schaaf, R., & Burke, J. P. (1997). What happens when we play? A neurodevelopmental explanation. In B. Chandler (Ed.), *The essence of play: A child's occupation* (pp. 79–105). Bethesda, MD: American Occupational Therapy Association.

Burke, J. P. (1996). Fundamental concepts of mental health practice. In M. Brinson & K. Kannenberg (Eds.), *Mental health service delivery guidelines* (pp. 3–8). Bethesda, MD: American Occupational Therapy Association.

Burke, J. P. (1996). Moving occupation into treatment: Clinical interpretation of legitimizing occupational therapy's knowledge. *American Journal of Occupational Therapy, 50*(8), 635–638.

Burke, J. P. (1996). Variations in childhood occupations: Play in the presence of chronic disability. In R. Zemke & F. Clark (Eds.), *Occupational science: The evolving discipline* (pp. 413–418). Philadelphia: F. A. Davis.

Burke, J. P. (1996, September). Videotape reviews. *Developmental Disabilities Special Interest Section Newsletter,* pp. 3, 4.

Burke, J. P., & Kern, S. B. (1996). The Issue Is—Is the use of life history and narrative in clinical practice reimbursable: Is it occupational therapy? *American Journal of Occupational Therapy, 50*(5), 389–392.

Hanft, B., Swenson-Miller, K., & Burke, J. P. (1996). Interdisciplinary training of occupational therapists working with infants and young children and their families. In D. Bricker & A. Widerstrom (Eds.), *Preparing personnel to work with infants and young children and their families* (pp. 115–134). Baltimore: Paul H. Brookes.

Burke, J. P. (1996). Foreword. In B. Cortellini Benamy (Ed.), *Developing clinical reasoning skills: Strategies for the occupational therapist* (pp. ix–x). San Antonio, TX: Therapy Skill Builders.

Kielhofner, G., Borell, L., Burke, J. P., Helfrich, C., & Nygard, L. (1995). Volition subsystem. In G. Kielhofner (Ed.), *A model of human occupation* (2nd ed., pp. 39–62). Philadelphia: Williams & Wilkins.

Schaaf, R., Swenson-Miller, K., & Burke, J. P. (1995). A collaborative approach to meeting the need for quality personnel training in early intervention. *Occupational Therapy in Health Care, 9*(2/3), 51–72.

Burke, J. P. (1993). Play—The life role of the infant and young child. In J. Case-Smith (Ed.), *Pediatric occupational therapy and early intervention* (pp. 198–224). Andover, MA: Andover Medical.

DePoy, E., & Burke, J. P. (1992). The Model of Human Occupation approach to cognition. In N. Katz (Ed.), *Cognitive rehabilitation: Models for occupational therapy* (pp. 240–257). Andover, MA: Andover Medical.

DePoy, E., Burke, J. P., & Sherwen, L. (1992). Training trainers: Evaluating services provided to children with HIV and their families. *Research on Social Work Practice, 2*(1), 39–55.

Hanft, B., Burke, J. P., Cahill, M., Swenson-Miller, K., & Humphry, R. (1992). *Working with families: A curriculum guide for pediatric occupational therapists.* Chapel Hill: Carolina Institute for Research on Infant Personnel Preparation.

Schaaf, R., & Burke, J. P. (1992). Clinical reflections on play and sensory integration. *Sensory Integration Special Interest Section Newsletter, 15*(1), 1.

Blanche, E., & Burke, J. P. (1991). Combining neurodevelopmental and sensory integration approaches in the treatment of the neurologically impaired child, Part I. *Sensory Integration Quarterly, 19*(1), 1–5.

Blanche, E., & Burke, J. P. (1991). Combining neurodevelopmental and sensory integration approaches in the treatment of the neurologically impaired child, Part II. *Sensory Integration Quarterly, 19*(2), 1–6.

Burke, J. P., & Cassidy, J. (1991). Disparity between reimbursement-driven practice and humanistic values in OT. *American Journal of Occupational Therapy, 45*(2), 173–176.

Burke, J. P., & DePoy, E. (1991). An emerging view of mastery, excellence, and leadership in occupational therapy practice. *American Journal of Occupational Therapy, 45*(11), 1027–1032.

Burke, J. P. (1989). Private practice in pediatric occupational therapy. In P. Pratt & A. Allen, (Eds.), *Occupational therapy for children: A pediatric text* (2nd ed., pp. 612–622). St. Louis, MO: Mosby.

Burke, J. P., & King-Thomas, L. (1989). The environment of the child: Assessment considerations, treatment/intervention implications. In *The AOTA Practice Symposium.* Rockville, MD: American Occupational Therapy Association.

Hamilton-Dodd, C., Kawamoto, T., Clark, F., Burke, J. P., & Fanchiang, S. (1989).The effects of an occupational therapy maternal role preparation program on mother–infant pairs: A pilot study. *American Journal of Occupational Therapy, 43*(8), 513–521.

Burke, J. P. (1988). Commentary—Combining the Model of Human Occupation with cognitive disability theory. *Occupational Therapy in Mental Health, 8*(1), xi–xiii.

Burke, J. P., Clark, F., Hamilton-Dodd, C., & Kawamoto, T. (1987). Maternal role preparation: A program using sensory integration, infant–mother attachment, and occupational behavior perspectives. *Occupational Therapy in Health Care, 4*(2), 9–22.

Burke, J. P. (1986). Theory development. In S. Vulpe (Ed.), *Proceedings of the Occupational Therapy for Maternal and Child Health Conference* (vol. 1). Los Angeles: Children's Hospital of Los Angeles, Center for Child Development.

Burke, J. P., & Kielhofner, G. (1985). Human occupation: Its components and determinants. In G. Kielhofner (Ed.), *Model of Human Occupation: Application of a conceptual approach* (pp. 12–36). Philadelphia: Williams & Wilkins.

Mailloux, Z., Knox, S., Burke, J. P., & Clark, F. (1985). Pediatric dysfunction. In G. Kielhofner (Ed.), *Model of Human Occupation: Application of a conceptual approach* (pp. 306–351). Philadelphia: Williams & Wilkins.

Burke, J. P. (1984). Occupational therapy: A focus for roles in practice. *American Journal of Occupational Therapy, 38*(1), 24–28.

Burke, J. P. (1984). Occupational therapy in health care: A perspective for our future. *Occupational Therapy in Health Care, 1*(1), 7–15.

Burke, J. P, Goldstein, N., & Skillman, A. (1984). Reviews from Superfest XII: A film festival on the exceptional individual. *Paedovita, 1.*

Burke, J. P. (1983). Defining occupation: Importing and organizing interdisciplinary knowledge. In G. Kielhofner (Ed.), *Health through occupation: A theory of practice* (pp. 125–138). Philadelphia: F. A. Davis.

Burke, J. P. (1983). *Readings for occupational therapists working in developmental disabilities* [Training Manual]. Los Angeles: University Affiliated Program.

Burke, J. P., Miyake, S., Kielhofner, G., & Barris, R.(1983). The demystification of health care and demise of the sick role: Implications for occupational therapy. In G. Kielhofner (Ed.), *Health Through occupation: A theory of practice* (pp. 197–210). Philadelphia: F. A. Davis.

Kielhofner, G., & Burke, J. P. (1983). The evolution of knowledge and practice in occupational therapy. In G. Kielhofner (Ed.), *Health through occupation: A theory of practice* (pp. 3–54). Philadelphia: F. A. Davis.

Parham, D., Burke, J. P., Clark, F., & Mack, W. (1983). *The theoretical roots of practice and research* [Training Manual]. Rockville, MD: American Occupational Therapy Foundation.

Burke, J. P. (1982). *Positioning and facilitation techniques for feeding self-instruction package* [Training Manual]. Los Angeles: University Affiliated Program.

Burke, J. P., Poulsen, M., & Rice, B. (Series Eds.). (1982). *School Nurse Self-Instruction Package* [Training Manual]. Los Angeles: University Affiliated Program.

Kielhofner, G., & Burke, J. P. (1980). A Model of Human Occupation, Part I. Conceptual framework and content. *American Journal of Occupational Therapy, 34*(9), 572–581.

Kielhofner, G., Burke, J. P., & Heard-Igi, C. (1980). A Model of Human Occupation, Part IV. Assessment and intervention. *American Journal of Occupational Therapy. 34*(12), 777–788.

Kielhofner, G., & Burke, J. P. (1977). Occupational therapy after sixty years: An account of changing identity and knowledge. *American Journal of Occupational Therapy, 31*(11), 675–689.

Burke, J. P. (1977). A clinical perspective on motivation: Pawn versus origin. *American Journal of Occupational Therapy, 31*(4), 254–258.

Burke, J. P. (1975). The need for ongoing evaluation in the handicapped individual. In *Mental Retardation Services Today and Tomorrow Conference Proceedings,* Los Angeles.

Charles H. Christiansen, EdD, OTR/L, FAOTA—1999

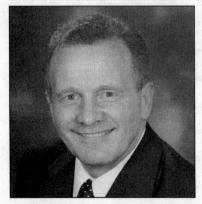

Charles H. Christiansen is executive director of the American Occupational Therapy Foundation (AOTF) in Bethesda, Maryland. Prior to his current position, he served as vice provost of health sciences and founding director of the Center for Allied Health Programs at the University of Minnesota. Earlier, and for nearly 14 years, he served as university chief academic officer, dean, and George T. Bryan Distinguished Professor in the College of Health Professions at the University of Texas Medical Branch (UTMB). He has also held administrative and academic appointments at the University of British Columbia, at the University of Texas Health Science Center at San Antonio, and at Texas Woman's University.

Christiansen was born in Panama and schooled in the United States and abroad. During his youth, he graduated from high school in Germany and returned to the United States to earn an undergraduate degree in occupational therapy at the School of Medicine, University of North Dakota. He later earned a master's degree in counseling psychology from Ball State University and a doctorate in educational administration from the University of Houston. He completed a post-doctoral administrative residency through Baylor College of Medicine in Houston.

Christiansen is an elected member of several honorary and professional societies, including Pi Theta Epsilon, Phi Kappa Phi, Sigma Xi, the American Congress of Rehabilitation Medicine, the Human Factors Society, and the Society for the Study of Occupation: USA (SSO:USA), and several international organizations, including the International Society on Quality of Life Studies. He has served as the vice president and treasurer of the American Occupational Therapy Association (AOTA) and as a board member for the SSO:USA and for the Texas Society of Allied Health Professions. He is a founding member of the International Society for Occupational Science.

Christiansen is the recipient of numerous awards, including selection as Occupational Therapist of the Year in 1984 by the Texas Occupational Therapy Association; recipient of the Ruth Zemke Lecture in Occupational Science in 2006; and recipient of the Eleanor Clarke Slagle Lectureship Award by AOTA in 1998, the association's highest academic honor. In 1997, he was presented with the Leone Award for Administrative Excellence and is the inaugural holder of the first endowed distinguished professorship established in the School of Health Professions at UTMB. Christiansen was appointed an honorary (adjunct) professor in the School of Health and Rehabilitation at the University of Queensland, Brisbane, Australia, and was honored as an outstanding alumnus of the University of North Dakota during its centennial homecoming celebrations in 2005.

Christiansen is the founding editor of the journal *OTJR: Occupation, Participation and Health* (now in its 28th year) and is senior editor and contributor to three major textbooks: *Occupational Therapy: Enabling Function and Well-Being; Ways of Living: Adaptive Strategies for Special Needs;* and *Introduction to Occupation: The Art and Science of Living.* He is coeditor of *Life Balance: Multidisciplinary Theories and Research.* He has been a consulting editor or content expert for the past six editions of *Taber's Cyclopedic Medical Dictionary* and has published over 100 articles, chapters, editorials, and abstracts in scholarly books and journals. He is a frequent international speaker who resides in Rockville, Maryland, and Rochester, Minnesota. He enjoys running, hiking, kayaking, fly-fishing, sailing, music, art collecting, and literature. He is passionate about his three children, sustainable development, and the civic responsibilities of academics and professionals.

On a Personal Note From a Phone Interview: Charles "Chuck" Christensen noted his professional mentor was Robert K. Bing, also a Slagle lecturer and a great historian of occupational therapy. Christiansen indicated that the printed version of the lecture as an article in the *American Journal of Occupational Therapy* could not capture the public lecture version, where video clips helped to highlight his points. He was inspired to write his 1999 Eleanor Clarke Slagle Lecture as he examined the personal projects he engaged in during the 1990s and drilled down to the characteristics of activities that contributed to his well-being using a concept called "personal projects analysis." Brian Little, a researcher from Canada, was a mentor for Christiansen with personal projects analysis. Also, Christiansen was very interested in literature about the use of narrative, or personal life stories, and utilized a term in his Slagle lecture coined by Dan McAdams of Northwestern University called *selfing.*

Christiansen valued this idea of what we do creating who we are and the reflective aspect of identity. He noted that his lecture was comes from a very Western Protestant view, and if he were to recast his lecture, he would qualify it saying that there are other viewpoints and orientations and that the concept discussed in his Slagle lecture about occupation and identity may be culturally specific.

Christiansen indicated that he would not change the essence of the lecture if he presented the same topic today. The stresses and changes in life seem similar to the early days of occupational therapy with urbanization and leads Christiansen to "lament that mental hygiene is not embraced in the profession as Adolph Meyer envisioned in the early days of occupational therapy with tremendous potential in the community and in public health." He notes that there is much potential for occupational therapists to work in public health and wellness, and he would continue to promote that today. Christiansen notes that being selected for the Eleanor Clarke Slagle Lectureship Award is a once-in-a-lifetime opportunity, and he savors the memories as he reflects back on the experience.

Linking Key Messages of the 1999 Eleanor Clarke Slagle Lecture to the AOTA *Centennial Vision*: When I wrote the Eleanor Clarke Slagle lecture for 1999, little did I know that some 5 years later I would be serving as AOTA vice president and charged with the responsibility for strategic planning and the development of the *Centennial Vision.* I feel honored to have had the opportunity to work with occupational therapy leaders across the United States (and abroad) to forge a set of ambitious and worthy goals for the profession to meet (and exceed) as it moves into its second century of service to humankind.

One key goal of the *Centennial Vision* is to establish occupational therapy is a powerful, widely recognized, science-based profession (AOTA, 2007, p. 613). The implication is that the identity of occupational therapy is important and that the profession's identity is related to public perceptions that are influenced by what practitioners do. Thus, the *Centennial Vision* and the Slagle Lecture I gave in Indianapolis both speak to the critical relationship between actions and identities. As I wrote in 1999, what people do on a daily basis establishes how they are known, both to themselves and to others. Ten years later, as health care reform continues to be seriously debated in the United States, we are reminded that what professions do can also influence their identities.

Being authentic and true to one's identity seems to be a key factor in how people flourish. What did occupational therapy's founders have in mind as the identity for occupational therapy when they created the profession 100 years ago? This seems to be a key question, because I asserted in 1999 that for activities to contribute to identity and well-being, they must have coherence. That is, they need to be understood by the doer in the context of a greater life story.

The "life story" of the profession of occupational therapy continues to be written, but whether the activities the profession is doing now are sufficiently understood and valued by the public at-large is very much an open question. The founders of occupational therapy would surely lament the assault on meaning that is occurring daily in the lives of people who are not able to participate in activities that add coherence and meaning to their lives. Evidence of an epidemic of "diseases of meaning" is everywhere. Depression, self-inflicted injury, substance abuse, and loneliness are common. Sleep disorders are widespread, and indicators of lives out of balance (such as burnout, obesity, and stress-related illnesses) seem to be ubiquitous.

The solution, it would seem, is to find a profession that realizes the relationship between all of these seemingly disparate signs and symptoms of disordered lives. Because health is not an outcome but an enabler for living, a person's ability to engage meaningfully in the activities of life should be central to efforts to address the public's health. Surely, healthy lifestyles must be understood in terms that go beyond concepts such as seat belt use, diets, and fitness regimens. Bringing coherence to lives through re-ordered lifestyles would be an important strategy for occupational therapy to undertake. But such efforts are vanishingly small, and their importance largely unappreciated by most practitioners. Of course, a focus on lives also helps people establish or reaffirm their identities. In stressful times, people are desperate to find reassurance that their lives matter.

Thus, as it celebrates a century of service, occupational therapy would do well in this age to recognize that reaffirming its identity involves going beyond the necessary but insufficient objectives inherent in strictly functional orientations of therapy. Yes, *enabling* people to do activities is important. But *to be able to do* activities is not the same thing as *doing them*. *Doing*, strictly speaking, is not the same as *participation*. To define occupational therapy practice in terms of functional enablement only leads to a professional identity that is not unique and that fails to realize the promise of the profession to attend to the *why* as well as the *what* and *how* of everyday activity. The consequence is that the question "What meaning does this activity have in the context of a person's life?" loses its relevance to practice.

In the same way, *imagining* an identity is not the same thing as *creating* one. The uniqueness of occupational therapy's rich historical identity is in recognizing the important links between activities and lives and meaning. A centennial proclamation of the profession's identity is likely to be fully realized only if these links are reaffirmed and enacted.

Note. My opinions are expressed as an independent scholar and observer and are not intended to represent the views of institutions or organizations with which I hold affiliations.

—*Charles Christiansen*

Reference

American Occupational Therapy Association. (2007). AOTA's *Centennial Vision* and executive summary. *American Journal of Occupational Therapy, 61,* 613–614.

Bibliography

Christiansen, C. H. (in press). Foreword. In K. Sladyk, K. Jacobs, & S. McRae (Eds.), *Occupational therapy: Principles of practice.* Thorofare, NJ: Slack.

Christiansen, C. H. (2011). The importance of everyday activities. In C. H. Christiansen & K. M. Matuska (Eds.), *Ways of living: Intervention strategies to enable participation in daily life* (4th ed., pp. 1–26). Bethesda, MD: AOTA Press.

Christiansen, C H., Haertl, K. L., & Rogers, S. (2011). Evaluation to plan intervention. In C. H. Christiansen & K. M. Matuska (Eds.), *Ways of living: Intervention strategies to enable participation in daily life* (4th ed., pp. 45–88). Bethesda, MD: AOTA Press.

Christiansen, C. H. (2009). Foreword. In S. Dunbar (Ed.), *An occupational therapy perspective on leadership: Theoretical and practical dimensions.* Thorofare, NJ: Slack.

Christiansen, C. H. (2009). Leadership. In E. Duncan (Ed.), *Skills for practice in occupational therapy.* London: Churchill Livingstone/Elsevier.

Christiansen, C. H., Haertl, K. L. & Rogers, S. (2009). Functional evaluation and management of self-care and other activities of daily living. In J. A. Delisa et. al. (Eds.), *Principles of rehabilitation medicine* (5th ed.). Philadelphia: Lippincott Williams & Wilkins.

Christiansen, C. H., & Matuska, K. M. (2009). Health promotion research in occupational therapy. In M. E. Scaffa, S. M. Reitz, & M. Pizzi (Eds.), *Occupational therapy in the promotion of health and wellness.* Philadelphia: F. A. Davis.

Christiansen, C. H., Matuska, K., Polatajko, H. J., & Davis, J. (2009). Life balance: Evolving the concept. In K. M. Matuska & C. H. Christiansen (Eds.), *Life balance: Multidisciplinary theories and research* (pp. 3–12). Thorofare, NJ, and Bethesda, MD: Slack & AOTA Press.

Christiansen, C. H., & Townsend, E. A. (2009). An introduction to occupation. In C. H. Christiansen & E. A. Townsend (Eds.), *Introduction to occupation: The art and science of living* (2nd ed., pp. 1–34). Upper Saddle River, NJ: Pearson.

Christiansen, C. H., & Townsend, E. A. (Eds.). (2009). *Introduction to occupation: The art and science of living* (2nd ed.). Upper Saddle River, NJ: Prentice Hall.

Christiansen, C. H., & Townsend, E. A. (2009). The occupational nature of social groups. In C. H. Christiansen & E. A. Townsend (Eds.), *Introduction to occupation: The art and science of living* (2nd ed., pp.175–206). Upper Saddle River, NJ: Pearson.

Matuska, K. M., & Christiansen, C. H. (Eds.). (2009). *Life balance: Multidisciplinary theories and research.* Thorofare, NJ, and Bethesda, MD: Slack & AOTA Press.

Matuska, K. M., & Christiansen, C. H. (2009). Theoretical model of lifestyle balance and imbalance. In K. M. Matuska & C. H. Christiansen (Eds.), *Life balance: Multidisciplinary theories and research* (pp. 163–178). Thorofare, NJ, and Bethesda, MD: Slack & AOTA Press.

Christiansen, C. (2008). The dangers of thin air: A commentary on exploring prayer as a spiritual modality. *Canadian Journal of Occupational Therapy, 75*(1), 14–15.

Christiansen, C. H. (2008). Envisioning a key role for occupational therapy to support healthy aging in the 21st century. In S. Coppola, S. J. Elliot, & P. E. Toto (Eds.), *Strategies to advance gerontological excellence: Promoting best practice in occupational therapy* (pp. 501–512). Bethesda, MD: AOTA Press.

Matuska, K. M., & Christiansen, C. H. (2008). A proposed model of Lifestyle Balance. *Journal of Occupational Science, 15*(1), 9–19.

Christiansen, C. H. (2007). Adolf Meyer revisited: Connections between lifestyle, resilience, and illness. *Journal of Occupational Science, 14*(2), 63–76.

Christiansen, C. H. (2006). Foreword. In M. Iwama (Ed.), *The Kawa model: Culturally relevant occupational therapy* (pp. ix–xii). Edinburgh, Scotland: Churchill Livingstone/Elsevier.

Christiansen, C. H. (2006). Foreword. In S. Rodger & J. Ziviani (Eds.), *Occupational therapy with children* (pp. ix–xii). Oxford, England: Blackwell.

Christiansen, C. H., & Matuska, K. M. (2006). Lifestyle balance: A review and synthesis. *Journal of Occupational Science, 13*(1), 49–61.

Baum, C. M., & Christiansen, C. H. (2005). Person–environment–occupation–performance: An occupation-based framework for practice. In C. Christiansen & C. Baum (Eds.), *Occupational therapy: Performance, participation, and well-being* (pp. 242–267). Thorofare, NJ: Slack.

Baum, C. M. , Haugen, J. B., & Christiansen, C. H. (2005). Person–environment–occupation–performance: A model for planning interventions for individuals and organizations. In C. Christiansen & C. Baum (Eds.), *Occupational therapy: Performance, participation, and well-being* (pp. 372–395). Thorofare, NJ: Slack.

Christiansen, C. H. (2005). Creating community: An essay on the social responsibility of health professionals. In R. B. Purtilo, G. M. Jensen, & C. B. Royeen (Eds.), *Educating for moral action: A sourcebook in health and rehabilitation ethics* (pp. 51–56). Philadelphia: F. A. Davis.

Christiansen, C. H. (2005). Functional evaluation and management of self-care and other activities of daily living. In J. A. Delisa et al. (Eds.), *Principles of rehabilitation medicine* (4th ed., vol. 2, pp. 975–1002). Philadelphia: Lippincott Williams & Wilkins.

Christiansen, C. H. (2005). Time use and patterns of occupation. In C. Christiansen & C. Baum (Eds.), *Occupational therapy: Performance, participation, and well-being* (pp. 70–91). Thorofare, NJ: Slack.

Christiansen, C. H., & Baum, C. M. (2005). The complexity of human occupation. In C. Christiansen & C. Baum (Eds.), *Occupational therapy: Performance, participation, and well-being* (pp. 2–23). Thorofare, NJ: Slack.

Christiansen, C. H., Baum, C. M., & Bass-Haugen, J. (Eds.). (2005). *Occupational therapy: Enabling participation and well-being* (3rd ed.). Thorofare, NJ: Slack.

Edwards, D., & Christiansen, C. H. (2005). Occupational development. In C. Christiansen & C. Baum (Eds.), *Occupational therapy: Performance, participation, and well-being* (pp. 42–69). Thorofare, NJ: Slack.

Ottenbacher, K. J., & Christiansen, C. H. (2005). Celebrating progress and creating the future: Reflections at the silver anniversary [Editorial]. *OTJR: Occupation, Participation and Health, 25*(1), 2–3.

Christiansen, C. H. (2004). Evaluation to plan intervention. In C. H. Christiansen & K. M. Matuska (Eds.), *Ways of living: Adaptive strategies for special needs* (pp. 37–70). Bethesda, MD: AOTA Press.

Christiansen, C. H. (2004). How does one develop and document the skills needed to assume a deanship in higher education? *Occupational Therapy in Health Care, 18*(1–2), 185–187.

Christiansen, C. H. (2004). Occupation and identity: Becoming who we are through what we do. In C. H. Christiansen & E. A. Townsend (Eds.), *Introduction to occupation: The art and science of living* (pp. 121–138). Upper Saddle River, NJ: Prentice Hall.

Christiansen, C. H., & Matuska, K. M. (2004). The importance of everyday activities. In C. H. Christiansen & K. M. Matuska (Eds.), *Ways of living: Adaptive strategies for special needs* (pp. 1–20). Bethesda, MD: AOTA Press.

Christiansen, C. H., & Townsend, E. A. (2004). Introduction to occupation. In C. H. Christiansen & E. A. Townsend (Eds.), *Introduction to occupation: The art and science of living* (pp. 1–27). Upper Saddle River, NJ: Prentice Hall.

Christiansen, C. H., & Townsend, E. A. (Eds.). (2004). *Introduction to occupation: The art and science of living.* Upper Saddle River, NJ: Prentice Hall.

Christiansen, C. H. & Matuska, K. M. (Eds.). (2004). *Ways of living: Adaptive strategies for special needs* (3rd ed.). Bethesda, MD: AOTA Press.

Christiansen, C. H., & Townsend, E. A. (2004). The occupational nature of communities. In C. H. Christiansen & E. A. Townsend (Eds.), *Introduction to occupation: The art and science of living* (pp. 141–167). Upper Saddle River, NJ: Prentice Hall.

Moyers, P. A., & Christiansen, C. H. (2004). Planning intervention. In C. H. Christiansen & K. M. Matuska (Eds.), *Ways of living: Adaptive strategies for special needs* (3rd ed., pp. 71–84). Bethesda, MD: AOTA Press.

Zhang, L, Abreu, B. C., Seale, G. S., Masel, B., Christiansen, C. H., Ottenbacher, K. J. (2003). A virtual reality environment for evaluation of a daily living skill in brain injury rehabilitation: Reliability and validity. *Archives of Physical Medicine and Rehabilitation, 84,* 1118–1124.

Stephenson, K., Peloquin, S., Richmond, S., Hinman, M., & Christiansen, C. H. (2002). Changing educational paradigms to prepare allied health professionals for the 21st century. *Education for Health: Change in Learning and Practice, 15*(1), 37–50.

Bonder, B., & Christiansen, C. H. (2001). Coming of age in challenging times [Editorial]. *Occupational Therapy Journal of Research*, *21*(1), 3–11.

Christiansen, C., & Lou, J. (2001). Ethical considerations related to evidence-based practice. *American Journal of Occupational Therapy*, *55*(3), 345–349.

Christiansen, C. H., Ottenbacher, K. J., & Abreu, B. A. (2001). Assessing cognitive functions related to ADL tasks after brain injury. *Clinical Neuropsychologist*, *15*(2), 276–276.

Zhang, L., Abreu, B. C., Masel, B., Scheibel, R. S., Christiansen, C. H., et al. (2001). Virtual reality in the assessment of selected cognitive function after brain injury. *American Journal of Physical Medicine and Rehabilitation*, *80*(8), 597–604.

Backman, C., & Christiansen, C. H. (2000). Evaluation of self-care skills. In C. H. Christiansen (Ed.), *Ways of living: Self-care strategies for special needs* (2nd ed., pp. 26–44). Bethesda, MD: American Occupational Therapy Association.

Christiansen, C. H. (2000). Identity, personal projects, and happiness: Self-construction in everyday action. *Journal of Occupational Science, 7*, 98–107.

Christiansen, C. H. (2000). Planning intervention for self care needs. In C. H. Christiansen (Ed.) *Ways of Living: Self-care strategies for special needs* (2nd ed., pp. 45–57). Bethesda, MD: American Occupational Therapy Association.

Christiansen, C. H. (2000). The social importance of self-care intervention. In C. H. Christiansen (Ed.), *Ways of living: Self-care strategies for special needs* (2nd ed., pp. 1–12). Bethesda, MD: American Occupational Therapy Association.

Christiansen, C. H. (Ed.). (2000). *Ways of living: Self-care strategies for special needs* (2nd ed.). Bethesda, MD: American Occupational Therapy Association.

Christiansen, C. H. (1999). Occupation as identity. Competence, coherence, and the creation of meaning (1999 Eleanor Clarke Slagle Lecture). *American Journal of Occupational Therapy*, *53*(6), 547–558.

Christiansen, C. H., Backman, C., Little, B., & Nguyen, A. (1999). Occupation and subjective well-being: A study of personal projects. *American Journal of Occupational Therapy*, *54*(1), 25–34.

Christiansen, C. H., Abreu, B., & Ottenbacher, K. (1998). Reliability of task performance in virtual environments used for cognitive rehabilitation following traumatic brain injury. *Archives of Physical Medicine and Rehabilitation*, *79*, 888–892.

Baum, C. M., & Christiansen, C. H. (1997). Person–environment occupational performance: A conceptual model for practice. In C. H. Christiansen & C. M. Baum (Eds.), *Occupational therapy: Enabling function and well-being* (pp. 46–71). Thorofare, NJ: Slack.

Christiansen, C. H. (1997). Acknowledging a spiritual dimension in occupational therapy practice. *American Journal of Occupational Therapy*, *51*(3), 169–172.

Christiansen, C. H., & Baum, C. M. (1997). The occupational therapy context: Philosophy–principles–practice: In C. H. Christiansen & C. M. Baum, (Eds.), *Occupational therapy: Enabling function and well-being* (pp. 26–46). Thorofare, NJ: Slack.

Christiansen, C. H., & Baum, C. M. (Eds.). (1997). *Occupational therapy: Enabling performance and well-being*. Thorofare, NJ: Slack.

Christiansen, C. H., & Baum, C. M. (1997). Understanding occupation: Definitions and concepts. In C. H. Christiansen & C. M. Baum, (Eds.), *Occupational therapy: Enabling function and well-being* (pp. 2–25). Thorofare, NJ: Slack.

Christiansen, C. H., Little, B. R., & Backman, C. (1997). Personal projects: A useful approach to the study of occupation. *American Journal of Occupational Therapy*, *52*(6), 439–446.

Ottenbacher, K., & Christiansen, C. H. (1997). Occupational performance assessment. In C. H. Christiansen & C. M. Baum, (Eds.), *Occupational therapy: Enabling function and well-being* (pp. 104–135). Thorofare, NJ: Slack.

Christiansen, C. H. (1996). Managed care: Challenges and opportunities for occupational therapy. *American Journal of Occupational Therapy*, *50*(6), 409–412.

Christiansen, C. H., Abreu, B., & Huffman, R. K. (1996). Creating a virtual environment for brain injury rehabilitation and research: A preliminary report. *Journal of Medicine and Virtual Reality*, *1*(2), 6–9.

Christiansen, C. H. (1994). Classification and study in occupation: A review and discussion of taxonomies. *Journal of Occupational Science*, *1*(3) 3–17.

Christiansen, C. H. (1994). Foreword. In C. Mattingly & M. Fleming (Eds.), *Clinical reasoning: Forms of inquiry in a therapeutic practice* (pp. vii–viii). Philadelphia: F. A. Davis.

Christiansen, C. H. (1994). A social framework for understanding self-care intervention. In C. H. Christiansen (Ed.), *Ways of living: Self-care strategies for special needs* (pp. 1–26). Rockville, MD: American Occupational Therapy Association.

Christiansen, C. H. (1994). Three perspectives on balance in occupation. In R. Zemke & F. Clark (Eds.), *Occupational science: The evolving discipline* (pp. 431–451). Philadelphia, F. A. Davis.

Christiansen, C. H. (Ed.). (1994). *Ways of living: Self-care strategies for special needs*. Rockville, MD: American Occupational Therapy Association.

Christiansen, C., & Christiansen, P. (1994, June 30). Canada, the OT's perspective. *OT Week*, pp. 20–23.

Christiansen, C., & Christiansen, P. (1994, June 30). What is the Canadian System? *OT Week*, pp. 16–19.

Christiansen, C. H. (1993). Continuing challenges of functional assessment in rehabilitation: Recommended changes. *American Journal of Occupational Therapy*, *47*(3), 258–259.

Christiansen, C. H., Schwartz, R. K., & Barnes, K. J. (1993). Self-care: Evaluation and management. In J. A. Delisa et al. (Eds.), *Principles of rehabilitation medicine* (2nd ed., pp. 178–200). Philadelphia: J. B. Lippincott.

Christiansen, C. H. (1991). Occupational performance assessment. In C. H. Christiansen & C. M. Baum (Eds.), *Occupational therapy: Overcoming human performance deficits* (pp. 343–387). Thorofare, NJ: Slack.

Christiansen, C. H. (1991). Occupational therapy: Intervention for life performance. In C. H. Christiansen & C. M. Baum (Eds.), *Occupational therapy: Overcoming human performance deficits* (pp. 2–43). Thorofare, NJ: Slack.

Christiansen, C. H. (1991). Performance deficits as sources of stress: Coping theory and occupational therapy. In C. H. Christiansen & C. M. Baum (Eds.), *Occupational therapy: Overcoming human performance deficits* (pp. 58–96). Thorofare, NJ: Slack.

Christiansen, C. H. (1991). Research: Looking back and ahead after four decades of progress. *American Journal of Occupational Therapy, 45*(5), 391–392.

Christiansen, C. H., & Baum, C. M. (Eds.). (1991). *Occupational therapy: Overcoming human performance deficits.* Thorofare, NJ: Slack.

Devereaux, E., Berger, J., & Christiansen, C. H. (1991). Pharmacological agents and their effect on performance. In C. H. Christiansen & C. M. Baum (Eds.), *Occupational therapy: Overcoming human performance deficits* (pp. 335–351). Thorofare, NJ: Slack.

Christiansen, C. H. (1990). The perils of plurality. *Occupational Therapy Journal of Research, 10*(5), 259–265.

Holcomb, J. D, Christiansen, C. H., & Roush, R. E. (1989). The scholarly productivity of occupational therapy faculty members: Results of a regional study. *American Journal of Occupational Therapy, 43*(1), 37–43.

Bruce, M. A., & Christiansen, C. H. (1988). The Issue Is—Advocacy in word as well as deed. *American Journal of Occupational Therapy, 42,* 189–191.

Christiansen, C. H., & Fritz, L. (1988). Matters of budget: Fiscal planning and management in the AOTA. *American Journal of Occupational Therapy, 42*(6).

Christiansen, C. H. (1987). Research: Its relationship to higher education. *American Journal of Occupational Therapy, 41,* 77–80.

Gilfoyle, E., & Christiansen, C. H. (1987). Research: The quest for truth and the key to excellence. *American Journal of Occupational Therapy, 41,* 7–9.

Christiansen, C. H. (1986). Facilitating collaborative research between faculty and practitioners. In *Target 2000: Promoting excellence in occupational therapy education* (pp. 199–202). Rockville, MD: American Occupational Therapy Association.

Christiansen, C. H. (1986). Research as reclamation. *Occupational Therapy Journal of Research, 6,* 323–328.

Christiansen, C. H. (1986). Specialized accreditation: Endangered species in an era of change? *American Journal of Occupational Therapy, 39,* 363–366.

Baldwin, L., & Christiansen, C. H. (1985). Self as known and self as knower: Testing an insight/empathy hypothesis. *Occupational Therapy Journal of Research, 5,* 125–128.

Christiansen, C. H. (1985). Evaluating studies for internal and external validity. In J. Morse (Ed.), *New dimensions in health professions research: A comprehensive instructional program* [audiocassette & workbook]. Laurel, MD: American Occupational Therapy Foundation & Ramsco.

Christiansen, C. H. (1983). Research: An economic imperative. *Occupational Therapy Journal of Research, 3,* 195–198.

Lanier, R. A., Hedl, J., & Christiansen, C. H. (1983). Faculty evaluation practices among occupational therapy chairpersons: a comparative study. *Occupational Therapy Journal of Research, 3,* 141–163.

Davidson, D. A., Christiansen, C. H., & Dillon, M. A. (1982). Personality process variables and their relationship to occupational therapy fieldwork performance. *Occupational Therapy Journal of Research, 2,* 50–53.

Christiansen, C. H. (1981). Toward resolution of crisis: Research requisites in occupational therapy. *Occupational Therapy Journal of Research, 1*(2), 113–120.

Christiansen, C. H. (1980). Biographical antecedents of empathic capacity in allied health students. *Texas Society of Allied Health Professions Newsletter, 2*(3), 18.

Christiansen, C. H. (1980). Educating for caring in the health professions: A critical appraisal from a social–psychological perspective. *Health Values Achieving High Level Wellness, 4*(3), 103–109.

Armitage, M. E., Christiansen, C. H., & Weinberg, A. D. (1977). Design of a medical record audit in continuing education. *Medical Record News, 48,* 71–84.

Christiansen, C. H. (1977). Measuring empathy in occupational therapy students. *American Journal of Occupational Therapy, 31,* 19–23.

Christiansen, C. H., & Weinberg, A. D. (1977). The effects of a geographical continuing education program on physician referral behavior. In *Proceedings of the 16th Annual Conference on Research in Medical Education* (pp. 97–99). Washington, DC: American Association of Medical Colleges.

Christiansen, C. H., Weinberg, A. D., & Ullian, L. (1977). Supply and demand: the basis for any film distribution program. *Biomedical Communications, 5,* 29–31.

Weinberg, A. D., Christiansen, C. H., & Armitage, M. E. (1977). Continuing medical and practitioner awareness: A country-wide program concerning congenital heart disease. *Journal of Hospital Medical Education, 2,* 6–8.

Weinberg, A. D., Christiansen, C. H., & Wise, D. J. (1977). Respiratory rate: Forgotten clue in the early detection of congenital heart disease. *Pediatric Nursing, 3,* 38–43.

Weinberg, A. D., Ullian, L., & Christiansen,. C. H. (1977). The accuracy of physician self-assessment. *Journal of the Association of Hospital Medical Education, 2,* 25–28.

Weinberg, A. D., Ullian, L., Christiansen, C. H., & Raizner, A. (1977). Perceived ability versus actual ability: A problem for continuing medical education. In *Proceedings of the 16th Annual Conference on Research in Medical Education* (pp. 79–83). Washington, DC: Association of American Medical Colleges.

Christiansen, C. H. (1975). Attitudes of graduates toward occupational therapy education. *American Journal of Occupational Therapy, 29,* 352–355.

Christiansen, C. H., & Davidson, D. A. (1974). A community health program with low achieving adolescents. *American Journal of Occupational Therapy, 28,* 346–349.

Christiansen, C. H. (1970). The male occupational therapist: Attitudes and trends. *American Journal of Occupational Therapy, 24,* 513–514.

Florence Clark, PhD, OTR, FAOTA—1993

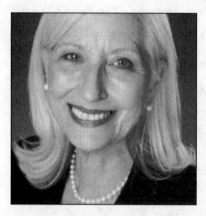

Florence Clark is professor and associate dean of the University of Southern California (USC) Division of Occupational Science and Occupational Therapy in Los Angeles.

Clark obtained a bachelor's degree in English and drama from the State University of New York at Albany, a master's degree in occupational therapy from the State University of New York at Buffalo, and a doctorate in education from USC. She also was awarded an honorary doctorate from the University of Indianapolis. Clark joined the USC faculty in 1976 and became chairperson of the Department of Occupational Science and Occupational Therapy in 1989. Her research interests include the development and dysfunction of sensory integration in children; maternal role behavior; the acquisition of independent living skills among adolescents with disabilities; health promotion in the elderly population; spinal cord injury; and occupational science. She is recognized for her roles in raising public awareness of occupational therapy and as lead investigator of the Well Elderly Study, the first occupational therapy study to be published in *JAMA (Journal of the American Medical Association)*.

Clark was appointed as a charter member of the Academy of Research of the American Occupational Therapy Association (AOTA) in 1986. She has served as special consultant to the U.S. Army Surgeon General and on the board of the National Center for Medical Rehabilitation Research.

Clark has received numerous awards. In 1999, she received the AOTA Award of Merit, and in 2001, she received a lifetime achievement award from the Occupational Therapy Association of California. In 2004, she received the Presidential Medallion from USC, which is awarded to academicians who have brought distinction and honor to the university. Clark's research and pedagogical interests over the past two decades have largely centered on the relationship between activity and lifestyle to health and wellness. Her recent scholarly activity focuses on the design of lifestyle intervention for various populations such as older adults, persons with weight concerns, and individuals with spinal cord injury. Clark became AOTA President in 2010.

Linking Key Messages of the 1993 Eleanor Clarke Slagle Lecture to the AOTA *Centennial Vision*: In my Eleanor Clarke Slagle lecture, I recounted the story of how Penny Richardson, a stroke survivor, through a process called Lifestyle Redesign®, became empowered and took her rightful place in society. To accomplish this, she needed to divest herself of self-limiting practices. Just as Penny conquered a world that did not know her true potential and worth, so too must the profession of occupational therapy break out of that which limits its scope, power, and ability to serve the public good. In 2017, occupational therapy will not be self-limiting. It will have achieved a stronger and clearer identity. It will be widely understood, powerful, and evidence-based. It will have rich, global connections and a workforce that is more diverse than ever before. Like Penny Richardson's metamorphosis, its transformation will be magnanimous.

—*Florence Clark*

Bibliography

Eakman, A. M., Carlson, M., & Clark, F. (2010). Factor structure, reliability, and convergent validity of the engagement in meaningful activities survey for older adults. *OTJR: Occupation, Participation and Health, 30*(3), 111–121.

Jackson, J., Carlson, M., Rubayi, S., Scott, M., Atkins, M., Blanche, E., Saunders-Newton, C., Mielke, S., & Clark, F. (2010). Qualitative study of principles pertaining to lifestyle and pressure ulcer risk in adults with spinal cord injury. *Disability and Rehabilitation, 32*(7), 567–578.

Clark, F., & Lawlor, M. (2009). The making and mattering of occupational science. In E. Crepeau, E. Cohn, & B. Schell (Eds.), *Willard and Spackman's occupational therapy* (11th ed.). Philadelphia: Lippincott Williams & Wilkins.

Dunn, C., Carlson, M., Jackson, J., & Clark, F. (2009). Response factors surrounding progression of pressure ulcers in community-residing adults with spinal cord injury. *American Journal of Occupational Therapy, 63*, 301–309.

Jackson, J., Mandel, D., Blanchard, J., Carlson, M., Cherry, B., Azen, S., Chou, C. P., Jordan-Marsh, M., Forman, T., White, B., Granger, D., Knight, B., & Clark, F. (2009). Confronting challenges in intervention research with ethnically diverse older adults: The USC Well Elderly II Trial. *Clinical Trials, 6*, 90–101.

Clark, F., Sanders, K., Carlson, M., Blanche, E., & Jackson, J. (2007). Synthesis of habit theory. *Occupational Therapy Journal of Research,* *27*(4).

Xie, B., Chou, C.-P., Spruijt-Metz, D., Reynolds, K., Clark, F., Palmer, P., et al. (2007). Socio-demographic and economic correlates of over-weight status in Chinese adolescents. *American Journal of Health Behavior, 31*(4), 339–352.

Clark, F. (2006). One person's thoughts on the future of occupational science. *Journal of Occupational Science, 13*(3), 167–179.

Clark, F., Jackson, J., Scott, M., Carlson, M., Atkins, M., Uhles-Tanaka, M., et al. (2006). Data-based models of how pressure ulcers develop in daily-living contexts of adults with spinal cord injury. *Archives of Physical Medicine and Rehabilitation, 87,* 1516–1525.

Clark, F., Jackson, J., & Carlson, M. (2004). Occupational science, occupational therapy, and evidence-based practice: What the Well Elderly Study has taught us. In M. Molineux (Ed.), *Occupation for occupational therapists* (pp. 200–218). Oxford, England: Blackwell.

Clark, F., Carlson, M., Jackson, F., & Mandel, D. (2003). Lifestyle Redesign improves health and is cost-effective. *OT Practice, 8*(2), 9–13.

Larson, E., Wood, W., & Clark, F. (2003). Occupational science: Building the science and practice of occupation through an academic discipline. In E. Crepeau, E. Cohn, & B. Schell (Eds.), *Willard and Spackman's occupational therapy* (10th ed., pp. 15–26). Philadelphia: Lippincott.

Hay, J., LaBbree, L., Luo, R., Clark, F., Carlson, M., Mandel, D., et al. (2002). Cost-effectiveness of preventive occupational therapy for independent-living older adults. *Journal of the American Psychiatric Society, 50,* 1381–1388.

Clark, F. (2001). Editorial. *Scandinavian Journal of Occupational Therapy, 8*(1), 3–6.

Clark, F., Azen, S. P., Carlson, M., Mandel, D., LaBree, L., Hay, J., et al. (2001). Embedding health-promoting changes into the daily lives of independent-living older adults: Long-term follow-up of occupational therapy intervention. *Journal of Gerontology: Psychological Sciences and Social Sciences, 56B*(1), 60–63.

Jackson, J., Mandel, D. R., Zemke, R., & Clark, F. (2001). Promoting quality of life in elders: An occupation-based occupational therapy program. *WFOT Bulletin, 43,* 5–12.

Clark, F. (2000). The concepts of habit and routine: A preliminary theoretical analysis. *Occupational Therapy Journal of Research, 20,* 123S–137S.

Azen, S. P., Palmer, J. M., Carlson, M., Mandel, D., Cherry, B. J., Fanchiang, S., Jackson, J., & Clark, F. (1999). Psychometric properties of a Chinese translation of the SF–36 Health Survey Questionnaire in the Well Elderly Study. *Journal of Aging and Health, 11*(2), 240–251.

Mandel, D., Jackson, J., Zemke, R., Nelson, L., & Clark, F. (1999). *Lifestyle redesign: Implementing the well elderly program.* Bethesda, MD: American Occupational Therapy Association.

Carlson, M., Clark, F., & Young, B. (1998). Practical contributions of occupational science to the art of successful ageing: How to sculpt a meaningful life in older adulthood. *Journal of Occupational Science, 5,* 107–118.

Harris, C., Brayman, S., Clark, F., Delaney, J., & Miller, R. (1998). COE recommends postbaccalaureate OT education. *OT Week, 12*(11), 18, 21.

Jackson, J., Carlson, M., Mandel, D., Zemke, R., & Clark, F. (1998). Occupation in lifestyle redesign: The well elderly study occupational therapy program. *American Journal of Occupational Therapy, 52,* 326–336.

Snyder, C., Clark, F., Masunaka-Noriega, M., & Young, B. (1998). Los Angeles street kids: New occupations for life program. *Journal of Occupational Science, 5,* 133–139.

Clark, F. (1997). Reflections on the human as an occupational being: Biological need, tempo, and temporality. *Journal of Occupational Science–Australia, 4*(3), 86–92.

Clark, F., Azen, S. P., Zemke, R., Jackson, J., Carlson, M., Mandel, D., et al. (1997). Occupational therapy for independent-living older adults: A randomized controlled trial. *JAMA, 278*(16), 1321–1326.

Clark, F., Carlson, M., & Polkinghorne, D. (1997). The Issue Is—The legitimacy of life history and narrative approaches in the study of occupation. *American Journal of Occupational Therapy, 51,* 313–317.

Carlson, M., Fanchiang, S. P., Zemke, R., & Clark, F. (1996). A meta-analysis of the effectiveness of occupational therapy for older persons. *American Journal of Occupational Therapy, 50,* 89–98.

Clark, F., Carlson, M., Zemke, R., Frank, G., Patterson, K., Ennevor, B. L., et al. (1996). Life domains and adaptive strategies of a group of low-income, well older adults. *American Journal of Occupational Therapy, 50,* 99–108.

Spitzer, S., Roley, S. S., Clark, F., & Parham, D. (1996). Sensory integration: Current trends in the United States. *Scandinavian Journal of Occupational Therapy, 3,* 123–138.

Zemke, R., & Clark, F. (1996). *Occupational science: The evolving discipline.* Philadelphia: F. A. Davis.

Christiansen, C., Clark, F., Kielhofner, G., Rogers, J., & Nelson, D. (1995). AOTA's 1995 Representative Assembly highlights: Occupation: A position paper. *OT Week, 9*(6), A11.

Christiansen, C., Clark, F., Kielhofner, G., Rogers, J., & Nelson, D. (1995). Position Paper—Occupation...An individual's performance of activities, tasks, and roles during daily occupations. *American Journal of Occupational Therapy, 49,* 1015–1018.

Clark, F. (1993). Occupation embedded in a real life: Interweaving occupational science and occupational therapy (1993 Eleanor Clarke Slagle Lecture). *American Journal of Occupational Therapy, 47,* 1067–1078.

Clark, F., Zemke, R., Frank, G., Parham, D., Neville, J. A., Hedricks, C., et al. (1993). The Issue Is—Dangers inherent in the partition of occupational therapy and occupational science. *American Journal of Occupational Therapy, 47,* 184–186.

Carlson, M. E., & Clark, F. (1991). The search for useful methodologies in occupational science. *American Journal of Occupational Therapy, 45*(3), 235–241.

Clark, F., Mailloux, Z., Parham, L. D., & Primeau, L. (1991). Statement—Occupational therapy provisions for children with learning disabilities and/or mild to moderate perceptual and motor deficits. *American Journal of Occupational Therapy, 45,* 1069–1074.

Wiss, T., & Clark, F. (1990). Validity of the Southern California Postrotary Nystagmus Test: Misconceptions lead to incorrect conclusions. *American Journal of Occupational Therapy, 44*, 658–660.

Clark, F., & Jackson, J. (1989). The application of the occupational science negative heuristic in the treatment of persons with human immunodeficiency infection. *Occupational Therapy in Health Care, 6*(4), 69–91.

Hamilton-Dodd, C., Kawamoto, T., Clark, F., Burke, J. P., & Fanchiang, S. P. (1989). The effects of a maternal preparation program on mother–infant pairs: A pilot study. *American Journal of Occupational Therapy, 43*, 513–521.

Jackson, J., Rankin, A., Siefken, S., & Clark, F. (1989). Options: An occupational therapy transition program for adolescents with developmental disabilities. *Occupational Therapy in Health Care, 6*(2/3), 197–214.

Primeau, L. A., Clark, F., & Pierce, D. (1989). Occupational therapy alone has looked upon occupation: Future applications of occupational science to pediatric occupational therapy. *Occupational Therapy in Health Care, 6*(4), 19–32.

Yerxa, E. J., Clark, F., Frank, G., Jackson, J., Parham, D., Pierce, D., et al. (1989). An introduction to occupational science, a foundation for occupational therapy in the 21st century. *Occupational Therapy in Health Care, 6*(4), 1–17.

Clark, F. (1988). *Transition needs assessment of high school students with severe disabilities and their parents and teachers.* Washington, DC: U.S. Department of Education, Office of Educational Research and Improvement, Educational Resources Information Center.

Parush, S., & Clark, F. (1988). The reliability and validity of a sensory developmental expectation questionnaire for mothers of newborns. *American Journal of Occupational Therapy, 42*, 11–16.

Burke, J. P., Clark, F., Hamilton-Dodd, C., & Kawamoto, T. (1987). Maternal role preparation: A program using sensory integration, infant–mother attachment, and occupational behavior perspectives. *Occupational Therapy in Health Care, 4*(2), 9–21.

Clark, F. (1986). The Foundation—A new concept: Research apprenticeships for occupational therapy researchers. *American Journal of Occupational Therapy, 40*, 639–641.

Clark, F., Sharrott, G., Hill, D. J., & Campbell, S. (1985). A comparison of impact of undergraduate and graduate occupational therapy education on professional productivity. *American Journal of Occupational Therapy, 39*, 155–162.

Saeki, K., Clark, F., & Azen, S. P. (1985). Performance of Japanese and Japanese American children on the Motor Accuracy–Revised and Design Copying Tests of the Southern California Sensory Integration Tests. *American Journal of Occupational Therapy, 39*, 103–109.

Bissell, J. C., & Clark, F. (1984). Dichotic listening performance in normal children and adults. *American Journal of Occupational Therapy, 38*, 176–183.

Clark, F., & Sharrott, G. W. (1984). Commentary—Toward an image of one's own: Sources of variation in the role of occupational therapy in psychosocial practice. *Occupational Therapy Journal of Research, 4*, 24–36.

Clark, F. (1983). Research on the neuropathophysiology of autism and its implications for occupational therapy. *Occupational Therapy Journal of Research, 3*, 3–22.

Allen, J., Clark, F., Gallagher, P., Scofield, F., & Prouty, R. (1982). *Classroom strategies for accommodating exceptional learners.* Minneapolis, MN: National Support Systems/U.S. Department of Education.

Benson, J., & Clark, F. (1982). A guide for instrument development and validation. *American Journal of Occupational Therapy, 36*, 789–800.

Clark, F. (1982). Research Instrumentation—The Illinois Test of Psycholinguistic Abilities: Considerations for its use in occupational and physical therapy practice. *Physical and Occupational Therapy in Pediatrics, 2*(4), 29–39.

Clark, F., & Staingold, L. P. (1982). A potential relationship between occupational therapy and language acquisition. *American Journal of Occupational Therapy, 36*, 42–44.

Shuer, J., Clark, F., & Azen, S. P. (1980). Vestibular function in mildly mentally retarded adults. *American Journal of Occupational Therapy, 34*, 664–670.

Clark, F., Miller, L. R., Thomas, J. A., Kurcherawy, D. A., & Azen, S. P. (1978). A comparison of operant and sensory integrative methods on development parameters in profoundly retarded adults. *American Journal of Occupational Therapy, 32*, 86–82.

Wendy J. Coster, PhD, OTR/L, FAOTA—2008

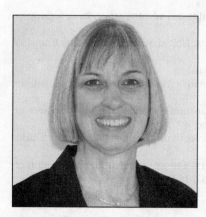

Wendy Coster moved to Boston with a background in psychology and mental health. After conversing with the head of the Occupational Therapy Department of a local mental health hospital, she was offered a position as an aide in that department. At Massachusetts Mental Health Center, she was able to learn about many clinical conditions. Her first occupational therapy supervisor was a strong, inspiring role model, demonstrating such pride in occupational therapy, assertiveness with opinions, and love of her work as an occupational therapist. The entry-level master's program in occupational therapy at Boston University (BU) had just begun, and in pursuing this degree Coster discovered how much she loved occupational therapy. After graduating, much of Coster's clinical practice up to 1986 included working with early childhood programs and school-age children and adolescents.

Coster noted the move into academia was natural, as she wanted to learn and understand more. The faculty members at BU were intellectually stimulating and inspiring. In addition, the faculty provided her very inquisitive nature with many different perspectives. She became a research assistant for Sharon Cermak and was intrigued by the research process. She had still so many questions and believed that she needed to pursue another graduate degree to explore the answers to these questions. Her classmates at BU had at one time voted Coster "the most likely to pursue a PhD" (personal communication, October 1, 2009).

In 1986, Coster graduated from Harvard University with a doctorate in psychology, concentrating on development and psychopathology. She started as an assistant professor at BU and was promoted to full professor. Additionally, she was a lecturer in the Department of Rehabilitative Medicine at Tufts University School of Medicine from 1991 to 2005. She also has assumed administrative positions at BU, including chair of the Department of Occupational Therapy, director of programs in occupational therapy and therapeutic studies, and acting chair of the Department of Physical Therapy and Athletic Training.

Coster is a conceptual leader in the field of occupational therapy and rehabilitation with her ground-breaking work considering developmental expectations and contextual influences for infants and children. Her early advocacy for an enablement perspective demonstrates foresight within the field of rehabilitation. In 2001, Coster received the American Occupational Therapy Foundation (AOTF) A. Jean Ayres Award for her sustained commitment to the development of theory in occupational therapy. Colleagues from other disciplines also recognize her expertise and have invited her to consult to their organization. These include the Centers for Disease Control and Prevention, the National Center on Birth Defects and Developmental Disabilities, the U.S. Department of Education, the American Physical Therapy Association, the National Association of State Directors of Special Education, the North Carolina Office of Disability, and the Frank Porter Graham Child Development Center in North Carolina.

Coster has an impressive background in research endeavors. From 1997 to 2002 she served on the Academic Development Committee of the Research Advisory Council of the AOTF. In that capacity she developed a monograph of curriculum materials that support the effective teaching of research in the occupational therapy field and coauthored a research competencies document published in the *American Journal of Occupational Therapy* in 2000.

In 2002, she became the project director for the AOTF International Conference on Evidence-Based Occupational Therapy. She saw a gap in the profession's knowledge base as she observed practitioners all over the world struggling to synthesize intervention outcome evidence to support the value of occupational therapy. Rather than passively observing, Coster took the initiative to mobilize international collaboration and wrote a grant to the Agency for Healthcare Research and Quality to fund an innovative conference for researchers from 13 countries to collaborate to achieve the common goal of demonstrating the value of occupational therapy. The conference focused on how researchers around the world were critically reviewing and synthesizing available evidence, educating practitioners, and developing coordinated clearinghouse efforts to disseminate findings. She continues to be involved with follow-up projects focused on synthesizing, organizing, and disseminating evidence to support occupational therapy intervention throughout the world. Most recently she contributed to the development of a Web-based portal to link evidence-based practice resources for occupational therapy educators worldwide.

Additionally, Coster has provided the occupational therapy profession with measurement tools that define problems and focus on the functional outcomes that are important to the profession's consumers. The conceptual frameworks of assessments Coster has developed—the Pediatric Evaluation of Disability Inventory (PEDI), the School Function Assessment (SFA), and the Late Life Function and Disability Instrument—encourage practitioners to look globally at performance situated in a context and identify both strengths and barriers to participation. She is involved in several other measurement development projects, including the development of a functional outcome measure for children with acquired brain injury and a measure of activity and participation for adults called the Activity Measure for Post Acute Care (AM–PAC). With the Late Life Function and Disability Instrument, practitioners and researchers now have a tool to help them provide and document occupation-centered interventions for community-dwelling older adults. Her prolific contributions in measurement enhance the services provided to occupational therapy's consumers around the world.

Coster also has been in the forefront of measurement development by using item response theory (IRT) models in test creation and validation, beginning with the ground-breaking work with the PEDI first published in 1992. The use of IRT methods, now considered state-of- the-art, has afforded new opportunities for making measures relevant to persons served, including developing flexible formats for specific settings and developing computer-adaptive testing models, which permits each examinee to be given only items tailored to that individual. Although prolific in this area of scholarship, Coster's research goes beyond measurement development and continues in the area of context on participation.

On a Personal Note From a Phone Interview: When asked about the inspiration for the topic of Coster's Eleanor Clarke Slagle Lecture, she noted that "The subject had been on my mind, especially the two measurements at the end of the lecture. A person should try to use knowledge and skill to influence for the better. It is important to recognize what we do not know and might be wrong, being humble in a sense of what you have researched . . . always keep in the back of your mind, What is missing?" (personal communication, October 1, 2009). Coster stated that there is a responsibility with measurement.

In exploring the impact of presenting the Eleanor Clarke Slagle Lecture, Coster said that "preparing the lecture, the process was enjoyable . . . more so than getting the award" (personal communication, October 1, 2009). She did want to acknowledge the influence of her mentor and colleague, Catherine Trombly. Coster indicated that Trombly is a shy person, and the thoughtfulness in the way she worked her ideas and disseminated her work was so influential on Coster. Trombly was as a role model as Coster worked on her own Slagle lecture. Coster preferred to present her lecture in a less-formal style, as if she were "just talking to people . . . telling them the story" (personal communication, October 1, 2009). This humble and compassionate style of presenting the lecture allowed those present in the Conference hall to be truly inspired.

Linking Key Messages of the 2008 Eleanor Clarke Slagle Lecture to the AOTA *Centennial Vision*: The *Centennial Vision* asks us to envision occupational therapy as a science-driven profession. The common perception of science is that it offers objective information. However, in reality, what makes an investigation or body of knowledge "science" is that it is replicable: The methods are openly known and will produce the same results if carried out by someone else. Science is a human enterprise and, as I discuss in my lecture, it is subject to the common biases, limitations in thought, and unconscious responses to which all people are susceptible. If we aspire to be science-driven, it is most important for us to be aware of and to check for these influences in the science we do and the science we use. Otherwise, we may be led by the language and instruments of science to accept ideas about "reality" that are not consistent with what we have learned from the clients, families, and communities we work with.

The *Centennial Vision* also asks us to envision occupational therapy as powerful, a theme I turn to in the final part of my lecture. I propose that we use the insight gained from clinical experience to challenge the limitations of current science and open new perspectives that better capture "the whole story" about people and their occupational lives. As I envision it, we must become "positive subversives."

Note. The biographical information in this section was written primarily by Ellen Cohen and Sue Berger, colleagues of Coster at Boston University, as part of their nomination essay for Coster for the Eleanor Clarke Slagle Lecture.

—*Wendy Coster*

Bibliography

Takahashi, K., Tickle-Degnen, L., Coster, W. J., & Latham, N. (in press). Expressive behavior in Parkinson's disease as a function of interview context. *American Journal of Occupational Therapy, 64,* 484–495.

Hwang, Y.-S., Lin, C.-H., Coster, W. J., Bigsby, R., & Vergara, E. (2010). Effectiveness of cheek and jaw support to improve feeding performance of preterm infants. *American Journal of Occupational Therapy, 64,* 886–894.

Dunn, M. L., Coster, W. J., Cohn, E. S., & Orsmond, G. I. (2009). Factors associated with participation of children with and without attention deficit hyperactivity disorder in household tasks. *Physical and Occupational Therapy in Pediatrics, 29,* 274–294.

Dunn, M. L., Coster, W. J., Orsmond, G. I., & Cohn, E. S. (2009). Household task participation of children with and without attentional problems. *Physical and Occupational Therapy in Pediatrics, 29,* 258–273.

Bedell, G., & Coster, W. J. (2008). Measuring participation of school-age children with traumatic brain injuries: Considerations and approaches. *Journal of Head Trauma Rehabilitation, 23,* 220–229.

Chou, Y.-H., Coster, W. J., Trombly Latham, C. A., Li, P.-L., Chung, M.-J., & Shie, J.-H. (2008). Rod bisection task: The roles of voluntary manual exploration and vision in perceptual judgment. *Perceptual and Motor Skills, 107,* 70–80.

Coster, W. J. (2008). Curricular approaches to professional reasoning for evidence-based practice. In B. A. Schell & J. W. Schell (Eds.), *Clinical and professional reasoning in occupational therapy* (pp. 311–334). Baltimore: Lippincott Williams & Wilkins.

Coster, W. J. (2008). Embracing ambiguity: Facing the challenge of measurement (2008 Eleanor Clarke Slagle Lecture). *American Journal of Occupational Therapy, 62,* 743–752.

Coster, W. J. (2008). Organizing the evidence to support practice. In S. Coppola, S. Elliott, & P. Toto (Eds.), *Strategies to advance gerontology excellence: Promoting best practice in occupational therapy* (pp. 513–524). Bethesda, MD: AOTA Press.

Coster, W., Haley, S. M., Ni, P. S., Dumas, H. M., & Fragala-Pinkham, M. A. (2008). Assessing self-care and social function using a computer adaptive testing version of the Pediatric Evaluation of Disability Inventory. *Archives of Physical Medicine and Rehabilitation, 89,* 622–629.

Coster, W., & Khetani, M. A. (2008). Measuring participation of children with disabilities: Issues and challenges. *Disability and Rehabilitation, 30,* 639–648.

Prvu Bettger, J. A., Coster, W. J., Latham, N. K., & Keysor, J. J. (2008). Analyzing change in recovery patterns in the year after acute hospitalization. *Archives of Physical Medicine and Rehabilitation, 89,* 1267–1275.

Tao, W., Haley, S. M., Coster, W. J., Ni, P., & Jette, A. (2008). An exploratory analysis of functional staging using an item response theory approach. *Archives of Physical Medicine and Rehabilitation, 89,* 1046–1063.

Haley, S. M., Gandek, B., Siebens, H., Black-Schaffer, R. M., Sinclair, S. J., Tao, W., Coster, W. J., et al. (2008). Computerized adaptive testing for follow-up after discharge from inpatient rehabilitation: II. Participation outcomes. *Archives of Physical Medicine and Rehabilitation, 89,* 275–283.

Coster, W., Haley, S. M., Jette, A., Tao, W., & Siebens, H. (2007). Predictors of basic and instrumental activities of daily living performance in persons receiving rehabilitation services. *Archives of Physical Medicine and Rehabilitation, 88,* 928–935.

Daunhauer, L., Coster, W. J., Tickle-Degnen, L., & Cermak, S. (2007). Effects of caregiver–child interactions on play occupations among young children institutionalized in Eastern Europe. *American Journal of Occupational Therapy, 61,* 429–440.

Coster, W. J. (2006). Evaluating the use of assessments in practice and research. In G. Kielhofner (Ed.), *Research in occupational therapy: Methods of inquiry for enhancing practice* (pp. 201–212). Philadelphia: F. A. Davis.

Coster, W. J. (2006). Guest Editorial—The road forward to better measures for practice and research. *OTJR: Occupation, Participation and Health, 26,* 131.

Coster, W. J., Haley, S. M., & Jette, A. J. (2006). Measuring patient-reported outcomes after discharge from inpatient rehabilitation. *Journal of Rehabilitation Medicine, 38,* 237–242.

Haley, S. M., Ni, P., Coster, W. J., Black-Shaeffer, R., Siebens, H., & Tao, W. (2006). Agreement in functional assessment: Graphical approaches to displaying respondent effects. *American Journal of Physical Medicine and Rehabilitation, 85,* 747–755.

Keysor, J. J., Jette, A. M., Coster, W. J., Bettger, J. P., & Haley, S. M. (2006). Association of environmental factors with levels of home and community participation in an adult rehabilitation cohort. *Archives of Physical Medicine and Rehabilitation, 87,* 1566–1575.

Haley, S. M., Siebens, H., Coster, W. J., Tao, W., Black-Shaffer, R. M., Gandek, B., et al. (2006). Computerized adaptive testing for follow-up after discharge from inpatient rehabilitation: I. Activity outcomes. *Archives of Physical Medicine and Rehabilitation, 87,* 1033–1042.

Latham, N., Jette, D. U., Coster, W., Richarts, L., Smout, R. J., James, R. A., et al. (2006). Occupational therapy activities and intervention techniques for clients with stroke in six rehabilitation hospitals. *American Journal of Occupational Therapy, 60,* 369–378.

Schenker, R., Coster, W. J., & Parush, S. (2006). Personal assistance, adaptation, and participation in students with cerebral palsy mainstreamed in elementary schools. *Disability and Rehabilitation, 28,* 1061–1069.

Coster, W. (2005). The Foundation—International Conference on Evidence-based Practice: A collaborative effort of the American Occupational Therapy Association, the American Occupational Therapy Foundation, and the Agency for Healthcare Research and Quality. *American Journal of Occupational Therapy, 59,* 356–358.

Haley, S. M., Raczek, A. E., Coster, W. J., Dumas, H. M., & Fragala-Pinkham, M. A. (2005). Assessing mobility in children using a computer adaptive testing version of the Pediatric Evaluation of Disability Inventory. *Archives of Physical Medicine and Rehabilitation, 86,* 932–939.

Jette, A. M., Keysor, J., Coster, W., Ni, P., & Haley, S. (2005). Beyond function: Predicting participation outcomes in a rehabilitation cohort. *Archives of Physical Medicine and Rehabilitation, 86,* 2087–2094.

Siebens, H., Andres, P., Ni, P., Coster, W. J., & Haley, S. M. (2005). Measuring physical function in patients with complex medical and post-surgical conditions. *American Journal of Physical Medicine and Rehabilitation, 84,* 741–748.

Kadlec, M. B., Coster, W., Tickle-Degnen, L., & Beeghly, M. (2005). Qualities of caregiver–child interaction during daily activities of children born very low birth weight with and without white matter disorder. *American Journal of Occupational Therapy, 59,* 57–66.

Lin, S. H., Cermak, S., Coster, W. J., & Miller, L. (2005). The relation between length of institutionalization and sensory integration in children adopted from Eastern Europe. *American Journal of Occupational Therapy, 59,* 139–147.

Schenker, R., Coster, W. J., & Parush, S. (2005). Neuroimpairments, activity performance, and participation in children with cerebral palsy mainstreamed in elementary schools. *Developmental Medicine and Child Neurology, 47,* 808–814.

Schenker, R., Coster, W., & Parush, S. (2005). Participation and activity performance of students with cerebral palsy within the school environment. *Disability and Rehabilitation, 27,* 539–552.

Coster, W. J., Haley, S. M., Andres, P., Ludlow, L., Bond, T., & Ni, P. (2004). Refining the conceptual basis for rehabilitation outcome measurement: Personal care and instrumental activities domain. *Medical Care, 42*(Suppl.), I62–I72.

Coster, W. J., Haley, S. M., Ludlow, L. H., Andres, P. L., & Ni, P. S. (2004). Development of an applied cognition scale for rehabilitation outcomes measurement. *Archives of Physical Medicine and Rehabilitation, 85,* 2030–2035.

Coster, W. J., & Haltiwanger, J. (2004). Social–behavioral skills of elementary children with physical disabilities included in general education classrooms. *Remedial and Special Education, 25,* 95–103.

Coster, W., & Schwarz, L. (2004, June). Facilitating transfer of evidence-based practice into practice. *Education Special Interest Section Quarterly, 14*(2), 1–3.

Coster, W. J., & Vergara, E. (2004, March 8). Finding resources to support evidence-based practice. *OT Practice, 9*(5), 10–15.

DeSantis, A., Coster, W., Bigsby, R., & Lester, B. (2004). Colic and fussing in infancy, and sensory processing at 3 to 8 years of age. *Infant Mental Health Journal, 25,* 522–539.

Dolva, A.-S., Coster, W. J., & Lilja, M. (2004). Functional performance in children with Down syndrome. *American Journal of Occupational Therapy, 58,* 621–629.

Egilson, S. T., & Coster, W. J. (2004). School Function Assessment: Performance of Icelandic students with special needs. *Scandinavian Journal of Occupational Therapy, 11,* 1–8.

Goldstein, D. N., Cohn, E., & Coster, W. J. (2004). Enhancing participation for children with disabilities—Application of the *ICF* enablement framework to pediatric physical therapist practice. *Pediatric Physical Therapy, 16,* 41–48.

Haley, S. M., Andres, P. L., Coster, W. J., Kosinski, M., Ni, P. S., & Jette, A. M. (2004). Short-form Activity Measures for Post-Acute Care (AM–PAC). *Archives of Physical Medicine and Rehabilitation, 85,* 649–660.

Haley, S. M., Coster, W. J., Andres, P. L. Kosinski, M., & Ni, P. S. (2004). Scoring comparability of short-forms and computerized adaptive testing: A simulation study with the Activity Measure for Post-Acute Care (AM–PAC). *Archives of Physical Medicine and Rehabilitation, 85,* 661–666.

Haley, S. M, Coster, W. J., Andres, P., Ludlow, L., Ni, P., Bond, T., et al. (2004). Activity outcome measurement for post-acute care. *Medical Care, 42*(Suppl.), I49–I61.

Mancini, M. C., & Coster, W. J. (2004). Functional predictors of school participation by children with disabilities. *Occupational Therapy International, 11,* 12–25.

Tarbell, M. H., Henry, A. D., & Coster, W. J. (2004). Psychometric properties of the Scorable Self-care Evaluation. *American Journal of Occupational Therapy, 58,* 324–332.

Bedell, G. M., Haley, S. M., Coster, W. J., & Smith, K. W. (2002). Developing a responsive measure of change for pediatric brain injury rehabilitation. *Brain Injury, 16,* 659–671.

Bedell, G. M., Haley, S. M., Coster, W. J., & Smith, K. W. (2002). Participation readiness at discharge from inpatient rehabilitation in children and adolescents with acquired brain injuries. *Pediatric Rehabilitation, 5,* 107–116.

Haley, S. M., Jette, A. M., Coster, W. J., Kooyoomjian, J. T., Levenson, S., Heeren, T., et al. (2002). Late Life Function and Disability Instrument: II. Development and evaluation of the function component. *Journal of Gerontology: Medical Sciences, 57A,* M217–M222.

Haley, S. M., Ludlow, L., Coster, W., & Langmuir, L. (2002). Reporting of capable versus typical functional activity performance in community-dwelling older adults: Is there a difference? *Journal of Geriatric Physical Therapy, 25*(1), 3–10.

Jette, A. M., Haley, S. M., Coster, W. J., Kooyoomjian, J. T., Levenson, S., Heeren, T., et al. (2002). Late Life Function and Disability Instrument: I. Development and evaluation of the disability component. *Journal of Gerontology: Medical Sciences, 57A,* M209–M216.

Mancini, M. C., Coster, W. J., Trombly, C. A., & Heeren, T. C. (2000). Predicting participation in elementary school of children with disabilities. *Archives of Physical Medicine and Rehabilitation, 81,* 339–347.

Mouradian, L., Als, H., & Coster, W. (2000). Neurobehavioral development of healthy preterm infants at varying gestational ages. *Developmental and Behavioral Pediatrics, 21,* 408–416.

Coster, W. J., Ludlow, L. H., & Mancini, M. C. (1999). Using IRT variable maps to enrich understanding of rehabilitation data. *Journal of Outcome Measurement, 3,* 123–133.

Coster, W. J., Mancini, M. C., & Ludlow, L. H. (1999). Factor structure of the School Function Assessment. *Educational and Psychological Measurement, 59,* 665–677.

Clark, G. C., & Coster, W.J. (1998). Evaluation/problem solving and program evaluation. In J. Case-Smith (Ed.), *Occupational therapy: Making a difference in school system practice* [AOTA Self-Paced Clinical Course]. Bethesda, MD: American Occupational Therapy Association.

Coster, W. J. (1998). Occupation-centered assessment of children. *American Journal of Occupational Therapy, 52,* 337–344.

Coster, W. J., Deeney, T., Haltiwanger, J., & Haley, S. (1998). *School Function Assessment.* San Antonio, TX: Psychological Corporation/ Therapy Skill Builders.

Cross, L., & Coster, W. J. (1997). Symbolic play language during sensory integration treatment. *American Journal of Occupational Therapy, 51,* 808–814.

Dunkerley, E., Tickle-Degnen, L., & Coster, W. J. (1997). Therapist–child interaction in the middle minutes of sensory integration treatment. *American Journal of Occupational Therapy, 51,* 799–805.

Henry, A. D., & Coster, W. J. (1997). Competency beliefs and occupational role behavior among adolescents: Explication of the personal causation construct. *American Journal of Occupational Therapy, 51,* 267–276.

Lin, K., Wu, C., Tickle-Degnen, L., & Coster, W. (1997). Enhancing occupational performance through occupationally embedded exercise: A meta-analytic review. *Occupational Therapy Journal of Research, 17,* 25–47.

Bigsby, R., Coster, W., Lester, B. M., & Peucker, M. R. (1996). Motor–behavioral cues of term and preterm infants at 3 months. *Infant Behavior and Development, 19,* 295–307.

Henry, A. D., & Coster, W. J. (1996). Predictors of functional outcome among adolescents and young adults with psychotic disorders. *American Journal of Occupational Therapy, 50,* 171–181.

Coster, W. J. (1995). Clinical interpretation of "The relationships among sensorimotor components, fine motor skills, and functional performance in preschool children." *American Journal of Occupational Therapy, 49,* 653–654.

Coster, W. (1995). Critique of the Alberta Infant Motor Scale (AIMS). *Physical and Occupational Therapy in Pediatrics, 15*(3), 53–64.

Coster, W. (1995) Development. In C. Trombly (Ed.), *Occupational therapy for physical dysfunction* (4th ed., pp. 255–264). Baltimore: Williams & Wilkins.

Coster, W. J. (1995). Developmental aspects of occupation. In C. B. Royeen, (Ed.), *The practice of the future: Putting occupation back into therapy* [AOTA Self-Study Series]. Bethesda, MD: American Occupational Therapy Association.

Coster, W. J., Tickle-Degnen, L., & Armenta, L. (1995). Therapist–child interaction during sensory integration treatment: Development and testing of a research tool. *Occupational Therapy Journal of Research, 15,* 17–35.

Tickle-Degnen, L., & Coster, W. J. (1995). Therapeutic interaction and the management of challenge during the beginning minutes of sensory integration treatment. *Occupational Therapy Journal of Research, 15,* 122–141.

Coster, W. J., Haley, S. M., & Baryza, M. J. (1994). Functional performance of young children after head injury: A six-month follow-up study. *American Journal of Occupational Therapy, 48,* 211–218.

Haley, S. M., Coster, W. J., & Binda-Sundberg, K. (1994). Measuring physical disablement: The contextual challenge. *Physical Therapy, 74,* 443–451.

Coster, W., & Cicchetti, D. (1993). Research on the communicative development of maltreated children: Implications for practice. *Topics in Language Disorders, 13*(4), 25–38.

Haley, S. M., & Coster, W. J. (1993). Response to Reid, D. T., et al. "Critique of the Pediatric Evaluation of Disability Inventory (PEDI)." *Physical and Occupational Therapy in Pediatrics, 13*(4), 89–93.

Haley, S. M., Ludlow, L. H., & Coster, W. J. (1993). Clinical interpretation of summary scores using Rasch Rating Scale methodology. In C. Granger & G. Gresham (Eds.), *New developments in functional assessment: Physical medicine and rehabilitation clinics of North America* (Vol. 4, No. 3). Philadelphia: W. B. Saunders.

Coster, W. J., & Haley, S. M. (1992). Conceptualization and measurement of disablement in infants and young children. *Infants and Young Children, 4,* 11–22.

Haley, S. M., Coster, W. J., & Ludlow, L. H. (1992). Development and validation of the Pediatric Evaluation of Disability Inventory (PEDI) [Abstract]. *Archives of Physical Medicine and Rehabilitation, 73,* 987–988.

Haley, S. M., Coster, W. J., Ludlow, L., Haltiwanger, J., & Andrellos, P. (1992). *Pediatric Evaluation of Disability Inventory (PEDI).* Boston: Boston University, Center for Rehabilitation Effectiveness.

Cicchetti, D., Beeghly, M., Carlson, V., Coster, W., Gersten, M., Rieder, C., et al. (1991). Development and psychopathology: Lessons from the study of maltreated children. In D. Keating & H. Rosen (Eds.), *Constructivist perspectives on developmental psychopathology and atypical development* (pp. 69–102). Hillsdale, NJ: Erlbaum.

Coster, W., & Jaffe, L. (1991). Current concepts of children's perceptions of control. *American Journal of Occupational Therapy, 45,* 19–25.

Haley, S. N., Coster, W. J., & Faas, R. (1991). A content validity study of the Pediatric Evaluation of Disability Inventory (PEDI). *Pediatric Physical Therapy, 3,* 177–184.

Haley, S. N., Coster W. J., & Ludlow, L. H. (1991). Pediatric functional outcome measures. In K. M. Jaffe (Ed.), *Pediatric rehabilitation: Physical medicine and rehabilitation clinics of North America* (Vol. 2, No. 4., pp. 689–723). Philadelphia: W. B. Saunders.

Haley, S., Coster, W., & Ludlow, L. (1991). Rasch scaling of functional items in a normative pediatric sample: Development of the Pediatric Evaluation of Disability Inventory [Abstract]. *Archives of Physical Medicine and Rehabilitation, 72,* 797.

Henderson, A., Cermak, S., Coster, W., Murray, E., Trombly, C., & Tickle-Degnen, L. (1991). The Issue Is—Occupational science is multidimensional. *American Journal of Occupational Therapy, 45,* 370–372.

Witt, A., Cermak, S., & Coster, W. (1990). Body part identification in 1 to 2 year-old children. *American Journal of Occupational therapy, 44,* 147–153.

Coster, W. (1989). Review of R. A. Barkley, "Defiant children—A clinician's manual for parent training." *Physical and Occupational Therapy in Pediatrics, 9*(1), 164–165.

Coster, W., Gersten, M., Beeghly, M., & Cichetti, D. (1989). Communicative functioning in maltreated toddlers. *Developmental Psychology, 25,* 1020–1029.

Ebb, E. W., Coster, W., & Duncombe, L. (1989). Comparison of normal and psychosocially dysfunctional male adolescents. *Occupational Therapy in Mental Health, 9*(2), 53–74.

Coster, W. J. (1988). Behavioral inhibition in young children: Implications of current research for occupational therapy. In *Proceedings of the Occupational Therapy for Maternal and Child Health Research and Leadership Development Conference* (Vol. 2., pp. 66–75). Rockville, MD: American Occupational Therapy Association.

Coster, W. (1988). [Review of *Evaluation and treatment of adolescents and children*]. *Disabilities Studies Quarterly, 8*(4), 19–20.

Coster, W. (1988). [Review of *Psychological Maltreatment of Children and Youth*]. *American Journal of Occupational Therapy, 42,* 617–618.

Gersten, M., Coster, W., Schneider-Rosen, K., Carlson, V., & Cicchetti, D. (1986). The socio-emotional bases of communicative functioning: Quality of attachment, language development, and early maltreatment. In M. Lamb, A. L. Brown, & B. Rogoff (Eds.), *Advances in developmental psychology* (Vol. 4, pp. 105–151). Hillsdale, NJ: Erlbaum.

Coster, W. J., & Miller, L. J. (1982). Guidelines for developmental evaluations. In E. Gilfoyle (Ed.), *Occupational therapy educational management in schools: A competency-based educational program (TOTEMS).* Rockville, MD: American Occupational Therapy Association.

Coster, W. J., & Miller, L. J. (1982). IEP and behavioral (performance) objectives. In E. Gilfoyle (Ed.), *Occupational therapy educational management in schools: A competency-based educational program (TOTEMS).* Rockville, MD: American Occupational Therapy Association.

Cermak, S., Coster, W., & Drake, C. (1980). Gestural representation in boys with learning disabilities. *American Journal of Occupational Therapy, 34,* 19–26.

Winifred Wiese Dunn, PhD, OTR, FAOTA—2001

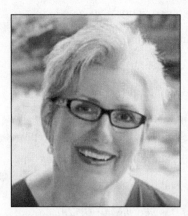

Winifred Wiese Dunn is a professor and chair at the University of Kansas Medical Center. Her practice expertise is with children and families in community settings, including early intervention and public school programs. She also has made significant contributions to the scholarship of knowledge integration and application of best practices based on interdisciplinary evidence for the profession of occupational therapy.

A graduate from the University of Missouri with a bachelor's degree in occupational therapy, Dunn holds a master's degree in education/learning disabilities from the University of Missouri in Columbia and a doctorate in applied neuroscience from the University of Kansas, Lawrence.

She received the Roster of Fellow of the American Occupational Therapy Association (AOTA) in 1982, the AOTA Award of Merit in 1991, and was inducted into the Academy of Research in 1993 by the American Occupational Therapy Foundation (AOTF). She also received the A. Jean Ayres Research Award for her contribution to knowledge about sensory processing. Dunn has served in various capacities with AOTA, AOTF, and the National Board for Certification of Occupational Therapy.

Dunn has been instrumental in developing and linking theory through practice. She developed the Ecology of Human Performance conceptual framework and is the author of Dunn's Model of Sensory Processing, which is based on her research and outlines how persons understand and use the sensory input for everyday life.

Linking Key Messages of the 2001 Eleanor Clarke Slagle Lecture to the AOTA *Centennial Vision:* One of the unique contributions that occupational therapy makes to global knowledge is an evidence-based conception of sensory processing. From early scholars in occupational therapy, we have demonstrated our focus on understanding the impact of sensory input and processing on the human body, the person's movement patterns, emotions, thinking, and problem solving. In my Slagle lecture, I provided a summary of the current evidence that informed our understanding about the impact of sensory processing on people's everyday life routines. Using interdisciplinary basic and applied science evidence, I outlined the known and hypothesized relationships among sensory, motor, cognitive, and emotional factors that contribute to both functional and maladaptive behavior. I proposed that sensory processing knowledge reflects the human condition and therefore affects everyone's occupational needs to live a satisfying life. Furthermore, I suggested that we might use this proposition to think more broadly about our impact on society, not only on those who have disabilities.

—Winnie Dunn

Bibliography

Dunn, W. (in press). Sensory processing: An important key to understanding learners with autism spectrum disorders. In K. D. Buron & P. Wolfberg (Eds.), *Educating learners on the autism spectrum: Translating theory into meaningful practice*. Kansas City, KS: Autism and Asperger Publishing.

Sigrkrist, S., Bjarnadotti, G., Townsend, E., & Dunn, W. (in press). Occupational performance and everyday sensations of preschool children in Iceland. *American Journal of Occupational Therapy*.

Nadon, G., Feldman, D., Dunn, W., & Gisel, E. (2010). Mealtime problems in children with autism spectrum disorder and their typically developing siblings: A comparison study. *Autism, 14*.

Dove, S., & Dunn, W. (2009). Sensory processing patterns in learning disabilities. *Occupational Therapy in Early Intervention, Preschool, and Schools, 2*(1), 1–11.

Dunn, W. (2009). Ecology of Human Performance Model. In S. Dunbar (Ed.), *Occupational therapy models for intervention with children and families*. Thorofare, NJ: Slack.

Dunn, W. (2009). Invited commentary on "Sensory Sensitivities in Gifted Children." *American Journal of Occupational Therapy, 63*(3), 296–300.

Dunn, W. (2009). Sensation and sensory processing. In E. Crepeau, E. Cohn, & B. Schell (Ed.), *Willard and Spackman's occupational therapy*. Philadelphia: Lippincott, Williams & Wilkins.

Dunn, W., & Foreman, J. (2009). Development of evidence-based knowledge. In M. Law (Ed.), *Evidence-based rehabilitation: A guide to practice* (2nd ed.). Thorofare, NJ: Slack.

Dunn, W. (2008). Harnessing teacher's wisdom for evidence-based practice: Standardization data from the Sensory Profile School Companion. *Journal of Occupational Therapy, Schools, and Early Intervention, 1*(3–4), 206–214.

Dunn, W. (2008). *Living sensationally: Understanding your senses*. London: Jessica Kingsley.

Mische-Lawson, L., & Dunn, W. (2008). Children's sensory processing patterns and play preferences. *Annals of Therapeutic Recreation, 17*, 1–14.

Dunn, W. (2007). *The Sensory Profile supplement*. San Antonio, TX: Psychological Corporation.

Dunn, W. (2007). Supporting children in everyday life using a sensory processing approach. *Infants and Young Children, 20*(2), 84–101.

Tomchek, S., & Dunn, W. (2007). Sensory processing in children with and without autism: A comparative study utilizing the Short Sensory Profile. *American Journal of Occupational Therapy, 61*(2), 190–200.

Dunn, W. (2006). *School Companion Sensory Profile manual*. San Antonio, TX: Psychological Corporation.

Dunn, W. (2006). *Sensory Profile School Companion*. San Antonio, TX: Psychological Corporation.

Dunn, W. (2006). *Sensory Profile supplement*. San Antonio, TX: Psychological Corporation.

Baum, C., Perlmutter, M., & Dunn, W. (2005). Establishing the integrity of measurement data: Identifying impairments that can limit occupational performance and threaten the validity of assessments. In M. Law, C. Baum, & W. Dunn (Eds.), *Measuring occupational performance: Supporting best practice in occupational therapy* (2nd ed.). Thorofare, NJ: Slack.

Dunn, W. (2005). Measurement issues and practices. In M. Law, C. Baum, & W. Dunn (Eds.), *Measuring occupational performance: Supporting best practice in occupational therapy* (2nd ed.). Thorofare, NJ: Slack.

Dunn, W. (2005). Sensory processing. In R. M. Simpson (Ed.), *Educating children and youth with autism*. San Antonio, TX: Pro-Ed.

Dunn, W. (2005). A sensory processing approach to supporting students with autism spectrum disorders. In R. M. Simpson (Ed.), *Educating children and youth with autism*. Austin, TX: Pro-Ed.

Law, M., Baum, C., & Dunn, W. (2005). Challenges and strategies in applying an occupational performance measurement approach. In M. Law, C. Baum, & W. Dunn (Eds.), *Measuring occupational performance: Supporting best practice in occupational therapy* (2nd ed.). Thorofare, NJ: Slack.

Law, M., Baum, C., & Dunn, W. (2005). *Measuring occupational performance: Supporting best practice in occupational therapy* (2nd ed.). Thorofare, NJ: Slack.

Coffelt, K., & Dunn, W. (2004). *The relationship between sensory processing patterns and expectations of students' performance in preschool teachers*. Master's thesis, University of Kansas, Kansas City.

Dunn, W. (2004). A sensory processing approach to supporting infant–caregiver relationships. In A. Sameroff, S. McDonough, & K. Rosenblum (Eds.), *Treating parent–infant relationship problems*. New York: Guilford Press.

Myles, B. S., Hagiwara, T., Dunn, W., Rinner, L., Reese, M., Huggins, A., et al. (2004). Sensory issues in children with Asperger syndrome and autism. *Education and Training in Developmental Disabilities, 3*(4), 283–290.

Dunn, W., Brown, C., & Youngstrom, M. (2003). Ecological Model of Occupation. In P. Kramer, J. Hinojosa, & C. B. Royeen (Eds.), *Perspectives in human occupation: Participation in life* (pp. 222–263). Philadelphia: Lippincott Williams & Wilkins.

Pohl, P., Dunn, W., & Brown, C. (2003). The role of sensory processing in the everyday lives of older adults. *Occupational Therapy Journal of Research, 23*, 99–106.

Brown, T., Cromwell, R., Filion, D., Dunn, W., & Tollefson, N. (2002). Sensory processing in schizophrenia: Missing and avoiding information. *Schizophrenia Research, 55*(1/2), 187–195.

Brown, C., & Dunn, W. (2002). *The Adult Sensory Profile*. San Antonio, TX: Psychological Corporation.

Daniels, D., & Dunn, W. (2002). Initial development of the Infant–Toddler Sensory Profile. *Journal of Early Intervention, 25*(1), 27–41.

Dunn, W. (2002). *The Infant Toddler–Sensory Profile*. San Antonio, TX: Psychological Corporation. '

Dunn, W., & Bennett, D. (2002). Patterns of sensory processing in children with attention deficit hyperactivity disorder. *Occupational Therapy Journal of Research, 22*, 4–15.

Dunn, W., Myles, B. S., & Orr, S. (2002). Sensory processing issues in Asperger syndrome: A preliminary investigation. *American Journal of Occupational Therapy, 56*, 97–102.

Dunn, W., Saiter, J., & Rinner, L (2002). Asperger syndrome and sensory processing: A conceptual model and guidance for intervention planning. *Focus on Autism and Other Developmental Disabilities, 17*(3), 172–185.

Brown, C., Tollefson, N., Dunn, W., Cromwell, R., & Filion, D. (2001). The Adult Sensory Profile: Measuring patterns of sensory processing. *American Journal of Occupational Therapy, 55*, 75–82.

Daniels, D., & Dunn, W. (2001). Development of the Infant–Toddler Sensory Profile. *Occupational Therapy Journal of Research, 20*(Suppl.), 86S–90S.

Dunn, W. (2001). The sensations of everyday life: Empirical, theoretical, and pragmatic considerations (2001 Eleanor Clarke Slagle Lecture). *American Journal of Occupational Therapy, 55*, 608–620.

Law, M., & Dunn, W. (2001). *Measuring occupational performance: Supporting best practice in occupational therapy*. Thorofare, NJ: Slack.

Dunn, W. (2000). *Best practice in occupational therapy: In community service with children and families*. Thorofare, NJ: Slack.

Dunn, W. (2000). Habit: What's the brain got to do with it? *Occupational Therapy Journal of Research, 20*(Suppl. 1), 6S–20S.

Huebner, R., & Dunn, W. (2000). Introduction and basic concepts of sensorimotor approaches to autism and related disorders. In R. Huebner (Ed.), *Autism and related disorders: A sensorimotor approach to management*. Gaithersburg, MD: Aspen.

Dunn, W. (1999). Making sense of the world. *Advance for Directors in Rehabilitation, 2*(2), 47–48.

Ermer, J., & Dunn, W. (1998). The Sensory Profile: A discriminant analysis of children with and without disabilities. *American Journal of Occupational Therapy, 52*(4), 283–290.

Dunn, W. (1997). The Sensory Profile: A discriminating measure of sensory processing in daily life. *Sensory Integration Special Interest Section Quarterly, 20*, 1–4.

Dunn, W., & Brown, C. (1997). Factor analysis on the sensory profile from a national sample of children without disabilities. *American Journal of Occupational Therapy, 51*, 490–495.

Dunn, W., & Cada, E. (1997). The national occupational therapy practice analysis: Findings and implications for competence. *American Journal of Occupational Therapy, 52*, 721–728.

Dunn, W., & Westman, K. (1997). The Sensory Profile: The performance of a national sample of children without disabilities. *American Journal of Occupational Therapy, 51*, 25–34.

Kemmis, B., & Dunn, W. (1997). A comparison of remedial and compensatory approaches to collaborative consultation in schools. *American Journal of Occupational Therapy, 9*, 23–35.

Kientz, M., & Dunn, W. (1997). A comparison of the performance of children with and without autism on the Sensory Profile. *American Journal of Occupational Therapy, 51*, 530–537.

Rondenelli, R., Dunn, W., Hassanein, K., Keesling, C., Meredith, S., Schulz, T., et al. (1997). A simulation of hand impairments: Effects on upper extremity function and implication towards medical impairment rating and disability determination. *Archive of Physical Medicine Rehabilitation, 78*, 1358–1363.

Kemmis, B., & Dunn, W. (1996). Collaborative consultation: The efficacy of remedial and compensatory interventions in school contexts. *American Journal of Occupational Therapy, 50*, 709–717.

Dunn, W. (1995). Current knowledge that affects school-based practice and an agenda for action. *School Systems Special Interest Section Quarterly, 2*, 3–4.

Dunn, W., & Westman, K. (1995). Current knowledge that affects school-based practice and an agenda for action, part 1 of 2. *School System Special Interest Section Quarterly, 2*, 1–2.

Dunn, W., & Westman, K. (1995). Current knowledge that affects school-based practice and an agenda for action, part 2 of 2. *School System Special Interest Section Quarterly, 2*, 3–4.

Dunn, W. (1994). Getting ready for the day. In C. Royeen (Ed.), *AOTA Self-study Series—The practice of the future: Putting occupation back into therapy.* Rockville, MD: American Occupational Therapy Association.

Dunn, W. (1994). Outsider trading. In C. Royeen (Ed.), *AOTA Self-study Series—The practice of the future: Putting occupation back into therapy.* Rockville, MD: American Occupational Therapy Association.

Dunn, W. (1994). Performance of typical children on the Sensory Profile: An item analysis. *American Journal of Occupational Therapy, 48*, 967–974.

Dunn, W. (1994). The rubber band. In C. Royeen (Ed.), *AOTA Self-study Series—The practice of the future: Putting occupation back into therapy.* Rockville, MD: American Occupational Therapy Association.

Dunn, W. (1994). The velveteen person: How human beings become real. In C. Royeen (Ed.), *AOTA Self-study Series—The practice of the future: Putting occupation back into therapy.* Rockville, MD: American Occupational Therapy Association.

Dunn, W., & Boyle, M. (1994). A comparison of funding patterns in professional occupational therapy education programs. *Occupational Therapy Journal of Research, 14*, 157–169.

Dunn, W., Brown, C., McClain, C., & Westman, K. (1994). The Ecology of Human Performance: A contextual perspective on human performance. In C. Royeen (Ed.), *AOTA Self-study Series—The practice of the future: Putting occupation back into therapy.* Rockville, MD: American Occupational Therapy Association.

Dunn, W., Brown, C., & McGuigan, A. (1994). The Ecology of Human Performance: A framework for thought and action. *American Journal of Occupational Therapy, 48*, 595–607.

Dunn, W. (1993). Grip strength of children ages 3–8 years using a modified sphygmomanometer: Comparison of typical children to children with rheumatic disorders. *American Journal of Occupational Therapy, 47*, 421–428.

Dunn, W. (1993). Measurement of function: Actions for the future. *American Journal of Occupational Therapy, 47*, 357–359.

Dunn, W. (1993). Useful research strategies for studying service provision in real-life contexts. *Developmental Disabilities Special Interest Section Quarterly, 16*(2), 1–3.

Law, M., & Dunn, W. (1993). Perspectives on understanding and changing environments for children. *Physical and Occupational Therapy in Pediatrics, 13*(3), 1–17.

Law, M., & Dunn, W. (1993). Response to commentary. *Physical and Occupational Therapy in Pediatrics, 13*(3), 23–24.

Dunn, W., DeGagi, G., & Royeen, C. (1992). Sensory integration and neurodevelopmental treatment for educational programming. In C. Royeen (Ed.), *AOTA Self-study Series—Classroom applications for school-based programming.* Rockville, MD: American Occupational Therapy Association.

Dunn, W., & Huss, A. J. (1992). Personal perspectives on career development: Interviews with occupational therapy leaders. *Occupational Therapy Practice, 3*(3), 1–6.

Dunn, W. (1991). Introduction to the spinal cord and brain stem. *Nautilus, 2*(6).

Dunn, W. (1991). Motivation. In C. Royeen (Ed.), *AOTA Self-study Series—Neuroscience: Foundations of human performance.* Rockville, MD: American Occupational Therapy Association.

Dunn, W. (Ed.). (1991). *Pediatric occupational therapy: Facilitating effective service provision.* Thorofare, NJ: Charles B. Slack.

Dunn, W., & Royeen, C. (Eds.). (1991). *AOTA Self-study Series—School-based practice for related services.* Rockville, MD: American Occupational Therapy Association.

Royeen, C., & Dunn, W. (Eds.). (1991). *AOTA Self-study Series—Assessing function.* Rockville, MD: American Occupational Therapy Association.

Boyle, M. A., Dunn, W., & Kielhofner, G. (1990). Funding for research and training in professional occupational therapy education program from 1985–1987. *Occupational Therapy Journal of Research, 10*, 334–342.

DiJoseph, L., Dunn, W., Lowenstein, P., Rabin, M., Strickland, L. R., & VanSchroeder, C. (1990). Entry-level role delineation for registered occupational therapists (OTRs) and certified occupational therapy assistants (COTAs). *American Journal of Occupational Therapy, 44*, 1091–1102.

Dunn, W. (1990). A comparison of service provision models in school-based occupational therapy services. *Occupational Therapy Journal of Research, 10*, 300–320.

Dunn, W. (1990). Establishing inter-rater reliability on a criterion-referenced developmental checklist. *Occupational Therapy Journal of Research, 10*, 377–380.

Dunn, W. (1989). Occupational therapy in early intervention: New perspectives create greater possibilities. *American Journal of Occupational Therapy, 43*, 717–721.

Dunn, W. (1989). Validity. *Physical and Occupational Therapy in Pediatrics, 9*(1), 149–168.

Dunn, W., & McGourty, L. (1989). Application of uniform terminology to practice. *American Journal of Occupational Therapy, 43*(12), 817–831.

Dunn, W., & Rask, S. (1989). Entry-level and specialized practice: A professional encounter. *American Journal of Occupational Therapy, 43*, 7–9.

Hughes, P., & Dunn, W. (1989). Preassessment: An effective tool for the rural therapist. *Development Disabilities Special Interest Section Quarterly.*

Dunn, W. (1988). Basic and applied neuroscience research provides a basis for sensory integration theory. *American Journal of Mental Retardation, 92*(5), 420–422.

Dunn, W. (1988). An educator's perspective. *Sensory Integration Special Interest Section Quarterly, 11*(4), 3–4.

Dunn, W. (1988). Integrated related services for preschoolers with neurological impairments: Issues and strategies. *Remedial and Special Education, 10*(3), 31–39.

Dunn, W. (1988). Models of occupational therapy service provision in the school system. *American Journal of Occupational Therapy, 42*, 718–723.

Dunn, W. (1988). Selecting a test to evaluate sensory integration. *Sensory Integration Special Interest Section Quarterly, 11*(4), 3–4.

Dunn, W., & Gray, B. (1988). *Managing occupational therapy in rural education (M.O.R.E.): Initial findings.* St. Louis, MO: American Consortium of Rural Educational Systems.

Calkins, C. F., Dunn, W., & Kultgen, P. (1986). A comparison of preschool and elderly community integration/demonstration projects at the University of Missouri Institute for Human Development. *Journal of the Association for Severely Handicapped, 11*(4), 276–285.

Dunn, W. (1986). Developmental and environmental contexts for interpreting clinical observations. *Sensory Integration Special Interest Section Quarterly, 9*(2), 4–7.

Dunn, W. (1986, Fall). Using structured play groups to facilitate interactive play skills at the preschool level. *Association for Persons With Severe Disabilities Newsletter*, p. 8.

Dunn, W. (1985). Occupational therapy's challenge: Caregiving and research. *American Journal of Occupational Therapy, 39*, 259–264.

Dunn, W. (1985). Therapists as consultants to educators. *Sensory Integration Special Interest Section Quarterly, 8*(1), 1–4.

Dunn, W. (1983). Critique of the Erhardt Developmental Prehension Assessment (EDPA). *Physical and Occupational Therapy in Pediatrics, 3*(4), 59–68.

Dunn, W., & Fisher, A. G. (1983). Sensory registration, autism, and tactile defensiveness. *Sensory Integration Special Interest Section Quarterly, 6*(2), 3–4.

Fisher, A. G., & Dunn, W. (1983). Tactile defensiveness: Historical perspectives, new research—A theory grows. *Sensory Integration Special Interest Section Quarterly, 6*(2), 1–2.

Dunn, W. (1982). Independence through activity: The practice of occupational therapy in pediatrics. *American Journal of Occupational Therapy, 36*, 745–747.

Dunn, W. (1981). Equipment development. *Sensory Integration Special Interest Section Quarterly, 4*(3), 3.

Dunn, W. (1981). *A guide to testing clinical observations in kindergartners.* Rockville, MD: American Occupational Therapy Association.

Dunn, W. (1981). A nontraditional recording system. In E. Gilfoyle (Ed.), *Training: Occupational therapy educational management in schools* (Mod. 4). Rockville, MD: American Occupational Therapy Association.

Dunn, W. (1980). Evaluation of preschoolers. *Sensory Integration Special Interest Section Quarterly, 3*(3).

Dunn, W. (1980). The parent component. *Sensory Integration Special Interest Section Quarterly, 2*(4), 4.

Dunn, W. (1979). Developing norms for charting classroom progress. *Journal of Learning Disabilities, 12*(3), 320–321.

Dunn, W. (1979). Games therapists play: Waterbeds as therapy aids. *Sensory Integration Special Interest Section Quarterly, 2*(1), 1.

Shereen Farber, PhD, OTR, FAOTA—1989

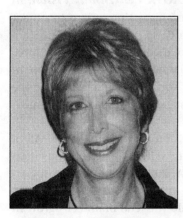

Shereen Farber is woman of many diverse talents. She is a consultant in private practice providing ortho–neuro–rehabilitation services to individuals with chronic pain and provides canine–equine rehabilitation to horses and dogs that are used in police work, patient services, search-and-rescue operations, and various other performance venues. She is a member of the Research Advisory Committee for Indiana University's Master's in Occupational Therapy Program; a board member and research consultant to a variety of private corporations, including the Integrative Learning Center of Mid-America (ILCMA), a 501(c) (3) organization. Farber currently is collaborating on a research project with ILCMA founder Cynthia Allen, FGCT, BFLP/P, and Carol Montgomery, MS, PT, FGCT, BFLP/P, studying the effect of Bones For Life® intervention on developing improved function in the elderly population. One of her passions is training her golden retrievers to participate in tracking (search and rescue), obedience, agility, field, and conformation performance venues. She occasionally breeds dogs under the kennel name of Arrowood Golden Retrievers.

Farber graduated with a bachelor of science in occupational therapy in 1967 from Ohio State University (OSU) and in 1972 earned a master's of science in special education and learning disabilities from Butler University in

Indianapolis, Indiana. In 1985, she earned a PhD in comparative anatomy/neurobiology from the Indiana University School of Medicine and in 1988 completed post-doctoral training in neurophysiology and neurotransplantation from the Indiana University School of Medicine, Department of Physiology and Biophysics. She also was a graduate teaching assistant for the Department of Anatomy and Physiology and Biophysics during her doctoral and post-doctoral training.

Farber was first employed in 1967 as a staff occupational therapist at the Cerebral Palsy Clinic at the Indiana University Medical Center and later became the chief occupational therapist at Riley Hospital Child Development Center in Indianapolis. She began her academic career as a part-time instructor at the Occupational Therapy Program, Division of Allied Health at the Indiana University School of Medicine. She later became a full-time faculty member in the occupational therapy program until 1982. She became assistant director of occupational therapy for administration of the occupational therapy clinics at the Indiana University Medical Center from 1988 to 1992. During this period, Farber also was an adjunct associate professor for the Department of Occupational Therapy, School of Allied Health Medicine within the School of Medicine. Since 1972, she has consulted to various universities and clinical units for program development and design of research programs.

Farber was inducted into the American Occupational Therapy Association (AOTA) Roster of Fellows in 1978. Her other awards include membership in the TAPS honor society (OSU), receiving the Award for Scientific Excellence in the area of sensory integration from Rush–Presbyterian St. Luke's Occupational Therapy Program in 1982, receiving the Eleanor Clarke Lecture in 1989, and presenting the Hite Symposium Speech at OSU in 2005.

Farber's research interests include (1) investigating the effects of mind–body, holistic craniosacral, and other alternative treatment on human, canine, and equine function; (2) promoting a wellness lifestyle; (3) studying all aspects of the human/animal/environmental interaction; (4) studying methods of canine/equine rehabilitation; and (5) examining consumer products and evaluating their impact on occupational performance.

On a Personal Note From a Phone Interview: Farber indicated that she adopted the occupational therapy philosophical base to organize her personal and professional behaviors. She noted, "Through occupational therapy, I learned numerous skills to enhance and evolve . . . where I could apply occupational therapy constructs to nontraditional environments. I go back and forth between my intuitive base, what one thinks of as right-brain skills, and being analytical, or more left-brain skills. This gives me a natural holistic perspective." She travels the United States doing animal seminars treating show dogs and show horses, still spreading occupational therapy's message in a unique way. Farber notes "occupational therapists need more choices and need to demonstrate courage by taking risks in new areas of practice and to be willing to change. Utilizing evidence-based occupational therapy applied to new and unique settings ensures quality service and promotes occupational therapy as a responsible health practice. Because of the influence of occupational therapy on my personal life, I keep evolving . . . seems like I am constantly on the edge of doing something different." Farber is an inspiration as she keeps envisioning new areas of practice.

Linking Key Messages of the 1989 Eleanor Clarke Slagle Lecture to the AOTA *Centennial Vision:* In 1967, when I started practicing occupational therapy, there were several "clinical experts" suggesting various treatment systems that one should use to treat given populations. These systems might have been based on some scientific readings, but they were not tested using the scientific method. Evidence-based therapy had not become standard at that time.

I was driven to understand how a treatment modality interacted with the brain and produced adaptive behavior in the animal model being studied. The main premise of my Eleanor Clarke Slagle Lecture was that by understanding the human brain, one could better interpret human behavior. Likewise, one needed to understand the effects of environment and specific therapeutic modalities on the brain.

The *Centennial Vision* has eight elements considered relevant to AOTA's shared vision for the profession. All of them "speak to me," and I consider them all important; however, the eighth element, "science-fostered innovation in occupational therapy practice," is the one in which I have deeply invested (AOTA, 2007, p. 614). My post-doctoral research (1985–1988) included fetal brain cell transplantation into a rat model with induced ischemia in the hippocampal area of the brain. We asked many basic science questions, such as would the fetal brain cells grow in the ischemic area, and if they grew, would they form synapses? We also wondered if we would see different functional behavioral changes between those with successful transplantations and sham-operated controls. Without undue details, the cells grew, formed synapses, and did produce functional differences. I then wondered, if I used enriched environmental conditions, would the transplants produce more synapses compared to those rats recovering without enrichment?

It was at that point that President George H. W. Bush imposed a ban on fetal stem cell research and so the National Institutes of Health could not fund grants in this area. The ban changed the future of my career as a neuroscientist–occupational therapist. I continued to do research, although it was for drug companies. In the past few years, I have been participating in a research project studying the effects of Bones for Life, a type of Feldenkrais movement (Foundation for Movement Intelligence, n.d.). We wanted to see if teaching Bones for Life processes to a group of 80-year-old healthy adults would improve their balance, posture, and activities of daily living status. The study has both qualitative and quantitative aspects that are currently being analyzed.

—Shereen Farber

References

American Occupational Therapy Association. (2007). AOTA's *Centennial Vision* and executive summary. *American Journal of Occupational Therapy, 61*, 613–614.

Foundation for Movement Intelligence. (n.d.). Home page. Available online at http://www.movementintelligence.org/

Bibliography

Farber, S. D. (1995, July/August). A tribute to William Worley. *Golden Retriever News*, pp. 6–8.

Farber, S. D. (1994, April/June). Conditioning your dog for improved gait. *Golden Retriever News*, pp. 125–127.

Farber, S. D. (1994). Values and beliefs. In C. B. Royeen (Ed.), *AOTA Self-Study Series: Human performance*. Bethesda, MD: American Occupational Therapy Association.

Farber, S. D., Koontz, S., & Van Fossen, R. (1994). Qualitative and quantitative video analysis of mothers and infants during feedings with angled and straight bottles. *Journal of Pediatrics, 136*, 332–338.

Farber, S. D. (1993, November/December). Conditioning your dog for improved performance and health. *Golden Retriever News*, pp. 94–96.

Farber, S. D. (1993). Neurobiology and occupational therapy: Functional relationships. In H. Hopkins & H. Smith (Eds.), *Willard and Spackman's occupational therapy* (8th ed., pp. 92–95). Philadelphia: Lippincott.

Farber, S. D., & Abreau, B. C. (1993). Understanding the brain and theories of learning related to cognitive function and rehabilitation. In C. B. Royeen (Ed.), *AOTA Self-Study Series: Cognitive rehabilitation*. Rockville, MD: American Occupational Therapy Association.

Farber, S. D. (1991). Evaluation of neuromotor performance. In C. Baum & C. Christensen (Eds.), *Occupational therapy: Overcoming human performance deficits* (pp. 259–282). Thorofare, NJ: Slack.

Farber, S. D. (1991). Principles of neuromotor performance. In C. Baum & C. Christensen (Eds.), *Occupational therapy: Overcoming human performance deficits* (pp. 507–521). Thorofare, NJ: Slack.

Farber, S. D., Magnes, C. J., Peterson, R. G., & Farber, M. O. (1991). 2,3 DPG and neuropathy. *Journal of Neurological Sciences, 101*, 204–207.

Farber, S. D., & Moore, J. C. (1990). Regional neuroanatomy of the nervous system. In C. B. Royeen (Ed.), *AOTA Self-Study Series: Neuroscience foundations of human performance*. Rockville, MD: American Occupational Therapy Association.

Farber, S. D., & Cool, S. J. (1990). Functional neurochemistry. In C. B. Royeen (Ed.), *AOTA Self-Study Series: Neuroscience foundations of human performance*. Bethesda, MD: American Occupational Therapy Association.

Moore, J. C., & Farber, S. D. (1990). Systemic neuroanatomy. In C. B. Royeen (Ed.), *AOTA Self-Study Series: Neuroscience foundations of human performance*. Rockville, MD: American Occupational Therapy Association.

Farber, S. D. (1989). Living with Meniere disease: An occupational therapist's personal perspective. *American Journal of Occupational Therapy. 43*, 341–343.

Farber, S. D. (1989). Neuroscience and occupational therapy: Vital connections (1989 Eleanor Clarke Slagle Lecture). *American Journal of Occupational Therapy, 43*, 637–646.

Farber, S. D., & Zoltan, B. (1989). Visual vestibular systems interaction: Therapeutic implication. *Journal of Head Trauma Rehabilitation, 4*, 9–16.

Low, W. C., Farber, S. D., Hill, T. G., Sattin, A., & Kubek, M. J. (1989). Evidence for extrinsic and intrinsic sources of thyrotropin-releasing hormone (TRH) in the hippocampal formation as determined by radioimmunoassay and immunocytochemistry. *Annals of New York Academy of Science, 553*, 574–578.

Low, W. C., Roepke, J., Farber, S. D., Hill, T. G., Sattin, A., & Kubek, M. J. (1989). Distribution of thyrotropin-releasing hormone (TRH) in the hippocampal formation as determined by radioimmunoassay. *Neuroscience Letters, 103*, 314–319.

Farber, S. D., Onifer, S. M., Murphy, S. H., Kaseda, Y., Wells, D., Vietje, B., et al. (1988). Neural transmission of embryonic hippocampus in an experimental model of cerebral ischemia. *Progress in Brain Research, 78*, 103–107.

Farber, S. D. (1985). *Effects of insulin on the morphology of peripheral nerve in alloxan-induced diabetic rats and their controls*. Doctoral dissertation, Indiana University School of Medicine Graduate School.

Farber, S. D. (1982). *Neurorehabilitation: A multisensory approach*. Philadelphia: W. B. Saunders.

Farber, S. D. (1981). Neurorehabilitation of the neonate. In J. Wilson (Ed.), *Comprehensive management of infants at risk for CNS dysfunction* (2nd ed., pp. 40–62). Chapel Hill: University of North Carolina, School of Medicine.

Farber, S. D. (1978). Olfaction in health and illness. *American Journal of Occupational Therapy, 32,* 155–160.

Farber, S. D. (1974). *Sensorimotor evaluation and treatment procedures for allied health personnel* (2nd ed.). Indianapolis: Indiana University Foundation.

Farber, S. D. (1974). Sensorimotor evaluation and treatment procedures for the high-risk neonate. In C. Heriza (Ed.), *Comprehensive management of infants at risk for CNS dysfunction* (pp. 119–134). Chapel Hill: University of North Carolina, School of Medicine.

Farber, S. D. (1973). *Sensorimotor evaluation and treatment procedures for allied health personnel.* Indianapolis: Indiana University Foundation.

Gail Fidler, OTR, FAOTA—1965

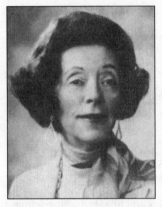

Gail Fidler earned her BA from Lebanon Valley College in 1938 with a double major in education and psychology. Her love for occupational therapy started at Wernersville State Hospital. In 1940, she enrolled in the occupational therapy certificate program at the University of Pennsylvania, graduating in 1942.

Fidler has a long history of contributions to the field of mental health. After graduating in 1942, she took a position as an occupational therapist at Norristown State Hospital, where she worked with Dr. Alfred Noyes, a renowned psychiatrist. She then moved to Walter Reed Army Medical Center in Washington, DC, and from 1944 to 1946 was the chief occupational therapist at the army hospital in Fort Story, Virginia. From 1946 to 1950 she was employed as a staff therapist at the veteran's hospital in Lyons, New Jersey.

Her career as instructor, administrator, and consultant began in 1952 when she took an instructor position with the Pennsylvania Department of Mental Health Training Programs until 1955. From 1955 to 1957 she was the coordinator of the AOTA Psychiatric Study Group, funded by the National Institute of Health. During this period, she also taught a summer session at the Philadelphia School of Occupational Therapy and lectured on occupational therapy theory in psychiatry at New York University (NYU). She served as member-at-large for the AOTA Board of Management from 1957 to 1963. From 1959 to 1968, Fidler served as the director of professional education for the Department of Occupational Therapy at the New York State Psychiatric Institute. In that position she developed and directed clinical fieldwork study for occupational therapy students; provided in-service education to physician residents, social workers, and nurses; supervised occupational therapy staff; initiated prevocational and work rehabilitation programs; developed patient evaluation and diagnostic measures; and collaborated with the Sociology Department to research and measure the nature and effect of change within institutional systems.

She later accepted a position as director of the Activities Therapy Department at Hillside Hospital, where she was responsible for the administration, coordination, and management of a staff consisting of occupational therapists, vocational counselors, therapeutic recreators, secondary school teachers, music and dance therapists, and volunteers. While working at the New York State Psychiatric Institute and Hillside Hospital, Fidler directed the master's-degree programs in psychiatric occupational therapy at NYU and at Columbia University. She also served as a consultant to several state and hospital programs. During this period, her civic duties included the League of Women Voters, United Fund Council, Visiting Nurses Association Homemakers Program, Education Committee for Teacher and Parents, Plainfield Public Schools, and Union County Aftercare Program. In her work with Union County, she was instrumental in developing the state's first psychiatric aftercare program.

Fidler was the interim executive director of the AOTA from March to October 1975 when she became coordinator of AOTA's Educator Training Institutes. During the 1970s and 1980s, she continued her consultative services to several psychiatric hospitals. Her work at the Department of Rehabilitation Services at Springfield Hospital in Maryland was used as a model for service delivery in mental health hospitals throughout the state.

From 1980 to 1982, she was assistant hospital administrator for programming at Greystone Park Psychiatric Hospital in New Jersey. Since 1980, she has acted as a consultant in curriculum development to the NYU Department of Occupational Therapy, and in 1982 she was appointed rehabilitation consultant to the New Jersey Division of Mental Health Hospitals. In 1984 she served as the chief executive officer of the Hagadorn Center for Geriatrics, a New Jersey state facility.

Throughout her career, Fidler has demonstrated a strong commitment and enthusiasm for the education of young professionals. She introduced occupational therapists to supervision as a tutorial learning process and offered the first workshop in supervision at Columbia University in the 1950s. During the 1970s, Fidler was a visiting professor at the University of California at San Jose, Kean College, the University of Pennsylvania, and Boston University. She taught and lectured on management, the meaning and uses of activities, group process, and program design. In 1990 she was asked by the College of Misericordia to assume the position of interim program director of occupational therapy.

Fidler received the AOTA Award of Merit in 1980 and was named AOTA Fellow in 1983. She died in 2005.

Bibliography

Hill, E. H., Vehlow, E. L., Fidler, G., Pleissner, E., & Gleave, M. (1947). Committee reports: Subcommittee on clinical field: Neuropsychiatry subcommittee of the research committee. *American Journal of Occupational Therapy, 1,* 250–252.

Fidler, G. S. (1948). Psychological evaluation of occupational therapy activities. *American Journal of Occupational Therapy, 2,* 284–287.

Fidler, G. S. (1953). Comments on a study of a task directed and free choice group. *American Journal of Occupational Therapy, 7,* 124–130.

Taber, F., Baron, S., Blackwell, A., Tucker, J. F., & Fidler, G. S. (1953). A study of a task directed and a free choice group: Comments. *American Journal of Occupational Therapy, 7,* 118–124.

Fidler, G. S. (1954). *Introduction to psychiatric occupational therapy.* New York: Macmillan.

Fidler, G. S. (1957). Nationally Speaking: Report on National Institute of Mental Health project. *American Journal of Occupational Therapy, 11,* 78–79, 81.

Fidler, G. S. (1957). The role of occupational therapy in a multi-discipline approach to psychiatric illness. *American Journal of Occupational Therapy, 11,* 8–12, 35.

Fidler, G. S. (1958). Some unique contributions of occupational therapy in the treatment of the schizophrenic. *American Journal of Occupational Therapy, 12,* 9–12.

Fidler, G. S., & Fine, S. B. (1962). The occupational therapist and psychotherapy. In R. Morehouse (Ed.), *Transitional programs in psychiatric occupational therapy* (pp. 14–20). Dubuque, IA: William Brown.

Fidler, G. S., & Fidler, J. W. (1963). *Occupational therapy: A communication process in psychiatry.* New York: Macmillan.

Fidler, G. S., & Spelbring, L. M. (1963). Nationally Speaking: The prescription in occupational therapy: The projected levels of function in occupational therapy departments in 1970. *American Journal of Occupational Therapy, 17,* 122–125.

Fidler, G. S. (1964). A guide to planning and measuring growth experience in the clinical affiliation. *American Journal of Occupational Therapy, 18,* 240–243.

Fidler, G. S. (1966). Learning as a growth process: A conceptual framework for professional education. (1965 Eleanor Clarke Slagle Lecture). *American Journal of Occupational Therapy, 20,* 1–8.

Fidler, G. S. (1966). A second look at work as primary force in rehabilitation. *American Journal of Occupational Therapy, 20,* 72–74.

Fidler, G. S. (1968). Diagnostic battery-scoring and summary of Grant No. 123-T-68. In Rehabilitation Services Administration (Ed.), *Field consultant in psychiatric rehabilitation* (pp. 10–27). Washington, DC: U.S. Government Printing Office.

Fidler, G. S., Kovalenko, L., Llorens, L., Mosey, A., Overly, K., Wilbarger, P., et al. (1968). Toward an integrated theory of occupational therapy: Proceedings of a seminar held August 26, 1967, at Albion, Michigan: Conference report. *American Journal of Occupational Therapy, 22,* 451–456.

Mazer, J. L., Fidler, G. S., Kovalenko, L. J., & Overly, K. (1968). *Exploring how a think feels: Selected portions of a workshop on object relations theory in occupational therapy held at Waldenwoods Conference Center, Hartland, Michigan, May 26–31, 1968.* Rockville, MD: American Occupational Therapy Association.

Crampton, M. W., Mosey, A. C., Talbot, N. H., Fidler, G. S., Newmann, F. M., & Solomon, L. F. (1969). *Development of teaching for occupational therapy assistants: Project report.* Boston: Medical Foundation.

Fidler, G. S. (1969). The task-oriented group as a context for treatment. *American Journal of Occupational Therapy, 23,* 43–48.

Fidler, G. S., & Fine, S. B. (1970). *Object history.* Unpublished manuscript.

Fidler, G. S. (1971). *Play/activity history.* Unpublished manuscript.

Clarke, D., Cromwell, F. S., Fanning, L., Fidler, G. S., Gillette, N., Hightower, M., et al. (1974). Association report: Task force on target populations. *American Journal of Occupational Therapy, 28,* 158–163.

Fidler, G. S. (1977). From plea to mandate. *American Journal of Occupational Therapy, 31,* 653–655.

Fidler, G. S., & Fidler, J. W. (1978). Doing and becoming: Purposeful action and self-actualization. *American Journal of Occupational Therapy, 32,* 305–310.

Fidler, G. S. (1978). Professional or non-professional. In American Occupational Therapy Association (Ed.), *Occupational Therapy: 2001 AD* (pp. 31–36). Rockville: MD: American Occupational Therapy Association.

Fidler, G. S. (1979). Specialization: Implications for education. *American Journal of Occupational Therapy, 33,* 34–35.

Fidler, G. S. (1981). From crafts to competence. *American Journal of Occupational Therapy, 35,* 567–573.

Fidler, G. S. (1981). *Overview of occupational therapy in mental health* (Prepared by the American Occupational Therapy Task Group of the American Psychiatric Association on Psychiatric Therapies). Rockville, MD: American Occupational Therapy Association.

Fidler, G. S. (1982). The activity laboratory: A structure for observing and assessing perceptual, integrative, and behavioral strategies. In B. Hemphill (Ed.), *The evaluation process in psychiatric occupational therapy* (pp. 195–207). Thorofoare, NJ: Slack.

Fidler, G. S., & Fidler, J. W. (1983). Doing and becoming: The occupational therapy experience. In G. Kielhofner (Ed.), *Health through occupation: Theory and practice in occupational therapy* (pp. 267–280). Philadelphia: F. A. Davis.

Fidler, G. S. (1984). *Design of rehabilitation services in psychiatric hospitals settings.* Laurel, MD: Ramsco.

Fidler, G. S. (1990). Reflections on choice. *Occupational Therapy in Mental Health, 10*(10), 77–84.

Fidler, G. S. (1991). The challenge of change to occupational therapy practice. *Occupational Therapy in Mental Health, 11*(1), 1–11.

Fidler, G. S. (1991). *Design of rehabilitation services in psychiatric hospital settings.* Rockville, MD: American Occupational Therapy Association.

Fidler, G. S., & Bristow, B. J. (1992). *Recapturing competence: A system's change for geropsychiatric care.* New York: Springer.

Fidler, G. S. (1993). Nationally Speaking: The quest for efficacy. *American Journal of Occupational Therapy, 47,* 583–586.

Fidler, G. S. (1995). AOTA's Representative Assembly: Highlights: The psychosocial core of occupational therapy. *OT Week, 9*(6), A12.

Fidler, G. (1995). Position paper: The psychosocial core of occupational therapy. *American Journal of Occupational Therapy, 49,* 1021–1022.

Fidler, G. S. (1996). Brief or new: Developing a repertoire of professional behaviors. *American Journal of Occupational Therapy, 50,* 583–587.

Fidler, G. S. (1996). Life-style performance: From profile to conceptual model. *American Journal of Occupational Therapy, 50,* 139–147.

Fidler, G. S. (1997). Position paper: The psychosocial core of occupational therapy. *American Journal of Occupational Therapy, 51,* 868–869.

Fidler, G. S. (1997). Viewpoint: An open letter to our elected leaders. *OT Week, 11*(21), 67.

Fidler, G. S., & Velde, B. P. (1999). *Activities: Reality and symbol.* Thorofare, NJ: Slack.

Fidler, G. S. (2000). The Issue Is: Beyond the therapy model: Building our future. *American Journal of Occupational Therapy, 54,* 99–101.

Fidler, G. S. (2001). Community practice: It's more than geography. *Occupational Therapy in Health Care, 13*(3/4), 7–9.

Velde, B. P., & Fidler, G. S. (2002). *Lifestyle performance: A model for engaging the power of occupation.* Thorofare, NJ: Slack.

Fidler, G. S. (2003). Editorial: What is the question? *OTJR: Participation and Health, 23,* 86–87.

Susan B. Fine, MA, OTR, FAOTA—1990

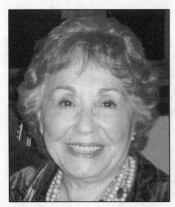

Susan Fine's 1990 Eleanor Clarke Slagle Lecture, "Resilience and Human Adaptability: Who Rises Above Adversity?" was written to heighten the occupational therapy profession's appreciation of the powerful interaction among a person's inner psychological life, his or her relationship to the surrounding world, and his or her emerging functional capacities: "The inner life (affective and cognitive processes and content) holds the potential for transforming traumas into varying degrees of triumph. Ironically, these same phenomena are often ignored in the clinical reasoning and practice of many health professions, including our own" (Fine, 1991).

This commitment to the power of "the inner life" and a deep belief that "the patient is more than the illness" have been dominant themes throughout Fine's multifaceted career as clinician, educator, researcher, author, public speaker, administrator, consultant, and advocate. They were, in fact, the driving force behind her decision to enter the field of occupational therapy. After completing undergraduate work in fine art and psychology at Brooklyn College in 1957, she went on to acquire her graduate certificate in occupational therapy in 1959 from Columbia University's College of Physicians and Surgeons and then began her 42-year career in mental health practice. She obtained a master's degree in developmental psychology from Columbia University in 1972, where she focused on the impact of activities on normal growth and development.

Fine's initial interest in the creative process and the ways in which art and other activities reflected "matters of the mind," as they were understood during the psychoanalytic era, were furthered by her collaboration with Gail Fidler, a significant role model and mentor at the New York State Psychiatric Institute. This premier teaching and research center provided extraordinary opportunities for professional and personal development when she entered the field. Among them, Fidler's notable abilities to promote critical thinking, challenge the status quo, and convey "the promise of OT and the promise of me: what I could perhaps become" (Fine, 1990). Their professional collaboration and shared admiration have been sustained over the years.

Ultimately, Fine became more than the therapist she initially set out to be. Her theoretical orientation expanded beyond the psychoanalytic model that first inspired her to a broader, integrated biopsychosocial perspective—while never losing sight of the importance of the inner-life on the outcome of occupational therapy's work in all areas of specialization. Her work in psychiatry at major teaching and research centers in New York City and her affiliations with many leading occupational therapy schools have provided opportunities to develop and promote new theories and strategies in psychosocial rehabilitation, collaborate in research, and influence the professional development of many disciplines. This has included the development of functional assessment instruments and innovative brief-focused and longer term rehabilitation programs addressing cognitive impairments and social disabilities in schizophrenia. She and her staff have been recipients of several research grants supporting these endeavors.

Fine's career has been grounded in an interdisciplinary approach. Her commitment to active collaboration with psychiatrists, psychologists, social workers, creative arts specialists, nurses, and rehabilitation counselors has been ongoing and evidenced in her leadership of interdisciplinary teams and programs. This also is reflected in the variety of roles she has played with national health care organizations. She served on the Joint Commission on Accreditation of Health Care Organizations (JCAHO), the Council on Accreditation of Rehabilitation Facilities (CARF), and the National Institute of Mental Health's (NIMH) Advisory Council and Ad-hoc Panel on Schizophrenia Research. She also served on the American Psychiatric Association's Hospital and Community Psychiatry Institute's Program Committee, as a member of their Consultation Service Team, as a consultant to their *DSM–IV* Task Force, and as advisor and reviewer for the *Psychiatric Services* journal.

Fine has rendered service to the profession in many capacities: first as chairperson of the Mental Health Special Interest Section of the American Occupational Therapy Association (AOTA), then as a member of AOTA's Mental Health Task Forces, as an editorial board member of the *Occupational Therapy in Mental Health* and the *American Journal of Occupational Therapy*, as chairperson of AOTA's Commission on Supervision, as a participant on the AOTA Registration Committee, and as a member of the Clinical Councils of New York and Columbia Universities' Schools of Occupational Therapy. She takes particular pride in the years spent on the Board of the American Occupational Therapy Foundation (AOTF) as member and vice president, promoting educational and research opportunities for the profession.

Fine has been acknowledged for her remarkable ability to demonstrate and articulate occupational therapy to persons and agencies in the mental health care and monitoring systems, thereby generating respect for the integrity and vitality of the profession. Her clinical knowledge, systems grasp, skill at dialogue, and conceptualization of occupational therapy are evident in her published works as well as in the many keynote and interdisciplinary conference presentations she has made. These efforts have benefited the profession, enhanced the quality of mental health services to patients and families, and contributed greatly to public awareness of occupational therapy. Her leadership skills and professional competencies have been recognized by many honors. In addition to awards for services rendered on many AOTA committees, she was named AOTA Fellow in 1978 and Eleanor Clarke Slagle Lecturer in 1990. She received the AOTA Merit Award and AOTF Meritorius Service Award in 2001. In addition, the Occupational Therapy Class of 1987 at the University of Texas Medical Branch at Galveston chose her as Class Mentor. She also was awarded the Annual Crawford Lectureship from the Toronto Hospital in 1991, the New York Health Chaplaincy Wholeness of Life Award in 1997, and New York University's Leadership and Excellence Award in Research in 1989.

At the time of her retirement in 2001, Fine was the director of psychiatric rehabilitation services at the Payne Whitney Clinic, New York Presbyterian Hospital–Weill-Cornell campus (a position she held for 25 years) and on the faculties of Columbia University's School of Occupational Therapy and Cornell Medical College's Department of Psychiatry. She and her husband Jerry, a psychologist/psychoanalyst who supported her many professional endeavors, are now enjoying their retirement in Charlotte, North Carolina, where she is involved in cultural and community activities while keeping up with their three children and three grandchildren. Although she has put aside formal professional roles, she continues to share her knowledge and skills with other Parkinson's caregivers (Jerry is a 20-year veteran of this challenging disease) and by serving as a mentor for a local family moving beyond homelessness and addiction.

Linking Key Messages of the 1990 Eleanor Clarke Slagle Lecture to the AOTA *Centennial Vision:* My purpose in 1990 was to awaken and/or remind all practitioners that "the patient is more than his/her illness"—and that the biopsychosocial model is key to successful approaches to health, treatment, and rehabilitation. I continue to believe that this mission must be central to our thinking about the occupational therapy process—if we are to assume meaningful and relevant roles in today's health care initiatives. In spite of the fact that much of the health care industry speaks to body parts (not the whole person) and is run by a hierarchy of professionals and insurers who play out their own visions of "health" and "care," courageous and creative professionals must take the initiative and define practice in more effective ways. My message not only addresses our consumers but also urges us to attend to and change the nature of our professional beliefs and actions. Resilience requires commitment—and the belief that we can marshal our assets as well as our liabilities. We should be vigorously influencing the strategic direction of the profession by re-examining and re-evaluating our principles and practices, by committing to a new generation of innovative practitioners, by educating other health care providers, the political network, and the public with more vigor than ever before.

No one needs to remind us that we are in a critical period of health care adversity. To rise above it, we must rapidly increase our visibility via leadership initiatives and renewed efforts to demonstrate our understanding and competence in managing the many factors that influence the outcome of our professional endeavors. Where have we been during the long and arduous 2009 debates over health care reform? Where will we be in the forthcoming decade as changes in health care delivery continue to reverberate on the national stage? While some may wonder "what else is new?" it is, in fact, the oldness of this mission that must command our attention and push us to seek more meaningful solutions to our perpetual hopes and visions for the future. The depth of our commitment, the speed with which we develop and implement proposals, and the wisdom with which we choose collaborators will surely determine the resilience of our profession and of those we seek to help. My efforts to define resilience and human adaptability in 1990 is an equally suitable challenge and goal for 2009 and beyond. Perhaps it can help serve as a call to action with which to rally the strengths and promise of the field.

—*Susan B. Fine*

Bibliography

Fine, S. B. (1999). Symbolization: Making meaning for self and society. In F. Fidler & B. Selby (Eds.), *Activities, realities, and symbols*. Thorofare, NJ: Slack.

Fine, S. B. (1998). Doing good work in bad times: A challenge to personal and professional resilience. In A. Scott (Ed.), *Occupational therapy in mental health*. New York: Haworth.

Fine, S. B. (1998). Surviving the health care revolution: Rediscovering the meaning of "good work." In A. Scott (Ed.), *New frontiers in psychosocial occupational therapy*. New York: Haworth.

Fine, S. B. (1994). Reframing rehabilitation: Putting skill acquisition and the mental health system into proper perspective. In W. Spaulding (Ed.), *Cognitive technology in treatment and the mental health system*. Lincoln: University of Nebraska Press.

Fine, S. B. (1994). The Slagle Lectureship: A legacy of leadership, achievement, and inspiration. *OT Week, 7*(43), 6–7.

Radomski, M. V., Dougherty, P. M., Fine, S. B., & Baum, C. (1994). Case studies in cognitive rehabilitation. In C. B. Royeen (Ed.), *AOTA Self-Study Series: Cognitive rehabilitation*. Rockville, MD: American Occupational Therapy Association.

Fine, S. B. (1993). Interaction between psychosocial variables and cognitive function. In C. Royeen (Ed.), *AOTA Self-Study Series: Cognitive rehabilitation*. Rockville, MD: American Occupational Therapy Association.

Fine, S. B. (1993). Psychosocial issues and adaptive capacities. *Mental Health Special Interest Section Newsletter, 16*(4), 1–4, 7.

Fine, S. B. (1992). Neurobehavioral perspectives on schizophrenia. In J. Van Deusen (Ed.), *Rehabilitation of adults with perceptual–motor dysfunction*. Orlando, FL: W. B. Saunders.

Fine, S. B. (1991). Resilience and human adaptability: Who rises above adversity? (1990 Eleanor Clarke Slagle Lecture). *American Journal of Occupational Therapy, 45*(6), 493–503.

Fine, S. B. (1990). Clinical case workbook II: Psychosocial issues and adaptive capacities. In C. B. Royeen (Ed.), *AOTA Self-Study Series: Assessing function* (pp. 3–20). Rockville, MD: American Occupational Therapy Association.

Fine, S. B. (1990). The promise of occupational therapy: Professional challenges, personal rewards. *Occupational Therapy in Mental Health, 10*(1), 63–75.

Fine, S. B. (1988). Nationally Speaking—Working the system: A perspective for managing change. *American Journal of Occupational Therapy, 42*, 417–419.

Greenberg, L., Fine, S. B., Cohen, C., Larson, K., Michaelson-Baily, A., Rubinton, P., et al. (1988). An interdisciplinary psychoeducation program for schizophrenic patients and their families in an acute care setting. *Hospital and Community Psychiatry, 39*(3), 277–282.

Good-Ellis, M., Fine, S. B., Spencer, J. H., & DiVittis, A. (1987). Developing the Role Activity Performance Scale. *American Journal of Occupational Therapy, 41*, 232–241.

Fine, S. B. (1987). Looking ahead: Opportunities for occupational therapy in the next decade. *Occupational Therapy in Mental Health, 7*(4), 3–12.

Fine, S. B. (1986). Trends in mental health. In S. Robertson (Ed.), *SCOPE curriculum manual* (pp. 19–32). Rockville, MD: American Occupational Therapy Association.

Fine, S. B., & Schwimmer, P. (1986). The effects of occupational therapy on independent living skills. *Mental Health Special Interest Section Newsletter, 9*(4), 2–3.

Good-Ellis, M., Fine, S. B., Haas, G. L., Spencer, J. H., & Glick, I. D. (1986). Quantitative role and performance assessment: Implications and application to treatment of major affective disorders. In *Depression: Assessment and treatment update, Proceedings of Preconference to APA Annual Institute on Hospital and Community Psychiatry*.

Fine, S. B., Bair, J., Hoover, S. P., & Aquaviva, J. D. (1985). Regulation and standard setting. In J. Bair & M. Gray (Eds.), *The occupational therapy manager*. Rockville, MD: American Occupational Therapy Association.

Fine, S. B. (1984). Book review of *Theory and Practice of Psychiatric Rehabilitation*, Fraser & Bennett (Eds.), N.Y.: Wiley & Sons. *Hospital and Community Psychiatry, 35*(10).

Fine, S. B. (1984). Occupational therapy. In T. B. Karasu (Ed.), *The psychiatric therapies*. Washington, DC: American Psychiatric Press.

Fine, S. B. (1983). Occupational therapy: The role of rehabilitation and purposeful activity in mental health practice. *Mental Health Special Interest Section Newsletter, 6*(4), 3–8.

Fine, S. B. (1982). Nationally Speaking—Mental health in Japan. *American Journal of Occupational Therapy, 36*, 157–162.

Fine, S. B. (1980–1981). Worth Repeating—Psychiatric treatment and rehabilitation: What's in a name? *Occupational Therapy in Mental Health, 1*(4).

Fine, S. B. (1980). Psychiatric treatment and rehabilitation: What's in a name? *Journal of the National Association of Private Psychiatric Hospitals, 11*(5).

Fine, S. B. (1978). The analytic model: Behavior is more than it appears to be. In *Proceedings of the Meeting of the World Federation of Occupational Therapy*, Jerusalem Israel.

Fine, S. B. (1968). Four concepts basic to the occupational therapy process. *American Journal of Occupational Therapy, 22*, 445–447.

Fidler, G., & Fine, S. B. (1962). The occupational therapist and psychotherapy: Transitional programs in psychiatric occupational therapy. In *Proceedings of the World Federation of Occupational Therapy Post-Congress Study Course*.

Geraldine L. Finn, MS, OTR/L, FAOTA—1971

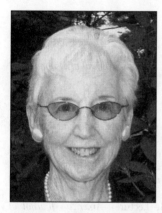

Geraldine Finn earned a bachelor of arts degree in 1953 in home economics from Regis College in Massachusetts. She graduated in 1955 with a certificate in occupational therapy from Tufts University. She earned a master of science degree with a specialization in human development and family relations from Simmons College in 1972.

Finn began working as a staff occupational therapist at Boston State Hospital, employed from 1955 to 1958, then later at the Fernald State School in Waverly, Massachusetts. Finn then moved to Cleveland and assumed the role of director of the occupational therapy department at Cleveland Psychiatric Institute from 1959 to 1964. She became a research associate in occupational therapy at the Cleveland State Hospital in 1964 and helped develop a day hospital for adult psychiatric clients. From 1967 to 1969, Finn worked as an occupational therapy consultant for the Hartford Rehabilitation Center in Connecticut, developing rehabilitation programs for the physically disabled, the mentally retarded, and adolescents with emotional distubances. From 1969 to 1979 she lectured in occupational therapy and human development at Boston University and at Tufts University.

From 1969 to 1976, Finn was director of occupational therapy at Boston State Hospital, focusing on community inter-agency coordination, community-based programs, and clinical student programming. She continued her work in department administration and program development at the Middlesex County Hospital from 1976 to 1980. Finn had the unique opportunity from 1981 to 1988 to be a member of the staff of the House of Affirmation, Inc., in Hopedale, Massachusetts, a residential therapeutic community and outpatient facility for Catholic priests and religious persons with emotional and psychiatric problems. During this period, she also was a lecturer in that organization's educational programs and summer institutes. From 1988 to 1992, Finn was the director of rehabilitation for Medfield State Hospital, overseeing occupational therapy, physical therapy, recreation therapy, speech–language pathology, and vocational rehabilitation.

Finn retired in 1992 and began volunteer work that she continues today. From 1992 to 1998, Finn was a certified ombudsman for the Massachusetts Long-Term Care Ombudsman Program, advocating for residents in nursing and rest homes. She is very proud of her work with the Massachusetts Women–Church, which is a group working toward educating and empowering women to claim their equality in church and society, as well as her work with the Lost Coin Women's Fund, Inc., a nonprofit organization providing opportunities for women with low incomes to pursue college and training.

The Eleanor Clarke Slagle Lectureship Award was bestowed in 1971 for her contributions to the profession. In 1973, Finn was inducted into the Roster of Fellows of the American Occupational Therapy Association (AOTA).

On a Personal Note From a Phone Interview: Finn identified Inez Huntting as her supervisor on her first affiliation, and she inspired Finn to publish, to develop programs, and to respect the importance of AOTA for the profession. Finn notes that her Slagle lecture would still be beneficial in reminding students and therapists to be aware of the larger environment and think creatively. Programs in the community, especially in prevention and wellness, are as needed as much today as in the 1970s. Those entering the occupational therapy field today must be aware of the greater society and pay attention to research and the quality of education for occupational therapists. Clinicians must be *active* members of AOTA, and students are especially encouraged to attend the AOTA Annual Conference to become inspired by experienced clinicians and scholars.

Linking Key Messages of the 1971 Eleanor Clarke Slagle Lecture to the AOTA *Centennial Vision:* There is the principle that as times change, professions also must change if they are to remain relevant. Although it is comfortable to stay in a known environment of knowledge and practice, change requires a willingness to expand one's boundaries and respond to the signs of the times. How to prevent or lessen the effect of illness or disabilities was gaining attention in the delivery of health services during the 1960s. My lecture addressed this trend and its impact on the occupational therapy profession.

We are now in a new century, and the occupational therapy profession needs to respond to today's signs of the times. AOTA is to be commended for its leadership in developing a vision statement. The *Centennial Vision* (AOTA, 2007) clearly describes the future the profession of occupational therapy wants to create. It also provides a framework for addressing individual issues arising in our society today. One of the most pressing issues is the reform of our health system, with significant attention being directed toward understanding the array of factors that influence a healthy lifestyle. It is an auspicious time for the occupational therapy profession to make a major contribution.

—*Geraldine Finn*

Reference

American Occupational Therapy Association. (2007). AOTA's *Centennial Vision* and executive summary. *American Journal of Occupational Therapy, 61,* 613–614.

Bibliography

Finn, G. L. (1977). Update of Eleanor Clarke Slagle Lecture: The occupational therapist in prevention programs. *American Journal of Occupational Therapy, 31,* 658–659.

Gardos, G. L., Orzach, M. H., Cole, J. O., & Finn, G. L. (1974). High and low dose thiothixene treatment in chronic schizophrenia. *Diseases of the Nervous System, 35,* 301–309.

Finn, G. L. (1973). Children's developmental workshop. In L. Llorens (Ed.), *Consultation in the community: Occupational therapy in child health* (pp. 45–57). Dubuque, IA: Kendall Hunt.

Finn, G. L. (1972). The occupational therapist in prevention programs (1971 Eleanor Clark Slagle Lecture). *American Journal of Occupational Therapy, 26,* 59–66.

Finn, G. L. (1968). Discussion—Four concepts basic to the occupational therapy process. *American Journal of Occupational Therapy, 22,* 447–448.

Finn, G. L. (1964). Severe character disorders: Treatment through occupational therapy. *American Journal of Occupational Therapy, 18,* 185–190.

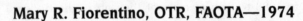

Mary R. Fiorentino, OTR, FAOTA—1974

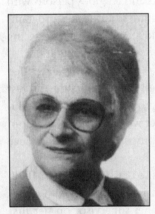

Mary R. Fiorentino was a self-employed occupational therapist. She graduated from Tufts University, School of Occupational Therapy with a postgraduate certificate in occupational therapy. Later she received a bachelor's degree in music from Boston University.

Fiorentino offered educational workshops in health-related fields in Hartford, Connecticut. She worked as a staff therapist, assistant director, and director of occupational therapy at the Newington Children's Hospital, Connecticut, retiring in 1978. After her retirement, Fiorentino worked as a consultant for the teaching staff at Mount Sinai Hospital, Hartford, and for the rehabilitation services of St. Francis Hospital and Medical Center and the Oakhill School for the Blind.

Her awards include Who's Who of American Women, 1968, and the Award of Merit, Connecticut Occupational Therapy Association, 1975. Fiorentino was named AOTA Fellow in 1973.

Bibliography

Mysak, E., & Fiorentino M. R. (1961). Neurophysiological considerations in occupational therapy for the cerebral palsied. *American Journal of Occupational Therapy, 15,* 112–117.

Fiorentino, M. R. (1963). *Reflex testing methods for evaluating CNS development.* Springfield, IL: Charles C Thomas.

Fiorentino, M. R., Nathan, C., & Kleinschmidt, K. (1963). Visual aid board. *American Journal of Occupational Therapy, 17,* 198–199.

Fiorentinto, M. R. (1966). The changing dimension of occupational therapy. *American Journal of Occupational Therapy, 20,* 251–252.

Fiorentino, M. R. (1972). *Normal and abnormal development: The influence of primitive reflexes on motor development.* Springfield, IL: Charles C Thomas.

Fiorentino, M. R. (1975). Occupational therapy: Realization to activation. (1974 Eleanor Clarke Slagle Lecture). *American Journal of Occupational Therapy, 29,* 15–29.

Fiorentino, M. R. (1981). *A basis of motor development: Normal and abnormal: The influence of primitive, postural reflexes on the development and distribution of tone* Springfield, IL: Charles C Thomas.

Anne Fisher, ScD, OTR, FAOTA—1998

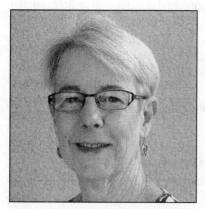

Anne Fisher is professor in the Division of Occupational Therapy, Department of Community Medicine and Rehabilitation, Umeå University, Sweden. She is also adjunct professor at both Dalhousie University, Halifax, Nova Scotia, Canada, and Colorado State University (CSU), Ft. Collins. Fisher obtained a bachelor's degree in occupational therapy at Western Michigan University in Kalamazoo, in 1969 and a master's degree in occupational therapy in 1977 and a doctorate in therapeutic science in 1984, both from Sargent College of Allied Health Professions in Boston.

Upon graduation in 1969, Fisher worked as an occupational therapist at the Mary Free Bed Hospital and Rehabilitation in Grand Rapids, Michigan. In 1970 she joined the Michigan Department of Public Health, Area Child Amputee Center in Grand Rapids, as a rehabilitation therapist and concomitantly taught at Northwestern University Medical School, Prosthetic–Orthotic Center in Chicago. By 1977, she had clearly defined her career as a professor, researcher, and consultant. As a researcher, she has received funding from the National Institutes of Aging, Swedish Research Council, and American Occupational Therapy Foundation (AOTF), among others. She serves of several editorial boards, including the *Journal of Applied Measurement,* the *Journal of Rehabilitation Medicine,* and the *Scandinavian Journal of Occupational Therapy.*

Fisher has consulted extensively nationally and internationally and has been an assistant professor of occupational therapy at Sargent College, Boston University; an assistant professor and then associate professor of occupational therapy at the University of Illinois at Chicago; a professor of occupational therapy at CSU, College of Applied Human Sciences; and a University Distinguished Professor at CSU. She also has been a visiting lecturer or guest professor at Curtin University of Technology, Perth, Western Australia; at Umeå University, Umeå, Sweden; at the University of Puerto Rico; and at Jyväskylä University, Jyväskylä, Finland.

Fisher is an internationally recognized expert in occupational therapy theory, functional assessment, and instrument development. She pioneered the use of Rasch analysis in occupational therapy and is now recognized internationally for her expertise in Rasch measurement. She developed the Assessment of Motor and Process Skills (AMPS) and is codeveloper of the School AMPS and the Evaluation of Social Interaction (ESI). The AMPS is an innovative, occupational therapy–specific, functional assessment used to test children, adults, and older persons who are experiencing or are at risk for problems with performance of self-care or home maintenance activities of daily living. The AMPS is now standardized on more than 150,000 people for use in more than 25 countries in North America, Scandinavia, Europe, Australasia, Asia, and the Middle East. The School AMPS is based on the AMPS methodology and provides the occupational therapist with the only existing observational assessment of a student's ability to perform schoolwork tasks assigned by the teacher and performed within the student's natural classroom milieu. The ESI is used to evaluate the quality of social interactions of persons ages 2 years or older when engaging in natural social exchanges, with typical partners, in natural settings.

Fisher has published more than 90 articles in refereed professional journals and more than 30 books or books chapters. She is a member of the AOTF's Academy of Research, and she was awarded the Foundation's A. Jean Ayres Award in 1991 in recognition of her efforts refining and synthesizing the theories of sensory integration and the Model of Human Occupation, for excellence in teaching, and for innovative research in measurement and functional assessment. She was the 1997 recipient of the Eleanor Clarke Slagle Lectureship Award for distinguished contributions to theory and functional assessment. In her lecture, Fisher first introduced the Occupational Therapy Intervention Process Model, a professional reasoning model that enables occupational therapists to implement client-centered, occupation-based, and true top-down assessment and intervention.

In November 2000, Fisher was awarded an honorary doctorate (*hedersdoktor*) from Umeå University, Sweden, and is the first occupational therapist ever to have been so honored by that institution. In 2001, she was named University Distinguished Professor at CSU, an honor bestowed on only 10 faculty who have made significant national and international contributions to their profession.

Linking Key Messages of the 1998 Eleanor Clarke Slagle Lecture to the AOTA *Centennial Vision:* My Eleanor Clark Slagle Lecture grew out of my belief in the value of occupation as a therapeutic agent, the need for each us to have a clear and strong professional identity that is based on our unique focus on occupation, and the importance of research that provides us with the evidence we need to support or refute current theory and practice and which can generate needed change that will prepare us for the future.

If we are to be widely recognized (AOTA, 2007), we must market ourselves based on that which makes us unique—occupation-based and client-centered services for all who experience or are at risk of experiencing diminished engagement in occupation. Marketing can occur at many levels. When we meet our clients and offer them services, we implicitly or explicitly market occupational therapy through the services we offer.

Whether our clients are a person, a constellation of persons, a company, or society at large, I believe that practice based on the Occupational Therapy Intervention Process Model (Fisher, 2009) is one way to ensure that what we do retains our focus on occupation. There remains a huge demand to become better at communicating to others what is we are able to offer in a manner that makes it clear that we are prepared to compliment, not duplicate, needed services that can be provided by our colleagues from other professions. There continues to be a need to make a philosophical change, to become more science driven, and to base our services on current and emerging evidence. AOTA's *Centennial Vision* is a grand one. May we all join to meet the challenge.

—Anne Fisher

References

American Occupational Therapy Association. (2007). AOTA's *Centennial Vision* and executive summary. *American Journal of Occupational Therapy, 61,* 613–614.

Fisher, A. G. (2009). *Occupational Therapy Intervention Process Model: A model for planning and implementing top–down, client-centered, and occupation-based interventions.* Ft. Collins, CO: Three Star Press.

Bibliography

Árnadóttir, S. A., Lundin-Olsson, L., Gunnardóttir, E. D., & Fisher, A. G. (2010). Application of Rasch analysis to validate the Activities-Specific Balance Confidence Scale when used in a new cultural context. *Archives of Physical Medicine and Rehabilitation, 91,* 156–163.

Munkholm, M., Berg, B., Löfgren, B., & Fisher, A. G. (2010). Cross-regional validation of the School Version of the Assessment of Motor and Process Skills. *American Journal of Occupational Therapy, 64,* 768–775.

Árnadóttir, G., & Fisher, A. G. (2009). Dimensionality of nonmotor neurobehavioral impairments when observed in the natural contexts of ADL task performance. *Neurorehabilitation and Neural Repair, 23,* 579–586.

Fisher, A. G. (2009). *Occupational Therapy Intervention Process Model: A model for planning and implementing top–down, client-centered, and occupation-based interventions.* Ft. Collins, CO: Three Star Press.

Fisher, A. G. & Griswold, L. A. (2009). *Evaluation of Social Interaction.* Ft. Collins, CO: Three Star Press.

Wæhrens, E. E., & Fisher, A. G. (2009). Developing linear ADL ability measures based on the ADL taxonomy: A Rasch analysis. *Scandinavian Journal of Occupational Therapy, 16,* 159–171.

Árnadóttir, G., & Fisher, A. G. (2008). Rasch analysis of the ADL scale of the A-ONE. *American Journal of Occupational Therapy, 62,* 51–60.

Granberg, M., Rydberg, A., & Fisher, A. G. (2008). Activities in daily living and schoolwork task performance in children with complex congenital heart disease. *Acta Pædiatrica, 97,* 1270–1274.

Munkholm, M., & Fisher, A. G. (2008). Differences in schoolwork performance between typically developing students and students with mild disabilities. *OTJR: Occupation, Participation and Health, 38,* 121–132.

Fischl, C., & Fisher, A. G. (2007). Development and Rasch analysis of the Assessment of Computer-Related Skills. *Scandinavian Journal of Occupational Therapy, 14,* 126–135.

Fisher, A. G., Atler, K., & Potts, A. (2007). Effectiveness of occupational therapy with frail community living older adults. *Scandinavian Journal of Occupational Therapy, 14,* 240–249.

Fisher, A. G., & Nyman, A. (2007). OTIPM: En model för ett professionellt resonemang som främjar bästa praxis I arbetsterapi (FOU-rapport 2007) [OTIPM: A model for professional reasoning that promotes best practice in occupational therapy]. Nacka, Sweden: Förbundet Sveriges Arbetsterapeuter.

Liu, K. P. Y., Chan, C. C. H., Chu, M. M. L., Ng, T. Y. L., Chu, L. W., Hui, S. L., Yuen, H. K., & Fisher, A. G. (2007). Activities of daily living performance in dementia. *Acta Neurologica Scandinavica, 116,* 91–95.

Lund, M. L., Fisher, A. G., Lexell, J., & Bernspång, B. (2007). Impact on Participation and Autonomy Questionnaire: Internal scale validity of the Swedish version for use in people with spinal cord injury. *Journal of Rehabilitation Medicine, 39,* 156–162.

Nilsson, I., Bernspång, B., Löfgren, B., & Fisher, A. (2007). Occupational engagement and life satisfaction in the oldest-old: The Umeå 85+ study. *OTJR: Occupation, Participation and Health, 27,* 131–139.

Nilsson, I., Löfgren, B., Fisher, A., & Bernspång, B. (2007). Focus on leisure repertoire in the oldest old, the Umeå 85+ study. *Journal of Applied Gerontology, 25,* 391–406.

Petersson, I., Fisher, A.G., Hemmingsson, H., & Lilja, M. (2007). The Client–Clinician Assessment Protocol (C–CAP): Evaluation of its psychometric properties for use with people aging with disabilities in need of home modifications. *OTJR: Occupation, Participation and Health, 27,* 140–148.

Wæhrens, E. E., & Fisher, A. G. (2007). Improving quality of ADL performance after rehabilitation among people with acquired brain injury. *Scandinavian Journal of Occupational Therapy, 14,* 250–257.

Fisher, A. G. (2006). *Assessment of Motor and Process Skills. Vol. 1: Development, standardization, and administration manual* (6th ed.). Fort Collins, CO: Three Star Press.

Fisher, A. G. (2006). *Assessment of Motor and Process Skills. Vol. 2: User manual* (6th ed.). Fort Collins, CO: Three Star Press.

Fisher, A. G. (2006). Overview of performance skills and client factors. In H. M. Pendleton & W. Schultz-Krohn (Eds.), *Pedretti's occupational therapy: Practice skills for physical dysfunction* (6th ed., pp. 372–402). St. Louis, MO: Mosby/Elsevier.

Fisher, A. G., Nilsson, I., & Widman-Lundmark, M. (2006, Nu. 6). Därfor är arbetsterapi unikt! [Therefore, occupational therapy is unique!]. *Arbetsterapeuten,* pp. 4–6.

Nilsson, I., & Fisher, A. G. (2006). Evaluating leisure activities in the oldest old. *Scandinavian Journal of Occupational Therapy, 13,* 31–37.

Fisher, A. G., Bryze, K., Hume, V., & Griswold, L. A. (2005). *School AMPS: School Version of the Assessment of Motor and Process Skills* (2nd ed.). Ft. Collins, CO: Three Star Press.

Hermansson, L. M., Fisher, A. G., Bernspång, B., & Elisson, A.-C. (2005). Assessment of capacity for myoelectric control: A new Rasch-built measure of prosthetic hand control. *Journal of Rehabilitation Medicine, 37,* 166–171.

Rexroth, P., Fisher, A. G., Merritt, B. K., & Gliner, J. (2005). ADL differences in individuals with unilateral hemispheric stroke. *Canadian Journal of Occupational Therapy, 72,* 212–221.

Fisher, A. G., & Duran, G. A. (2004). Schoolwork task performance of students at risk for delays. *Scandinavian Journal of Occupational Therapy, 11,* 191–198.

Hayase, D., Mosenteen, D. A., Thimmaiah, D., Zemke, S., Atler, K., & Fisher, A. G. (2004). Age-related changes in activities of daily living ability. *Australian Occupational Therapy Journal, 51,* 192–198.

Bernspång, B., Kottorp, A., & Fisher, A. G. (2003, Nu. 7). Välkommen debatt om arbetsterapi och AMPS. *Arbetsterapeuten,* pp. 5–6.

Fisher, A. G. (2003). Why it is so hard to practice as an occupational therapist? [Guest Editorial]. *Australian Occupational Therapy Journal, 50,* 193–194.

Kottorp, A., Bernspång, B., & Fisher, A. G. (2003). Activities of daily living in persons with intellectual disability: Strengths and limitations in specific motor and process skills. *Australian Occupational Therapy Journal, 50,* 195–204.

Kottorp, A., Bernspång, B., & Fisher, A. G. (2003). Validity of a performance assessment of activities of daily living for persons with developmental disabilities. *Journal of Intellectual Disability Research, 47,* 597–605.

Kottorp, A., Hällgren, M., Bernspång, B., & Fisher, A. G. (2003). Client-centred occupational therapy for persons with mental retardation: Implementation of an intervention programme in activities of daily living tasks. *Scandinavian Journal of Occupational Therapy, 10,* 51–60.

Merritt, B. K., & Fisher, A. G. (2003). Gender differences in performance of activities of daily living. *Archives of Physical Medicine and Rehabilitation, 84,* 1872–1877.

Oakley, F., Duran, L., Fisher, A.G., & Merritt, B. (2003). Differences in activities of daily living motor skills of persons with and without Alzheimer's disease. *Australian Occupational Therapy Journal, 50,* 72–78.

Bray, K., Fisher, A. G., & Duran, L. (2001). The validity of adding new tasks to the Assessment of Motor and Process Skills. *American Journal of Occupational Therapy, 55,* 409–415.

Derrickson, J. P., Fisher, A. G., & Anderson, J. E. L. (2001). An assessment of various household food security measures in Hawai?i has implications for national food security research and monitoring. *Journal of Nutrition, 131,* 749–757.

Ellison, S., Fisher, A. G., & Duran, L. (2001). The alternate forms reliability of the new tasks added to the Assessment of Motor and Process Skills. *Journal of Applied Measurement, 2,* 120–133.

McNulty, M. C., & Fisher, A. G. (2001). Validity of using the Assessment of Motor and Process Skills to estimate overall home safety in persons with psychiatric conditions. *American Journal of Occupational Therapy, 55,* 649–655.

Sellers, S. W., Fisher, A. G., & Duran, L. (2001). Validity of the Assessment of Motor and Process Skills with students who are visually impaired. *Journal of Visual Impairment and Blindness, 95,* 164–167.

Tham, K., Ginsburg, E., Fisher, A. G., & Tegnér, R. (2001). Training to improve awareness of disabilities in clients with unilateral neglect. *American Journal of Occupational Therapy, 55,* 46–54.

Cooke, K. Z., Fisher, A. G., Mayberry, W., & Oakley, F. (2000). Differences in activities of daily living process skills of persons with and without Alzheimer's disease. *Occupational Therapy Journal of Research, 20,* 87–104.

Derrickson, J. P., Anderson, J. E. L., & Fisher, A. G. (2000). *Concurrent validity of a face valid food security measure* (Discussion Paper DP-1206-00). Madison: University of Wisconsin, Institute for Research on Poverty. Available online at http://www.ssc.wisc.edu/irp/dplist.htm

Derrickson, J. P., Fisher, A. G., & Anderson, J. E. L. (2000). The Core Food Security Module scale measure is valid and reliable when used with Asians and Pacific Islanders. *Journal of Nutrition, 130,* 2666–2674.

Fisher, A. G., Bryze, K, & Atchison, B. T. (2000). Naturalistic assessment of functional performance in school settings: Reliability and validity of the School AMPS scales. *Journal of Outcome Measurement, 4,* 504–522.

Stauffer, L. M., Fisher, A. G., & Duran, L. (2000). ADL performance of Black and White Americans on the Assessment of Motor and Process Skills. *American Journal Occupational Therapy, 54,* 607–613.

Duran, L., & Fisher, A. G. (1999). Evaluation and intervention with executive functions impairment. In C. Unsworth (Ed.), *Cognitive and perceptual dysfunction: A clinical reasoning approach to evaluation and intervention* (pp. 209–255). Philadelphia: F. A. Davis.

Fisher, A. G. (1999). Uniting practice and theory: Author's response [Letter to the Editor]. *American Journal of Occupational Therapy, 53,* 403–404.

Girard, C., Fisher, A. G., Short, M. A., & Duran, L. (1999). Occupational performance differences between psychiatric groups. *Scandinavian Journal of Occupational Therapy, 6,* 119–126.

Hartman, M. L., Fisher, A. G., & Duran, L. (1999). Assessment of functional ability of people with Alzheimer's disease. *Scandinavian Journal of Occupational Therapy, 6,* 111–118.

Kirkley, K., & Fisher, A. G. (1999). Alternate forms reliability of the Assessment of Motor and Process Skills. *Journal of Outcome Measurement, 3,* 53–70.

Robinson, S. E., & Fisher, A. G. (1999). Functional and cognitive differences between cognitively-well people and people with dementia. *British Journal of Occupational Therapy, 62,* 466–471.

Tham, K., Bernspång, B., & Fisher, A.G. (1999). Development of the Assessment of Awareness of Disability. *Scandinavian Journal of Occupational Therapy, 6,* 184–190.

Atchison, B. T., Fisher, A. G., & Bryze, K. (1998). Rater reliability and internal scale and person response validity of the School Assessment of Motor and Process Skills. *American Journal of Occupational Therapy, 52,* 843–850.

Darragh, A. R., Sample, P. L., & Fisher, A. G. (1998). The effect of the environment on functional task performance: Use of the Assessment of Motor and Process Skills with adults with acquired brain injuries. *Archives of Physical Medicine and Rehabilitation, 79,* 418–423.

Doble, S. E., & Fisher, A. G. (1998). The dimensionality and validity of the Older Americans Resources and Services (OARS) activities of daily living (ADL) scale. *Journal of Outcome Measurement, 2,* 2–23.

Fisher, A. G. (1998). Uniting practice and theory in an occupational framework (1998 Eleanor Clarke Slagle Lecture). *American Journal of Occupational Therapy, 52,* 509–521.

Fisher, A. G., Murray, E. A., & Bundy, A. C. (1998). *Sensorische integrationstherapie: Theorie und praxis* [Sensory integration: Theory and practice] (M. Schlegtendal & M. Wittlich, Trans.). Berlin: Springer-Verlag.

Dickerson, A. E., & Fisher, A. G. (1997). The effects of familiarity of task and choice on the functional performance of young and old adults. *Psychology and Aging, 12,* 247–254.

Doble, S. E., Fisk, J. D., MacPherson, K. M., Fisher, A. G., & Rockwood, K. (1997). Measuring functional competence in older persons with Alzheimer's disease. *International Psychogeriatrics, 9,* 25–38.

Fisher, A. G. (1997). Multifaceted measurement of daily life task performance: Conceptualizing a test of instrumental ADL and validating the addition of personal ADL tasks. *Physical Medicine and Rehabilitation: State of the Art Reviews, 11,* 289–303.

Goldman, S. L., & Fisher, A. G. (1997). Cross-cultural validation of the Assessment of Motor and Process Skills (AMPS). *British Journal of Occupational Therapy, 60,* 77–85.

Stahl, J., Shumway, R., Bergstrom, B., & Fisher, A. G. (1997). On-line performance assessment using rating scales. *Journal of Outcome Measurement, 1,* 173–191.

Duran, L., & Fisher, A. G. (1996). Male and female performance on the Assessment of Motor and Process Skills. *Archives of Physical Medicine and Rehabilitation, 77,* 1019–1024.

Goto, S., Fisher, A. G., & Mayberry, W. L. (1996). AMPS applied cross-culturally to the Japanese. *American Journal of Occupational Therapy, 50,* 798–806.

Lai, J. S., Fisher, A. G., Magalhaes, L. C., & Bundy, A. C. (1996). Construct validity of the praxis tests on the Sensory Integration and Praxis Tests. *Occupational Therapy Journal of Research, 16,* 75–97.

Magalhães, L., Fisher, A. G., Bernspång, B., & Linacre, J. M. (1996). Cross-cultural assessment of functional ability. *Occupational Therapy Journal of Research, 16,* 45–63.

Robinson, S. E., & Fisher, A. G. (1996). A study to examine the relationship of the Assessment of Motor and Process Skills (AMPS) to other tests of cognition and function. *British Journal of Occupational Therapy, 59,* 260–263.

Bernspång, B., & Fisher, A. G. (1995). Differences between persons with right or left CVA on the Assessment of Motor and Process Skills. *Archives of Physical Medicine and Rehabilitation, 76,* 1144–1151.

Bernspång, B., & Fisher, A. G. (1995). Validation of the Assessment of Motor and Process Skills for use in Sweden. *Scandinavian Journal of Occupational Therapy, 2,* 3–9.

Bryze, K., & Fisher, A. G. (1995). Diane: The use of the Assessment of Motor and Process Skills in treatment planning for as adult with developmental disabilities. In G. Kielhofner (Ed.), *A model of human occupation: Theory and application* (2nd ed., pp. 286–295). Baltimore: Williams & Wilkins.

Dickerson, A. E., & Fisher, A. G. (1995). Culture-relevant functional performance assessment of the Hispanic elderly. *Occupational Therapy Journal of Research, 15,* 50–68.

Englund, B., Bernspång, B., & Fisher, A. G. (1995). Development of an instrument for assessment of social interaction skills in occupational therapy. *Scandinavian Journal of Occupational Therapy, 2,* 17–23.

Fisher, A. G., & Kielhofner, G. (1995). Mind–brain–body performance subsystem. In G. Kielhofner (Ed.), *A model of human occupation: Theory and application* (2nd ed., pp. 83–89). Baltimore: Williams & Wilkins.

Fisher, A. G., & Kielhofner, G. (1995). Skill in occupational performance. In G. Kielhofner (Ed.), *A model of human occupation: Theory and application* (2nd ed., pp. 113–137). Baltimore: Williams & Wilkins.

Kottorp, A., Bernspång, B., Fisher, A .G., & Bryze, K. (1995). IADL ability measured with the AMPS: Relation to two classification systems of mental retardation. *Scandinavian Journal of Occupational Therapy, 2*, 121–128.

Doble, S. E., Fisk, J. D., Fisher, A. G., Ritvo, P. G., & Murray, T. J. (1994). Functional competence of community-dwelling persons with multiple sclerosis using the Assessment of Motor and Process Skills. *Archives of Physical Medicine and Rehabilitation, 75*, 843–851.

Fisher, A. G. (1994). Development of a functional assessment that adjusts ability measures for task simplicity and rater leniency. In M. Wilson (Ed.), *Objective measurement: Theory into practice,* (Vol. 2, pp. 145–175). Norwood, NJ: Ablex.

Fisher, A. G. (1994). Functional assessment and occupation: Critical issues for occupational therapy. *New Zealand Journal of Occupational Therapy, 45*(2), 13–19.

Fisher, A. G., Bryze, K. A., Granger, C. V., Haley, S. M., Hamilton, B. B., Heineman, A. W., et al. (1994). Applications of conjoint measurement to the development of functional measures. *International Journal of Educational Research, 21*, 579–593.

Nygård, L., Bernspång, B., Fisher, A. G., & Winblad, B. (1994). Comparing motor and process ability of persons with suspected dementia in home and clinic settings. *American Journal of Occupational Therapy, 48*, 689–696.

Pan, A. W., & Fisher, A. G. (1994). The Assessment of Motor and Process Skills of persons with psychiatric disorders. *American Journal of Occupational Therapy, 48*, 775–780.

Park, S., Fisher, A. G., & Velozo, C. A. (1994). Using the Assessment of Motor and Process Skills to compare occupational performance between clinic and home settings. *American Journal of Occupational Therapy, 48*, 697–709.

Campbell, S. K., Osten, E. T., Kolobe, T. H. A., & Fisher, A. G. (1993). Development of the Test of Infant Motor Performance. *Physical Medicine and Rehabilitation Clinics of North America: New Developments in Functional Assessment, 4*, 541–550.

Dickerson, A. E., & Fisher, A. G. (1993). Age differences in functional performance. *American Journal of Occupational Therapy, 47*, 686–692.

Fisher, A. G. (1993). The assessment of IADL motor skills: An application of many-faceted Rasch analysis. *American Journal of Occupational Therapy, 47*, 319–329.

Fisher, W. P., & Fisher, A. G. (1993). Applications of Rasch analysis to studies in occupational therapy. *Physical Medicine and Rehabilitation Clinics of North America: New Developments in Functional Assessment, 4*, 551–569.

Fisher, A. G., & Short-DeGraff, M. (Eds.). (1993). Critical issues in functional assessment [Special issue]. *American Journal of Occupational Therapy, 47*(3).

Fisher, A. G., & Short-DeGraff, M. (1993). Nationally Speaking—Improving functional assessment in occupational therapy: Recommendations and philosophy for change. *American Journal of Occupational Therapy, 47*, 199–201.

Short-DeGraff, M., & Fisher, A. G. (Eds.). (1993). Alternative strategies for functional assessment [Special issue]. *American Journal of Occupational Therapy, 47*(4).

Short-DeGraff, M. A., & Fisher, A. G. (1993). Nationally Speaking—A proposal for diverse research methods and a common research language. *American Journal of Occupational Therapy, 47*, 295–297.

Bundy, A. C., & Fisher, A. G. (1992). Evaluation of sensory integrative dysfunction. In H. Forssberg & H. Hirschfeld (Eds.), *Series in Medicine and Sport Science: Vol. 36. Movement Disorders in Children.* Basel, Switzerland: Karger.

Fisher, A. G. (1992). Commentary [Haley, S.M., & Ludlow, L.H., Applicability of the hierarchical scales of the Tufts Assessment of Motor Performance for school-aged children and adults with disabilities]. *Physical Therapy, 72*, 202–203.

Fisher, A. G. (1992). Functional measures, Part I: What is function, what should we measure, and how should we measure it? *American Journal of Occupational Therapy, 46*, 183–185.

Fisher, A. G. (1992). Functional measures, Part II: Selecting the right test, minimizing the limitations. *American Journal of Occupational Therapy, 46*, 278–281.

Fisher, A. G., & Bundy, A. C. (1992). Sensory integration theory. In H. Forssberg & H. Hirschfeld (Eds.), *Series in Medicine and Sport Science: Vol. 36. Movement Disorders in Children.* Basel, Switzerland: Karger.

Fisher, A. G., Liu, Y., Velozo, C. V., & Pan, A. W. (1992). Cross-cultural assessment of process skills. *American Journal of Occupational Therapy, 46*, 876–885.

Puderbaugh, J. K., & Fisher, A. G. (1992). Assessment of motor and process skills in normal young children and children with dyspraxia. *Occupational Therapy Journal of Research, 12*, 195–216.

Fisher, A. G. (1991). Vestibular–proprioception and bilateral integration and sequencing disorders. In A. G. Fisher, E. M. Murray, & A. C. Bundy (Eds.), *Sensory integration: Theory and practice.* Philadelphia: F. A. Davis.

Fisher, A. G. & Bundy, A. C. (1991). The interpretation process. In A. G. Fisher, E. M. Murray, & A. C. Bundy (Eds.), *Sensory integration: Theory and practice.* Philadelphia: F. A. Davis.

Fisher A. G. & Murray, E. M. (1991). Sensory integration theory. In A. G. Fisher, E. M. Murray, & A. C. Bundy (Eds.), *Sensory integration: Theory and practice.* Philadelphia: F. A. Davis.

Fisher, A. G., Murray, E. M. & Bundy, A. C. (Eds.). (1991). *Sensory integration: Theory and practice.* Philadelphia: F. A. Davis.

Kielhofner, G., & Fisher, A. G. (1991). The mind-body problem. In A. G. Fisher, E. M. Murray, & A. C. Bundy (Eds.), *Sensory integration: Theory and practice.* Philadelphia: F. A. Davis.

Morrison, C. D., Bundy, A. C., & Fisher, A. G. (1991). The contribution of motor skills and playfulness to play performance of preschool-aged children. *American Journal of Occupational Therapy, 45*, 687–694.

Case-Smith, J., Fisher, A. G., & Bauer, D. (1989). An analysis of the relationship of proximal and distal motor control. *American Journal of Occupational Therapy, 43*, 657–662.

Fisher, A. G. (1989). Amputation and prosthetics. In C. A. Trombly (Ed.), *Occupational therapy for physical dysfunction* (3rd ed.). Baltimore: Williams & Wilkins.

Fisher, A. G. (1989). Objective assessment of the quality of response during two equilibrium tasks. *Physical and Occupational Therapy in Pediatrics, 9*(3), 57–78.

Fisher, A. G., & Bundy, A. C. (1989). Vestibular stimulation in the treatment of postural and related deficits. In O. Payton, R. P. Di Fabio, S. V. Paris, E. J. Protas, & A. F. Vansant (Eds.), *Manual of physical therapy*. New York: Churchill Livingstone.

Fisher, A. G., Kielhofner, G., & Davis, C. (1989). Research values of occupational and physical therapists. *Journal of Allied Health, 18*, 143–155.

Fisher, A. G., Wietlisbach, S. E., & Wilbarger, J. L. (1988). Adult performance on three tests of equilibrium. *American Journal of Occupational Therapy, 42*, 30–35.

Bundy, A. C., Fisher, A. G., Freeman, M., Lieberg, G., & Izraelevitz, T. E. (1987). Concurrent validity among tests of equilibrium for learning disabled boys with and without vestibular dysfunction. *American Journal of Occupational Therapy, 41*, 28–34.

Hung, S., Fisher, A. G., & Cermak, S. A. (1987). Performance of learning-disabled and normal male young adults on the Test of Visual–Perceptual Skills. *American Journal of Occupational Therapy, 41*, 790–797.

MacWhinney, K., Cermak, S., & Fisher, A. G. (1987). Body part identification in 1-to 4-year-old children. *American Journal of Occupational Therapy, 41*, 454–459.

Menken, C., Cermak, S. A., & Fisher, A. (1987). Evaluation of visual–perceptual skills in normal and cerebral palsied children. *American Journal of Occupational Therapy, 41*, 646–651.

Schulmann, D. L., Godfrey, B., & Fisher, A. G. (1987). Effect of eye movements in dynamic equilibrium. *Physical Therapy, 67*, 1054–1057.

Fisher, A. G., Mixon, J., & Herman, R. (1986). The validity of the clinical diagnosis of vestibular dysfunction. *Occupational Therapy Journal of Research, 6*, 3–20.

Herman, R., Mixon, J., Fisher, A., Maulucci, R., & Stuyck, J. (1985). Idiopathic scoliosis and the central nervous system: A motor control problem. *Spine, 10*, 1–14.

Izraelevitz, T. A., Fisher, A. G., & Bundy, A. C. (1985). Equilibrium reactions in preschoolers. *Occupational Therapy Journal of Research, 5*, 154–169.

Fisher, A. G. (1982). Amputation and prosthetics. In C. A. Trombly (Ed.), *Occupational therapy for physical dysfunction* (2nd ed.). Baltimore: Williams & Wilkins.

Fisher, A. G., & Bundy, A. C. (1982). Equilibrium reactions in normal children and in boys with sensory integrative dysfunction. *Occupational Therapy Journal of Research, 2*, 171–183.

Bundy, A. C., & Fisher, A. G. (1981). The relationship of prone extension to other vestibular functions. *American Journal of Occupational Therapy, 35*, 782–787.

Fisher, A. G. (1977). Initial prosthetic fitting of the congenital below elbow amputee: Are we fitting them early enough? *Inter-Clinic Information Bulletin, 15*(11/12), 7–9.

Fisher, A. G. (1977). *Parental attitudes toward juvenile amputees* [Video]. Kalamazoo, MI: University Television.

Fisher, A. G. (1976). Functional results with electrically powered devices for children. *Minutes on a Workshop for Children's Prosthetics*. Washington, DC: National Academy of Sciences.

Aitken, G. T., Fisher, A. G., & Spagnuolo, W. (1975). *Wendy* [Film]. Grand Rapids: Michigan Department of Public Health, Area Child Amputee Center.

Fisher, A. G., & Childress, D. (1973). The Michigan Electric Hook: A preliminary report on a new electrically powered hook for children. *Inter-Clinic Information Bulletin, 12*(9), 1–10.

Elnora M. Gilfoyle, DSc, OTR, FAOTA—1984

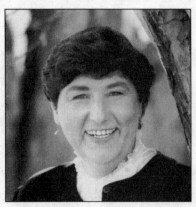

Elnora M. Gilfoyle, professor emeritus, was named the first female provost and academic vice-president at a major research university. She was an associate professor and head of the Department of Occupational Therapy at Colorado State University in Fort Collins. A graduate of the State University of Iowa with a degree in occupational therapy, she holds an honorary doctor of science degree from Colorado State University.

Gilfoyle served as project coordinator for the Training: Occupational Therapy Education Management in Schools project funded by the Department of Education; consultant and faculty member for the John F. Kennedy Child Development Center, University of Colorado; director of occupational therapy, the Denver Children's Hospital; and staff therapist at Craig Rehabilitation Center and Denver General Hospital.

Gilfoyle served as AOTA president from 1986 to 1989. She also served in various capacities in the Occupational Therapy Association of Colorado. She was named to the AOTA Roster of Fellows in 1973. Other awards include the Marjorie Ball Lectureship Award from the Occupational Therapy Association of Colorado and listing in Who's Who in America Certificate of Appreciation.

Bibliography

Young, L., Gordon, G., & Gilfoyle, E. M. (1961). Functional use of "nylon" muscle in severe quadriplegia. *Archives of Physical Medicine and Rehabilitation, 42*, 739–743.

Gilfoyle, E. M. (1962). Functional hand bracing. *Children's Hospital Medical Journal, 12*(3), 11–17.

Gilfoyle, E. M. (1965). Functional bracing in the treatment of cerebral palsy. In W. West (Ed.), *Occupational therapy for the multiply handicapped child* (pp. 58–92). Chicago: University of Illinois Press.

Gilfoyle, E. M. (1966). The three faces of evaluation. In W. West (Ed.), *Evaluation and treatment of perceptual–motor dysfunction* (pp. 235–250). Madison: University of Wisconsin Press.

Martin, H., & Gilfoyle, E. M. (1969). Assessment of perceptual development. *American Journal of Occupational Therapy, 23*, 1–14.

Gilfoyle, E. M., & Grady, A. (1970). Cognitive–perceptual–motor development. In H. S. Willard & C. S. Spackman (Eds.), *Occupational therapy* (4th ed., pp. 178–202). Philadelphia: Lippincott.

Gilfoyle, E. M., & Grady, A. (1971). A developmental theory of sensory–motor reactions and spontaneous integrative behavior. In *Symposium for Somatosensory Perceptual Deficits.* Boston: Boston University Press.

Gilfoyle, E. M. (1973). Research in sensory integrative development: An introduction. *American Journal of Occupational Therapy, 27*, 189–190.

Henderson, A., Llorens, L., & Gilfoyle, E. M. (1976). *The development of sensory integrative theory and practice: A collection of the works of A. Jean Ayres.* Dubuque, IA: Kendall/Hunt.

Yerxa, E., & Gilfoyle, E. M. (1976). Research seminar. *American Journal of Occupational Therapy, 30*, 509–514.

Price, A., Gilfoyle, E. M., & Myers, C. (1976). *Research in sensory-integrative development.* Rockville, MD: American Occupational Therapy Association.

Gilfoyle, E. M. (1978). BEH project report. *Occupational Therapy Newspaper, 32*(10), 1.

Gilfoyle, E. M., & Grady, A. (1978). Posture and movement development: Minimal brain dysfunction. In H. D. Smith & H. L. Hopkins (Eds.), *Willard and Spackman's occupational therapy* (5th ed., pp. 218–230). Philadelphia: Lippincott.

Gilfoyle, E. M., & Hays, C. (1979). Occupational therapy roles and functions in the education of the school-based handicapped student. *American Journal of Occupational Therapy, 33*, 565–576.

Gilfoyle, E. (1980). Caring: A philosophy for practice. *American Journal of Occupational Therapy, 34*, 517–521.

Gilfoyle, E. M., & Hays, C. (1980). *Training: Occupational therapy educational management in schools: A competency-based educational program* (Vols. 1, 2, 3, & 4). Rockville, MD: American Occupational Therapy Association.

Gilfoyle, E. M. (1981). *Occupational therapy in the school systems.* Rockville, MD: American Occupational Therapy Association.

Gilfoyle, E. M., & Farace, J. (1981). Official position paper: The role of occupational therapy as an education-related service. *American Journal of Occupational Therapy, 35*, 811.

Gilfoyle, E. M., Grady, A., & Moore, J. (1981). *Children adapt.* Thorofare, NJ: Slack.

Gilfoyle, E. M., & Hays, C. (1981). *The final report on the AOTA competency-based project entitled "Advanced training for occupational therapists in (public) school systems," Grant No. G 007801499.* Rockville, MD: American Occupational Therapy Association.

Gilfoyle, E. M., & Grady, A. (1983). Spatiotemporal adaptation. In H. D. Smith & H. L. Hopkins (Eds.), *Willard and Spackman's occupational therapy* (6th ed., pp. 212–227). Philadelphia: Lippincott.

Hinojosa, J., Goldstein, P. K., Becker-Lewin, M., Gilfoyle, E. M., Rosen, M., & Reeves, G. D. (1983). Draft: Occupational therapy for sensory integrative dysfunction. *Occupational Therapy News, 36*(4), 6.

Gilforyle, E. M. (1984). Transformation of a profession. (1984 Eleanor Clarke Slagle Lecture). *American Journal of Occupational Therapy, 38*, 575–584.

Gilfoyle, E. M., & Gliner, J A. (1985). Attitudes toward handicapped children: Impact of an educational program. *Physical and Occupational Therapy in Pediatrics, 5*(4), 27–41.

Gilfoyle, E. M. (1986). From the President. *Mental Health Special Interest Section Newsletter, 10*(1), 1.

Gilfoyle, E. M. (1986). Nationally Speaking: Professional directions: Management in action. *American Journal of Occupational Therapy, 40*, 593–596.

Gilfoyle, E. M. (1986). Nationally Speaking: Taking care of ourselves as health care providers. *American Journal of Occupational Therapy, 40*, 387–389.

Gilfoyle, E. M. (1987). Letter from the President. *Administration & Management Special Interest Section Newsletter, 10*(1), 1.

Gilfoyle, E. M. (1987). Letter from the President. *Developmental Disabilities Special Interest Section Newsletter, 10*(1), 1.

Gilfoyle, E. M. (1987). Letter from the President. *Gerontology Special Interest Section Newsletter, 10*(1), 1.

Gilfoyle, E. M. (1987). Letter from the President. *Physical Disabilities Special Interest Section Newsletter, 10*(1), 1.

Gilfoyle, E. M. (1987). Letter from the President. *Sensory Integration Special Interest Section Newsletter, 10*(1), 1.

Gilfoyle, E. M. (1987). Nationally Speaking: Creative partnerships: The profession's plan. *American Journal of Occupational Therapy, 41*, 779–781.

Gilfoyle, E. M. (1987). Nationally Speaking: Leadership and management. *American Journal of Occupational Therapy, 41*, 281–283.

Gilfoyle, E. M. (1987). Research topics chosen for developmental disabilities symposium. *Developmental Disabilities Special Interest Section Newsletter, 10*(1), 4.

Gilfoyle, E. M., & Christiansen, C. (1987). Nationally Speaking: Research: The quest for truth and the key to excellence. *American Journal of Occupational Therapy, 41*, 7–9.

Gilfoyle, E. M. (1988). Nationally Speaking: Partnerships for the future. *American Journal of Occupational Therapy, 42*, 485–488.

Gilfoyle, E. M. (1989). Nationally Speaking: Leadership and occupational therapy. *American Journal of Occupational Therapy, 43*, 567–570.

Gilfoyle, E. M., Grady, A. P., & Moore, J. C. (1990). *Children adapt: A theory of sensorimotor–sensory development* (2nd ed.). Thorofare, NJ: Slack.

Ann P. Grady, PhD, OTR—1994

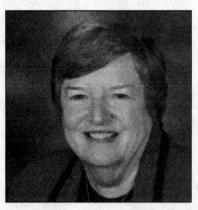

Ann P. Grady was assistant professor of pediatrics, University of Colorado Health Science Center in Denver and director of Interdisciplinary Education and Occupational Therapy Discipline Director at JFK Partners. She received a bachelor's degree in sociology from the College of New Rochelle (New York), a certificate in occupational therapy from Columbia University, and a master's degree in human communication studies and a doctorate in communication studies from the University of Denver.

Grady has more than 30 years of experience working in the field of developmental disabilities, including teaching, research, development, and implementation of demonstration projects and policy advocacy at the state and national levels in early intervention services. She has particular expertise in the area of early intervention services and supports. Her research interests include the development of leadership in women and the effectiveness of services delivered in context to children and families.

She has been associate professor of occupational therapy at Colorado State University, director of Occupational and Physical Therapy at the Children's Hospital in Denver, and founder and Director of the AccessAbility Resource Center at the Children's Hospital. Grady has served the profession several capacities on state and national levels. She is a charter Fellow, former speaker of the Representative Assembly, and past-president of the AOTA. She previously served as vice president of the American Occupational Therapy Foundation and chair of its Research Development Committee. She has provided leadership in Colorado and on a national level in early intervention and related-service personnel preparation, team and leadership development, and principles of family-centered care. Her current research interests include development of leadership practices.

Her passion focuses on the inclusion of all people in their community of choice for living, working, and playing. Her love of the mountains and outdoors frequently takes her to her mountain home in Dillon, Colorado, for hiking, cross-county skiing, and contemplating.

She received the AOTF's Meritorious Service Award.

Bibliography

Gilfoyle, E. M., Grady, A. P., & Moore, J. C. (1981). *Children adapt: A theory of sensorimotor–sensory development.* Thorofare, NJ: Slack.

Grady, A. P. (1985). The effect of DRGs in a pediatric setting. *Administration & Management Special Interest Section Newsletter, 1*(2), 1–2, 4.

Grady, A. P. (1987). Nationally Speaking: Research: Its role in enhancing the professional image. *American Journal of Occupational Therapy, 41,* 347–349.

Grady, A. P. (1988). Nationally Speaking: AOTA organizational planning: Focus on the future. *American Journal of Occupational Therapy, 42,* 143–145.

Gilfoyle, E. M., Grady, A. P., & Moore, J. C. (1990). *Children adapt: A theory of sensorimotor–sensory development* (2nd ed.). Thorofare, NJ: Slack.

Grady, A. P. (1990). Nationally Speaking: Collaborative relationships: Opportunities for occupational therapy in the 1990s and beyond. *American Journal of Occupational Therapy, 44,* 105–108.

Grady, A. P. (1990). Nationally Speaking: Leadership is everybody's practice. *American Journal of Occupational Therapy, 44,* 1065–1068.

Grady, A. (1990). Recruitment is everybody's business. *Occupational Therapy News, 44*(2), 193-C.

Grady, A. P. (1991). Nationally Speaking: Directions for the future: Opportunities for leadership. *American Journal of Occupational Therapy, 45,* 7–9.

Grady, A., & Timms, J. (1991, September 12). Focus: School-based practice: Computers in the classroom–A winning combination. *OT Week,* pp. 12–13.

Grady, A. P. (1992). Brief or new: Highlights of AOTA presidents' terms, 1961–1989. *American Journal of Occupational Therapy, 46,* 1123–1125.

Grady, A. P. (1992). Nationally Speaking: Occupation as vision. *American Journal of Occupational Therapy, 46,* 1062–1065.

Grady, A. P., Kivach, T., Lange, M. L., & Shannon, L. (1993). "Consumer knows best": Promoting choice in assistive technology. *PT: Magazine of Physical Therapy, 1*(2), 50–56.

Grady, A. P. (1994). From the guest editor. *Technology Special Interest Section Newsletter, 4*(3), 1.

Tougher, M., Kyler-Hutchinson, P., Howard, D., Mu-oz, J., Hansen, R. A., & Grady, A. P. (1995). *Everyday ethics.* Bethesda, MD: American Occupational Therapy Association.

Grady, A. P. (1995). Building inclusive community: A challenge for occupational therapy (1994 Eleanor Clarke Slagle Lecture). *American Journal of Occupational Therapy, 49,* 300–310.

Grady, A. P. (1999). *Voices of change: Development of leadership practices in women.* Denver, CO: University of Denver.

Jacobs, K., Grady, A. P., Loukas, K., Thonpson, L. K., Fine, S., Hoover, S., et al. (2000 March 27). "Tenacity, energy, spirit, and savvy": Jeannette Bair's colleagues celebrate her contributions. *OT Practice 5*(7), 10–12.

Betty Risteen Hasselkus, PhD, OTR, FAOTA—2006

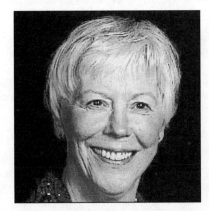

Betty Risteen Hasselkus is emeritus professor of occupational therapy/kinesiology, University of Wisconsin–Madison (UW–Madison). She grew up in the small Midwestern town of Baraboo, Wisconsin. Over the span of 30 years, Hasselkus earned an undergraduate degree in occupational therapy, a master of science degree in physical education, and a doctor of philosophy degree in adult education—all at UW–Madison.

Hasselkus started her professional career as an occupational therapist in general medicine and surgery at a large teaching hospital in Madison. While her two children were young, she held a succession of part-time community-based therapy positions: an outpatient children's clinic, a community hospital outpatient program, and a nonprofit neighborhood program elderly people. After earning her master's degree in 1974, she served for 7 years as the occupational therapist with a Veterans Administration interdisciplinary geriatric home care program. These early years of practice helped nurture and develop her deep interest in and commitment to geriatric practice, teaching, and research. Hasselkus ultimately returned to graduate school and completed her doctoral work in 1987; her dissertation was titled *Family Caregivers for the Elderly at Home: An Ethnography of Meaning and Informal Learning.* At that point she accepted a faculty position as assistant professor at the UW–Madison and subsequently was promoted to associate professor and then full professor before her retirement in 1999.

Throughout her over 40 years of research, teaching, and practice, Hasselkus has focused on the everyday experience of occupation for people in the community, with a special emphasis on caregiving by family members, physicians, day care staff, and occupational therapists. She has over 90 publications in journals and texts and published her first book, *The Meaning of Everyday Occupation*, in 2002 (a 2nd edition is due to be released in late 2010). She served as the first scholar–editor of the *American Journal of Occupational Therapy* from 1998 to 2003. As editor, she created the *AJOT* feature "From the Desk of the Editor," a journal offering that continues to this day.

Hasselkus's international reputation as a scholar has taken her to Australia, Canada, Denmark, Sweden, Wales, and Northern Ireland; in these countries, she has served as dissertation opponent, visiting professor, conference presenter, and qualitative research workshop leader. While on faculty at UW–Madison, she hosted visiting scholars from Japan, South Africa, Australia, and Sweden. Hasselkus considers her many international friends and opportunities—including the WFOT Congresses held in Montreal and Stockholm—to be highlights of her career.

Hasselkus was elected to the Roster of Fellows of the American Occupational Therapy Association in 1986 and the Academy of Research of the American Occupational Therapy Foundation in 1999; she received the Wisconsin Occupational Therapy Association Lifetime Achievement Award in 1999. In 2003, she was awarded the Wilma West Lecture from the University of Southern California. Hasselkus received the Eleanor Clarke Slagle Lectureship Award in 2005.

Hasselkus's message to all occupational therapy personnel is to encourage careers filled with knowledge and awareness of the compelling issues of the profession at home and abroad, deepening understandings about the nature of occupation as it is embodied in human beings, and the continual nurturance of intellectual growth.

Linking Key Messages of the 2006 Eleanor Clarke Slagle Lecture to the AOTA *Centennial Vision:* In her Eleanor Clarke Slagle Lecture, Hasselkus states that she hopes to "promote understandings of everyday occupation as a therapeutic entity, as a focus for teaching and training, and as an area of research inquiry with vast potential." The aim of the key message is to encourage awareness of the complexity, beauty, and importance of everyday occupation in the lives of all people, worldwide. Everyday occupation is a primary means by which we organize the worlds in which we live and by which we build meaning and community in our lives. In Hasselkus's lecture, the importance and power of occupation in people's lives is recognized and made visible; its global relevance and application are voiced. The universality of the occupational needs of all the world's communities and cultures is supported.

—Betty Hasselkus

Bibliography

Hasselkus, B. R. (2010). *The meaning of everyday occupation* (2nd ed.). Thorofare, NJ: Slack.

Hasselkus, B. R., & Murray, B. J. (2007). Everyday occupation, well-being, and identity: The experience of caregivers in families with dementia. *American Journal of Occupational Therapy, 61*, 9–20.

Hasselkus, B. R. (2006). The world of everyday occupation: Real people, real lives (2006 Eleanor Clarke Slagle Lecture). *American Journal of Occupational Therapy, 60*, 627–640.

Rosa, S., & Hasselkus, B. R. (2005). Finding common ground with patients: The centrality of compatibility. *American Journal of Occupational Therapy, 59*, 198–208.

Hasselkus, B. R. (2004). Deeper into the heart of the matter. *American Journal of Occupational Therapy, 58*, 476–479.

Hasselkus, B. R. (2004). Foreword. In R. Watson & E. Schwartz (Eds.), *Transformation and occupation*. London: Whurr.

Jacques, N., & Hasselkus, B. R. (2004). The nature of occupation surrounding dying and death. *OTJR: Occupation, Participation and Health, 24*, 44–53.

Hasselkus, B. R. (2003). From the Desk of the Editor—The sense of an ending. *American Journal of Occupational Therapy, 57*(3), 247–249.

Hasselkus, B. R. (2003). From the Desk of the Editor—Voices of qualitative researchers. *American Journal of Occupational Therapy, 57*(1), 7–8.

Hasselkus, B. R. (2003). From the Desk of the Editor—The world of occupational therapy. *American Journal of Occupational Therapy, 57*(2), 127–128.

Hasselkus, B. R. (2003). Introduction to adult and older adult populations. In E. Crepeau, B. Schell, & E. Cohn (Eds.), *Willard and Spackman's occupational therapy* (10th ed.). Philadelphia: Lippincott Williams & Wilkins.

Hasselkus, B. R. (2002). From the Desk of the Editor—Keeping body and soul together. *American Journal of Occupational Therapy, 56*(4), 367–369.

Hasselkus, B. R. (2002). From the Desk of the Editor—Unmasking the reviewers. *American Journal of Occupational Therapy, 56*(1), 7–8.

Hasselkus, B. R. (2002). From the Desk of the Editor—Unspeakable occupations. *American Journal of Occupational Therapy, 55*(6), 606–607.

Hasselkus, B. R. (2002). From the Desk of the Editor—The use of "race" in research. *American Journal of Occupational Therapy, 56*(2), 127–128.

Hasselkus, B. R. (2002). *The meaning of everyday occupation*. Thorofare, NJ: Slack.

Hasselkus, B. R., Ottenbacher, K. J., & Tickle-Degnen, L. (2002). From the Desk of the Editor—Therapists awake! The challenge of evidence-based occupational therapy. *American Journal of Occupational Therapy, 56*(3), 247–249.

Bonder, B. R., & Hasselkus, B. R. (2001). Families and professionals: Therapeutic considerations. In B. R. Bonder & M. B. Wagner (Eds.), *Functional performance in older adults* (2nd ed., pp. 487–499). Philadelphia: F. A. Davis.

Hasselkus, B. R. (2001). From the Desk of the Editor—Author's guide: Revised. *American Journal of Occupational Therapy, 55*(1), 7–8.

Hasselkus, B. R. (2001). From the Desk of the Editor—Dear Ann Landers. *American Journal of Occupational Therapy, 55*(3), 247–248.

Hasselkus, B. R. (2001). From the Desk of the Editor—It's great to be in the fifties! *American Journal of Occupational Therapy, 55*(4), 367–368.

Hasselkus, B. R. (2001). From the Desk of the Editor—Occupation: On the rocks. *American Journal of Occupational Therapy, 55*(5), 487–488.

Hasselkus, B. R. (2001). From the Desk of the Editor—Writing the abstract: The most important part of the manuscript? *American Journal of Occupational Therapy, 55*(2), 127–128.

Hasselkus, B. R. (2000). From the Desk of the Editor—Habits of the heart. *American Journal of Occupational Therapy, 54*(3), 247–248.

Hasselkus, B. R. (2000). From the Desk of the Editor—It was a very good year. . .or was it? *American Journal of Occupational Therapy, 54*(4), 359–360.

Hasselkus, B. R. (2000). From the Desk of the Editor—New Offerings in *AJOT*. *American Journal of Occupational Therapy, 54*(1), 7.

Hasselkus, B. R. (2000). From the Desk of the Editor—Reaching consensus. *American Journal of Occupational Therapy, 54*(2), 127–128.

Hasselkus, B. R. (2000). From the Desk of the Editor—What makes an editor groan. *American Journal of Occupational Therapy, 54*(5), 455–456.

Hasselkus, B. R. (1999). From the Desk of the Editor—Incentives for change. *American Journal of Occupational Therapy, 53*(1), 7–8.

Hasselkus, B. R. (1999). From the Desk of the Editor—More about writing for *AJOT*. *American Journal of Occupational Therapy, 53*(5), 427–428.

Hasselkus, B. R. (1999). From the Desk of the Editor—No "student section" in *AJOT*. *American Journal of Occupational Therapy, 53*(4), 331–332.

Hasselkus, B. R. (1999). From the Desk of the Editor—Writing for AJOT. *American Journal of Occupational Therapy, 53*(2), 127–128.

Hasselkus, B. R., & Jacobs, K. (1999). From the Desks of the Editor and President—The guide to occupational therapy practice. *American Journal of Occupational Therapy, 53*(3), 246.

Chang, L.-H., & Hasselkus, B. R. (1998). Occupational therapists' expectations in rehabilitation following stroke: Sources of satisfaction and dissatisfaction. *American Journal of Occupational Therapy, 52*, 629–637.

Hasselkus, B. R. (1998). From the Desk of the Editor—Starting the journey. *American Journal of Occupational Therapy, 52*(9), 698.

Hasselkus, B. R. (1998). From the Desk of the Editor—WFOT '98: Reflections on the experience. *American Journal of Occupational Therapy, 52*(10), 783–784.

Hasselkus, B. R. (1998). Occupation and well-being in dementia: The experience of day care staff. *American Journal of Occupational Therapy, 52*, 423–434.

Hasselkus, B. R., & Borell, L. (1998). Editorial. *Scandinavian Journal of Occupational Therapy, 5*, 107–108.

Hasselkus, B. R., & LaBelle, A. (1998). Dementia day care endings: The uncertain limits of care. *Journal of Applied Gerontology, 17*, 3–24.

Hasselkus, B. R. (1997). Everyday ethics in dementia care: Narratives of crossing the line. *The Gerontologist, 37*, 640–649.

Hasselkus, B. R. (1997). In the eye of the beholder: The researcher in qualitative research. *Occupational Therapy Journal of Research, 17*, 81–83.

Hasselkus, B. R. (1997). Introduction to adult and older adult populations. In M. Neistadt & E. Crepeau (Eds.), *Willard and Spackman's occupational therapy* (9th ed., pp. 651–659, 756–758). Philadelphia: J. B. Lippincott.

Hasselkus, B. R., Dickie, V. A., & Gregory, C. (1997). Geriatric occupational therapy: The uncertain ideology of long-term care. *American Journal of Occupational Therapy, 51,* 132–139.

Hasselkus, B. R., & Rosa, S. A. (1997). Meaning and occupation. In C. Christiansen & C. Baum (Eds.), *Occupational therapy: Achieving human performance needs in daily living* (2nd ed., pp. 362–377). Gaithersburg, MD: Aspen.

Rosa, S., & Hasselkus, B. R. (1996). Connecting with patients: The personal experience of professional helping. *Occupational Therapy Journal of Research, 16,* 245–260.

Hasselkus, B. R. (1995). Beyond ethnography: Expanding our understandings and criteria for qualitative research [Editorial]. *Occupational Therapy Journal of Research, 15,* 75–84.

Hasselkus, B. R. (1994). Commentary—Occupational programming in a day hospital for patients with dementia. *Occupational Therapy Journal of Research, 14,* 239–243.

Hasselkus, B. R. (1994). From hospital to home: Family–professional relationships in geriatric rehabilitation. *Gerontology and Geriatric Education, 15,* 91–100.

Hasselkus, B. R. (1994). Three-track care: Older patient, family member, and physician in the medical visit. *Journal of Aging Studies, 8,* 291–307.

Hasselkus, B. R. (1994). Working with family caregivers: The therapeutic alliance. In B. Bonder & M. Wagner (Eds.), *Functional performance in the elderly* (pp. 339–351). Philadelphia: F. A. Davis.

Hasselkus, B. R., & Dickie, V. A. (1994). Doing occupational therapy: Dimensions of satisfaction and dissatisfaction. *American Journal of Occupational Therapy, 48,* 145–154.

Hasselkus, B. R. (1993). Aging and health. In H. Smith & H. Hopkins (Eds.), *Willard and Spackman's occupational therapy* (8th ed., pp. 733–741). Philadelphia: J. B. Lippincott.

Hasselkus, B. R. (1993). Death in very old age: A personal journey of caregiving. *American Journal of Occupational Therapy, 47,* 717–723.

Hasselkus, B. R. (1993). Functional disability in older adults. In H. Smith & H. Hopkins (Eds.), *Willard and Spackman's occupational therapy* (8th ed., pp. 742–752). Philadelphia: J. B. Lippincott.

Hasselkus, B. R. (1992). Family caregiver as interpreter in the geriatric medical interview. *Medical Anthropology Quarterly, 6,* 288–304.

Hasselkus, B. R. (1992). The meaning of activity in Alzheimer day care. *American Journal of Occupational Therapy, 46,* 199–206.

Hasselkus, B. R. (1992). Staff helping behaviors: Alzheimer day care. *American Journal of Alzheimer's Care and Related Disorders and Research, 7*(5), 9–16.

Cooper, B. A., & Hasselkus, B. R. (1992). Independent living and the physical environment: Aspects that matter to residents. *Canadian Journal of Occupational Therapy, 59,* 6–15.

Hasselkus, B. R. (1992). Physician and family caregiver in the medical setting: Negotiation of care? *Journal of Aging Studies, 6,* 67–80.

Cooper, B. A., Ahrentzen, S., & Hasselkus, B. R. (1991). Post-occupancy evaluation: An environment behavior technique for assessing the built environment. *Canadian Journal of Occupational Therapy, 58,* 181–188.

Cooper, B., Cohen, U., & Hasselkus, B. (1991). Barrier-free design: A review and critique of the occupational therapy perspective. *American Journal of Occupational Therapy, 45,* 344–351.

Hasselkus, B. R. (1991). Ethical dilemmas in family caregiving for the elderly: Implications for occupational therapy. *American Journal of Occupational Therapy, 45,* 206–213.

Hasselkus, B. R. (1991). Ethnographic interviewing: A tool for practice with family caregivers for the elderly. *Occupational Therapy Practice, 2*(1), 9–16.

Hasselkus, B. R. (1991). Qualitative research: Not another orthodoxy [Editorial]. *Occupational Therapy Journal of Research, 11,* 3–7.

Hasselkus, B. R., & Kiernat, J. M. (1991). Education for empowerment. In J. M. Kiernat (Ed.), *Occupational therapy and the older adult: A clinical manual* (pp. 61–74). Gaithersburg, MD: Aspen.

Hasselkus, B. R., & Stetson, S. A. (1991). Ethical dilemmas: The organization of family caregiving for the elderly. *Journal of Aging Studies, 5,* 99–110.

Hasselkus, B. R., & Dickie, V. A. (1990). Themes of meaning: Occupational therapists' perspectives on practice. *Occupational Therapy Journal of Research, 10,* 195–207.

Hasselkus, B. R. (1989). The meaning of daily activity in family caregiving for the elderly. *American Journal of Occupational Therapy, 43,* 649–656.

Hasselkus, B. R. (1989). Occupational and physical therapy in geriatric rehabilitation. *Physical and Occupational Therapy in Geriatrics, 7*(3), 3–20.

Hasselkus, B. R., & Kiernat, J. M. (1989). Nationally Speaking—Not by age alone: Gerontology as a specialty in occupational therapy. *American Journal of Occupational Therapy, 43,* 77–79.

Hasselkus, B. R. (1988). Commentary—Value acquisition in an occupational therapy curriculum. *Occupational Therapy Journal of Research, 8,* 275–279.

Hasselkus, B. R. (1988). Meaning in family caregiving: Perspectives on caregiver/professional relationships. *The Gerontologist, 28,* 686–691.

Hasselkus, B. R. (1988). Rehabilitation: The family caregiver's view. *Topics in Geriatric Rehabilitation, 4,* 60–70.

Hasselkus, B. R., & Maguire, G. H. (1988). Functional assessments used with older adults. In B. Hemphill (Ed.), *The evaluative process: An integrative approach to occupational therapy assessments used in mental health* (pp. 165–177). Charles B. Slack.

Hasselkus, B. R., & Ray, R. O. (1988). Informal learning and family caregiving: A worm's eye view. *Adult Education Quarterly, 39,* 31–40.

Ottenbacher, K. J., & Hasselkus, B. R. (1988). Research and practice: An evolving synthesis [Editorial]. *Occupational Therapy Journal of Research, 8,* 67–74.

Hasselkus, B. R. (1986). Assessment. In L. J. Davis & M. Kirkland (Eds.), *The role of occupational therapy with the elderly*. Bethesda, MD: American Occupational Therapy Association.

Hasselkus, B. R. (1986). Patient education. In L. J. Davis & M. Kirkland (Eds.), *The role of occupational therapy with the elderly.* Bethesda, MD: American Occupational Therapy Association.

Hasselkus, B. R. (1985). Changing trends in geriatric health care. *Gerontology Special Interest Section Quarterly, 8*(2).

Hasselkus, B. R. (1985). The occupational therapist. In G.A. Maguire (Ed.), *Care of the elderly: A health team approach* (pp. 145–158). Boston: Little, Brown & Co.

Hasselkus, B. R. (1983). Patient education and the elderly. *Physical and Occupational Therapy in Geriatrics, 2,* 55–70.

Hasselkus, B. R., & Brown, M. (1983). Respite care for community elderly. *American Journal of Occupational Therapy, 37,* 83–88.

Hasselkus, B. R. (1982). Barthel Self-care Index and geriatric home care patients. *Physical and Occupational Therapy in Geriatrics, 1*(4), 11–22.

Hasselkus, B. R. (1982). Commentary—Service provision and the elderly: Attitudes of three generations of urban women. *Occupational Therapy Journal of Research, 1,* 53–55.

Hasselkus, B. R. (1982). Service learning as it benefits the aging client. In *Service learning in aging: Implications for occupational therapy.* Washington, DC: National Council on Aging.

Hasselkus, B. R. (1982). Use of a monthly newsletter for life review. *Physical and Occupational Therapy in Geriatrics, 2,* 53–55.

Hasselkus, B. R., & Bauwens, S. (1982). Occupational therapy and pharmacy: Adapting drug regimens for older people. *Gerontology Special Interest Section Quarterly, 5*(4), 1–2.

Hasselkus, B. R., Kshepakaran, K. K., Houge, J. C., & Plautz, K. A. (1981). Rheumatoid arthritis: A two-axis goniometer to measure metacarpophalangeal lateral mobility. *Archives of Physical Medicine and Rehabilitation, 62,* 137–139.

Hasselkus, B. R., Kshepakaran, K. K., & Safrit, M. J. (1981). Handedness and hand joint changes in rheumatoid arthritis. *American Journal of Occupational Therapy, 35,* 705–710.

Hasselkus, B. R. (1981). Occupational behavior in the frail elderly. In G. Reidel, A. H. Kutscher, & J. A. Downey (Eds.), *Bereavement of physical disability: Recommitment to life, health, and function.* New York: Arno Press.

Hasselkus, B. R. (1978). Relocation stress and the elderly. *American Journal of Occupational Therapy, 32,* 631–636.

Hasselkus, B. R. (1977). A small group home for the elderly. *American Journal of Occupational Therapy, 31,* 525–529.

Hasselkus, B. R., & Safrit, M. J. (1976). Measurement in occupational therapy. *American Journal of Occupational Therapy, 30,* 429–436.

Hasselkus, B. R., & Shambes, G. M. (1975). Aging and postural sway in women. *Journal of Gerontology, 30,* 661–667.

Hasselkus, B. R. (1974). Aging and the human nervous system. *American Journal of Occupational Therapy, 28,* 16–21.

Hasselkus, B. R., & Kiernat, J. M. (1973). Independent living for the elderly. *American Journal of Occupational Therapy, 27,* 181–188.

Hasselkus, B. R. (1970). Occupational therapy in a small town. *American Journal of Occupational Therapy, 24,* 506–507.

Anne Henderson, PhD, OTR, FAOTA—1988

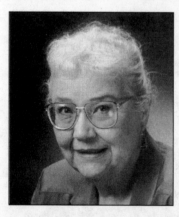

Anne Henderson is professor emeritus and founder of the doctoral program at Sargent College, Boston University, in Boston. She was born September 28, 1924. Her education includes an associate's degree from the University of California, Berkeley, in 1944; a bachelor's degree in occupational therapy from the University of Southern California, in 1946; a master's degree in education from the University of Pennsylvania in 1963; and a doctorate in educational psychology from the University of Pennsylvania in 1971. She has written in the areas of spatial abilities, hand function, and activities of daily living.

Henderson was assistant professor from 1963 to 1964 at Richmond Professional Institute. At the University of New Hampshire, she was assistant professor and supervisor of the occupational therapy curriculum from 1957 to 1961. At the University of Pennsylvania, she was instructor in occupational therapy from 1961 to 1962 and part-time from 1964 to 1967.

Henderson's academic appointments at Boston University, Sargent College of Allied Health Professions in occupational therapy began as an assistant professor from 1967 to 1970, associate professor from 1970 to 1983 and full professor from 1983 to 1990. She was the coordinator in the Interdisciplinary Doctoral Program (OT/PT) from 1979 to 1990; chairman of the occupational therapy department from 1984 to 1987; and coordinator of the advanced master's program in occupational therapy from 1970 to 1977 and 1979 to 1984.

Henderson's professional appointments include research coordinator, Occupational Therapy Department, Kennedy Memorial Hospital for Children, from 1980 to 1985; occupational therapy consultant, Infant Stimulation Project, Horace Mann School, Boston, from 1974 to 1975; director of training in occupational therapy, Fernald State School, from 1967 to 1969; research associate, American Occupational Therapy Association (AOTA) Curriculum Study Project, from 1962 to 1963; occupational therapist working with cerebral palsy, New York State Rehabilitation Hospital, from 1956 to 1957; therapy coordinator, Society for Crippled Children and Adults, Camp for Handicapped Children,

1956; director of occupational therapy, American British Cowdray Hospital, Mexico, from 1952 to 1956; occupational therapist, Sunrise School, Hayward, California, from 1950 to 1951; and occupational therapist, the Jefferson School, Oakland, California, from 1947 to 1950.

Among the honors Henderson has received are Pi Theta Epsilon, 1959; Pi Lambda Theta, 1970; AOTA Fellow, 1974; Award for Service to Sargent College, 1980; Certificate of Appreciation, Massachusetts Association for Occupational Therapy, 1987; Evelyn Kirrane Award, Sargent College, May 1989; Wilma West Lecturer, University of Southern California, 1990; Ayres Lectureship, Sensory Integration International, 1992; and AOTA Award of Merit, 1993.

Linking Key Messages of the 1988 Eleanor Clarke Slagle Lecture to the AOTA *Centennial Vision:* The key message of my lecture was directly linked to a central tenet of the *Centennial Vision*, that the profession be science driven and evidenced based. This comment addresses neuroscience as a driving force. Neuroscience has long driven occupational therapy practice with individuals with neurological dysfunction: specialized knowledge of the nervous system has guided the skilled observation and clinical judgment of practitioners and provided clues for new procedures. Our practice knowledge tells us what works and what does not work, and efficacy research will refine and verify that knowledge. Neuroscience will continue to suggest new approaches, but neuroscience also can tell us how and why our intervention works. Brain imaging is showing us how and why long-held occupational therapy principles of motor intervention work. Brain imaging also contributes to our understanding of occupation and its value by showing responses to occupation in the normal brain.

It is essential that entry-level occupational therapy practitioners be literate in neuroscience and that there be continual upgrading of the neuroscience curriculum. Post-professional education with an emphasis on neuroscience is needed to prepare therapists to read and understand brain research. Then, with the unique perspective that only an occupational therapist can bring, they can glean and organize the emerging neuroscience knowledge to support the development of occupational science.

—Anne Henderson

Bibliography

Henderson, A., & Eliasson, A. C. (2008). Self-care and hand function. In A. C. Eliasson & P. A. Burtner (Eds.), *Improving hand function in cerebral palsy.* London: MacKeith Press.

Henderson, A., & Pehoski, C. (2006). *Hand function in the child: Foundations for remediation* (2nd ed.). St. Louis, MO: Mosby.

Tseng, M. H., Henderson, A., Chow, S. M., & Yao, G. (2004). Relationship between motor proficiency, attention, impulse, and activity in children with ADHD. *Developmental Medicine and Child Neurology, 46*(6), 381–388.

Marr, D., Cermak, S. A., Cohn, E. S., & Henderson, A. (2003). Fine motor activities in Head Start and kindergarten classrooms. *American Journal of Occupational Therapy, 57,* 550–557.

Henderson, A., Pehoski, C., & Murray, E. (2002). Visual–spatial abilities. In A. C. Bundy, S. J. Lane, & E. Murray (Eds.), *Sensory integration: Theory and practice.* Philadelphia: F. A. Davis.

Sudsawad, P., Trombly, C. A., Henderson, A., & Tickle-Degnen, L. (2002). Testing the effect of kinesthetic training on handwriting performance in first-grade students. *American Journal of Occupational Therapy, 56,* 26–33.

Sudsawad, P., Trombly, C. A., Henderson, A., & Tickle-Degnen, L. (2001). The relationship between the evaluation tool of children's handwriting and teachers' perceptions of handwriting legibility. *American Journal of Occupational Therapy, 55,* 518–523.

Chen, C. C., Cermak, S. A., Murray, E. A., & Henderson, A. (1999). The effect of strategy on the recall of the Rey–Osterrieth complex figure in children with or without learning disabilities. *Occupational Therapy Journal of Research, 19,* 258–279.

Pehoski, C., Henderson, A., & Tickle-Degnen, L. (1997). In-hand manipulation in young children: Rotation of an object in the fingers. *American Journal of Occupational Therapy, 51,* 544–552.

Pehoski, C., Henderson, A., & Tickle-Dengen, L. (1997). In-hand manipulation in young children: Transition movements. *American Journal of Occupational Therapy, 51,* 719–728.

Henderson, A., & Cermak, S. (1995). *Pediatric occupational therapy: Challenges for the future in education and research.* Boston: Boston University.

Henderson, A., & Pehoski, C. (1995). *Hand function in the child: Foundations for remediation.* St. Louis, MO: Mosby/Year Book.

Chen-Sea, M., & Henderson, A. (1994). The reliability and validity of visuospatial inattention tests with stroke patients. *Occupational Therapy International, 1*(1), 36–48.

Chen-Sea, M., Henderson, A., & Cermak, S. A. (1993). Patterns of visual–spatial inattention and their functional significance in stroke patients. *Archives of Physical Medicine and Rehabilitation, 74*(4), 355–360.

Henderson, A., Cermak, S., Coster, W., Murray, E., Trombly, C., & Tickle-Dengen, L. (1991). The Issue Is—Occupational science is multidimensional. *American Journal of Occupational Therapy, 45,* 370–372.

Schneck, C. M., & Henderson, A. (1990). Descriptive analysis of the developmental progression of grip position for pencil and crayon control in nondysfunctional children. *American Journal of Occupational Therapy, 44,* 893–900.

Lawlor, M., & Henderson, A. (1989). A descriptive study of the clinical practice patterns of occupational therapists working with infants and young children. *American Journal of Occupational Therapy, 43,* 755–764.

Henderson, A. (1988). Occupational therapy knowledge: From practice to theory (1988 Eleanor Clarke Slagle Lecture). *American Journal of Occupational Therapy, 42,* 567–576.

Henderson, A. (1987). Selected bibliography review of research in developmental disabilities. *Developmental Disabilities Special Interest Section Newsletter, 10*(3), 7–8.

Henderson, A., Lawlor, M., & Pehoski, C. (1986). *Pediatric occupational therapy: Challenges for the future.* Medford, MA: Boston University.

Watemberg, J., Cermak, S. A., & Henderson, A. (1986). Right–left discrimination in blind and sighted children. *Physical and Occupational Therapy in Pediatrics, 6*(1), 7–19.

Haron, M., & Henderson, A. (1985). Active and passive touch in developmentally dyspraxic and normal boys. *Occupational Therapy Journal of Research, 5,* 101–112.

Bailey, D., MacDonald, J., & Henderson, A. (1984). Position paper in the support of changing entry-level education for occupational therapists from the baccalaureate-degree level to the post-baccalaureate-degree level. *Occupational Therapy News, 38*(3), 10–11.

Coryell, A., Henderson, A., & Liederman, J. (1982). Factors influencing the asymmetrical tonic neck reflex in normal infants. *Physical and Occupational Therapy in Pediatrics, 2*(2/3), 51–65.

Henderson, A., & Duncombe, L. (1982). Development of kinesthetic judgments of angle and distance. *Occupational Therapy Journal of Research, 2,* 131–144.

Henderson, A. (1981). Research in occupational therapy and in physical therapy with children. *Advances in Behavioral Pediatrics, 2*(1), 33–59.

Coryell, J., & Henderson, A. (1979). Role of the asymmetric tonic neck reflex in hand visualization in normal infants. *American Journal of Occupational Therapy, 33,* 255–260.

Ayers, A. J., Henderson, A., Llorens, L. A., Gilfoyle, E. M., Myers, C., & Prevel, S. (1974). *The development of sensory integrative theory and practice: A collection of works of A. Jean Ayers.* Dubuque, IA: Kendall/Hunt.

Henderson, A., & Coryell, A. (Eds.). (1973, March). The body senses and perceptual deficit. In *Proceedings of the Occupational Therapy Symposium on Somatosensory Aspects of Perceptual Deficit.* Boston: Boston University.

Jim Hinojosa, PhD OT, FAOTA—2007

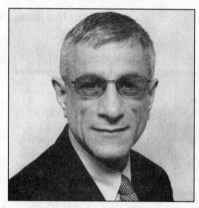

Jim Hinojosa grew up in Fort Collins, Colorado, in a traditional Mexican American family. He received a scholarship to Colorado State University (CSU), where he originally majored in chemistry. He found chemistry to be uninteresting or too competitive and desired to do something more creative. Part of the scholarship he received was a work–study position to provide tours of the campus. While giving a tour to a family in the home economics department, Hinojosa was given a brochure on occupational therapy. He decided to enroll in an occupational therapy course as an elective in his junior year in college and fell in love with the profession.

CSU was a very large program with many students to place for fieldwork and often sent students long distances for fieldwork. Hinojosa agreed to go to New York and was placed at Letchworth Developmental Center. Once he finished his fieldwork in Thiells, New York, he continued there as a staff occupational therapist for a year. However, Hinojosa states that "working at Blythedale Children's Hospital is where I received most of my real clinical experience" (personal communication, October 1, 2009). He decided to pursue a master's degree in special education, which he earned from Colombia University Teachers' College in 1977. He focused on the area of pediatrics as a practice specialty.

Hinojosa's academic career began by conducting workshops and being invited to teach a course at New York University (NYU). Early in his academic career when he was hired, it was made clear to him that he needed to pursue a doctorate; publish 2–3 times a year, preferably in refereed journals; and work on a portfolio of work. This wise advice set the tone for the rest of his career. Hinojosa noted that most of his scholarly written work and research has been a result of collaborating with others, and he enjoys this style of working on projects. He has been a prolific scholar, researching interests such as the therapist–parent relationship, homework and family life, and children's handwriting. He has written numerous books and articles focusing on topics such as theory, assessment, and pediatrics. He also is on the editorial boards of the *American Journal of Occupational Therapy;* the *Journal of Occupational Therapy, Schools, and Early Intervention;* and Miller and Keane's *Encyclopedia and Dictionary of Medicine, Nursing, and Allied Health.*

Hinojosa has been honored with numerous awards, including the American Occupational Therapy Association's (AOTA's) Award of Merit and Roster of Fellows in 1984, as well as numerous service awards from AOTA for serving on the Executive Board; chairing the Commission on Practice; and working on various other committees, task groups, and projects. He also has received a Meritorious Service Award from the American Occupational Therapy Foundation in 2000. He has been recognized in New York with the Award of Merit for Service (1980) from the New York State Occupational Therapy Association; the Abreu Award for Service (1987); New York State/United University Professions Excellence Award (1990); and the Ailanthus Award, Downstate Medical Center's highest honor for leadership in allied health (2005) from the State University of New York. He has been included in the Marquis Who's Who in Rehabilitation (1985), Who's Who in the East (1998), and Who's Who in the World (1999). He has been honored with awards from various universities and colleges, including the Research Scholar (1997) award from Texas Women's University in Dallas; Visiting Scholar (1997) from Dominican University in Orangeburg, New York; and the Barbara A. Rider Endowed Lectureship from Western Michigan University in Kalamazoo.

On a Personal Note From a Phone Interview: When asked about the motivation and inspiration for the 2007 Eleanor Clarke Slagle Lectureship, Hinojosa noted that the "first thing I did was go back and read all of the past Eleanor Clarke Slagle Lectures that I had not read and categorize the lectures. The one that always stuck out was Mary Reilly's. I wanted to look at what was *my* contribution. What would I recommend for the next decade? . . . We have to do things differently" (personal communication, October 1, 2009). He considered all of the documents he had helped write, his service on boards and committees, and his leadership of various groups. Hinojosa also had attended a lecture on hyperchange and pondered that, as professions needed to change and adapt, why was occupational therapy resisting change for so many years? He believed the structures within AOTA had become very rigid: "We needed to think about what it is we are going to do and how do we want to create the future we want? How can we use monies to change the profession for the positive? What are we creating leaders for, as leadership is situational? What are we going to empower the therapists to do?" (personal communication, October 1, 2009).

Hinojosa also examined how occupational therapy education needs to change and be different. He was chair of the faculty council at NYU at the time he received the Eleanor Clarke Slagle Lecture, and so he was attuned to the politics of higher education and kept hearing the same messages that if universities are to survive in the future, then these institutions need to do things differently. This was the inspiration for focusing his Slagle lecture on hyperchange and prompting others to think about the future of occupational therapy.

Hinojosa noted that as a result of presenting the Eleanor Clarke Slagle Lecture, he gained recognition and was a part of a special group of individuals. He believes that his messages are listened to more than before the lecture. He stated that the process of writing and giving the lecture was a growth experience in itself. He decided to not use PowerPoint slides and to go back to the old days of just talking to the audience. This was a powerful presentation, as he stood in a single spotlight next to the podium sharing his message to the profession.

Linking Key Messages of the 2007 Eleanor Clarke Slagle Lecture to the AOTA *Centennial Vision*: The *Centennial Vision* for AOTA identifies what it needs to do to prepare the profession for the future. In my lecture, I talked about what I felt occupational therapy needed to do for it to control its evolution to meet the needs of current American society. Professions change and adapt to changes in society, expansion of knowledge, and advances in technology. The rate of change has increased dramatically. AOTA's *Centennial Vision* is a response to these changes. To achieve some of the identified priorities in the *Centennial Vision*, occupational therapists and occupational therapy assistants must examine their roles, responsibilities, and traditions in education, practice, and research. In my Slagle lecture, I outlined my views of how occupational therapists and occupational therapy assistants can engage in changes that will support shaping occupational therapy's future. Many changes are consistent with the *Centennial Vision*. I propose that occupational therapy's future will be supported by developing innovative, reflective occupational therapists and occupational therapy assistants who embrace life in an era of hyperchange.

—Jim Hinojosa

Bibliography

Hinojosa, J., & Segal, R. (in press). Legos and Tinkertoys: Building intervention from theory. In S. J. Lane & A. C. Bundy (Eds.), *Kids can be kids: Supporting the occupations and activities of childhood*. Philadelphia: F. A. Davis.

Cohen, M., Hinojosa, J., & P. Kramer (2010). Administration of evaluation and assessments. In J. Hinojosa, P. Kramer, & P. Crist (Eds.), *Evaluation: Obtaining and interpreting data* (3rd ed., pp. 103–121). Bethesda, MD: AOTA Press.

Hinojosa, J., & Kramer, P. A. (2010). Frames of reference in the real world. In P. Kramer & J. Hinojosa (Eds.), *Frames of reference for pediatric occupational therapy* (3rd ed., pp. 571–581). Baltimore: Lippincott Williams & Wilkins.

Hinojosa, J., Kramer, P., & Crist, P. (2010). *Evaluation: Obtaining and interpreting data* (3rd ed.). Bethesda, MD: AOTA Press.

Hinojosa, J., Kramer, P., & Crist, P. (2010). Evaluation: Where do we begin? In J. Hinojosa, P. Kramer, & P. Crist (Eds.), *Evaluation: Obtaining and interpreting data* (3rd ed., pp. 1–20). Bethesda, MD: AOTA Press.

Hinojosa, J., Kramer, P., & Leubben, A. (2010). Structure of the frame of reference. In P. Kramer & J. Hinojosa (Eds.), *Frames of reference for pediatric occupational therapy* (3rd ed., pp. 3–22). Baltimore: Lippincott Williams & Wilkins.

Kramer, P., & Hinojosa, J. (2010). Philosophical and theoretical influences on evaluation. In J. Hinojosa, P. Kramer, & P. Crist (Eds.), *Evaluation: Obtaining and interpreting data* (3rd ed., pp. 21–39). Bethesda, MD: AOTA Press.

Kramer, P., Hinojosa, J., & Leubben, A. (2010). Contemporary legitimate tools of pediatric occupational therapy. In P. Kramer & J. Hinojosa (Eds.), *Frames of reference for pediatric occupational therapy* (3rd ed., pp. 51–66). Baltimore: Lippincott Williams & Wilkins.

Kramer, P., & Hinojosa, J. (2010). Developmental perspective: Fundamentals of developmental theory. In P. Kramer & J. Hinojosa (Eds.), *Frames of reference for pediatric occupational therapy* (3rd ed., pp. 23–30). Baltimore: Lippincott Williams & Wilkins.

Kramer, P., & Hinojosa, J. (Eds.). (2010). *Frames of reference for pediatric occupational therapy* (3rd ed.). Baltimore: Lippincott Williams & Wilkins.

Leubben, A., Kramer, P., & Hinojosa, J. (2010). Domain of concern of occupational therapy: Relevance to pediatric practice. In P. Kramer & J. Hinojosa (Eds.), *Frames of reference for pediatric occupational therapy* (3rd ed., pp. 31–49). Baltimore: Lippincott Williams & Wilkins.

Moyers Cleveland, P. A., & Hinojosa, J. (2010). Continuing competence and competency. In K. Jacobs & G. L. McCormack (Eds.), *The occupational therapy manager* (5th ed., pp. 485–501). Bethesda, MD: AOTA Press.

Wang, T., Hinojosa, J., & Kramer, P. (2010). Applying the evidence-based practice approach. In P. Kramer & J. Hinojosa (Eds.), *Frames of reference for pediatric occupational therapy* (3rd ed., pp. 582–591). Baltimore: Lippincott Williams & Wilkins.

Blount, M. L. B., Blount, W., & Hinojosa, J. (2009). Perspectives. In J. Hinojosa, & M. L. Blount (Eds.), *The texture of life* (3rd., pp. 21–48). Bethesda, MD: AOTA Press.

Blount, M. L., Hinojosa, J., & Kramer, P. (2009). Preparing for the future: How activities relate to human occupation. In J. Hinojosa, & Blount (Eds.). *The texture of life* (3rd ed., pp. 523–546). Bethesda, MD: AOTA Press.

Cohen Podvey, M., & Hinojosa, J. (2009) Transition from early intervention to preschool services: An example of family-centered care. *Journal of Occupational Therapy, Schools, and Early Intervention, 2,* 73–83.

Hinojosa, J., & Blount, M. L. (2009). Occupation, purposeful activities, and occupational therapy. In J. Hinojosa & M. L. Blount (Eds.), *The texture of life* (3rd ed., pp. 1–19). Bethesda, MD: AOTA Press.

Hinojosa, J., & Blount, M. L. (Eds.). (2009). *The texture of life: Purposeful activities in occupational therapy* (3rd ed.). Bethesda, MD: AOTA Press.

Hinojosa, J., & Cleveland-Moyers, P. (2009). Perspectives on advance practice from occupational therapy. *Topics in Clinical Nutrition, 24*(3), 200–205.

Kramer, P., & Hinojosa, J. (2009). Activity synthesis as a means to occupation. In J. Hinojosa & M. L. Blount (Eds.), *The texture of life* (3rd ed., pp. 165–190). Bethesda, MD: AOTA Press.

Bose, P., & Hinojosa, J. (2008). Reported experiences of occupational therapists on interacting with teachers in inclusive early childhood classrooms. *American Journal of Occupational Therapy, 62*(3), 289–297.

Hinojosa, J. (2008). Foreword. In B. J. Hemphill-Pearson (Eds.), *Assessments in occupational therapy mental health: An integrative approach* (3rd ed., pp. xvii–xviii). Thorofare, NJ: Slack.

Hinojosa, J., & Kramer, P. (2008). Integrating children with disabilities into family play. In D. L. Parham & L. S. Fazio (Ed.), *Play in occupational therapy for children* (2nd ed., pp. 321–334). St. Louis, MO: Mosby/Year Book

Roston, K. L., Hinojosa, J., & Kaplan, H. (2008). Using the Minnesota Handwriting Assessment and Handwriting Checklist in screening first and second graders' handwriting legibility. *Journal of Occupational Therapy, Schools, and Early Intervention, 1*(1), 100–115.

Gutman, S. A., Mortera, M., Hinojosa, J., & Kramer, P. (2007). The Issue Is—Revision of the *Occupational Therapy Practice Framework*. *American Journal of Occupational Therapy, 61,* 119–126.

Hinojosa, J. (2007). Becoming innovators in an era of hyperchange (2007 Eleanor Clarke Slagle Lecture). *American Journal of Occupational Therapy, 61*(6), 629–637.

Howe, T., Sheu, C., Holzman, I. R., Hinojosa, J., & Lin, J. (2007). Multiple factors related to bottle-feeding performance in preterm infants. *Nursing Research, 56*(5), 307–311.

Hinojosa, J. (2006). Professional development planning: Establishing clarity, focus, meaning, and relevance to client outcomes. *OT Practice, 11*(11), 7–8.

Kramer, P., & Hinojosa J. (2006). The need for academic doctorates in occupational therapy. *Philippine Journal of Occupational Therapy. 2*(1/2), 62–64.

Segal, R., & Hinojosa, J. (2006). The activity setting of homework: An analysis of three cases and implications for occupational therapy. *American Journal of Occupational Therapy, 60,* 50–59.

Cohen, M. E., Hinojosa, J., & Kramer, P. (2005). Administration of evaluation and assessment. In. J. Hinojosa, P. Kramer, & P. Crist, (Eds.), *Occupational therapy evaluation: Obtaining and interpreting data* (2nd ed., pp. 81–99). Bethesda, MD: AOTA Press.

Hinojosa, J., Kramer, P., & Crist, P. (Eds.). (2005). *Evaluation: Obtaining and interpreting data* (2nd ed.). Bethesda, MD: AOTA Press.

Hinojosa, J., Kramer, P., & Crist, P. (2005). Evaluation: Where do we begin. In. J. Hinojosa, P. Kramer, & P. Crist, (Eds.), *Evaluation: Obtaining and interpreting data* (2nd ed., pp. 1–17). Bethesda, MD: AOTA Press.

Kramer, P., & Hinojosa, J. (2005). Philosophical and theoretical influences on evaluation. In. J. Hinojosa, P. Kramer, & P. Crist, (Eds.), *Evaluation: Obtaining and interpreting data* (2nd ed., pp. 19–36). Bethesda, MD: AOTA Press.

Segal, R., Hinojosa, J., Addonizio, C., Borisoff, D., Inderwies, L., & Lee, J. (2005). Homework strategies for a child with attention deficit hyperactivity disorder. *OT Practice, 10*(7), 9–12.

Dooley, N. R., & Hinojosa, J. (2004). Improving quality of life for people with Alzheimer's disease and their family caregivers: Brief occupational therapy intervention. *American Journal of Occupational Therapy, 58,* 561–569.

Blount, M. L. B., Blount, W., & Hinojosa, J. (2004). Perspectives. In J. Hinojosa & M. L. Blount (Eds.), *The texture of life* (2nd ed., pp. 17–38). Bethesda, MD: AOTA Press.

Blount, M. L., Chen, S., & Hinojosa, J. (2004). Preparing for the future: How activities relate to human occupation. In J. Hinojosa & M. L. Blount (Eds.), *The texture of life* (2nd ed., pp. 460–481). Bethesda, MD: AOTA Press.

Goverover, Y., & Hinojosa, J. (2004). Interrater reliability and discriminant validity of the Deductive Reasoning Test. *American Journal of Occupational Therapy, 58,* 104–108.

Hinojosa, J. (2004). AOTA Standards for Continuing Competence: Proposed revision. *OT Practice. 9*(22), 12–13.

Hinojosa, J. (2004). Developing personal professional competencies. *OT Practice. 9*(1), 7–8.

Hinojosa, J., & Blount, M. L. (2004). Purposeful activities within the context of occupational therapy. In J. Hinojosa & M. L. Blount (Eds.), *The texture of life* (2nd ed., pp. 1–16). Bethesda, MD: AOTA Press.

Hinojosa, J., & Blount, M. L. (Eds.). (2004). *The texture of life: Purposeful activities in occupational therapy* (2nd ed.). Bethesda, MD: AOTA Press.

Hinojosa, J., & Foto, M. (2004, December). Occupational therapy documentation for reimbursement. *Sensory integration Special Interest Section Quarterly, 27,* 1–3.

Kramer, P., & Hinojosa, J. (2004). Activity synthesis as a means to occupation. In J. Hinojosa & M. L. Blount (Eds.), *The texture of life* (2nd ed., pp. 136–158). Bethesda, MD: AOTA Press.

Weinstock-Zlotnick, G., & Hinojosa, J. (2004). The Issue Is—Bottom-up or top-down evaluation: Is one better then the other? *American Journal of Occupational Therapy,58,* 594–599.

Hinojosa, J. (2003). Developing a professional developing plan. *OT Practice, 8*(1), 7–8.

Hinojosa, J. (2003). Occupation and continuing competence—Part I. *OT Practice, 8*(12), 9–10.

Hinojosa, J. (2003). Occupation and continuing competence—Part II. *OT Practice, 8*(14), 11–12.

Hinojosa, J. (2003). [Review of *Infants and Young Children*]. *American Journal of Occupational Therapy, 57*(5), 599.

Hinojosa, J. (2003). The Issue Is—Therapist or scientist? How do these roles differ? *American Journal of Occupational Therapy, 57,* 225–226.

Hinojosa, J., Bedell, G., & Kaplan, M. (2003). Children with HIV/AIDS and their families. In E. B. Crepeau, E. Cohn, & B. Schell (Eds.), *Willard and Spackman's occupational therapy* (10th ed., pp. 725–729). Philadelphia: Lippincott Williams & Wilkins.

Hinojosa, J., Kramer, P., Royeen, C. B., & Luebben, A. (2003). The core concept of occupation. In P. Kramer, J. Hinojosa, & C. B. Royeen (Eds.), *Perspectives in human occupation: Participation in life* (pp. 1–17). Philadelphia: Lippincott Williams & Wilkins.

Hinojosa, J., & Poole, S. (2003). Modalities and domain of concern. In D. M. Bailey & S. L. Schwartzberg (Eds.), *Ethical and legal dilemmas in occupational therapy* (2nd ed., pp. 98–111). Philadelphia: F. A. Davis.

Kramer, P., Hinojosa, J., & Royeen, C. (Eds.). (2003). *Perspectives in human occupation: Participation in life.* Philadelphia: Lippincott Williams & Wilkins.

Kramer, P., Luebben, A., Royeen, C. B., & Hinojosa, J. (2003). Reaffirming the importance of occupation. In P. Kramer, J. Hinojosa, & C. B. Royeen (Eds.) *Perspective in human occupation: Participation in life* (pp. 312–216). Philadelphia: Lippincott Williams & Wilkins.

Moyers, P., & Hinojosa, J. (2003). Continuing competence and competency. In G. McCormack, E. Jaffe, & M. Goodman-Lavey (Eds.), *The occupational therapy manager* (4th ed., pp. 463–487). Bethesda, MD: AOTA Press.

Goverover, Y., & Hinojosa, J. (2002). Categorization and deductive reasoning: Can they serve as predictors of instrumental activities of daily living performance in adults with brain injury? *American Journal of Occupational Therapy, 56,* 509–516.

Goverover, Y., & Hinojosa, J. (2002). *Functional status based on categorization and deductive reasoning of individuals with brain injuries* [CD-ROM]. 13th World Congress of Occupational Therapists, School of Health Sciences, Occupational Therapy Programme, Jonkoping University, Sweden.

Goverover, Y., & Hinojosa, J. (2002). *Inter-rater reliability and discriminate validity of the Deductive Reasoning Test (DR)* [CD-ROM]. 13th World Congress of Occupational Therapists, School of Health Sciences, Occupational Therapy Programme, Jonkoping University, Sweden.

Hinojosa, J. (2002). [Review of *Best Practice in Occupational Therapy: Community Service for Children and Families*]. *American Journal of Occupational Therapy, 56,* 477–478.

Hinojosa, J., & Sproat, C. (2002). *Shifts in parent–therapist relationships: Twelve years of change* [CD-ROM]. 13th World Congress of Occupational Therapists, School of Health Sciences, Occupational Therapy Programme, Jonkoping University, Sweden.

Hinojosa, J., Sproat, C., Mankhetwit, S., & Anderson, J. (2002). Shifts in parent–therapist partnerships: Twelve years of change. *American Journal of Occupational Therapy, 56,* 556–563.

Kramer, P., & Hinojosa, J. (2002). *Frames of reference in the age of occupation* [CD-ROM]. 13th World Congress of Occupational Therapists, School of Health Sciences, Occupational Therapy Programme, Jonkoping University, Sweden.

Moyers, P., & Hinojosa, J. (2002, December). Assuring continuing competence in the practice of work programs. *Work Programs Special Interest Section Quarterly, 16*(4), 1–4.

Fertel-Daly, D., Bedell, G., & Hinojosa, J. (2001). Effects of a weighted vest on attention to task and self-stimulatory behaviors in preschoolers with pervasive developmental disorders. *American Journal of Occupational Therapy, 55,* 629–640.

Hinojosa, J., Bedell, G., Buchholz, E. S., Charles, J., Shigaki, I. S., & Bicchieri, S. M. (2001). Team collaboration: A case study of an early intervention team. *Qualitative Health Research, 11,* 206–220.

Blount, M. L, Kramer, P., & Hinojosa, J. (2000). Preparing for activity in the future. In J. Hinojosa & M. L. Blount (Eds.), *The texture of life: Purposeful activities in occupational therapy* (pp. 420–432). Bethesda, MD: American Occupational Therapy Association.

Cardona, M. D. P., Martinez, A. L., & Hinojosa, J. (2000). Effectiveness of using a computer to improve attention to visual analysis activities of five preschool children with disabilities. *Occupational Therapy International, 7,* 42–56.

Elenko, B. K., Hinojosa, J., Blount, M. L., & Blount W. (2000). Perspectives. In J. Hinojosa & M. L. Blount (Eds.), *The texture of life: Purposeful activities in occupational therapy* (pp. 16–34). Bethesda, MD: American Occupational Therapy Association.

Hinojosa, J., & Blount. M. L. (2000). Purposeful activities within the context of occupational therapy. In J. Hinojosa & M. L. Blount (Eds.), *The texture of life: Purposeful activities in occupational therapy* (pp. 1–5). Bethesda, MD: American Occupational Therapy Association.

Hinojosa, J., & Blount, M. L. (Eds.). (2000). *The texture of life: Purposeful activities in occupational therapy*. Bethesda, MD: American Occupational Therapy Association.

Hinojosa, J., Bowen, R., Case-Smith, J., Epstein, C. F., Moyers, P., & Schwope, C. (2000). Self-initiated continuing competence [Self-study]. *OT Practice, 5*(24), CE1–CE8.

Hinojosa, J., Bowen, R., Case-Smith, J., Epstein, C. F., Moyers, P., & Schwope, C. (2000). Standards for continuing competence for occupational therapy practitioners [Self-study]. *OT Practice, 5*(7), CE1–CE8.

Kramer, P., & Hinojosa, J. (2000). Activity synthesis. In J. Hinojosa & M. L. Blount (Eds.), *The texture of life: Purposeful activities in occupational therapy* (pp. 91–105). Bethesda, MD: American Occupational Therapy Association.

Dirette, D., & Hinojosa, J. (1999). The effects of a compensatory intervention on processing deficits of adults with acquired brain injuries. *Occupational Therapy Journal of Research, 19,* 223–240.

Dirette, D. K., Hinojosa, J., & Carnevale, G. J. (1999). Comparison of remedial and compensatory intervention for adults with acquired brain injuries. *Journal of Brain Injury Research, 14,* 595–601.

Hinojosa, J., & Kramer, P. (1999). Developmental perspective: Fundamentals of developmental theories. In P. Kramer & J. Hinojosa (Eds.), *Frames of reference for pediatric occupational therapy* (2nd ed., pp. 3–8). Baltimore: Lippincott Williams & Wilkins.

Hinojosa, J., & Kramer, P. (1999). Frames of reference in the real world. In P. Kramer & J. Hinojosa (Eds.), *Frames of reference for pediatric occupational therapy* (2nd ed., pp. 519–532). Baltimore: Lippincott Williams & Wilkins.

Kramer, P., & Hinojosa, J. (1999). Domain of concern of occupational therapy: Relevance to pediatric practice. In P. Kramer & J. Hinojosa (Eds.), *Frames of reference for pediatric occupational therapy* (2nd ed., pp. 9–26). Baltimore: Lippincott Williams & Wilkins.

Kramer, P., & Hinojosa, J. (Eds.). (1999). *Frames of reference for pediatric occupational therapy* (2nd ed.). Baltimore: Williams & Wilkins.

Kramer, P., & Hinojosa, J. (1999). Structure of the frame of reference. In P. Kramer & J. Hinojosa (Eds.), *Frames of reference for pediatric occupational therapy* (2nd ed., pp. 83–118). Baltimore: Lippincott Williams & Wilkins.

Luebben A. J., Hinojosa, J., & Kramer, P. (1999). Legitimate tools of pediatric occupational therapy. In P. Kramer & J. Hinojosa (Eds.), *Frames of reference for pediatric occupational therapy* (2nd ed., pp. 27–40). Baltimore: Lippincott Williams & Wilkins.

Muhlenhaupt, M., Hinojosa, J., & Kramer, P. (1999). Perspective of context as related to frame of reference. In P. Kramer & J. Hinojosa (Eds.), *Frames of reference for pediatric occupational therapy* (2nd ed., pp. 41–66). Baltimore: Lippincott Williams & Wilkins.

Hinojosa, J. (1998, March 19). NBCOT lacks requisite authority [Letter to the Editor]. *OT Week,* p. 48.

Hinojosa, J., Bedell, G., & Kaplan, M. (1998). In M. E. Neistadt & E. B. Crepeau (Eds.), *Willard and Spackman's occupational therapy* (9th ed., pp. 618–621). Philadelphia: J. B. Lippincott/Raven.

Hinojosa, J., & Blount, M. L. (1998). National Speaking—Professional competence. *American Journal of Occupational Therapy, 52,* 699–701.

Hinojosa, J., & Kramer, P. (1998). Evaluation—Where do we begin? In J. Hinojosa & P. Kramer (Eds.), *Evaluation: Obtaining and interpreting data* (pp. 1–15). Bethesda, MD: American Occupational Therapy Association.

Hinojosa, J., & Kramer, P. (Eds.). (1998). *Evaluation: Obtaining and interpreting data.* Bethesda, MD: American Occupational Therapy Association.

Kramer, P., & Hinojosa, J. (1998). Theoretical basis of evaluation. In J. Hinojosa & P. Kramer (Eds.), *Evaluation: Obtaining and interpreting data* (pp. 17–28). Bethesda, MD: American Occupational Therapy Association.

Hinojosa, J., & Kramer, P. (1997). Continuum of services. In *Occupational therapy services for children and youth under the Individual with Disabilities Education Act.* Bethesda, MD: American Occupational Therapy Association.

Hinojosa, J., & Kramer, P. (1997). Integrating children with disabilities into family play. In D. L. Parham & L. S. Fazio (Ed.), *Play in occupational therapy for children* (pp. 159–170). St. Louis, MO: Mosby/Year Book.

Hinojosa, J. (1997, March 13). Who gave NBCOT their mandate? [Letter to the Editor]. *OT Week,* p. 60.

Hinojosa, J. (1997, February 6). Defining competency [Letter to the Editor]. *OT Week,* p. 64.

Hinojosa, J., Blount, M. L., & Labovitz, D. R. (1996). *AOTA: Asserting its responsibility to society.* Bethesda, MD: American Occupational Therapy Association.

Bell, P., & Hinojosa, J. (1996). Perception of the impact of assistive devices on daily life of three individuals with quadriplegia. *Assistive Technology, 7,* 87–94.

Hinojosa, J., Kramer, P., & Pratt, P. N. (1996). Theoretical foundations of practice: Developmental principles, theories, and frames of reference. In J. Case-Smith, A. Allen, & P. Pratt (Eds.), *Occupational therapy for children* (3rd ed., pp. 25–45). Baltimore: Mosby.

Moryosef-Ittah, S., & Hinojosa, J. (1996). Discriminant validity of the DTVP-2 for children with learning disabilities. *Occupational Therapy International, 3,* 204–211.

Hinojosa, J. (1996). Practice makes perfect. *OT Practice, 1,* 34–38.

Clerico, C., Hansen, R., Hinojosa, J., Mitchell, M., & Manoly, B. (1995, March 9). Occupational therapy and cross-training initiatives [White Paper]. *OT Week,* pp. 32–33.

Hinojosa, J., & Poole, S. (1995). Modalities and domain of concern. In D. M. Bailey & S. L. Schwartzberg (Eds.), *Ethical and legal dilemmas in occupational therapy* (pp. 95–111). Philadelphia: F. A. Davis.

Kramer, P., & Hinojosa, J. (1995). Epiphany of human occupation. In C. B. Royeen (Ed.), *Human occupation* (AOTA Self-Study Series, pp. 5–17). Bethesda, MD: American Occupational Therapy Association.

Shimelman, A., & Hinojosa, J. (1995). Gross motor activity and attention in three adults with brain injury. *American Journal of Occupational Therapy, 49,* 973–979.

Dirette, D., & Hinojosa, J. (1994). The effects of continuous passive motion on the edematous hands of two individuals with flaccid hemiplegia. *American Journal of Occupational Therapy, 48,* 403–409.

Hinojosa, J. (1994). The just-right challenge. *Work: A Journal of Prevention, Assessment, and Rehabilitation, 14,* 253–258.

Hinojosa, J., & Kramer, P. (1994). *Defining multiculturalism for occupational therapy* [Summary]. 11th International Congress of the World Federation of Occupational Therapists.

Hinojosa, J., Moore, D. S., Sabari, J., & Doctor, R. G. (1994). Competency-based training program in early intervention. *American Journal of Occupational Therapy, 48*, 361–366.

Kramer, P., & Hinojosa, J. (1994). Frames of reference: Blueprints for practice [Summary]. 11th International Congress of the World Federation of Occupational Therapists.

Hinojosa, J., & Kramer, P. (1993). Defining multiculturalism for occupational therapy. *Education Special Interest Section Newsletter, 2*(4), 1.

Hinojosa, J., & Kramer, P. (1993). Developmental perspective: Fundamentals of developmental theories. In P. Kramer & J. Hinojosa (Eds.), *Frames of reference for pediatric occupational therapy* (pp. 3–8). Baltimore: Williams & Wilkins.

Hinojosa, J., & Kramer, P. (1993). From frames of reference to actual intervention. In P. Kramer & J. Hinojosa (Eds.), *Frames of reference for pediatric occupational therapy* (pp. 439–447). Baltimore: Williams & Wilkins.

Hinojosa, J., & Kramer, P. (1993). Influence of the human context on the application of frames of reference. In P. Kramer & J. Hinojosa (Eds.), *Frames of reference for pediatric occupational therapy* (pp. 475–482). Baltimore: Williams & Wilkins.

Hinojosa, J., & Kramer, P. (1993). Legitimate tools of pediatric occupational therapy. In P. Kramer & J. Hinojosa (Eds.), *Frames of reference for pediatric occupational therapy* (pp. 25–33). Baltimore: Williams & Wilkins.

Kramer, P., & Hinojosa, J. (1993). Alternative applications of frames of reference. In P. Kramer & J. Hinojosa (Eds.), *Frames of reference for pediatric occupational therapy* (pp. 447–454). Baltimore: Williams & Wilkins.

Kramer, P., & Hinojosa, J. (1993). Domain of concern of occupational therapy relevant to pediatric practice. In P. Kramer & J. Hinojosa (Eds.), *Frames of reference for pediatric occupational therapy* (pp. 9–24). Baltimore: Williams & Wilkins.

Kramer, P., & Hinojosa, J. (Eds.). (1993). *Frames of reference for pediatric occupational therapy.* Baltimore: Williams & Wilkins.

Kramer, P., & Hinojosa, J. (1993). Structure of frames of reference. In P. Kramer & J. Hinojosa (Eds.), *Frames of reference for pediatric occupational therapy* (pp. 37–48). Baltimore: Williams & Wilkins.

Abreu, B. C., & Hinojosa, J. (1992). Process approach for cognitive–perceptual and postural control dysfunction for adults with brain injury. In N. Katz (Ed.), *Cognitive rehabilitation: Models for intervention in occupational therapy* (pp. 167–194). Stoneham, MA: Andover Press.

Hansen, R., Hinojosa, J., Schroeder, C., & Sands, M. (1992). *Advanced practice review: A preliminary examination of the practice of experienced occupational therapist registered and certified occupational therapy assistants.* Rockville, MD: American Occupational Therapy Association.

Hinojosa, J. (1992). Be prepared. *Healthcare Trends and Transitions, 3*, 34–35.

Hinojosa, J. (1992). Using case management to improve services to children. In C. B. Royeen (Ed.), *School-based practice for related services* [AOTA Self-Study Series]. Rockville, MD: American Occupational Therapy Association.

Hinojosa, J., & Anderson, J. (1991). Home programs for preschool children with cerebral palsy: Mothers' perceptions. *American Journal of Occupational Therapy, 45*, 273–279.

Anderson, J., Hinojosa, J., Bedell, G., & Kaplan, M. T. (1990). Occupational therapy for children with perinatal HIV infection. *American Journal of Occupational Therapy, 44*, 249–255.

Hinojosa, J. (1990). How mothers of preschool children with cerebral palsy perceive occupational and physical therapists and their influence on family life. *Occupational Therapy Journal of Research, 10*, 144–162.

Hinojosa, J., & Anderson, J. (1990). *Occupational therapy: Early intervention preservice training program.* Brooklyn: SUNY Health Science Center.

Hinojosa, J. (1988). MultiMate Advantage II, version 4.0. In J. V. Seidel, R. Kjolseth, & E. Seymour (Eds.), *The ethnograph* (pp. A6–A8). Littleton, CO: Qualis Research.

Hinojosa, J. (1988). *Procedures for the review of therapy services regarding the use of neurodevelopmental treatment techniques.* Van Nuys: Blue Cross of California.

Hinojosa, J., Anderson, J., & Ranum, G. W. (1988). Relationships between therapists and parents of preschool children with cerebral palsy: A survey. *Occupational Therapy Journal of Research, 8*, 285–297.

Hinojosa, J., Anderson, J., & Strauch, C. (1988). Pediatric occupational therapy in the home. *American Journal of Occupational Therapy, 42*, 17–22.

Hinojosa, J. (1987). [Review of *Occupational Therapy for Children*]. *American Journal of Occupational Therapy, 41*.

Anderson, J., Hinojosa, J., & Strauch, C. (1987). Integrating play in neurodevelopmental therapy (NDT). *American Journal of Occupational Therapy, 41*, 421–426.

Hinojosa, J., & Anderson, J. (1987). Brief—Working relationships between therapists and parents of children with cerebral palsy: A survey of attitudes. *Occupational Therapy Journal of Research, 7*, 123–126.

Hinojosa, J. (1985). Defining sensory integration—Current terminology [Letter to the Editor]. *Occupational Therapy Journal of Research, 5*(1), 74.

Hinojosa, J. (1985). Implications for occupational therapy of a competency-based orientation. *American Journal of Occupational Therapy, 39*, 539–541.

Hinojosa, J., & Scott, A. (1985). Meeting educators' needs. *Education Bulletin, Occupational Therapy Newspaper, 39*(10)

Anderson, J., & Hinojosa, J. (1984). Parents in a professional partnership. *American Journal of Occupational Therapy, 38*, 451–461.

Hinojosa, J. (1984). *Procedures for the review of therapy services regarding sensory integrative dysfunction.* Van Nuys: Blue Cross of California.

Hinojosa, J., Cohen, L., & Kramer, P. (1984). Development and implementation of a non-traditional Fieldwork II administrative experience. *Education Bulletin, Occupational Therapy Newspaper, 38*(10).

Hinojosa, J., & Anderson, J. (1983). Living skills: Teaching learning units. *Education Bulletin, Occupational Therapy Newspaper, 37*(10).

Hinojosa, J., Anderson, J., Becker-Lewin, M., & Goldstein, P. K. (1982). Occupational therapy for sensory integrative dysfunction. *American Journal of Occupational Therapy, 36*, 831–832.

Hinojosa, J., Anderson, J., Becker-Lewin, M., & Goldstein, P. K. (1982). The roles and functions of the occupational therapist in the treatment of sensory integrative dysfunction. *American Journal of Occupational Therapy, 36*, 832–834.

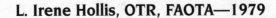

L. Irene Hollis, OTR, FAOTA—1979

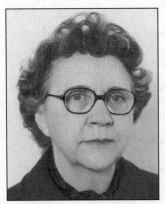

Irene Hollis, an accomplished occupational therapy practitioner, presented her Eleanor Clarke Slagle Lecture after dedicating 35 years to the treatment of individuals with physical disabilities.

Among her accomplishments are threading looms for the U.S. Army in 1944, training under Margaret Rood at the University of Southern California, conducting occupational therapy services at centers for amputees in Texas, and working at various hospitals in the physical disability unit.

In 1947, before the use of antibiotics, she began working with burns. Hollis also developed a cerebral palsy treatment unit for dependents of the armed forces personnel. In 1952, she worked with patients with polio, and after the polio vaccine came out, she treated hand patients. After a year of treating hand patients, she received a position with AOTA as a field consultant in physical disabilities. After fulfilling her duties at AOTA, she traveled to Switzerland, where she spent time mending and sewing clothing for a cerebral palsy treatment center.

On returning from Europe, she settled in North Carolina as a hand therapist and practiced there for 15 years. In 1979, Hollis used her Eleanor Clarke Slagle Lecture to explain her career as an occupational therapist, reminding all that many of the problems we have today are the same ones we had as when she was a consultant. In reflection on the numerous jobs she held, she stated, "With our broad basic preparation in occupational therapy, if, in the drama of our professional lives, the casting director should put us in one particular role or another, we can perform adequately!" She reminded us that the flexibility of our broad humanistic base enables us to build peaks of professional excellence or specialization. Specialties in occupational therapy are nothing more than special arrangements of things that are already familiar to us. The therapist's special competence must be combined with compassion at all times!

Hollis calls for continuing education, whether it be reading extensively, attending workshops and courses, or communicating with others personally. This must be an active ongoing process. Every single day one should give oneself a chance to be a good occupational therapist—the very best! In wrapping up her speech, Hollis stated, "All I did was to do the common things uncommonly well." Occupational therapy is commonplace and unsophisticated often, but we should take pride in this when we bring out desired results and more sophisticated modalities have failed.

Bibliography

Sniderman, M., & Hollis, L. I. (1954). The use of self-curing acrylic in the making of a mouthpiece to aid the upper extremity paralytic patient. *American Journal of Occupational Therapy, 8*, 115–116.

Robinson, R. A., Fish, M., Kilburn, V. T., & Hollis, I. (1958). Nationally Speaking: From the national executive director: From the director of education: From the field consultant. *American Journal of Occupational Therapy, 12*, 180–183.

Willard, H. S., Kilburn, V. T., & Hollis, L. I. (1959). Nationally Speaking: From the president: From the director of education: From Puerto Rico Conference. *American Journal of Occupational Therapy, 13*, 173–175.

Hollis, L. I. (1961). Nationally Speaking: Reports from the White House Conference on Aging. *American Journal of Occupational Therapy, 15*, 164–169, 176.

Hollis, L. I. (1963). Five-year summary report: Field consultant in rehabilitation of the physically disabled. *American Journal of Occupational Therapy, 17*, 128–130.

Hollis, L. I. (1967). Splint substitutes. *American Journal of Occupational Therapy, 21*, 139–145.

Hollis, L. I., & Harrison, E. (1970). An improved surface electrode for monitoring myopotentials. *American Journal of Occupational Therapy, 24*, 28–30.

Hollis, L. I. (1974). Skinnerian occupational therapy. *American Journal of Occupational Therapy, 28*, 208–213.

Hollis, L. I. (1979). Remember? (1979 Eleanor Clarke Slagle Lecture). *American Journal of Occupational Therapy, 33*, 493–499.

Hollis, L. I. (1986, December). Identifying occupational therapy: The use of purposeful activities. *Physical Disabilities Special Interest Section Newsletter, 9*(4), 2–3.

Hollis, L. I., & Hollis E. J. (1995, March 9). Teaching what you know. *OT Week, 9*(10), 18–19.

Margo B. Holm, PhD, OTR/L, FAOTA, ABDA—2000

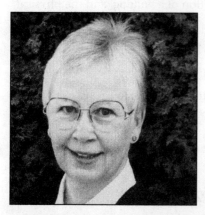

Margo Holm earned a bachelor of science at the University of Minnesota in 1968 and in 1977 completed a master's degree at Pacific Lutheran University in Tacoma, Washington. She earned a doctor of philosophy at the University of Nebraska–Lincoln in 1980 and completed post-doctoral fellowships at the Woodrow Wilson Foundation at Princeton, New Jersey, as well as the University of Pittsburgh.

Holm first worked as a staff occupational therapist at the University Hospital in Minneapolis, Minnesota, in 1968 and later at the Day Hospital Program at the Minneapolis VAMC in 1969. She became the field supervisor for a Mobilization of Resources Grant until 1971, then was employed as a staff therapist with the United Hospitals in St. Paul. She continued as a senior staff therapist with the Golden Valley Health Center until 1975.

Holm's career in academia began at the University of Puget Sound, spanning from 1975 through 1987. During this period, she also consulted with the Colonial Institute of Newport News, Virginia, and conducted institutional research as a Woodrow Wilson Postdoctoral Fellow at the Hampton Institute. From 1984 to 1992, she was the program director in the Department of Occupational Therapy at the University of Puget Sound and was promoted to full professor in 1987. She continued to teach at the University of Puget Sound until 1996. From 1990 through 1997, she also was an adjunct assistant professor with the School of Medicine, Department of Psychiatry, at the University of Pittsburgh. In addition, from 1996 to 1999, she was a professor in occupational therapy, Division of Health Sciences, with the College Misericordia in Dallas, Pennsylvania.

Holm is currently professor with the School of Health and Rehabilitation Sciences at the University of Pittsburgh. She is an occupational therapist with the Pittsburgh VAMC, focusing on geriatric research, education, and clinical care. She also is a professor emeritus at the University of Puget Sound.

Holm's awards include the Academy of Research, American Occupational Therapy Foundation, 2001; the 1999 Eleanor Clarke Slagle Lectureship Award, awarded for exemplary contributions to occupational therapy research and education; Diplomate, American Board of Disability Analysts, 1998; Distinguished Professorship, University of Puget Sound, 1992–1997; Post-Doctoral Fellowship in Rehabilitation Research, University of Pittsburgh School of Medicine, Department of Psychiatry, 1988–1990; Burlington–Northern Foundation Outstanding Faculty Award, University of Puget Sound, 1987; Roster of Fellows of the American Occupational Therapy Association, 1987; Phi Kappa Phi Honor Society, 1987; John Lantz Senior Faculty Fellowship, 1986; and Woodrow Wilson Post-Doctoral Fellowship, 1980–1981.

On a Personal Note:*

Wilma West characterized Eleanor Clarke Slagle as "a very strong woman with very definite opinions about many things." Everyone who knew her said she could be very forceful, which as it evolved, benefited the profession and the association greatly. Similarly, everyone who knows Dr. Holm knows that this description could apply to her as well.

Margo Holm's credentials for encouraging the profession to practice differently includes her excellence in teaching and learning, research achievements, and excellence in advocacy. Unlike most scholars in occupational therapy who have achieved prominence by devising conceptual models to guide practice, Holm took the "road less traveled" by focusing on testing existing models. Early in her research career she recognized that the proliferation of conceptual models would fail to advance the science of occupational therapy unless there was a simultaneous effort to test scientifically their usefulness for patient care.

Despite her considerable scholarship and research achievements, Holm is humble in that she is most proud of the students that she advised on research projects who have become published authors and of the junior faculty that she has "mentored to publication." The following accolade is from the College of Misericordia Occupational Therapy Class

*Based on an introduction graciously provided by Joan Rogers at Holm's Eleanor Clarke Slagle Lecture.

at its January 2000 commencement. They aptly described Margo Holm as having demonstrated "the patience of a saint, the compassion of Mother Theresa, the integrity of Elliot Ness, the determination of a bulldog, and the physical resilience of a long-distance runner."

Bibliography

Christianson, M. A., Mills, T., & Holm, M. B. (n.d.). *Responses of the public to residential universal design features.* Available online at http://www.lifease.com/lifease-universaldesign-responses.html

Shih, M.-M., Rogers, J. C., Skidmore, E. R., Irrgang, J. J., & Holm, M. B. (2009). Measuring stroke survivors' functional status independence: Five perspectives. *American Journal of Occupational Therapy, 64,* 600–608.

Rogers, J. C., & Holm, M. B. (2008). The occupational therapy process. In E. B. Crepeau, E. S. Cohn & B. A. B. Schell (Eds.), *Willard and Spackman's occupational therapy* (11th ed., pp. 47–50). Philadelphia: Lippincott Williams & Wilkins.

Tomycz, N. D., Holm, M. B., Horowitz, M. B., Wechsler, L. R., Raina, K., Gupta R., et al. (2008). Extensive brainstem ischemia on neuroimaging does not preclude meaningful recovery from locked-in syndrome: Two cases of endovascularly managed basilar thrombosis. *Journal of Neuroimaging, 18,* 1–3.

Brininger, T. L., Rogers, J. C., Holm, M. B., Baker, N. A., Li, Z.-M., & Goitz, R. J. (2007). Efficacy of a fabricated customized splint and tendon and nerve-gliding exercises for the treatment of carpal tunnel syndrome: A randomized controlled trial. *Archives of Physical Medicine and Rehabilitation, 88,* 1429–1435.

Crane, B. A., Holm, M. B., Hobson, D., Cooper, R. A., & Reed, M. P. (2007). A dynamic seating intervention for wheelchair seating discomfort. *American Journal of Physical Medicine and Rehabilitation, 12,* 988–993.

Crane, B., Holm, M. B., Hobson, D., Cooper, R. A., & Reed, M. P. (2007). Responsiveness of the TAWC tool for assessing wheelchair discomfort. *Disability and Rehabilitation: Assistive Technology, 2*(2), 97–103.

Gildengers, A. G., Butters, M. A., Chisholm, D., Rogers, J. C., Holm, M. B., Bhalla, R. K., et al. (2007). Cognitive functioning and instrumental activities of daily living in late-life bipolar disorder. *American Journal of Geriatric Psychiatry, 15*(2), 174–179.

Mills, T. L., Holm, M. B., & Schmeler, M. (2007). Test–retest reliability and cross-validation of the functioning everyday with a wheelchair instrument. *Assistive Technology, 19*(2), 61–77.

Raina, K. D., Rogers, J. C., & Holm, M. B. (2007). Influence of the environment on activity performance in older women with heart failure. *Disability and Rehabilitation, 29*(7), 545–557.

Skidmore, E. R., Rogers, J. C., Chandler, L. S., Jovin, T. G., & Holm, M. B. (2007). A precise method for linking neuroanatomy to function after stroke: A pilot study. *Topics in Stroke Rehabilitation, 14*(5), 12–17.

Breland, H. L., Rogers, J. C., Holm, M. B., & Starz, T. W. (2006). Triggers of fibromyalgia (FM) flares in subgroups with fibromyalgia: A mixed-methods study. *Arthritis and Rheumatism, 54*(9), S503.

Skidmore, E. R., Rogers, J. C., Chandler, L. S., & Holm, M. B. (2006). Developing empirical models to enhance stroke rehabilitation. *Disability and Rehabilitation, 28*(16), 1027–1034.

Skidmore, E. R., Rogers, J. C., Chandler, L. S., & Holm, M. B. (2006). Dynamic interactions between impairment and activity after stroke: Examining the utility of decision analysis methods. *Clinical Rehabilitation, 20*(6), 523–535.

Crane, B. A., Holm, M. B., Hobson, D., Cooper, R. A., Reed, M. P., & Stadelmeier, S. (2005). Test–retest reliability, internal item consistency, and concurrent validity of the Wheelchair Seating Discomfort Assessment Tool. *Assistive Technology, 17*(2), 98–107.

Gildengers, A. G., Butters, M. A., Chisholm, D., Holm, M. B., Rogers, J. C., Bhalla, R. K., et al. (2005). Cognitive functioning and IADLs in older adults with bipolar disorder. *Bipolar Disorders, 7,* 59.

Raina, K., Callaway, C., Rittenberger, J., & Holm, M. (2005). Neurological and functional status following cardiac arrest: Method and tool utility. *Resuscitation, 79*(2), 249–256.

Rogers, J. C., Holm, M. B., Breland, H. L., Johnson, B. D., Shih, M. M., & Starz, T. W. (2005). Subjective and objective parameters of fibromyalgia (FM). *Arthritis and Rheumatism, 52*(9), S415.

Rogers, J. C., Holm, M. B., Johnson, B. D., Breland, H. L., Shih, M. M., & Starz, T. W. (2005). Meds, METs, and fibromyalgia. *Arthritis and Rheumatism, 52*(9), S436.

Crane, B., Holm, M. B., Hobson, D., Cooper, R. A., Reed, M., & Stadelmeier, S. (2004). Development of a consumer-driven Wheelchair Seating Discomfort Assessment Tool (WcS–DAT). *International Journal of Rehabilitation Research, 27,* 85–90.

Desai, K., Rogers, J. C., Skidmore, E. R., & Holm, M. B. (2004). Use of the Mini-mitter Actiwatch–64 to identify functional use of the affected and unaffected upper extremities poststroke. *Circulation, 109*(20), E238.

Gwinn, S. M. G., Rogers, J. C., Starz, T. W., Vogt, M. T., & Holm, M. B. (2004). Understanding pain and functioning in knee osteoarthritis (KOA): How do patient and rheumatologist's ratings compare? *Arthritis and Rheumatism, 50*(9), S79.

Holm, M. B., Rogers, J. C., Breland, H. L., Johnson, D., & Starz, T. (2004). Understanding nocturnal pain medication dynamics in fibromyalgia. *Arthritis and Rheumatism, 50*(9), S473.

Rogers, J. C., Desai, K., Jovin, T., & Holm, M. B. (2004). Cross-sectional performance-based functional outcomes of patients receiving and not receiving IV tPA. *Circulation, 109*(20), E238.

Finlayson, M., Havens, B., Holm, M. B., & Van Denend, T. (2003). Integrating a performance-based observation measure of functional status into a population-based longitudinal study of aging. *Canadian Journal on Aging, 22,* 185–195.

Holm, M. B. (2003, February 10). Top 10 reasons for becoming an evidence-based practitioner. *OT Practice, 8*(3), 9–11.

Holm, M. B., Rogers, J. C., & James, A. (2003). Interventions for activities of daily living. In E. B. Crepeau, E. S. Cohn, & B. A. B. Schell (Eds.), *Willard and Spackman's occupational therapy* (10th ed., pp. 491–533). Philadelphia: Lippincott Williams & Wilkins.

Holm, M. B., Rogers, J. C., & Stone, R. G. (2003). Person–task–environment interventions: A decision-making guide. In E. B. Crepeau, E. S. Cohn, & B. A. B. Schell (Eds.), *Willard and Spackman's occupational therapy* (10th ed., pp. 460–490). Philadelphia: Lippincott Williams & Wilkins.

Lenze, E., Holm, M. B., Rogers, J. C., & Reynolds, C. F. (2003). Combining pharmacotherapy and psychotherapy in the rehabilitative and maintenance treatment of late-life depression. *Directions in Psychiatry, 23*, 43–54.

Rogers, J. C., & Holm, M. B. (2003). Evaluation of activities of daily living (ADL) and instrumental activities of daily living (IADL). In E. B. Crepeau, E. S. Cohn, & B. A. B. Schell (Eds.), *Willard and Spackman's occupational therapy* (10th ed., pp. 315–339). Philadelphia: Lippincott Williams & Wilkins.

Rogers, J. C., Holm, M. B., Beach, S., Schulz, R., Cipriani, J., Fox, A., et al. (2003). Concordance of four methods of disability assessment using performance in the home as the criterion method. *Arthritis and Rheumatism, 49*, 640–647.

Holm, M. B., & Rogers, J. C. (2002). Preventing functional disability: Change your MODE of operation! *Aging Upbeat, 3*(3), 1–2.

Mills, T., Holm, M. B., Schmeler, M., Trefler, E., Fitzgerald, S., Boninger, M., et al. (2002). Cross-validation of the Functional Evaluation in a Wheelchair (FEW) instrument with consumer goals. In *Proceedings of the 8th International Seating Symposium* (pp. 237–241). British Columbia, Canada.

Mills, T., Holm, M. B., Schmeler, M., Trefler, E., Fitzgerald, S., Boninger, M., et al. (2002). The Functional Evaluation in a Wheelchair (FEW) instrument: Test–retest reliability and cross-validation with consumer goals. In *Proceedings of the Rehabilitation Engineering and Assistive Technology Society of North America 25th International Conference* (pp. 245–247).

Mills, T., Holm, M. B., Trefler, E., Schmeler, M., Fitzgerald, S., & Boninger, M. (2002). Development and consumer validation of the Functional Evaluation in a Wheelchair (FEW) instrument. *Disability and Rehabilitation, 24*(1–3), 38–46.

Rogers, J. C., Holm, M. B., & Perkins, L. (2002). The trajectory of assistive device usage and user and non-user characteristics: Long-handled bath sponge. *Arthritis Care and Research, 47*, 645–650.

Banford, M., Kratz, M., Brown, R., Emick, K., Ranck, J., Wilkins, R., & Holm, M. B. (2001). Stroke survivor caregiver education: Methods and effectiveness. *Physical and Occupational Therapy in Geriatrics, 19*(1), 37–52.

Basante, J., Bentz, E., Heck-Hackley, J., Kenion, B., Young, B., & Holm, M. B. (2001). Falls risk among older adults in long-term care facilities: A focused literature review. *Physical and Occupational Therapy in Geriatrics, 16*(2), 63–85.

Brandthill, S., Duczeminski, J., Surak, E., Erdly, A., Bayer, S., & Holm, M. B. (2001). Coping strategies that elicit psychological well-being and happiness among older Catholic nuns with physical impairments and disabilities. *Physical and Occupational Therapy in Geriatrics, 16*(2), 87–98.

Holm, M. B. (2001). Authorship contribution declaration. In E. B. Crepeau (Ed.), *Research across the curriculum: A guide for occupational therapy educators* (pp. 125–130). Bethesda, MD: American Occupational Therapy Foundation.

Holm, M. B. (2001). Our mandate for the new millennium: Evidence-based practice. *OT Practice, 6*(12), CE1–CE16.

Kirchner, G., Stone, R. G., & Holm, M. B. (2001). Validation of the fieldwork evaluation for the occupational therapist. *Occupational Therapy in Health Care, 14*(1), 39–46.

Mills, T., Holm, M. B., & Christianson, M. (2001). Public opinion of universal design in housing. In *Proceedings of the Rehabilitation Engineering and Assistive Technology Society of North America 24th International Conference* (pp. 112–114).

Mills, T., Holm, M. B., Trefler, E., Schmeler, M., Fitzgerald, S., & Boninger, M. (2001). Development of an outcome measure tool for wheelchair seating and mobility interventions: A work in progress. In *Proceedings of the Rehabilitation Engineering and Assistive Technology Society of North America 24th International Conference* (pp. 245–247).

Porter, J., Franklin, T., Pieninck, M., Springer, C., & Holm, M, B. (2001). Quality of follow-through with feeding interventions for long-term care facility residents. *Physical and Occupational Therapy in Geriatrics, 19*(1), 77–90.

Rogers, J. C., Gwinn, S., & Holm, M. B. (2001). Comparing activities of daily living assessment instruments: FIM,' MDS, OASIS, MDS–PAC. *Physical and Occupational Therapy in Geriatrics, 18*(3), 1–25.

Rogers, J. C., & Holm, M. B. (2001). Behavioral rehabilitative activities of daily living intervention. *Alzheimer's Care Quarterly, 2*(4), 66–69.

Rogers, J. C., Holm, M. B., Beach, S., Schulz, R., & Starz, T. (2001). Task independence, safety, and adequacy among nondisabled and OAK-disabled older women. *Arthritis Care and Research, 45*, 410–418.

Cipriani, J., Hess, S., Higgins, H., Resavy, D., Sheon, S., Szychowski, M., & Holm, M. B. (2000). Collaboration in the therapeutic process: Older adults' perspectives. *Physical and Occupational Therapy in Geriatrics, 17*(1), 43–54.

George, K., DiJiacomo, R., Neely-Aurandt, J., Dworak, P., & Holm, M. B. (2000). Patterns of referral and intervention for persons with AIDS. *Occupational Therapy in Health Care, 13*(2), 25–39.

Harkleroad, A., Schirf, D., Volpe, J., & Holm, M. B. (2000). Critical pathway development: An integrative literature review. *American Journal of Occupational Therapy, 54*, 148–154.

Holm, M. B. (2000). Our mandate for the new millennium: Evidence-based practice (2000 Eleanor Clarke Slagle Lecture). *American Journal of Occupational Therapy, 54*, 575–585.

Holm, M. B., Santangelo, M. A., Fromuth, D. J., Brown, S. O., & Walter H. (2000). Effectiveness of everyday occupations for changing client behaviors in a community living arrangement. *American Journal of Occupational Therapy, 54*, 361–371.

Kirchner, G., Stone, R. G., & Holm, M. B. (2000). Use of admission criteria to predict performance of students in an entry-level master's program on fieldwork placements and in academic courses. *Occupational Therapy in Health Care, 13*(1), 1–11.

McAndrew, E., McDermott, S., Vitzakovich, S., Warunek, M., & Holm, M. B. (2000). Therapists and patient perceptions of the occupational therapy goal setting process: A pilot study. *Physical and Occupational Therapy in Geriatrics, 17*(1), 55–63.

Rogers, J. C., & Holm, M. B. (2000). Daily living skills and habits of older women with depression. *Occupational Therapy Journal of Research, 20*(Suppl.), 68S–85S.

Rogers, J. C., Holm, M. B., Burgio, L. D., Hsu, C., Hardin, J. M., & McDowell, B. J. (2000). Excess disability during morning care in nursing home residents with dementia. *International Psychogeriatrics, 12*(2), 267–282.

Holm, M. B., & Rogers, J. C. (1999). Functional assessment: The Performance Assessment of Self-Care Skills (PASS). In B. J. Hemphill (Ed.), *Assessments in occupational therapy mental health: An integrative approach* (pp. 117–124). Thorofare, NJ: Slack.

Holm, M. B., Rogers, J. C., Burgio, L. D., Hardin, J. M., Hsu, C., & McDowell, B. J. (1999). Observational data collection using computer and manual methods: Which informs best? *Topics in Health Information Management, 19*, 15–25.

Mayhan, Y. D., Holm, M. B., & Fawcett, L. (Eds.), & National Commission on Continued Competency in Occupational Therapy. (1999). *Continued competency in occupational therapy: Recommendations to the profession and key stakeholders*. Gaithersburg, MD: National Board for Certification in Occupational Therapy.

Rogers, J. C., & Holm, M. B. (1999). Role Change Assessment: An interview tool for older adults. In B. Hemphill-Pearson (Ed.), *Assessments in occupational therapy mental health* (2nd ed., pp. 73–86). Thorofare, NJ: Slack.

Rogers, J. C., Holm, M. B., Burgio, L. D., Granieri, E., Hsu, C., Hardin, J. M., et al. (1999). Improving morning care routines of nursing home residents with dementia. *Journal of the American Geriatrics Society, 47*, 1049–1057.

Holm, M. B., & Mayhan, Y. D. (1998). How can we measure clinical competency? *Advance for Occupational Therapy Practitioners, 14*(32), 7.

Holm, M. B., & Mayhan, Y. D. (1998). When does competency need to be tested? *Advance for Occupational Therapy Practitioners, 14*(38), 7.

Holm, M. B., & Rogers, J. C. (1998). Assessment and rehabilitation of adult brain function: The focus of occupational therapy research. In G. Goldstein & S. R. Beers (Eds.), *Handbook of human brain function: Assessment and rehabilitation* (pp. 9–31). New York: Plenum.

Holm, M. B., Rogers, J. C., & Kwoh, C. K. (1998). Predictors of functional disability in patients with rheumatoid arthritis. *Arthritis Care and Research, 11*, 346–355.

Nakamura, M., Holm, M. B., & Wilson, A. (1998). Measures of balance and fear of falling in the elderly. *Physical and Occupational Therapy in Geriatrics, 15*(4), 17–32.

Rogers, J. C., & Holm, M. B. (1998). Assessment and rehabilitation of adult brain function: The focus of geriatric research. In G. Goldstein & S. R. Beers (Eds.), *Handbook of human brain function: Assessment and rehabilitation* (pp. 89–109). New York: Plenum.

Glauner, J., Ekes, A., James, A., & Holm, M. B. (1997). A pilot study of the theoretical and technical competence and appropriate education for the use of nine physical agent modalities in occupational therapy practice. *American Journal of Occupational Therapy, 51*, 767–774.

Holm, M. B., Rogers, J. C., & James, A. (1997). Treatment of activities of daily living. In M. E. Neistadt & E. B. Crepeau (Eds.), *Willard and Spackman's occupational therapy* (9th ed., pp. 323–364). Philadelphia: Lippincott.

Holm, M. B., Rogers, J. C., & Stone, R. G. (1997). Person–task–environment interventions: A decision-making guide. In M. E. Neistadt & E. B. Crepeau (Eds.), *Willard and Spackman's occupational therapy* (9th ed., pp. 471–498). Philadelphia: Lippincott.

Holm, M. B., Rogers, J. C., & Stone, R. G. (1997). Referral, evaluation and intervention in home health. In M. J. Youngstrom & M. Steinhauer (Eds.), *Occupational therapy in home health: Preparing for best practice* (pp. 136–157). Bethesda, MD: American Occupational Therapy Association.

Kirchner, G., & Holm, M. B. (1997). Prediction of academic and clinical performance of occupational therapy students in an entry-level master's program. *American Journal of Occupational Therapy, 51*, 775–779.

Nuismer, B., Ekes, A., & Holm, M. B. (1997). The use of low-load prolonged stretch devices in rehabilitation programs in the pacific northwest. *American Journal of Occupational Therapy, 51*, 538–543.

Rogers, J. C., & Holm, M. B. (1997). Diagnostic reasoning: The process of problem identification. In C. H. Christiansen & C. M. Baum (Eds.), *Occupational therapy: Achieving human performance needs in daily living* (2nd ed., pp. 136–156). Thorofare, NJ: Slack.

Rogers, J. C., & Holm, M. B. (1997). Evaluation of activities of daily living (ADL) and home management. In M. E. Neistadt & E. B. Crepeau (Eds.), *Willard and Spackman's occupational therapy* (9th ed., pp. 185–208). Philadelphia: Lippincott.

Rogers, J. C., & Holm, M. B. (1997). Occupational therapy in the home. *Home Healthcare Consultant, 4*(4), 15–33.

Rogers, J. C., Holm, M. B., & Stone, R. G. (1997). Evaluation of daily living tasks: The home care advantage. *American Journal of Occupational Therapy, 51*, 410–422.

Rogers, J. C., & Holm, M. B. (1996). Performance Assessment of Self-Care Skills (PASS). In I. E. Asher (Ed.), *An annotated index of occupational therapy evaluation tools* (2nd ed.). Bethesda, MD: American Occupational Therapy Association.

Tomlin, G., Holm, M. B., Rogers, J. C., & Kwoh, C. K. (1996). Comparison of standard and alternative HAQ scoring procedures for documenting functional outcomes in patients with rheumatoid arthritis. *Journal of Rheumatology, 23*, 1524–1530.

Williams, A., Agho, A. O., & Holm, M. B. (1996). Perceptions of computer literacy among occupational therapy students. *American Journal of Occupational Therapy, 50*, 217–222.

Atwood, S., Holm, M. B., & James, A. (1994). Activities of daily living capabilities and values of long-term care facility residents. *American Journal of Occupational Therapy, 48*, 710–716.

Brodie, J., Holm, M. B., & Tomlin, G. (1994). Cerebrovascular accident: Relationship of demographic, diagnostic, and occupational therapy antecedents to rehabilitation outcomes. *American Journal of Occupational Therapy, 48*, 906–913.

Casby, J., & Holm, M. B. (1994). The effect of music on repetitive disruptive vocalizations of persons with dementia. *American Journal of Occupational Therapy, 48*, 883–889.

Furth, H., Holm, M. B., & James, A. (1994). Reinjury prevention follow-through for clients with cumulative trauma disorders. *American Journal of Occupational Therapy, 48*, 890–898.

Holm, M. B. (1994, June 15). *Current and needed research in occupational therapy*. Bethesda, MD: Agency for Health Care Policy and Research.

Kirchner, G., Holm, M. B., Ekes, A., & Williams, R. (1994). Predictors of success in an entry-level master in physical therapy program. *Journal of Physical Therapy Education, 8*, 76–79.

Rogers, J. C., & Holm, M. B. (1994). Assessment of self-care. In B. Bonder & M. B. Wagner (Eds.), *Functional performance in older adults* (pp. 181–202), Philadelphia: F. A. Davis.

Rogers, J. C., & Holm, M. B. (1994). Nationally Speaking—Accepting the challenge of outcome research: Examining the effectiveness of occupational therapy practice. *American Journal of Occupational Therapy, 48*, 871–876.

Rogers, J. C., Holm, M. B., Goldstein, G., & Nussbaum, P. D. (1994). Stability and change in functional assessment of patients with geropsychiatric disorders. *American Journal of Occupational Therapy, 48*, 914–918.

Carlson, J., & Holm, M. B. (1993). Effectiveness of occupational therapy for reducing restraint use in a psychiatric setting. *American Journal of Occupational Therapy, 47*, 885–889.

Holm, M. B., Manoly, B., & Tomlin, G. (1993). American Occupational Therapy Association Accreditation Committee reliability study. *American Journal of Occupational Therapy, 47,* 561–567.

Settle, C., & Holm, M. B. (1993). Program planning: The clinical utility of three activities of daily living assessment tools. *American Journal of Occupational Therapy, 47,* 911–918.

Rogers, J. C., Hill, D. J., Holm, M. B., & Wasser, T. (1992). Educational level and professional activities of occupational therapists. *Occupational Therapy Journal of Research, 12,* 148–158.

Rogers, J. C., & Holm, M. B. (1992). Assistive technology device use in patients with rheumatic disease. *American Journal of Occupational Therapy, 46,* 120–127.

Holm, M. B. (1991). Guest editor's introduction. *International Journal of Technology and Aging, 4,* 87–88.

Holm, M. B., & Rogers, J. C. (1991). High, low, or no assistive technology devices for older adults undergoing rehabilitation? *International Journal of Technology and Aging, 4,* 153–162.

Rogers, J. C., & Holm, M. B. (1991). Occupational therapy diagnostic reasoning: A component of clinical reasoning. *American Journal of Occupational Therapy, 45,* 1045–1053.

Rogers, J. C., & Holm, M. B. (1991). Task performance of older adults and low assistive technology devices. *International Journal of Technology and Aging, 4,* 93–106.

Rogers, J. C., & Holm, M. B. (1991). Teaching older persons with depression: Educational issues. *Topics in Geriatric Rehabilitation, 6*(3), 27–44.

Holm, M. B. (1990). Allied health research priorities for medical treatment effectiveness studies. In *Conference Proceedings of the Agency for Health Care Policy and Research Allied Health Medical Treatment Effectiveness Program Research Issues Conference.* Bethesda, MD: Agency for Health Care Policy and Research.

Holm, M. B. (1989). *Adapting new electronic technologies to serve the frail elderly living at home* [Communications and Society Forum Report 10]. Truro, MA: Aspen Institute.

Holm, M. B., & Heires, G. (1989). Northwest Therapy, Inc.: A model program. In L. Ogden-Niemeyer & K. Jacobs (Eds.), *Work hardening: State of the art* (pp. 357–372). Thorofare, NJ: Slack.

Holm, M. B., & Mizoguchi, J. (1989). Professional services for the injured: A model program. In L. Ogden-Niemeyer & K. Jacobs (Eds.), *Work hardening: State of the art* (pp. 336–356). Thorofare, NJ: Slack.

Holm, M. B., & Rogers, J. C. (1989). The therapist's thinking behind functional assessment. In C. Royeen (Ed.), *Assessment of function: An action guide* (pp. 1–36). Rockville, MD: American Occupational Therapy Association.

Iwasaki, K., & Holm, M. B. (1989). Sensory treatment for the reduction of stereotypic behaviors in persons with severe multiple disabilities. *Occupational Therapy Journal of Research, 9*(3), 1–14.

Holm, M. B. (1986). External funding and the grant proposal writing process. *Administration and Management Newsletter, 2*(1), 1, 7.

Holm, M. B. (1986). Frames of reference: Guides for action—Occupational therapist. In H. Schmid (Ed.), *Project for independent living in occupational therapy (PILOT)* (pp. 69–78). Rockville, MD: American Occupational Therapy Association.

Holm, M. B. (1986). Frames of reference: Guides for action—Occupational therapy assistant. In H. Schmid (Ed.), *Project for independent living in occupational therapy (PILOT)* (pp. 79–85). Rockville, MD: American Occupational Therapy Association.

Holm, M. B. (1986). *A "hands on" introduction to microcomputers as therapeutic, administrative, and research tools in occupational therapy.* Tacoma, WA: University of Puget Sound.

Holm, M. B., LaVesser, P., & Shealey, S. (1986). Implementing programs for adolescents and young adults with severe disabling conditions. In H. Schmid (Ed.), *Project for independent living in occupational therapy (PILOT)* (pp. 125–144). Rockville, MD: American Occupational Therapy Association.

Holm, M. B. (1983, Fall). Student selection for practice of the profession. *OT Education Bulletin,* pp. 14–16.

Holm, M. B. (1983). Video as a medium in occupational therapy. *American Journal of Occupational Therapy, 37,* 531–534.

Holm, M. B. (1980). The pragmatics of extracurricular activities: Planning, organizing, and evaluating. *Extracurricular Education: Policies, Pragmatics, Legal Issues, 7,* 11–14.

Holm, M. B. (1969). The open-ended task group in psychiatry. *AOTA Bulletin on Practice, 4*(6), 1.

Joy Huss, MS, OTR, RPT, FAOTA—1976

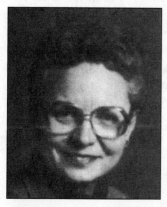

Joy Huss was an associate professor, Occupational Therapy Program, at the University of Minnesota, Minneapolis. A graduate of Whittier College with a degree in sociology, Huss holds a certificate in occupational therapy from the University of Southern California, a certificate in physical therapy from the University of Michigan, and a master of science degree in educational psychology from Butler University.

Huss served as staff occupational therapist at Crippled Children's Hospital School, Sioux Falls, South Dakota, and at the Cerebral Palsy Clinic at Indiana University. She was an occupational therapy and physical therapy consultant for Crippled Children's Services, Indiana; supervisor of occupational therapy at Riley Children's Hospital, Indiana. She was on the occupational therapy faculties at Indiana University, at the University of Wisconsin–Eau Claire, and at the University of Minnesota, as well as on the honorary occupational therapy faculty at the University of St. Catherine in St. Paul, Minnesota.

Huss conducted many workshops on a neurophysiological approach to central nervous system dysfunction throughout the United States and Canada. Her awards include Fellow of the American Occupational Therapy Association; Mentor, Occupational Therapy Class of 1983 at the University of Texas Medical Branch; Who's Who of American Women; and World's Who's Who of Women.

Linking Key Messages of the 1976 Eleanor Clarke Slagle Lecture to the AOTA *Centennial Vision:* This lecture addressed the need for understanding and use of therapeutic touch/tactile inputs and its effects on therapist–client interactions. This understanding also is important in daily life at work and in the community at large.

Although progress has been made in many areas, the need is still there and always will be, as we are humans of diverse cultures and needs. Hopefully, practitioners will continue to recognize this by continuing to back it up with "science-driven and evidence-based practice" as stipulated in the *Centennial Vision* statement (AOTA, 2007). It still needs to be addressed at all levels of education and cultural contexts.

—*Joy Huss*

Reference

American Occupational Therapy Association. (2007). AOTA's *Centennial Vision* and executive summary. *American Journal of Occupational Therapy, 61,* 613–614.

Bibliography

Dunn, W., & Huss, A. J. (1992). Personal perspectives on career development: Interviews with occupational therapy leaders. *OT Practice, 3*(3), 1–6.

Huss, A. J. (1984). Whither thou goest? *American Journal of Occupational Therapy, 35,* 574–580.

Huss, A. J. (1983). Basis for sensorimotor approaches—Neuroanatomy and neurophysiology. Overview of sensorimotor approaches. In H. Smith & H. Hopkins (Eds.), *Willard and Spackman's occupational therapy* (6th ed.). Philadelphia: Lippincott.

Huss, A. J. (1981). From kinesiology to adaptation. *American Journal of Occupational Therapy, 35,* 574–580.

Huss, A. J. (1978). Neuroanatomy and neurophysiology and sensorimotor approaches. In H. Smith & H. Hopkins (Eds.), *Willard and Spackman's occupational therapy* (5th ed.). Philadelphia: Lippincott.

Huss, A. J. (1977). Touch with care or a caring touch? (1976 Eleanor Clarke Slagle Lecture). *American Journal of Occupational Therapy, 31,* 11–18.

Farber S., & Huss, A. J. (1974). *Sensorimotor evaluation and treatment procedures for allied health personnel* (2nd ed.). Indianapolis: Indiana University Foundation.

Huss, A. J. (1971). Sensorimotor treatment approaches. In H. Willard & C. Spackman (Eds.), *Occupational therapy* (4th ed.). Philadelphia: Lippincott.

Huss, A. J. (1971). An introduction to treatment techniques developed by Margaret Rood. In S. Perlmutter (Ed.), *Neuroanatomy and neurophysiology underlying current treatment techniques for sensorimotor dysfunction.* Chicago: University of Illinois Press.

Huss, A. J. (1969). Clinical application of sensorimotor treatment techniques in physical dysfunction, and clinical aspects of controversy and confusions in physical dysfunction treatment techniques. In L. Zamir (Ed.), *Expanding dimensions in rehabilitation: A guide for therapists, counselors, and rehabilitation specialists.* Springfield, IL: Charles C Thomas.

Huss, A. J. (1965). Application of Rood techniques to the treatment of the cerebral palsied. In W. West (Ed.), *Occupational Therapy for the multiply handicapped child.* Chicago: University of Illinois Press.

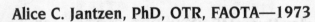

Alice C. Jantzen, PhD, OTR, FAOTA—1973

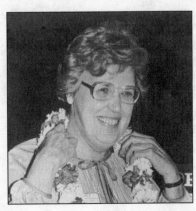

During her 31 years as an occupational therapist, Alice C. Jantzen had a distinguished career in health care, both as a practitioner and as an educator. She began her occupational therapy career in 1952 as a staff therapist in the Cerebral Palsy Department of New York State Rehabilitation Hospital; her career in education came 2 years later with an assistant professorship at Western Michigan University.

In 1956, Jantzen became a National Foundation Teaching Fellow and founded the Department of Occupational Therapy at the University of Florida in 1958; she served as its chair for 18 years. The department became the first of its kind in southeastern United States. She was committed to occupational therapy education, practice, and research until she retired in 1978.

Jantzen served on many AOTA committees and as vice-president; she also was the first president of the American Occupational Therapy Foundation and vice-president and president of the Florida Occupational Therapy Association. Her honors include AOTA's Roster of Fellows and Award of Merit and listings in Who's Who in America, Who's Who of American Women, and Leaders in American Science.

Jantzen graduated with honors from Wellesley College and Boston School of Occupational Therapy, where she received her certificate. She received a master's degree in education from the University of Pennsylvania and a doctorate in counseling psychology from Boston College. She died in October 1983.

Bibliography

Miller, A. S., Steward, M. D., Murphy, M. A., & Jantzen, A. C. (1955). An evaluation method for cerebral palsy. *American Journal of Occupational Therapy, 11*, 105–111.

Jantzen, A. C. (1958). Proposed revision of the education of occupational therapists. *American Journal of Occupational Therapy, 12*, 314–321, 329.

Jantzen, A. C. (1960). The contribution of occupational therapy to patient care. *Journal of the Florida Medical Association, 46*, 1360–1362.

Jantzen, A. C. (1962). Some strengths of occupational therapy. *American Journal of Occupational Therapy, 16*, 124–126.

Jantzen, A. C. (1963). Some strengths of occupational therapy. *Canadian Journal of Occupational Therapy, 30*, 64–66.

Jantzen, A. C., Pershing, R., Bates, E., Booth, M., Burns, C., Hoffman, C., et al. (1964). Graduate degrees held by occupational therapists, March 1962. *American Journal of Occupational Therapy, 18*, 152–157

Anderson, H. E., & Jantzen, A. C. (1965). A prediction of clinical performance. *American Journal of Occupational Therapy, 19*, 76–78.

Anderson, H. E., Jantzen, A. C., Shelton, M. J., & Dunteman, G. H. (1965). The effects of response sets in questionnaire studies. *American Journal of Occupational Therapy, 19*, 348–350.

Jantzen, A. C., & Anderson, H. E. (1965). Patient evaluation of occupational therapy programs. *American Journal of Occupational Therapy, 19*, 19–22.

Jantzen, A. C., & Yerxa, E. J. (1966). *The clinical experience.* New York: American Occupational Therapy Association.

Jantzen, A. C. (1967). Theses and dissertations: 1963–1966. *American Journal of Occupational Therapy, 21*, 166–170.

Bailey, J. P., Jantzen, A. C., & Dunteman, G. H. (1969). Relative effectiveness of personality, achievement, and interest measures in the predication of a performance criterion. *American Journal of Occupational Therapy, 23*, 27–29.

Jantzen, A. C. (1969). Definitions of mental health and mental illness. *American Journal of Occupational Therapy, 23*, 249–253.

Jantzen, A. C. (1971). *Some characteristics of female occupational therapists.* Boston: Boston University.

Jantzen, A. C. (1972). Some characteristics of female occupational therapists, 1970, Part 1: Descriptive study. *American Journal of Occupational Therapy, 26*, 19–26.

Jantzen, A. C. (1972). Some characteristics of female occupational therapists, 1970, Part 2: Employment patterns. *American Journal of Occupational Therapy, 26*, 67–77.

Jantzen, A. C. (1972). Some characteristics of female occupational therapists, 1970, Part 3: A comparison: Faculty and clinical practitioners. *American Journal of Occupational Therapy, 26*, 150–154.

Jantzen, A. C. (1973). Some characteristics of male occupational therapists, 1970. *American Journal of Occupational Therapy, 27*, 388–391.

Jantzen, A. C. (1974). Academic occupational therapy: A career specialty (1973 Eleanor Clarke Slagle Lecture). *American Journal of Occupational Therapy, 28*, 73–81.

Jantzen, A. C., Aanderson, R. L., & Sieg, K. W. (1975). *The occupational therapist as consultant to community agencies: Proceedings from consultation in the community: A conference for occupational therapists.* Gainesville: University of Florida.

Jantzen, A. C. (1977). A proposal for occupational therapy education. *American Journal of Occupational Therapy, 31*, 660–662.

Jantzen, A. C. (1981). *Research: The practical approach for occupational therapy.* Laurel, MD: RAMSCO.

Jerry A. Johnson, MBA, EdD, OTR, FAOTA—1972

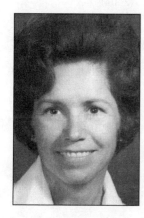

Jerry A. Johnson is a graduate of Texas Woman's University with a BS in occupational therapy. She has an MBA from Harvard University and a doctoral degree in educational administration from Boston University.

Johnson was founder, professor, and director of the Department of Occupational Therapy at Boston University, where she also served as chairman of the Graduate Division and then as associate dean for academic affairs. Later, she served as director of graduate education and research in the Occupational Therapy Department at Colorado State University. In 1976, she assumed the chairmanship and also served as professor in occupational therapy at Washington University in St. Louis until 1982, when she moved to Colorado. There she was president and director of the Resource Center for Health and Well-Being, Inc.

Johnson served as AOTA president from 1973 to 1978. Her awards include serving as visiting professor at Queensland University, Brisbane, Australia, and the AOTA Award of Merit and Roster of Fellows. She also was named a Distinguished Alumna of Texas Women's University in 1984.

Bibliography

Johnson, J. A. (1965). Guest Editorial: The emerging role of occupational therapy in psychiatry. *American Journal of Occupational Therapy, 19,* 215–218.

Johnson, J. A., & Smith, M. (1966). Changing concepts of occupational therapy in a community rehabilitation center. *American Journal of Occupational Therapy, 20,* 267–273.

Johnson, J. A. (1968). Occupational therapy techniques applicable to the stroke patient in the rehabilitation center and general hospital. *Journal of Medical Science, 5,* 34–38.

Johnson, J. A. (1971). Consideration of work as therapy in the rehabilitation process. *American Journal of Occupational Therapy, 25,* 303–308.

Johnson, J. A. (1972). Report of the task force on social issues. *American Journal of Occupational Therapy, 26,* 332–359.

Johnson, J. A. (1973). Occupational therapy: A model for the future (1972 Eleanor Clarke Slagle Lecture). *American Journal of Occupational Therapy, 27,* 1–7.

Johnson, J. A. (1974). Allied health professions—Proliferation or restraint. *Israel Journal of Medical Science, 10,* 96–104.

Johnson, J. A. (1974). Annual review of occupational therapy education. *Annual Review of Allied Health Education.*

Johnson, J. A. (1975). Nationally Speaking: No more waiting. *American Journal of Occupational Therapy, 29,* 519–532.

Johnson, J. A. (1976). Nationally Speaking: Commitment to action. *American Journal of Occupational Therapy, 30,* 135–148.

Johnson, J. A. (1977). Challenges confronting occupational therapy. *Canadian Journal of Occupational Therapy, 44,* 113–117.

Johnson, J. A. (1977). Nationally Speaking: Humanitarianism and accountability: A challenge for occupational therapy in its 60th anniversary. *American Journal of Occupational Therapy, 31,* 631–637.

Johnson, J. A. (1977). Nationally Speaking: Mission alpha: A new beginning. *American Journal of Occupational Therapy, 31,* 143–149.

Johnson, J. A. (1978). Nationally Speaking: Issues in education. *American Journal of Occupational Therapy, 32,* 355–258.

Johnson, J. A. (1978). Nationally Speaking: Sixty years of progress: Questions for the future. *American Journal of Occupational Therapy, 34,* 209–213.

Johnson, J. A. (1979). Reorganization in relation to the issues. In *Occupational Therapy 2001 AD.* Rockville, MD: American Occupational Therapy Association.

Johnson, J. A. (1981). Old values—New directions: Competence, adaptation, integration. *American Journal of Occupational Therapy, 35,* 589–598.

Johnson, J. A. (1982). Commentary: Application of role and role conflict theory to administration in occupational therapy education. *Occupational Therapy Journal of Research, 2,* 39–41.

Johnson, J. A. (1984). Occupational therapy and the patient in pain. *Occupational Therapy in Health Care, 1*(3), 1–27.

Johnson, J. A. (1985). Wellness: Its myths, realities, and potential for occupational therapy. *Occupational Therapy in Health Care, 2,* 117–138.

Johnson, J. A. (1986). *New dimensions in wellness: A context for living.* Thorofare, NJ: Slack.

Johnson, J. A. (1986). Wellness and occupational therapy. *American Journal of Occupational Therapy, 40,* 753–758.

Johnson, J. A. (Ed.). (1988). *Certified occupational therapy assistants: Opportunities and challenges.* New York: Haworth Press.

Johnson, J. A. (1988). Certified occupational therapy assistants: Reflections on their thirtieth anniversary. *Occupational Therapy in Health Care, 5,* 213–220.

Johnson, J. A., & Ethridge, D. A. (Eds.). (1989). *Developmental disabilities: A handbook for occupational therapists.* New York: Haworth Press.

Johnson, J. A., & Jaffe, E. (Eds.). (1989). *Occupational therapy: Program development for health promotion and preventive services.* New York: Haworth Press.

Johnson, J. A., & Jaffe, E. (1989). Thoughts on leadership: An interview with Ruth Brunyate Wiemer and Wilma L. West. *Occupational Therapy in Health Care, 6*(1), 5–16.

Johnson, J. A., & Yerxa, E. (Eds.). (1989). *Occupational science: The foundation for new models of practice.* New York: Haworth Press.

Johnson, J. A. (1990). Introduction . . . the treatment of individuals with brain injuries. *Occupational Therapy in Health Care, 7*(1), 5–6.

Johnson, J. A. (1990). Productive living strategies for people with AIDS. *Occupational Therapy in Health Care, 7*(2/3/4), 1–2.

Johnson, J. A., & Krefting, L. (Eds.). (1990). *Occupational therapy approaches to traumatic brain injury.* New York: Haworth Press.

Johnson, J. A., & Pizzi, M. (Eds.). (1990). *Productive living strategies for people with AIDS.* New York: Harrington Park Press.

Jones, W. J., Johnson, J. A., Beasley, L. W., & Johnson, J. P. (1996). Allied health workforce shortages: The systemic barriers to response. *Journal of Allied Health, 25*(3), 219–232.

Johnson, J. A., & Schkade, J. K. (2001). Effects of an occupation-based intervention on mobility problems following a cerebral vascular accident. *Journal of Applied Anthropology, 20,* 91–110.

Lorna Jean King, OTR, FAOTA—1978

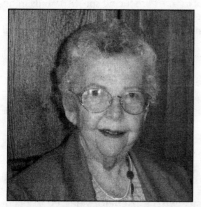

Lorna Jean King was born in Denver, Colorado, and was married to William Warren King. She completed a BS in occupational therapy from Milwaukee–Downer College in 1944. She also completed graduate studies at the University of Southern California (USC) in 1950 and at the University of Arizona in 1958.

King began her career in occupational therapy as an instructor in occupational therapy at USC from 1945 to 1947. She also worked as a staff therapist at the Brentwood Veteran's Administration Hospital in Los Angeles from 1947 to 1949. She worked with delinquent and emotionally disturbed adolescents as a staff therapist with the Downey School for Girls in California from 1949 to 1950. She moved to Arizona and became director of occupational therapy at the Square and Compass Crippled Children's Clinic in Tucson from 1950 to 1953.

From 1964 to 1966, King was employed as a staff therapist at the Arizona State Hospital in Phoenix and later became the director of rehabilitative therapies for Arizona State Hospital until 1974. She consulted for the Phoenix School Districts and the Community Foundation for Mental Health from 1974 to 1978. She was the founder and director of the Center for Neurodevelopmental Studies in Phoenix from 1978 to 1988 and 1990 to 1995. She became director and chief executive officer of the Children's Center for Neurodevelopmental Studies from 1995 to 1998. Since 1974, she has lectured in the United States and internationally, including in Canada, Australia, New Zealand, and South Africa.

King was inducted into the AOTA Roster of Fellows in 1973 and was awarded the Eleanor Clarke Slagle Lectureship in 1978. She died November 4, 2006 in Phoenix, AZ.

On a Personal Note From a Phone Interview: King reflected on writing her Eleanor Clarke Slagle Lecture and was concerned about the various directions the profession was heading. She wanted to bring focus to the profession and considered adaptation as a unifying theory. Interestingly, some wanted King to change the title of her lecture, saying the one she chose ("Toward a Science of Adaptive Responses") was too informal. The Eleanor Clarke Slagle Lectureship was the pinnacle of her career, and she was honored to receive a standing ovation from the audience in San Diego. King encourages therapists and students today to read her 1978 lecture, as she believes her message is still relevant and needed now.

Bibliography

King, L. J. (1974). A sensory integrative approach to schizophrenia. *American Journal of Occupational Therapy, 28,* 529–536.

King, L. J. (1978). *Object Manipulation Speed Test.* Phoenix, AZ: Center for Neurodevelopmental Studies.

King, L. J. (1978). *Theory and application of sensory integrative treatment for residents of long-term-care facilities with histories of chronic schizophrenia.* Phoenix, AZ: Greenroom Publications.

King, L. J. (1978). Toward a science of adaptive responses (1978 Eleanor Clarke Slagle Lecture). *American Journal of Occupational Therapy, 32,* 429–437.

King, L. J. (1980). Creative caring. *American Journal of Occupational Therapy, 34,* 522–528.

King, L. J. (1982). The person symbol as an assessment tool. In B. J. Hemphill (Ed.), *The evaluative process in psychiatric occupational therapy.* Thorofare, NJ: Slack.

King, L. J. (1983). Occupational therapy and neuropsychiatry. *Occupational Therapy in Mental Health, 3,* 1–14.

King, L. J. (1984, June). Current schizophrenia research: Implications for occupational therapy practice. *Mental Health Special Interest Section Newsletter, 7*(4), 1–2, 5.

King, L. J., Fowler R. H., & Snow, B. A. (1984, March). The use of dance in therapy. *Sensory Integration Special Interest Section Newsletter, 7*(2), 1–8.

King, L. J. (1987). A sensory integrative approach to the education of the autistic child. *Occupational Therapy in Health Care, 4,* 77–85.

Paracheck, J. F., & King, L. J. (1987). *Paracheck Geriatric Rating Scale and treatment manual* (3rd ed.). Phoenix, AZ: Center for Neuropdelevelopmental Studies.

Ray, T. C., King, L. J., & Grandin, T. (1988). The effectiveness of self-initiated vestibular stimulation in producing speech sounds in an autistic child. *Occupational Therapy Journal of Research, 8,* 186–190.

Cabay, M., & King, L. J. (1989, December). Sensory integration and perception: The foundation for concept formation. *Occupational Therapy Practice,* pp. 18–27.

King, L. J. (1990, September). Moving the body to change the mind: Sensory integration therapy in psychiatry. *Occupational Therapy Practice,* pp. 12–22.

King, L. J. (1991). Sensory integration: An effective approach to therapy and education. *Autism Research Review International, 5*(3), 6.

King, L. J. (1991). When the therapist encounters 'behavior' problems. *Occupational Therapy Forum, 4,* 3–5.

Cabay, M., King, L. J., & Wojten, C. (1999, March). The efficacy of sensory integration–based occupational therapy on conceptual development and academic readiness in preschoolers. *OT Practice,* pp. 55.

Lela A. Llorens, PhD, OTR, FAOTA—1969

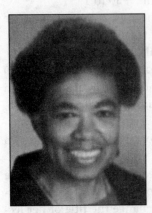

Lela Llorens is a graduate of Western Michigan University with a bachelor's degree in occupational therapy and holds a master's degree in vocational rehabilitation as well as an earned doctorate from Walden University. Llorens worked as a staff therapist at Wayne County General Hospital and at Northville State Hospital and as supervisor of occupational therapy services of Lafayette Clinic in Michigan (Denegan & Walker, 1993). During this period, she also served as instructor of the Department of Occupational Therapy at Wayne State University. She held a consultant position with the Comprehensive Child Care Project at Mount Zion Hospital in San Francisco. Llorens's academic career includes serving as professor, chair, and graduate coordinator at the University of Florida and San Jose State University in California. In 1990, she was appointed co-director of the Division of Health Professions in addition to her role as department chair. As a core faculty member of the Geriatric Education Center at Stanford University School of Medicine, she helped write and develop a clearinghouse for ethnogeriatric literature and curricula (Denegan & Walker, 1993). From 1993 to 1996, Llorens held the position of associate academic vice-president for faculty at San Jose State University. She is a professor emeritus at San Jose State and has consulted extensively for the U.S. Maternal and Child Health Services, demonstrating how occupational therapy can make a difference in community health. Since retiring in 1996, she has continued contributing to the field of occupational therapy as a guest lecturer and consultant to the department chair at the University of Southern California (USC). At USC, she participates in graduate seminars in occupational therapy and helps create a developmental cross-cultural therapy perspective.

Llorens has an impressive list of awards in her career. She was named to the Roster of Fellows of the American Occupational Therapy Association (AOTA) in 1973, received the Award of Excellence from the Florida Occupational Therapy Association (FOTA) in 1977, and received the AOTA Award of Merit in 1986 and a Service Award in 1989. The American Occupational Therapy Foundation has granted her the following awards: Certificate of Appreciation and Honorary Life Membership in 1981, A. Jean Ayres Award for research in 1988, and a Meritorious Service Award in 1989 (AOTF, n.d.). Other honors include the Sadie Philcox Lecture (1981) from the University of Queensland, Brisbane, Australia; Outstanding Young Woman of America in 1966; Outstanding Educators of America; Wall of Distinction, Western Michigan University; and Mentor, Class of 1976, University of Texas Medical Branch. She also has been honored as a visiting scholar at Western Michigan University in 1987; at Medical University of South Carolina in 1990; and at Wayne State University at Texas Women's University , and the University of Wisconsin–Madison in 1991. In 1991, she also received a Certificate of Merit from the Michigan State Senate and was invited to submit her written work for preservation in the Women's Collection at Texas Women's University (Denegan & Walker, 1993). Llorens was awarded the AOTA/AOTF Presidential Commendation in Honor of Wilma L. West in 1997. Currently, Western Michigan University has initiated the Lela Williams Llorens Scholarship to recognize outstanding student leadership and diversity.

Linking Key Messages of the 1969 Eleanor Clarke Slagle Lecture to the AOTA *Centennial Vision:* AOTA's *Centennial Vision* (AOTA, 2007) articulates the goal to ensure that occupational therapy's practice will enable people to improve their physical and mental health and to overcome obstacles to participation in activities that they value. In the paper "Facilitating Growth and Development: The Promise of Occupational Therapy" (Llorens, 1970), it was my intent to articulate an understanding of how occupational therapy could be utilized to affect individuals in the sensory, perceptual, cognitive, and environmental spheres of their development throughout their lifespan. While "growth and development" issues often are restricted to thinking in terms of children, it was my contention that occupational therapy had the potential to view our work as facilitating growth and development for adolescents, adults, and elders as well. The 10 premises presented in the lecture resonated with this idea.

This notion was further presented and discussed in a little book entitled *Application of a Developmental Theory for Health and Rehabilitation* (Llorens, 1976), last published by AOTA. In this book, the schematic that was presented in the original lecture was expanded to show how this concept could, in fact, be understood relative to the lifespan. Further discussion of the applicability of the "facilitating growth and development" theory was presented in several editions of *Occupational Therapy for Children* (Pratt, 1989) and in the first edition of *Occupational Therapy: Overcoming Human Performance Deficits* by Christiansen and Baum (1991). Most recently, LaCorte (2009) has published *New and Expanded Neuropsychosocial Concepts Complementary to Llorens' Developmental Theory*, in which she presents further applicable indications of the efficacy of concepts presented in the lecture. The promise continues.

—Lela Llorens

References and Resources

American Occupational Therapy Association. (2007). AOTA's *Centennial Vision* and executive summary. *American Journal of Occupational Therapy, 61*, 613–614.

American Occupational Therapy Foundation. (n.d.). Past award recipients. Last accessed September 28, 2010, at http://www.aotf.org/awardshonors/pastawardrecipients.aspx

Christiansen, C., & Baum, C. (1991). *Occupational therapy: Overcoming human performance deficits*. Thorofare, NJ: Slack.

Denegan, S., & Walker, K. (1993). Lela A. Llorens. In R. Miller & K. Walker (Eds.), *Perspectives on theory for the practice of occupational therapy*. Gaithersburg, MD: Aspen.

LaCorte, L. F. (2009). *New and expanded neuropsychosocial concepts complementary to Llorens' development theory*. London: Routledge/Taylor & Francis Group.

Llorens, L. A. (1970). Facilitating growth and development: The promise of occupational therapy. *American Journal of Occupational Therapy, 25*, 1–9.

Llorens, L. A. (1976). *Application of a developmental theory for health and rehabilitation*. Rockville, MD: American Occupational Therapy Association.

Pratt, P. N. (1989). *Occupational therapy for children*. St. Louis, MO: Mosby.

Stanford School of Medicine. (n.d.). *Welcome to the Stanford Geriatric Education Center*. Last accessed September 28, 2010, at http://www.stanford.edu/dept/medfm/fac.html

University of Southern California. (n.d.). *Faculty and research*. Last accessed September 28, 2010, at http://www.usc.edu/assets/ot/faculty/LelaLlorens.html

Bibliography

Llorens, L. A. (2009). Foreword. In L. F. LaCorte (Ed.), *New and expanded neuropsychosocial concepts complementary to Llorens' developmental theory* (pp. x–xii). London: Routledge/Taylor & Francis Group.

Llorens, L. A., Burton, G., & Still, J. R. (1999). Achieving occupational role: Accommodations for students with disabilities. *Occupational Therapy in Health Care, 11*(4), 1–8.

Llorens, L. A. (1997). Foreword. In D. Watson (Ed.), *Task analysis: An occupational performance approach* (pp. v–vii). Bethesda, MD: American Occupational Therapy Association.

Llorens, L. A. (1997). Foreword. In G. Gilkenson (Ed.), *Occupational therapy leadership* (pp. iii–v). Philadelphia: F. A. Davis.

Llorens, L. A., Umphred, D. B., Burton, G. U., & Glogoski-Williams, C. (1993). Ethnogeriatrics: Implications for occupational therapy and physical therapy. *Physical and Occupational Therapy in Geriatrics, 11*(3), 59–69.

Llorens, L. A. (1993). Activity analysis: Agreement between participants and observers on perceived factors in occupation components. *Occupational Therapy Journal of Research, 13*, 198–211.

Shiotsuka, W., Burton, G. U., Pedretti, L. W., & Llorens, L. A. (1992). An examination of performance scores on activities of daily living between elders with right and left cerebrovascular accident. *Physical and Occupational Therapy in Geriatrics, 10*(4), 47–57.

McCormack, G. L., Llorens, L. A., & Glogoski, C. (1991). Culturally diverse elders. In J. M. Kiernat (Ed.), *Occupational therapy and the older adult: A clinical manual* (pp. 11–25). Gaithersburg, MD: Aspen.

Bolding, D. J., & Llorens, L. A. (1991). The effects of habilitative hospital admission on self-care, self-esteem, and frequency of physical care. *American Journal of Occupational Therapy, 45*, 796–800.

Llorens, L. A. (1991). Performance tasks and roles throughout the life span. In C. Christiansen & C. Baum (Eds.), *Occupational therapy: Overcoming human performance deficits* (pp. 69–96). Thorofare, NJ: Slack.

Llorens, L. A. (1990). Research utilization: A persona/professional responsibility [Guest Editorial]. *Occupational Therapy Journal of Research, 10*, 3–6.

Kibele, A., & Llorens, L. A. (1989). Going to the source: The use of qualitative methodology in a study of the needs of adults with cerebral palsy. *Occupational Therapy in Health Care, 6*(2/3), 27–40.

Hames-Han, C. S., & Llorens, L. A. (1989). Impact of a multisensory occupational therapy program on components of self-feeding behavior in the elderly. *Physical and Occupational Therapy in Geriatrics, 6*(3/4), 63–86.

Llorens, L. A. (1989). Health care system models and occupational therapy. *Occupational Therapy in Health Care, 5*(4), 25–37.

Hardison, J., & Llorens, L. A. (1988). Structured craft group activities for adolescent delinquent girls. *Occupational Therapy in Mental Health, 8*(3), 101–117.

Oyster, C. K., Hanten, W. P., & Llorens, L. A. (1987). *Introduction to research: A guide for the health science professional*. Philadelphia: Lippincott Williams & Wilkins.

Llorens, L. A., & Snyder, N. V. (1987). Nationally Speaking—Research initiatives for occupational therapy. *American Journal of Occupational Therapy, 41*, 491–493.

Llorens, L. A. (1986). Activity analysis: Agreement among factors in a sensory processing model. *American Journal of Occupational Therapy, 40*, 103–110.

Llorens, L. A., & Gillette, N. P. (1985). Nationally Speaking—The challenge for research in a practice profession. *American Journal of Occupational Therapy, 39*, 143–145.

Llorens, L. A., Ward, J. M., Still, J., & Eyler, R. (1984). Education Bulletin—Professional education for occupational therapy. *Occupational Therapy News, 38*(4), 6–9.

Llorens, L. A. (1984). Theoretical conceptualizations of occupational therapy: 1960–1982. *Occupational Therapy in Mental Health, 4*(2), 1–14.

Llorens, L. A. (1984). Changing balance: Environment and individual. *American Journal of Occupational Therapy, 38*, 29–34.

Llorens, L. A., & Donaldson, K. (1983). Documentation of occupational therapy services: A process model. *Canadian Journal of Occupational Therapy, 50*, 171–175.

Llorens, L. A. (1983). Educating for professional competency: Accountability theory in practice. *Journal of the New Zealand Association of Occupational Therapists, 34*(1), 22, 24.

Llorens, L. A. (1983). The DSM-III, sensory integration, and child psychiatry: Implication for treatment and research. *Sensory Integration Special Interest Section Newsletter, 6*(1), 2.

Llorens, L. A. (1981). The role of occupational therapy in vocational rehabilitation of psychiatric patients. *Mental Health Special Interest Section Newsletter, 4*(3), 1–2.

Llorens, L. A. (1981). OT Education Bulletin—Maintaining credibility: The academic occupational therapist and practice. *Occupational Therapy News, 35*(9), 10–13.

Llorens, L. A. (1981). On the meaning of activity in occupational therapy. *Journal of the New Zealand Association of Occupational Therapists, 32*(1), 3–6.

Llorens, L. A. (1981). A journal of research in occupational therapy: The need, the response [Guest Editorial]. *Occupational Therapy Journal of Research, 1*, 3–6.

Llorens, L. A. (1979). Thinking research in occupational therapy. *Developmental Disabilities Special Interest Section Newsletter, 2*(3), 1.

Llorens, L. A., & Adams, S. P. (1978). Learning style preferences of occupational therapy students. *American Journal of Occupational Therapy, 32*, 161–164.

Llorens, L. A., & Shuster, J. J. (1977). Occupational therapy sequential client care recording system: A comparative study. *American Journal of Occupational Therapy, 31*, 367–371.

Llorens, L. A. (1977). A developmental theory revisited. *American Journal of Occupational Therapy, 31*, 656–657.

Llorens, L. A. (1976). *Evaluation of a client care recording system fir occupational therapy*. Fort Collins: Colorado State University.

Llorens, L. A. (1976). *Application of developmental theory for health and rehabilitation*. Rockville, MD: American Occupational Therapy Association.

Llorens, L. A., & Sieg, K. W. (1975). A profile for managing sensory integrative test data. *American Journal of Occupational Therapy, 29*, 205–208.

Ayers, A. J., Henderson, A., Llorens, L. A., Gilfoyle, E. M., Myers, C., & Prevel, S. (1974). *The development of sensory integrative theory and practice: A collection of works of A. Jean Ayers*. Dubuque, IA: Kendall/Hunt.

Llorens, L. A. (1974). The effects of stress on growth and development. *American Journal of Occupational Therapy, 28*, 82–86.

Llorens, L. A. (1973). *Consultation in the community: Occupational therapy in child health*. Dubuque, IA: Kendall/Hunt.

Llorens, L. A. (1972). Problem-solving the role of occupational therapy in a new environment. *American Journal of Occupational Therapy, 26*, 234–238.

Llorens, L. A. (1971). Occupational therapy in community child health. *American Journal of Occupational Therapy, 25*, 335–339.

Llorens, L. A. (1971). Black culture and child development. *American Journal of Occupational Therapy, 25*, 144–149.

Llorens, L. A. (1970). Facilitating growth and development: The promise of occupational therapy (1969 Eleanor Clark Slagle Lecture). *American Journal of Occupational Therapy, 24*, 93–101.

Llorens, L. A., Rubin, E. Z., Braun, J. S., Beck, G. R., & Beal, C. D. (1969). The effects of a cognitive–perceptual–motor training approach on children with behavior maladjustment. *American Journal of Occupational Therapy, 23*, 502–512.

Llorens, L. A., & Rubin, E. Z. (1968). *Developing ego functions in disturbed children: Occupational therapy in milieu*. Detroit, MI: Wayne State University Press.

Fidler, G. S., Kivalenko, L., Llorens, L. A., Mosey, A. C., Overly, K., Wilbarger, P., et al. (1968). Toward an integrated theory of occupational therapy: Proceedings of seminar held August 26–31, 1967, at Albion, Michigan: Conference report. *American Journal of Occupational Therapy, 22*, 451–456.

Llorens, L. A. (1968). Identification of the Ayres' syndromes in emotionally disturbed children: An exploratory study. *American Journal of Occupational Therapy, 22*, 286–288.

Llorens, L. A. (1968). Changing methods in treatment of psychosocial dysfunction. *American Journal of Occupational Therapy, 22*, 19–22.

Llorens, L. A., & Johnson, P. A. (1967). Occupational therapy in an ego-centered milieu. *American Journal of Occupational Therapy, 21*, 178–181.

Llorens, L. A. (1967). Projective technique in occupational therapy. *American Journal of Occupational Therapy, 21*, 226–229.

Llorens, L. A. (1967). An evaluation procedure for children 6–10 years of age. *American Journal of Occupational Therapy, 21,* 64–69.

Llorens, L. A. (1965). *Techniques and procedures of psychiatric occupational therapy: A study guide.* Detroit, MI: Wayne State University Press.

Llorens, L. A., Rubin, E. X., Braun, J., Beck, G., Mottley, N., & Beall, D. (1964). Cognitive–perceptual–motor functions: A preliminary report on training in occupational therapy. *American Journal of Occupational Therapy, 18,* 202–207.

Llorens, L. A., Levy, R., & Rubin, E. Z. (1964). Work adjustment program: A pre-vocational experience. *American Journal of Occupational Therapy, 18,* 15–19.

Llorens, L. A., & Bernstein, S. P. (1963). Finger-painting with an obsessive–compulsive organically-damaged child. *American Journal of Occupational Therapy, 17,* 120–121.

Llorens, L. A., & Rubin, E. Z. (1962). A directed activity program for disturbed children. *American Journal of Occupational Therapy, 16,* 287–290.

Llorens, L. A., & Toung, G. G. (1960). Case History—Finger-painting for the hostile child. *American Journal of Occupational Therapy, 14,* 306–307.

Llorens, L. A. (1960). Psychological tests in planning therapy goals. *American Journal of Occupational Therapy, 14,* 243–246.

Josephine C. Moore, PhD, OTR, DSc—1975

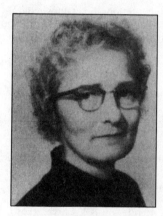

Josephine C. Moore was born in Ann Arbor, Michigan, in 1925. She earned a bachelor's degree in geology from the University of Michigan in 1947. In 1955, she completed her bachelor's degree in occupational therapy from the Michigan State Normal College, now known as Eastern Michigan University. She earned a master's degree and a doctoral degree in anatomy from the University of Michigan in 1964.

In 1955, Moore accepted the position of instructor in anatomy, kinesiology, medical lectures, and adaptive equipment and appliances in the Department of Special Education and Occupational Therapy at Eastern Michigan University in Ypsilanti. Next, as an instructor at the University of Michigan, Department of Anatomy, Moore taught a variety of courses such as dental gross anatomy, physical therapy gross anatomy, dental hygiene, and neuroanatomy. From 1966 to 1970, she was an assistant professor in the Department of Anatomy at the University of South Dakota Medical School. In the period of 1970 to 1976, she was promoted to associate professor and later became a full professor and the head of the Neuroanatomy Section. She also was the vice chairman of anatomy at the University of South Dakota Medical School from 1978 to 1984.

Moore chose to be "semi-retired" in 1991 and retired fully in 1993. She "finished lecturing forever" in 1995. Today, she is enjoying life as a retiree and pursuing her interests in genealogy and oil painting.

Moore has received numerous honors and awards, including being one of the few occupational therapists in the United States who was asked to attend or send materials to the World Federation Occupational Therapy Conference in Copenhagen in 1957. In 1967, Moore was 1 of 30 occupational therapists in the United States invited to an OT/PT Research Conference in Puerto Rico and 1 of 4 occupational therapists in the United States asked to write a paper from this research conference. She was recognized by the students at the University of South Dakota with awards for outstanding teaching from 1970 to 1972. She was chosen by the medical school class of 1974 as one of the most outstanding professors in the basic sciences for the years 1972–1974; in addition, she was selected by the students for the Hyden Award, which is awarded each year "to the all-over best professor at the University of South Dakota School of Medicine.

In 1973, Moore was inducted into the Roster of Fellows of the American Occupational Therapy Association, the first year that the honor was awarded. She is listed in the Who's Who in American Women; the American Men and Women of Science Medical and Health Services; the Dictionary of International Biography, Men of Achievement; the World's Who's Who of Women in Education; and the Community Leaders and Noteworthy Americans. In 1975, Moore was awarded the Eleanor Clarke Slagle Lectureship Award at the AOTA National Conference in Milwaukee, Wisconsin.

Moore has received certificates of appreciation from the South Dakota Occupational Therapy Association and the New Hampshire Occupational Therapy Association. In 1982, she received an Award of Merit from Quinnipiac College, School of Allied Health and Natural Sciences and the Connecticut Occupational Therapy Association. In 1982, she received an honorary doctor of science degree from Eastern Michigan University, College of Health and Human Services. A few years later, she received another honorary doctor of science degree from the University of Indianapolis.

On a Personal Note From a Phone Interview: Moore identified her father, a professor at the University of Michigan in electrical engineering, and her mother as her inspiration mentors. Her parents held high standards for Moore and encouraged her to pursue science and higher education as career interests. Moore presented her lecture focused on neuroscience and encouraged other occupational therapists to seek graduate degrees in science and to share our expertise as occupational therapists.

Bibliography

Moore, J. C. (1984). Recovery potentials following CNS lesions. *American Journal of Occupational Therapy, 40,* 459–463.

Moore, J. C. (1984). The Golgi tendon organ: A review and update. *American Journal of Occupational Therapy, 38,* 227–236.

Moore, J. C. (1982). Sensory system's influence on movement and muscle tone. *Proceedings of the 10th Annual Sensorimotor Symposium* (pp. 2–41). San Diego: Office of Continuing Education in the Health Sciences, University of California School of Medicine.

Moore, J. C. (1981). Oral and related vital functions. *Proceedings of the 8th Annual Sensorimotor Symposium* (pp. 5–39). San Diego: Office of Continuing Education in the Health Sciences, University of California School of Medicine.

Grady, A., Gilfoyle, E., & Moore, J. C. (1981). We hold these truths to be self evident re adaptation and the spiraling continuum. In E. Gilfoyle (Ed.), *Children adapt* (pp. 233–276). New York: Charles Slack.

Grady, A., Gilfoyle, E., & Moore, J. C. (1981). Nervous system development in relation to pediatric rehabilitation. In E. Gilfoyle (Ed.), *Children adapt* (pp. 15–31). New York: Charles Slack.

Bunger, P. C., Neufeld, D. A., Moore, J. C., & Carter, G. A. (1981). Persistent left superior vena cava and associated structural and functional considerations. *Journal of Angiology, 32,* 601–608.

Moore, J. C. (1981). Hemispheric specialization and integration syllabus. *Proceedings of the 9th Annual Sensorimotor Symposium* (pp. 1–38). San Diego: Office of Continuing Education in the Health Sciences, University of California School of Medicine.

Moore, J. C. (1981). Foreword. In M. R. Fiorentino (Ed.), *A basis for sensorimotor development—Normal and abnormal* (p. viii). Springfield, IL: Charles C Thomas.

Moore, J. C. (1980). Neuroanatomical considerations relative to recovery of function following brain injury. In P. Bachyrita, (Ed.), *Recovery of function following brain injury: Theoretical considerations.* Bern, Switzerland: Verlag Hans Huber.

Moore, J. C. (1977). Individual differences and the art of therapy. *American Journal of Occupational Therapy, 31,* 663–665.

Moore, J. C. (1976). Behavior, bias, and the limbic system (1975 Eleanor Clarke Slagle Lecture). *American Journal of Occupational Therapy, 30,* 11–19.

Moore, J. C. (1975). Excitation overflow: An EMG investigation. *Archives of Physical Medicine and Rehabilitation, 56,* 115–119.

Moore, J. C. (1973). Terminology today. *American Journal of Occupational Therapy, 27,* 149–155.

Moore, J. C. (1973). Cranial nerves and their importance in current rehabilitation techniques. In A. Henderson & J. Coryell (Eds.), *The body senses and perceptual deficit* (pp. 102–120). Boston: Sargent College of Allied Health Professions.

Moore, J. C. (1973). *Concepts from the neurobehavioral sciences in relation to the mentally/physically handicapped.* Dubuque, IA: Kendall/Hunt.

Moore, J. C. (1972). A review of the nervous system in chart form. *American Journal of Occupational Therapy, 26,* 305–308.

Moore, J. C. (1972). Physiological properties of nerve fibers. *American Journal of Occupational Therapy, 26,* 244–248.

Moore, J. C. (1971). Difference in electrical activity of the biceps brachii and brachioradialis muscles performing isometric like supination and pronation exercises. *American Journal of Occupational Therapy, 25,* 391–397.

Moore, J. C. (1971). Active resistive stretch and isometric exercise in strengthening wrist flexion in normal adults. *Archives of Physical Medicine and Rehabilitation 52,* 264–269.

Moore, J. C. (1969). Structure and function of the nervous system in relation to treatment techniques. In L. Zamir (Ed.), *Expanding dimensions in rehabilitation* (pp. 21–41). Springfield, IL: Charles C Thomas.

Moore, J. C. (1969). The neuron concluded, Part II, Section C. The location of cell bodies in the central nervous system. *American Journal of Occupational Therapy, 23,* 232–243.

Moore, J. C. (1969). *Neuroanatomy simplified: Some basic concepts for understanding rehabilitation techniques.* Dubuque, IA: Kendall/Hunt.

Moore, J. C. (1969). The developing nervous system in relationship to techniques in treating physical dysfunction. In L. Zamir (Ed.), *Expanding dimensions in rehabilitation* (pp. 3–20). Springfield, IL: Charles C Thomas.

Moore, J. C. (1969). Confusion and controversy concerning treatment techniques utilized in physical dysfunction. In L. Zamir (Ed.), *Expanding dimensions in rehabilitation* (pp. 42–51). Springfield, IL: Charles C Thomas.

Moore, J. C. (1968). A new look at the nervous system in relation to rehabilitation techniques. *American Journal of Occupational Therapy, 22,* 489–501.

Moore, J. C. (1967). *Part II, Structure and function of the nervous system in relation to treatment techniques.* Cleveland, OH: Case Western Reserve University.

Moore, J. C. (1967). *Part I, The developing nervous system in relation to treatment techniques used in physical disabilities.* Cleveland, OH: Case Western Reserve University.

Moore, J. C. (1967). *Medical abbreviations: A crossreference dictionary* (2nd ed.). Ann Arbor: Michigan Occupational Therapy Association.

Moore, J. C. (1967). *Confusion and controversy concerning treatment techniques utilized in physical disabilities.* Cleveland, OH: Case Western Reserve University.

Moore, J. C. (1967). Changing methods in the treatment of physical dysfunction. *American Journal of Occupational Therapy, 21,* 18–28.

Moore, J. C. (1967). Basic research in occupational therapy. *Proceedings of the Occupational and Physical Therapy Conference on Research, Puerto Rico* (p. 42). Washington, DC: U.S. Department of Health, Education and Welfare.

Moore, J. C. (1966). Perceptual motor dysfunction in rehabilitation personnel [Editorial]. *American Journal of Occupational Therapy, 20,* 7.

Moore, J. C. (1966). Facilitation of a forearm flexor response: Utilization of active resistive stretch in normal adults. *Journal of Applied Physiology. 21*, 649–665.

Moore, J. C. (1966). Fabrication of suction cup electrodes for electromyography. *Journal of Electroencephalography and Clinical Neurophysiology. 20*, 405–406.

Moore, J. C. (1965). Neuroanatomy simplified, Part II, Section A, the neuron. *American Journal of Occupational Therapy, 20*, 130–143.

Moore, J. C. (1965). Neuroanatomy simplified, Part I. *American Journal of Occupational Therapy, 19*, 208–212.

Moore, J. C. (1965). Neuroanatomical and neurophysiological factors basic to the use of neuromuscular facilitation techniques. In W. West (Ed.), *Occupational therapy for the multiple handicapped child* (pp. 31–85). Chicago: University of Illinois.

Moore, J. C. (1964). *Utilization of active resistive stretch to obtain an improved response in the forearm flexors of normal adults.* Unpublished dissertation, University of Michigan, Rackham Graduate School, Ann Arbor.

Moore, J. C. (1963). Are we halfbreeds? *American Journal of Occupational Therapy, 18*, 8.

Moore, J. C. (1961). *Medical abbreviations: A cross-reference dictionary*. Ann Arbor: Michigan Occupational Therapy Association.

Moore, J. C. (1960). Dura-form. *American Journal of Occupational Therapy, 14*, 256–257.

Moore, J. C., & Champaign, I. (1959). The wheelchair sideboard. *American Journal of Occupational Therapy, 13*, 66.

Moore, J. C. (1959). Bending jigs and dies. *American Journal of Occupational Therapy, 12*, 13–15.

Moore, J. C. (1958). *Rehabilitation equipment and supplies directory*. Ann Arbor, MI: Cushing Malloy.

Moore, J. C. (1957). *Simplified neurological review for students and therapists*. Ann Arbor, MI: Overbeck.

Moore, J. C. (1957). *Adaptive equipment and appliances (for the handicapped)*. Ann Arbor, MI: Overbeck.

Moore, J. C. (1956). Reading aids for a quadriplegic patient. *American Journal of Occupational Therapy, 10*, 133.

Moore, J. C. (1956). *The occupational therapy glossary*. Ypsilanti: Eastern Michigan University.

Moore, J. C. (1956). Adjustable reading rack for the visually handicapped. *American Journal of Occupational Therapy, 10*, 82–84.

Anne Cronin Mosey, PhD, OT, FAOTA—1985

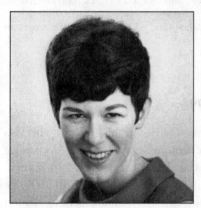

Anne Cronin Mosey retired in 2002 as professor of occupational therapy at New York University (NYU). A prominent educator, researcher, and leader in the occupational therapy discipline, she joined occupational therapy department at NYU as a faculty member in 1969 and served as its second chair from 1972 to 1980. She earned a bachelor's degree in occupational therapy from the University of Minnesota in 1961 and a master's degree (1965) and a doctorate in human relations and community studies (1968), both from NYU.

After graduation in 1961, Mosey worked at Glenwood Hills Hospital in Minneapolis. She later moved to New York City to work with and learn from Gail Fidler. She joined the New York State Psychiatric Institute, where she remained for 5 years until August 1966. From 1966 to 1968, she was on the faculty of Columbia University as an instructor in occupational therapy. During this period, she developed and wrote *Three Frames of Reference for Mental Health* and completed her dissertation. She then joined NYU, serving as the department chairperson from 1972 to 1980. In 1977, she was named the acting head of the Division of Health.

Mosey served as a consultant to several hospitals and state mental health systems, including the Massachusetts Department of Mental Health, the Division of Rehabilitation Education at NYU, Hillside Hospital Professional Examination Services, the Family-Centered Research Project, the Institute of Pennsylvania Hospital, the Greater Trenton Mental Health Center, and Christopher House. She also was a faculty member for the AOTA Regional Institutes from 1966 to 1967.

Mosey served AOTA in several leadership positions on the state and national levels. She was a member of the Panel of Experts of the AOTA Continuing Education Programs in Mental Health from 1984 to 1988; a member of the Scholars Group for the Directions for the Future Project of AOTA/American Occupational Therapy Foundation (AOTF) from 1988 to 1991; a member of the Panel for the Review of Research Proposals of AOTF; an AOTF research consultant; and in 1992 participated in the development of the AOTA Self-Study Series on Cognitive Rehabilitation.

Among the honors she has received are AOTA Fellow, 1973; Distinguished Service Award from the National Association of Activity Therapy, 1975; and the Anne Cronin Mosey Lectureship, presented annually by NYU.

Bibliography

Mosey, A. C. (1968). *Occupational therapy: Theory and practice*. Medford, MA: Pothier Brothers Press.

Mosey, A. C. (1968). Recapitulation of ontogenesis: A theory for the practice of occupational therapy. *American Journal of Occupational Therapy, 22*, 426–432.

Crampton, M. W., Mosey, A. C., Talbot, N. H., Fidler, G. S., Newmann, F. M., & Solomon, L. F. (1969). *Development of teaching materials for occupational therapy assistants: Project report.* Boston: Medical Foundation.

Mosey, A. C. (1969). Treatment of pathological distortion of body image. *American Journal of Occupational Therapy, 23,* 413–416.

Mosey, A. C. (1970). The concept and use of developmental groups. *American Journal of Occupational Therapy, 24,* 272–275.

Mosey, A. C. (1970). *Three frames of reference for mental health.* Thorofare, NJ: Slack.

Mosey, A. C. (1971). Involvement in the rehabilitation movement 1942–1960. *American Journal of Occupational Therapy, 25,* 234–236.

Mosey, A. C. (1973). *Activities therapy.* New York: Raven Press.

Mosey, A. C. (1973). Meeting health needs. *American Journal of Occupational Therapy, 27,* 14–17.

Mosey, A. C. (1974). An alternative: The biopsychosocial model. *American Journal of Occupational Therapy, 28,* 137–140.

Corry, S., Sebastian, V., & Mosey, A. C. (1974). Acute short-term treatment in psychiatry. *American Journal of Occupational Therapy, 28,* 401–406.

Mosey, A. C. (1976). The night of January twenty-seven. *American Journal of Occupational Therapy, 30,* 648–649.

Katz, G. M., & Mosey, A. C. (1980). Fieldwork performance, academic grades, and pre-selection criteria of occupational therapy students. *American Journal of Occupational Therapy, 34,* 794–800.

Mosey, A. C. (1980). A model of occupational therapy. *Occupational Therapy in Mental Health, 1,* 11–32.

Mosey, A. C. (1981). The art of practice. In B. C. Abreu (Ed.), *Physical disabilities manual* (pp. 1–3). New York: Raven Press.

Mosey, A. C. (1981). *Occupational therapy: Configuration of a profession.* New York: Raven Press.

Mosey, A. C. (1985). A monistic or a pluralistic approach to professional identity? (1985 Eleanor Clarke Slagle Lecture). *American Journal of Occupational Therapy, 39,* 504–509.

Mosey, A. C. (1985). *Psychosocial components of occupational therapy.* New York: Raven Press.

Mosey, A. C. (1989). The proper focus of scientific inquiry in occupational therapy: Frames of reference. *Occupational Therapy Journal of Research, 9,* 195–201.

Mosey, A. C. (1991). Letter to the Editor: Common vocabulary. *Occupational Therapy Journal of Research, 11,* 67–68.

Mosey, A. C. (1992). *Applied scientific inquiry in the health professions: An epistemological orientation.* Rockville, MD: American Occupational Therapy Association.

Mosey, A. C. (1993). The Issue Is: Partition of occupational science and occupational therapy: Sorting out some issues. *American Journal of Occupational Therapy, 46,* 851–853.

Mosey, A. C. (1996). *Applied scientific inquiry in the health professions: An epistemological orientation* (2nd ed.). Bethesda, MD: American Occupational Therapy Association.

Mosey, A. C. (1998). The competent scholar. *American Journal of Occupational Therapy, 52,* 760–764.

David Nelson, PhD, OTR, FAOTA—1996

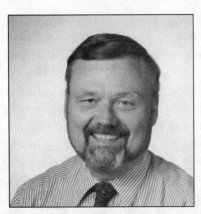

David Nelson was born in Minneapolis, Minnesota, where he grew up with two sisters in a quiet residential area. After high school, he served in the U.S. Air Force from 1964 to 1968. He attended New York University, earning a BS in occupational therapy in 1973 and an MS in occupational therapy in 1976. In 1978, he earned a PhD in human development from Union Graduate School, Union Institute and University in Cincinnati.

Nelson began his occupational therapy career at the Queens Children's Psychiatric Center in Bellerose, New York, working with institutionalized children and adolescents who had mental retardation and autism. From 1975 to 1976, he was a senior occupational therapist at Brooklyn Developmental Center. He spent summers from 1976 to 1979 as the co-director of an intensive program for children with autism as part of the National Society for Autistic Children.

In 1978, Nelson began a career in academia as an assistant professor at Boston University, Sargent College of Allied Health Professions. He participated in the development of doctoral programs in occupational therapy and physical therapy at Boston University. In 1984, he became an associate professor and later professor at Western Michigan University in Kalamazoo, Michigan (until 1992). From 1992 to 1995, he continued his occupational therapy practice at the Medical College Rehabilitation Hospital of Toledo and St. Francis Health Care Centre of Green Springs, Ohio. From 2006 to 2008, he provided occupational therapy services at the University of Toledo Parkinson's Disease Interdisciplinary Clinic. He is a tenured professor in the Department of Occupational Therapy, College of Health Science and Human Service, University of Toledo (formerly the Medical College of Ohio).

Nelson was inducted into the Roster of Fellows of the American Occupational Therapy Association (AOTA) in 1987. He received a Certificate of Recognition from the Michigan Occupational Therapy Association (MOTA) in 1988. The College of Health and Human Services at Western Michigan University bestowed the Certificate of Appreciation "for distinguished scholarship" to Nelson in 1989 and 1990. In June 1991, he was designated a Fellow of the Academy of Research, which is the highest research award of the American Occupational Therapy Foundation (AOTF). In October 1991, he also was chosen as an MOTA Fellow. AOTF recognized Nelson with a Certificate for Contributions to the *OTJR* Editorial Board in December 1991.

In 1993, the AOTA Developmental Disabilities Special Interest Section honored Nelson with a Certificate of Recognition for his work in this area. Of special note, the Eleanor Clarke Slagle Lectureship Award, the highest AOTA academic award, was awarded to Nelson in Denver, Colorado, April 11, 1995, Later that year, the School of Allied Health at the Medical College of Ohio selected Nelson for the Dean's Award for Teaching Excellence. In 1997, he was honored with the Award of Merit from the Ohio Occupational Therapy Association.

Nelson has an impressive background of refereed, competitive grants. His research interests include testing functional approaches to subacute rehabilitation, movement analysis, development of assessments for skilled nursing facilities, therapeutic summer programs for children with autism, measuring the effects of occupation, falls prevention with the elderly population, and home-based programming for people with Parkinson's disease

On a Personal Note From a Phone Interview: Nelson spoke about the large differences between the actual lecture and the printed article in the *American Journal of Occupational Therapy*. The published article could not truly capture the personal meanings and flavor of the lecture due to the many video clips and other bits of humor integrated into the live presentation. Nelson brought his children up on the stage at the end of the lecture, and this was a poignant moment, as many of the video clips used as exemplars of concepts in his lecture featured his children. The lecture brought occupational therapy history to life, adding the sentiment and meaning sometimes words cannot communicate.

The year before the actual lecture, Nelson was inspired by two women who happened to share a cab with him to the airport after receiving the Eleanor Clarke Slagle Lectureship Award, who urged him to talk about something "inspiring." Nelson noted the lecture is a snapshot in occupational therapy history.

Linking Key Messages of the 1996 Eleanor Clarke Slagle Lecture to the AOTA *Centennial Vision:* My Slagle lecture (what a wonderful opportunity, as I think back) was also a "centennial vision," in that the lecture provided reasons why occupational therapy as a profession will thrive 100 years in the future. Like the AOTA *Centennial Vision*, my lecture posited that the profession of occupational therapy will flourish because occupation is such a powerful force in human nature. Our advocacy of occupation is the key to enhancing the reputation of the field, so that occupational therapy can gain *recognition* and power as one of society's leading professions. My lecture also emphasized scientific research, both basic research into the nature of occupation as well as applied research providing an evidence base for occupation-based interventions.

As a theoretician, however, I must quibble with some of the language in the *Centennial Vision*. The phrase *society's occupational needs* (AOTA, 2007) is unfortunate. According to the terminology used in my lecture, which is based on my reading of the founders, only a human being can have an occupational need; technically and precisely, a society cannot have an occupational need. In my opinion, occupational therapy is not and should not be a branch of population-based public health, even though our individualized occupational interventions can improve the public's health. The profession is most likely to fulfill its great promise by shunning distracting fads and building its knowledge base at its core: synthesis of an occupational form by an occupational therapist in order to provide the challenge and/or the assistance needed by a unique person to achieve that person's personal and social success and adaptation.

In summary, the recommendations made in my Slagle lecture are remarkably parallel to the *Centennial Vision*. However, as we go forward with visions and revisions, it is essential that we critically evaluate our language and its implications for fidelity to our core in occupation.

—*David Nelson*

Reference

American Occupational Therapy Association. (2007). AOTA's *Centennial Vision* and executive summary. *American Journal of Occupational Therapy, 61*, 613–614.

Bibliography

Hearns, M. K., Kopp Miller, B., & Nelson, D. L. (2010). Hands-on learning versus learning by demonstration at three recall points in university students. *OTJR: Occupation, Participation and Health, 30*(4).

Johnson, C. J., & Nelson, D. L. (2010). Convergent validity of three occupational self-assessments. *Physical and Occupational Therapy in Geriatrics, 28*(1), 13–21.

Norton-Mabus, J. C., & Nelson, D. L. (2008). Reporting of randomized controlled trials in occupational therapy and speech therapy: Evaluation using an expansion of the CONSORT Statement. *Occupational Therapy Journal of Research, 28,* 64–71.

Butts, D. S., & Nelson, D. L. (2007). Agreement between *Occupational Therapy Practice Framework* classifications and occupational therapists' classifications. *American Journal of Occupational Therapy, 61,* 512–518.

Moberg-Mogren, E., & Nelson, D. L. (2006). Evaluating the quality of reporting occupational therapy randomized trials by expanding the CONSORT criteria. *American Journal of Occupational Therapy, 60,* 226–235.

Nelson, D. L. (2006). Critiquing the logic of the *Domain* section of *Occupational Therapy Practice Framework: Domain and Process. American Journal of Occupational Therapy, 60,* 511–523.

Nelson, D. L. (2006). Group comparison designs: Quantitative research design. In G. Kielhofner (Ed.), *Research in occupational therapy: Methods of inquiry for enhancing practice* (pp. 65–90). Philadelphia: F. A. Davis.

Kopp Miller, B., & Nelson, D. L. (2004). Constructing a program development proposal for community-based practice: A valuable learning experience for occupational therapy students. *Occupational Therapy in Health Care, 18,* 137–150.

Nelson, D. L., & Mathiowetz, V. (2004). Randomized controlled trials to investigate occupational therapy research questions. *American Journal of Occupational Therapy, 58,* 24–34.

Nelson, D. L., & Thomas, J. J. (2003). Occupational form, occupational performance, and a conceptual framework for therapeutic occupation. In P. Kramer, J. Hinojosa, & C. Royeen (Eds.), *Perspectives on human occupation: Participation in life* (pp. 87–155). Philadelphia: Lippincott Williams & Wilkins.

Peterson, C. Q., & Nelson, D. L. (2003). Effect of an occupational intervention on printing in children with economic disadvantages. *American Journal of Occupational Therapy, 57,* 152–160.

Melville, L. L., Baltic, T. A., Bettcher, T., & Nelson, D. L. (2002). Patients' perspectives on the Self-Identified Goals Assessment. *American Journal of Occupational Therapy, 56,* 650–659.

Nelson, D. L., Melville, L. L., Wilkerson, J. D., Fogle, R. A., Grech, J. L., & Rosenberg, J. A. (2002). Interrater reliability, concurrent validity, responsiveness, and predictive validity of the Melville–Nelson Self-Care Assessment. *American Journal of Occupational Therapy, 56,* 51–59.

Eakman, A. M., & Nelson, D. L. (2001). The effect of hands-on occupation on recall memory in men with traumatic brain injury. *Occupational Therapy Journal of Research, 21,* 109–114.

Nelson, D. L., Cipriani, D. J., & Thomas, J. J. (2001). Physical therapy and occupational therapy: Partners in rehabilitation for persons with movement impairments. *Occupational Therapy in Health Care, 15*(3–4), 35–57.

Hartman, B. A., Kopp Miller, B., & Nelson, D. L. (2000). The effects of hands-on occupation versus demonstration on children's recall memory. *American Journal of Occupational Therapy, 54,* 477–483.

Nelson, D. L. (2000). Conceptual framework of therapeutic occupation. In P. Crist, C. B. Royeen, & J. K. Schade (Eds.), *Infusing occupation into practice* (2nd ed., pp. 114–118, 122–128, 132–135, 138–141, 144–145, 147–148). Bethesda, MD: American Occupational Therapy Association.

Ross, L. M., & Nelson, D. L. (2000). Comparing materials-based occupation, imagery-based occupation, and rote movement through kinematic analysis of reach. *Occupational Therapy Journal of Research, 20,* 45–60.

Thomas, J. J., & Nelson, D. L. (2000). Moving toward a scientific base for one of the oldest and most important ideas in the profession of occupational therapy. In J. Hinojosa & M. L. Blount (Eds.), *The texture of life: Purposeful activities in occupational therapy* (pp. 394–419). Bethesda, MD: American Occupational Therapy Association.

Nelson, D. L. (1999). Occupational form (contribution to "Occupational Terminology Interactive Dialogue"). *Journal of Occupational Science, 6,* 76–78.

Nelson, D. L., & Glass, L. M. (1999). Occupational therapists' involvement with the Minimum Data Set in skilled and intermediate care facilities. *American Journal of Occupational Therapy, 53,* 348–352.

Nelson, D. L., & Jonsson, H. (1999). Occupational terms across languages and countries. *Journal of Occupational Science, 6,* 42–47.

Beauregard, R., Thomas, J. J., & Nelson, D. L. (1998). Quality of reach during a game versus a rote movement in children with cerebral palsy. *Physical and Occupational Therapy in Pediatrics, 18*(3/4), 67–84.

Hall, B. A., & Nelson, D. L. (1998). The effect of materials on performance: A kinematic analysis of eating. *Scandinavian Journal of Occupational Therapy, 5,* 69–81.

Nelson, D. L. (1998). Positioning to enhance occupational performance in developmentally disabled adults. *OT Practice, 3,* 49.

Moyer, J. A., & Nelson, D. L. (1998). Replication and resynthesis of an occupationally embedded exercise with adult rehabilitation patients. *Israel Journal of Occupational Therapy, 7,* 57–75.

Sakemiller, L. M., & Nelson, D. L. (1998). Eliciting functional extension in prone through the use of a game. *American Journal of Occupational Therapy, 52,* 150–157.

Sass, P. L., & Nelson, D. L. (1998). Pilot study of the Inpatient Rehabilitation Scales of Therapeutic Occupation. *Occupational Therapy International, 5,* 66–81.

Munich, H., Cipriani, D., Hall, C., Nelson, D. L., & Falkel, J. (1997). The test–retest reliability of an inclined squat strength test protocol. *Journal of Orthopaedic and Sports Physical Therapy, 26,* 209–213.

Nelson, D. L. (1997, April). Positioning to enhance occupational performance in developmentally disabled adults. *Clinical Facts: Occupational Therapy, 4.*

Nelson, D. L. (1997). Why the profession of occupational therapy will continue to flourish in the twenty-first century (1996 Eleanor Clarke Slagle Lecture). *American Journal of Occupational Therapy, 51,* 11–24.

Nelson, D. L., & Jonsson, H. (1997). Comment—Connotations of the works "occupation" and "occupational therapy" in different languages and countries. *Journal of Occupational Science: Australia, 4,* 39–42.

Nelson, D. L., & Schau, E. M. (1997). Effects of a standing table on work productivity and posture in an adult with developmental disabilities. *Work: A Journal of Prevention, Assessment, and Rehabilitation, 9,* 13–20.

Hsieh, C. L., Nelson, D. L., Smith, D. A., & Peterson, C. Q. (1996). A comparison of performance in added-purpose occupation and rote exercise for dynamic standing balance in persons with hemiplegia. *American Journal of Occupational Therapy, 50,* 10–16.

Nelson, D. L. (1996). Therapeutic occupation: A definition. *American Journal of Occupational Therapy, 50,* 775–782.

Nelson, D. L., Konosky, K., Fleharty, K., Webb, R., Newer, K., Hazboun, V. P., et al. (1996). The effects of an occupationally embedded exercise on bilaterally assisted supination in persons with hemiplegia. *American Journal of Occupational Therapy, 50,* 639–646.

Nelson, D. L., & Lenhart, D. A. (1996). Resumption of outpatient occupational therapy for a young woman five years after traumatic brain injury. *American Journal of Occupational Therapy, 50,* 223–228.

Schmidt, C. L., & Nelson, D. L. (1996). A comparison of three occupational forms in rehabilitation inpatients receiving upper extremity strengthening. *Occupational Therapy Journal of Research, 16,* 200–215.

Zimmerer-Branum, S., & Nelson, D. L. (1995). Occupationally embedded exercise versus rote exercise: A choice between forms by elderly nursing home residents. *American Journal of Occupational Therapy, 49,* 397–402.

Nelson, D. L. (1994). Foreword. In E. Breines (Ed.), *Occupational therapy activities from clay to computers.* Philadelphia: F. A. Davis.

Nelson, D. L. (1994). Occupational form, occupational performance, and therapeutic occupation. In C. B. Royeen (Ed.), *AOTA Self-Study Series—The practice of the future: Putting occupation back into therapy* (pp. 9–48). Rockville, MD: American Occupational Therapy Association.

Yuen, H. K., Nelson, D. L., Peterson, C. Q., & Dickinson, A. (1994). Prosthesis training as a context for studying occupational forms and motoric adaptation. *American Journal of Occupational Therapy, 48,* 55–61.

Borst, M. J., & Nelson, D. L. (1993). Usage of *Uniform Terminology* by occupational therapists. *American Journal of Occupational Therapy, 47,* 611–618.

DeKuiper, W. P., Nelson, D. L., & White, B. E. (1993). Materials-based occupation versus imagery-based occupation versus rote exercise: A replication and extension. *Occupational Therapy Journal of Research, 13,* 183–197.

LaMore, K., & Nelson, D. L. (1993). The effects of options on performance of an art project in adults with mental disabilities. *American Journal of Occupational Therapy, 47,* 397–401.

Nelson, D. L. (1993). The experimental analysis of therapeutic occupation. *Developmental Disabilities Special Interest Section Newsletter, 16*(2), 7–8.

Nelson, D. L. (1993). [Review of information searching in health care]. *Occupational Therapy Journal of Research, 13,* 62–63.

Sietsema, J. M., Nelson, D. L., Mulder, R. M., Mervau-Scheidel, D., & White, B. E. (1993). The use of a game to promote arm reach in persons with traumatic brain injury. *American Journal of Occupational Therapy, 47,* 19–24.

Lang, E. M., Nelson, D. L., & Bush, M. A. (1992). Comparison of performance in materials-based occupation, imagery-based occupation, and rote exercise in nursing home residents. *American Journal of Occupational Therapy, 46,* 607–611.

Nelson, D. L., & Stucky, C. (1992). The roles of occupational therapy in preventing further disability of elderly persons in long-term care facilities. In J. Rothman & R. Levine (Eds.), *Prevention practice: Strategies for physical and occupational therapy* (pp.19–35). Philadelphia: W. B. Saunders.

Nelson, D. L., & Peterson, C. Q. (1991). The effects of competitive versus cooperative structures on subsequent productivity in boys with psychosocial disorders. *Occupational Therapy Journal of Research, 11,* 714–719.

Licht, B. C., & Nelson, D. L. (1990). The adding of meaning to a design copy task through representational stimuli. *American Journal of Occupational Therapy, 44,* 408–413.

Nelson, D. L. (1990). The experimental analysis of occupations: Applications in mental health. *Mental Health Special Interest Section Newsletter, 13*(2), 5–7.

Riccio, C. M., Nelson, D. L., & Bush, M. A. (1990). Adding purpose to the repetitive exercise of elderly women through imagery. *American Journal of Occupational Therapy, 44,* 714–719.

Bloch, M. R., Smith, D. A., & Nelson, D. L. (1989). Heart rate, activity, duration, and affect in added-purpose versus single-purpose jumping activities. *American Journal of Occupational Therapy, 43,* 25–30.

Nelson, D. L., & Peterson, C. Q. (1989). Enhancing therapeutic exercise through purposeful activity: A theoretic analysis. *Topics in Geriatric Rehabilitation, 4*(4), 12–22.

Yoder, R. M., Nelson, D. L., & Smith, D. A. (1989). Added-purpose versus rote exercise in female nursing home residents. *American Journal of Occupational Therapy, 43,* 581–586.

Nelson, D. L. (1988). Occupation: Form and performance. *American Journal of Occupational Therapy, 42,* 633–641.

Nelson, D. L., Peterson, C. Q., Smith, D. A., Boughton, J. A., & Whalen, G. M. (1988). Effects of project versus parallel groups on social interaction and affective responses in senior citizens. *American Journal of Occupational Therapy, 42,* 23–29.

Rice, M. S., & Nelson, D. L. (1988). Effect of choice making on a self-care activity in mentally retarded males. *Occupational Therapy Journal of Research, 8,* 176–185.

Banning, M. R., & Nelson, D. L. (1987). The effects of activity-elicited humor and group structure on group cohesion and affective meanings. *American Journal of Occupational Therapy, 41,* 510–514.

Hatter, J. K., & Nelson, D. L. (1987). Altruism and task participation in the elderly. *American Journal of Occupational Therapy, 41,* 379–381.

Kahn-D'Angelo, L., & Nelson, D. L. (1987). Habituation of the flexion and glabella reflexes in normal one- and two-month-old infants. *Physical and Occupational Therapy in Pediatrics, 7,* 39–56.

Miller, L., & Nelson, D. L. (1987). Dual-purpose activity versus single-purpose activity in terms of duration on task, exertion level, and affect. *Occupational Therapy in Mental Health, 7,* 55–67.

Mullins, C. S., Nelson, D. L., & Smith, D. A. (1987). Exercise through dual-purpose activity in the institutionalized elderly. *Physical and Occupational Therapy in Geriatrics, 5*(3), 29–39.

Rocker, J. D., & Nelson, D. L. (1987). Affective responses to keeping and not keeping an activity product. *American Journal of Occupational Therapy, 41*, 152–157.

Steffan, J. A., & Nelson, D. L. (1987). The effects of tool scarcity on group climate and affective meaning within the context of a stenciling activity. *American Journal of Occupational Therapy, 41*, 449–453.

Froehlich, J., & Nelson, D. L. (1986). Affective meanings of life review through activities and discussion. *American Journal of Occupational Therapy, 40*, 27–33.

Laskas, C. A., Mullen, S. L., Nelson, D. L., & Willson-Broyles, M. L. (1985). Enhancement of two motor functions of the lower extremity in a child with spastic quadriplegia. *Physical Therapy, 65*, 11–16.

Blumenkopf, M., Levangie, P. K., & Nelson, D. L. (1985). Perceived role responsibilities of physical therapists and adapted physical educators in the public school setting. *Physical Therapy, 65*, 1046–1051.

Pelletier, J. M., Short, M. A., & Nelson, D. L. (1985). Immediate effects of waterbed flotation on approach and avoidance behaviors of premature infants. *Physical and Occupational Therapy in Pediatrics, 5*, 81–92.

Adelstein, L. A., & Nelson, D. L. (1985). Effects of sharing versus non-sharing on affective meaning in collage activities. *Occupational Therapy in Mental Health, 5*, 29–45.

Opara, C. U., Levangie, P. K., & Nelson, D. L. (1985). Effects of selected assistive devices on normal distance gait characteristics. *Physical Therapy, 65*, 1188–1191.

Palisano, R. J., Short, M. A., & Nelson, D. L. (1985). Chronological vs. adjusted age in assessing motor development of healthy twelve-month-old premature and full-term infants. *Physical and Occupational Therapy in Pediatrics, 5*, 1–16.

Davidson, D. A., Short, M. A., & Nelson, D. L. (1984). The measurement of empathic ability in normal and atypical five- and six-year-old boys. *Occupational Therapy in Mental Health, 4*, 13–24.

Henry, A. D., Nelson, D. L., & Duncombe, L. W. (1984). Choice-making in group and individual activity. *American Journal of Occupational Therapy, 38*, 245–251.

Kremer, E. R. H., Nelson, D. L., & Duncombe, L. W. (1984). Effects of selected activities on affective meaning in psychiatric clients. *American Journal of Occupational Therapy, 38*, 522–528.

Mandell, R. J., Nelson, D. L., & Cermak, S. A. (1984). Differential laterality of hand function in right-handed and left-handed boys. *American Journal of Occupational Therapy, 38*, 114–120.

Nelson, D. L. (1984). *Children with autism and other pervasive disorders of development and behavior: Therapy through activities.* Thorofare, NJ: Charles B. Slack.

Nelson, D. L., Anderson, V. G., & Gonzales, A. D. (1984). Music activities as therapy for children with autism and other pervasive developmental disorders. *Journal of Music Therapy, 21*, 100–116.

Nelson, D. L., Weidensaul, N. K., Shing-Ru Shih, L., & Anderson, V. G. (1984). The Southern California Postrotary Nystagmus Test and electronystagmography under different conditions of visual input. *American Journal of Occupational Therapy, 38*, 535–540.

Schuster, N. D., Nelson, D. L., & Quisling, C. (1984). Burnout among physical therapists. *Physical Therapy, 64*, 299–303.

Shing-Ru Shih, L., Nelson, D. L., & Duncombe, L. W. (1984). Mood and affect following success and failure in two cultural groups. *Occupational Therapy Journal of Research, 4*, 213–230.

Smith, C. M., Cermak, S. A., & Nelson, D. L. (1984). Sequential versus simultaneous graphesthesia tasks in 6- and 10-year-old children. *American Journal of Occupational Therapy, 38*, 377–381.

Carter, B. A., Nelson, D. L., & Duncombe, L. W. (1983). The effect of psychological type on the mood and meaning of two collage activities. *American Journal of Occupational Therapy, 37*, 688–693.

Lydic, J. S., Short, M. A., & Nelson, D. L. (1983). Comparison of two scales for assessing motor development in infants with Down's syndrome. *Occupational Therapy Journal of Research, 3*, 213–221.

Ray, S. A., Bundy, A. C., & Nelson, D. L. (1983). Decreasing drooling through techniques to facilitate mouth closure. *American Journal of Occupational Therapy, 37*, 749–753.

Reilly, C., Nelson, D. L., & Bundy, A. C. (1983). Sensorimotor versus fine motor activities in eliciting vocalizations in autistic children. *Occupational Therapy Journal of Research, 3*, 199–212.

Ingolia, P., Cermak, S. A., & Nelson, D. L. (1982). The effect of choreoathetoid movements on the Quick Neurological Screening Test. *American Journal of Occupational Therapy, 36*, 801–807.

Nelson, D. L., Thompson, G., & Moore, J. A. (1982). Identification of factors of affective meaning in four selected activities. *American Journal of Occupational Therapy, 36*, 381–387.

Hsu, Y. T., & Nelson, D. L. (1981). Adult performance on the Southern California Kinesthesia and Tactile Perception Tests. *American Journal of Occupational Therapy, 35*, 788–791.

Nelson, D. L. (1980–1981). Evaluating autistic clients. *Occupational Therapy in Mental Health, 1*(4), 1–22.

Nelson, D. L., Gergenti, E., & Hollander, A. C. (1980). Extra prompts vs. no extra prompts in self-care training of autistic children and adolescents. *Journal of Autism and Developmental Disorders, 10*, 311–321.

Nelson, D. L., Nitzberg, L., & Hollander, A. C. (1980). Visually monitored postrotary nystagmus in seven autistic children. *American Journal of Occupational Therapy, 34*, 382–386.

Suzanne M. Peloquin, PhD, OTR, FAOTA—2005

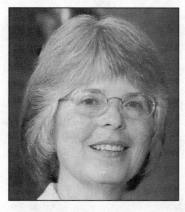

Suzanne Peloquin is a tenured professor in the Department of Occupational Therapy in the School of Health Professions at the University of Texas Medical Branch (UTMB) in Galveston, where she has been on faculty since 1989. She is also the occupational therapist at the Alcohol and Drug Abuse Women's Center in Galveston, where she has led occupational therapy groups since 2006. Prior to these positions she worked in mental health settings in Texas and West Virginia, both as staff therapist and manager.

Before becoming an occupational therapist, Peloquin engaged in various occupations that continue to inform her practice: nanny, religious sister in a teaching order, counselor in a halfway house, nursery school teacher, recruiter and admissions director in a northeastern college, troubleshooter in a Boys' and Girls' Club, teacher of art and languages at junior high and high school levels, and farm hand in tomato fields in Massachusetts.

Peloquin's decision to become an occupational therapist turned closely on the implementation of Chapter 766 legislation in Massachusetts. This law, which predated federal legislation, mainstreamed children and youth with physically and emotionally disabling conditions into public school classrooms. Hoping to learn more about how to work well with such youngsters, she researched various fields and found occupational therapy.

At the time, the University of Pennsylvania offered a certificate in occupational therapy through a rigorous program. After earning her certificate, Peloquin worked in mental health settings. She simultaneously earned a master's degree in counseling to develop interpersonal skills so needed among her patients. She relocated to Texas to serve as a clinical specialist in psychiatry at UTMB. She moved from the clinic to the classroom within that same institution when Donald Davidson, then chair of the Department of Occupational Therapy, suggested that she might convey her passion for the therapeutic use of self more widely as an educator. She pursued a doctoral degree in the medical humanities while teaching as a way of deepening her understanding of illness and disability. Peloquin enjoys teaching and has received numerous awards for teaching excellence.

Peloquin's published work in occupational therapy reflects the influences of her diverse life and educational experiences. She has written several book chapters in occupational therapy, physical therapy, and physician assistant textbooks. She has numerous published articles in the *American Journal of Occupational Therapy* on topics related to the history and service of the profession; the nature, character, and art of occupational therapy practice; and the unique manifestations of empathy and spirituality in occupational therapy. Her work on innovative and confluent approaches to education also has been published, both inside and outside of occupational therapy.

A constant theme coursing through her inquiry is the affective dimension of practice. Considered provocative by some and evocative by others, Peloquin's work prompts a reflective response. The American Occupational Therapy Association (AOTA) has recognized her work through the Roster of Fellows and the Eleanor Clarke Slagle Lecture.

Peloquin was raised in the country town of Easthampton, Massachusetts, on an acre of land surrounded by cow pastures, apple orchards, and chicken farms. Her mother was a hairdresser who worked out of their home, and her father was a factory worker who had served in World War II. Both parents were the youngest in very large families who had come to the United States from Canada. Both were avid readers. Her one brother, two years her junior, resides in California, where he works in structural design and development. Although Peloquin considers herself a Texan and Galveston islander by choice, she retains fond memories of the mountains surrounding her native New England town.

Linking Key Messages of the 2005 Eleanor Clarke Slagle Lecture to the AOTA *Centennial Vision:* A professional association's vision statement invokes an image of best practice for the future. A successful vision turns the collective gaze of practitioners from what is not yet realized to what could be. When ascribing to any individual the characteristic of being *visionary*, one compliments that person's imagination and foresight. A profession that would thrive must be visionary. As important as the visionary capacity is, it complements others that are vital to leadership. When a leader possesses *vision* alongside what most call *character*, others are inspired to follow. That leader has foresight as well as insight. The profession's ethos, or character, which is the subject of my Slagle lecture, stands in a complementary relationship to the *Centennial Vision*. The profession needs its vision and ethos in equal measure.

The term *perspective* comes to mind. In the world of art, the depth that emerges when a person sees the world in perspective comes from *binocular vision*—looking with both eyes. When considered together, the vision and ethos yield a helpful perspective. Occupational therapy will thrive if we see it as "a powerful, widely recognized, and evidence-based" (AOTA, 2007, p. 613) practice, but only if we also see ourselves as pathfinders who reach for hearts as well as hands. Occupational therapy will thrive if we see it as science-driven to meet occupational needs, but only if we know that we will co-create lives if we are artists and scientists at once. Only in tandem with its ethos can a vision achieve its depth.

—*Suzanne M. Peloquin*

Reference

American Journal of Occupational Therapy. (2007). AOTA's *Centennial Vision* and executive summary. *American Journal of Occupational Therapy, 61,* 613–614.

Bibliography

Peloquin, S. M. (2010). An ethos that transcends borders. In F. Kronenberg, N. Pollard, & K. Sakellariou (Eds.), *Occupational therapy without borders: Toward and ecology of occupation-based practice* (Vol. 2). Edinburgh, Scotland: Churchill Livingstone/Elsevier.

Peloquin, S. M. (2008). Foreword. In R. Taylor (Eds.), *The intentional relationship: Occupational therapy and the use of self.* Philadelphia: F. A. Davis.

Peloquin, S. M. (2008). The profession's ethos as a guide to professional identity. *Revista de Terapia Ocupacional, 5.*

Peloquin, S. M. (2007). Beliefs of the founders of the National Society for the Promotion of Occupational Therapy. *Revista de Terapia Ocupacional.*

Peloquin, S. M. (2007). History matters. *Revista de Terapia Ocupacional.*

Peloquin, S. M. (2007). A reconsideration of occupational therapy's core values. *American Journal of Occupational Therapy, 61,* 474–478.

Peloquin, S. M. Cavazos, H., Marion, R., Stephenson, K. S., & Pearrow, D. (2007). Report on an interdisciplinary program for allied health. *Education for Health.*

Misch, D. A., & Peloquin, S. M. (2006). Developing empathy through confluent education. *Journal of Physical Therapy Education, 3,* 41–52.

Peloquin, S. M. (2006). Occupations: Strands of coherence in a life. *American Journal of Occupational Therapy, 60,* 236–239.

Abreu, B. C., & Peloquin, S. M. (2005). The quadraphonic approach holistic: Rehabilitation for brain injury. In N. Katz (Ed.), *Cognitive and occupation across the life span: Models for intervention in occupational therapy* (2nd ed.). Bethesda, MD: AOTA Press.

Ledet, L., Kaufman C. E., & Peloquin, S. M. (2005). Conceptualization, formative evaluation, and design of a process for student professional development. *American Journal of Occupational Therapy, 59,* 457–466.

Peloquin, S. M. (2005). Affirming empathy as a moral disposition. In R. B. Purtilo, G. M. Jensen, & C. B. Royeen (Eds.), *Educating for moral action: A sourcebook in health and rehabilitation ethics.* Philadelphia: F. A. Davis.

Peloquin, S. M. (2005). The art of practice. In F. Kronenberg, S. Algado, & N. Pollard (Eds.), *Occupational therapy without borders: The spirit of survivors.* Edinburgh, Scotland: Churchill Livingstone/Elsevier.

Peloquin, S. M. (2005). Embracing our ethos, reclaiming our heart (2005 Eleanor Clarke Slagle Lecture). *American Journal of Occupational Therapy, 59,* 611–625.

Peloquin, S. M. (2005). Ethics in research. In D. Blessing (Ed.), *Physician assistant's guide to research and medical literature.* Philadelphia: F. A. Davis.

Peloquin, S. M. (2005). Foreword. In R. Padilla (Ed.), *A professional legacy: The Eleanor Clarke Slagle Lectures in occupational therapy, 1955–2004* (p. xiii). Bethesda, MD: AOTA Press.

Abreu, B. C., & Peloquin, S. M. (2004). Affirming diversity within occupational therapy. *American Journal of Occupational Therapy, 33,* 353–359.

Peloquin, S. M. (2003, June). Creating a practice climate: Elaboration on the first three strategies. *Education Special Interest Section Quarterly, 13,* 3–4.

Peloquin, S. M. (2003, September). Creating a practice climate: Elaboration on the next three strategies. *Education Special Interest Section Quarterly, 13,* 3–4.

Peloquin, S. M. (2003, December). Creating a practice climate: Elaborations on the last three strategies. *Education Special Interest Section Quarterly, 13,* 6–7.

Peloquin, S. M. (2003, March). Creating a practice climate in academic settings. *Education Special Interest Section Quarterly, 13,* 1–4.

Peloquin, S. M. (2003). Historical reflections. In E. Crepeau, E. Cohn, & B. Schell (Eds.), *Willard and Spackman's occupational therapy* (10th ed.). Philadelphia: Lippincott Williams & Wilkins.

Peloquin, S. M. (2003). Spirituality: Meanings related to occupational therapy. In E. Crepeau, E. Cohn, & B. Schell (Eds.), *Willard and Spackman's occupational therapy* (10th ed.). Philadelphia: Lippincott Williams & Wilkins.

Peloquin, S. M. (2003). The therapeutic relationship: Manifestations and challenges. In E. Crepeau, E. Cohn, & B. Schell (Eds.), *Willard and Spackman's occupational therapy* (10th ed.). Philadelphia: Lippincott Williams & Wilkins.

Peloquin, S. M., & Osborne, K. A. (2003). Establishing a practice climate in classroom settings. *Journal of Allied Health, 32,* 78–85.

Peloquin, S. M. (2002). Confluence: Moving forward with affective strength. *American Journal of Occupational Therapy, 56*(1), 69–77.

Peloquin, S. M. (2002). Reclaiming the vision of *Reaching for Heart as Well as Hands. American Journal of Occupational Therapy, 56*(5), 517–525.

Stephenson, K. S., Peloquin, S. M., Richmond, S. A., Hinman, M. R., & Christiansen, C. H. (2002). Changing educational paradigms to prepare allied health professionals. *Education for Health, 15*(1), 37–49.

Froman, R., & Peloquin, S. M. (2001). Rethinking the use of the Hogan Empathy Scale. *American Journal of Occupational Therapy, 55*(5), 566–572.

Peloquin, S. M. (2001). Ethics in research. In D. Blessing (Ed.), *Physician assistant's guide to research and medical literature.* Philadelphia: F. A. Davis.

Peloquin, S. M. (2001). Integrating ethics and research. In E. Crepeau (Ed.), *Integrating research into occupational therapy education.* Bethesda, MD: American Occupational Therapy Association.

Peloquin, S. M. (2000, January). Do we *really* want to call them consumers? *OT Practice,* pp. 26–28.

Peloquin, S. M. (2000). Expanding the utility of scholarly activity: Establishing links with continued education. In P. Crist (Ed.), *Innovations in occupational therapy education* (pp. 157–165). Bethesda, MD: American Occupational Therapy Association.

Punwar, A., & Peloquin, S. (2000). *Occupational therapy principles and practice.* Baltimore: Lippincott Williams & Wilkins.

Babola, K., & Peloquin, S. M. (1999). Making a clinical climate: An assessment. *American Journal of Occupational Therapy, 53*(4), 373–380.

Abreu, B., Peloquin, S., & Ottenbacher, K. (1998). Competence in scientific inquiry and research. *American Journal of Occupational Therapy, 52*(9), 751–759.

Davidson, D., & Peloquin, S. (1998). *Making connections with others: A handbook on interpersonal practice.* Bethesda, MD: American Occupational Therapy Association.

Peloquin, S. M. (1998). Historical reflections. In E. Crepeau & M. Neistadt (Eds.), *Willard and Spackman's occupational therapy* (9th ed.). Philadelphia: Lippincott Williams & Wilkins.

Peloquin, S. M. (1998). The therapeutic relationship. In E. Crepeau & M. Neistadt (Eds.), *Willard and Spackman's occupational therapy* (9th ed.). Philadelphia: Lippincott Williams & Wilkins.

Peloquin, S. M. (1997). Should we trade person-centered care for a consumer-based model? *American Journal of Occupational Therapy, 51*(7), 612–615.

Peloquin, S. M. (1996). Art: An occupation with promise for developing empathy. *American Journal of Occupational Therapy, 50*(8), 655–661.

Peloquin, S. M. (1996). Nationally Speaking—The spiritual depth of occupation: Making worlds and making lives. *American Journal of Occupational Therapy, 51*(3), 167–168.

Peloquin, S. M. (1996). Now that we have managed care, shall we inspire it? *American Journal of Occupational Therapy, 50*(6), 455–459.

Peloquin, S. M. (1996). Using the arts to enhance confluent learning. *American Journal of Occupational Therapy, 50*(2), 148–151.

Peloquin, S. M., & Abreu, B. A. (1996). The academic and clinical worlds: Shall we make meaningful connections? *American Journal of Occupational Therapy, 50*(7), 588–591.

Peloquin, S. M., & Babola, K. B. (1996). Making a clinical climate in the classroom. *American Journal of Occupational Therapy, 50*(10), 894–898.

Peloquin, S. M. (1995). Communication skills: Why not turn to a training model? *American Journal of Occupational Therapy, 49*(7), 721–723.

Peloquin, S. M. (1995). The fullness of empathy: Reflections and illustrations. *American Journal of Occupational Therapy, 49*(1), 24–31.

Peloquin, S. M. (1994). Moral treatment: How a caring practice lost its rationale. *American Journal of Occupational Therapy, 48*(2), 167–173.

Peloquin, S. M. (1994). Occupational therapy as art and science: Should the older definition be reclaimed? *American Journal of Occupational Therapy, 48*(11), 1093–1096.

Peloquin, S. M. (1993). The depersonalization of patients: A profile gleaned from narratives. *American Journal of Occupational Therapy, 47*(9), 830–837.

Peloquin, S. M. (1993). The patient–therapist relationship: Beliefs that shape care: Reflections from narratives. *American Journal of Occupational Therapy, 47*(10), 935–942.

Peloquin, S. M., & Davidson, D. A. (1993). Interpersonal skills for practice: An elective course. *American Journal of Occupational Therapy, 47*(3), 260–264.

Peloquin, S. M. (1991). Occupational therapy service: Individual and collective understanding of the founders, part I. *American Journal of Occupational Therapy, 45*(4), 352–359.

Peloquin, S. M. (1991). Occupational therapy service: Individual and collective understanding of the founders, part II. *American Journal of Occupational Therapy, 45*(8), 733–744.

Peloquin, S. M. (1991). Time as a commodity: Implications and reflections. *American Journal of Occupational Therapy, 45*(2), 147–154.

Peloquin, S. M. (1990). AIDS: Toward a compassionate response. *American Journal of Occupational Therapy, 44*(3), 271–278.

Peloquin, S. M. (1990). Helping through touch: The embodiment of caring. *Journal of Religion and Health, 28*(4), 299–322.

Peloquin, S. M. (1990). The patient–therapist relationship in occupational therapy: Understanding visions and images. *American Journal of Occupational Therapy, 44*(1), 13–21.

Peloquin, S. M. (1989). Moral treatment: Contexts considered. *American Journal of Occupational Therapy, 43*(8), 537–544.

Peloquin, S. M. (1989). Sustaining the art of practice. *American Journal of Occupational Therapy, 43*(4), 219–226.

Peloquin, S. M. (1988). Linking purpose to procedure during interactions with patients. *American Journal of Occupational Therapy, 42*(12), 775–781.

Peloquin, S. M. (1987, March). Continued learning: An adaptive response. *Mental Health Special Interest Section Quarterly.*

Peloquin, S. M. (1986). Uniform Terminology as a basis for goal formulation. *Occupational Therapy in Mental Health, 6*(4), 49–62.

Peloquin, S. M. (1983). The development of an occupational therapy interview/therapy set procedure. *American Journal of Occupational Therapy, 37*(7), 457–461.

Kathlyn Louise Reed, PhD, OTR, FAOTA, MLIS, AHIP—1986

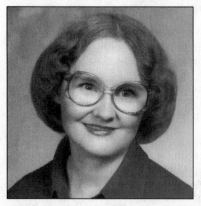

Kathlyn L. Reed is a visiting Professor at Texas Woman's University. She was born June, 2, 1940, in Detroit, Michigan, to Herbert Curtis Reed and Jessie Ruth Krehbiel Reed. She had only one sibling, who died at early age from bronchiolitis. Her father worked as research chemist in aviation and furniture finishes from 1931 to 1958 and as a store owner (paint, wallpaper, and hobbies) from 1958 to 1975. Her mother was an executive secretary with Hartford Insurance in Kansas City, Missouri, from 1930 to 1937, a housewife from 1938 to 1958, and co-owner of family business from 1958 to 1975.

Due to her father's profession, the family moved around the United States often. She lived in Detroit until 1940; in Stoneham (Boston), Massachusetts, from 1940 to 1942; in Louisville, Kentucky, from 1942 to 1946; in Rocky River (Cleveland), Ohio, from 1946 to 1950; in Grand Rapids, Michigan, from 1950 to 1956; in Rockford, Illinois, from 1956 to 1958, where she graduated from East Rockford High School in 1958; and in Beloit, Wisconsin starting in 1958.

Upon high school graduation, Reed attended the University of Wisconsin, Madison, completing 90 credits and then transferring to the University of Kansas, Lawrence, where she obtained a bachelor's degree in occupational therapy. She holds two master's degrees, one in organization and administration of occupational therapy from Western Michigan, Kalamazoo, and the second in library and information studies from the University of Oklahoma, Norman. In 1973, she received a doctorate in special education from the University of Washington in Seattle.

Reed worked as a staff therapist in psychiatric services at the Kansas University Medical Center and later served as a supervisor of psychiatric occupational therapy services at the University of Washington Hospital in Seattle. Throughout Reed's career, she has served a consultant in areas of occupational therapy, public health, research, developmental disabilities, Medicare, and pediatric orthopedics. Her academic career includes serving as professor at University of Oklahoma; Western Michigan University; and Texas Woman's University, Houston Center, as well as a graduate coordinator the University of Washington. Today, she remains active as a publicist, educator, and consultant for occupational therapy.

Reed was named to the Roster of Fellows of the American Occupational Therapy Association (AOTA) in 1975 and received the AOTA Award of Merit in 1983, the Award of Merit from the Canadian Occupational Therapy Association in 1988, and the AOTA Service Award in 1986 and 2001. The American Occupational Therapy Foundation has granted her the following awards: certificate of appreciation for work in developing the *Occupational Therapy Thesaurus* (1987) and certificate of appreciation for reviewing grant proposals (1990). She also has been honored with a certificate of appreciation from the American Occupational Therapy Certification Board (1989), was named Senior Member of the Academy of Health Information Professionals of the Medical Library Association (1993) and Distinguished Member (1998), received the Colby Award as outstanding professional from Sigma Kappa Social Sorority (1994), and received the Roster of Merit Award from the Texas Occupational Therapy Association (2002).

Linking Key Messages of the 1986 Eleanor Clarke Slagle Lecture to the AOTA *Centennial Vision:* My message was and is that occupational therapists and assistants must make a concerted effort to study and better understand the conceptual and theoretical heritage of occupational therapy. If we do not know and do not adequately articulate what occupational therapy is as a discipline, why should we expect others to understand? Occupational therapy is not a typical profession. It did not come from an existing academic discipline (it selected knowledge and skills from several) or from the advances in one new technology (it embraced several). The profession came from studying the needs of different marginalized groups of people (those with diseases, disabilities, and injuries) to enable them to engage and participate more fully in daily occupations and everyday activities and tasks. My lecture focused on how media and methods have been selected over the years to enhance people's abilities to engage and participate in daily occupation and everyday activities. My point was and is that media and methods will continue to change because the needs of the people we serve will change in response to environmental and contextual factors (physical, personal, social, political, economic, cultural, historical, and virtual). If a better understanding of our own professional heritage is subsumed under the rubrics of "science-driven" and "evidence-based," then my message is concurrent with the *Centennial Vision*, but I'm not sure that the concept of a theory-driven profession is included.

—Kathlyn Reed

Bibliography

Davidson, H., & Reed, K. L. (2008). Community adaptive planning assessment. In B. J. Hemphill-Pearson (Ed.), *Assessments in occupational therapy mental health* (2nd ed., pp. 127–143). Thorofare, NJ: Slack.

Reed, K. L. (2008). Stay focused on solutions in EI. *Advance for Occupational Therapy Practitioners, 24*(18), 5, 12.

Reed, K. L., & Peters, C. (2008). Occupational therapy values and beliefs, part IV: A time of professional identify, 1970–1985—Would the real therapist please stand up? *OT Practice, 13*(18), 15–18.

Reed, K. L., & Slater, D. Y. (2008). Ethics in governance. In D. Y. Slater (Ed.), *Reference guide to the occupational therapy ethics standards* (2008 ed., pp. 97–99). Bethesda, MD: AOTA Press.

White, V. K., & Reed, K. L. (2008). A summary of assessments in wellness. In B. J. Hemphill-Pearson (Ed.), *Assessments in occupational therapy mental health* (2nd ed., pp. 331–345). Thorofare, NJ: Slack.

Reed, K. L. (2007). Assessments of roles, habits, and routines. In I. E. Asher (Ed.), *Occupational therapy assessment tools: An annotated index* (3rd ed., pp. 619–532). Bethesda, MD: AOTA Press.

Reed, K. L., & Peters, C. (2007). Occupational therapy values and beliefs, part III: A new view of occupation and the profession: 1950–1969. *OT Practice, 12*(22), 17–21.

Reed, K. L. (2006). Occupational therapy values and beliefs: The formative years: 1904–1929. *OT Practice, 11*(7), 21–25.

Reed, K. L., & Peters, C. (2006). Occupational therapy values and beliefs, part II: The Great Depression and war years: 1930–1949. *OT Practice, 11*(18), 17–22.

Reed, K. L. (2005). Dr. Hall and the work cure. *Occupational Therapy in Health Care, 19*(3), 33–50.

Pauls, J., & Reed, K. L. (2004). *Quick reference to physical therapy* (2nd ed.). Austin, TX: Pro-Ed.

Reed, K. L. (2004). Concepts for the 21st century. In C. Christensen & C. Baum (Eds.), *Occupational therapy: Performance, participation, and well-being* (3rd ed., pp. 568–625). Thorofare, NJ: Slack.

Reed, K. L. (2000). *Quick reference to occupational therapy* (2nd ed.). Gaithersburg, MD: Aspen.

Pore, S. G., & Reed, K. L. (1999). *Quick reference to speech–language pathology.* Gaithersburg, MD: Aspen.

Reed, K. L. (1999). Mapping the literature of occupational therapy. *Bulletin of the Medical Library Association, 87*(3), 298–304.

Reed, K. L. (1999). The model of personal adaptation through occupation. In C. Jerosch-Herold, U. Maratzki, B. M. Hack, & P. Weber (Eds.), *Ergotherapie–reflexion und anlyse: Konzeptionelle modelle fur die ergotherapeutische praxis* (pp. 83–125). Berlin: Springer.

Reed, K. L., & Sanderson, S. N. (1999). *Concepts of occupational therapy* (4th ed.). Baltimore: Williams & Wilkins.

Reed, K. L. (1997). Theory and frame of reference. In M. E. Neistadt & E. E. Crepeau (Eds.), *Willard and Spackman's occupational therapy* (9th ed., pp. 521–524). Philadelphia: J. B. Lippincott.

Reed, K. L., & Cunningham, S. (1997). *Internet for rehabilitation professionals.* Philadelphia: Lippincott-Raven.

Cohen, H., & Reed, K. L. (1996). The historical development of neuroscience in physical rehabilitation. *American Journal of Occupational Therapy, 50*, 561–568.

Pauls, J., & Reed, K. L. (1996). *Quick reference to physical therapy.* Gaithersburg, MD: Aspen.

Reed, K. L. (1996). *Medical library research—A down and dirty approach* (Audiovisual). Houston, TX: Medical–Legal Consulting Institute.

Reed, K. L. (1995, Fall). Action research hypothesis. *Newsletter of the Library Research Section of MLA*, pp. 5, 8.

Reed, K. L. (1995). Citation analysis of faculty publication: Beyond Science Citation Index and Social Science Citation Index. *Bulletin of the Medical Library Association, 83*(4), 503–508.

Reed, K. L. (1995). Ready to surf the Internet? *Medico–Legal Newsletter, 7*(1), 1, 5–7.

Reed, K. L. (1995). Turf wars in the clinic. *Advance for Physical Therapists, 6*(43), 10–11.

Reed, K. L. (1994). History of neuroscience in rehabilitation. *Synapse: Neurosciences Division Newsletter of the Canadian Physiotherapy Association, 14*(2), 7–9.

Reed, K. L. (1994). Locating information on psychological and educational tests. *Medical Reference Service Quarterly, 13*(3), 27–36.

Reed, K. L. (1993). The beginning of occupational therapy. In H. Hopkins & H. Smith (Eds.), *Willard and Spackman's occupational therapy* (8th ed., pp. 26–43). Philadelphia: J. B. Lippincott.

Reed, K. L. (1992). History of federal legislation for persons with disabilities. *American Journal of Occupational Therapy, 46*, 397–418.

Reed, K. L. (1992). Not just a plain old library anymore. *Library Lines of the Houston Academy of Medicine–Texas Medical Center Library, 5*(4), 1–2.

Reed, K. L., & Sanderson, S. N. (1992). *Concepts of occupational therapy* (3rd ed.). Baltimore: Williams & Wilkins.

Reed, K. L. (1991). *Quick reference to occupational therapy.* Gaithersburg, MD: Aspen.

Reed, K. L. (1990). CD-ROM discs in the HAM–TMC Library. *Library Lines of the Houston Academy of Medicine–Texas Medical Center Library, 4*(4), 1–2.

Reed, K. L. (1990). Chronology of publication dates: From newspapers to the professional literature. *Library Lines of the Houston Academy of Medicine–Texas Medical Center Library, 4*(8), 2.

Reed, K. L. (1989, Spring). Research bibliography. *Hypothesis: The Newsletter of the Library Research Section of MLA.*

Reed, K. L. (1988). Focus on nursing and allied health resources. *Library Lines of the Houston Academy of Medicine–Texas Medical Center Library, 1*(12), 1–2.

Reed, K. L. (1988). Occupational therapy articles in serial publications: An analysis of sources. *Medical Library Association Bulletin, 76*(2), 125–130.

Reed, K. L. (1986). "The Making of Rehabilitation" [Book Review]. *American Journal of Occupational Therapy, 40*, 437–438.

Reed, K. L. (1986). The role of the COTA in work and productive occupational programs. In S. Ryan (Ed.), *The Certified Occupational Therapy Assistant: Roles and responsibilities* (pp. 265–293). Thorofare, NJ: Slack.

Reed, K. L. (1986). Tools of practice: Heritage or baggage? (1986 Eleanor Clarke Slagle Lecture). *American Journal of Occupational Therapy, 40*, 597–695.

Reed, K. L. (1985). The functions of professional ethics. *Occupational Therapy News, 39*(6).

Reed, K. L. (1985). Values orientation in occupational therapy and vocational readiness. In M. Kirkland (Ed.), *Planning and implementing vocational readiness in occupational therapy* (pp. 35–43). Rockville, MD: American Occupational Therapy Association.

Reed, K. L. (1984). *Models of practice in occupational therapy*, Baltimore: Williams & Wilkins.

Reed, K. L. (1984). Understanding theory: A first step in research. *American Journal of Occupational Therapy, 38*, 677–682.

Reed, K. L. (1983). The occupational therapy library: A professional resource. *American Journal of Occupational Therapy, 37*, 412–413.

Reed, K. L., & Sanderson, S. R. (1983). *Concepts of occupational therapy* (2nd ed.). Baltimore: Williams & Wilkins.

Reed, K. L. (1982). Did you know—Do you remember? *American Journal of Occupational Therapy, 36*, 630.

Reed, K. L. (1980). Therapy for learning disabilities. *Newsletter of the Oklahoma Division for Children With Learning Disabilities, 3*(2), 2–3.

Reed, K. L., & Sanderson, S. R. (1980). *Concepts of occupational therapy*. Baltimore: Williams & Wilkins.

Reed, K. L. (Ed.). (1975). *Fieldwork experience manual for supervisors, coordinators, and students*. Rockville, MD: American Occupational Therapy Association.

Reed, K. L. (1972). Certification of occupational therapists in public schools. *American Journal of Occupational Therapy, 26*, 406–409.

Mary Reilly, EdD, OTR—1961

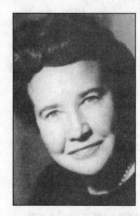

Mary Reilly is professor emeritus at the University of Southern California (USC), where she retired as professor and graduate coordinator of occupational therapy in 1977. She obtained a certificate in occupational therapy from Boston School of Occupational Therapy in 1940, a bachelor's degree from USC in 1951, and a master's degree from San Francisco State College in California in 1951. She earned her doctor of education degree from the University of California at Los Angeles in 1959.

Reilly was an occupational therapy consultant at the Service Command Surgeon's Office, Fourth Service Command, in Atlanta, Georgia, from 1944 to 1946. Her work in the Fourth Service Command included supervising occupational therapy programs in 11 general, 2 convalescent, and 6 regional and station hospitals, for which she received the Meritorious Civilian Service Award. Before World War II, she was director of occupational therapy in the Sigma Gamma Hospital School, Detroit, Michigan.

Reilly is recognized for developing a frame of reference for occupational behavior that describes the biopsychosocial nature of the human occupations of work, play, and self-care. Major influences on her work came from social science, psychology, vocational theorists, and the founders of occupational therapy.

Since her retirement, Reilly has served as a consultant for USC, as well as for programs at Oxford and Kent Universities, England, and at the University of Madrid. She was guest lecturer at selected tutorial sessions at Oxford.

Bibliography

Licht, S., & Reilly, M. (1943). The correlation of physical and occupational therapy. *Occupational Therapy and Rehabilitation, 22*, 171–175.

Reilly, M. (1943). Organization of an occupational therapy section in an Army or Navy hospital. *War Medicine 3*, 512–531.

Reilly, M. (Ed.). (1944). Army issue. *Occupational Therapy and Rehabilitation, 25*, 163–187.

Reilly, M., & Barton, W. E. (1944). Dos and donts in military occupational therapy. *Occupational Therapy and Rehabilitation, 23*, 121–123.

Reilly, M. (1946). *Technical manual 8-291 occupational therapy*. Washington, DC: U.S. War Department.

Reilly, M. (1949). Ruth A. Robinson, a biographical sketch. *American Journal of Occupational Therapy, 3*, 316.

Reilly, M. (1956). The role of the therapist in protective and functional devices. *American Journal of Occupational Therapy, 10*, 118–132.

Reilly, M., & Ryerson, A. M. (1956). Session on neurology: Therapeutically influenced recovery. *American Journal of Occupational Therapy, 10*, 229–232.

Reilly, M. (1958). An occupational therapy curriculum for 1965. *American Journal of Occupational Therapy, 12*, 293–299.

Reilly, M. (1959). *Occupational therapy: Report of coordinated training in rehabilitation*. Phoenix, AZ: Western Interstate Commission for Higher Education.

Reilly, M. (1960). Research potentiality of occupational therapy. *American Journal of Occupational Therapy, 14*, 206–209.

Reilly, M. (1961). In Memoriam: H. Elizabeth Messick. *American Journal of Occupational Therapy, 15*, 24–25.

Reilly, M. (1961). Planning curriculum revisions in physical therapy. *Physical Therapy Review, 41*, 302–330.

Reilly, M. (1962). Occupational therapy can be one of the great ideas of 20th-century medicine (1961 Eleanor Clarke Slagle Lecture). *American Journal of Occupational Therapy, 16*, 1–9.

Reilly, M. (1963). The Eleanor Clarke Slagle Lecture. *Canadian Journal of Occupational Therapy, 30*, 5–19.

Reilly, M. (1965). Medical information in the occupational therapy curriculum. In *Studies in Rehabilitation Counselor Training, Monograph* 4.

Reilly, M. (1966). The challenge of the future to an occupational therapist. *American Journal of Occupational Therapy, 20*, 221–225.

Reilly, M. (1966). A psychiatric occupational therapy program as a teaching model. *American Journal of Occupational Therapy, 22*, 61–67.

Reilly, M. (1966). Role of parent as model for child as future wage earner. *Today's Child.*

Reilly, M. (1967). The mental health team: Occupational therapy. In *Proceedings of the AMA 13th Annual Conference of State Mental Health Representatives of State Medical Associations,* Chicago.

Reilly, M. (1968). Introduction of scientific method into clinical practice. In *Proceedings of the Northern and Southern California Joint Occupational Therapy Association Conference,* Morro Bay.

Reilly, M. (1968). *Needed: A revolution in the care of chronic patients.* Medford, MA: Tufts University.

Reilly, M. (1969). The educational process. *American Journal of Occupational Therapy, 23,* 299–307.

Reilly, M. (1969). Selecting human development knowledge for occupational therapy. In W. L. West (Ed.), *Occupational therapy functions in interdisciplinary programs for children* (pp. 64–75). Rockville, MD: U.S. Department of Health, Education, and Welfare.

Reilly, M. (1971). The modernization of occupational therapy. *American Journal of Occupational Therapy, 25,* 243–246.

Reilly, M. (1971). Occupational therapy: A historical perspective: The modernization of occupational therapy. *American Journal of Occupational Therapy, 23,* 299–307.

Reilly, M. (1974). Defining a cobweb. In M. Reilly (Ed.), *Play as exploratory learning* (pp. 57–116). Beverly Hills, CA: Sage.

Reilly, M. (1974). An explanation of play. In M. Reilly (Ed.), *Play as exploratory learning* (pp. 117–149). Beverly Hills, CA: Sage.

Reilly, M. (1974). *Play as exploratory learning: A study of curiosity behavior.* Beverly Hills, CA: Sage.

Reilly, M. (1977). A Response To: Defining occupational therapy: The meaning of therapy and the virtues of occupation. *American Journal of Occupational Therapy, 31,* 673–674.

Reilly, M. (1984). The challenge of the future to an occupational therapist. *Occupational Therapy in Health Care, 1*(1), 89–98.

Reilly, M. (1984). The Issue Is: The importance of the client vs. patient issue for occupational therapy. *American Journal of Occupational Therapy, 38,* 404–406.

Joan C. Rogers, PhD, OTR, FAOTA—1983

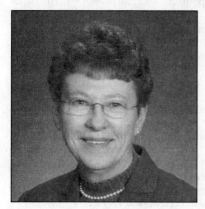

Joan Rogers was born in Buffalo, New York. She earned a BS in biology in 1966 from Canisius College, a master's degree in occupational therapy from the University of Southern California (USC) in 1968, and a doctor of philosophy in educational psychology and gerontology from the University of Illinois at Urbana–Champaign in 1975.

Rogers worked at the Edward J. Meyer Memorial Hospital in Buffalo and in other programs as a clinician. She is most associated with academia and began her academic career at the State University of New York (SUNY) at Buffalo in 1969 as an assistant clinical professor of occupational therapy. Rogers then assumed several positions at the USC, including assistant professor of occupational therapy, director of graduate studies, and interim chair of the College of Letters, Arts, and Sciences. In 1977, she moved back to Buffalo and became a research associate and professor of occupational therapy at SUNY. From 1978 to 1984, Rogers held academic appointments at the University of North Carolina–Chapel Hill in occupational therapy and medicine. She was employed as a faculty associate from 1985 to 1991 at the Geriatric Education Center of Pennsylvania at Temple University as part of a U.S. Public Health Service Grant. She later was director of geropsychiatric occupational therapy, clinical, educational, and research services at the Western Psychiatric Institute and Clinic of the University of Pittsburgh Medical Center until 1998.

Currently, Rogers is a professor and department chairperson at the University of Pittsburgh and a faculty member of the McGowan Institute for Regenerative Medicine. She was inducted into the AOTA Roster of Fellows in 1981 and awarded the Eleanor Clarke Slagle Lectureship in 1983. She was awarded several service awards from the association and in 1984 was elected to the Academy of Research as a charter member from the American Occupational Therapy Foundation for exemplary and distinguished contribution toward the science of occupational therapy. She has been selected as a visiting scholar to Queens University in Ontario, Canada, and a distinguished invited lecturer to several universities in the United States. In 1990, she received the AOTA Award of Merit. She was recognized as a Research Fellow by the Arthritis Health Professions in 1991 and elected a Fellow of the Gerontological Society of America in 2000.

Rogers's research interests include strategies for community practice, clinical reasoning of occupational therapists, self-care capacity of older adults, functional outcomes of treatment, validity of functional assessment methodologies, quality of life in patients with rheumatoid arthritis, and neuropsychology. Her research interests are extensive and include numerous other areas.

On a Personal Note From a Phone Interview: Rogers credits colleagues, students, and another Slagle lecturer, Irene Hollis, as inspirations for her lecture. Rogers's desire to highlight how students build thinking skills was eloquently translated into her lecture. She notes that, as the profession is thrust toward evidenced-based practice, her comments are still relevant today with the three-part message of science, art, and ethics. She encourages the profession and the association to honor scholarship and respect the Eleanor Clarke Slagle Lectureship as the highest academic award recognizing quality research and academic performance.

Bibliography

Published Honorary Lectures

Rogers, J. C. (1983). Clinical reasoning: The ethics, science, and art (1983 Eleanor Clarke Slagle Lecture). *American Journal of Occupational Therapy, 37*, 601–616.

Rogers, J. C. (1984). *From independence to interdependence: Functional capacity of the elderly. The 1983–1984 Brookdale Lecture.* Columbia University, NY: Brookdale Institute on Aging and Human Development.

Peer-Reviewed Articles

Rogers, J. C., & Figone J. J. (1978). The avocational pursuits of rehabilitants with traumatic quadriplegia. *American Journal of Occupational Therapy, 32*, 571–576.

Rogers J. C., Weinstein J. M., & Figone J. J. (1978). The interest check list: An empirical assessment. *American Journal of Occupational Therapy, 32*, 628–630.

Rogers J. C., & Figone J. J. (1979). Psychosocial parameters in treating the person with quadriplegia. *American Journal of Occupational Therapy, 33*, 432–439.

Rogers J. C. (1980). Advocacy: The key to assessing the older client. *Journal of Gerontological Nursing, 6*, 33–36.

Rogers J. C. (1980). The design of the master's degree in occupational therapy: Part 1: A logical approach. *American Journal of Occupational Therapy, 34*, 113–118.

Rogers J. C. (1980). The design of the master's degree in occupational therapy: Part 2: An empirical approach. *American Journal of Occupational Therapy, 34*, 176–184.

Rogers J. C., & Figone, J. J. (1980). Traumatic quadriplegia: A follow-up study of self-care skills. *Archives of Physical Medicine and Rehabilitation, 61*, 316–321.

Rogers J. C., & Hill, D. J. (1980). Learning style preferences of bachelor's and master's students. *American Journal of Occupational Therapy, 34*, 789–793.

Rogers J. C., & Mann, W. C. (1980). The relationship between professional productivity and educational level, part I: Review of literature and methodology. *American Journal of Occupational Therapy, 34*, 387–392.

Rogers J. C., & Mann W. C. (1980). The relationship between professional productivity and educational level, part II: Results and discussion. *American Journal of Occupational Therapy, 34*, 460–468.

Rogers, J. C. (1981). Gerontic occupational therapy. *American Journal of Occupational Therapy, 35*, 663–666.

Rogers J. C. (1982). Order and disorder in medicine and occupational therapy. *American Journal of Occupational Therapy, 36*, 28–35.

Rogers J. C. (1982). Terminology quandary in education. *American Journal of Occupational Therapy, 36*, 188–192.

Rogers J. C. (1982). Sponsorship: Developing leaders for occupational therapy. *American Journal of Occupational Therapy, 36*, 309–313.

Rogers J. C. (1982). The spirit of independence: Evolution of a philosophy. *American Journal of Occupational Therapy, 36*, 709–715.

Rogers J. C. (1982). Teaching clinical reasoning for practice in geriatrics. *Physical and Occupational Therapy in Geriatrics, 1*, 29–37.

Rogers J. C., & Masagatani, G. (1982). Clinical reasoning of occupational therapists during the initial assessment of physically disabled patients: A pilot study. *Occupational Therapy Journal of Research, 2*, 195–219.

Rogers J. C., & Snow T. (1982). An assessment of the feeding behaviors of the institutionalized elderly. *American Journal of Occupational Therapy, 36*, 375–380.

Sparling, J, & Rogers, J. C. (1985). Feeding assessment: Development of a biopsychosocial instrument. *Occupational Therapy Journal of Research, 5*, 3–23.

Sparling, J, & Rogers, J. C. (1985). Intergenerational interventions: A reciprocal service delivery system for preschoolers, adolescents, and older persons. *Educational Gerontology, 11*, 41–46.

Rogers, J. C. (1986). Occupational therapy assessment for older adults with depression: Asking the right questions. *Physical and Occupational Therapy in Geriatrics, 5*, 13–33.

Bynum, H. S., & Rogers, J. C. (1987). The use and effectiveness of assistive devices possessed by patients seen in home care. *Occupational Therapy Journal of Research, 7*, 181–191.

Jackoway, I. S., Rogers, J. C, & Snow, T. L. (1987). The Role Change Assessment: An interview tool for evaluating older adults. *Occupational Therapy in Mental Health, 7*, 17–37.

Rogers, J. C., Marcus, C. L., & Snow, T. L. (1987). Maude: A case of sensory deprivation. *American Journal of Occupational Therapy, 41*, 673–676.

Rogers, J. C., Brayley, C. R., & Cox, R. C. (1988). Educational level and professional activities. *American Journal of Occupational Therapy, 42*, 642–646.

Rogers, J. C., & Dodson, S. C. (1988). Burnout in occupational therapists. *American Journal of Occupational Therapy, 42*, 787–792.

Skurla, E., Rogers, J., & Sunderland, T. (1988). Direct assessment of patients with Alzheimer's disease. *Journal of the American Geriatrics Society, 36*, 97–103.

Cheng, S., & Rogers, J. C. (1989). Changes in occupational role performance after a severe burn: A retrospective study. *American Journal of Occupational Therapy, 43*, 17–24.

Rogers, J. C. (1989). The occupational therapy home assessment: The home as a therapeutic environment. *Journal of Home Health Care Practice, 273–281.*

Rogers, J. C. (1989). Therapeutic activity and health status. *Topics in Geriatric Rehabilitation, 4*(4), 1–11.

McCue, M., Rogers, J. C., & Goldstein, G. (1990). Relationship between neuropsychological and functional assessment in elderly neuropsychiatric patients. *Rehabilitation Psychology, 35,* 91–99.

Holm, M. B., & Rogers, J. C. (1991). High, low or no assistive technology devices for older adults undergoing rehabilitation? *International Journal of Technology and Aging, 4,* 153–162.

Rogers, J. C., & Holm, M. B. (1991). Occupational therapy diagnostic reasoning: A component of clinical reasoning. *American Journal of Occupational Therapy, 45,* 1045–1053.

Rogers, J. C., & Holm, M. B. (1991). Task performance of older adults and low assistive technology devices. *International Journal of Technology and Aging, 4,* 93–106.

Rogers, J. C., & Holm, M. B. (1991). Teaching older persons with depression. *Topics in Geriatric Rehabilitation, 6*(3), 27–44.

Goldstein, G., McCue, M., Rogers, J. C., & Nussbaum, P. D. (1992). Diagnostic differences in memory test based predictions of functional capacity in the elderly. *Neuropsychological Rehabilitation, 2,* 307–317.

Rogers, J. C., Hill, D. J., Holm, M. B., & Wasser, T. (1992). Educational level and professional activities of occupational therapists. *Occupational Therapy Journal of Research, 12,* 148–158.

Rogers, J. C., & Holm, M. B. (1992). Assistive technology device usage in patients with rheumatic disease. *American Journal of Occupational Therapy, 46,* 120–127.

Haley, P. B., Brancati, F., Rogers, J. C., Hanusa, B. H., & Kapoor, W. N. (1993). Measuring functional change in community acquired pneumonia: A pilot study using the Sickness Impact Profile. *Medical Care, 31,* 649–657.

Rogers, J. C., Holm, M. B., Goldstein, G., & Nussbaum, P. D. (1994). Stability and change in functional assessment of patients with geropsychiatric disorders. *American Journal of Occupational Therapy, 48,* 914–918.

Rogers, J. C., & Salta, J. (1994). Documenting functional outcomes. *American Journal of Occupational Therapy, 48,* 939–945.

Tomlin, G. S., Holm, M. B., Rogers, J. C., & Kwoh, C. K. (1996). Comparison of standard and alternative HAQ scoring procedures for documenting functional outcomes in patients with rheumatoid arthritis. *Journal of Rheumatology, 23,* 1524–1530.

DeSantis, J., Engberg, S., & Rogers, J. C. (1997). Geropsychiatric restraint use. *Journal of the American Geriatrics Society, 45,* 1515–1518.

Rogers, J. C., Holm, M. B., & Stone, R. S. (1997). Evaluation of daily living tasks: The home care advantage. *American Journal of Occupational Therapy, 51,* 410–422.

Rosen, J., Rogers, J. C., Marin, R. S., Mulsant, B. H., Shahar, A., & Reynolds, C. F. (1997). Control-relevant interventions in the treatment of minor and major depression in a long-term-care facility. *American Journal of Geriatric Psychiatry, 5,* 247–257.

Holm, M. B., Rogers, J. C., & Kwoh, C. K. (1998). Predictors of functional disability in patients with rheumatoid arthritis. *Arthritis Care and Research, 11,* 346–355.

Holm, M. B., Rogers, J. C., Burgio, L. D., Hardin, J. M., Hsu, C., & McDowell, B. J. (1999). Observational data collection using computer and manual methods: Which informs best? *Topics in Health Information Management, 19,* 15–25.

Rogers, J. C., Holm, M., Burgio, L. D., Granieri, E., Hsu, C., Hardin, J. M., et al. (1999). Improving morning care routines of nursing home residents with dementia. *Journal of the American Geriatrics Society, 47,* 1049–1057.

Rogers, J. C., & Holm, M. B. (2000). Daily-living skills and habits of older women with depression. *Occupational Therapy Journal of Research, 20*(Suppl. 1), 68S–85S.

Rogers, J. C., Holm, M. B., Burgio, L. D., Hsu, C., Hardin, J. M., & McDowell, B. J. (2000). Excess disability during morning care in nursing home residents with dementia. *International Psychogeriatrics, 12,* 267–282.

Lenze, E., & Rogers, J. C. (2001). The association of late-life depression and anxiety with physical disability. *American Journal of Geriatric Psychiatry, 9,* 113–135.

Rogers, J. C., & Dolhi, C. (2001). Dementia, nutrition, and self-feeding: A systematic review of the literature. *Occupational Therapy in Health Care, 15*(3/4), 59–87.

Rogers, J. C., Gwinn, S., & Holm, M. B. (2001). Comparing activities of daily living assessment instruments: FIM™, MDS, OASIS, MDS–PAC. *Physical and Occupational Therapy in Geriatrics, 18*(3), 1–25.

Rogers, J. C., Holm, M. B., Beach, S., Schulz, R., & Starz, T. W. (2001). Task independence, safety, and adequacy among nondisabled and OAK-disabled older women. *Arthritis Care and Research, 45,* 410–418.

Rogers, J. C. (2002). Understanding Alzheimer's disease: From diagnosis to rehabilitation. *Physical and Occupational Therapy in Geriatrics, 20,* 103–123.

Rogers, J. C., Holm, M. B., & Perkins, L. (2002). The trajectory of assistive device usage and user and non-user characteristics: Long-handled bath sponge. *Arthritis Care and Research, 47,* 645–650.

Lenze, E., Holm, M. B., Rogers, J. C., & Reynolds, C. F. (2003). Combining pharmacotherapy and psychotherapy in the rehabilitative and maintenance treatment of late-life depression. *Directions in Psychiatry, 23,* 43–54.

Rogers, J. C., Holm, M. B., Beach, S., Schulz, R., Cipriani, J., Fox, A., et al. (2003). Concordance of four methods of disability assessment using performance in the home as the criterion method. *Arthritis and Rheumatism, 49,* 640–647.

Rogers, J. C., & Irrgang, J. J. (2003). Measures of adult lower extremity function. *Arthritis and Rheumatism, 49*(Suppl.), S67–S84.

Lenze, E. J., Munin, M. C., Dew, M. A., Rogers, J. C., Seligman, K., Mulsant, B. H., et al. (2004). Adverse effects of depression and cognitive impairment on rehabilitation participation and recovery from hip fracture. *International Journal of Geriatric Psychiatry, 19,* 472–478.

Lenze, E. J., Munin, M. C., Quear, T., Dew, M. A., Rogers, J. C., Begley, A. E., et al. (2004). The Pittsburgh Rehabilitation Participation Scale: Reliability and validity of a clinician-rated measure of participation in acute rehabilitation. *Archives of Physical Medicine and Rehabilitation, 85,* 380–384.

Lenze, E. J., Munin, M. C., Ferrell, R. E., Pollock, B. G., Skidmore, E., Lotrich, F., Rogers, J. C., et al. (in press). Association of the serotonin transporter gene-linked polymorphic region (5-HTTLPR) genotype with depressive symptoms in elderly persons after hip fracture. *American Journal of Geriatric Psychiatry.*

Invited Published Papers

Rogers, J. C. (1982). Editorial. The occupational needs of older persons: A focus of occupational therapy practice. *Physical and Occupational Therapy in Geriatrics, 2,* 1–3.

Rogers, J. C. (1982). Guest Editorial: Educating the inquisitive practitioner. *Occupational Therapy Journal of Research, 2,* 3–11.

Rogers, J. C., & Snow, T. L. (1982). *Service-learning in aging: Implications for occupational therapy.* Washington, DC: National Council on Aging.

Rogers, J. C. (1983). Assistive devices: Aids to functional independence. *American Health Care Association Journal, 9*(2), 31–34, 36.

Rogers, J. C. (1983). Position Paper: Role and functions of occupational therapy in long-term care: Occupational therapy and activity programs. *American Journal of Occupational Therapy, 37,* 807–810.

Rogers, J. C. (1984). "I Can": Restoring courage through occupational therapy. *Generations, 8,* 20–22.

Rogers, J. C. (1984). Why study human occupation? *American Journal of Occupational Therapy, 38,* 47–49.

Rogers, J. C. (1985). Low technology devices: Helping impaired elders experience the challenge of retaining self-control. *Generations, 10,* 59–61.

Rogers, J. C. (1986). Nationally Speaking: Mentoring for career achievement and advancement. *American Journal of Occupational Therapy, 40,* 79–82.

Rogers, J. C. (1986). Position Paper: Occupational therapy services for Alzheimer's disease and related disorders. *American Journal of Occupational Therapy, 40,* 822–824.

Rogers, J. C. (1986). Rehabilitation philosophy for individuals with Alzheimer's disease. *Physical and Occupational Therapy in Geriatrics, 4,* 3–4.

Rogers, J. C. (1994). Position Paper: Occupational therapy services for persons with Alzheimer's disease and other dementias. *American Journal of Occupational Therapy, 48,* 1029–1031.

Rogers, J. C., & Holm, M. B. (1994). Nationally Speaking: Accepting the challenge of outcome research: Examining the effectiveness of occupational therapy practice. *American Journal of Occupational Therapy, 48,* 871–876.

Rogers, J. C., & Holm, M. B. (1997). Functional outcomes of occupational therapy. *Home Healthcare Consultant: Journal of Alternate Site Medicine and Management, 4,* 15–35.

Rogers, J. C. (2000). Habits: Do we practice what we preach? *Occupational Therapy Journal of Research, 20*(Suppl. 1), 119S–122S.

Rogers, J. C., & Holm, M. B. (2001). Behavioral rehabilitative activities of daily living intervention. *Alzheimer's Care Quarterly, 2,* 66–69.

Rogers, J. C., Holm, M. B., Beach, S., Schulz, R., & Starz, T. (2001). Task independence, safety, and adequacy among nondisabled and OAK-disabled older women. *Arthritis Care and Research, 45,* 410–418.

Books/Chapters

Rogers, J. C. (1983). The study of human occupation. In G. Kielhofner (Ed.), *Occupational therapy: Toward a definition of practice for the future* (pp. 93–124). Philadelphia: F. A. Davis.

Snow, T., Snow, D., & Rogers, J. (1984). Data-based articles in *AJOT.* In American Occupational Therapy Foundation (Ed.), *Bibliography of completed research in occupational therapy* (pp. A1–A137). Rockville, MD: Editor.

Rogers, J. C. (1985). Articulating a frame of reference in occupational therapy. In M. Kirkland & S. Robertson (Eds.), *Planning and implementing vocational readiness in occupational therapy* (pp. 137–145). Rockville, MD: American Occupational Therapy Association.

Rogers, J. C. (1985). Roles and functions of occupational therapy. In L. Davis & M. Kirkland (Eds.), *Roles of occupational therapy with the elderly* (pp. 75–79). Rockville, MD: American Occupational Therapy Association.

Rogers, J. C., & Kielhofner, G. (1985). Treatment planning. In G. Kielhofner (Ed.), *The model of human occupation: Theory and application* (pp. 136–146). Baltimore, MD: Williams & Wilkins.

Rogers, J. C., & Poole, J. (1985). The relationship between theory and research. In J. Morse (Ed.), *New dimensions in research for health professionals* (pp. 14–36). Laurel, MD: American Occupational Therapy Foundation & Ramsco.

Rogers, J. C., & Snow, T. (1985). Later adulthood. In G. Kielhofner (Ed.), *The model of human occupation: Theory and application* (pp. 123–133). Baltimore, MD: Williams & Wilkins.

Snow, T., & Rogers, J. C. (1985). Dysfunctional older adults In G. Kielhofner (Ed.), *The model of human occupation: Theory and application* (pp. 352–370). Baltimore, MD: Williams & Wilkins.

Rogers, J. C. (1987). Selection of evaluation instruments. In L. King Thomas & B. Hacker (Eds.), *A therapist's guide to pediatric assessment* (pp. 19–33). Boston: Little, Brown.

Rogers, J. C. (1988). The assessment of interests: The interest checklist. In B. Hemphill (Ed.), *The evaluative process: An integrated approach to occupational therapy assessments in mental health* (pp. 95–114). Thorofare, NJ: Slack.

Holm, M. B., & Rogers, J. C. (1989). The therapist's thinking behind the process of functional assessment II. In C. Royeen (Ed.), *AOTA's Self Study Series on Assessing Function.* Rockville, MD: American Occupational Therapy Association.

Rogers, J. C., & Holm, M. B. (1989). The therapist's thinking behind the process of functional assessment I. In C. Royeen (Ed.), *AOTA's Self Study Series on Assessing Function.* Rockville, MD: American Occupational Therapy Association.

Rogers, J. C. (1990). Improving the ability to perform daily tasks. In B. Kemp, K. Brummel-Smith, & J. Ramsdell (Eds.), *Geriatric rehabilitation* (pp. 137–155). Boston: Little, Brown.

Rogers, J. C., & Wood, W. (1992). Consultative models in geriatric psychiatry. In E. G. Jaffe & C. F. Epstein (Eds.), *Occupational therapy consultation: Theory, principles, and practice* (pp. 293–310). Hanover, MD: Mosby.

Rogers, J. C. (1993). Geriatric psychiatry. In H. L. Hopkins & H. D. Smith (Eds.), *Willard and Spackman's occupational therapy* (8th ed., pp. 753–764). Philadelphia: Lippincott.

Rogers, J. C., & Holm, M. B. (1994). Assessment: Self-care. In B. Bonder & M. B. Wagner (Eds.), *Functional performance of older adults* (pp. 181–202). Philadelphia: F. A. Davis.

Rogers, J. C. (1995). Assistive technology. In A. Romaine-Davis (Ed.), *Encyclopedia of home care for the elderly* (pp. 74–80). Westport, CT: Greenwood.

Rogers, J. C. (1995). Occupational therapy. In W. B. Abrams & R. Berkow (Eds.), *The Merck manual of geriatrics* (pp. 388–396). West Point, PA: Merck.

Rogers, J. C. (1996). Occupational role performance in late life. In AOTA (Ed.), *Role of occupational therapy with the elderly (ROTE)*. Bethesda, MD: American Occupational Therapy Association.

Holm, M. B., Rogers, J. C, & James, A. B. (1997). Treatment of activities of daily living. In M. E. Neistadt & E. B. Crepeau (Eds.), *Willard and Spackman's occupational therapy* (9th ed., pp. 323–364). Philadelphia: Lippincott.

Holm, M. B., Rogers, J. C., & Stone, R. G. (1997). Module 4: Referral, evaluation, and intervention in home health. In M. J. Youngstrom & M. Steinhauer (Eds.), *Occupational therapy in home health: Preparing for best practice*. Bethesda, MD: American Occupational Therapy Association.

Holm, M. B., Rogers, J. C., & Stone, R. G. (1997). Person–task–environment interventions: Decision-making guide. In M. E. Neistadt & E. B. Crepeau (Eds.), *Willard and Spackman's occupational therapy* (9th ed., pp. 471–499). Philadelphia: Lippincott.

Rogers, J. C., & Holm, M. B. (1997). Diagnostic reasoning: Decision-making for intervention. In C. Christiansen & C. Baum (Eds.), *Occupational therapy: Achieving human performance needs in daily living* (pp. 136–156). Thorofare, NJ: Slack.

Rogers, J. C., & Holm, M. B. (1997). Evaluation of activities of daily living. In M. E. Neistadt & E. B. Crepeau (Eds.), *Willard and Spackman's occupational therapy* (9th ed., pp. 185–208). Philadelphia: Lippincott.

Holm, M. B., & Rogers, J. C. (1998). Assessment and rehabilitation of adult brain function: The focus of occupational therapy. In G. Goldstein & S. R. Beers (Eds.), *Handbook of human brain function* (Vol. IV, pp. 9–31). New York: Plenum.

Rogers, J. C., & Holm, M. B. (1998). Assessment and rehabilitation of adult brain function: Geriatric rehabilitation. In G. Goldstein & S. R. Beers (Eds.), *Handbook of human brain function* (Vol. IV, pp. 87–109). New York: Plenum.

Fine, M. J., Stone, R. A., Singer, D. E., &Rogers, J. C. (1999). Pneumonia Outcomes Research Team (PORT): Processes and outcomes of care for patients with community-acquired pneumonia. In J. E. Dalen (Ed.), *The best of archives of internal medicine*. Washington, DC: American Medical Association.

Holm, M. B., & Rogers, J. C. (1999). Functional assessment: The Performance Assessment of Self-Care Skills. In B. J. Hemphill-Pearson (Ed.), *Mental health assessment in occupational therapy: An integrative approach to the evaluative process* (pp. 113–124). Thorofare, NJ: Slack.

Rogers, J. C., & Holm, M. B. (1999). The Role Change Assessment: An interview tool for older adults. In B. J. Hemphill-Pearson (Ed.), *Mental health assessments in occupational therapy: An integrative approach to the evaluative process* (pp. 73–82). Thorofare, NJ: Slack.

Rogers, J. C., & Dolhi, C. (2002). Dementia, nutrition, and self-feeding: A systematic review of the literature. In S. Paul & C. Q. Peterson (Eds.), *Interprofessional collaboration in occupational therapy* (pp. 59–87). New York: Hawthorn Press.

Rogers, J. C., & Gwinn, S. M. G. (2002). Functional assessment and outcomes. In D. Weiner, K. Herr, & T. E. Rudy (Eds.), *Persistent pain in older adults: An interdisciplinary guide for treatment* (pp. 133–159). New York: Springer.

Holm, M. B., Rogers, J. C., & James, A. B. (2003). Interventions for activities of daily living. In E. B. Crepeau, E. S. Cohn, & B. A. B. Schell (Eds.), *Willard and Spackman's occupational therapy* (10th ed., pp. 491–533). Philadelphia: Lippincott Williams & Wilkins.

Holm, M. B., & Rogers, J. C. (2003). Activities of daily living and instrumental activities of daily living. In E. B. Crepeau, E. S. Cohn, & B. A. B. Schell (Eds.), *Willard and Spackman's occupational therapy* (10th ed., pp. 315–339). Philadelphia: Lippincott Williams & Wilkins.

Holm, M. B., Rogers, J. C., & Stone R. G. (2003). Person–task–environment interventions: A decision making guide. In E. B. Crepeau, E. S. Cohn, & B. A. B. Schell (Eds.), *Willard and Spackman's occupational therapy* (10th ed., pp. 460–490). Philadelphia: Lippincott Williams & Wilkins.

Rogers, J. C. (2004). Occupational diagnosis. In M. Molineux (Ed.), *Occupation for occupational therapists*. Oxford, UK: Blackwell.

Margaret S. Rood, OTR, RPT, MA, FAOTA—1958

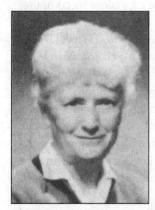

Margaret S. Rood was professor emeritus, University of Southern California (USC). She was recognized for her development of a neurophysiological approach in the treatment of central nervous system disorders, which has been used internationally by various therapy professions and medical fields. She presented numerous workshops, lectures, and symposia on this treatment approach.

Rood received a bachelor's degree (1932) and a diploma in occupational therapy (1933) from Downer College, Milwaukee, Wisconsin. She earned a master's degree and a certificate in physical therapy from Stanford University.

Registered as both an occupational therapist and a physical therapist, Rood was chair of the Department of Physical Therapy at USC from 1959 until 1966, where she initiated the second physical therapy master's degree program in the United States. She established the Department of Occupational Therapy in 1943 and served as professor and department chairperson and director of programs until 1952. While at USC, she developed a method of therapeutic exercise known as the Rood System.

731

Rood also worked with the Elks Major Project at Riverside County, California, from 1952 until 1955 and spent the next year investigating swallowing and speech procedures with bulbar poliomyelitis patients at Ranchos Los Amigos Hospital, Hondo, California. She was staff occupational therapist for the Asylum for Chronic Insane, Wauwatosa, Wisconsin (1933–1936) and therapy supervisor in the Cerebral Palsy Clinic, Indiana University Medical Center, Indianapolis (1937–1943).

Rood received the Mary McMillan Lectureship Award from the American Physical Therapy Association in 1969. She was elected AOTA Fellow in 1973. She received the Distinguished Emeriti Award from USC in March 1984, 6 months before her death in September 1984.

Bibliography

Rood, M. S. (1938) Project for treatment of cerebral palsy. *Occupational Therapy and Rehabilitation, 17,* 93–96.

Rood, M. S., McNary, H., Ness, J., Theiss, H., Kahmann, W. C., Myers, J., et al. (1938). Committee reports: Report of committee on research and efficiency. *Occupational Therapy and Rehabilitation, 17,* 412–414.

Morse, L. G., Rood, M. S., Wade, B. D., & Barnes, S. (1941). Reports of committees: Report of the committee on scientific study and research. *Occupational Therapy and Rehabilitation, 20,* 409–412.

Moore, M. S. (1941). Reports of committees on the study of cerebral palsy. *Occupational Therapy and Rehabilitation, 20,* 413.

Rood, M. S., & Merrill, A. (1943). Summary of minutes of the house of delegates meeting: Indianapolis Athletic Club, Indianapolis, Indiana, October 14, 1943. *Occupational Therapy and Rehabilitation, 22,* 310–312.

Rood, M. S. (1947). A program for paraplegics. *American Journal of Occupational Therapy, 1,* 22–25.

Rood, M. S. (1947). School section: University of Southern California Occupational Therapy Department; Columbia University Division of Occupational Therapy. *American Journal of Occupational Therapy, 1,* 285–261.

Rood, M. S. (1952). Occupational therapy in the treatment of cerebral palsied. *Physical Therapy Review, 32,* 76–82.

Rood, M. S. (1954). Neurophysiological reactions as a basis for therapy. *Physical Therapy Review, 34,* 444–449.

Rood, M. S. (1956). Session on neurology: Neurophysiological mechanisms utilized in the treatment of neuromuscular dysfunction. *American Journal of Occupational Therapy, 10,* 220–225.

Rood, M. S. (1958). Everyone counts (1958 Eleanor Clarke Slagle Lecture). *American Journal of Occupational Therapy, 12,* 326–329.

Charlotte Royeen, PhD, OTR/L, FAOTA—2003

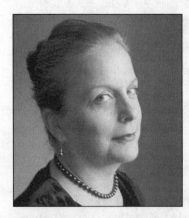

Charlotte Royeen is currently dean of the Edward and Margaret Doisy School of Allied Health Professions at St. Louis University. In her undergraduate work, she concentrated on fine arts, painting, psychology, and anatomy. She graduated with a bachelor of science in occupational therapy from Tufts University in 1976. A master's degree in occupational therapy was earned at Washington University School of Medicine in 1980. She also was a graduate teaching assistant at St. Louis University from 1978 to 1980. In 1983, she received a doctoral fellowship jointly awarded from the American Occupational Therapy Association (AOTA) and the American Occupational Therapy Foundation (AOTF). Royeen earned a doctor of philosophy from Virginia Polytechnic Institute and State University in 1986, focusing on educational research and evaluation and statistics. She completed post-doctoral work as a U.S. West Fellow in computer technology and higher education at Creighton University in 2000.

Royeen was recognized in 1986 with the Quality Step Increase, an award for outstanding service in the federal government. In 1988, she was inducted into the AOTA Roster of Fellows based on her work in research and scholarly activity in pediatric occupational therapy and research methodology. She was granted the status of professor emeritus from Sensory Integration International in 1989. She served as editor of the AOTA Self-Study Series and was honored with the Outstanding Innovation in Continuing Education award by the American Society of Association Executives. In 1992, she received a Certificate of Appreciation for Leadership in NDT research by the Neurodevelopmental Treatment Association. The Jean Ayres Research Award, a scholarly award presented by AOTF for exemplary and sustained contributions in the development and application of theory, was given to Royeen in 1998. The profession honored Royeen by bestowing the Eleanor Clarke Slagle Lectureship Award in 2003. The Nebraska Occupational Therapy Association honored Royeen with the Contributor of the Year Award in 2003.

On a Personal Note From a Phone Interview: In her Eleanor Clarke Slagle Lecture, Royeen also was inspired to focus on chaos and complexity theory "because this is life . . . we deal with chaos and complexities in real life so this makes sense for occupational therapy." The unique use of fractals in the slides accompanying the lecture added dimension and visual appeal to the lecture. These could not be captured in the published article in the *American Journal of Occupational Therapy*.

Royeen is a bold pioneer of the clinical doctoral degree in occupational therapy education stating that "this is the vision of the future . . . clinical doctoral-degree programs must deliver graduates with bona fide clinical skills and need to build an in-depth clinical management in order to compare to other professional doctorates in law, pharmacy, and optometry."

Royeen conducted considerable historical research in preparing her 2002 Eleanor Clarke Slagle Lecture and was surprised by the strong feminist perspective of the prior Slagle lecturers. As a predominantly female profession, Royeen recommends therapists and students review the November 1992 issue of *AJOT*, which focused on the feminism and the ideologies of occupational therapy, especially examining the history of occupational therapy from the context of women.

Linking Key Messages of the 2003 Eleanor Clarke Slagle Lecture to the AOTA *Centennial Vision*: My Eleanor Clarke Slagle Lecture attempted to shift occupational therapy's vision from linear models to dynamical systems and chaos theory and to include an emphasis of the art of practice from the heart. The *Vision* statement focuses on evidence-based decision making and science fostered innovation as reflected in current trends in health care. It fails, however, to incorporate our traditional strength in theory development and application and in our exceptional creative and intuitive practice art. It also fails to come to terms with a main issue holding back occupational therapy: Our ambivalence about power and how to use it.

—*Charlotte Royeen*

Bibliography

Royeen, C. B. (in press). Confessions of an occupational therapist who became an artist (ode to Yerxa, 2000) [Keynote Speech]. *Irish Journal of Occupational Therapy*.

Royeen, C. B. (in press). Reflections on education and learning in occupational therapy for the 21st century. *Occupational Therapy in Health Care*.

Cassini, T., Royeen, C. B., Barney, K., & Royeen, M. (2010). The occupation of city walking: Crossing the invisible line. In F. Kronenberg, N. Pollard, & D. Sakellariou (Eds.), *Occupational therapy without borders: Toward an ecology of occupation-based practice* (vol. 2). Edinburgh, Scotland: Churchill Livingstone/Elsevier.

Harvan, R., Royeen, C. B., & Jensen, G. M. (2009). Grounding interprofessional education in theory. In C. B. Royeen, G. M. Jensen, & R. Harvan (Eds.), *Leadership in interprofessional health education and practice*. Sudbury, MA: Jones & Bartlett.

Jensen, G. M., Harvan, R., & Royeen, C. B. (2009). Interprofessional education: Context, complexity, and challenge. In C. B. Royeen, G. M. Jensen, & R. Harvan (Eds.), *Leadership in interprofessional health education and practice*. Subury, MA: Jones & Bartlett.

Royeen, C. B., Jensen, G. M., & Harvan, R. (2009). Where do we go from here? In C. B. Royeen, G. M. Jensen, & R. Harvan (Eds.), *Leadership in interprofessional health education and practice*. Sudbury, MA: Jones & Bartlett.

Royeen, C. B., & Luebben, A. J. (Eds.). (2009). *Sensory integration: A compendium of leading scholarship*. Bethesda, MD: AOTA Press.

Royeen, C. B., Terharre, E., & Walsh, S. (2009). Interprofessional education: History, review, and recommendations for professional accreditation agencies. In C. B. Royeen, G. M. Jensen, & R. Harvan (Eds.), *Leadership in interprofessional health education and practice*. Sudbury, MA: Jones & Bartlett.

Royeen, C. B., & Lavin, M. A. (2007). A contextual and logical analysis of the clinical doctorate for health practitioners: Dilemma, delusion, or defacto. *Journal of Allied Health, 36*(2), 101–106.

Royeen, C. B., & Luebben, A. J. (2007). Toward verstehen: An etymological and historical wave of the terms *habit, routine, occupation,* and *participation. OTJR: Occupation, Participation and Health, 27*(Suppl.), 865S–866S.

Siler, W. L., & Royeen, C. B. (2007). Guiding principles in a merger of allied health and nursing schools. *Journal of Allied Health, 36*(1), 24–29.

Luebben, A., & Royeen, C. B. (2005). Nonstandardized testing. In J. Hinojosa & P. Kramer (Eds.), *Evaluation: Obtaining and interpreting data* (2nd ed.). Bethesda, MD: AOTA Press.

Royeen, C. B. (2005). The ephemeral ethics of evidence-based practice. In R. B. Purtilo, G. M. Jensen, & C. B. Royeen (Eds.), *Ethics for moral action: A sourcebook for health and rehabilitation ethics*. Philadelphia: F. A. Davis.

Royeen, C. B. (2005). Ongoing wisdom after the lecture: "Her-story": A polemic for action, or a pink-collar call for feminist development in occupational therapy. In R. Padilla (Ed.), *A professional legacy: The Eleanor Clarke Slagle Lectures in occupational therapy, 1955–2004* (2nd ed., pp. 810–819). Bethesda, MD: AOTA Press.

Houtz, L. E., Kosoko-Lasaki, O., Zardetto-Smith, A., Mu, K., & Royeen, C. B. (2004). Teacher education professionals as partners in health science outreach. *Journal of Allied Health, 33*(3), 174–177.

Mu, K., Chao, C. C., Jensen, G. M., & Royeen, C. B. (2004). Effects of interprofessional rural training on students' perceptions of interprofessional health care services. *Journal of Allied Health, 33*(2), 125–131.

Mu, K., & Royeen, C. B. (2004). Facilitating participation of students with severe disabilities: Aligning school-based occupational therapy practice with best practices in severe disabilities. *Physical and Occupational Therapy in Pediatrics, 24*(3), 5–22.

Mu, K., & Royeen, C. B. (2004). Interprofessional or transprofessional services in school-based occupational therapy practice. *Occupational Therapy International, 11*(4), 244–247.

Royeen, C. B. (2004). Trajectory towards the strange attractor of academic administration: Top ten vectors for plotting. *Occupational Therapy in Health Care, 18,* 188–190.

Kramer P., Hinojosa, J., & Royeen, C. B. (Eds.). (2003). *Perspectives in human occupation: Participation in life.* Philadelphia: Lippincott Williams & Wilkins.

Royeen, C.B. (2003). Chaotic occupational therapy: Collective wisdom for a complex profession (2003 Eleanor Clarke Slagle Lecture). *American Journal of Occupational Therapy, 57,* 609–624.

Royeen, C., & Mu, K. (2003). Stability of tactile defensiveness across cultures: European and American children's responses to the Touch Inventory for Elementary School Aged Children (TIE). *Occupational Therapy International, 10,* 166–175.

Galt, K. A., Barr, C. C., Young, W., & Royeen, C. (2002). Are doctor of pharmacy students prepared for high technology learning? *Pharmacy Education, 1,* 145–157.

Lohman, H., & Royeen, C. B. (2002). Post traumatic stress disorder and traumatic hand injuries: A neuro-occupational view. *American Journal of Occupational Therapy, 56,* 527–537.

Royeen, C. B. (2002). Occupation reconsidered. *Occupational Therapy International, 9,* 112–121.

Royeen, C. B., & Luebben, A. J. (2002). Annotation of literature on chaos. *Occupational Therapy in Health Care, 16*(1), 63–80.

Zardetto-Smith, A., Mu, K., Phillips, C., Houtz, L. E., & Royeen, C. B. (2002). Brains rule! Fun = learning = neuroscience literacy. *The Neuroscientist, 8,* 396–404.

Crabtree, J. L., Royeen, C. B., & Mu, K. (2001). The effects of learning through discussion in a course in occupational therapy: A search for deep learning. *Journal of Allied Health, 30,* 243–247.

Jensen, G. M., & Royeen, C. B. (2001). Analysis of academic–community partnerships using the integration matrix. *Journal of Allied Health, 30,* 168–175.

Mu, K., Royeen, C. B., Paschal, K., & Zardetto-Smith, A. (2001). Promoting awareness and understanding of occupational therapy and physical therapy in young school-aged children: An interdisciplinary approach. *Occupational Therapy in Health Care, 15*(3/4), 89–99.

Reistetter, T., & Royeen, C. B. (2001). A needs assessment for doctoral-level education in occupational therapy. *Education Special Interest Section Quarterly, 11*(1), 1–4.

Royeen, C. B. (2001). "I saw a bald eagle fly" [Foreword]. In S. Schwartzberg (Ed.), *Interactive reasoning in the practice of occupational therapy* (pp. v–vii). Upper Saddle River, NJ: Prentice Hall.

Royeen, C. B., Duncan, M., & McCormack, G. (2001). Reconstruction of the Rood approach for occupation-based treatment. In L. Pedretti (Ed.), *Occupational therapy: Practice skills for physical dysfunction* (5th ed., pp. 567–587). St. Louis, MO: Mosby.

Royeen, C. B., Zardetto-Smith, A., Duncan, M., & Mu, K. (2001). What do young school-age children know about occupational therapy? An evaluation study. *Occupational Therapy International, 8,* 263–272.

Crist, P. A., Royeen, C. B., & Schkade, J. K. (2000). *Infusing occupation into practice* (2nd ed.). Bethesda, MD: American Occupational Therapy Association.

Royeen, C. B. (2000). Theory to practice in occupational therapy education [Foreword]. In P. Crist (Ed.), *Innovations in occupational therapy education 2000* (pp. vii–viii). Bethesda, MD: American Occupational Therapy Association.

Royeen, C. B., Duncan, M., Crabtree, J., Richards, J., & Frolek Clark, G. (2000). Effects of billing Medicaid for occupational therapy services in the schools: A pilot study. *American Journal of Occupational Therapy, 54,* 429–433.

Royeen, C. B., Mu, K., Barrett, K., & Luebben, A. (2000). Problem-based learning: Pilot investigation: Evaluation of a clinical reflective reasoning before and after workshop intervention. In P. Crist (Ed.), *Innovations in occupational therapy education 2000* (pp. 107–115). Bethesda, MD: American Occupational Therapy Association.

Zardetto-Smith, A., Mu, K., Ahmad, S. O., & Royeen, C. B. (2000). A model program for bringing neuroscience to children: An informal neuroscience education program bridges a gap. *The Neuroscientist, 6,* 165–174.

Cochran, T., Jensen, G. M., Duncan, M., & Royeen, C. (1999). Cultural incompetence: When your best efforts are challenged. *Physical Therapy, 79,* S78.

Hammel J., Royeen C., Bagatell N., Chandler S., Jensen G., Loveland J., et al. (1999). Student perspectives on problem-based learning in an occupational therapy curriculum: A qualitative study. *American Journal of Occupational Therapy, 53,* 199–206.

Royeen, C. B. (1999). From the chairperson. *Education Special Interest Section Quarterly, 9*(3), 1.

Royeen, C. B. (1999). Scholarship revisited: Expanding horizons and guidelines for evaluation of the scholarship of teaching [Foreword]. In P. Crist (Ed.), *Innovations in occupational therapy education 1999* (pp. x–xi). Bethesda, MD: American Occupational Therapy Association.

Royeen, C. B., & Duncan, M. (1999). Acquisitional frame of reference. In P. Kramer & J. Hinojosa (Eds.), *Frames of reference for pediatric occupational therapy* (2nd ed., pp. 377–400). Philadelphia: Lippincott Williams & Wilkins.

Royeen, C. B., & Stohs, S. (1999). Should the clinical doctoral degree be the standard of entry into the practice of occupational therapy? In P. Crist (Ed.), *Innovations in occupational therapy education 1999* (pp. 171–177). Bethesda, MD: American Occupational Therapy Association.

Royeen, C. B., Zardetto-Smith, A. M., & Duncan, M. E. M. (1999). Preliminary study of learning through discussion in occupational therapy education. In P. Crist (Ed.), *Innovations in occupational therapy education 1999* (pp.13–26). Bethesda, MD: American Occupational Therapy Association.

Threlkeld, A. J., Jensen, G., & Royeen, C. B. (1999). The clinical doctorate: A framework for analysis in physical therapist education. *Physical Therapy, 79,* 567–581.

Hotz, S. D., & Royeen, C. B. (1998). Perception of behaviors associated with tactile defensiveness: An exploration of the differences between mothers and their children. *Occupational Therapy International, 5,* 281–291.

Royeen, C. B. (1998). Four areas of sensory integrative scholarship for the next millennium [Editorial]. *Occupational Therapy International, 5,* 249–251.

Royeen, C. B., & Richards, J. (1998). Nonstandardized assessment tools. In J. Hinojosa & P. Kramer (Eds.), *Evaluation: Obtaining and interpreting data.* Bethesda, MD: American Occupational Therapy Association.

Stephens, C., & Royeen, C. B. (1998). Investigation and tactile defensiveness and self-esteem typically developing in children. *Occupational Therapy International, 5*, 273–280.

Crist, P., & Royeen, C. B. (Eds.). (1997). *Infusing occupation into practice: A comparison of three clinical approaches in occupational therapy.* Bethesda, MD: American Occupational Therapy Association.

Royeen, C. B. (Ed.). (1997). *Neuroscience and occupation: Links to practice.* Bethesda, MD: American Occupational Therapy Association.

Royeen, C. B. (1997). Play as an indicator of health and wellness. In B. E. Chandler (Ed.), *The essence of play: A child's occupational therapy.* Bethesda, MD: American Occupational Therapy Association.

Royeen, C. B. (1997). *A research primer.* Bethesda, MD: American Occupational Therapy Association.

Royeen, C. B., & Salavatori, P. (1997). Comparison of problem-based learning curricula in two occupational therapy programs. *Canadian Journal of Occupational Therapy, 64,* 197–202.

Royeen, C. B. (Ed.). (1996). *Stroke.* Bethesda, MD: American Occupational Therapy Association.

Royeen, C. B. (1996). Third-party prescription for school-based occupational therapy. *American Journal of Occupational Therapy, 50,* 750–751.

Royeen, C. B. (1996). Viewpoints—20 years of occupational therapy: As much as things change, some things stay the same. *OT Week, 10*(45), 60.

Royeen, C. B., & Furbush, R. (1996). A pilot study of needs assessment for school-based practice. *American Journal of Occupational Therapy, 50,* 747–749.

Royeen, C. B. (Ed.). (1995). *Hands on: A guide to rehabilitation of the hand.* Bethesda, MD: American Occupational Therapy Association.

Royeen, C. B. (1995). A new focus in occupational therapy education. *American Journal of Occupational Therapy, 49,* 338–346.

DeGangi, G. A., & Royeen, C. B. (1994). Current practice among neurodevelopmental treatment association members. *American Journal of Occupational Therapy, 48,* 803–809.

DeGangi, G. A., Wietlisbach, S., & Royeen, C. B. (1994). A look at cross-cultural issues in early intervention. *Topics in Early Childhood Special Education, 14,* 503–520.

Royeen, C. B. (1994). Problem-based learning in action: Key points for practical use. *Education Special Interest Section Quarterly, 4*(4), 1–2.

Royeen, C. B. (Ed.). (1994). *Putting occupation back into therapy.* Bethesda, MD: American Occupational Therapy Association.

Royeen, C. B. (Ed.). (1993). *Cognitive rehabilitation.* Bethesda, MD: American Occupational Therapy Association.

DeGangi, G., Royeen, C. B., & Wietlisbach, S. (1992). How to examine the individualized family service plan process: Preliminary findings and a procedural guide. *Infants and Young Children, 5*(2), 42–56.

Royeen, C. B. (Ed.). (1992). *Classroom applications for school based practice.* Bethesda, MD: American Occupational Therapy Association.

Royeen, C. B. (1992). A glimpse of the human experience: Parenting infants and toddlers who are disabled. *Infants and Young Children, 5*(2), 65–67.

Royeen, C. B. (1992). Viewpoint: A personal experience with family-centered care. In E. Vergara (Ed.), *Foundations for practice in the neonatal intensive care unit and early intervention: A self-guided practice manual.* Rockville, MD: American Occupational Therapy Association.

Royeen, C. B., DeGangi, G., & Poisson, S. (1992). Development of the individualized family service plan anchor guide. *Infants and Young Children, 5*(2), 57–64.

Hanft, B., & Royeen, C. B. (1991). Commentary—Efficacy of therapeutic intervention intensity with infants and young children with cerebral palsy. *Infants and Young Children, 4*(2), 8–10.

Royeen, C. B. (Ed.). (1991). *School-based practice for related services.* Bethesda, MD: American Occupational Therapy Association.

Royeen, C. B., & Coutinho, M. (1991). What special education administrators need to know about occupational therapy. In W. Dunn (Ed.), *Pediatric occupational therapy: Facilitating effective service provision* (pp. 307–317). Thorofare, NJ: Slack.

Royeen, C. B., & Gorga, D. (1991). Occupational therapy in pediatric rehabilitation. *Pediatrician, 17,* 278–282.

Royeen, C. B., Koomar, J., Cromack, R., & Fortune, J. (1991). Development of the sensory integration and praxis tests competency exam: Exploration of validity and reliability. *Occupational Therapy Journal of Research, 11,* 1–6.

Royeen, C. B., & Lane, S. (1991). Tactile functions. In A. Fisher & B. Murrey (Eds.), *Sensory integration theory and practice* (pp. 109–136). Philadelphia: F. A. Davis.

Royeen, C. B., Slavik, B., & Garreton, I. (1991). *Handbook of sensory integration for parents.* Cincinnati, OH: Southpaw.

Royeen, C. B. (Ed.). (1990). *Neuroscience foundations of human performance.* Bethesda, MD: American Occupational Therapy Association.

Royeen, C. B. (1990). Occupational therapy in a nontraditional setting. *American Journal of Occupational Therapy, 44,* 172–174.

Royeen, C. B., & Fortune, J. C. (1990). TIE: Tactile inventory for school-aged children. *American Journal of Occupational Therapy, 44,* 155–160.

Royeen, C. B. (Ed.). (1989). *Assessing function.* Bethesda, MD: American Occupational Therapy Association.

Royeen, C. B. (Ed.). (1989). *Clinical research handbook: An analysis for the service professions.* Thorofare, NJ: Slack.

Royeen, C. B. (1989). Commentary on "Tactile functions in learning disabled and normal children: Reliability and validity considerations." *Occupational Therapy Journal of Research, 9,* 16–23.

Royeen, C. B. (1989). Program evaluation in pediatric occupational therapy. In P. N. Clark (Ed.), *Occupational therapy for children* (2nd ed.). New York: Mosby.

Royeen, C. B. (1988). Nationally Speaking—Occupational therapy in the schools. *American Journal of Occupational Therapy, 42,* 697–700.

Royeen, C. B. (1988). *Research tradition in occupational therapy: Process, philosophy, and status.* Thorofare, NJ: Slack.

Royeen, C. B. (1988). Review of the Degangi–Berk test of sensory integration. *Physical and Occupational Therapy for Pediatrics, 8*(2/3), 71–75.

Royeen, C. B., & Marsh, D. M. (1988). Promoting occupational therapy in the schools. *American Journal of Occupational Therapy, 42,* 713–717.

Royeen, C. B. (1987). Test–retest reliability of touch inventory for elementary school-aged children. *Physical and Occupational Therapy in Pediatrics, 7*(3), 45–52.

Royeen, C. B. (1987). TIP: Touch inventory for preschoolers. *Physical and Occupational Therapy in Pediatrics, 7*(1), 29–40.

Royeen, C. B. (1986). The boxplot: A test for screening research data. *American Journal of Occupational Therapy, 40*, 569–571.

Royeen, C. B. (1986). Commentary on "Preliminary report of a methodology for determining tactile localization in adults." *Occupational Therapy Journal of Research, 6*, 207–210.

Royeen, C. B. (1986). Development of a touch scale for elementary school-aged children. *American Journal of Occupational Therapy, 40*, 414–419.

Royeen, C. B. (1986). Entry-level education in occupational therapy. *American Journal of Occupational Therapy, 40*, 425–427.

Royeen, C. B. (1986). Evaluation of school-based occupational therapy programs: Need, strategy, and dissemination. *American Journal of Occupational Therapy, 40*(12), 811–813.

Royeen, C. B., & Seaver, W. F. (1986). Promise in nonparametrics. *American Journal of Occupational Therapy, 40*, 191–193.

Neville, P., Royeen, C. B., & Kielhofner, K. (1985). Childhood. In G. Kielhofner (Ed.), *A model of human occupation: Theory and application*. Baltimore: Williams & Wilkins.

Royeen, C. B. (1985). Adaptation of Likert scaling for use with children. *Occupational Therapy Journal of Research, 5*, 59–69.

Royeen, C. B. (1985). Domain specification of the construct tactile defensiveness. *American Journal of Occupational Therapy, 39*, 596–599.

Royeen, C. B., & Fortune, J. F. (1985). Data modification commands for summated scale reliability analysis using SPSS. *Journal of Occupational Therapy Research, 5*(4), 257–258.

Royeen, C. B., & Little, L. (1985). Autistic adolescents: Developmental milestones and a model program. *Occupational Therapy in Health Care, 2*(3), 59–69.

Royeen, C. B. (1984). Incidence of atypical responses to vestibular stimulation among behavioral-disordered children. *Occupational Therapy Journal of Research, 4*, 59–60.

Royeen, C. B. (1984). Initial profile of therapists seeking certification in sensory integrative testing. *American Journal of Occupational Therapy, 38*, 44–45.

Royeen, C. B., & Kannegieter, R. A. (1984). Fingertip textural perception in normal children. *Occupational Therapy Journal of Research, 4*, 261–270.

Royeen, C. B. (1982). Comments upon "The Southern California Postrotary Nystagmus Test: Test–retest reliability for preschool children" [Letter to the Editor]. *Occupational Therapy Journal of Research, 2*, 125–126.

Royeen, C. B. (1982). Roughness perception in children. *Perceptual and Motor Skills, 54*, 323–330.

Royeen, C. B., Lesinski, G., Ciani, S., & Schneider, D. (1981). The Southern California Sensory Integration Tests, the Southern California Postrotary Nystagmus Test, and clinical observations accompanying them to evaluations in otolaryngology, ophthalmology, and audiology. *American Journal of Occupational Therapy, 35*, 443–450.

Royeen, C. B. (1980). Test–retest reliability of the Southern California Postrotary Nystagmus Test. *American Journal of Occupational Therapy, 34*, 37–39.

Kay Barker Schwartz, EdD, OTR/L, FAOTA—2009

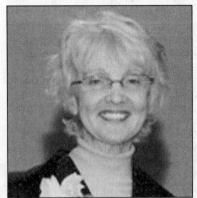

Kay Barker Schwartz earned a bachelor's degree in English literature from the University of Massachusetts in 1969 and an master of science degree in occupational therapy from Boston Sargent University in 1975. Her first job as an occupational therapy educator was with Tufts University, Boston School of Occupational Therapy, in Medford, Massachusetts, as the academic coordinator of field programs. She later became a lecturer in occupational therapy as well at Tufts University (1980–1985) and assistant professor in the occupational therapy program at Worchester State College in Worchester, Massachusetts (1986–1987). In 1986, she earned an EdD from Harvard University.

Schwartz began her academic career at San Jose State University in San Jose, California, in 1987. She has held various academic appointments at the university for over 20 years, including department chair from 1996 to 2000, graduate coordinator from 2000 to 2004, and professor from 1994 to the present. She also was a faculty associate with Stanford Geriatric Education Center, part of the Stanford University Medical School, from 1994 to 2000. Her clinical experience focused on physical rehabilitation and administration.

Schwartz's work as a historical scholar began with her doctoral studies at Harvard University, where she learned historical inquiry. At the time of her graduation in 1986, there was a growing interest in systematically recording occupational therapy history. She has published numerous articles on this history and has contributed to various committees of the American

Occupational Therapy Association focused on preserving and fostering appreciation for the early years of occupational therapy. She became the contributing editor of the "Looking Back" department of the *American Journal of Occupational Therapy* in 1988, a position she held for the next 10 years. From that position she solicited manuscripts and mentored colleagues desiring to write occupational therapy history. Indeed, a review of the literature shows that most of the published articles on occupational therapy history appeared in "Looking Back" while Schwartz was contributing editor. She has consistently conveyed the message of the importance of occupational therapy history throughout the past several decades.

Schwartz was the first person at San Jose State University to be awarded the title of "teacher–scholar" from the Chancellor's Institute for Teaching and Learning and is considered a leader in curriculum and educational design in the Occupational Therapy Department. Furthermore, her leadership is exemplified by her receiving the President's Special Recognition Award. She has a remarkable record of service, including editorial roles and national and university committees, as well as being actively involved in the landmark Clinical Reasoning Study sponsored by the American Occupational Therapy Foundation.

It is not surprising that Schwartz would be influenced by her love of the history of the profession and would choose this as the focus of her Eleanor Clarke Slagle Lecture in 2009. In a phone interview, Schwartz stated that she has returned to her love of teaching, is currently completing work on two books, and is documenting the history of the California Occupational Therapy Association.

Note. Some of the biographical information was written Ann MacRae in 2008.

Linking Key Messages of the 2009 Eleanor Clarke Slagle Lecture to the AOTA *Centennial Vision:* In my 2009 Slagle lecture, I examined the historical connection between the vision that the founders of occupational therapy proposed and that is expressed in the *Centennial Vision*. I proposed that the *Centennial Vision* builds on values that the profession has held since its inception in 1917. One major thread that connects the visions is a profound belief in the healing nature of occupation. The other major thread is the emphasis on the importance of scientific research to validate the profession's effectiveness. Like the founders, in today's society occupational therapy is confronted with inequities that affect people's health, quality of life, and participation. Through occupational therapy's commitment to participation for all and an innovative, evidence-based practice, we can successfully implement the profession's *Centennial Vision* and help change the 21st century.

—*Kathleen Baker Schwartz*

Bibliography

Schwartz, K. (2009). Reclaiming our heritage: Connecting the *Founding Vision* to the *Centennial Vision* (2009 Eleanor Clarke Slagle Lecture). *American Journal of Occupational Therapy, 63*(6), 681–690.

Richardson, P., MacRae, A., & Schwartz, K. (2008). Student outcomes in a post-professional online master's-degree program. *American Journal of Occupational Therapy, 62,* 600–610.

Schwartz, K. (2006). History of the treatment of individuals with physical disability in occupational therapy. In H. Pendleton & W. Schultz-Krohn (Eds.), *Pedretti's occupational therapy for physical dysfunction* (6th ed.). St Louis, MO: Elsevier.

Schwartz, K. (2005). The history and philosophy of psychosocial occupational therapy. In L. Cara & A. MacRae (Eds.), *Psychosocial occupational therapy: A clinical practice* (2nd ed.). Clifton Park, NY: Delmar.

Miller, R., & Schwartz, K. (2004). What is theory and why does it matter? In F. A. Ludwig, K. F. Walker, & R. J. Miller (Ed.), *Contemporary occupational therapy practice theorists*. Gaithersburg, MD: Aspen.

Southam, M., & Schwartz, K. (2004). Laugh and learn: Humor as a teaching strategy in occupational therapy education. *Occupational Therapy in Health Care, 18,* 57–70.

Schwartz, K. (2003). The history of occupation. In J. Hinojosa, P. Kramer, & C. B. Royeen (Eds.), *Current perspectives in human occupation: Participation in life*. Philadelphia: Lippincott Williams & Wilkins.

Schwartz, K. (2003). The history of occupational therapy. In E. Crepeau, E. Cohn, & B. Schell (Eds.), *Willard and Spackman's occupational therapy* (10th ed.). Philadelphia: Lippincott Williams & Wilkins.

Schwartz, K. (2001). History and practice trends in the treatment of physical dysfunction. In L. W. Pedretti & M. B. Early (Eds.), *Occupational therapy: Practice skills for physical dysfunction* (5th ed.). St Louis, MO: Mosby.

Schwartz, K. (1998). History of occupational therapy. In E. Crepeau & M. Neistadt (Eds.), *Willard and Spackman's occupational therapy* (9th ed.). Philadelphia: Lippincott.

Schwartz, K. (1997). An approach to supervision of students on fieldwork. In C. R. Privott (Ed.), *The fieldwork anthology: A classic research and practice collection*. Bethesda, MD: American Occupational Therapy Association.

Schwartz, K. (1997). Clinical reasoning and new ideas on intelligence: Implications for teaching and learning. In C. R. Privott (Ed.), *The fieldwork anthology: A classic research and practice collection*. Bethesda, MD: American Occupational Therapy Association.

Schwartz, K., & Engle-Ramirez, J. (1996). Health reform and occupational therapy. In L. Pedretti (Ed.), *Occupational therapy: Practice skills for physical disabilities* (4th ed.). St Louis, MO: Mosby.

Ambrosi, E., & Schwartz, K. (1995). The profession's expressed image, 1917–1925: Occupational therapy as represented in the media. *American Journal of Occupational Therapy, 49*, 828–832.

Ambrosi, E., & Schwartz, K. (1995). The profession's expressed image, 1917–1925: Occupational therapy as represented by the profession. *American Journal of Occupational Therapy, 49*, 715–719.

Schwartz, K. (1993). San Jose State University: Its place in occupational therapy history. In *Proceedings of the 50th Anniversary Symposium.* San Jose, CA: San Jose State University, Department of Occupational Therapy.

Cooperstein, K., & Schwartz, K. (1992). Reasons for choosing occupational therapy as a profession: Implications for recruitment. *American Journal of Occupational Therapy, 46*, 534–539.

Schwartz, K. (1992). Education and occupational therapy: A shared vision. *American Journal of Occupational Therapy, 46*, 12–18.

Schwartz, K. (1992). Nationally Speaking—Examining the profession's legacy. *American Journal of Occupational Therapy, 46*, 9–10.

Schwartz, K. (1991). Clinical reasoning and new ideas on intelligence: Implications for teaching and learning. *American Journal of Occupational Therapy, 45*, 1033–1037.

Schwartz, K. (1991). The legacy of Mary Parker Follett: Implications for school reform. *Journal of Educational Administration and History, 23*(1), 33–41.

Wittman, P., & Schwartz, K. (1991). Identifying the developmental needs of students. In *SPICES: Self-instructional package to improve clinical education and supervision.* Rockville, MD: American Occupational Therapy Association.

Schwartz, K. (1990). Creating excellence in patient care. *American Journal of Occupational Therapy, 44*, 816–821.

Schwartz, K. (1988). Productivity through excellence: A promising approach to hospital management. *Hospital Topics, 66*(6), 16–18.

Schwartz, K., & Colman, W. (1988). Historical research methods in occupational therapy. *American Journal of Occupational Therapy, 42*, 239–244.

Cooper, R., Schwartz, K., Brooks, B., Christie, B., Crist, P., & Shapiro, D. (1987). *The fieldwork evaluation for the occupational therapist.* Rockville, MD: American Occupational Therapy Association.

Schwartz, K. (1986). Scientific management and administrative reform in education, 1900–1920: One specializes in science, the other in practice. *Dissertation Abstracts International, 47A*, 2056.

Schwartz, K. (1984). An approach to supervision of occupational therapy students. *American Journal of Occupational Therapy, 38*, 393–397.

Schwartz, K. (1984). Balancing objectives of efficient and effective occupational therapy services. *American Journal of Occupational Therapy, 38*, 198–200.

June Sokolov, MA, OTR, FAOTA, DHL (Hon.)—1956

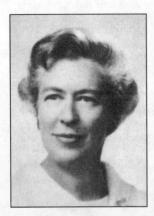

June Sokolov was the founding director of the Hartford (Connecticut) Easter Seal Rehabilitation Center, where she served from 1949 to 1978. She retired, closing a distinguished career of service to the center and individuals with disabilities.

Sokolov received a BS, graduating magna cum laude, from New York University (NYU). She completed her clinical training at Belleview Hospital in New York City; Sheppard and Enoch Pratt Hospital in Baltimore, Maryland; and Bridgeport Rehabilitation Center in Bridgeport, Connecticut. She completed her master's degree at NYU while serving as acting director of its School of Occupational Therapy.

During her early years, Sokolov danced professionally with the Martha Graham and Agnes de Mille companies and conducted dance classes for children. After graduating from college, she joined the Connecticut Society for Crippled Children and Adults for 2 years as chief occupational therapist.

Sokolov was active in both state and national occupational therapy associations. She served on the AOTA Executive Board, the Committee on Student Affiliation, and the Advisory Panel for the Office of Vocational Rehabilitation. She was program chairperson of AOTA's 1956 Annual Conference.

Among the awards received are the AOTA Roster of Fellows in 1973 and an honorary doctor of human letters from the University of Hartford in 1978.

From her retirement until her death in October 1983, Sokolov managed the Grist Mill Gallery in Hartford and taught English to illiterate people through the Hartford Literacy Volunteer Program.

Bibliography

McNary, H., Fish, M., Jameson, E., Sokolov, J., & Heermans, M. F. (1954). Nationally Speaking: From the Executive Director: Report on CCI Conference: From the Education Secretary. *American Journal of Occupational Therapy, 8,* 214–217.

Sokolov, J. (1955). Working as a team: The occupational therapist in a rehabilitation center. *American Journal of Occupational Therapy, 9,* 270–271, 296.

Sokolov, J. (1956). Therapist into administrator: Ten inspiring years (1956 Eleanor Clarke Slagle Lecture). *American Journal of Occupational Therapy, 11,* 13–19, 34.

Sokolov, J. (1965). The occupational therapist of the future: Planning for. *American Journal of Occupational Therapy, 19,* 1–4.

Florence M. Stattel, MA, OTR, FAOTA—1955

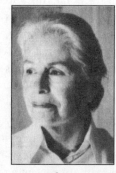

Florence M. Stattel was associate professor and coordinator of the occupational therapy program at the Texas Woman's University, Institute of Health Sciences, Denton, and associate professor of occupational therapy at the University of Florida, Gainesville.

Born and raised in Kings Park, New York, she was 1 of 7 children descended from the early German farm families who came to Long Island in the 19th century. She began her career in 1939 after receiving a certificate from the Philadelphia School of Occupational Therapy. After graduation, she got her first job in the field, earning $1,200 a year, at the Kings County Hospital in Brooklyn, treating patients with tuberculosis and mental health, neurological, and orthopedic problems. In 1945, after receiving her bachelor's degree in occupational therapy at New York University (NYU), she began helping injured soldiers returning from World War II readapt to daily life. Four years later, after completing her master's degree in vocational rehabilitation, she joined the Kessler Institute for Rehabilitation in West Orange, New Jersey. Stattel coordinated the rehabilitation services for the Regional Interdepartmental Rehabilitation Committee of the New York City Medical and Health Research Association, Inc. She also was a consultant for the National Society for Crippled Children and Adults, Inc., NYU School of Education; the American Public Health for Chest Disease, Jersey City, New Jersey; and the Rehabilitation Shops, Bridgeport, Connecticut.

Among the awards Stattel received are the AOTA Fellow in 1973 and the Award of Merit in 1998. She also was a charter member of the World Federation of Occupational Therapists. In 1997, she was the commencement speaker for the first graduating class of occupational therapists at Nova Southeastern University in Florida.

Before her death on May 13, 2002, at the age of 85, she was active with the American Association of University Women; with the East Hampton, New York, town health committee and Meals on Wheels; and with the Kings Park Heritage Museum, spurred by her love of family history.

Bibliography

Stattel, F. (1948). The student occupational therapist. *American Journal of Occupational Therapy, 2,* 162.

Stattel, F. (1952). Featured occupational therapy departments: Kessler Institute. *American Journal of Occupational Therapy, 6,* 29.

Stattel, F. (1954). The painful phantom limb. *American Journal of Occupational Therapy, 8,* 156.

Stattel, F. (1954, August). *Treatment of the (congenital) arm amputee.* Presented at the First International Congress of the World Federation of Occupational Therapists, Edinburgh, Scotland.

Stattel, F. (1955). People you should know: Frances L. Shuff: A biographical sketch; Aloise C. Parker: A biographical sketch. *American Journal of Occupational Therapy, 9,* 71–72.

Stattel, F. (1956). Equipment designed for occupational therapy (1955 Eleanor Clarke Slagle Lecture). *American Journal of Occupational Therapy, 10,* 195–198.

Stattel, F. (1966). The occupational therapist in rehabilitation: Projections toward the future. *American Journal of Occupational Therapy, 20,* 144

Stattel, F. (1967, May). *The occupational therapy consultant.* Presented at the 1st Manpower Conference for Health Related Professions, State University of New York, School of Health-Related Professions, Buffalo.

Stattel, F., & Koestler, F. A. (1968). Regional coordination and planning in an urban setting. *Rehabilitation Literature, 29,* 354–362.

Stattel, F. (1969). *A profile of state-designed comprehensive rehabilitation centers in New York City.* Report to the New York State Commissioner of Health.

Catherine A. Trombly Latham, ScD, OTR/L, FAOTA, AR—1995

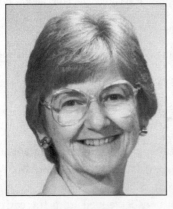

In recognition of her outstanding and sustained contributions to occupational therapy theory, research, and practice, particularly in the area of physical dysfunction, the Eleanor Clarke Slagle Lectureship Award was presented to Catherine Trombly in 1995.

Over a period spanning 42 years, both while a clinician at Highland View Cuyahoga County Hospital in Cleveland, Ohio, and on the faculty of Boston University, she articulated a model of occupational therapy practice for use with persons with physical dysfunction and designed and implemented research consistent with this theory. As an educator and mentor, Trombly Latham's scholarship and research have influenced students who have gone on to develop research programs that contribute to the evidence base of the field. Through clinical practice, teaching, and research, Trombly Latham sought to define the boundaries of occupational therapy practice and challenged both students and practitioners to research the questions that must be addressed to ensure the future of the profession.

Trombly Latham has been professor emerita with Boston University from 2001 to the present. Her service to the profession includes work as a member of numerous editorial boards, chair of the American Occupational Therapy Foundation's (AOTF's) Grant Review Committee, and participation in the annual AOTF Research Colloquium. In retirement she continues to contribute to the American Occupational Therapy Association (AOTA) by providing systematic literature reviews to support the Occupational Therapy Practice Guidelines for stroke and traumatic brain injury, reviewing for the *American Journal of Occupational Therapy*, and reviewing abstracts for conference presentations. In addition, she reviews for several rehabilitation and neurorehabilitation journals and serves as a grant reviewer for the National Institute on Disability and Rehabilitation Research.

Linking Key Messages of the 1995 Eleanor Clarke Slagle Lecture to the AOTA *Centennial Vision:* Trombly Latham's Eleanor Clarke Slagle Lecture, although delivered long before AOTA's *Centennial Vision* was articulated, actually addressed two elements of the vision: occupational therapy is a *science-driven* and as an *evidence-based* profession. The lecture examined the concept of occupation scientifically as the primary intervention and the ultimate goal of occupational therapy. It presented the research available at the time to support the concepts of meaningfulness and purposefulness that Trombly Latham had identified as the therapeutic mechanisms of both occupation-as-means (intervention) and occupation-as-end (goal). The goal of the lecture was to "spark an explosion of research" concerning therapeutic occupation, both the basic science of occupation and the effectiveness of occupation as therapy.

—*Catherine Trombly*

Bibliography

Radomski, M. V., & Trombly Latham, C. A. (2008). *Occupational therapy for physical dysfunction* (6th ed.). Philadelphia: Lippincott Williams & Wilkins.

Ma, H.-I., & Trombly, C. A. (2004). Effects of task complexity on reaction time and movement kinematics in elderly people. *American Journal of Occupational Therapy, 58,* 150–158.

Ma, H.-I., Trombly, C. A., Wagenaar, R. C., & Tickle-Degnen, L. (2004). Effect of one single auditory cue on movement kinematics in patients with Parkinson's disease. *American Journal of Physical Medicine and Rehabilitation, 83,* 530–536.

Fasoli, S., Trombly, C. A., Tickle-Degnen, L., & Verfaellie, M. H. (2002). Context and goal-directed movement: The effect of materials-based occupation. *Occupational Therapy Journal of Research, 22,* 119–128.

Fasoli, S., Trombly, C. A., Tickle-Degnen, L., & Verfaellie, M. H. (2002). Effect of instructions on functional reach in person with and without cerebrovascular accident. *American Journal of Occupational Therapy, 56,* 380–390.

Ma, H.-I., & Trombly, C. A. (2002). A synthesis of the effects of occupational therapy for persons with stroke, Part II: Remediation of impairments. *American Journal of Occupational Therapy, 56,* 260–274.

Sudsawad, P., Trombly, C. A., & Henderson, A. (2002). Testing the effect on kinesthetic training on handwriting performance in first-grade students. *American Journal of Occupational Therapy, 56,* 26–33.

Trombly, C. A., & Ma, H.-I. (2002). A synthesis of the effects of occupational therapy for persons with stroke: Part I: Restoration of roles, tasks, and activities. *American Journal of Occupational Therapy, 56,* 250–259.

Trombly, C. A., & Radomski, M. V. (Eds.). (2002). *Occupational therapy for physical dysfunction* (5th ed.). Philadelphia: Lippincott Williams & Wilkins.

Trombly, C. A., Radomski, M. V., Troxel, C., & Burnett-Smith, S. E. (2002). Occupational therapy and achievement of self-identified goals by adults with acquired brain injury: Phase II. *American Journal of Occupational Therapy, 56,* 489–498.

Ma, H.-I., & Trombly, C. A. (2001). The comparison of motor performance between part and whole tasks in elderly persons. *American Journal of Occupational Therapy, 55,* 62–67.

Sudsawad, P., Trombly, C. A., Henderson, A., & Tickle-Degnen, L. (2001). The relationship between the evaluation tool of children's handwriting and teacher's perceptions of handwriting legibility. *American Journal of Occupational Therapy, 55,* 518–523.

Mancini, M. C., Coster, W. J., Trombly, C. A., & Herren, T. C. (2000). Predicting elementary school participation in children with disabilities. *Archives of Physical Medicine and Rehabilitation, 81,* 339–347. ·

Tickle-Degnen, L., & Trombly, C. (2000). The concept of habit: A research synthesis. *Occupational Therapy Journal of Research, 20*(Suppl. 1), 138S–143S.

Wu, C.-Y., Trombly, C. A., Lin, K.-C., & Tickle-Degnen, L. (2000). A kinematic study of contextual effects on reaching performance in persons with and without stroke: Influences of object availability. *Archives of Physical Medicine and Rehabilitation, 81,* 95–101.

Baker, N. A., Jacobs, K., & Trombly, C. A. (1999). The effect of video display (VDT) mouse use on muscle contractions in the neck and forearm. *Work: A Journal of Prevention, Assessment, and Rehabilitation, 12,* 109–116.

Ma, H.-I., Robinson-Podolski, C., & Trombly, C. A. (1999). The effect of context on skill acquisition and transfer. *American Journal of Occupational Therapy, 53,* 138–144.

Murphy, S., Jacobs, K., Tickle-Degnen, L., & Trombly, C. A. (1999). The effect of keeping an end-product on intrinsic motivation. *American Journal of Occupational Therapy, 53,* 153–158.

Trombly, C. A., & Wu, C.-Y. (1999). Effect of rehabilitation tasks on organization of movement after stroke. *American Journal of Occupational Therapy, 53,* 333–344.

Cope, S. M., & Trombly, C. A. (1998). Grasping in children with and without cerebral palsy: A kinematic analysis. *Scandinavian Journal of Occupational Therapy, 5,* 59–68.

Kelly-Hayes, M., Robertson, J. T., Broderick, J. P., Duncan, P. W., Hershey, L. A., Roth, E. J., Thies, W. H., & Trombly, C. A. (1998). The American Heart Association stroke outcome classification [AHA Scientific Statement]. *Stroke, 29,* 1274–1280.

Lin, K.-C., Wu, C.-Y., & Trombly, C. A. (1998). Effects of task goal on movement kinematics and line bisection performance in adults without disabilities. *American Journal of Occupational Therapy, 52,* 179–187.

Trombly, C. A. (1998). Invited editorial. *Scandinavian Journal of Occupational Therapy, 5,* 3–5.

Trombly, C. A., Radomski, M. V., & Davis, E. S. (1998). Achievement of self-identified goals by adults with traumatic brain injury: Phase I. *American Journal of Occupational Therapy, 52,* 810–818.

Wu, C.-Y., Trombly, C. A., Lin, K.-C., & Tickle-Degnen, L. (1998). Effects of object affordances on reaching performance in persons with and without cerebrovascular accident (CVA). *American Journal of Occupational Therapy, 52,* 447–456.

Wu, C.-Y., Trombly, C. A., Lin, K.-C., & Tickle-Degnen, L. (1998). Effects of object affordances on movement performance: A meta-analysis. *Scandinavian Journal of Occupational Therapy, 5,* 83–92.

Ferguson, J. M., & Trombly, C. A. (1997). Effects of added purpose and meaningful occupation on motor learning. *American Journal of Occupational Therapy, 51,* 508–515.

Fuller, Y., & Trombly, C. A. (1997). Effects of object characteristics on female grasp patterns. *American Journal of Occupational Therapy, 51,* 481–487.

Gresham, G. E., Alexander, D., Bishop, D. S., Giuliana, C., Goldberg, G., Holland, A., Kelly-Hayes, M., Linn, R. T., Roth, E. J., Stason, W. B., & Trombly, C. A. (1997). AHA Prevention Conference IV: Stroke—Rehabilitation. *Stroke, 28,* 1522–1526.

Lin, K.-C., Cermak, S. A., Kinsbourne, M., & Trombly, C. A. (1996). Effects of left-sided movements on line bisection in unilateral neglect. *Journal of the International Neuropsychological Society, 2,* 404–411.

Gresham, G. E., Duncan, P. W., Stason, W. B., Adams, H. P., Adelman, A. M., Alexander, D. N., Bishop, D. S., Diller, L., Donaldson, N. E., Granger, C. V., Holland, A. L., Kelly-ayes, M., McDowell, F. H., Myers, L., Phipps, M. A., Roth, E. J., Siebens, H. C., Tarvin, G. A., & Trombly, C. A. (1995). *Clinical Practice Guideline 16: Post-stroke rehabilitation* (AHCPR Pub. No. 95-662). Rockville, MD: U.S. Department of Health and Human Services, Agency for Health Care Policy and Research.

Trombly, C. A. (1995). Health policy: Clinical practice guideline for post-stroke rehabilitation and occupational therapy practice. *American Journal of Occupational Therapy, 49,* 711–714.

Trombly, C. A. (1995). Occupation: Purposefulness and meaningfulness as therapeutic mechanisms (1995 Eleanor Clarke Slagle Lecture). *American Journal of Occupational Therapy, 49,* 960–972.

Trombly, C. A. (Ed.). (1994). *Occupational therapy for physical dysfunction* (4th ed.). Baltimore: Williams & Wilkins.

Wu, C.-Y., Trombly, C. A., & Lin, K.-C. (1994). The relationship between occupational form and occupational performance: A kinematic perspective. *American Journal of Occupational Therapy, 48,* 679–687.

Trombly, C. A. (1993). The Issue Is—Anticipating the future: Assessment of occupational function. *American Journal of Occupational Therapy, 47,* 253–257.

Trombly, C. A. (1993). Observations of improvement in reaching in five subjects with left hemiparesis. *Journal of Neurology, Neurosurgery, and Psychiatry, 56,* 40–45.

Trombly, C. A. (1992). Deficits of reaching in subjects with left hemiparesis: A pilot study. *American Journal of Occupational Therapy, 45,* 887–897.

Cermak, S. A., Trombly, C. A., Hausser, J., & Tiernan, A. M. (1991). Effects of lateralized tasks on unilateral neglect after right cerebrovascular accident. *Occupational Therapy Journal of Research, 11,* 271–291.

Henderson, A., Cermak, S., Coster, W., Murray, E., Trombly, C. A., & Tickle-Dengen, L. (1991). The Issue Is—Occupational science is multidimensional. *American Journal of Occupational Therapy, 45,* 370–372.

Dortch, H. L., & Trombly, C. A. (1990). The effects of education on hand use with industrial workers in repetitive jobs. *American Journal of Occupational Therapy, 44,* 777–782.

Iammatteo, P. A., Trombly, C. A., & Luecke, L. (1990). The effect of mouth closure on drooling and speech. *American Journal of Occupational Therapy, 44,* 689–691.

Trombly, C. A. (Ed.). (1989). *Occupational therapy for physical dysfunction* (3rd ed.). Baltimore: Williams & Wilkins.

Trombly, C. A. (1987). Caution advised in using predictors for at-risk workers [Letter to the Editor]. *American Journal of Occupational Therapy, 41,* 194.

Jette, D. U., Falkel, J. E., & Trombly, C. A. (1986). Effect of intermittent, supine traction on the myoelectric activity of the upper trapezius muscle in subjects with neck pain. *Physical Therapy, 40,* 1173–1176.

Trombly, C. A., Thayer-Nason, L., Bliss, G., Girard, C. A., Lyrist, L. A., & Brexa-Hooson, A. (1986). The effectiveness of therapy in improving finger extension in stroke patients. *American Journal of Occupational Therapy, 40,* 612–617.

Opila-Lehman, J., Short, M. A., & Trombly, C. A. (1985). Kinesthetic recall of children with athetoid and spastic cerebral palsy and of non-handicapped children. *Developmental Medicine and Child Neurology, 27,* 223–230.

Trombly, C. A., & Quintana, L. A. (1985). Differences in response to exercise by post-CVA and normal subjects. *Occupational Therapy Journal of Research, 5,* 39–58.

Trombly, C. A., & Neuhaus, B. E. (1984). Graduate education for the physical disabilities specialist. *Physical Disabilities Special Interest Section Newsletter, 7,* 1–2.

Wilson, B. N., & Trombly, C. A. (1984). Proximal and distal function in children with and without sensory integrative dysfunction. *Canadian Journal of Occupational Therapy, 51,* 11–17.

Carlson, J. D., & Trombly, C. A. (1983). The effect of wrist immobilization on performance of the Jebsen Hand Function Test. *American Journal of Occupational Therapy, 37,* 167–175.

Mathiowetz, W., Bolding, D. J., & Trombly, C. A. (1983). Immediate effects of positioning devices on the normal and spastic hand measured by electromyography. *American Journal of Occupational Therapy, 37,* 247–254.

Trombly, C. A. (Ed.). (1983). *Occupational therapy for physical dysfunction* (2nd ed.). Baltimore: Williams & Wilkins.

Trombly, C. A., & Quintana, L. A. (1983). Activity analysis: Electromyographic and electrogoniometric verification. *Occupational Therapy Journal of Research, 3,* 104–120.

Trombly, C. A., & Quintana, L. A. (1983). The effects of exercise on finger extension of CVA patients. *American Journal of Occupational Therapy, 37,* 195–202.

Trombly, C. A. (1982). Include exercise in "purposeful activity" [Letter to the Editor]. *American Journal of Occupational Therapy, 36,* 467–468.

Trombly, C. A., & Cole, J. M. (1979). Electromyographic study of four hand muscles during selected activities. *American Journal of Occupational Therapy, 33,* 440–449.

Trombly, C. A., & Scott, A. (Eds.). (1977). *Occupational therapy for physical dysfunction.* Baltimore: Williams & Wilkins.

Long, C., & Trombly, C. A. (1968). Clinical applications of myoelectric control in upper extremity orthotics: A preliminary report. *Archives of Physical Medicine and Rehabilitation, 39,* 661–664.

Trombly, C. A. (1968). Myoelectric control of orthotic devices for the severely paralyzed. *American Journal of Occupational Therapy, 22,* 385–389.

Trombly, C. A., Prentke, E., & Long, C. (1967). Myoelectrically controlled electrical torque motor for the flexor hinge hand splint. *Orthopedic and Prosthetic Appliance Journal, 21,* 39–43.

Trombly, C. A. (1966). Principles of operant conditioning: Related to orthotic training of quadriplegic patients. *American Journal of Occupational Therapy, 20,* 217–220.

Trombly, C. A. (1964). Effects of selected activities on finger extension of adult hemiplegic patients. *American Journal of Occupational Therapy, 18,* 233–239.

Lilian B. Wegg, OTR, FAOTA—1959

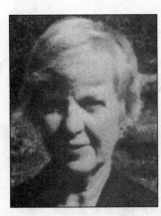

Lilian B. Wegg was born July 1, 1924, in Ontario, Canada. Wegg attended high school and secretarial school in Toronto for 5 years and later graduated from the University of Toronto, where she obtained a diploma in occupational therapy in 1946. She also attended the University of San Francisco, receiving a certificate in rehabilitation administration. In her career, she developed various rehabilitation workshops and work training centers for adults with developmental delays and a variety of other illnesses. Some of her jobs included working (1) as a vocational counselor a private rehabilitation counseling center in California called Work Wise; (2) at a workers' compensation center in 1948, in Toronto, Canada, duplicating occupations that people previously engaged in or might face when returning to work (work therapy); (3) at the Morrison Rehabilitation Center in San Francisco from 1948 to 1959, treating a young population between the ages of 16 and 17 who suffered from post polio; and (4) as a work evaluator for the Goodwill Industries at the Pacific Career Center from 1981 to 1983 (L. Wegg, personal communication, June 2004).

Wegg noted that the Pacific Career Center was one of the first places to recognize her work as an occupational therapist. When asked what was the hallmark of her life she stated, "OT as a career was the most important thing in my life" (L. Wegg, personal communication, June 2004). Wegg became a fellow of the American Occupational Therapy Association in 1973. She is retired and currently living in California.

Linking Key Messages of the 1959 Eleanor Clarke Slagle Lecture to the AOTA *Centennial Vision:* In reflecting about her Eleanor Clarke Slagle Lecture, Wegg believed, "It was not a time when people were really interested in work therapy and that [her] message was not accepted nor truly recognized by both the association and by therapists at the time" (L. Wegg, personal communication, June 2004). Wegg noted that today's therapists and students should remember how important it is to see the client's actual workplace and engage clients in work therapy in the actual work setting. She spoke passionately about the young veterans returning from war and how occupational therapy will allow the person to return to work. Wegg noted that it is significant that returning veterans are really absorbed back into the world of work (L. Wegg, personal communication, October 2009). As the *Centennial Vision* describes meeting societal needs and articulating the profession's value to society, this example with returning veterans is one area in which occupational therapists can truly make a difference.

Bibliography

Wegg, L. (1977). The essentials of work evaluation. *American Journal of Occupational Therapy, 31,* 651–652.

Wegg, L. (1960). The essentials of work evaluation (1959 Eleanor Clarke Slagle Lecture). *American Journal of Occupational Therapy, 14,* 65–69, 79.

Wegg, L. (1957). The role of the occupational therapist in vocational rehabilitation. *American Journal of Occupational Therapy, 11,* 252–254.

Wilma L. West, MA, OTR, FAOTA—1967

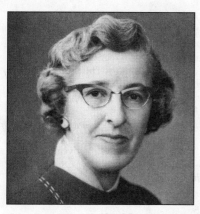

Wilma L. West graduated from Mount Holyoke College in 1939. She received a certificate in occupational therapy from Tufts University and a master's degree from the University of Southern California.

Long active in AOTA, West's roles included educational field secretary, executive director, treasurer, and president. She also served as president of the American Occupational Therapy Foundation from 1972 to 1982 and was named president emeritus in 1982. Her major clinical interests were in physical disabilities and pediatrics, while her experience included positions in administration, education, research, and consultation. In 1977, she retired from the U.S. Department of Health, Education, and Welfare (HEW) after 10 years as consultant in occupational therapy with the agency's Children's Bureau and Maternal and Child Health Service. She also served 4 years as chief, Health Services Research and Training, HEW.

Her honors include the Bernard Baruch Fellowship for Graduate Study, 1946; the AOTA Award of Merit, 1951; the AOTA Roster of Fellows, 1973; and the HEW Superior Service Award, 1972. She received the Army Surgeon General's Meritorious Civilian Service Award in 1946 and served as a consultant to the Surgeon General from 1958 to 1964. She served on the Professional Advisory Council of the National Easter Seal Society for Crippled Children and Adults and on the Advisory Council on Physical Therapy Education for the American Physical Therapy Association. She died in 1996.

Bibliography

West, W. L. (1947). The future of occupational therapy in the army. *American Journal of Occupational Therapy, 1,* 89–91.

West, W. L. (1947). The future of occupational therapy in the army. *American Journal of Occupational Therapy, 1,* 155–157.

West, W. L., & Kahmann, W. C. (1947). Occupational therapy in the United States Army hospitals: World War II. In H. S. Willard & H. S. Spackman (Eds.), *Principles of occupational therapy* (pp. 329–375). Philadelphia: Lippincott.

West, W. L. (1948). Report of the executive director. *American Journal of Occupational Therapy, 2,* 303–205.

West, W. L. (1949). Annual report of the executive director. *American Journal of Occupational Therapy, 3,* 252–255.

West, W. L. (1949). The need for graduate study in occupational therapy. *American Journal of Occupational Therapy, 3,* 309.

West, W. L. (1949). Report on the performance of war emergency course graduates. *American Journal of Occupational Therapy, 4,* 199–205.

West, W. L. (1950). Annual report of the executive director. *American Journal of Occupational Therapy, 4,* 274.

West, W. L. (1950). The need for an international association of OTs. *American Journal of Occupational Therapy, 4,* 23–25.

West, W. L. (1950). People you should know: Hyman Brandt. *American Journal of Occupational Therapy, 4,* 75–76

West, W. L. (1950). The principles of occupational therapy in the rehabilitation of the physically handicapped. In H. Kessler (Ed.), *Principles and practices of rehabilitation* (pp. 141–174). Philadelphia: Lea & Febriger.

West, W. L. (1951). Annual report of the executive director. *American Journal of Occupational Therapy, 5,* 258.

West, W. L. (1951). The profession's stand against licensure for OTs. *American Journal of Occupational Therapy, 5,* 60–62.

West, W. L. (1951). Report of the Mid-century White House Conference on Children and Youth. *American Journal of Occupational Therapy, 5,* 31–35.

West, W. L., & Clark, A. W. (1951, September). Planning the complete occupational therapy service. *Hospitals, 25,* 3–23.

West, W. L. (1955). Evaluation of the institute. In *Proceedings of the Occupational Therapy Institute: A reassessment of professional education and practice in occupational therapy as related to rehabilitation* (p. 199). New York: American Occupational Therapy Association.

West, W. L., & McNary, H. (1956). The present and potential role of occupational therapy in rehabilitation. *American Journal of Occupational Therapy, 10,* 103–107, 150.

West, W. L. (1957). Nationally speaking. *American Journal of Occupational Therapy, 11,* 190–191.

West, W. L. (1958). Essentials of treatment. In *Proceedings of the 1956 Regional Occupational Therapy Institutes and Annual Institute* (pp. 165–169). New York: American Occupational Therapy Association.

West, W. L. (1958). The present status of graduate education in occupational therapy. *American Journal of Occupational Therapy, 12,* 291–292, 299.

West, W. L. (1958). The present status of graduate education in occupational therapy. In *Changing concepts and practice in psychiatric occupational therapy.* New York: American Occupational Therapy Association.

West, W. L. (1958). The specific role of the occupational therapist in implementing group goals. In *Proceedings of the 1956 Regional Occupational Therapy Institutes and Annual Institute* (pp. 16–22, 121–126, 136–138). New York: American Occupational Therapy Association.

West, W. L. (1958). Synthesis. *American Journal of Occupational Therapy, 12,* 225–230.

Willard, H. S., Killburn, V. T., & West, W. L. (1958). Nationally Speaking: New officers: From the president: From the education office: Curriculum study plans. *American Journal of Occupational Therapy, 12,* 330–333.

West, W. L. (Ed.). (1959). *Changing concepts and practices in psychiatric occupational therapy: Proceedings of the Allenberry Workshop Conference on the Function and Preparation of the Psychiatric Occupational Therapist, Allenberry Inn, Boiling Springs, Pennsylvania, November 13–19, 1956.* New York: American Occupational Therapy Association.

West, W. L. (1962). Nationally speaking. *American Journal of Occupational Therapy, 16,* 90–91.

West, W. L. (1962). Nationally speaking. *American Journal of Occupational Therapy, 16,* 194–195.

West, W. L. (1962). Nationally Speaking: From the president. *American Journal of Occupational Therapy, 16,* 146–148.

West, W. L. (1963). Nationally speaking. *American Journal of Occupational Therapy, 17,* 64–66.

West, W. L. (1963). The president's address: 1962 annual conference. *American Journal of Occupational Therapy, 17,* 26–28.

West, W. L. (1963). The president's address: 1963 annual conference. *American Journal of Occupational Therapy, 17,* 252–253.

West, W. L., Fidler, G. S., & Spelbring, L. M. (1963). Nationally Speaking: The prescription in occupational therapy: The projected levels of function in occupational therapy departments in 1970. *American Journal of Occupational Therapy, 17,* 122–125.

West, W. L. (1964). Graduate education as a requisite for status and advancement. *American Journal of Occupational Therapy, 18,* 68.

West, W. L. (1964). Nationally Speaking: From the president. *American Journal of Occupational Therapy, 18,* 116.

West, W. L. (1964). The role of occupational therapy in work adjustment. In W. C. Brown (Ed.), *Work adjustment as a function of occupational therapy* (Study Course V, pp. 49–68). Dubuque, IA: Kendall/Hunt.

West, W. L., & Helmig, F. (1964). Board of management: American Occupational Therapy Association minutes: Midyear meeting, Indianapolis, Indiana, April 12/13, 1964. *American Journal of Occupational Therapy, 18,* 165–172.

West, W. L. (Ed.). (1965). *Occupational therapy for the multiply handicapped child: Proceedings of the Conference on Occupational Therapy for the Multiply Handicapped Child, Center for Continuing Education, Chicago, Illinois, April 28–May 2, 1965.* Chicago: University of Illinois.

West, W. L. (1965). The president's address. *American Journal of Occupational Therapy, 19,* 31–33.

West, W. L. (1966). Occupational therapy in neuropsychiatry. In *Neuropsychiatry in World War II* (Vol. 1, pp. 157–198). Washington, DC: Office of the Surgeon General, U.S. Department of the Army.

West, W. L. (1967). The occupational therapist's changing responsibility to community. *American Journal of Occupational Therapy, 21,* 312–316.

West, W. L. (1968). Occupational therapy: Philosophy and perspective. *American Journal of Nursing, 68,* 322–340.

West, W. L. (1968). Professional responsibility in times of change (1967 Eleanor Clarke Slagle Lecture). *American Journal of Occupational Therapy, 22,* 9–15.

West, W. L. (1968). *Professional services of occupational therapists, World War II: Army Medical Specialist Corps.* Washington, DC: Office of the Surgeon General.

West, W. L. (1968). Statement to the Committee on Health Manpower: American Medical Association, Chicago, September 15, 1967. *American Journal of Occupational Therapy, 22,* 89.

West, W. L. (1968). *Training in World War II: Army Medical Specialist Corps.* Washington, DC: Office of the Surgeon General.

West, W. L. (1968). *Wartime organization and administration: Army Medical Specialist Corps.* Washington, DC: Office of the Surgeon General.

West, W. L. (1969). The growing importance of prevention. *American Journal of Occupational Therapy, 23,* 226–231.

West, W. L. (Ed.). (1969). *Occupational therapy functions in interdisciplinary programs for children: Proceedings of the conference, the Training Function of Occupational Therapy in University-Affiliated Centers, Ramada Inn, Los Angeles, California, August 25–27, 1969.* Washington, DC: U.S. Department of Health, Education, and Welfare.

West, W. L. & Wiemer, R. B. (1970). Occupational therapy in community health care. In *Occupational therapy today—tomorrow* (pp. 187–204). Basel, Switzerland: Karger.

Wiemer, R. B., & West, W. L. (1970). Occupational therapy in community health care. *American Journal of Occupational Therapy, 24,* 323–328.

West, W. L. (1973). The principles and process of consultation. In L. Llorens (Ed.), *Consultation in the community: Occupational therapy in child health.* Dubuque, IA: Kendall/Hunt.

West, W. L. (1975). The foundation: The first decade. *American Journal of Occupational Therapy, 29,* 636.

West, W. L. (1976). Problems and policies in licensure of occupational therapists. *American Journal of Occupational Therapy, 30,* 40–43.

West, W. L. (1976). Research seminar. *American Journal of Occupational Therapy, 30,* 477–478.

West, W. L. (1977). The Foundation: Open letter to Jerry A. Johnson, AOTA President. *American Journal of Occupational Therapy, 31,* 10.

West, W. L. (1978). Reflections at retirement: Address of AOTF president at AOTA's 60th anniversary conference. *American Journal of Occupational Therapy, 32,* 9–12.

West, W. L. (1979). Historical perspectives. In American Occupational Therapy Association (Ed.), *Occupational therapy: 2001 AD.* Rockville, MD: Editor.

West, W. L. (1979). Professional unity. *American Journal of Occupational Therapy, 33,* 40–49.

Hightower-Vandamm, M., & West, W. L. (1980). Helen S. Willard Scholarship planned. *Occupational Therapy Newspaper, 34*(8), 2.

West, W. L. (1980). Fifteenth-anniversary celebration: American Occupational Therapy Foundation. *American Journal of Occupational Therapy, 34,* 683–685.

West, W. L. (1980). The Foundation: The $5 annual giving fund. *American Journal of Occupational Therapy, 33,* 823.

West, W. L. (1980). Foundation to publish *OT Journal of Research. Occupational Therapy Newspaper, 34*(12), 1.

West, W. L. (1981). Commentary: A journal of research in occupational therapy: The response, the responsibility. *Occupational Therapy Journal of Research, 1,* 7–12.

Cox, R. C., & West, W. L. (1982). *Fundamentals of research for health professionals.* Laurel, MD: Ramsco.

West, W. L. (1982). The Foundation: Message from the president: The need, the response: "Occupational Therapy Journal of Research." *American Journal of Occupational Therapy, 36,* 44.

West, W. L. (1982). In memoriam: Winifred Conrick Kahmann. *American Journal of Occupational Therapy, 36,* 472–475.

West, W. L. (1984). A reaffirmed philosophy and practice of occupational therapy for the 1980s. *Journal of Occupational Therapy, 38,* 15–23.

Cox, R. C., & West, W. L. (1986). *Fundamentals of research for health professionals* (2nd ed.). Laurel, MD: Ramsco.

West, W. L. (1989). In memoriam: Ruth A. Robinson, 1909–1989. *American Journal of Occupational Therapy, 42,* 481–482.

West, W. L. (1989). Nationally Speaking: Perspectives on the past and future, part 1. *American Journal of Occupational Therapy, 42,* 787–790.

West, W. L. (1990). Nationally Speaking: Perspectives on the past and future, part 2. *American Journal of Occupational Therapy, 44,* 9–10.

West, W. L. (1991). A tribute to Lela Llorens. *OT Week, 5*(5), 10–11.

West, W. L., & Wiemer, R. B. (1991). The Issue Is: Should the Representative Assembly have voted as it did, when it did, on occupational therapists' use of physical agent modalities? *American Journal of Occupational Therapy, 45,* 1143–1147.

West, W. L. (1992). Ten milestone issues in AOTA history. *Amercian Journal of Occupational Therapy, 46,* 1066–1074.

Elizabeth J. Yerxa, ED, OTR, FAOTA—1966

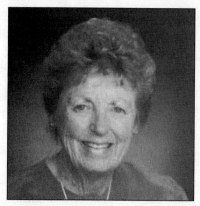

Elizabeth "Betty" Yerxa is a Distinguished Professor Emerita for the Department of Occupational Therapy at the University of Southern California (USC). She began her education at USC with a Bachelor of Science in Occupational Therapy in 1952. She later earned a Master of Education and a Doctor of Education in Educational Psychology from Boston University.

Yerxa was first employed as a staff occupational therapist at Orthopedic Hospital in Los Angeles, California, in 1953. She then worked with children with cerebral palsy in Lancaster, California, before her long and illustrious career in academia. Yerxa also was a research coordinator in occupational therapy at Rancho Los Amigos Hospital from 1971 to 1976. She was a faculty member at the College of Puget Sound in Tacoma, Washington, from 1955 to 1956 and the Sargent College of Allied Health Professions at Boston University from 1969 to 1971. She became an associate professor in the USC School of Medicine, Department of Community Medicine and Public Health, from 1971 to 1979, and a joint appointment as chairperson of the Department of Occupational Therapy, from 1976 to 1982. Yerxa was promoted to professor at USC from 1982 to 1987 and from 1988 to the present is an emeritus professor in the Department of Occupational Therapy. She has been a visiting professor or fellow traveling the world to such places as England, Sweden, Australia, Canada, and Finland.

Her awards have been numerous, including recipient of the Eleanor Clarke Slagle Lectureship Award in 1966 and being inducted into the Roster of Fellows of the American Occupational Therapy Association (AOTA) in 1973. Yerxa was a charter member of the Academy of Research for the American Occupational Therapy Foundation (AOTF) in 1983. She received several other recognitions and honors from the AOTF, including an Award of Appreciation in 1986 and the A. Jean Ayres Award in 1990. AOTA has also given Yerxa a Service Award in 1984 and bestowed the Award of Merit, the highest award from the association, in 1987. She received an Honorary Doctor of Humane Letters from Thomas Jefferson University in 1988 and an Honorary Doctor of Science from Exeter University in Exeter, England, in 1995. She also was the recipient of the Killiam Memorial Lectureship, Dalhousie University in Halifax, Nova Scotia, and of the Wilma West Lectureship, Occupational Science Symposium, from USC.

Yerxa's research interests include community adaptation of disabled persons, organization and use of time, occupational therapy philosophical base, instrument development, and occupational behavior of persons with chronic disability. She currently is retired but still is actively engaged in scholarly projects.

On a Personal Note From a Phone Interview: Betty Yerxa noted that 1966 was a very stimulating time of her life and in writing her lecture she wanted to be true to the spirit of the Eleanor Clarke Slagle Lecture. She believes that her message is as timely today as it was in 1966.

Linking Key Messages of the 1966 Eleanor Clarke Slagle Lecture to the AOTA *Centennial Vision:* In regard to the *Centennial Vision*, Yerxa states, because of a market-based work environment that pressures practitioners to be technical and reductionistic, there has never been a more important need for authentic occupational therapy provided by ethical professionals than in the 21st century. For more on this position see Yerxa (2009).

—*Elizabeth Yerxa*

Bibliography

Yerxa, E. J. (2009). Infinite distance between the *I* and the *it*. *American Journal of Occupational Therapy, 63,* 490–497.

Yerxa, E. J. (2005). Learning to love the questions. *American Journal of Occupational Therapy, 59,* 108–112.

Yerxa, E. J. (2002). Habits in context: A synthesis, with implications for research in occupational science. *Occupational Therapy Journal of Research, 22,* 104S–110S.

Yerxa, E. J. (2000). Occupational science: A renaissance of service to humankind through knowledge. *Occupational Therapy International, 7,* 87–98.

Yerxa, E. J. (2000). Confessions of an occupational therapist who became a detective. *British Journal of Occupational Therapy, 63,* 192–199.

Yerxa, E. J. (1998). Occupation: The keystone of a curriculum for a self-defined profession. *American Journal of Occupational Therapy, 52,* 365–372.

Yerxa, E. J. (1998). Health and the human spirit for occupation. *American Journal of Occupational Therapy, 52,* 412–418.

Yerxa, E. J. (1996). The social and psychological experience of having a disability: Implications for occupational therapists. In L. W. Pedretti (Ed.), *Occupational therapy practice skills for physical dysfunction* (4th ed., pp. 253–274). St. Louis, MO: Mosby.

Yerxa, E. J. (1995). Who is the keeper of occupational therapy's practice and knowledge? *American Journal of Occupational Therapy, 29,* 295–299.

Yerxa, E. J. (1994). In search of good ideas for occupational therapy. *Scandinavian Journal of Occupational Therapy, 1,* 7–15.

Yerxa, E. J. (1994). Dreams, dilemmas, and decisions for occupational therapy practice in a new millennium: An American perspective. *American Journal of Occupational Therapy, 48,* 586–589.

Yerxa, E. J. (1993). Occupational science: A source of power for participants in occupational therapy. *Journal of Occupational Science Australia, 1,* 3–10.

Yerxa, E. J. (1992). Some implications of occupational therapy's history for its epistemology, values, and relation to medicine. *American Journal of Occupational Therapy, 46,* 79–83.

Yerxa, E. J. (1992). Foreword. In N. Katz (Ed.), *Cognitive rehabilitation: Models for intervention in occupational therapy* (pp. v–vii). Fort Washington, PA: Ruttle, Shaw, & Wetherill.

Titus, M. N., Gall, N. G., Yerxa, E. J., Robertson, T. A., & Mack, W. (1991). Correlation of perceptual performance and activities of daily living in stroke patients. *American Journal of Occupational Therapy, 45,* 410–418.

Yerxa, E. J. (Guest Ed.). (1991). Special Issue on qualitative research. *American Journal of Occupational Therapy, 45.*

Yerxa, E. J. (1991). Seeking a relevant, ethical, and realistic way of knowing for occupational therapy. *American Journal of Occupational Therapy, 45,* 199–204.

Yerxa, E. J. (1991). Occupational therapy: An endangered species or an academic discipline in the 21st century? *American Journal of Occupational Therapy, 45,* 680–685.

Yerxa, E. J., & Locker, S. B. (1990). Quality of time use by adults with spinal card injuries. *American Journal of Occupational Therapy, 44,* 318–326.

Stein, C., & Yerxa, E. J. (1990). A test of fine finger dexterity. *American Journal of Occupational Therapy, 44,* 499–504.

Yerxa, E. J. (1990). A mind is a precious thing [Guest Editorial]. *Australian Occupational Therapy Journal, 37,* 170–171.

Yerxa, E. J., & Johnson, J. A. (Eds.). (1989). *Occupational science: The foundation for new models of practice.* New York: Haworth Press.

Yerxa, E. J., Clark, F., Frank, G., Jackson, J., Parham, D., Pierce, D., et al. (1989). An introduction to occupational science, a foundation for occupational therapy in the 21st century. *Occupational Therapy in Health Care, 6*(3/4), 1–17.

Yerxa, E. J., Burnett Beaulieu, S., Stocking, S., & Azen, S. (1988). Development of the satisfaction with performance scaled questionnaire (SPSQ). *American Journal of Occupational Therapy, 42,* 215–221.

Yerxa, E. J. (1988). Oversimplification: The hobgoblin of theory and practice in occupational therapy. *Canadian Journal of Occupational Therapy, 55,* 5–6.

Yerxa, E. J., & Baum, S. (1987). The physical environment of the older person. *Topics in Geriatric Rehabilitation, 3,* 718.

Yerxa, E. J. (1987). Review of "Occupational Therapy in Health Care: Origins and Adaptations: A Philosophy of Practice." *Occupational Therapy in Health Care, 4,* 186–187.

Yerxa, E. J. (1987). Research: The key to the development of occupational therapy as an academic discipline. *American Journal of Occupational Therapy, 41,* 415–419.

Yerxa, E. J., & Sharrott, G. W. (1986). Liberal arts: The foundation for occupational therapy. *American Journal of Occupational Therapy, 40,* 153–159.

Yerxa, E. J., & Baum, S. (1986). Occupational therapy in rehabilitation: Reduction of patient incapacity across the lifespan. *Annual Review of Rehabilitation, 5,* 39–66.

Yerxa, E. J., & Baum, S. (1986). Engagement in daily occupations and life satisfaction among people with spinal cord injuries. *Occupational Therapy Journal of Research, 6,* 271–283.

Cooper, C., & Yerxa, E. J. (1986). Denial: Implications of a pilot study on activity level related to sexual competence in burned adults. *American Journal of Occupational Therapy, 38,* 529–534.

Sharrott, G. W., & Yerxa, E. J. (1985): Promises to keep: Implications of the referent "patient" versus "client" or those served by occupational therapy. *American Journal of Occupational Therapy, 39,* 401–405.

Yerxa, E. J. (1985). *Putting it all together by evaluating a research article* (AOTF Audiotapes, Module 10). Rockville, MD: Ramsco.

Yerxa, E. J. (1985). *Preparing to read a research study* (AOTF Audiotapes, Module 1). Rockville, MD: Ramsco.

Su, R. V., & Yerxa, E. J. (1984). Comparison of the test–retest reliability between the motor tests of the Southern California Sensory Integration Tests (SCSIT) and the Luria–Nebraska Neuropsychological Battery: Children's Version (L–NNBC) in 30 dysfunctional children aged 8 years. *Occupational Therapy Journal of Research, 4,* 96–108.

Gregory, J. L., & Yerxa, E. J. (1984). Standardization of the prone extension postural test on children ages four through eight. *American Journal of Occupational Therapy, 38,* 187–194.

Cooper, C., & Yerxa, E. J. (1984). Activity level related to sexual competence in burned adults. *American Journal of Occupational Therapy, 38,* 187–194.

Yerxa, E. J. (1984). The role of the occupational therapist. In G. K. Riggs & E. Gall (Eds.), *Rheumatic diseases: Rehabilitation and management* (pp. 19–21). Boston: Butterworth.

Yerxa, E. J. (1984). Evaluation versus research: Outcomes or knowledge? *American Journal of Occupational Therapy, 38,* 407–408.

Yerxa, E. J., Barber, L. M., Diaz, O., Black, W., & Azen, S. P. (1983). Development of a hand sensitivity test for use in desensitization of the hypersensitive hand. *American Journal of Occupational Therapy, 37,* 176–181.

Yerxa, E. J. (1983). Research priorities. *American Journal of Occupational Therapy, 37,* 699.

Yerxa, E. J. (1983). The occupational therapist as researcher. In H. Smith & C. Hopkins (Eds.), *Willard and Spackman's occupational therapy* (6th ed., pp. 869–875). Philadelphia: J. B. Lippincott.

Yerxa, E. J. (1983). Audacious values, the energy source for occupational therapy practice. In G. Kielhofner (Ed.), *Health through occupation: Theory and practice in occupational therapy* (pp. 149–162). Philadelphia: F. A. Davis.

Yerxa, E. J. (1982). A response to testing and measurement in occupational therapy: A review of current practice with special emphasis on the Southern California Sensory Integration Tests. *American Journal of Occupational Therapy, 36,* 399–404.

Tickle, L., & Yerxa, E. J. (1981). Need satisfaction of older persons living in the community and in institutions: Part II, role of activity. *American Journal of Occupational Therapy, 35,* 650–655.

Tickle, L., & Yerxa, E. J. (1981). Need satisfaction of older persons living in the community and in institutions: Part I, the environment. *American Journal of Occupational Therapy, 35,* 644–649.

Chaparro, C. J., Yerxa, E. J., Nelson, J., & Wilson, L. (1981). The incidence of sensory integrative dysfunction among children with orofacial cleft. *American Journal of Occupational Therapy, 35,* 96–100.

Yerxa, E. J. (1981). Review of *Children Adapt. Occupational Therapy Journal of Research, 1,* 99–101.

Yerxa, E. J. (1981). Basic or applied: A "developmental assessment" of occupational therapy research. *American Journal of Occupational Therapy, 35,* 820–821.

Yerxa, E. J. (1980). Occupational therapy's role in creating a future climate of caring, *American Journal of Occupational Therapy, 34,* 529–534.

Burnett, S., & Yerxa, E. J. (1980). Community based and college based needs assessment of physically disabled persons. *American Journal of Occupational Therapy, 34,* 201–207.

Mazur, H., Beeston, J., & Yerxa, E. J. (1979). Clinical interdisciplinary health team care: An educational experiment. *Journal of Medical Education, 54,* 703–713.

Furgang, N., & Yerxa, E. J. (1979). Expectations of teachers for physically handicapped and normal first grade students. *American Journal of Occupational Therapy, 33,* 697–704.

Yerxa, E. J. (1979). The philosophical base of occupational therapy. In *Occupational therapy: 2001 A.D.* (pp. 26–30). Rockville, MD: American Occupational Therapy Association.

Yerxa, E. J. (1978). The profession of occupational therapy: Today and tomorrow. In H. Smith & C. Hopkins (Eds.), *Willard and Spackman's occupational therapy* (5th ed., pp. 697–703). Philadelphia: J. B. Lippincott.

Yerxa, E. J. (1978). The occupational therapist as consultant and researcher: Autonomous change agentry. In H. Smith & C. Hopkins (Eds.), *Willard and Spackman's occupational therapy* (5th ed., pp. 689–693). Philadelphia: J. B. Lippincott.

Yerxa, E. J. (1976). On being a member of a feminine profession. *American Journal of Occupational Therapy, 30,* 597–598.

Yerxa, E. J. (1974). *Human interaction and physical differences* (Vols. I & II). Costa Mesa, CA: Concept Media.

Yerxa, E. J. (1970). Attitude development in childhood education toward foreign people. *Boston University Journal of Education, 4,* 37–41.

Yerxa, E. J. (1967). Authentic occupational therapy (1966 Eleanor Clark Slagle Lecture). *American Journal of Occupational Therapy, 21,* 1–9.

Ruth Zemke, PhD, OTR (ret.), FAOTA—2004

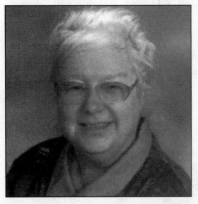

Ruth Zemke is a professor emerita in the Department of Occupational Therapy and Occupational Science at the University of Southern California (USC) in Los Angeles. She also was a visiting professor and graduate program development consultant in the Department of Occupational Therapy at Sapporo Medical University in Sapporo, Japan. She is a grant reviewer for the American Occupational Therapy Foundation (AOTF).

Zemke received a bachelor's degree in occupational therapy from the University of Wisconsin in 1965 and a master's degree and a PhD in human development from Iowa State University (ISU) in 1974 and 1977, respectively. She began her career in 1966 in Madison, Wisconsin, working as a staff therapist. During the late 1960s and mid-1970s she held various clinical positions in St. Louis, Missouri, and Ames, Iowa. Concomitantly, in the early 1970s she pursued a teaching career at the ISU and later in the Occupational Therapy Program at the University of Wisconsin–Milwaukee. She moved to USC, from where she recently retired, in 1983.

Over the years, Zemke's practice experience has included inpatient evaluation and treatment of children with mental health problems, including childhood schizophrenia, as well as children with autism. She has done home-based evaluation and community-based programming for people with mental retardation. In addition, she has performed pre-vocational evaluations for persons with developmental disabilities and mental illnesses as well as helped develop sheltered work programs. Zemke participated in hospital-based and outpatient work on neurorehabilitation units, with a focus on adults who have had a stroke. She has been a daily living supervisor in a community home for adolescents with behavioral problems, a small general hospital therapist, an administrator, a consultant, a service provider for both psychiatric and physically disabled in- and outpatients, and a service provider to older adults in skilled nursing facilities.

Zemke's career in research is vast and exemplary. She was the co-principal investigator on the USC Well Elderly Project, one of the most laureate studies in the history of occupational therapy. She used her interest in applying concepts of occupational science to occupational therapy practice. Her basic focus remains on understanding the characteristics of occupation, especially the temporal and spatial ones.

Zemke was inducted into the Roster of Fellows from the American Occupational Therapy Association (AOTA) in 1988. She also received the AOTF Distinguished Service Award in 1992; Omicron Nu from the National Honor Society in1972; the PACE (Premium for Academic Excellence) Award from ISU for 1973–1974; Phi Kappa Phi from the National Honor Society in 1975; the U.S. Department of Health, Education, and Welfare [HEW]/AOTA Health Traineeship Grant Award for doctoral studies in 1974–1976; the HEW Traineeship for the Institute on the Role of Occupational Therapists in Public Schools in 1979; the Award of Appreciation from the Wisconsin Occupational Therapy Association in 1981; the Award of Excellence from the Occupational Therapy Association of California (OTAC) in 1994; an Honorary Membership in the Pi Theta Epsilon National Honor Society in 1995; the Faculty Appreciation Award at the USC International Student Assembly in 1995; Honored Lecturer for the California Foundation for Occupational Therapy in 1996; the Caroline G. Thompson Lecture in the Department of Occupational Therapy at the University of Wisconsin–Madison in 1996; the Thelma Caldwell Lecture in the Department of Occupational Therapy at the University of Toronto in 1999; the Lifetime Achievement Award from OTAC in 2002; and the Ruth Zemke Lecture for Society for the Study of Occupation: USA, in Galveston, Texas, in 2002. Other awards include the USC International Student Assembly Faculty Appreciation Award and the Award of Excellence from OTAC.

On a Personal Note From a Phone Interview: One thing that Zemke values most about occupational therapy as a professional field is the breath of options it offers practitioners. Occupational therapists can become salaried service providers, entrepreneurs, consultants, administrators, and educators. Within these roles, occupational therapists also have a large variety of directions in which to provide service. In traditional hospital/rehabilitation settings, practitioners may work with any age group, from premature infants to older adults. In community-based service, practitioners emphasize wellness and prevention of occupational dysfunction.

"In the last 35 years, as my life changed, with marriage, parenting, and moving between urban and rural environments in several states, I always knew that there would be an exciting opportunity in occupational therapy wherever I lived," said Zemke. "I knew it would not only fit my needs but also provide the opportunity to meet the needs of others. I thrive in problem solving around helping diverse clients develop an appropriate balance of daily occupations in spite of disease, disability, or life changes."

Linking Key Messages of the 2004 Eleanor Clarke Slagle Lecture to the AOTA *Centennial Vision:* In contrast to cosmic, evolutionary, and human levels of understanding time and space, the AOTA membership has selected a visionary level, one in which occupational therapy can be envisioned in its centennial year. The time, 2017, and the space, that of American practice, seem clear-cut and specific. But the perception of time, which is our sense of temporality, and perception of space, our sense of place, is far less precise. It is through our engagement in occupation that we develop the appropriate perceived temporality and spatiality to make the vision a reality.

I stated in my Slagle lecture, "As an occupational scientist, I find culture interesting mainly as a group's view of what occupations are important to engage in and why, when, where and how we do them" (Zemke, 2004, 616). I asked, "If we look through the lenses of Here and Now, . . . what do we see for our role as occupational therapists, given our focus on occupation?" (pp. 617–618) Our *Vision* statement indicates that the culture of occupational therapy is changing. The importance of occupation-centered research to our practice, as its base and its evidence for practice, is clear. Our global connections are supporting the development of local as well as universal theories of occupation for use by occupational therapists. An increasing awareness of the needs of society have focused our answers to my question "What is a healthy society?" and our *Vision* suggests that the "political" practice of occupational therapy is a part not only of our past but also of our future in reaching our goal.

—*Ruth Zemke*

Reference

Zemke, R. (2004). Time, space, and the kaleidoscopes of occupation (2004 Eleanor Clarke Slagle Lecture). *American Journal of Occupational Therapy, 58*, 608–620.

Bibliography

Frank, G., Block, P., & Zemke, R. (2008). Anthropology, occupational therapy, and disability studies: Collaborations and prospects. *Applied Anthropology, 30*(3), 2–5.

Frank, G., & Zemke, R. (2008). Occupational therapy foundations for political engagement and social transformation. In N. Pollard, F. Kronenberg, & D. Sakellariou (Eds.), *Political practice of occupational therapy* (pp. 111–136). Oxford, England: Churchill Livingstone/Elsevier.

Zemke, R. (2007). Preface to the first volume. *Japanese Journal of Occupational Science.*

Minato, M., & Zemke, R. (2004). Occupational choices of persons with schizophrenia living in the community. *Journal of Occupational Science, 11*(1), 31–39.

Minato, M., & Zemke, R. (2004). Time use of people with schizophrenia living in the community. *Occupational Therapy International, 11*, 177–191.

Zemke, R. (2004). Time, space, and the kaleidoscopes of occupation (2004 Eleanor Clarke Slagle Lecture). *American Journal of Occupational Therapy, 58*, 608–620.

Larson, E., & Zemke, R. (2003). Shaping the temporal patterns of our lives: The social coordination of occupation. *Journal of Occupational Science, 10*, 80–89.

Yoshida, M., Sonoda, T., & Zemke, R. (2003). Validation of Urdu Interaction With Disabled Persons Scale. *International Journal of Rehabilitation Research, 26*, 229–233.

Hay, J., LaBree, L., Luo, R., Clark, F., Carlson, M., Mandel, D., Zemke, R., et al. (2002). Cost-effectiveness of preventive occupational therapy for independent-living older adults. *Journal of the American Geriatrics Society, 50*, 1381–1388.

Jackson, J., Gray, J., & Zemke, R. (2002). Optimizing abilities and capacities: Range of motion, strength, and endurance. In C. Trombly & M. Radomski (Eds.), *Occupational therapy for physical dysfunction* (5th ed., pp. 463–480). Baltimore: Lippincott Williams & Wilkins.

Clark, F., Azen, S., Hay, J., Carlson, M., Mandel, D., LaBree, L., Hay, J., Zemke, R., et al. (2001). Embedding health-promoting changes into the daily lives of independent-living older adults: Long-term follow-up of occupational therapy intervention. *Journal of Gerontology: Psychological Sciences, 56B*(1), 60–63.

Jackson, J., Mandel, D., Zemke, R., & Clark, F. (2001). Promoting quality of life in elders: An occupation-based occupational therapy program. *WFOT Bulletin, 43*, 5–12.

Jackson, J., Kennedy, B. L., Mandel, D., Carlson, M., Cherry, B., Fanchiang, S.-P., Ding, L., Zemke, R., et al. (2000). Derivation and pilot assessment of a health promotion program for Mandarin-speaking Chinese older adults. *International Journal of Aging and Human Development, 50*(2), 127–149.

Mandel, D., Jackson, J. M., Zemke, R., Nelson, L., & Clark, F. A. (1999). *Lifestyle redesign: Implementing the well elderly program.* Bethesda, MD: American Occupational Therapy Association.

Jackson, J., Carlson, M., Mandel, D., Zemke, R., & Clark, F. (1998). Occupation in lifestyle redesign: The USC Well Elderly Study occupational therapy program. *American Journal of Occupational Therapy, 52,* 326–336.

Zemke, R., & Clark, F. A. (1998). *Occupational science: The evolving discipline* (T. Sato, trans.). Tokyo: Miwa.

Clark, F., Azen, S., Zemke, R., Jackson, J., Carlson, M., Mandel, D., et al. (1997). Occupational therapy for independent-living older adults: A randomized controlled trial. *JAMA, 278,* 1321–1328.

Lo, J. L., & Zemke, R. (1997). The relationship between affective experiences during daily occupations and subjective well-being measures: A pilot study. *Occupational Therapy in Mental Health, 13*(3), 1–21.

Parham, L. D., & Zemke, R. (1997). Research activities survey of professional programs. *American Journal of Occupational Therapy, 51,* 622–626.

Zemke, R. (1997). Cultural issues in occupational science and occupational therapy. *Japanese Journal of Occupational Therapy, 31,* 962–967.

Carlson, M., Fanchiang, S.-P., Zemke, R., & Clark, F. (1996). A meta-analysis of the effectiveness of occupational therapy for the elderly. *American Journal of Occupational Therapy, 50,* 89–98.

Clark, F., Carlson, M., Zemke, R., Frank, G., Patterson, K., Ennevor, B. L., et al. (1996). Life domains and adaptive strategies of a group of low-income, well older adults. *American Journal of Occupational Therapy, 50,* 99–108.

Clark, F., Carlson, M., Zemke, R., Frank, G., Patterson, K., Larson, B., et al. (1996). A qualitative study of the life domains and adaptive strategies of the low-income well elderly. *American Journal of Occupational Therapy, 50,* 99–108.

Clark, F., & Zemke, R. (1996). Introduction: The nature of the discipline and the concept of occupation. In R. Zemke & F. Clark (Eds.), *Occupational science: The evolving discipline* (pp. vii–xviii). Philadelphia: F. A. Davis.

McLaughlin-Gray, J., Kennedy, B., & Zemke, R. (1996). Application of dynamic systems theory to occupation. In R. Zemke & F. Clark (Eds.), *Occupational science: The evolving discipline* (pp. 309–324). Philadelphia: F. A. Davis.

McLaughlin-Gray, J., Kennedy, B., & Zemke, R. (1996). Dynamic systems theory: An overview. In R. Zemke & F. Clark (Eds.), *Occupational science: The evolving discipline* (pp. 297–308). Philadelphia: F. A. Davis.

Zemke, R. (1996). Brain, mind, and meaning. In R. Zemke & F. Clark (Eds.), *Occupational science: The evolving discipline* (pp. 163–170). Philadelphia: F. A. Davis.

Zemke, R., & Clark, F. A. (Eds.). (1996). *Occupational science: The evolving discipline.* Philadelphia: F. A. Davis.

Zemke, R., & Fraits-Hunt, D. (1996). Games mothers and their full-term or pre-term infants play. In R. Zemke & F. Clark (Eds.), *Occupational science: The evolving discipline* (pp. 217–226). Philadelphia: F. A. Davis.

Zemke, R., & Horger, M. M. (1996). Hands: Tools for crafting human adaptation. In C. Royeen (Ed.), *AOTA Self-study Series—Hands on: Practical interventions for the hand.* Bethesda, MD: American Occupational Therapy Association.

Zemke, R. (1995). Habits. In C. Royeen (Ed.), *AOTA Self-study Series—The practice of the future.* Bethesda, MD: American Occupational Therapy Association.

Zemke, R. (1995). Remediating biomechanical and physiological impairments of motor performance. In C. Trombly (Ed.), *Occupational therapy for physical dysfunction* (4th ed., 405–422). Baltimore: Williams & Wilkins.

Zemke, R. (1994). Task skills, problem solving, and social interaction. In C. Royeen (Ed.), *AOTA Self-study Series—Cognitive rehabilitation.* Rockville, MD: American Occupational Therapy Association.

Clark, F., Zemke, R., Frank, G., Parham, D., Neville-Jan, A., Hedricks, C., et al. (1993). The Issue Is—Dangers inherent in the partition of occupational therapy and occupational science. *American Journal of Occupational Therapy, 47,* 184–186.

Koehn, D., Winistorfer, W. L., & Zemke, R. (1993). Career laddering for certified occupational therapy assistants. *Administration and Management Special Interest Section Quarterly, 9*(3), 6.

Zemke, R. (1992). Integrating computers into occupational therapy education. *Education Special Interest Section Quarterly, 2*(1), 3–4.

Clark, F. A., Parham, D., Carlson, M. E., Frank, G., Jackson, J., Pierce, D., Wolfe, R. J., & Zemke, R. (1991). Occupational science: Academic innovation in the service of occupational therapy's future. *American Journal of Occupational Therapy, 45,* 300–310.

Hoffman, M., & Zemke, R. (1990). Developmental assessment. In D. Van Dyke (Ed.), *Clinical perspectives in the management of Down syndrome* (pp. 202–228). New York: Springer.

Van Dyke, D., Hoffman, M., Van Duyne, S., Heidi, F., & Zemke, R. (1990). Development and behavior. In D. Van Dyke (Ed.), *Clinical perspectives in the management of Down syndrome* (pp. 171–180). New York: Springer.

Zemke, R. (1990). Preface. In G. Arnadottir (Ed.), *The brain and behavior: Assessing cortical dysfunction through ADL* (pp. v–vii). St. Louis, MO: Mosby.

Iberall, T., Preti, M., & Zemke, R. (1989). Task influence on timing and grasping patterns in human prehension. *Abstracts of the Society for Neuroscience, 15*(Pt. 1), 397.

Yerxa, E., Clark, F., Frank, G., Jackson, J., Parham, D., Pierce, D., Stein, C., & Zemke, R. (1989). An introduction to occupational science: A foundation for occupational therapy in the 21st century. *Occupational Therapy in Health Care, 6*(4), 1–17.

Zemke, R. (1989). Computer-assisted occupational therapy of visual–perceptual dysfunction. In *Technology review.* Rockville, MD: American Occupational Therapy Association.

Zemke, R. (1989). The Foundation—The continua of scientific research designs. *American Journal of Occupational Therapy, 43,* 551–553.

Zemke, R. (1988). *Curriculum unit: Gerontic occupational therapy.* Los Angeles: Pacific Geriatric Education Center.

Zemke, R. (1988). *Hand splinting: Principles and methods, 2nd ed.,* by E. Fess and C. Philips [Book Review]. *Occupational Therapy in Health Care, 5*(2/3), 205–206.

Zemke, R. (1986). An apple for the teacher: Microcomputer applications for OT educators. *Occupational Therapy in Health Care, 3*(3/4), 133–140.

Zemke, R. (1986). Taking a byte of the apple: Computers in a senior day care center. *Physical and Occupational Therapy in Geriatrics, 4*(2), 39–47.

Zemke, R. (1985). Application of an ATNR Rating Scale to preschool children. *American Journal of Occupational Therapy, 39,* 178–181.

Zemke, R. (1985). Microcomputer applications in a senior day care program. In C. Smith (Ed.), *Technology for disabled persons.* Menomonie: University of Wisconsin, Stout Materials Development Center.

Frank, G., & Zemke, R. (1984). OT Education Bulletin—Work-related disability: A teaching module. *Occupational Therapy News, 38*(10), 12–14.

Zemke, R. (1984). Notes on the measurement of magnitude of the asymmetrical tonic neck reflex response in normal preschool children. *Journal of Motor Behavior, 16*(3), 336–343.

Zemke, R., Knuth, S., & Chase, J. (1984). Change in self-concepts of children with learning difficulties during a residential camp experience. *Occupational Therapy in Mental Health, 4*(4), 1–12.

Zemke, R. (1983). The consistency of the magnitude of the ATNR response in normal preschool children. *Physical and Occupational Therapy in Pediatrics, 3*(3), 57–62.

Zemke, R. (1983). Microcomputer study of the ATNR. *Newsletter of the Center for the Study of Sensory Integrative Dysfunction, 10*(2), 1, 6.

Zemke, R., & Gratz, R. R. (1982). The role of theory: Erikson and occupational therapy. *Occupational Therapy in Mental Health, 2*(3), 45–63.

Zemke, R., & Zemke, W. (1982). Research Instrumentation—Electrogoniometry: A proposed research tool for measurement of the asymmetrical tonic neck reflex. *Physical and Occupational Therapy in Pediatrics, 2*(1), 51–59.

Gratz, R. R., & Zemke, R. (1980). Piaget, preschoolers, and pediatric practice. *Physical and Occupational Therapy in Pediatrics, 1*(1), 3–9.

Zemke, R. (1980). Incidence of ATNR response in normal preschool children. *Physical and Occupational Therapy in Pediatrics, 1*(2), 31–37.

Zemke, R. (1968). Operant conditioning. *Bulletin on Practice, 3*(5), 1.

Muriel E. Zimmerman, MA, OTR, FAOTA—1960

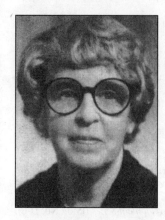

Muriel E. Zimmerman worked at the Institute of Rehabilitation Medicine at the New York University (NYU) Medical Center since the early 1950s. She was the associate director of occupational therapy and assistant professor of clinical rehabilitation medicine at the NYU School of Medicine.

A 1939 graduate of the Philadelphia School of Occupational Therapy, Zimmerman received a BS in 1960 and a MA in 1966 from NYU. From 1956 to 1974, she was an instructor of occupational therapy at NYU in the area of adaptive equipment. She was an active participant of all in-services and special courses at the Institute of Rehabilitation and Medicine of NYU.

She completed and directed extensive research on self-help devices. She also contributed to numerous exhibitions and demonstrations of self-help devices and equipment in the United States and abroad. She also pioneered and authored several films in this area.

Zimmerman chaired several international and national committees since 1957 and was a member of the International Society for Rehabilitation of the Disabled's advisory committee to the International Center on Technical Aids, Transportation, and Housing. She directed the research committee of the Clothing Research and Development Foundation.

Zimmerman served the AOTA as chairman of the Special Studies Committee and as contributing editor to the *American Journal of Occupational Therapy.* She was named an AOTA Fellow in 1973 and was listed in International Who's Who in Education and in International Who's Who of Intellectuals.

Bibliography

Morrisey, A., & Zimmerman, M. E. (1953). Helps for the handicapped. *American Journal of Nursing, 53,* 316–318.

Rusk, H., Taylor, E. J., Zimmerman, M. E., & Judson, J. (1953). *Living with a disability.* New York: McGraw-Hill.

Zimmerman, M. E. (1954). Adapted equipment for rehabilitation, Part 6. In H. Willard & C. Spackman (Eds.), *Principles of occupational therapy* (2nd ed., pp. 330–339). Philadelphia: Lippincott.

Rusk, H. A., Kristeller, R. L., Judson, J. S., Hunt, G. M., & Zimmerman, M. E. (1955). *A manual for training the disabled homemaker.* New York: Institute pf Physical Medicine and Rehabilitation.

Zimmerman, M. (1955). Accent on progress. *Institute of Physical Medicine and Rehabilitation, 1*(3), 19–23.

Zimmerman, M. (1957). Session on physical disabilities: Analysis of adapted equipment. *American Journal of Occupational Therapy, 4,* 229–237.

Robinson, R. A., & Zimmerman, M. E. (1958). Nationally Speaking: From the President: From the National Special Studies Committee: Summary report of the student report form. *American Journal of Occupational Therapy, 12*, 75–83.

Zimmerman, M. (1958). Principles in the training of the disable homemaker. In H. Rusk (Ed.), *Rehabilitaiton medicine* (pp. 177–197). Saint Louis, MO: Mosby.

Zimmerman, M. (1958). *Self-help devices for rehabilitation: Part 1.* Dubuque, IA: William C. Brown.

Zimmerman, M. (1959). Modern materials and methods for splinting. Self-help devices. In E. Lowman et al. (Eds.), *Arthritis: General principles, physical medicine, and rehabilitation* (pp. 135–164). Boston: Little Brown.

Zimmerman, M., & Hicks, T. (1959). Clamp device to aid in placement of tunnel pin of bilateral amputee with cineplastic operated prosthesis. *American Orthotic and Prosthetic Journal, 13*(4), 55–58.

Rusk, H., Lawton, E., Elvin, F., Judson, J., & Zimmerman, M. (1960). *The functional home for easier living.* New York: New York University, Medical Center Institute of Rehabilitation Medicine.

Zimmerman, M. (1960). Devices: Development and direction (1960 Eleanor Clarke Slagle Lecture). In *Proceedings of the American Occupational Therapy Association 1960 Annual Conference, Los Angeles, California, November 14–17, 1960: Theme, reflections, and projections* (pp. 17–24). New York: American Occupational Therapy Association.

Zimmerman, M. (1960). Independence through equipment. *Orthopedic and Prosthetic Appliance Journal, 4*, 71–77.

Cookman, H., & Zimmerman, M. (1961). *Functional fashions for the physically handicapped.* New York: New York University Medical Center, Institute of Rehabilitation Medicine.

Rusk, H., Kristeller, E., Judson, J., Hunt, G., & Zimmerman, M. E. (1961). *Rehabilitation monograph no. VIII, A manual for training the disabled homemaker.* New York: New York University Medical Center, Institute of Rehabilitation Medicine.

Zimmerman, M. (1961, October). *The disabled homemaker and their problems: Summary disabled and their environment.* Proceedings, International Society for Rehabilitation of the Disabled Conference, Stockholm, Sweden.

Zimmerman, M. (1961). A model home for the disabled. *Rehabilitation Record, 2*(6), 17–20.

Judson, J., Wagner, E., & Zimmerman, M E. (1962). *Homemaking and housing for the disabled in the USA.* New York: New York University Medical Center, Institute of Rehabilitation Medicine.

Zimmerman, M. E. (1962). Current concepts and use of self-help devices. In E. Wagner & M. E. Zimmerman (Eds.), *Approaches to independent living, Post Congress Study Course IV* (pp. 1–3). New York: World Federation of Occupational Therapists/American Occupational Therapy Association.

Zimmerman, M. E. (1962). Architectural planning. In E. Wagner & M. E. Zimmerman (Eds.), *Approaches to independent living, Post Congress Study Course IV* (pp. 38–40). New York: World Federation of Occupational Therapists/American Occupational Therapy Association.

Zimmerman, M. E. (1962). Homemaking training units for rehabilitation centers. *American Journal of Occupational Therapy, 20*, 226–235.

Zimmerman, M. E. (1962). Problems in clothing and dressing and their solutions. In E. Wagner & M. E. Zimmerman (Eds.), *Approaches to independent living, Post Congress Study Course IV* (pp. 63–64). New York: World Federation of Occupational Therapists/American Occupational Therapy Association.

Zimmerman, M. E. (1963). Occupational therapy in the ADL program. In H. S. Willard & C. Spackman (Eds.), *Occupational therapy* (3rd ed., pp. 320–357). Philadelphia: Lippincott.

Zimmerman, M. E. (1964). Principles of homemaking and housing. In H. A. Rusk (Ed.), *Rehabilitation medicine* (2nd ed, pp. 189–228). St. Louis, MO: Mosby.

Zimmerman, M. E. (1965). *Self-help devices for rehabilitation* (Part II). Dubuque, IA: William C. Brown.

Zimmerman, M. E. (1966). Homemaking training units for rehabilitation centers. *American Journal of Occupational Therapy, 10*, 226–235.

Zimmerman, M. E. (1966). Overcoming architectural barriers in the USA. In R. L. Kleinman (Ed.), *Proceedings of the 4th International Congress of the World Federation of Occupational Therapists* (pp. 330–333). New York: Excerpta Medica Foundation.

Zimmerman, M. E. (1967). The tasks of an information center of technical aids. *International Program Development Series* (ISRD No. D-6).

Zimmerman, M. E. (1968). *Bibliography on self-help devices and orthotics, Rehabilitation Monograph (1950–1967).* New York: New York University Medical Center, Institute of Rehabilitation Medicine.

Zimmerman, M. E. (1969). The functional motion test as an evaluation tool for patients with lower motor neuron disturbances. *American Journal of Occupational Therapy, 23*, 49–56.

Zimmerman, M. E. (1969). A learning experience in occupational therapy using 8-mm loop films. In *Methods and media for academic and clinical teaching* (AOTA Workshop, pp. 55–60). Salt Lake City: University of Utah.

Zimmerman, M. E. (1971). Occupational therapy in the ADL program. In H. S. Spackman & C. Spackman (Eds.), *Occupational therapy* (4th ed, pp. 217–256), Philadelphia: Lippincott.

Zimmerman, M. E. (1971). Principles of self-help devices. Principles of homemaking. Principles of housing. In H. Rusk et al. (Eds.), *Rehabilitation medicine* (3rd ed., pp. 152–198). St. Louis, MO: Mosby.

Zimmerman, M. E. (1976). Principles of self-help devices. Principles of homemaking. Principles of housing. In H. Rusk et al. (Eds.), *Rehabilitation medicine* (4th ed.). St. Louis, MO: Mosby.

Zimmerman, M. E. (1977). Role of special equipment in the rehabilitation of the spinal cord-injured. In J. Cull & R. E. Hardy (Eds.), *Physical medicine and rehabilitation medicine approaches in spinal cord injury* (pp. 224–278). Springfield, IL: Charles C Thomas.

Youdin, M., Sell, G. H., Clagnaz, M., Louie, H., Stratford, C., & Zimmerman, M. E. (1978). Initial evaluation of the IRM–NYU voice controlled powered wheelchair and environmental control system for the severely disabled. *Proceedings of the 5th Annual Conference on Systems and Devices for the Disabled* (pp. 177–182). Houston, TX.

Sell, H., Stratford, C., Zimmerman, M. E., Youdin, M., & Milner, D. (1979). Environmental and typewriter control systems for the high level quadriplegic patient: Evaluation and prescription. *Archives of Physical Medicine and Rehabilitation, 60*, 57–63.

Stratford, C. D., Dickey, R., Zimmerman, M. E., Sell, G. H., & Youdin, M. (1980). Voice control: Clinical evaluation by persons with severe physical disabilities with and without speech impairments. *Proceedings of International Conference on Rehabilitation Engineering* (pp. 98–101). Toronto, Canada.

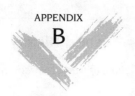

Bibliography:
U.S. and World History

Editor's Note

Many excellent publications can provide a thorough understanding of the United States and world historical context within which occupational therapy evolved and the Eleanor Clarke Slagle lecturers developed their thoughts. Caution must be used, however, in the interpretation of the influence that historical events might have had on the lecturers—that influence ultimately is up to the lecturers to decipher for us. However, our understanding of the lecturers' remarks is greatly enhanced when we realize their timeliness. The works listed here provide large overviews of history and were selected because their authors linked historical events across time.

U.S. History

Abraham, H. (2008). *Justices, presidents, and senators: A history of U.S. Supreme Court appointments from Washington toe Bush II.* Lanham, MD: Rowman & Littlefield.

Baxandall, R., & Gordon, L. (1995). *America's working women: A documentary history 1600 to the present.* New York: W. W. Norton.

Bender, T. (2006). *A nation among nations: America's place in world history.* New York: Hill & Wang.

Brogan, H. (1999). *The Penguin history of the United States of America* (2nd ed.). New York: Penguin Books.

Chomsky, N. (2003). *Hegemony or survival: America's quest for global dominance.* New York: Henry Holt.

Davis, K. (2003). *Don't know much about history: Everything you need to know about American history but never learned.* New York: HarperCollins.

Faragher, M. (Ed.). (1998). *The American Heritage encyclopedia of American history.* New York: Henry Holt.

Goldfield, D., Abbot, C., Anderson, V., & Argensinger, J. (2008). *The American journey: A history of the United States* (Vols. I and II). Upper Saddle River, NJ: Prentice Hall.

Hullar, L., & Nelson, S. (2006). *The United States: A brief history* (2nd ed.). Wheeling, IL: Harlan Davidson.

Hyser, R., & Arndt. J. (2007). *Voices of the American past: Documents in U.S. history* (4th ed.). Belmont, CA: Wadsworth.

Johnson, M. (1999). *A history of the American people.* New York: HarperCollins.

Loewen, J. (2007). *Lies my teacher told me: Everything your American history textbook got wrong.* New York: Touchstone.

Morris, R. (1996). *Encyclopedia of American history* (7th ed.). New York: Harper Resource.

Nelson, M. (2009). *The elections of 2008.* Washington, DC: CQ Press.

Rosenbaum, R. (2003). *The Penguin encyclopedia of American history.* New York: Penguin Putnam.

Schlesinger, A. M. (Ed.). (1993). *The almanac of American history.* Greenwich, CT: Brompton Books.

Urdang, L. (Ed.). (2001). *The timetables of American history.* Westport, CT: Touchstone.

Wilentz, S. (2008). *The age of Reagan: A history 1974–2008.* New York: Harper.

Zakaria, F. (2008). *The post American world.* New York: W. W. Norton.

Zinn, H. (2003). *A people's history of the United States: 1492–present.* New York: HarperCollins.

World History

Baylis, J., Smith, S. & Owens, P. (2008). *Globalization of world politics: An introduction to international relations.* New York: Oxford University Press.

Beck, R., Black, L. & Krieger, L. (2002). *World history: Patterns of interaction.* Orlando, FL: Holt Rinehart Winston.

Best, A., Hanhimaki, J., Maiolo, J., & Schulze, K. (2008). *International history of the twentieth century and beyond (2nd ed.).* New York: Routledge.

Brakeman, L., & Gall, S. (1996). *Chronology of women worldwide: People, places, and events that shaped women's history.* Farmington Hills, MI: Gale Group.

Christian, D. (2004). *Maps of time: An introduction to big history.* Berkeley: University of California Press.

Clifton, D. (2000). *20th century day by day.* New York: DK Publishing.

Coll, S. (2004). *Ghost wars: The secret history of the CIA, Afghanistan, and Bin Laden, from the Soviet invasion to September 10, 2001.* New York: Penguin Books.

Cook, M. (2003). *A brief history of the human race.* New York: W. W. Norton.

Daniels, P. Y., & Hyslop, S. (2002). *The National Geographic almanac of world history.* Washington, DC: National Geographic Society.

Eitzen, D. & Zinn, M. (2008). *Globalization: The transformation of social worlds (2nd ed.).* Belmont, CA: Wadsworth.

Farah, M. & Karls, A. (2001). *World history: The human experience (7th ed).* New York: McGraw-Hill.

Friedman, T. (2007). *The word is flat: A brief history of the 21st century.* New York: Picador.

Greenville, J. (2005). *A history of the world: From the 20th to the 21st century.* New York: Routledge.

Grun, B. (1991). *The timetables of history: A horizontal linkage of people and events* (3rd ed.). Westport, CT: Touchstone.

Haliday, F. (2005). *The Middle East in international relations: Power, politics, and international relations.* New York: Cambridge University Press.

Hellmans, A. & Bunch, B. (Eds.). (2004). *The history of science and technology: A browser's guide to the great discoveries, inventions, and people who made them from the dawn of time to today.* New York: Houghton Mifflin.

Maning, P. (Ed.). (2005). *World history: Global and local interactions.* Princeton, NJ: Markus Wiener.

Mazlish, B. & Iriye, A. (2004). *The global history reader.* New York: Routledge.

National Council on Economic Education. (2001). *World history: Focus on economics.* New York: Author.

O'Brien, P. (2001). *Atlas of world history.* Oxford, UK: Oxford University Press.

Organization for Economic Cooperation and Development. (2008). *International migration outlook.* Paris, France: Author.

Palmer, R. R., Colton, J., & Kramer, L. (2002). *A history of the modern world* (9th ed.). New York: Knopf.

Roberts, J. (1997). *A short history of the world.* Oxford, UK: Oxford University Press.

Roberts, J. (2003). *The new history of the world* (4th ed.). Oxford, UK: Oxford University Press.

Ross, D. (2004). *The missing peace: The inside story of the fight for Middle East peace.* New York: Farrar, Straus, & Giroux.

Scheuer, M. (2007). *Imperial hubris: Why the West is losing the war on terror.* Dulles, VA: Potomac Books.

Stearns, P. (Ed.). (2001). *The encyclopedia of world history* (6th ed.). Boston: Houghton Mifflin.

Steger, M. (2009). *Globalization: A very short introduction.* New York: Oxford University Press.

Teeple, J. (2002). *Timelines of world history.* New York: DK Publishing.

Trager, J. (1994). *The people's chronology: A year-by-year record of human events from prehistory to the present.* New York: Henry Holt.

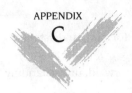

Bibliography:
History of Occupational Therapy
in the United States

Editor's Note

Colleagues and students have frequently commented in the past that "there just aren't many writings about occupational therapy in the United States." While indeed the proportion of such writings may be small in comparison to other practice issues, there is not a complete void. To date no comprehensive history of occupational therapy has been undertaken, but the works listed below cover the entire span of the profession's existence. In addition, the Wilma West Library of the American Occupational Therapy Foundation houses many official documents such as meeting minutes and letters that can help fill any gaps.

Bibliography

Adams, E. (2008). *Women professional workers: A study made for the women's educational and industrial union.* Charleston, NC: BiblioLife.

Ambrosi, E. M., & Schwartz, K. B. (1995). Looking back. The profession's image, 1917–1925, part I: Occupational therapy as represented in the media. *American Journal of Occupational Therapy, 49,* 715–719.

Ambrosi, E., & Schwartz, K. B. (1995). The profession's image, 1917–1925, part II: Occupational therapy as represented by the profession. *American Journal of Occupational Therapy, 49,* 828–832.

American Occupational Therapy Association. (1980). In memoriam: Helen Willard. *American Journal of Occupational Therapy, 34,* 497.

American Occupational Therapy Association. (1992). Special 75th anniversary issue. *American Journal of Occupational Therapy, 46,* 9–85.

American Occupational Therapy Association. (2000). The Foundation. A twenty-year history of research funding in occupational therapy. *American Journal of Occupational Therapy, 54,* 441–442.

Anthony, S. (2005a). Dr. Herbert J. Hall: Originator of honest work for occupational therapy 1904–1923 [Part I]. *Occupational Therapy in Health Care, 19*(3), 3–19.

Anthony, S. (2005b). Dr. Herbert J. Hall: Originator of honest work for occupational therapy 1904–1923 [Part II]. *Occupational Therapy in Health Care, 19*(3), 21–32.

Applebaum, A. H., & Munich, R. L. (1989). Reinventing moral treatment: The effects upon patients and staff members of a program of psychosocial rehabilitation. *Occupational Therapy in Mental Health, 9,* 69–86.

Baum, C. M. (1983). A look at our strengths in the '80s. *American Journal of Occupational Therapy, 37,* 451–455.

Baum, C. M., & Gray, M. S. (1988). Certification: Serving the public interest. *American Journal of Occupational Therapy, 42,* 77–79.

Bing, R. (1983). Professional nationalism. *American Journal of Occupational Therapy, 37,* 301–304.

Bing, R. (1983). Nationally Speaking: The industry, the art, and the philosophy of history. *American Journal of Occupational Therapy, 37,* 800–801.

Bing, R. K. (1984). Nationally Speaking: Living forward, understanding backwards, part I. *American Journal of Occupational Therapy, 38,* 363–366.

Bing, R. K. (1984). Nationally Speaking: Living forward, understanding backwards, part II. *American Journal of Occupational Therapy, 38,* 435–439.

Bing, R. K. (1987). Who originated the term *occupational therapy?* Author's response. *American Journal of Occupational Therapy, 41,* 192–194.

Bing, R. K. (1992). Point of departure (A play about founding the profession). *American Journal of Occupational Therapy, 46,* 27–32.

Bing, R. K. (1997). "And teach agony to sing": An afternoon with Eleanor Clarke Slagle. *American Journal of Occupational Therapy, 51,* 220–227.

Black, R. M. (2002). Occupational therapy's dance with diversity. *American Journal of Occupational Therapy, 56,* 140–148.

Bockoven, J. S. (1971). Occupational therapy—A historical perspective. Legacy of moral treatment—1800s to 1910. *American Journal of Occupational Therapy, 25,* 223–225.

Bone, C. D., Jeffers, L. S., Catterton, M. M., Levine, B., & Meyers, C. (1971). The *American Journal of Occupational Therapy.* Official publication of the American Occupational Therapy Association. *American Journal of Occupational Therapy, 25,* 47–59.

Brainerd, W. (1967). OT and me: Early days at the Sanitarium, Clifton Springs, New York. *American Journal of Occupational Therapy, 21,* 278–280.

Breines, E. (1987). Pragmatism as a foundation for occupational therapy curricula. *American Journal of Occupational Therapy, 41,* 522–525.

Breines, E. (1987). Who originated the term *occupational therapy? American Journal of Occupational Therapy, 41,* 192.

Breines, E. B. (1992). Rabbi Hirsch influenced the Chicago School of Civics and Philanthropy. *American Journal of Occupational Therapy, 46,* 567–568.

Breines, T. I. (1988). Redefining professionalism for occupational therapy. *American Journal of Occupational Therapy, 42,* 55–57.

Brown, K. M. (1987). Wellness: Past visions, future roles. *Occupational Therapy in Mental Health, 4*(1), 155–164.

Case-Smith, J., & Powell, C. (2008). Concepts in clinical scholarship: Research literature in occupational therapy, 2001–2005. *American Journal of Occupational Therapy, 62,* 480–486.

Christiansen, C. (1991). Research: Looking back and ahead after four decades of progress. *American Journal of Occupational Therapy, 45,* 391–393.

Cohen, H., & Reed, K. L. (1996). The historical development of neuroscience in physical rehabilitation. *American Journal of Occupational Therapy, 50,* 561–568.

Cole, M., & Tufano, R. (2008). Occupational therapy's broadening horizons. In M. Cole & R. Tufano (Eds.), *Applied theories in occupational therapy: A practical approach* (pp. 3–21). Thorofare, NJ: Slack.

Colman, W. (1988). The evolution of occupational therapy in the public schools: The laws mandating practice. *American Journal of Occupational Therapy, 42,* 701–705.

Colman, W. (1990). The curriculum directors: Influencing occupational therapy education, 1948–1964. *American Journal of Occupational Therapy, 44,* 357–362.

Colman, W. (1990). Evolving educational practices in occupational therapy: The war emergency courses, 1936–1954. *American Journal of Occupational Therapy, 44,* 1028–1036.

Colman, W. (1990). Recruitment standards and practices in occupational therapy, 1900–1930. *American Journal of Occupational Therapy, 44,* 742–748.

Colman, W. (1992). Exploring educational boundaries: Occupational therapy and the multiple-entry-route system, 1970–1982. *American Journal of Occupational Therapy, 46,* 260–266.

Colman, W. (1992). Maintaining autonomy: The struggle between occupational therapy and physical medicine. *American Journal of Occupational Therapy, 46,* 63–70.

Coppard, B., Dickerson, A., Fazio, L., Costa, D., Musselman, L., Haynes, D., et al. (2007). A descriptive review of occupational therapy education. *American Journal of Occupational Therapy, 61,* 672–677.

Cottrell, R. P. (2000). COTA education and professional development: A historical review. *American Journal of Occupational Therapy, 54,* 407–412.

Creighton, C. (1992). The origin and evolution of activity analysis. *American Journal of Occupational Therapy, 46,* 45–48.

Creighton, C. (1993). Graded activity: Legacy of the sanatorium. *American Journal of Occupational Therapy, 47,* 745–748.

Cromwell, F. S. (1974). Proceedings: The development of the occupational therapy assistant: History and status report. *ASHA, 16,* 671–676.

Cromwell, F. S. (1977). Eleanor Clarke Slagle, the leader, the woman. In retrospect on the 60th anniversary of the founding of the AOTA. *American Journal of Occupational Therapy, 31,* 645–648.

Custard, C. (1998). Tracing research methodology in occupational therapy. *American Journal of Occupational Therapy, 52,* 676–683.

DeBeer, F. (1987). Major themes in occupational therapy: A content analysis of the Eleanor Clarke Slagle Lectures, 1955–1985. *American Journal of Occupational Therapy, 41,* 527–531.

Devereaux, E. B. (1990). American Occupational Therapy Foundation: Milestones of a quarter century. *American Journal of Occupational Therapy, 44,* 295–297.

Diasio, K. (1971). The modern era—1960 to 1970. *American Journal of Occupational Therapy, 25,* 237–242.

Eldar, R., & Jelic, M. (2003). The association of rehabilitation and war. *Disability and Rehabilitation, 25,* 1019–1023.

Ellenberg, D. D. (1996). Outcomes research: The history, debate, and implications for the field of occupational therapy. *American Journal of Occupational Therapy, 50,* 435–441.

Ellsworth, P. D. (1983). Army psychiatric occupational therapy from the past and into the future. *Occupational Therapy in Mental Health, 3*(2), 1–6.

Engelhardt, H. T. (1977). Defining occupational therapy: The meaning of therapy and the virtues of occupation. *American Journal of Occupational Therapy, 31,* 666–672.

Fess, E. E. (2002). A history of splinting: To understand the present, view the past. *Journal of Hand Therapy, 15,* 97–132.

Fidler, G. S., & Fidler, J. W. (1994). A retrospective view of the affiliation of occupational therapy and psychiatry. *Hospital and Community Psychiatry, 45,* 978–980.

Friedland, J. (1998). Occupational therapy and rehabilitation: An awkward alliance. *American Journal of Occupational Therapy, 52,* 373–380.

Friedland, J., & Silva, J. (2008). Evolving identities: Thomas Bessell Kidner and occupational therapy in the United States. *American Journal of Occupational Therapy, 62,* 349–360.

Gainer, R. (2008). History of ergonomics and occupational therapy. *Work, 31*(1), 5–9.

Gillette, N., & Kielhofner, G. (1979). The impact of specialization on the professionalization and survival of occupational therapy. *American Journal of Occupational Therapy, 33,* 20–28.

Gillette, N. (2008). A Firm Persuasion in Our Work—Mentors I have known (and loved). *American Journal of Occupational Therapy, 62,* 487–490.

Gillette, N. (1998). A vision for our future. *American Journal of Occupational Therapy, 52,* 318–319.

Gilligan, M. B. (1976). Developmental stages of occupational therapy and the feminist movement. *American Journal of Occupational Therapy, 30,* 560–567.

Goldberg, J. (2009). *Social aspects of the treatment of the insane.* Charleston, NC: BiblioLife.

Grant, H. K. (1991). Education then and now: 1949 and 1989. *American Journal of Occupational Therapy, 45,* 295–299.

Gritzer, G., & Arluke, A. (1985). *The making of rehabilitation: A political economy of medical specialization, 1890–1980.* Berkeley: University of California Press.

Gutman, S. A. (1995). Influence of the U.S. military and occupational therapy reconstruction aides in World War I on the development of occupational therapy. *American Journal of Occupational Therapy, 49,* 256–262.

Gutman, S. A. (1997). Looking back. Occupational therapy's link to vocational reeducation, 1910–1925. *American Journal of Occupational Therapy, 51,* 907–915.

Hamlin, R. B. (1992). Embracing our past, informing our future: A feminist re-vision of health care. *American Journal of Occupational Therapy, 46,* 1028–1035.

Hanson, C. S., & Walker, K. F. (1992). The history of work in physical dysfunction. *American Journal of Occupational Therapy, 46,* 56–62.

Harvey-Krefting, L. (1985). The concept of work in occupational therapy: A historical review. *American Journal of Occupational Therapy, 39,* 301–307.

Hightower-Vandamm, M. D. (1981). The role of occupational therapy in vocational evaluation, part 1. *American Journal of Occupational Therapy, 35*, 563–565.

Hightower-Vandamm, M. D. (1981). The role of occupational therapy in vocational evaluation, part 2. *American Journal of Occupational Therapy, 35*, 631–633.

Hinojosa, J., & Moyers Cleveland, P. (2009). Perspectives on advanced practice from occupational therapy. *Topics in Clinical Nutrition, 24*, 200–205.

Hodges, J. M. (1976). Reflections: Occupational therapy. *American Journal of Occupational Therapy, 30*, 409–410.

Hooper, B. (2006). Epistemological transformation of occupational therapy. Educational implications and challenges. *OTJR: Occupation, Participation and Health, 26*(1), 15–24.

Hooper, B., & Wood, W. (2002). Pragmatism and structuralism in occupational therapy: The long conversation. *American Journal of Occupational Therapy, 56*, 40–50.

Hoover, J. A. B. (1996). Looking back. Diversional occupational therapy in World War I: A need for purpose in occupations. *American Journal of Occupational Therapy, 50*, 881–885.

Jackson, B. N. (1992). Home-based occupational therapy: Then and now. *American Journal of Occupational Therapy, 46*, 84–85.

Jaffe, E. (1985). Transition in health care—Critical planning for the 1990s: Part I. *American Journal of Occupational Therapy, 39*, 431–435.

Johnson, J. A. (1974). An overview of AOTA. *American Journal of Occupational Therapy, 28*, 516–521.

Johnson, J. A. (1976). Commitment to action. *American Journal of Occupational Therapy, 30*, 135–148.

Johnson, J. A. (1988). Certified occupational therapy assistants: Reflections on their thirtieth anniversary. *Occupational Therapy in Health Care, 5*(2/3), 213–220.

Jones, J. L. (1988). Early occupational therapy education in Wisconsin: Elizabeth Upham Davis and Milwaukee-Downer College. *American Journal of Occupational Therapy, 42*, 27–33.

Jones, J. L. (1992). Therefore be it resolved: 25 years of Delegate Assembly/Representative Assembly legislation. *American Journal of Occupational Therapy, 46*, 72–78.

Kahmann, W. C. (1967). Fifty years in occupational therapy. *American Journal of Occupational Therapy, 21*, 281–283.

Kellegrew, D. H., & Allen, D. (1996). Occupational therapy in full-inclusion classrooms: A case study from the Moorpark model. *American Journal of Occupational Therapy, 50*, 718–724.

Kielhofner, G., & Burkem, J. P. (1977). Occupational therapy after 60 years: An account of changing identity and knowledge. *American Journal of Occupational Therapy, 31*, 675–689.

Laurencelle, P. (1968). Facio, ergo cogito, ergo sum: Some classical antecedents to a theory of occupational therapy. *American Journal of Occupational Therapy, 22*, 275–277.

Levine, R. E. (1983). A historical perspective on professional values. *Journal of Allied Health, 12*, 183–191.

Levine, R. E. (1987). The influence of the arts-and-crafts movement on the professional status of occupational therapy. *American Journal of Occupational Therapy, 41*, 248–254.

Licht, S. (1967). The founding and founders of the American Occupational Therapy Association. *American Journal of Occupational Therapy, 21*, 269–277.

Licht, S. (1983). The early history of occupational therapy: An outline. *Occupational Therapy in Mental Health, 3*(1), 67–88.

Litterst, T. A. (1992). Occupational therapy: The role of ideology in the development of a profession for women. *American Journal of Occupational Therapy, 46*, 20–25.

Loomis, B. (1992). The Henry B. Favill School of Occupations and Eleanor Clarke Slagle. *American Journal of Occupational Therapy, 46*, 34–37.

Low, J. F. (1992). The reconstruction aides. *American Journal of Occupational Therapy, 46*, 38–43.

Marble, H. (2009). Application of curative therapy in the ward, 1920. *Clinical Orthopaedics and Related Research, 467*(6), 1398–1399.

Marshall, E. M. (1985). Looking back: The beginnings of occupational therapy: Work evaluation. *American Journal of Occupational Therapy, 39*, 297–300.

McDaniel, M. L. (1971). Forerunners of the American Journal of Occupational Therapy. *American Journal of Occupational Therapy, 25*, 41–46.

Metaxas, V. A. (2000). Eleanor Clarke Slagle and Susan E. Tracy: Personal and professional identity and the development of occupational therapy in Progressive Era America. *Nursing History Review, 8,* 39–70.

Meyer, A. (1977). The philosophy of occupation therapy. *American Journal of Occupational Therapy, 31,* 639–642.

Mosey, A. C. (1971). Involvement in the rehabilitation movement—1942–1960. *American Journal of Occupational Therapy, 25,* 234–236.

Mu, K., & Coppard, B. (2007). The development of an entry-level occupational therapy doctorate in the USA: A case illustration. *WFOT Bulletin, 56,* 45–53.

Pasquinelli, S. (1996). History and trends in treatment methods. In L. W. Pedretti (Ed.), *Occupational therapy: Practice skills for physical dysfunction* (pp. 3–21). St. Louis, MO: Mosby/YearBook.

Peloquin, S. M. (1989). Moral treatment: Contexts considered. *American Journal of Occupational Therapy, 43,* 537–544.

Peloquin, S. (1991). Occupational therapy service: Individual and collective understandings of the founders. *American Journal of Occupational Therapy, 45,* 352–360.

Peloquin, S. (1991). Occupational therapy service: Individual and collective understandings of the founders, part 2. *American Journal of Occupational Therapy, 45,* 733–744.

Peloquin, S. (1994). Moral treatment: How a caring practice lost its rationale. *American Journal of Occupational Therapy, 48,* 167–173.

Peloquin, S. (1995). The fullness of empathy: Reflections and illustrations. *American Journal of Occupational Therapy, 49,* 24–31.

Peloquin, S. (2007). A reconsideration of occupational therapy's core values (Eleanor Clarke Slagle Lecture). *American Journal of Occupational Therapy, 61,* 474–478.

Phillips, M. S. (1996). Looking back. The use of drama and puppetry in occupational therapy during the 1920s and 1930s. *American Journal of Occupational Therapy, 50,* 229–233.

Pierce, D., & Peyton, C. (1999). A historical cross-disciplinary perspective on the professional doctorate in occupational therapy. *American Journal of Occupational Therapy, 52,* 64–71.

Pollock, H. (1942). Eleanor Clarke Slagle: 1876–1942. *American Journal of Psychiatry, 99,* 472–474.

Powell, J. (1986). Historical perspective on entry-level discussion. *American Journal of Occupational Therapy, 40,* 719–720.

Quiroga, V. (1995). *Occupational therapy: The first 30 years: 1900–1930.* Bethesda, MD: American Occupational Therapy Association.

Reed, K. L. (1988). Occupational therapy articles in serial publications: An analysis of sources. *Bulletin of the Medical Librarian Association, 76,* 125–130.

Reed, K. L. (1992). History of federal legislation for persons with disabilities. *American Journal of Occupational Therapy, 46,* 397–408.

Reed, K. (2005). Dr. Hall and the work cure. *Occupational Therapy in Health Care, 19*(3), 33–50.

Reed, K. (2006). Occupational therapy values and beliefs—The formative years: 1904–1929. *OT Practice, 11*(7), 21–25.

Reed, K., & Peters, C. (2006). Occupational therapy values and beliefs, part II—The Great Depression and war years: 1930–1949. *OT Practice, 11*(18), 17–22.

Reed, K., & Peters, C. (2007). Occupational therapy values and beliefs, part III—A new view of occupation and the profession: 1950–1969. *OT Practice, 12*(22), 17–21

Reed, K., & Peters, C. (2008). Occupational therapy values and beliefs, part IV—A time of professional identity: 1970–1985—Would the real therapist please stand up? *OT Practice, 13*(18), 15–18.

Reilly, M. (1971). The modernization of occupational therapy. *American Journal of Occupational Therapy, 25,* 243–246.

Reitz, S. M. (1992). A historical review of occupational therapy's role in preventive health and wellness. *American Journal of Occupational Therapy, 46,* 50–55.

Rerek, M. D. (1971). The depression years—1929–1941. *American Journal of Occupational Therapy, 25,* 231–233.

Schemm, R. L. (1994). Bridging conflicting ideologies: The origins of American and British occupational therapy. *American Journal of Occupational Therapy, 48,* 1082–1088.

Schwartz, K. B. (1992). Examining the profession's legacy. *American Journal of Occupational Therapy, 46,* 9–10.

Schwartz, K. B. (1992). Nationally Speaking: Establishing the profession's legacy. *American Journal of Occupational Therapy, 46,* 9–10.

Schwartz, K. B. (1992). Occupational therapy and education: A shared vision. *American Journal of Occupational Therapy, 46,* 12–18.

Serrett, K. D. (1985). Another look at occupational therapy's history: Paradigm or pair-of-hands? *Occupational Therapy in Mental Health, 5*(3), 1–31.

Serret, K. (1985). Eleanor Clarke Slagle: Founder and leader in occupational therapy. *Occupational Therapy in Mental Health, 5*(3), 101–108.

Shannon, P. D. (1977). The derailment of occupational therapy. *American Journal of Occupational Therapy, 31,* 229–234.

Silva, D. (1977). John Dewey: Implications for schooling. *American Journal of Occupational Therapy, 31,* 40–43.

Spackman, C. S. (1968). A history of the practice of occupational therapy for restoration of physical function: 1917–1967. *American Journal of Occupational Therapy, 22,* 67–71.

Spaights, E., & Krippendorf, C. E. (1967). Ten years of the *American Journal of Occupational Therapy:* 1956–1965. *American Journal of Occupational Therapy, 21,* 61–63.

Stattel, F. M. (1977). Occupational therapy: Sense of the past—Focus on the present. *American Journal of Occupational Therapy, 31,* 649–650.

Stein, F. (2008). Reflections on 50 years as an occupational therapist. *Occupational Therapy International, 15*(1), 1–3.

Stein, F., & Tallant, B. K. (1988). Applying the group process to psychiatric occupational therapy: Part 1: Historical and current use. *Occupational Therapy in Mental Health, 8*(3), 9–28.

Strickland, L. R. (1991). Directions for the future—Occupational therapy practice then and now, 1949–the present. *American Journal of Occupational Therapy, 45,* 105–107.

Swarbrick, M. (2009). Historical perspective—From institution to community. *Occupational Therapy in Mental Health, 25*(3), 201–223.

West, W. L. (1978). Reflections at retirement. *American Journal of Occupational Therapy, 32,* 9–12.

West, W. L. (1979). Professional unity. *American Journal of Occupational Therapy, 33,* 40–49.

West, W. L. (1982). Winifred Conrick Kahmann 1895–1982. *American Journal of Occupational Therapy, 36,* 472–475.

West, W. L. (1989). Nationally Speaking: Perspectives on the past and future, part 1. *American Journal of Occupational Therapy, 43,* 787–790.

West, W. L. (1990). Nationally Speaking: Perspectives on the past and future, part 2. *American Journal of Occupational Therapy, 44,* 9–10.

West, W. L. (1992). Ten milestone issues in AOTA history. *American Journal of Occupational Therapy, 46,* 1066–1074.

Willard, H. S., & Spackman, C. S. (1977). Willard and Spackman: Viewpoints of change. Role of the occupational therapist. Interview by Marsha Bassett. *American Journal of Occupational Therapy, 31,* 7–9.

Wish-Baratz, S. (1989). Bird T. Baldwin: A holistic scientist in occupational therapy's history. *American Journal of Occupational Therapy, 43,* 257–260.

Wood, W. (1995). Weaving the warp and weft of occupational therapy: An art and science for all times. *American Journal of Occupational Therapy, 49,* 44–52.

Wood, W. (1998). Nationally Speaking: The genius within. *American Journal of Occupational Therapy, 52,* 320–325.

Wood, W. (2004). The heart, mind, and soul of professionalism in occupational therapy. *American Journal of Occupational Therapy, 58*(3), 249–257.

Woodside, H. H. (1971). The development of occupational therapy 1910–1929. *American Journal of Occupational Therapy, 25,* 226–230.

Yerxa, E. J. (1992). Some implications of occupational therapy's history for its epistemology, values, and relation to medicine. *American Journal of Occupational Therapy, 46,* 79–83.

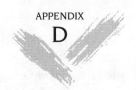

APPENDIX
D

Bibliography:
History of Occupational Therapy
Around the World

Editor's Note

Occupational therapy in the United States evolved within a global context. The works that appear below make reference (sometimes minor, sometimes substantial) to people and events of American occupational therapy or provide a sense of the timeline of development of the profession around the world. A quick glance at these works will make readers realize that the issues raised by the Eleanor Clarke Slagle lecturers have resonance around the globe.

Bibliography

Alsop, A. (1996). The origins of our species: A brief history of our time. *British Journal of Occupational Therapy, 59,* 155.

Anderson, B., & Bell, J. (1991). Recording the past for the future. *Australian Occupational Therapy Journal, 38,* 207–210.

Bourne, R. (1991). From the past: 50 years of achievement. *Australian Occupational Therapy Journal, 38,* 183–184.

Bracegirdle, H. (1991). Two hundred years of therapeutic occupations for women hospital patients. *British Journal of Occupational Therapy, 54,* 231–232.

Burnette, N. L. (1986). The status of occupational therapy in Canada (reprinted from 1923). *Canadian Journal of Occupational Therapy, 53,* 6–8.

Busuttil, J. (1992). Psychosocial occupational therapy: From myth and misconception to multidisciplinary team member. *British Journal of Occupational Therapy, 55,* 457–461.

Canadian Occupational Therapy Association. (1972). A tribute to Muriel Driver. *Canadian Journal of Occupational Therapy, 39,* 71–72.

Carswell-Opzoomer, A. (1990). Occupational therapy—Our time has come. *Canadian Journal of Occupational Therapy, 57,* 197–204.

Clouston, T., & Whitcombe, S. (2008). The professionalisation of occupational therapy: A continuing challenge. *British Journal of Occupational Therapy, 71*(8), 314–320.

Cockburn, L. (2005). Canadian occupational therapists' contributions to prisoners of war in World War II. *Canadian Journal of Occupational Therapy, 72*(3), 183–188.

Cockburn, L. (2001). Change, expansion, and reorganization: CAOT in the 1970s. *Occupational Therapy Now, 3*(4), 3–6.

Cockburn, L. (2001). The greater the barrier, the greater the success: CAOT during the 1940s. *Occupational Therapy Now, 3*(2), 15–18.

Cockburn, L. (2001). The professional era: CAOT in the 1950s and 1960s. *Occupational Therapy Now, 3*(3), 5–9.

Craik, C. (1998). Pioneers for the next century. *British Journal of Occupational Therapy, 61,* 185.

De La Charite, J. (1986). The neglected phase of rehabilitation (reprinted from 1962). *Canadian Journal of Occupational Therapy, 53,* 28–33.

Do Rozario, L., & Ross, M. (1991). A step in Western Australia's history: Creating a professional strategic directions plan for the 21st century. *Australian Occupational Therapy Journal, 38,* 201–206.

Driver, M. F. (1968). A philosophic view of the history of occupational therapy in Canada. *Canadian Journal of Occupational Therapy, 35,* 52–60.

Driver, M. F., & Robinson, I. M. (1967). Tribute: Helen P. LeVesconte. *Canadian Journal of Occupational Therapy, 34,* 103–105.

Elkin, S. (2002). Health care ethics and the practice of occupational therapy—Past, present, and future. *New Zealand Journal of Occupational Therapy, 49,* 22–25.

Ellis, M. (1987). The Casson Memorial Lecture, 15 May 1987. Quality: Who cares? *British Journal of Occupational Therapy, 50,* 195–200.

Ellis, M., Monteath, H. G., Henson, C. R., & Lock, S. J. (1987). BJOT: Fifty years of publication. *British Journal of Occupational Therapy, 50,* 348–349.

Friedland, J. (2001). Knowing from whence we came: Reflecting on return-to-work and interpersonal relationships. *Canadian Journal of Occupational Therapy, 68,* 266–271.

Friedland, J. (2003). Muriel Driver Memorial Lecture: Why crafts? Influences on the development of occupational therapy in Canada from 1890 to 1930. *Canadian Journal of Occupational Therapy, 70,* 204–212.

Friedland, J., Robinson, I., & Cardwell, T. (2001). In the beginning: CAOT from 1926–1939. *Occupational Therapy Now, 3*(1), 15–18.

Gonzalves, S. M., & Faias, J. (2003). Occupational therapy education in Portugal. *WFOT Bulletin, 48,* 5–8.

Grayson, R. (1993). Footprints on the sands of time—Reflecting on the impact of attitude: 1993 Sylvia Docker Lecture. *Australian Occupational Therapy Journal, 40,* 55–66.

Green, M. C., Lertvilai, M., & Bribriesco, K. (2001). Prospering through change: CAOT from 1991 to 2001. *Occupational Therapy Now, 3*(6), 13–19.

Grove, E. (1988). Working together: The Casson Memorial Lecture, 15 April 1988. *British Journal of Occupational Therapy, 51,* 150–156.

Hocking, C. (2005). The 2004 Frances Rutherford Lecture—Evidence from the past. *New Zealand Journal of Occupational Therapy, 52*(1), 4–16.

Hocking, C. (2007a). Early perspective of patients, practice and the profession. *British Journal of Occupational Therapy, 70*(7), 284–291.

Hocking, C. (2007b). The romance of occupational therapy. In J. Creek & A. Lawson-Porter (Eds.), *Contemporary issues in occupational therapy: Reasoning and reflection* (pp. 23–40). New York: John Wiley & Sons.

Hocking, C. (2008a). The Way We Were—The ascendance of rationalism . . . Last in a series articles. *British Journal of Occupational Therapy, 71*(6), 226–233.

Hocking, C. (2008b). The Way We Were—Romantic assumptions of pioneering occupational therapists in the United Kingdom . . . First in a series. *British Journal of Occupational Therapy, 71*(4), 146–154.

Hocking, C. (2008c). The Way We Were—Thinking rationally . . . Second of three articles. *British Journal of Occupational Therapy, 71*(5), 185–195.

Howland, G. (1986). Presidential address (reprinted from 1939). *Canadian Journal of Occupational Therapy, 53,* 16–17.

Howland, G. (1986). Occupational therapy across Canada (reprinted from 1944). *Canadian Journal of Occupational Therapy, 53,* 18–26.

Hume, C. A. (1992). 1930s: Ourselves as others saw us: Occupation therapy for mental patients. *British Journal of Occupational Therapy, 55,* 260–262.

Jackson, M. (1993). From work to therapy: The changing politics of occupation in the twentieth century. *British Journal of Occupational Therapy, 56,* 360–364.

Jay, P., Mendez, A., & Monteath, H. G. (1992). The Diamond Jubilee of the professional association, 1932–1992: An historical review. *British Journal of Occupational Therapy, 55,* 252–256.

Jonsson, H. (1998). Ernst Westerlund—A Swedish doctor of occupation. *Occupational Therapy International, 5,* 155–171.

Lall, A., Klein, J., & Brown, G. T. (2003). Changing times: Trials and tribulations of the move to master's entry-level education in Canada. *Canadian Journal of Occupational Therapy, 70,* 152–162.

Law, M. (1992). Michel Foucault's historical perspective on normality and restrictive environments. *Canadian Journal of Rehabilitation, 5,* 193–203.

LeVesconte, H. P. (1986). Expanding fields of occupational therapy (reprinted from 1935). *Canadian Journal of Occupational Therapy, 53,* 9–15.

Macdonald, M., Rush, M., Parras, G., Goodwin, G., & Lovell, R. (1991). Fifty years of occupational therapy at Heidelberg Repatriation Hospital. *Australian Occupational Therapy Journal, 38,* 211–215.

Mayers, C. A. (2000). The Casson Memorial Lecture 2000: Reflect on the past to shape the future. *British Journal of Occupational Therapy, 63,* 358–366.

McKay, E. (2008). What have we been 'doing'? A historical review of occupational therapy. In E. McKay, C. Craik, K. Lim, & Y. G., Richards (Eds.), *Advancing occupational therapy in mental health practice* (pp. 3–16). Boston: Wiley-Blackwell.

Mocellin, G. (1992). An overview of occupational therapy in the context of the American influence on the profession: Part 1. *British Journal of Occupational Therapy, 55,* 7–12.

Mocellin, G. (1992). An overview of occupational therapy in the context of the American influence on the profession: Part 2. *British Journal of Occupational Therapy, 55,* 55–60.

Molke, D. (2009). Outlining a critical ethos for historical work in occupational science and occupational therapy. *Journal of Occupational Science, 16*(2), 75–84.

Moubnter, C. R., & Ilott, L. (2000). Occupational science: Updating the United Kingdom journey of discovery. *Occupational Therapy International, 7,* 111–120.

Park, K. (1998). The development of occupational therapy in Korea. *WFOT Bulletin, 38,* 44–45.

Paterson, C. F. (1994). The First International Congress of the World Federation of Occupational Therapists—Edinburgh, 1954. *British Journal of Occupational Therapy, 57,* 116–120.

Paterson, C. F. (1997). Rationales for the use of occupation in 19th-century asylums. *British Journal of Occupational Therapy, 60,* 179–183.

Paterson, C. F. (1998). Occupational therapy and the National Health Service, 1948–1998. *British Journal of Occupational Therapy, 61,* 311–315.

Paterson, C. F. (2003). Focus on research: The development of occupational therapy in Scotland 1900–1960. *British Journal of Occupational Therapy, 66,* 518.

Philcox, S. (1991). A personal memoir—"How it was." *Australian Occupational Therapy Journal, 38,* 193–194.

Polatajko, H. J. (2001). The evolution of our occupational perspective: The journey from diversion through therapeutic use to enablement. *Canadian Journal of Occupational Therapy, 68,* 203–207.

Punwar, A. (1994). Current trends in international occupational therapy practice. *Occupational Therapy International, 1,* 1–12.

Precin, P. (Ed.). (2003). *Surviving 9/11: Impact and experiences of occupational therapy practitioners.* New York: Routledge.

Robinson, I. M. (1981). Muriel Driver Memorial Lecture 1981: The mists of time. *Canadian Journal of Occupational Therapy, 48,* 145–152.

Sachs, D., & Sussman, N. (1995). Historical research: The first decade of occupational therapy in Israel: 1946–1956. *Occupational Therapy International, 2,* 241–256.

Salvatori, P. (2001). The history of occupational therapy assistants in Canada: A comparison with the United States. *Canadian Journal of Occupational Therapy, 68,* 217–227.

Sedgwick A., Cockburn, L., & Trentham, B. (2007). Exploring the mental health roots of occupational therapy in Canada: A historical review of primary texts from 1925–1950. *Canadian Journal of Occupational Therapy, 74*(5), 407–417.

Sinclair, K. (2000). Overview of the profession: An historical perspective. *WFOT Bulletin, 42,* 29.

Soechting, E., Glennon, T., Miller-Kuhaneck, H., Erwin, B., Henry, D., Basaraba, C. et al. (2009). The history, development, and purpose of the Sensory Integration Global Network. *Sensory Integration Special Interest Section Quarterly, 32*(1), 1–2.

Thibeault, R. (2002). Muriel Driver Memorial Lecture: In praise of dissidence: Anne Lang-Etienne (1932–1991). *Canadian Journal of Occupational Therapy, 69,* 197–204.

Tompson, M., & Tompson, C. (1987). The evolution of standards for the fieldwork component of the curriculum. *Canadian Journal of Occupational Therapy, 54,* 237–241.

Trentham, B. (2001). Diffident no longer: Building structures for a proud profession: CAOT in the 1980s. *Occupational Therapy Now, 3*(5), 3–7.

Van Iterson, L. (2009). OT then. An inspiring 25+ years of international occupational therapy fieldwork. *Occupational Therapy Now, 11*(2), 24–25.

Waddell, M. A. (1998). Renewed beginnings for occupational therapy in Bangladesh. *WFOT Bulletin, 38,* 50–56.

Wallis, M. A. (1987). "Profession" and "professionalism" and the emerging profession of occupational therapy: Part 1. *British Journal of Occupational Therapy, 50,* 264–265.

Wallis, W. A. (1987). "Profession" and "professionalism" and the emerging profession of occupational therapy: Part 2. *British Journal of Occupational Therapy, 50,* 300–302.

Wilcock, A. A. (2001). Occupation for health: Re-activating the *Regimen Sanitatis. Journal of Occupational Science, 8,* 20–24.

Wilcock, A. (2003). Making sense of what people do: Historical perspectives. *Journal of Occupational Science, 10,* 4–6.

Wilcock, A. (2003). A science of occupation: Ancient or modern? *Journal of Occupational Science, 10,* 115–119.

Wilcock, A. A., & Steeden, B. (1999). Reflecting the creative roots of the profession. *British Journal of Occupational Therapy, 62,* 1.

Wilson, L. H. (2002). A review of the journals of the New Zealand Association of Occupation Therapists, 1949–2002. *New Zealand Journal of Occupational Therapy, 49,* 5–13.

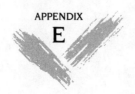

Presidents of the
American Occupational Therapy Association

Name	Date
George E. Barton, AIA	1917
William R. Dunton, MD	1917–1919
Eleanor Clarke Slagle, OTR	1919–1920
Herbert J. Hall, MD	1920–1923
Thomas B. Kidner	1923–1928
C. Floyd Haviland, MD	1928–1930
Joseph C. Doane, MD	1931–1939
Everett S. Elwood	1939–1947
Winifred C. Kahmann, OTR	1947–1952
Henrietta W. McNary, OTR	1952–1955
Ruth A. Robinson, OTR, FAOTA	1955–1958
Helen S. Willard, OTR, FAOTA	1958–1961
Wilma L. West, MA, OTR, FAOTA	1961–1964
Ruth Brunyate Wiemer, MEd, OTR, FAOTA	1964–1967
Florence S. Cromwell, MA, OTR, FAOTA	1967–1973
Jerry A. Johnson, EdD, MBA, OTR, FAOTA	1973–1978
Mae D. Hightower-Vandamm, OTR, FAOTA	1978–1982
M. Carolyn Baum, PhD, OTR/C, FAOTA	1982–1983
Robert K. Bing, EdD, OTR, FAOTA	1983–1986
Elnora M. Gilfoyle, ScD (Hon), OTR, FAOTA	1986–1989
Ann P. Grady, PhD, OTR, FAOTA	1989–1992
Mary M. Evert, MBA, OTR, FAOTA	1992–1995
Mary Foto, OTR, FAOTA	1995–1998
Karen Jacobs, EdD, OTR/L, CPE, FAOTA	1998–2001
Barbara L. Kornblau, JD, OT/L, FAOTA, DAAPM, ABDA, CCM, CDMS	2001–2004
M. Carolyn Baum, PhD, OTR/C, FAOTA	2004–2007
Penelope A. Moyers Cleveland, EdD, OTR/L, BCMH, FAOTA	2007–2010
Florence Clark, PhD, OTR/L, FAOTA	2010–

Index

Note. page numbers in italics indicate figures, tables and photographs.

9/11 attacks, 472–474

A

academic occupational therapy programs, 162–171
    see also training
Ackley, Naida, biography of, 638, *638*
acquired immune deficiency syndrome (AIDS), 227
activity, as a treatment method, 309–322, *313*, *314*
adaptation, defined, 417
adaptive equipment
    development of, 58–67, *62*
    tables, *10*, 10–15, *12*, *13*, *14*
adaptive processes, 201–210
administrators, role of, 16–24
adversity, overcoming, 357–367
Age of Enlightenment, 244–245
Allen, Claudia. K., 423, *638*, 638–640
allied health professionals, 232
    see also health care system
alternative explanations, 320
    see also activity, as a treatment method
Americans With Disabilities Act (ADA) (1990), 356
animal behavior, and mankind, 187–189
AOTA
    during an era of change, 583
    founders, *603*, 603–609, *606*, *607*
    presidents, 765
    Standards of the National Society for the
        Promotion of Occupational Therapy, 511, *512*
apraxia, hypothesized development of, 92–93
Arab–Israeli conflict, 139–140

arts and crafts, as media and methods, 300–303, *301*, *303*
assessments, 267–270, 276, 590–599
    see also clinical reasoning
assisted suicide, 355
audiovisual metronome, 13–14
authentic practice, 105–114
Ayres Baker, A. Jean, biography of, *640*, 640–642

B

Baldwin. B. T., model of practice for the restoration of
    movement, 421
Barton, George Edward, 251–252, *606*, 606–607
Baum, M. Carolyn, biography of, *642*, 642–647
bilateral tilt tables, 12–15, *13*, *14*
    see also adaptive equipment
Bing, Robert Kendall, biography of, *648*, 648–649
biomedical model, 289
Bowen v. American Hospital Association, 227
brain, functional aspects in relation to the limbic
    system, 180–183, *181*, *182*, *183*
Burke, Janice Posatery, biography of, *650*, 650–654

C

Centennial Vision, connecting with the *Founding Vision*,
    602–612, *603*
cerebral palsy, and object manipulation, 330–332
change
    innovation during, 579–588
    professional resistance to, 122
    therapeutic adaptation to, 207–209

About the Editors

Yolanda Griffiths, OTD, OTR/L, FAOTA, is an associate professor of occupational therapy and director of the post professional distance OTD program at Creighton University. Yolanda graduated with a BSOT from the University of Puget Sound, an MHR with an emphasis in counseling from the University of Oklahoma, and an OTD from Creighton University. She also has a certificate as an advanced master practitioner in neurolinguistic programming. Yolanda has primarily worked in the area of mental health since 1977 and began her career in academia in 1993. Her research interests include the scholarship of teaching and learning, occupational therapy education, distance learning, active learning, and generational learning styles. Yolanda has served AOTA from 1999 to 2009 as Fieldwork Subsection Coordinator and later Chairperson for the Education Special Interest Section, member of the Commission on Education and member of the Recognition and Awards Committee. She has three adult daughters and lives in Omaha with her husband and two dogs.

René Padilla, PhD, OTR/L, FAOTA, LMHP, is associate dean for academic and student affairs at Creighton University in Omaha, Nebraska. René has worked in mental health, rehabilitation, administration, and education throughout the world. He has consulted for various nongovernmental organizations involved in international efforts of community development in Latin America, the Middle East, and Africa. He conducts research on health and social disparities of refugees and immigrants and maintains a private practice in psychotherapy with an emphasis on issues of disability and migration trauma. He is past chairperson of the AOTA Education Special Interest Section and of the Commission on Education.